Core Concepts in Health

Sixth Edition

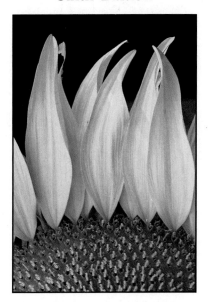

Paul M. Insel · Walton T. Roth

Stanford University

Mayfield Publishing Company

Mountain View, California
London · Toronto

Library of Congress Cataloging-in-Publication Data

Core concepts in health / [compiled by] Paul M. Insel,
    Walton T. Roth.—6th ed.
        p.   cm.
    Includes bibliographical references and index.
    ISBN 0-87484-967-5
    1. Health.   I. Insel, Paul M.   II. Roth, Walton T.
RA776.C83   1991
613—dc20   90-13277
                                                                CIP

Manufactured in the United States of America
10 9 8 7 6 5 4

Mayfield Publishing Company
1240 Villa Street
Mountain View, California 94041

Sponsoring editor, James Bull; *developmental editors,* Kathleen Engelberg, Kirstan Price, and Joan Pendleton; *managing editor,* Linda Toy; *art director,* Jeanne M. Schreiber; *text and cover designer,* Gary Head; *cover photographer* Ray Ellis/Photo Researchers, Inc.; *illustrators,* Natalie Hill, Judith Ogus, and Robin Mouat. The text was set in 10/12 Palatino by Waldman Graphics and printed on 45# Mead Publishers Thinbulk by Von Hoffmann Press, Inc.

Text and Photo Credits

Sources

Page 149   Human Life and Natural Family Planning Foundation

Page 178   Statistics from *Family Planning Perspectives,* vol. 19, no. 2, March/April 1987.

Page 180   *Facts in Brief: Abortion in the United States.* November 1, 1989. ©The Alan Guttmacher Institute.

Page 356   Source: G. A. Bray, 1978, Definitions, measurements, and classification of the syndrome of obesity. *International Journal of Obesity* 2:99–112.

Page 362   From F. Grands, "Nutrition and Energy Balance in Body Composition Studies," in *Techniques for Measuring Body Composition.* National Research Council, Washington, D.C., 1961.

Page 466   Reprinted from the *San Francisco Chronicle,* July 14, 1989.

Page 531   Centers for Disease Control.

Page 509   Copyright 1986 Time, Inc. Reprinted by permission.

Page 531   Adapted from: Ken Dychtwald and Joe Flower. 1989. *Age Wave.* (Los Angeles: Jeremy P. Tarcher), and Washington Post Health. Sept. 19, 1989.

Page 608   Reprinted from June 1988 *Mayo Clinic Health Letter* with permission of Mayo Foundation for Medical Education and Research, Rochester, Minnesota 55905.

Page 670   Excerpted from *In Health.* Copyright ©1988 (for 1) 1989(for 2, 3, 4) Hippocrates Partners.

Photo Credits

Chapter 1
pg1, Sam Forencich; pg5, ©1979 Joe Baraban; pg9, ©Billy E. Barnes/Stock Boston; pg 15, Shepard Sherbell/Stock Boston; pg17, ©Suzanne Arms Wimberley; pg19, Sam Forencich ©1987

Chapter 2
pg23, ©Daemmrich/Stock Boston; pg25, ©Bernard Giani/Photo Researchers, Inc.; pg26, © Daemmrich/Stock Boston; pg28, ©1984 Jay Maisel; pg36, Jim Weiner ©1985/Photo Researchers, Inc.; pg38, ©Bill Gallery/Stock Boston; pg41, Photograph ©Suzanne Arms Wimberley

Chapter 3
pg49, Sam Forencich; pg53, Elizabeth Crews; pg54, ©MCMLXXXVI Charles Gupton/Stock Boston; pg62, ©Bill Gallery 1982/Stock Boston; pg67, Sam Forencich; pg72, Rick Brown/Stock Boston

(Photo credits continue on p. viii)

Preface

Now in its sixth edition, *Core Concepts in Health* has maintained its leadership in the field of health education for over 15 years. Since we pioneered the concept of self-responsibility for personal health in 1976, hundreds of thousands of students have used our book to become active, informed participants in their own health care. Each edition of *Core Concepts* has brought improvements and refinements, but the principles underlying the book have remained the same. Our commitment to these principles has never been stronger than it is today.

Our Goals

Our goals in writing this book can be stated simply:

- To present scientifically based, accurate, up-to-date information in an accessible format
- To involve students in taking responsibility for their health
- To instill a sense of competence and personal power in students

The first of these goals means making expert knowledge about health and health care available to the individual. *Core Concepts* brings scientifically based, accurate, up-to-date information to students about topics and issues that concern them—nutrition, weight control, contraception, exercise, intimate relationships, stress, AIDS, drugs, alcohol, and a multitude of others. Current, complete, and straightforward coverage is balanced with "user-friendly" features designed to make the text appealing. Written in an engaging, easy-to-read style and presented in a colorful, open format, *Core Concepts* invites the student to read, learn, and remember. Boxes, tables, artwork, photographs, and many other features highlight areas of special interest throughout the book.

The second of our goals is to involve students in taking responsibility for their health. *Core Concepts* uses innovative pedagogy and unique interactive features to get students thinking about how the material they're reading relates to their own lives. We invite them to examine their emotions about the issues under discussion, to consider their personal values and beliefs, and to analyze their health-related behaviors. Beyond this, for students who want to change behaviors that detract from a healthy lifestyle, we offer guidelines and tools, ranging from samples of health diaries and personal contracts to detailed behavior change strategies.

Perhaps our most important goal in writing *Core Concepts in Health* is to instill a sense of competence and personal power in the students who read the book. Everyone has the ability to monitor, understand, and affect his or her own health. Although the medical and health professions possess impressive skills and have access to a huge body of knowledge that benefits everyone in our society, people can help to minimize the amount of professional care they actually require in their lifetimes by taking care of their health—taking charge of their health—from an early age. Our hope is that *Core Concepts* will continue to help young people make this exciting discovery—that they have the power to shape their own futures.

Content and Organization of the Sixth Edition

For this edition, all chapters were carefully reviewed, revised, and updated. The latest information from scientific and health-related research is incorporated in the text, and newly emerging topics and issues are discussed. The following list gives a sample of some of the current concerns addressed in the sixth edition:

- The changing profile of the AIDS epidemic and the latest approaches to treatment
- Opposing views on abortion
- Anger, hostility, and cardiovascular disease
- Crack cocaine, why it is so widely used, and how it affects babies before birth
- The effect of passive smoking on cardiovascular health
- Seasonal affective disorder
- Female condoms
- Marketing strategies of the tobacco industry
- Changing social attitudes toward smoking and drinking
- The drug legalization debate

- The newest Recommended Dietary Allowances
- The relationship between cervical cancer and papillomavirus
- Sunscreens demystified and their importance today
- Lyme disease
- Living wills

Of all these current health concerns, the most important, of course, is AIDS. Approximately half of Chapter 17 (Sexually Transmissible Diseases) is now devoted to a discussion of this disease, and four new boxes address related issues—AIDS Milestones, Who Needs an AIDS Test? Preventing AIDS Infection, and Reflections on AIDS (a selection by Robert Gallo of the National Cancer Institute). Another box on AIDS in Chapter 18 (Immunity and Infection) explains why HIV infections are so deadly.

An especially volatile current health concern is abortion. As in the fifth edition, we devote a separate chapter to abortion to reflect both the importance of this issue and our belief that abortion is not a form of contraception and should not be included in the chapter on that topic. Continuing our balanced treatment of this controversial issue, we include in this edition statements representing opposing views on abortion, one by Kate Michelman of the National Abortion Rights Action League and the other by J. C. Willke of the National Right to Life Committee. Also included in this chapter are a new box on adoption, an updated account of the latest Supreme Court and state rulings, a section on the "abortion pill" RU-486, and a sensitive discussion of the decision-making processes involved when abortion is being considered.

An area of particular concern and the subject of a great deal of recent research is cardiovascular disease, the number-one killer of Americans. Chapter 15 reports the latest findings on the role of anger and hostility (as the crucial components of the global "Type A" personality) in the development of heart disease. The chapter also examines the complex and controversial role played by cholesterol in cardiovascular health and disease. Five new boxes address related topics, such as how to lower the risk of heart disease through diet and how to interpret cardiovascular health claims by food manufacturers.

Of course, the health field is dynamic, with new discoveries, advances, trends, and theories reported every week. Ongoing research—on the genetic links in Alzheimer's disease, for example, or the effect of human growth hormone on aging—continually changes our understanding of the human body and how it works. For this reason, no health book can claim to have the final word on every topic. Yet within these limits, *Core Concepts* does present the latest available information and scientific thinking on innumerable topics.

In addition to being brought up to date for this edition, all chapters were reexamined for clarity and coherence. A number of chapters were completely reorganized to ensure that explanations and discussions were as clear as possible. The chapter outlines at the beginning of each chapter reflect this sharper focus.

The organization of the book as a whole was revised as well, so that there are now eight parts instead of six. The first four parts treat the same topics as in the corresponding parts of the fifth edition—Establishing a Basis for Wellness (including chapters on taking charge of your health, stress, and mental health), Understanding Sexuality (covering physical sexuality, intimate relationships, contraception, abortion, and pregnancy and childbirth), Making Responsible Decisions: Substance Use and Abuse (dealing with tobacco, alcohol, and other psychoactive drugs), and Getting Fit (covering nutrition, weight control, and exercise).

The remaining chapters of the book have been reorganized into new parts. Part Five, Protecting Yourself from Disease, brings together four chapters dealing with the most serious health problems facing people today—cardiovascular disease, cancer, and sexually transmissible diseases—and with the body's impressive defense system against disease. Part Six, Accepting Physical Limits, explores aging and dying and death. Part Seven, Making Choices in Health Care, provides information about medical self-care and the health-care system. Part Eight, Improving Your Chances: Personal Safety and Environmental Health, expands the boundaries of health care to include accident prevention and the effects of the environment on personal health. Taken together, the parts of the book provide students with a complete guide to managing and protecting their health, now and through their entire lives, as individuals, as participants in a health care community and system, and as citizens of a planet that also needs to be protected if it is to continue providing human beings with the means to healthy lives.

Features of the Sixth Edition

This edition of *Core Concepts in Health* builds on the features that attracted and held our readers' interest in the previous five editions. One of the most popular features has always been the **boxes**, which allow us to explore a wide range of current topics in greater detail than is possible in the text itself. In this edition, over half of the boxes are new; the rest are revised, expanded, or updated versions of the best boxes from the fifth edition. A few titles will suggest their range and currency:

- Premenstrual Syndrome—Still a Mystery (Chapter 4)
- Dealing with Rape (Chapter 5)
- How Much Does a Child Cost? (Chapter 8)
- What to Do Instead of Drugs (Chapter 11)
- Fat Substitutes: Good News for Mayonnaise Lovers (Chapter 12)

- Carbohydrate Loading—Does It Work? (Chapter 14)
- Getting to the Heart of Type A's (an interview with Redford Williams) (Chapter 15)
- The Selling of Cardiovascular Health to Americans (Chapter 15)
- Genital Self-Examination Guide (Chapter 17)
- Dental Self-Care (Chapter 21)
- When the Cure Becomes Part of the Problem (Chapter 21)
- Ten Ways to Avoid Being Quacked (Chapter 22)
- Drive Like a Pro (Chapter 23)
- What You Can Do to Save the Ozone Layer (Chapter 24)

Also included in this edition are two new features, which we have called Tactics and Tips and Vital Statistics. **Tactics and Tips** boxes distill from each chapter the practical advice students need in order to apply information to their own lives. Although such advice has always been in the book, in this edition we have made a point of presenting it in this clearer, more accessible way. By referring to these boxes, students can easily find specific suggestions on ways to drink less, for example; to improve the effectiveness of contraceptive methods; to reduce the amount of fat in their diets; to support their immune systems; to protect themselves from drunk drivers; to derail "Type A" behavior; to improve interpersonal communication; and so on.

Vital Statistics boxes, figures, and tables highlight important facts and figures in a memorable format that often reveals surprising contrasts and connections. From boxes, tables, and figures marked with the Vital Statistics label, students can learn about the prevalence of various types of cardiovascular disease among different populations; the incidence of various types of cancer in men and women; the trends in abortion since the Supreme Court decision of 1973; world population growth and world energy use; facts about accidents; and a wealth of other information. For students who grasp a subject best when it is displayed graphically, numerically, or in a list or table, the Vital Statistics feature provides an alternative way of approaching and understanding the text.

Making Connections is another new feature in this edition, designed to facilitate learning by getting students personally involved in specific health-related issues. Each chapter opens with several scenarios that describe situations involving concerns treated in the following pages. In each situation, someone has to make a decision, choose a course of action, or use information. We ask students to imagine themselves in the situations and consider what they would do, both before and after reading the chapter. The Making Connections scenarios demonstrate ways students can use material in the chapter to address issues and solve problems in their lives.

In addition to these new features, the most popular and useful features of *Core Concepts*—Exploring Your Emotions, Take Action, and Behavior Change Strategies—have been retained and revised for this edition. **Exploring Your Emotions**, appearing at appropriate points throughout each chapter, asks open-ended questions designed to inspire self-examination and heighten students' awareness of their feelings, values, beliefs, and thought processes. With such awareness, students are better able to take control of their lives and make healthy behavior changes. Most of the Exploring Your Emotions questions in this edition are new. We have taken care to formulate them in a nonjudgmental way to encourage honest self-analysis.

Take Action, appearing at the end of every chapter, suggests exercises and projects that students can undertake to extend and deepen their grasp of the material. Many suggestions involve the Health Diary, which we recommend each student keep while using *Core Concepts*. Other suggestions involve more elaborate activities, such as interviews, hands-on research projects, and investigations of community resources. Again, many Take Action entries are new to this edition; special care has been taken to ensure that the projects are both feasible and worthwhile.

The **Behavior Change Strategies** that conclude many chapters offer specific behavior management/modification plans relating to the chapter's topic. Based on the principles of behavior management that are carefully explained in Chapter 1, these strategies will help students change unhealthy or counterproductive behaviors. Included are strategies for dealing with test anxiety, quitting smoking, developing responsible drinking habits, planning a personal exercise program, phasing in a healthier diet, and many other practical plans for change.

Core Concepts has always set the standard in the field for innovative graphics and illustrations. This edition is much more abundantly illustrated than previous editions; nearly all of the photos are new, and nearly all are in color. A compelling photographic image appears on each chapter opening page, suggesting an important theme of that chapter. New drawings and improved renderings of the best art from the fifth edition create a fresh and exciting look. Those who learn best from visual images will benefit from illustrations showing, for example, how to rescue someone who is choking or how to lift a weight without sustaining a back injury.

In addition to the many photos, drawings, and charts in this edition, new and revised tables add interest to the text. From the tables students can quickly learn about such topics as the supposed and actual effects of selected drugs on sexual functioning, the most commonly used generic prescription drugs and their possible side effects, where to complain or seek help about health care fraud, and how the popular diet programs compare.

Also designed for quick reference are this edition's **appendixes**. A *Fast Food Eating Guide,* located following Chapter 12 (Nutrition Facts and Fallacies), provides students with a handy guide to the nutritional content of the most commonly ordered menu items at six popular fast food restaurants. Especially useful is the information about the fat and sodium content of each item and its proportion of fat calories to total calories. A new *Red Cross First Aid Chart* appears inside the back cover of the text, providing information that can save lives. Revised and updated appendixes on self-care follow Chapter 21, entitled *Home Medical Tests, Self-care Guide for Common Medical Problems,* and *Resources for Self-care.* These guides offer students the kind of information they can keep and use for years to come.

Learning Aids

Although all the features of *Core Concepts in Health* are designed to facilitate learning, several specific learning aids have also been incorporated into the text. **Chapter outlines** provide an overview of the contents of the following pages, orienting students at the outset of each new subject area. Important terms appear in boldface type in the text and are defined on the same page in a **running glossary,** helping students handle a large and complex new vocabulary.

New to this edition are **chapter summaries,** which offer students a concise review and a way to make sure they have grasped the most important concepts in the chapter. Also found at the end of every chapter are **selected bibliographies** and annotated **recommended readings,** carefully updated for this edition. Students can use these lists to extend and broaden their knowledge of particular topics or pursue subjects of interest to them. A complete **index** at the end of the book includes references to glossary terms in boldface type.

Ancillary Package

Available with *Core Concepts in Health* is a comprehensive package of supplementary materials that enhance teaching and learning. Included in the package are the following items:

- Instructor's Resource Guide
- Transparency acetates
- Videotapes
- Health Risk Appraisal Software
- Student Study Guide
- Brownstone academic management system

The **Instructor's Resource Guide** that accompanies the sixth edition has been produced as a three-ring binder to allow instructors maximum flexibility in using these materials. In the guide the instructor will find a variety of teaching aids: (1) Teaching Tips, consisting of learning objectives for each chapter, extended chapter outlines, suggestions for student activities, and listings of additional resources, including films, books, and periodicals; (2) Wellness Worksheets, suitable for duplication and designed for student self-assessment and exploration; (3) a complete set of over 3,000 examination questions, also available on Brownstone software; and (4) more than fifty transparency masters, providing additional lecture resources for instructors.

The set of **transparency acetates,** many in full color, provides material suitable for lecture and discussion purposes. These acetates do not duplicate the transparency masters in the Instructor's Resource Guide, and many of them are from sources other than the text.

Our exciting **videotapes** give instructors the opportunity to illustrate and extend coverage of the most current and compelling health-related topics treated in the text. For information about the videos, instructors should contact their Mayfield representative or call 1 (800) 433–1279.

The completely new computerized **Health Risk Appraisal** software package provides students with a self-assessment tool that alerts them to their personal risk areas and advises them on how to improve their risk profile. Designed for IBM-compatible computers, the program provides a detailed two-page report for each user.

The **Student Study Guide,** prepared by Thomas M. Davis and Susan Koch of the University of Northern Iowa, is designed to help students understand and assimilate the material in the text. The guide includes learning objectives, key terms, major concepts, and sample test questions for students.

The **Brownstone academic management system** gives instructors a powerful, easy-to-use method of handling time-consuming tasks such as creating tests and calculating and entering grades. Examination items are provided on computer disk for IBM-compatible and Apple computers. Instructors can select, add, or edit questions, randomize them, and print tests appropriate for their individual classes. The system also includes a convenient "gradebook" that enables the instructor to keep detailed performance records for individual students and for the entire class; maintain averages; graph each student's progress; and set the desired grade distribution, maximum score, and weight for every test.

A Note of Thanks

The efforts of innumerable people have gone into producing this sixth edition of *Core Concepts in Health*. The book has benefited immensely from their thoughtful commentaries, expert knowledge and opinions, and many helpful suggestions. We are deeply grateful for their participation in the project.

Academic Contributors

Stephen Barrett, M.D., consumer advocate and Editor, *Nutrition Forum Newsletter*
The Health-care System

Roger Baxter, M.D., Internist and Infectious Disease Specialist, Kaiser Permanente Medical Center, Oakland, California
Immunity and Infection

Boyce Burge, Ph.D., Triton Bioscience, Inc.
Cancer: A Closer Look

Thomas Fahey, Ed.D., California State University, Chico
Exercise for Health, Fitness, and Performance

Michael R. Hoadley, Ph.D., University of South Dakota
Accident Prevention

Marcia Seyler Insel, M. Phil.
Sexual Behavior and Intimate Relationships; Becoming a Parent: Pregnancy and Childbirth; Aging; Dying and Death

Paul Insel, Ph.D., Stanford University
Taking Charge of Your Health; Toward a Tobacco-free Society; Cardiovascular Health

Bea Mandel, R.N., M.P.H., Director, Education Services, Seton Medical Center
Sexually Transmissible Diseases

Joyce D. Nash, Ph.D., Pacific Graduate School of Psychology
Weight Control

David Quadagno, Ph.D., Florida State University
Sex and Your Body

Walton T. Roth, M.D., Stanford University School of Medicine
Mental Health

James H. Rothenberger, M.P.H., University of Minnesota
Environmental Health

David Sobel, M.D., M.P.H., Director of Patient Education and Health Promotion, Kaiser Permanente Medical Care Program, Northern California Region
Medical Self-care: Skills for the Health-care Consumer

Edward C. Suarez, Ph.D., Duke University Medical Center
Stress: The Constant Challenge

Jared R. Tinklenberg, M.D., Palo Alto Veterans Administration Medical Center and Stanford University
The Responsible Use of Alcohol; The Use and Abuse of Psychoactive Drugs

Mae V. Tinklenberg, R.N., N.P., M.S., Fair Oaks Family Health Center
Contraception; Abortion

Gordon Wardlaw, Ph.D., R.D., Ohio State University
Nutrition Facts and Fallacies

Academic Advisors and Reviewers

Daniel D. Adame, Emory University

Evelyn E. Ames, Western Washington University

Rebecca Banks, Mankato State University

W. Henry Baughman, Western Kentucky University

Fay R. Biles, Kent State University (emeritus)

Jeffrey E. Brandon, New Mexico State University

Michael S. Davidson, Montclair State College

Thomas S. Davis, University of Northern Iowa

Judy C. Drolet, Southern Illinois University

David F. Duncan

Sherry N. Filby, American River College

Michael R. Hoadley, University of South Dakota

Cornelia B. McCaskill, Northeastern University

Warren L. McNab, University of Nevada, Las Vegas

Martha Milk, California State University, Fresno

Roberta J. Ogletree, Indiana University

Larry K. Olsen, The Pennsylvania State University

Marion Pollock, California State University, Long Beach (emeritus)

James H. Rothenberger, University of Minnesota

Marty Siegel

Myra Sternlieb, De Anza College

Richard W. Wilson, Western Kentucky University

Finally, the book could not have been published without the efforts of the staff at Mayfield Publishing Company and the *Core Concepts* book team: Jim Bull, Sponsoring Editor; Kate Engelberg, Kirstan Price, and Joan Pendleton, Developmental Editors; Linda Toy, Managing Editor; Jeanne Schreiber, Art Director; Pam Trainer, Permissions Editor; and Julie Rovesti, Product Manager. To all, we express our deep appreciation.

Paul M. Insel

Walton T. Roth

Chapter 4

pg79, ©Frank Siteman 1988/Stock Boston; pg81, ©Daemmrich/Stock Boston; pg87, ©1987 Lawrence Migdale/Stock Boston; pg94, Photograph ©Suzanne Arms Wimberley; pg95, Elizabeth Crews; pg100, ©1985 James Lester/Photo Researchers, Inc.

Chapter 5

pg105, ©1987 Lawrence Migdale All Rights Reserved/Stock Boston; pg107, ©Chris Brown/Stock Boston; pg111, ©Liane Enkelis 1985/Stock Boston; pg115, John Lei/Stock Boston; pg120, ©Willie L. Hill Jr./Stock Boston; pg127, ©Suzanne Arms Wimberley

Chapter 6

pg133, ©Ray Ellis/Photo Researchers, Inc.; pg136, ©'86 by Blair Seitz All Rights Reserved/Photo Researchers, Inc.; pg143, Russ Kinne ©/Photo Researchers, Inc.; pg146, ©John Lei/Stock Boston; pg153, Hank Morgan/Science Source/Photo Researchers; pg 157,©Suzanne Goldstein/Photo Researchers, Inc.

Chapter 7

pg165, ©Van Bucher 1983/Photo Researchers, Inc.; pg167, Newsweek Arthur Grace/Stock Boston; pg172, ©Vernon Doucette/Stock Boston; pg173, ©Stephen J. Krasemann/Photo Researchers, Inc.

Chapter 8

pg 191, Photograph ©Suzanne Arms Wimberley; pg195, Alexander Tsiaras/Stock Boston; pg 201, Mike Malysko ©/Stock Boston; pg205a, b, c, Nestle Science Source/Photo Researchers, Inc.; pg214, Photograph ©Suzanne Arms Wimberley; pg215, Elizabeth Crews

Chapter 9

pg223, ©1986 Peter Menzel; pg229, ©Spencer Grant/Stock Boston; pg233, Richard Hutchings/Photo Researchers, Inc.; pg236, CNRI/Science Photo Library/Photo Researchers, Inc.; pg242, ©David Austen/Stock Boston

Chapter 10

pg249, ©F.B. Grunzweig/Photo Researchers, Inc.; pg251, ©Jon Feingersh 1988/Stock Boston; pg254, ©Daemmrich/Stock Boston; pg258, Dagmar Fabricius/Stock Boston; pg262, ©Larry Mulvehill/Photo Researchers, Inc.

Chapter 11

pg271, ©Barbara Alper/Stock Boston; pg274, ©Billy E. Barnes/Stock Boston; pg277, ©Lawrence Migdale/Photo Researchers, Inc.; pg283, ©Owen Franken/Stock Boston; pg291, Adam Hart-Davis/Science Photo Library/Photo Researchers, Inc.

Chapter 12

pg295, ©Bob Daemmrich/Stock Boston; pg301, ©Bob Daemmrich/Stock Boston; pg303, ©L. Dardelet/Photo Researchers, Inc.; pg309, ©1984 John Neubauer; pg320, ©Bob Daemmrich/Stock Boston; pg323, Elizabeth Crews/Stock Boston; pg330, ©1984 John Neubauer

Chapter 13

pg341, ©David Madison 1989; pg343, Illusration: Richard Hess; pg349, Photo by Jerry La Rocca for Nike; pg355, ©Bob Daemmrich/Stock Boston; pg361, ©MCMLXXXVIII Charles Gupton/Stock Boston; pg366, Gregg Mancuso/Stock Boston

Chapter 14

pg375, ©Bob Daemmrich/Stock Boston; pg377, ©David Madison 1989; pg382, Sam Forencich ©1987; pg389, ©David Madison 1987; pg397, ©David Madison 1990

Chapter 15

pg405, ©Will and Deni McIntyre 1985/Photo Researchers, Inc.; pg410, ©Suzanne Arms Wimberley; pg418, ©MCMLXXXVI Charles Gupton/Stock Boston; pg421, Sam Forencich; pg421, Sam Forencich; pg423, ©Josephus Daniels/Photo Researchers, Inc.; pg425, ©David Madison 1989

Chapter 16

pg433, ©Cecil Fox/Science Source/Photo Researchers, Inc.; pg437, David Austen/Stock Boston; pg457, ©Larry Mullvehill/Photo Researchers, Inc.; pg458, ©'87 Blair Seitz/Photo Researchers, Inc.

Chapter 17

pg463, ©David Weintraub/Photo Researchers, Inc.; pg467, ©Charles Daguet/Photo Researchers, Inc.; pg477, ©Hank Morgan/Photo Researchers, Inc.; pg479, David Toy; pg483, ©John Kaprielian/Photo Researchers, Inc.; pg485, Roswell Angier/Stock Boston

Chapter 18

pg493, ©Will and Deni McIntyre/Photo Researchers, Inc.; pg496, Dr. Andrejs Liepins/Science Photo Library/Photo Researchers, Inc.; pg500, ©Daemmrich/Stock Boston; pg508, John Durham/Photo Researchers, Inc.

Chapter 19

pg521, Sam Forencich; pg523, ©Jon Feingersch 1988/Stock Boston; pg527, ©Richard Hutchings/Photo Researchers, Inc.; pg529, Elizabeth Crews; pg536, Elizabeth Crews; pg539, ©Mark Shaw/Photo Researchers, Inc.

Chapter 20

pg543, ©David Madison 1981; pg545, Painting by Fred Burell; pg549, ©Hank Morgans/Photo Researchers, Inc.; pg551, ©Ellis Herwig/Stock Boston; pg558, ©John Moss/Photo Researchers, Inc.; pg561, ©Michael Grecco/Stock Boston

Chapter 21

pg565, ©Ray Ellis/Photo Researchers, Inc.; pg568, David Toy; pg576, ©'86 Blair Seitz/Photo Researchers, Inc.; pg577, ©Suzanne Arms Wimberley; pg582, NIH Science Source/Photo Researchers, Inc.; pg587, ©Suzanne Arms Wimberley

Chapter 22

pg607, ©Joseph Nettis/Photo Researchers, Inc.; pg610, ©Joseph Nettis 1989/Photo Researchers, Inc.; pg612, ©Art Stein/Photo Researchers, Inc.; pg614, Tim Malyon and Paul Biddle/Photo Researchers, Inc.; pg621, Suzanne Arms Wimberley

Chapter 23

pg629, ©David Madison; pg631, ©Gary Ladd 1984/Photo Researchers, Inc.; pg633, ©Jon Feingersh 1987/Stock Boston; pg634, ©MCMLXXXVIII Charles Gupton/Stock Boston; pg640, Cary Wolinsky/Stock Boston; pg648, ©Daemmrich/Stock Boston

Chapter 24

pg657, ©NASA/Stock Boston; pg661, ©David Madison 1990; pg662, ©James R. Fischer 1982/Photo Researchers, Inc.; pg664, ©Eunice Harris 1983/Photo Researchers, Inc.; pg667, ©Ellis Herwig/Stock Boston; pg672, ©Tom and Pat Leeson/Photo Researchers, Inc.

Contents

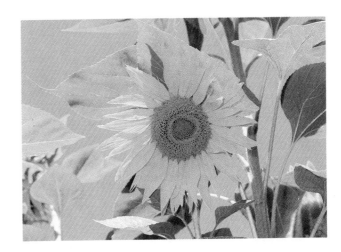

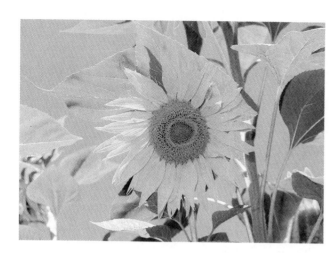

Chapter 10
The Responsible Use of Alcohol 249

Chapter 11
The Use and Abuse of Psychoactive Drugs 271

Part Four
Getting Fit

Chapter 12
Nutrition Facts and Fallacies 301

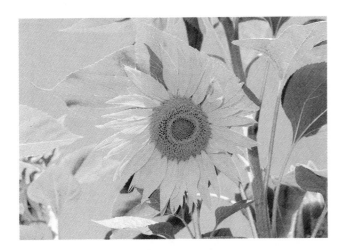

**Part Five
Protecting Yourself from Disease**

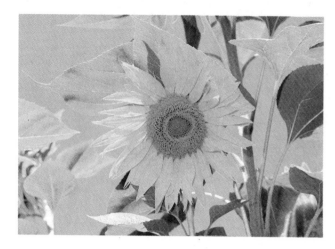

Part Eight
Improving Your Chances: Personal Safety and Environmental Health

Boxes

Core Concepts in Health

Sixth Edition

Contents

Making Connections

The years of transition from adolescent to adult life present a unique opportunity for change. Old patterns of behavior are being discarded, and new ones—some to become lifelong habits—are being adopted. The challenge is to make the right decisions and choices as you take charge of your health. The scenarios presented on these pages describe health-related situations in which people have to use information, make a decision, or choose a course of action. As you read them, imagine yourself in each situation and consider what you would do. After you've finished the chapter, read the scenarios again and see if what you've learned has changed how you would think, feel, or act in each situation.

You've never had so many wonderfully interesting and exciting experiences as you've had since coming to college. The only thing is, your everyday routines have become haphazard now that you're on your own for the first time. At first it was just a matter of skipping meals and staying up late. Now you've started sleeping in and missing classes. Even though you're having a good time, you know deep down that you're treading on thin ice. You want to establish some reasonable habits, but you're not sure where to start. What can you do to get your life under control?

1
Taking Charge of Your Health

One of your roommates never eats any pizza when you order it at night, even though she joins in with the socializing. You thought she just didn't like it, but in the course of talking with her the other day you found out otherwise. She happened to mention that three of her four grandparents had died of cancer at an early age. Her family doctor advised her and her parents to modify their diets to lower their risks of getting cancer themselves. "I try not to eat very many high-fat foods like cheese," she said. "That's why I usually don't eat pizza." You're puzzled—you thought no one knew what caused cancer. And if cancer is inherited, what difference does it make what you eat? Is your roommate being an extremist, or does she know what she's talking about?

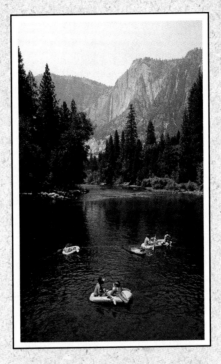

You started smoking as a sophomore in high school and finally managed to quit last summer. You'd like to convince your parents to stop smoking too, especially your dad, who's been smoking for 25 years and has a terrible cough. Armed with information about the hazards of smoking, you plan to mount a campaign over Christmas vacation to get them to quit. You tried to enlist your brother's help, but he says you'll never persuade them to change their ways, at least not just with facts. "Don't you think they know it's bad for them?" he asks you. Does he have a point? If so, what *can* you do?

You recently stayed up all night typing a paper and at 6 o'clock were astonished to see one of your housemates coming downstairs in her jogging clothes. When you told her you like jogging too but could never do it at that hour, she said she couldn't either if it wasn't for her jogging buddy. "We meet at the corner five mornings a week. We make each other feel guilty if we miss a day. In the winter, when it's still dark at 6, we don't feel safe going alone, so if one of us doesn't show, the other one can't go at all. It's the buddy system—and it really works." Ordinarily you like to jog alone, but lately, you've been slacking off. Could the buddy system work for you?

An overweight college freshman gives up snacking between meals. A sedentary executive asks a friend to run with her at noon. A former smoker anticipates her impulse to start smoking again and joins a stop-smoking support group. What do these people have in common? Each has made a commitment to take charge of his or her health. In addition, these actions reflect the assumption that the power to change behavior lies within oneself. We are our own resource. What we can do for ourselves will, over the long run, have the greatest impact on our health.

Today, many people are striving for optimal health. A hundred or even fifty years ago, such a goal was unknown. If you were born in 1890, for example, you could have expected to live about 40 years. As a child, you might have contracted polio, smallpox, or diphtheria. If you survived, you still might not have escaped tuberculosis, typhus, or dysentery. These diseases were the price paid for unrefrigerated, spoiled food, poor sanitary conditions, and air polluted by coal-burning furnaces and factories. Chances are high you would have died of an infectious disease, perhaps in the flu epidemic of 1918, which took 20 million lives.

Living in the last years of the twentieth century means you can expect to celebrate your seventieth birthday and more. As a baby you were vaccinated against the common childhood diseases, and antibiotics and other drugs help you recover quickly from the infections and illnesses you do contract. The most serious health threats you will face in your lifetime are chronic illnesses such as heart disease. Not only have life spans nearly doubled in 100 years, but medical research has also provided information and guidelines that you can use to avoid disease, live longer, and enjoy a quality of life unimagined by your grandparents.

The message of this book is that good health—even optimal health—is something everyone can have. Achieving it requires knowledge, self-awareness, motivation, and effort, but the benefits last a lifetime. Optimal health comes mostly from a healthy lifestyle—patterns of behavior that promote and support your health now and as you get older. In the pages that follow, you'll find current information about topics in health that you can use to build a better lifestyle. Besides information, you'll also learn things about yourself that will help you make healthy choices. There are tools for assessing yourself, for exploring your inner experiences, and for planning and carrying out specific behavior changes. Questions and suggestions appear frequently as you read about each major topic. You can use this book in a very real way to take charge of your health and improve the quality of your life.

What Is Health?

What exactly is meant by the term *health*? Today's ideas about health are very different from those held in 1890. How people saw health then influenced how they led their lives. To see how we got where we are today, let's look briefly at how the concept of health has evolved in a century.

Health as the Absence of Illness   In the past, a person who was born without a congenital defect, who had no symptoms of disease, and who was free of discomfort, pain, and disability was considered healthy. Throughout most of history, this was the best that one could hope for. More often than not, people died from infectious diseases that periodically swept around the world, ravaging whole populations. Bubonic plague, for example, took over 25 million lives in Europe in the fourteenth century. This was the worst outbreak of plague in history, but it was only one of more than 100 major outbreaks, dating back to biblical times. Whole tribes of native Americans were wiped out by infectious diseases brought to this country by European colonizers. No age was immune from the terrors of epidemic, whether of malaria, measles, syphilis, cholera, or some other contagious disease. No wonder health was defined as simply the absence of illness.

As medical science began to unravel the mystery of these diseases and bring them under control, patterns of life and death began to change. Life expectancies began to rise and death rates began to fall. (For a description of the important medical discoveries of the nineteenth and twentieth centuries, see the box entitled "Ages of Health Advancement.") Notions about health began to change too.

Health as Longevity: Is Longer Better?   As the average age at death rose dramatically, people began to wonder if the human life span could be increased indefinitely. The age-old dream of superlongevity—living to a ripe old age of 150 or so—was renewed. Once antibiotics were introduced for widespread use in the 1940s, people speculated that all diseases might soon be conquered by modern medicine. An age of medical miracles seemed just around the corner. Health began to be defined in terms of longevity—how long people could expect to live.

■ **Exploring Your Emotions**

How do you feel about your health now and in the future? What would your ideal state of health be at 30, 40, 50, 60, and 70 years of age?

Ages of Health Advancement

A study of death rates over the last century illustrates the dramatic changes that have taken place in the nature of health problems and solutions to these problems. The figure below shows overall death rates in the United States (age-adjusted) from 1885 to 1985, with the times at which major medical innovations became available.

- Over 70 percent of the decline in death rate between 1885 and 1985 occurred *before* the most significant medical innovations were introduced, in a period dominated by improvements in the environment and in our public health policies.
- The discovery of antibiotics in the 1930s ushered in what might be called the Age of Medicine and did noticeably accelerate the decline in the U.S. death rate. For about 20 years substantial progress was made via this route.
- The decline slid to a stop in the early 1950s as the problems still responsive to this approach began to disappear. For the next 20 years there was almost no reduction in the death rate or corresponding increase in life expectancy. Ironically, this was the same period in which many of our most expensive medical innovations were introduced— intensive care units, open heart surgery, and all the rest. The cost of medical care rose dramatically in this period.
- Finally, in the early 1970s, death rates again began to decline at a significant rate. This continuing decline reflects a drop in the deaths due to heart attacks and stroke. It coincides with reduced use of tobacco, less saturated fat and cholesterol in the diet, and increased exercise among American adults. This could be called the beginning of the Age of Life-Style in health.

Thus the "miracles of modern medicine" have had little to do with the long-term declines in the death rate. The two things simply do not go together historically. Furthermore, we appear to be in an era where lifestyle, rather than medicine, will be the dominant factor in further gains in health.

Source: Donald M. Vickery. 1978. *Life Plan for Your Health* (Reading, Mass.: Addison-Wesley), pp. 17–18.

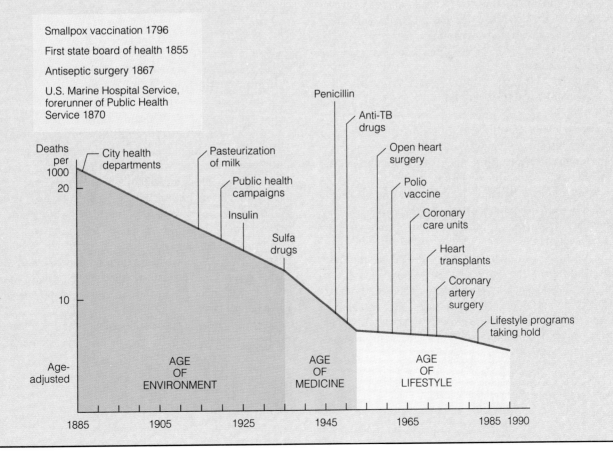

Communicable diseases yielded to public health campaigns, vaccines, and antibiotics. But this progress was interrupted when a different set of diseases emerged as major health threats and a new pattern of death took shape. By the 1950s, degenerative diseases like coronary heart disease, cancer, stroke, diabetes, atherosclerosis, and cirrhosis replaced pneumonia and influenza as the leading causes of death in the United States.

Degenerative diseases spawned new treatments—open heart surgery, chemotherapy and radiation, organ transplants, and others—but they were less successful than earlier innovations had been. They were also enormously expensive and raised a whole new set of social and ethical questions. Many people began to question the value of some of the most advanced procedures, such as heart-lung transplants, which seem to lead to incapacitating strokes, and life support systems, which sometimes are used to keep people alive in a permanent vegetative state. Merely being alive—with minimal physical and mental functions, supported by machines or in a coma—was seen in these terms as a kind of living death.

It became apparent that the best treatment for the new killers was prevention—people taking care of their bodies before degeneration and disease could set in. A number of habits and behaviors were identified as culprits in the development of disease; others seemed to promote health. Many of the factors contributing to disease turned out to be popular aspects of the lifestyle enjoyed by many Americans—our diet, our work and play habits, our recreational choices, and the environment in which we live. We're in control of these factors—not our doctors or the health establishment.

Wellness: The New Health Goal   The focus on lifestyle and the role of the individual has helped redefine health. No longer do we consider health as simply the absence of disease; instead, today we view health as the presence of vitality and overall well-being—a concept known as optimal health, or **wellness.** Health is not a static condition but rather a dynamic process that changes from day to day and from year to year with changes in our bodies and minds, our attitudes and beliefs, and our habits and behaviors.

One of the best-known definitions of health in modern times comes from the United Nations World Health Organization, which defines health as "a state of complete physical, mental, and social well-being and not merely the absence of disease or infirmity." Health today is seen as being multidimensional, encompassing many interre-lated areas—physical, emotional, intellectual, spiritual, interpersonal, societal, environmental, even planetary. A person who is physically healthy but who fails in intimate relationships, for example, isn't really in optimal health, nor is someone who buckles under everyday stress or who can't find a purpose in life. Good health extends to living in harmony with oneself and others, balancing inner demands with those of the world, being in tune with nature.

■ **Exploring Your Emotions**

What makes you feel exuberant? How often do you feel this way, and what are the circumstances?

The concept of **vitality** can help shed light on this broad (and perhaps overly idealistic) definition of health. Vitality is defined as the ability to function with vigor, to live life actively, energetically, and fully. It is considered by some to be the very essence of health. People of all types can experience vitality at different stages of life—children, adults of every age, and people with physical and mental disabilities. Most people are capable of leading vital, energetic lives. Good health begins with the absence of disease and the chance for a long life; it also is a state of energy, vitality, and well-being—a meaningful life lived to its fullest.

Choosing Wellness

This wellness model of health has a far-reaching effect on how we view ourselves and live our lives. We now have greater control over our health than human beings have ever had before—and greater responsibility for it as well. Being healthy and maintaining vitality are not just matters of getting immunizations and taking medications. Although these are still important, living a certain way and adopting a number of habits and behaviors, major and minor, are the keys to a truly healthy lifestyle. Healthy people eat well, get enough exercise and sleep, make responsible decisions about sex, choose not to smoke, and make many other crucial decisions about their daily lives.

Scientific research is continually revealing new connections between our habits and the level of health we

---

Wellness   Optimal health and vitality, encompassing physical, emotional, intellectual, spiritual, interpersonal, and environmental well-being.

Vitality   The ability of an organism to function with vigor.

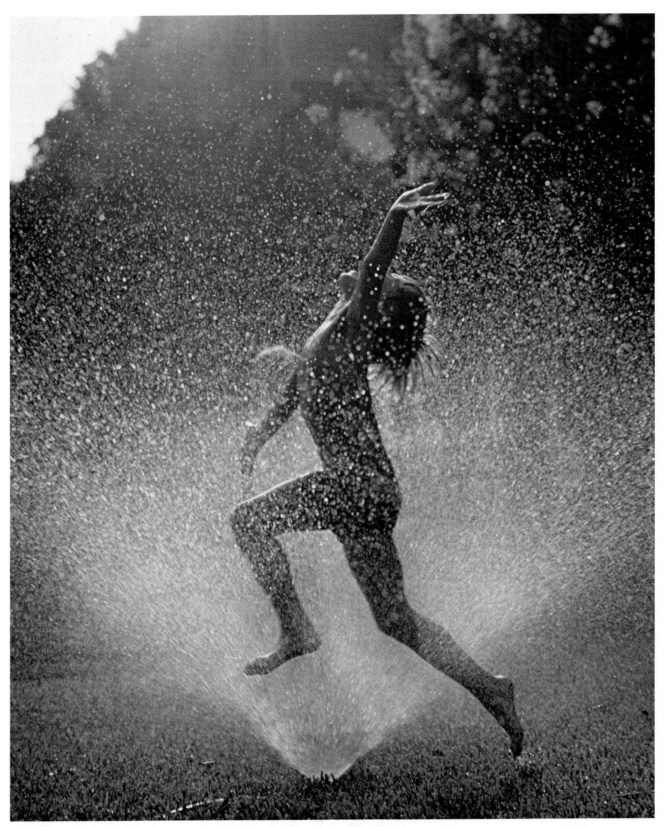

With wellness comes vitality, exuberance, a capacity for joy—and for fun. Do you remember what it feels like to run through a cold sprinkler on a hot day? What makes you feel that vital today?

> ## VITAL STATISTICS
>
> **Table 1-1** Estimated total deaths and percent of total deaths for the ten leading causes of death: United States, 1987
>
> | Rank | Cause of Death | Number | Percent of Total Deaths |
> |------|----------------|--------|-------------------------|
> | 1 | Heart disease*‡ | 759,400 | 35.7 |
> | 2 | Cancers*‡ | 476,700 | 22.4 |
> | 3 | Strokes*‡ | 148,700 | 7.0 |
> | 4 | Accidents† | 92,500 | 4.4 |
> | | (Motor vehicle) | (46,800) | (2.2) |
> | | (All others) | (45,700) | (2.2) |
> | 5 | Chronic obstructive lung diseases‡ | 78,000 | 3.7 |
> | 6 | Pneumonia and influenza‡ | 68,600 | 3.2 |
> | 7 | Diabetes mellitus* | 37,800 | 1.8 |
> | 8 | Suicide† | 29,600 | 1.4 |
> | 9 | Chronic liver disease and cirrhosis† | 26,000 | 1.2 |
> | 10 | Atherosclerosis* | 23,100 | 1.1 |
> | ... | All causes[1] | 2,125,100 | 100.0 |
>
> *Cause of death in which diet plays a part.
> †Cause of death in which excessive alcohol consumption plays a part.
> ‡Causes of death in which smoking plays a part.
> [1]AIDS was number 15 on this list in 1987, the latest year for which statistics are available.
> Source: National Center for Health Statistics, *Monthly Vital Statistics Report,* vol. 37, no. 1, April 25, 1988.

enjoy. For example, heart disease, the number one killer in the United States today, is associated with cigarette smoking, high levels of stress, a hostile personal style, a high-fat diet, and a sedentary way of life (see Table 1-1). Regular exercise, on the other hand, seems to correlate with health maintenance, whether in terms of weight control, a healthier cardiovascular system, or improved mental functioning. As we learn more about how our actions affect our bodies and minds, we can use the information to make choices for a healthier life.

Our behavior—our lifestyle, the choices we make—isn't the only factor involved in health, of course; our heredity and the environment we live in play important roles too. A person born with cystic fibrosis or an inherited tendency for mental illness won't have the same control over his or her destiny as someone without those congenital problems. And a person living in poverty or breathing powerful cancer-causing chemicals on the job has a more difficult course to follow to achieve good health. But in many cases, behavior can tip the balance toward health even where inheritance or environment are negative factors. For example, breast cancer can run in

families, but it also seems to be associated with overweight and with a diet high in animal fats, among other things. A woman with a family history of breast cancer is less likely to become a victim of the disease if she controls her weight, keeps fat intake low, does breast self-exams, and has regular mammograms taken.

Similarly, a young man with a family history of obesity can maintain a normal weight by being careful to balance calorie intake against activities that burn calories. If your life is highly stressful, you can lessen the chances of heart disease and stroke by learning ways to manage and cope with stress. If you live in an area with severe air pollution, you can reduce the risk of lung disease by not smoking. Going beyond this first step in improving your chances, you can also take an active role in improving your environment. Behaviors like these allow you to make a difference in how great an impact heredity and environment will have on your health.

A Wellness Profile   What does it mean to be healthy today? A basic list of important behaviors and habits would include the following:

- Having a sense of responsibility for your own health and taking an active rather than passive stance toward your life
- Learning to manage stress in effective ways
- Maintaining high self-esteem and mentally healthy ways of interacting with other people
- Understanding your sexuality and having satisfying intimate relationships
- Avoiding tobacco and drugs and using alcohol wisely, if at all
- Eating well, exercising, and maintaining normal weight
- Knowing when to treat your illnesses yourself and when to seek help
- Understanding the health system and using it intelligently
- Knowing the facts about cardiovascular disease, cancer, infections, sexually transmitted diseases, and accidents and using your knowledge to protect yourself against them
- Understanding the natural processes of aging and dying and accepting the limits of human existence
- Understanding how the environment affects your health and taking appropriate action to improve it

This may seem like a tall order, and in a sense it *is* the work of a lifetime. But the habits that you establish between the ages of 18 and 24 are crucial: They tend to set lifelong patterns. Some behaviors do more than set up patterns—they produce permanent changes in your health. If you become addicted to drugs or alcohol at age 20, for example, you may be able to kick the habit, but you will never again be a nonaddict; you will always face the struggle of a recovered addict. If you contract gonorrhea, you may discover later that your reproductive organs were damaged without your realizing it, making you infertile or sterile. If you ruin your knees doing the wrong exercises or hurt your back in an automobile accident, you won't have them to count on when you're older. Some things just can't be undone.

What Do You Need to Know?   Nothing can be achieved instantly. It's easier to make choices and changes once you set up your own system. It requires:

- *Facts and information about topics and issues in health.* You will have many questions about your health status. How much fat should you eat? How much exercise will keep your heart and lungs healthy? How can you protect yourself against unwanted pregnancy and sexually transmissible disease? What do you risk when you don't wear a seat belt? If you don't have basic facts, you can't make good decisions.
- *Knowledge about yourself.* You are a unique individual, with a unique way of being in the world. What are your strengths and your weaknesses? What characteristics or tendencies have you inherited from your family? What beliefs, attitudes, and values guide you as you interact with other people and the world? Just exactly how healthy—or unhealthy—are you? To make decisions for yourself, you have to know where you fit into the health picture. You have to know what your strengths are and what makes you resist. You need tools for knowing yourself as you really are. True insight can be obtained only by being honest with yourself, by tuning in to your innermost thoughts, feelings, and sensations.
- *A plan of action.* Once you've recognized the way you're dealing (or not dealing) with a health issue, you may decide that you can do better in that area. However, just wanting to make a change is not the same as actually making the change—you still need a plan of action. How can you quit smoking? What's the best way to work exercise into your busy life? How can you learn to relax? How can you achieve your ideal weight and, more important, maintain it? You need to take specific, concrete steps to make your plan for health improvement successful.

Taking big steps toward health may at first seem like too much work, but as you make progress toward wellness it gets easier. At first you'll be rewarded with a greater sense of control over your life, a feeling of empowerment, higher self-esteem, and more joy in life. These benefits will encourage you to make further improvements. Over time, you'll come to know what wellness feels like—more energy; greater vitality; deeper feelings of curiosity, interest, and enjoyment; and a higher quality of life.

Getting Down to Basics: How Do You Reach Wellness?

The picture drawn here of wellness may seem out of reach to you right now. Your life may not resemble the Wellness Profile at all. You probably have a number of healthy habits and some others that place your health at risk. Maybe your life is more like this:

> It's Tuesday. Rob wakes up feeling blue, not really wanting to get out of bed. He wishes he knew what he wanted to do with his life. He wishes he'd meet someone new and fall in love. No time for breakfast so he grabs a cup of coffee to drink during his first class. He hasn't done the reading and stares blankly at the teacher during the lecture. Later he goes to the student union and has a sugary doughnut and some more coffee; he lights up his first cigarette of the day. Lunch is a fast-food cheeseburger, french fries, and a shake. He spends the afternoon at the library desperately researching a paper that's due the next day, finally quitting at 6 o'clock and heading to the student union for a beer. He meets up with some buddies and joins them for pizza instead of having dinner at the dorm. They offer him a toke of marijuana, but he passes it up because he needs to finish that paper. By 11 o'clock he's tired, but he's written only one page, so he takes a little "speed" to keep going. It makes his heart race and floods his head with so many ideas he has difficulty sorting them all out. He works feverishly and finally finishes at 4 o'clock the next morning. Exhausted, he falls asleep in his clothes. The next thing he knows, it's Wednesday morning, time to start a new day.

This is hardly an ideal lifestyle, but it's not unusual. Rob functions okay, comes through on his commitments, and shows some self-discipline. On the other hand, time gets away from him, he doesn't get much exercise, doesn't eat as well as he could, and flirts with the dangers of taking drugs. Overall, he seems low on energy and has little control over his life. He could be living a lot better.

Rob isn't alone in neglecting or abusing his health; many people fall into a lifestyle that puts their health at risk. Some aren't aware of the damage they're doing to themselves; others are aware but aren't motivated or don't know how to change; and still others want to change but can't seem to get started. All of these are very real problems, but they're not insurmountable. If they were, there would be no ex-smokers, recovered alcoholics, or successful Weight Watchers graduates around. People can and do make difficult changes in their lives.

Taking Charge of Your Health: Motivation, Commitment, and Sense of Control   What makes you act the way you do? Countless factors come into play, both internal and external, both rational and irrational—knowledge, emotions, values, ideals, habit, circumstances, beliefs, and perceptions about yourself and the world.

Changing your behavior can be complicated by the many factors involved. Knowledge is a necessary ingredient, for example, but knowledge alone isn't usually enough to make you act. Millions of smokers stick to their habit even though they know it's bad for their health.

More important than knowing what is right is being motivated to change. People are motivated primarily by their desires and their fears—things they want to have and things they want to avoid. In theory, people might be motivated to make healthy choices because they want to be more fit, have more energy, or longer life; on the other hand, they might be motivated by fear of getting cancer or having a heart attack at 50. In fact, most people aren't provoked to action by long-term goals like avoiding disease that will hit them twenty or thirty years from now. They're motivated more by shorter-term, more personal goals, such as looking better, being more popular with the opposite sex, doing better in school, getting a good job, improving at a sport or game, and gaining higher self-esteem. When it comes to particularly risky behaviors, what motivates them to change may be fear for their lives, fear of contracting a sexually transmissible disease like AIDS.

Some things we want are good, and others are bad; often we choose those things that give us more immediate satisfaction. You might want to lose weight so you'll look good in a bathing suit next month, but you may also be sorely tempted by a hot fudge sundae right now. When it's right in front of you, you'll probably choose immediate gratification over a long-term goal. Motivation alone is usually no more effective at breaking a long-standing habit than knowledge alone is.

Motivation has to be built on commitment, the resolve to stick with a plan no matter what temptations you encounter. Commitment provides a turning point when you bring the full force of your resolve to change a particular situation. With deeply rooted habits, it often takes a while to build up to the level of commitment you need to conquer a habit. Many smokers, for example, don't succeed in quitting until their third or fourth try, when their commitment is fueled by frustration and disgust over earlier failures, anger at cigarette manufacturers, and a burning desire to succeed.

Whether or not you succeed in changing behaviors is rooted in how strongly you believe you will succeed, what you unconsciously intend, the kind of support you can draw from family and friends, and so on. Perhaps the most crucial factor of all is how active or passive you want to be about your life. Consider the question, Who is controlling your life? Is it your parents, your friends, your school, circumstances, the stars? Or is it you? When you succeed in making changes it is because *you* have taken charge of your life and you have come to see that what you do is within your control. Recognizing that you're in charge of your own life will eventually free you from the bonds of the past and mobilize you to create your own life.

■ Exploring Your Emotions

How do you feel about the idea of putting together and carrying out a plan for changing some part of your behavior? Have you ever taken this kind of deliberate action before? Do you feel uneasy about the idea? Does it excite you?

Most of your behaviors are habits you've learned. They may be deeply ingrained, long-standing habits, but they're still habits, and you can unlearn them the same way you learned them. The key is to approach them in a systematic way. The approach recommended in this book is based on principles of behavioral self-management that have proven effective in helping people make changes in their lives. Once you have the motivation and the commitment, behavioral self-management techniques will give you the means to change your behavior. As you read about different areas of health in the chapters that follow, you can apply the self-management model to your own behaviors to help you plan and carry out changes in your life.

A Plan for Action: Behavior Self-Management   Your behaviors and actions don't happen in a vacuum. They take place as you are surrounded by sights, sounds, and other sensations from both within and without. You can trace your behaviors to the circumstances that trigger them, and you can also recognize the consequences that follow from them. The heart of the behavior self-management model is isolating a **target behavior** that you wish to change and identifying its circumstances and consequences. Once you know these, you can intervene to break the chain of habit.

Behaviors can be triggered or stimulated by many different circumstances. **External stimuli**, or cues, are events or sensations in the environment—the sound of your name being called in class, the smell of bacon cooking, the sight of a sexy person. **Internal stimuli** are thoughts, feelings, and other inner sensations and experiences that trigger an action—hunger, low levels of nicotine in the blood, exhaustion.

Behaviors can also have different kinds of consequences, or "payoffs." Consequences that tend to make you repeat a behavior are known as reinforcers. Some reinforcers, known as **positive reinforcers**, encourage you to repeat a behavior by adding something positive that makes you feel good. For example, drinking a few glasses of wine at a party may give you feelings of pleasure, excitement and fun, at least temporarily, and

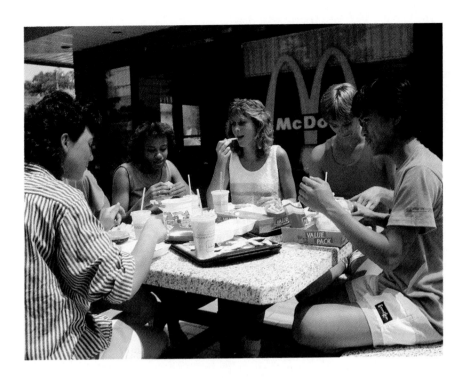

Many actions and behaviors are triggered by external stimuli, or cues in the environment. Once these students saw a popular fast food restaurant and decided to eat there, their choice of burgers, sodas, and fries for lunch was practically inevitable. If they wanted to change their diet, they would probably have to begin by choosing a different restaurant.

make it more likely you will drink again at the next party.

Other reinforcers, known as **negative reinforcers**, encourage a behavior by covering up or removing something unpleasant that was making you feel bad. When a person is addicted to nicotine, for example, smoking a cigarette removes the unpleasant feelings of nicotine craving. Both kinds of reinforcers help a behavior remain a habit, one by adding something and increasing your pleasure, the other by removing something and decreasing your discomfort. Sometimes a behavior is supported by both positive and negative reinforcers; for example, taking a drink makes you feel good and at the same time lowers your inhibitions and your anxiety around people. (Consequences that make a behavior less likely to happen are known as punishers, and for a variety of reasons they aren't particularly effective in self-management programs.)

Intervening in the chain of events that occur before and after a behavior is the basis of behavior self-management. This approach provides surprisingly powerful tools that you can use to make the changes you want in your life. Let's consider now the actual steps involved in putting together a behavior management program.

Putting Together a Behavior Management Program   If your lifestyle is more like Rob's than the ideal, there may be several changes you could make to improve it. The worst thing you could do would be to try to change everything at once—quit smoking, give up high-fat foods, eat a good breakfast, start jogging, do sit-ups, plan your study time better, avoid drugs, get enough sleep. Overdoing it leads to burnout. Concentrate on one behavior that you want to change and work on it systematically until you gain some control over it. To start with something simple, substitute margarine for butter in your diet, if you use a lot of butter, or skim milk for whole milk. Or you might concentrate on a minor but potentially deep-seated habit like biting your fingernails. Working on even one behavior will make high demands on your energy. Once you've decided on a behavior you want to change, following the six steps we discuss next will help you succeed.

Your key to success in this methodical six-step approach is to be consistent and to persist. Don't skip steps or rush through the plan. You may think you know everything there is to know about your target behavior, but people are almost always surprised by patterns that

Target behavior   An isolated behavior selected as the object of a behavior change program.

External stimuli (cues)   Factors from outside the person that arouse activity.

Internal stimuli   Factors from within the person that arouse activity.

Positive reinforcer   Something added to the environment following a behavior that results in an increase in the frequency of the behavior.

Negative reinforcer   Something removed from the environment following a behavior that results in an increase in the frequency of the behavior.

emerge from carefully recorded daily accounts of their thoughts and actions.

1. **Monitor your behavior and gather data.** Begin your program by keeping careful records of the behavior you wish to change (your target behavior) and the circumstances surrounding it. You can keep these records in a health diary, a notebook in which you write the details of your behavior along with observations and comments. Note exactly what the activity was, when and where it happened, what you were doing, and what your feelings were at the time. In a diary for a weight loss program, for example, you would typically record how much food you ate, the time of day, the situation, the location, your feelings, and how hungry you were (see Figure 1–1).

   This record helps you identify and get information about the circumstances of the behavior—the internal and external stimuli that lead to it—and about any related factors that may be present, supporting the behavior or making it difficult to resist. In a weight loss program, related factors might be the presence of candy in the house, for example, or rainy weather that discourages you from exercising outdoors. Keep your diary for a week or two to get some solid information about the behavior you want to change.

2. **Analyze the data and identify patterns.** After you have collected data on the behavior, analyze the data to identify patterns in stimuli and responses. When are you most hungry? When are you most likely to overeat? What events seem to trigger your appetite? Perhaps you are especially hungry at mid-morning or when you put off eating dinner until 9 P.M. Perhaps you overindulge in food and drink when you go to a particular restaurant or when you're with certain friends. Be sure to note the connections between your feelings and such external stimuli as time of day, location, situation, and the actions of others around you. Do you always think of having a cigarette when you read the newspaper? Do you always bite your fingernails when you're studying?

3. **Set specific goals.** Whatever your ultimate goal, it's a good idea to break it down into a few small steps, or "chunks." Your plan will seem less overwhelming and more manageable, increasing the chances that you'll stick to it. You'll also build in more opportunities to reward yourself (and reinforce the changes you've made so far) as well as milestones you can use to measure your progress.

   If you plan to lose 30 pounds, for example, you'll find it easier to take off 10 pounds at a time. If you want to quit smoking, plan a series of steps that takes you to the day you'll quit, such as asking yourself how ready you are to quit, listing your reasons for quitting, looking at patterns from when you tried be-

fore to quit, then cutting your daily smoking in half, and, three days later, quitting altogether. Take the easier steps first and work up to the harder steps. If you think through your goals carefully, you'll probably succeed.

4. **Make a personal contract.** Once you have set your goals and developed a plan of action, make your plan into a personal contract. A serious personal contract clearly states your objective and your commitment to reach it. You may add details of your plan—the date you'll begin; the completed steps you'll use to measure your progress; the date you expect to reach your final goal; and perhaps the time, resources, and energy you've committed to the plan. A nearby box gives more details. It often helps to have another person witness the contract especially someone who may be actively involved in the behavior or who may serve as an umpire or a banker.

   You can write a series of small contracts or one big one with a number of checkpoints. Either way, start by identifying your first goal and then lay out your subgoals to reach that goal. Be sure your first subgoal has a start and stop date and a clear description of what you hope to accomplish.

5. **Devise a strategy or plan of action.** As you fill in your health diary, you gather quite a lot of information about your target behavior—the times it typically occurs; the situations in which it usually happens; the ways sight, smell, mood, situation, and accessibility trigger it. You can probably trace the chains of events that lead to the behavior and also how you can make other choices at various points in the chain.

   You can be more effective in modifying behavior if you control the environmental stimuli that provoke it. This might mean not having cigarettes or certain foods or drinks in the house, not going to parties where you're tempted to overindulge, or not spending time with particular people, at least for a while. If you always get a candy bar at a certain vending machine, change your route so you don't pass by it. If you enjoy certain foods so much that you can't resist having seconds, cook only enough for single portions. If you always end up taking a coffee break and chatting with friends when you go to the library to study, choose a different place to study, such as your room.

   It's also helpful to control other behaviors or habits that seem to be linked to the target behavior. You may give in to an urge to eat when you have a beer (alcohol increases the appetite) or when you watch TV. Try substituting some other activities for habits that seem to be linked with your target behavior, such as exercising to music instead of plopping down in front of the TV with a beer and a bag of chips. Or, if possible, put an exercise bicycle in front of your TV and burn calories while you watch your favorite show.

Date _November 5_   **Day** M (TU) W TH F SA SU

Time of day	M/S	Food Eaten	Cals.	H	Where did you eat?	What else were you doing?	How did someone else influence you?	What made you want to eat what you did?	Emotions and feelings?	Thoughts and concerns?
7:30	M	1 C Crispix cereal	110	3	dorm cafeteria	reading newspaper	eating w/ roommates, but I ate what I usually eat	I always eat cereal in the morning	a little excited and worried	thinking about quiz in class today
		1/2 C skim milk	40							
		coffee	—							
		2 t sugar	25							
		2 T milk	10							
		1 C orange juice	120							
10:30	S	1 apple	90	1	library	studying	alone	felt tired and wanted to wake up	tired and fuzzy; slight headache	worried about next class
12:30	M	1 cheeseburger		2	cafeteria terrace	talking	eating with friends, we all ordered the same thing	didn't want to feel left out	excited and happy	anxious to hear the latest gossip
		meat patty	200							
		cheese	95							
		lettuce	10							
		tomato	20							
		bun	120							
		10 french fries	125							
		2 oatmeal cookies	100							
		diet soda	—							
3:00	S	package of M and M's	120	1	at work	shelving books	alone	needed a break; went to candy machine	bored	thinking about party coming up this weekend
6:30	M	salad		3	student union	talking with friends	we all got ice cream for dessert	best thing offered for dinner	relaxing with friends	thinking about paper to write this evening
		lettuce	15							
		tomato	40							
		cucumber	5							
		1 T Italian dressing	90							
		4 oz roast chicken	205							
		3/4 C mashed potatoes	150							
		1/2 C ice cream	125							
		diet soda	—							
10:30	S	hot chocolate	100	1	living room	watching TV w/ roommates	didn't want to be left out	it was already fixed	tired of studying; wanted a break	nothing really
		1 c plain popcorn	25							
		Total for day	1940							

M/S = Meal or Snack   H = Hunger Rating (0–3)

Figure 1-1 Daily Eating Behavior Record

A Personal Contract for Change

All of us are familiar with the power of signed contracts. Documentation in black and white that commits our word, money, and/or property carries a strong impact and results in a higher chance of follow-through than do casual, off-hand assurances or promises. Contracts can be used to try to change a health behavior if they include the time, date, and details of the change program. Some target behaviors, such as quitting smoking or losing extra pounds, lend themselves to contracts with very specific goals. Often a witness is also asked to sign the contract; this helps to set in motion the support and encouragement of a social network. Contracts reduce procrastination by specifying the dates and other details of the behavioral tasks and goals. They also act as reminders of a personal commitment to change. Here is an example of a behavioral contract for smoking.

Contract for Stopping by Yourself

Many people can stop smoking with little difficulty. In fact, they may have considerable experience with quitting in the past. If this corresponds to your smoking history, then you should follow the rules presented here.

Rule 1 Set a specific date and time for quitting, and write this in your personal contract. The time could be as early as three days from now or as far away as next week, whichever you prefer. This date and time (early in the morning or in the evening) should be listed in the target date box. Of course, you should follow through with

the date, once chosen, and actually stop smoking at that time.

Rule 2 Three days before your target date, you should cut your daily smoking in half. For example, if you smoke 20 cigarettes per day, then you should reduce that total to only 10 cigarettes daily for the three-day period. Do NOT try to gradually reduce your smoking down to zero, however, because this will actually increase the value of each remaining cigarette and make your attempt to quit extremely frustrating. This rule is based on strong clinical evidence, so we urge you not to gradually go to zero cigarettes per day.

Rule 3 When you reach your target date, you may want to throw away all your cigarettes. Some people like to make a ceremony out of this event. If you feel that you will panic unless you have cigarettes available somewhere (even if they are in the garage, the trunk of the car, or the attic), then you should follow your own inclinations. That is particularly true if these methods have been at least temporarily helpful to you in the past.

Rule 4 Try not to make too much out of quitting. Do not magnify it out of proportion because this may make you experience more stress and other withdrawal effects.

Rule 5 Once you have reached your target date and have successfully stopped smoking, remember to continue keeping track of smoking urges in your smoking diary.

Contract for Stopping with Help from Others

The second method for stopping smoking involves arranging a contract with yourself and another person, preferably a trusted friend. The contract would involve a commitment on your part to stop smoking as of a particular date and hour following three days of reduced smoking—half the usual level—as was described in the previous section. In this case, however, you also build in an added incentive—the possible loss of money. The contract states

---

My Personal Contract for Quitting

I agree to stop all smoking on _____ *at* _____. *I understand that it*
                                    (target date)   *(target time)*
is important for me to make a strong personal effort at this particular time so that I can become a permanent ex-smoker. I sign this contract as an indication of my personal commitment to stop smoking on target.

_____   _____
                    (your signature)   *(date of signing)*

A Personal Contract for Change (continued)

that you deposit a specified sum of money, which you will forfeit if you fail to stop smoking. But you will receive portions of the deposit back as "payment" if you become an ex-smoker.

This contract arrangement can work without the help of others; you may act as your own banker for the agreement. But many people find that asking assistance of a friend helps them stick to their contract. This friend, the "banker" in your contract, should not be a smoker and should not attempt to tell you how to quit.

There are several rules for developing a contract with the help of others as a method for stopping smoking.

Rule 1   Risk an amount of money that would hurt you if it were forfeited. Five dollars would very likely be small and insignificant to you if it were lost; $20 or $50 is more significant.

Rule 2   Choose the banker with great care. He or she can be any nonsmoker you trust, who is willing to help by taking responsibility for keeping your deposit.

Rule 3   Once the contract is signed, stick to it. There should be no changes made in the target date and the monetary agreement, because changes undermine the effectiveness of this entire procedure.

Rule 4   Decide with great care what will be done with any forfeited money. The money must *not* go to your banker. Instead, it should be payable to either a favorite charity or, even better, your least favorite organization— one you would hate to see get your good money. Write checks in advance with the name of the least favorite organization for the banker to hold, so that payment is almost automatic if you smoke. These strategies provide a powerful incentive for you to uphold the contract.

Rule 5   Use the contract presented here. One side should be signed by you and become your copy. The other copy is kept by the trusted banker as his or her copy of the contract.

B. G. Danaher and E. Lichtenstein
Become an Ex-Smoker

(Your copy)   **Two-Party Contract for Quitting**

I agree to stop smoking on _____ at _____. I have given the sum of
                              (target date)   *(target time)*
$ _____ to _____ with the understanding that he/she will send the money
              (banker's name)
to _____ if I am unable to stop smoking according to this agreement. If I am
     (organization)
able to stop smoking completely for the first week after the target date specified above, I will at that time receive half of the deposit back. The remaining portion of the deposit will be returned after the second week of nonsmoking (two weeks from the target date).

_____   _____
(your signature)   *(date)*

_____   _____
(banker's signature)   *(date)*

(Banker's copy)   **Two-Party Contract for Quitting**

I agree to stop smoking on _____ at _____. I have given the sum of
                              (target date)   *(target time)*
$ _____ to _____ with the understanding that he/she will send the money
              (banker's name)
to _____ if I am unable to stop smoking according to this agreement. If I am
     (organization)
able to stop smoking completely for the first week after the target date specified above, I will at that time receive half of the deposit back. The remaining portion of the deposit will be returned after the second week of nonsmoking (two weeks from the target date).

_____   _____
(your signature)   *(date)*

_____   _____
(banker's signature)   *(date)*

You can change the cues in your environment so they trigger the new behavior you want instead of the old one. Put a picture of a gymnast on your refrigerator door or a picture of a cyclist speeding down a hill on your television set. Chart your progress and have it in a special place at home to make your goals highly visible and inspire you to keep at it. When you're trying to change a strong habit, small cues can play an important part in keeping you on track.

A second very powerful way to affect your target behavior is by taking control of its effects on you—by setting up a reward system that will reinforce your efforts. Think about how you get yourself to tackle any difficult job. How much are you motivated by the long-range payoff? How much are you motivated by the rewards and good feelings you get as you go along? Sometimes when you make healthy choices there are **intrinsic rewards** that lie very far in the future or are very hard to measure, such as improved chances you will avoid cancer or heart disease. We have seen that most people find it difficult to change long-standing habits for rewards they can't see right away. Giving yourself instant, real rewards for good behavior along the way will help you stick with a plan to change your behavior.

If your target behavior is something you want to stop doing, the behavior you'll be rewarding is the new, desirable behavior you want to substitute for it—eating moderately instead of overeating, not smoking instead of smoking, making good use of your time instead of putting things off, and so on. Carefully plan your reward payoffs and what they will be. In most cases, rewards should be collected when you reach specific objectives or subgoals in your plan. For example, you might treat yourself to a movie after a week of avoiding extra snacks. Don't forget to reward yourself for good behavior that is consistent and persistent—if you simply stick with your program week after week—because that behavior is moving you toward your goal. Decide on a reward for yourself after you reach a certain goal or mark off the sixth month of a valiant effort. Write it down in your health diary and remember it as you follow your plan—especially when the going gets rough.

Make a list of your activities and favorite events to use as rewards. They should be special, inexpensive, and preferably unrelated to food or alcohol. Depending on what you like to do, you might treat yourself to a concert, a ball game, a new tape or CD, a long-distance phone call to a friend, a day off from studying for a long hike in the woods—whatever is rewarding to you. Everyone has a different "reinforcement menu"; find out what will work best to support your good behavior. And don't forget to reward yourself with a pat on the back—congratulate yourself, notice how much better you look or feel, and feel good about how far you've come and how you've gained control of your behavior.

Rewards and support can also come from your family and friends. Tell them about your plan and ask for their help. Get them to be active, interested participants in what you're doing. Ask them to support you when you set aside time to go running or avoid second helpings at Thanksgiving dinner. You may have to remind them not to do things that make you "break training" and not to be hurt if you have to refuse something when they forget. Getting encouragement, support, praise, and good wishes from important people in your life can powerfully reinforce the new behavior you're trying to adopt.

Your strategy or plan for action should be tailored to the behavior you want to change. You might want to give up a dangerous or reckless habit, fit in 30 minutes of exercise every day, manage your time better, learn more about safety and first aid, overcome test anxiety, or change any one of a vast number of behaviors. Whatever you want to change, you can build a self-management program that makes the circumstances as well as the consequences of your behavior work for rather than against you.

6. **Keep track of your progress; revise your plan if necessary**. Use your health diary to keep track of how well you are doing in achieving your ultimate goal. Record your daily activities and any relevant details, such as how far you walked, how many calories you ate, and so on. Each week chart your progress on a graph and see how it lines up against the subgoals you listed on your contract. You may want to track more than one behavior, especially if they are related, such as the time you spend in working out each week and your weight.

If you don't seem to be making progress, analyze your plan to see what might be causing the problem. A number of possible barriers to success are listed in the section titled "Keeping on Track," along with suggestions for addressing them. Once you've identified

---

Intrinsic rewards   Personal satisfaction or benefits achieved as a result of improved behavior.

the problem, revise your plan so that it has a better chance of working, and keep at it. Be faithful about keeping your health diary, about signing a contract, about implementing your plan. The more effort you put into your program, the greater the benefits for you.

Making Sure You Succeed   Once you've started a program, there are many things you can do to increase your chances of success. Some have already been discussed—recruiting support from your family and friends, changing the cues in your environment, and so on. A list of other strategies follows, some involving further environmental changes and others involving important changes in your thinking.

- *Make your efforts cost-effective.* Think about how to get the best return, the biggest health benefit, from the effort you'll be devoting to your plan. As you launch your program, you may tend to overdo or to try things that take more work than the potential gain is worth. To avoid this pitfall, be sure, first of all, that the new behavior you want has a real and lasting value for you personally. Unless it's right for you, no behavior change project can succeed. Then be realistic about the amount of time and energy you can put into it. The best program is usually one that you can keep following over a long time.

  You may choose any of a number of strategies to reach your goal—just make sure you choose one that works for you. Many activities lead to physical fitness, for example, ranging from walking to bicycle racing. Some of them will appeal to you more than others. If you can fit your new activity smoothly into your existing schedule, you're more likely to succeed. If you plan to take two hours that you would have spent getting together with friends and spend them exercising every day, you may resent the loss of time with friends and your commitment may crumble. With some planning, you can find an activity that works for you in more than one way—both lowering your weight and lifting a mild depression. You can create a self-tailored system to move toward your goal.

- *Find a buddy.* Using the "buddy system" has many advantages. Ask the people around you, and you're likely to find someone who wants to make the same changes you do. You may find a buddy in your roommate, classmate, or your brother or sister. Recruit one or more of them to join your plan. If you can't find someone this way, try joining a group that forms a ready made set of buddies, such as Weight Watchers.

  Having a buddy makes it easier to stay with your program. You can give each other encouragement, support, motivation, sympathy, and information. You'll

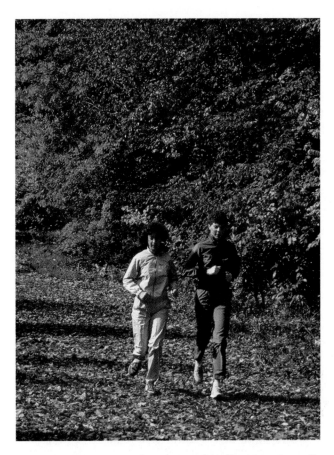

A beautiful day, a spectacular setting, a friendly companion—all conspire to make jogging a satisfying and pleasurable experience for these people. Choosing the right activity and doing it the right way are important elements in a successful health behavior strategy.

have a stake in each other's progress. The fear of letting your buddy down makes it less likely that you'll take a day off. And in a crisis, you can be there to help your buddy overcome the urge to smoke, gorge on snacks, take drugs, or slip in any other way. You'll come to count on your buddy's help, too. For some problems, such as alcoholism, the buddy system (used in Alcoholics Anonymous) is the most successful of all methods that have been tried.

- *Use a role model.* Find someone who reached the goal you're striving for—a celebrity who overcame a disability, a sports hero, a family member, a friend who quit smoking, an acquaintance. Consider how this person got to where he or she is today. How would your role model deal with what you're struggling against? Once you start looking, you may be surprised at the number of people you know who have stopped smoking, kept with an aerobic fitness program or lost weight, or broken a drug habit. Talk to them about how they did it. What strategies worked for them? What can you borrow from their experience?

- *Expect success.* Shakespeare wrote, "There is nothing either good or bad, but thinking makes it so." What you expect and the attitude you take can have a powerful effect on your behavior change program. Expect success and you will dramatically increase your chances of actually succeeding. Drop your old self-image and take on a new one. Picture yourself as a nonsmoker, a jogger, an A student, a thin person. Very often, people keep an old self-image even after they've taken big steps toward a new self. This inner image is always ready to say "I told you so" when you slip. Avoid this trap by changing your ideas about yourself as you change your behavior.

- *Realize that lasting change takes time.* Fad diets promise you'll lose weight instantly; but, in reality, weight loss and other major life changes are long-term projects that take weeks or months. They involve giving up a familiar and comfortable part of your life in exchange for something new and unknown. To be deep and long-lasting, changes have to take time. They happen one day at a time, with lots of ups and downs. At first you may notice a significant change, but then your progress levels off and you reach a plateau. Don't be discouraged—plateaus are a natural part of all learning processes. They give you a chance to settle into the changes you've made so far and prepare for the next step forward. Be persistent and you'll work your way through the doldrums.

- *Forgive and forget.* Every time you try to change your behavior you'll make slips—start on an eating binge, accept a cigarette from a friend, miss a workout. Slips aren't catastrophes—they're problems to be solved. Instead of berating yourself, try to discover what triggered the slip and decide how you'll deal with it next time.

  One way to prevent slips is to rehearse what you would do differently in those situations where you know your target behavior will be triggered. If you don't want to drink too much at a party, decide on your drink limit ahead of time and switch to a soft drink when you hit your limit. If you want to go out to eat, decide ahead of time what you will order and stick to your decision once you're in the restaurant. If you feel you need a break from the program you've set for yourself, go ahead and indulge yourself, but do it outside your regular environment. Go out for ice cream—don't buy a half gallon and put it in your freezer.

When you do slip, be easy on yourself. Feeling guilty, putting yourself down, and blaming yourself are all self-destructive and will work against you. Keeping up your self-esteem will help you stay with your plan; negative feelings will get in your way. Try to understand your slips without judging yourself. See what you can learn from them. Don't use them as a reason to give up or to doubt you can succeed. Remember, most ex-smokers tried and failed many times before they finally succeeded. This may be the time you succeed!

Keeping on Track: Some Troubleshooting Tips As you continue with your program, don't be surprised when you run up against problems and obstacles—they're inevitable. In fact, it's a good idea to expect problems and to give yourself time out to step back, see how you're doing, and make some changes before going on again. If you find that your program is grinding to a halt, try to identify what it is that's blocking your progress. Look at what's going on and be honest about what's causing the problem. It may come from one of these sources:

- *Social influences.* A sibling or a close friend can be very helpful when they're "with you," but they can also cause problems. Perhaps they were part of the problem to begin with, and they may not be willing or able to change. This family member may even be benefiting from the very behavior that you're trying so hard to change. Obviously, such an individual is best avoided until the conflicts have been resolved. Take a hard look at the reactions of the people you're counting on and see if they're really supporting you. If they come up short, try connecting and networking with others who will be more supportive.

  A related trap you should watch out for is trying to get your friends or members of your family to change *their* behaviors. No matter how much you care about them, no matter how much you think they're hurting themselves, you can't make other people change. The decision to make a major behavior change, as you've seen, is something people come to only after intensive self-examination. You may be able to influence someone by tactfully giving them facts or support, but any effort you make to change someone else's life will backfire by wasting your time and energy. Focus on yourself—if you succeed, you may become a role model for someone else.

- *Levels of motivation and commitment.* You won't make real progress until an inner drive leads you to make a personal commitment to the goal. If commitment is your problem, you may need to wait until the behavior you're dealing with makes your life more miserable; then your desire to change it will be stronger. Or you may find that changing your goal will inspire you to keep going. If you really want to change but your motivation comes and goes, look at your support system and at your confidence that you will succeed. Building these up may be the key to pushing past a barrier.

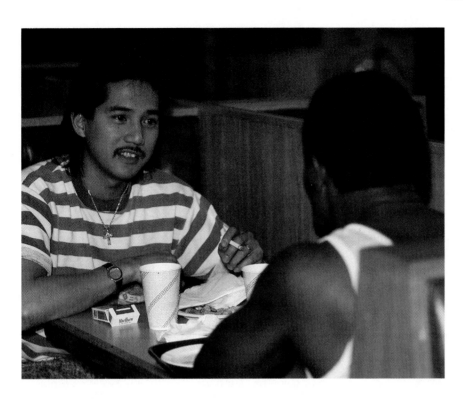

No facts, warnings, or advice from his friend will persuade this young man to quit smoking until he decides to quit himself. Behavior changes, especially those involving powerful habits, usually come from self-examination and deeply felt personal decisions.

• *Choice of techniques and level of effort.* Your techniques may not be working as well as you thought they would in your original plan. Check them against your experience and make changes where you're having the most trouble. If you've lagged on your running schedule, for example, maybe it's because you really don't like doing it. Maybe you would exercise more regularly if you took an aerobics class that offered more structure and group support. There are many ways to move toward your goal. Another pitfall is that your techniques may be right but you may not be trying hard enough. "No pain, no gain" shouldn't be overdone, but you do have to push toward your goal. If it were easy, you wouldn't need to have a plan for change!

• *Stress barrier.* When you're stressed out by crisis or even by everyday living, your behavior change program can derail. Stress isn't something you can remove from your life; you have to find ways to deal with it. Very often, people use overeating, drinking, or smoking as ways to manage their stress. If they try to give up one of these habits, they lose an important coping mechanism. Even if they're successful at first, tension builds, making it more and more difficult to continue.

If you've hit a wall in your program, look at the sources of stress in your life and see how they feed the behavior you're trying to change. Chapter 2 discusses stress and lists common, stressful life events. If there is a temporary stressor in your life, such as catching a cold or having a term paper due, you may want to wait until it's over before stepping up your effort. If stress is a fact of life for you, try to find some healthier ways to deal with it. For example, you may find that sitting in a movie or taking a half-hour walk after lunch are effective things you can do to manage stress. You may even want to make stress management your highest priority for behavior change.

• *Games people play:* procrastinating, rationalizing, and blaming. Even when they want to change, people hold on fiercely to what they know and love (or know and hate). You may have very mixed feelings about the change you're trying to make, and your underlying motives may sabotage your conscious ones if you keep them hidden from yourself. Try to detect the games you might be playing with yourself, so you'll have the opportunity to change them.

If you're procrastinating ("It's Friday already; I might as well wait until Monday to begin"), try breaking your program down into still smaller steps that you can knock off one day at a time. If you're rationalizing or making excuses ("I wanted to go swimming today, but I wouldn't have had time to wash my hair afterwards"), remember that the only one you're fooling is yourself and that when you "win" by deceiving yourself, it's not much of a victory. If you're wasting time blaming yourself or others ("Everyone in that class talks so much that I don't get a chance to say my piece"), recognize that blaming is a way of taking your focus off the real problem and denying responsibility for your actions. Try refocusing by taking a positive attitude and renewing your determination to succeed.

Getting Outside Help   When you hit a snag in your behavior change program, or even before you do, go ahead and take advantage of all the resources around you. Outside help is often needed to change behavior that seems to be too deeply rooted for a self-management approach. Drug and alcohol addictions, excessive overeating, and other conditions or behaviors that put you at a serious health risk, and behaviors that interfere with the ability to function fall into this category. Many communities have programs that help people deal with these problems; Weight Watchers, Alcoholics Anonymous, Smoke Enders, and Coke Enders are only a few of the better known ones.

On campus, you will find courses in physical fitness, stress management, and weight control. The student health center or campus counseling center may also be sources of assistance. Most communities offer a wide variety of low-cost services through adult education, school programs, health departments, and private agencies. Consult the Yellow Pages, your local health department, or the referral service often sponsored by the United Way. Whatever you do, don't be stopped by a problem when you can tap into resources to help you solve it.

Being Healthy for Life

Your first few behavior management projects may never go beyond the project stage and those that do may not all succeed. But as you taste success and begin to see progress and changes, something will probably happen. You'll start to experience new and surprising positive feelings about yourself. You'll probably find that you're less likely to buckle under stress. You may begin opening doors to a new world of enjoyable physical and social events and different types of people. You may surprise yourself by accomplishing things you never thought possible—winning a race, climbing a mountain, breaking a nicotine habit, having a lean, muscular body. Your new way of life will help sustain you for life. Being healthy takes extra effort, but the paybacks in energy and vitality are priceless.

■ **Exploring Your Emotions**

Are you as healthy as you want to be? If not, in what ways would you like to improve?

Once you've started, don't stop. Assume that health improvement is forever. Tackle one area at a time, but make a careful inventory of your health strengths and weaknesses and lay out a long-range plan. Take on the easier problems first and then use what you have learned to attack more difficult areas. Look over your shoulder at your past problems to make sure you don't fall into old habits. Keep yourself informed about the latest health news and trends; research is constantly providing new information that directly affects daily choices and habits.

Making Changes In Your World   You're probably aware that you can't completely control every aspect of your health. At least two other factors—heredity and environment—play important roles in your well-being. After you quit smoking, for example, you may still be inhaling the smoke from other people's cigarettes—smoke that is actually more poisonous to you. Your resolve to eat better foods may suffer a setback when you can't find any healthy choices in vending machines—only an endless array of chips, pretzels, candy, gum, soda, and coffee.

Some things in the environment can be changed, and as an individual you can make a difference. You can use what you have learned to help create an environment around you that supports a healthy lifestyle. You can help support nonsmoking areas in public places by not shying away from asking people to follow the rules. You can speak up in favor of more nutritious foods and better physical fitness facilities, such as a pool, indoor track, and bicycle lanes or trails. You can include a choice of nonalcoholic drinks at your parties and show constraint in your drinking. You can join in special events, such as fun runs and health fairs.

On a broader scale, you can also get involved in working on the environmental challenges facing all of us: air and water pollution, traffic congestion, overcrowding and overpopulation, depletion of the ozone layer of the atmosphere, toxic and nuclear waste disposal, and many others. These difficult issues need the attention and energy of people who are informed and who care about health. On every level, from personal to planetary, individuals can take an active role in shaping their environment.

In fact, Americans have made many changes in recent years as they've gained greater awareness of healthy and unhealthy behaviors and of the power of individuals to change their behavior and take a stand on health issues. Smoking is a prime example. Until recently, the image of the smoker was one of elegance and glamor. Today, people are more likely to see smokers as victims of a dangerous addiction and as adding to a public health threat. As millions of people quit smoking, as more and more nonsmoking areas are created, people's opinions about smoking and smokers are changing. The physical and the social environment have both changed, along with individual awareness and attitudes.

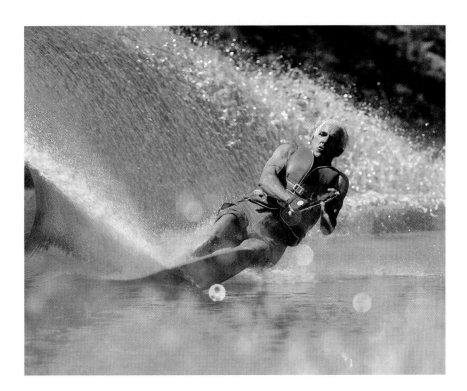

A 60-year-old man who water-skis like a 30-year-old gets his strength from years of vigorous activity. If you want to enjoy vigor and health in *your* middle and old age, begin now to make the choices that will give you life-long vitality.

What Does the Future Hold?   Statistics show that sweeping changes in lifestyle have resulted in healthier Americans in recent years and could have even greater positive effects in the years to come. Coronary heart attack rates, although still high, are down from ten years ago. Stroke rates are down by an amazing 40 percent. Average blood pressure and cholesterol levels are down by small but significant amounts. Problems remain, of course—children seem to be less fit, more people are using drugs, sexually transmissible diseases are on the rise, and AIDS looms as an immense challenge for all of us. What these problems have in common is a strong behavioral component; without question, the direction of the future is toward greater individual responsibility for health.

In your lifetime, you can choose an active role in the movement toward increased awareness, greater individual responsibility and control, and healthier lifestyles. You live in a world in which your own choices and actions will have a tremendous impact on your present and future health. You have the opportunity to reach levels of wellness that your ancestors could only imagine. The door is open, and the time is now—you simply have to begin.

Summary

- A healthy lifestyle promotes optimal health. Through knowledge, self-awareness, motivation, and effort, everyone can achieve good health.

What Is Health?

- Ideas about health have changed over the years. Whereas once it was considered to be the absence of disease and disability, advances in medical science in the twentieth century led people to start thinking of health in terms of longevity.

- As degenerative diseases like coronary heart disease and cancer became the leading causes of death in the United States, people recognized that merely being alive is not the same as health.

- Today, health is perceived as a matter of *wellness*—having a sense of vitality and overall well-being in life. Health is dynamic and multidimensional; it incorporates physical, emotional, intellectual, spiritual, and interpersonal well-being, among other factors.

Choosing Wellness

- People today have greater control over their health than ever before. Being responsible for one's health means making choices, adopting habits and behaviors that will ensure wellness.
- Scientific research regularly makes connections between diseases and certain lifestyles or behaviors and between wellness and other lifestyles or behaviors. Although heredity and environment both play roles in wellness and disease, behavior can mitigate their effects.
- Behaviors and habits that reinforce wellness include (1) taking an active, responsible role in one's health, (2) managing stress, (3) maintaining self-esteem and good interpersonal relationships, (4) understanding sexuality and having satisfying intimate relationships, (5) avoiding tobacco and drugs and restricting alcohol intake, (6) eating well, exercising, and maintaining normal weight, (7) knowing about illnesses and help for them, (8) understanding and wisely using the health system, (9) knowing about diseases and accidents and protecting yourself against them, (10) understanding the processes of aging and dying, and (11) understanding the environment and its effects on your health and working to improve it.
- The habits established during young adulthood tend to become lifelong; some even permanently change health.
- People who make the choices that assure wellness (1) are well-informed on health issues and topics, (2) have self-knowledge and self-insight, (3) know how to set up plans for behavior change.

Getting Down to Basics: How Do You Reach Wellness?

- Many people practice lifestyles that put their health at risk; some aren't aware, others are aware but aren't motivated, and others are aware but don't know how to start on a behavior change program.
- Motivation is one of the most important factors in behavior change. Most people are motivated most strongly by short-term, personal goals.
- Commitment is the second necessary factor in behavior change. It involves the full force of the resolve to change.
- The third and perhaps most important factor in behavior change is taking control of one's life, taking an active role in living and maintaining health. With motivation and commitment, habits that have been learned can be unlearned through behavioral self-management.
- Behavior can be traced to the circumstances that trigger

it; the consequences of behavior can also be identified. The circumstances that trigger behavior include internal and external stimuli; the consequences of behavior can be positive and negative reinforcers. Reinforcers are the basis of behavior self-management.
- The best way to begin a behavior self-management program is to choose one target behavior and follow a systematical six-step program to change. Consistency and persistence are highly important.
- The six steps to behavior management are (1) monitoring behavior, often through a diary, (2) analyzing the recorded data, (3) setting specific goals, usually broken down into small steps, (4) making a personal contract, sometimes with a witness, (5) devising a strategy based on information gathered during the monitoring stage, and (6) keeping track of progress, constantly revising the strategy if barriers arise.
- Strategies for change include controlling environmental stimuli—finding new habits to replace those linked with your target behavior and changing external cues. Setting up a reward system—using instant, real rewards—is an important part of strategy; it reinforces motivation.
- Chances of success in behavior management increase if efforts are cost effective, if the change in behavior would have a real and lasting value. The best programs are those that can be followed over a long time.
- Other strategies for success include having a buddy help, looking for role models, expecting success through adopting a new self-image, recognizing that change takes time, and learning to forgive oneself. Keeping up self-esteem helps; negative feelings undermine the plan.
- Obstacles sometimes come in the form of nonsupportive people, a low level of commitment, inappropriate techniques, too much stress, and procrastinating, rationalizing, and blaming.
- Taking advantage of outside sources and programs can help; some behavior is too deeply rooted to be changed by self-management techniques alone.

Being Healthy for Life

- Each small success in a behavior-management program leads to increased self-esteem and increased motivation to continue.
- Although people can't control every aspect of their health, individuals can make a difference in improving the environment—from insisting on nonsmoking areas in local restaurants to working on planetary issues like nuclear waste disposal and depletion of the ozone layer.
- Changes in lifestyle have resulted in healthier Americans in recent years; this trend will continue.

Take Action

1. Purchase a small notebook to use as your health diary throughout this course. On the first page make a list of the positive behaviors that help you enhance your health (such as jogging and getting enough sleep). Consider what additions you can make to the list or how you can strengthen or reinforce these behaviors. (Don't forget to congratulate yourself for these positive aspects of your life.) Next, list the behaviors that block you from achieving wellness (such as smoking and eating a lot of candy). Consider which of these behaviors you might be able to change. Use these lists as the basis for self-evaluation as you proceed through this book.

2. Think about what troubled you most during the past week. In your health diary, write down the names of three or four people who might be able to help you with whatever troubled you. If the problem persists, consider starting at the top of your list and talking to this person about it.

3. Think of the last time you did something you knew to be unhealthy primarily because those around you were doing it. How could you have restructured the situation or changed the environmental cues so that you could have avoided the behavior? In your health diary, describe several possible actions that will help you

avoid the behavior the next time you're in a similar situation.

4. Choose a person you consider a role model and interview him or her. What do you admire about this person? What can you borrow from his or her experiences and strategies for success?

5. Make a list in your health diary of rewards that are meaningful to you. Add to the list as you think of new things to use. Refer to this list of rewards when you're developing plans for behavior change.

Selected Bibliography

Barsky, Arthur J. 1988. *Worried Sick: Our Troubled Quest for Wellness.* Boston: Little, Brown.

Fries, James F., and Lawrence M. Crapo. 1981. *Vitality and Aging.* New York: W. H. Freeman.

Healthy People: The Surgeon General's Report on Health Promotion and Disease Prevention. U.S. Department of Health Services, DHEW Pub. 79–55071.

Justice, Blair. 1988. *Who Gets Sick: How Beliefs, Moods, and Thoughts Affect Your Health.* Los Angeles: Jeremy Tarcher.

Hiatt, Howard H. 1987. *America's Health in the Balance: Choice or Chance?* New York: Harper and Row.

Recommended Readings

The following are highly readable monthly or bimonthly newsletters and magazines filled with the latest research and thinking on health-related topics.

Harvard Medical School Health Letter (P.O. Box 10944, Des Moines, IA 50340)

Healthline (The C. V. Mosby Company, 11830 Westline Industrial Drive, St. Louis, MO 63146–3318)

In Health (formerly *Hippocrates*) (Hippocrates Partners, 475 Gate Five Rd., Suite 225, Sausalito, CA 94965)

Mayo Clinic Health Letter (Mayo Foundation for Medical Education and Research, 200 First Street SW, Rochester, MN 55905)

University of California, Berkeley Wellness Letter (P.O. Box 420148, Palm Coast, FL 32142)

Contents

Making Connections

P eople in our society are continually enduring daily hassles, making major changes in their lives, and balancing the flow of money, time, and energy. Developing ways to cope with the inevitable stress of life is an important task of early adulthood and a challenge not always met successfully. The scenarios presented on these pages describe stress-related situations in which people have to use information, make a decision, or choose a course of action. As you read them, imagine yourself in each situation and consider what you would do. After you've finished the chapter, read the scenarios again and see if what you've learned has changed how you would think, feel, or act in each situation.

At the beginning of the year, your roommate was rowdy and unpredictable, often overreacting to trivial incidents. Then someone got him involved in jogging every day. Lately, you haven't noticed as many incidents of explosive behavior. In fact, his personality definitely seems to have improved. Now he's encouraging you to take up jogging too, saying it helps him chill out when he's feeling stressed. Could jogging really have that effect?

You've been at college for a month now, and the initial thrill is starting to wear off. You got a D on your first English paper, you don't seem to be able to get all your course work done, and you haven't hit it off with some of the people you live with. Lately, your stomach has been hurting, you feel a little shaky, and you're having trouble sleeping. You've even wondered if you're getting sick. Should you see a doctor at the student health center? Drop out and go home? Just wait for things to get better? How can you figure out what to do?

2

Stress: The Constant Challenge

Your father recently achieved a goal you know he'd dreamed of for years—the vice presidency of his company. To celebrate, your mother planned a huge party for friends and relatives, and you and your brothers and sisters all came home for the occasion. But you were surprised by how drained and even depressed your father seemed when you saw him. He was drinking too much and, worst of all, had started smoking again after five years without cigarettes. You keep trying to figure out what's going on—if this is what he's always wanted, why does he seem to be falling apart?

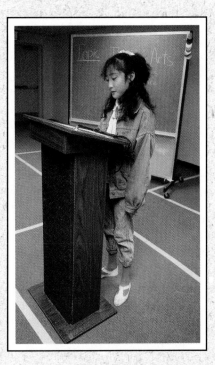

One of your instructors has you intimidated with his harsh criticism, sarcastic comments, and hostile attitude. He seems to expect the worst of people and be angry at the whole world. When you were home recently, you described him to your family and your grandmother commented, "He's digging his own grave." But your sister said, "It's normal. That's how ambitious people have to be to get ahead. If you want to succeed, you'll be tough too." You're not sure you want to be as cynical as he is. Is your sister right?

You were complaining about your tension headaches to the resident advisor in your dorm, a person you admire for his air of calm authority. He says he used to be tense all the time too, but then he read something about meditation and decided to try it. Now he meditates every day for 20 minutes. He says it quiets his mind, relaxes his body, and gives him a feeling of being "centered." He also says his blood pressure is lower since he started meditating. You're having a hard time accepting all of this and think he's a little weird, but he does seem to have it all together. He offers to lend you one of his books on how to meditate. If you tried it, would people think you're strange too, or is there something to it that might be helpful?

Everybody talks about **stress.** People say they're "over-stressed" or "stressed out." They may blame a headache or an ulcer on stress, and they may take an aerobics class—or drugs—to help them deal with stress. But what is stress? And why is it important to manage it wisely?

Although most people have experienced periods of higher-than-normal stress, they often associate these times with negative events such as the death of a close relative or friend, financial problems, or significant changes in their lives that lead to nervous tension. But stress isn't merely nervous tension, and it isn't something that should be avoided at all costs. As a matter of fact, complete freedom from stress is death. Before we explore more fully what stress is, consider this list of common stressful situations or events:

Interviewing for a job
Running in a race
Christmas
Going out on a date
Watching a football game
Getting a promotion

Obviously, stress doesn't arise just from unpleasant situations. From this list it's apparent that stress can be associated with physical challenges and even with success and the achievement of personal goals. Physical and psychological stress-producing factors can be either pleasant or unpleasant. The crucial factor is how the individual responds to them, whether in positive, life-enhancing ways or in negative, counterproductive ways.

As a young adult, you are probably in one of the most stressful periods of your whole life. You may be on your own for the first time, meeting new people, exploring different activities, and trying to establish yourself as an independent person in the world. All of these events and challenges are likely to have a powerful effect on your physical and psychological states. Ineffective responses to stress eventually take their toll on your sense of well-being and overall health, but effective responses enhance your health and give you a feeling of control over your life. How can you tell when your stress level is getting dangerously high? And how can you develop techniques to cope positively with the stress that is part of your life? This chapter will help you discover answers to these questions.

What Is Stress?

With the broad range of stress-eliciting situations in mind, how can we arrive at a clear definition of stress? No one has more thoroughly explored the biochemical and environmental facets of stress than Dr. Hans Selye, an endocrinologist and biologist. Selye defines stress as "the nonspecific response of the body to any demand." "Nonspecific response" refers to the body's total biological response to stress-producing factors, such as increases in heart rate and blood pressure and the release of stress **hormones.** The body's response may be larger or smaller, but it is limited to these physiological changes, no matter what the stressful situation.

Selye coined the word **eustress** for stress that is pleasant and beneficial, the stimulation that keeps the mind and body functioning properly, such as exercise. **Distress,** on the other hand, is unpleasant and can have negative effects if not handled well. Distress arises in such situations as getting a poor grade, hearing bad news, or being rejected for a date or a job. Both eustress and distress are characterized by such familiar physiological reactions as sweaty palms, a pounding heart, and cold hands and feet.

■ Exploring Your Emotions

Whether you're skidding on an icy road, giving an oral presentation in class, asking someone out on a date, or reading an exciting murder mystery, the basic stress reaction is the same. Your heart beats faster, your hands and feet get cold, your mouth gets dry, your bladder and intestines relax, your hair even stands on end. Watch for these physical changes when you're in a stressful situation. Keep track of how often in a day you experience the stress reaction to some degree. Is there much stress in your life?

In common usage, the word *stress* is used to refer to two different things—the situations and events that produce physiological changes and the physiological changes themselves. Strictly speaking, stress-producing factors are more accurately referred to as **stressors,** and the physiological changes are more accurately called the **stress response.** Because of this common usage, we often use the word *stress* broadly in this book, referring to both stressors and the stress response. The exact meaning of the word will be apparent from the context.

The Stress Response What's happening when we feel that surge of alarm or excitement in a stressful situation, and why does it happen? The answers to these questions can be found by taking a closer look at what we think of as normal, everyday functioning. Life is dependent on ceaseless **metabolic activity,** the internal processes of change, growth, deterioration, and replacement. The body is continually trying to maintain a dynamic steady state, or **homeostasis.** Anything, internal or external, that disrupts this steady state stresses the organism. If homeo-

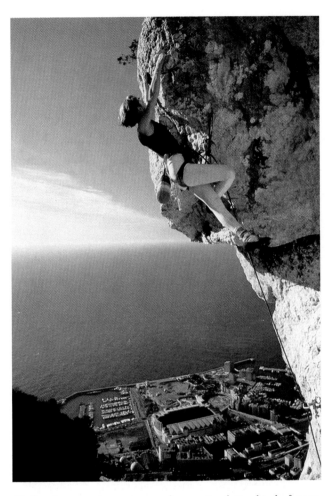

Challenging experiences can produce a stimulating kind of stress known as eustress. This young woman seeks out and thrives on the thrills of rock climbing.

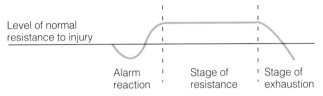

Figure 2-1   In Selye's experiments, rats subjected to cold at first exhibited the hormonal changes typical of the alarm reaction but then adapted to life at lower temperatures. After several months, however, they lost their acquired resistance, and exhaustion set in.

stasis is to be restored, **adaptive reactions**—adjustments of hormone levels or heart rate, for example—have to be made. In a sense, life is just one adaptation after another. We don't consciously notice the smaller adaptations that our bodies are making all the time, but we're acutely aware of the larger ones.

Selye used the term **general adaptation syndrome (GAS)**, or stress response, to describe the totality of adjustments in the body in response to internal and external changes. The GAS develops in three stages: alarm, resistance, and exhaustion. People typically go through the first two stages quite often in the course of adapting to their various everyday activities and to the demands made on them. The energy used to make these adjustments is replenished when people eat, sleep, relax, exercise, and so on. Exhaustion sets in if the stress is long lasting and the person's response to the stress is counterproductive—drinking and smoking, for example, instead of exercising and relaxing. In extreme situations, exhaustion can lead to death (see Figure 2-1).

The entire stress response is under the control of the **autonomic nervous system.** This nervous system functions in many respects independently of conscious thought and controls the organs and glands (as opposed to the somatic nervous system, which controls the muscles attached to the skeleton). The autonomic nervous

---

Stress   The sum of the biological reactions to any stimulus—pleasant or unpleasant; physical, mental, or emotional; internal or external—that tends to disturb the organism's homeostasis.

Hormones   Chemical messengers produced in the body and transported by the bloodstream to target cells or organs for specific regulation of their activities.

Eustress   A stress state believed to be pleasant, even beneficial.

Distress   An unpleasant stress state believed to cause illness.

Stressor   Any physical or psychological event or condition that produces stress.

Stress response   The physiological changes associated with stress.

Metabolic activity   Chemical and physical processes that involve the body's use of food to convert nutrients into energy.

Homeostasis   A state of stability and consistency in the physiological functioning of an organism.

Adaptive reaction   The organism's attempt to readjust its activities and restore homeostasis when the demands of stress have disturbed the body's equilibrium.

GAS (general adaptation syndrome)   A pattern of stress responses described by Hans Selye as having three stages: alarm, resistance, and exhaustion.

Autonomic nervous system   The branch of the peripheral nervous system that, largely without conscious thought, controls basic body processes; subdivided into the sympathetic and parasympathetic systems.

Heavy traffic on a rain-slicked highway is a recipe for stress. Some of the people involved in this series of collisions are still unnerved; others show signs of readjustment to normal functioning.

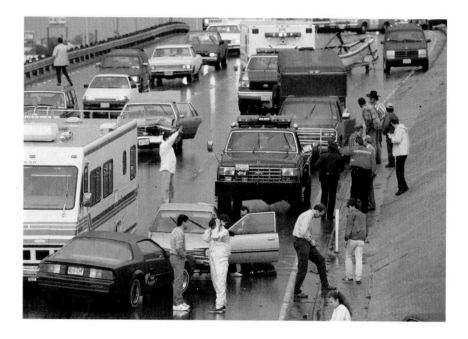

system is made up of two parts, the **sympathetic** and the **parasympathetic** branches. The sympathetic branch mobilizes the body for action during times of increased awareness, danger, or excitement; the parasympathetic branch calms it down when the excitement subsides, restoring normal functions. The two branches are constantly interacting in a complex system of checks and balances to keep the body functioning effectively.

GAS: Alarm   During the alarm stage of the GAS, the alerted body prepares for physical action—the familiar **fight-or-flight reaction.** Though often absurdly inappropriate, this reaction is part of our biological heritage. It can be triggered by stumbling over a doorstep, going to a party, being insulted, hearing the telephone ring, get-

ting a bill, or any of countless other experiences, mild or intense, mundane or monumental. We all know the feeling—the surge of emotion, the rush of adrenaline, the heightened sense of surroundings. We may mask emotional turmoil to be socially acceptable, but our aroused physiological processes are indifferent to such niceties.

Once the threat is perceived and the brain signals "Danger!" a complex series of chemical reactions takes place. The **hypothalamus,** a remarkable control center nestled in the lower brain and capable of sending messages both to and from the brain, stimulates the **pituitary gland** (the "master gland" at the base of the brain) to send **adrenocorticotropic hormone (ACTH)** into the bloodstream. When the ACTH reaches the **adrenal glands,** located just above the kidneys, it stimulates the

---

Sympathetic nervous system   A division of the autonomic system that reacts to danger or other challenges by almost instantly putting the body processes in high gear.

Parasympathetic nervous system   A division of the autonomic system that tones down the excitatory effect of the sympathetic system, slowing metabolism and restoring energy supplies.

Fight-or-flight reaction   A defense reaction that prepares the organism for conflict or escape by triggering hormonal, cardiovascular, metabolic, and other changes.

Hypothalamus   A part of the brain that activates, controls, and integrates the autonomic mechanisms, endocrine activities, and many body functions.

Pituitary gland   The "master gland," closely linked with the hypothalamus, that controls other endocrine glands and secretes hormones that regulate growth, maturation, and reproduction.

Adrenocorticotropic hormone (ACTH)   A hormone, formed in the pituitary gland, that stimulates the outer layer of the adrenal gland to secrete its hormones.

Adrenal glands   Two glands, one lying atop each kidney, their outer layer (cortex) producing steroid hormones such as cortisol, and their inner core (medulla) producing the hormones epinephrine and norepinephrine.

Cortisol   A steroid hormone secreted by the cortex (outer layer) of the adrenal gland; also called *hydrocortisone.*

Epinephrine   A hormone secreted by the medulla (inner core) of the adrenal gland; also called *adrenaline,* the "fear hormone."

Norepinephrine   A hormone secreted by the medulla (inner core) of the adrenal gland; also called *noradrenaline,* the "anger hormone."

Adaptive energy   Limited body reserves that are activated when the body feels exhausted.

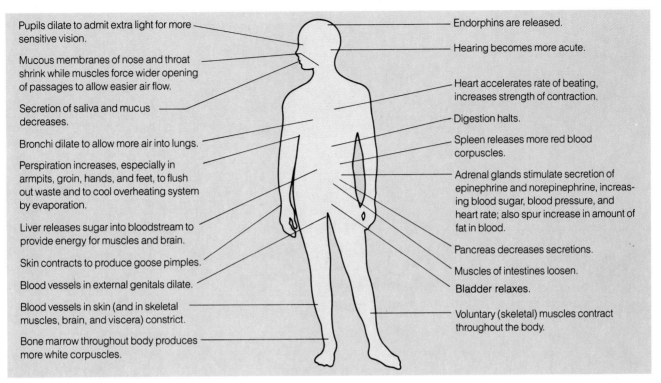

Pupils dilate to admit extra light for more sensitive vision.

Mucous membranes of nose and throat shrink while muscles force wider opening of passages to allow easier air flow.

Secretion of saliva and mucus decreases.

Bronchi dilate to allow more air into lungs.

Perspiration increases, especially in armpits, groin, hands, and feet, to flush out waste and to cool overheating system by evaporation.

Liver releases sugar into bloodstream to provide energy for muscles and brain.

Skin contracts to produce goose pimples.

Blood vessels in external genitals dilate.

Blood vessels in skin (and in skeletal muscles, brain, and viscera) constrict.

Bone marrow throughout body produces more white corpuscles.

Endorphins are released.

Hearing becomes more acute.

Heart accelerates rate of beating, increases strength of contraction.

Digestion halts.

Spleen releases more red blood corpuscles.

Adrenal glands stimulate secretion of epinephrine and norepinephrine, increasing blood sugar, blood pressure, and heart rate; also spur increase in amount of fat in blood.

Pancreas decreases secretions.

Muscles of intestines loosen.

Bladder relaxes.

Voluntary (skeletal) muscles contract throughout the body.

Figure 2-2 The Body's Response to Stress

cortex (outer layer) of the adrenal glands to rush **cortisol** and other "stress hormones" into the bloodstream.

Sympathetic nerves stimulate the medulla (inner core) of the adrenals to release **epinephrine,** or adrenaline, the "fear hormone," and **norepinephrine,** or noradrenaline, the "anger hormone." These events, all orchestrated by the hypothalamus, cause various useful changes in the body's organs and tissues, such as dilation of the bronchi to allow more air into the lungs, acceleration of the heart rate to pump oxygen through the body, increase in perspiration to cool the skin, and, happily, release of endorphins to relieve pain in case of injury (see Figure 2-2).

GAS: Resistance During the resistance (or adaptive) stage, the body readjusts, regulating body systems and beginning to repair any damage that may have been sustained during the alarm reaction. When the stressful situation ends, the parasympathetic branch of the autonomic nervous system calms the body down, slowing rapid heartbeat, drying sweaty palms, and adjusting skin temperature. As the stress symptoms diminish, normal functioning gradually returns. The body readjusts and resumes "housekeeping" functions, such as digestion, temperature regulation, and normal circulation. As you might imagine, both the mobilization of forces during the alarm reaction and the restoration of homeostasis

during the adaptive stage require a considerable amount of energy.

GAS: Exhaustion If the stressful situation doesn't end and the alarm reaction continues for a long time, the body's ability to adjust diminishes. Energy is being used to keep the body in a state of vigilance, prepared to fight or run for survival. In our present circumstances, of course, this response is rarely necessary. As the body's energy is depleted, reserves of **adaptive energy** can be activated, but these reserves are also limited. If they are spent, the result is general exhaustion—characterized by such symptoms as distorted perceptions and disorganized thinking—and, as mentioned earlier, even death. The body's reserves of adaptive energy can be restored to some extent through proper diet and exercise, adequate sleep, and other behaviors, but there is no evidence that they can be fully controlled. In fact, they may be genetically determined. Clearly, it's in our best interest not to overreact to the normal stresses of everyday life.

Mobilized for Survival in a Civilized World The stress response gets you all revved up for physical action, but most of the stressors of modern life can't be handled with physical means. You're expected to deal with job interviews, arguments with friends, confrontations with

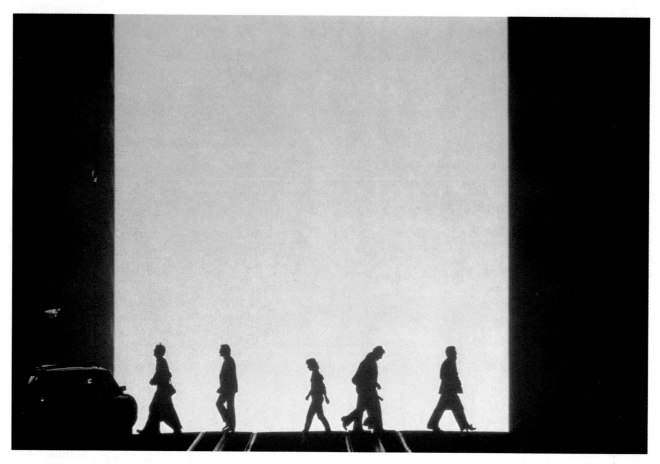

Cities, with their crowds, noise, dirt, and impersonality, offer an unrelentingly stressful environment to millions of people. Yet many individuals thrive there, finding excitement, challenge, and glamour. How do you react to cities?

authority figures, and other stressful situations in rational, verbal ways. If you're stopped for driving too fast when you're late for an important track meet, for example, you may feel like screaming at the police officer, but it would be unwise of you to do so. If you're unable to console a crying baby, you may feel like hitting it, but you have to do something else instead.

■ Exploring Your Emotions

How do you respond when you're in a frustrating situation such as a traffic jam? Do you find that such situations really bother you sometimes but not other times? What else is going on when you stay calm? When you fly off the handle?

Additionally, some of the stressors of modern life—noise, overcrowding, overwork, competition, economic pressures, and so on—go on not just for a few minutes but for days, weeks, months, or years. The body may try to stay mobilized indefinitely to deal with them, and its system of checks and balances may go awry. The result is a more or less constant state of arousal that depletes energy and can lead to nervous tension, aches and pain, and disease. If the body's mobilization for combat occurs too often over a period of years or is too prolonged, irreparable damage can occur. The person may develop what Selye calls "diseases of adaptation," which include cardiovascular, kidney, and glandular diseases, ulcers, mental disorders, and possibly cancer. These unsuccessful adaptations are discussed more fully later in the chapter.

How do you know when you are overmobilizing? Table 2-1 highlights the danger signals of stress. Of course, you don't have to experience them all to realize that you're overstressed. And some of the signals may be symptoms of a medical problem rather than stress. In general, though, such signals are distinct warnings about a problem that requires your attention. Ignoring or worrying about such symptoms will only increase your stress. If your body is trying to tell you something, it's important

Table 2-1 Signals of stress	
Emotional and Behavioral Signs	**Physical Signs**
Tendency to be irritable, hyperexcited, or depressed	Pounding heart
Impulsiveness, aggressiveness, emotional instability	Trembling, with nervous tics
Overpowering urge to cry or to run and hide	Grinding of teeth
Inability to concentrate, general disorientation, flight of thoughts	Dry mouth
Weakness, dizziness, or sense of unreality	Excessive perspiration
Fatigue and loss of the joy of living	Gastrointestinal problems (diarrhea, constipation, indigestion, queasy stomach, perhaps vomiting)
"Floating anxiety" (fear without an obvious reason)	Aching of neck or lower back
Keyed-up feeling	Migraine or tension headaches
Tendency to be easily startled by small sounds	Frequent colds or low-grade infections
Nervous, high-pitched laughter	Cold hands and feet
Tendency to move about or gesture for no apparent reason	Allergy or asthma attacks
Increased smoking	
Increased use of prescription drugs, especially tranquilizers and pep pills (e.g., amphetamines)	
Addiction to alcohol or drugs	
Addiction to TV	
Frequent feelings of boredom	
Sleep disturbances (insomnia, nightmares) or excessive sleep	
Speech difficulties (e.g., stuttering)	
Overeating or undereating	
Sexual problems	

Source: Partially based on Selye, 1979, pp. 66–68.

to listen and figure out what the message is. Then you can take action to relieve the discomfort before it gets worse.

Emotional and Behavioral Responses to Stress

Physiologically, everyone responds to stress in a basically similar and fairly predictable way. But emotionally and behaviorally, people vary widely in their responses to stress, depending on a broad range of factors. A situation that might be very stressful to you could leave someone else utterly calm. You may do better in sports and public performance when the competition is stiff and the pressure is on, while your roommate may perform poorly under pressure and excel only in a relaxed atmosphere. You may feel comfortable flying in a plane but be nervous about talking to members of the opposite sex, while your roommate may love challenging social situations and be terrified of flying. What accounts for these differences?

To answer this question, let's consider the example of two students, Laurel and Stacey, in a familiar situation—taking the first exam of the semester. As the exam is passed out, Laurel feels anxious and agitated. Scanning the questions, she sees a few on a subject she didn't study. She becomes more anxious and finds she can't recall some of the material she did study. The more she blanks out, the more upset she gets, all the time thinking about the possible consequences of failing the course and kicking herself mentally for not preparing better. She answers as many questions as she can and then turns in her paper without checking her answers or going back to the ones she skipped. She's almost in tears as she hurries from the classroom.

Stacey also feels agitated as the test is passed out, and she also finds she doesn't know some of the answers. But after an initial moment of concern, she takes a deep breath and starts writing the answers she knows. Then she does a second pass through the exam, concentrating intently on the wording of the questions. Some material comes back to her, and she makes some educated guesses on other items. She spends the whole hour writing as much as she can. At the end of the test she thinks she did fairly well and feels exhilarated as she leaves the room.

Laurel and Stacey responded to the same stressor in very different ways. Laurel got flustered, blanked out, and concluded that she was a failure. Stacey took a deep breath, concentrated, and fulfilled her expectation of success. Their responses are influenced by a complex set of factors, both innate and learned—their intelligence, their temperaments and predispositions, their ideas and beliefs about themselves, their prior experience with situations of this sort, the techniques they habitually use to cope with challenges. Research indicates that two of the most important factors in how different individuals respond to stress are personality traits and experience. Personality traits are the stable set of characteristics that underlie a person's psychological behavior, including thoughts and actions. Personality affects how the individual perceives situations and how he or she habitually responds to them. Experience with similar situations further influences the response.

In our example, it may be that Laurel is less confident of her academic abilities or her likelihood of success than Stacey. She may respond anxiously to many situations in her life and especially to tests. If she had had a bad test experience before, in which she blanked out, she may have been worried that it would happen again. She may not have been able to study very effectively because of worry and anxiety, which interfere with thinking. Stacey, on the other hand, may be a calmer, more relaxed person who doesn't get easily upset by things. She may be more confident of her academic abilities and have more prior experiences of success. She may be able to focus her attention and study effectively despite distractions.

■ **Exploring Your Emotions**

How did the people in your family cope with stress when you were growing up? Were their methods successful? Do you use the same methods (or nonmethods) they did? Are there people around you who use different methods that you could try?

Whatever the exact reasons for the differences in the two women's experiences, it's clear that what made the situation so stressful for Laurel was not the test itself so much as how she interpreted and responded to it. The test itself was basically neutral. Sometimes people have such intense emotional and behavioral responses to situations that they need professional assistance in learning how to cope.

Most people don't experience reactions of this severity, however; more often, people have stress-related problems that they themselves can learn to handle. Like Laurel, they may habitually respond to situations in maladaptive ways, ways that make it harder for them to cope rather than easier. Some behavioral responses to stress, such as drinking alcohol, drinking coffee, and smoking cigarettes, actually accentuate the stress response, increasing blood pressure and heart rate. Later in this chapter we describe a number of successful coping methods that can be used to modify emotional and behavioral responses to stress.

The Role of Stress in Disease

Stress clearly produces extensive changes in the functioning of the body, ranging from imperceptible adjustments in hormone levels to full-blown fight-or-flight responses. Does stress also play a role in sickness and disease? Most researchers no longer doubt that stress contributes to the occurrence, course, and deadliness of diseases. They are beginning to accept the idea that even susceptibility to infectious diseases can be profoundly influenced by how the individual habitually handles the stresses of daily living, both emotionally and behaviorally.

In the short term, a chronic and prolonged stress response may lead to a stiff neck, a queasy stomach, or a tension headache. In the long term, it may lead to lowered resistance to disease and a damaged cardiovascular system. There seems to be a stress-related component in a number of conditions and diseases, including heart disease, hypertension, headaches, asthma, arthritis, digestive problems such as ulcers and colitis, skin conditions such as eczema and hives, and possibly even cancer. Although the mechanisms by which stress translates into physical illness are not all known, research is actively going on in several areas.

Stress and the Immune System   Sometimes it seems that you get sick at the very times you need all your energy reserves to deal with events in your life—when your car is in the garage, your bicycle has been stolen, you're snowed under with work, your apartment is a mess, and your parents are coming for a visit. In fact, observations that people tended to get sick when their lives were particularly stressful led some researchers to suggest that life events and changes were a major contributing factor in illness. (For a more complete discussion of this issue, see the box entitled, "Life Events and Disease: Is There a Link?")

Now it seems that the role of stress in disease is more complex than was previously thought. Whether you actually become sick depends not just on the number of events that occur but also on other factors such as the qualities of the events themselves, how you perceive the events, how you respond emotionally to them, how effective your coping techniques are, and so on. As pointed out earlier, much depends on the individual and the situation.

When stress and illness are related, a possible mechanism may be the effect of stress on the immune system. Although preliminary, evidence suggests that stressful situations may lead to a diminished immune response. For example, researchers in the field of **psychoneuroimmunology** (a scientific field investigating mind-body interactions) have found that medical students have decreased immune responses during times of increased academic pressures. Other studies have shown that when individuals experience emotional stressors, such as anxiety, depression, or anger, or physical stressors, such as overexertion or sleep deprivation, there is a decline in the number of their helper T-cells, the white blood cells that are in charge of the body's immune response (see Chapter 18). When stress diminishes, the helper T-cell count rises. In other words, our emotional reactions can have a direct bearing on our ability to fight off disease agents (such as cold and flu viruses) and other threats to the body.

In more general terms, we could say that resistance to disease may be lowered as a person tries to cope with stress and that resistance becomes even lower when the person uses ineffective coping techniques. Everyone has a finite amount of energy. If too much is expended dealing with the environment, there is less reserve for preventing disease. The crucial point once again, however, is that it's not the stressor itself that causes the problem; it's how the individual responds to the stressor emotionally and behaviorally.

Stress and Heart Disease: Personality Types   A link between stress and heart disease has been the subject of research for many years. In the 1970s cardiologists reported that people with certain personality characteristics had a higher incidence of heart disease than people with other characteristics. They described people with "Type A personalities" as energetic, mentally alert, productive, and apparently rarely depressed. Type A's often hold responsible managerial jobs and engage in a host of wide-ranging activities. Typically aggressive, competitive, easily angered, impatient, and controlling, Type A's hate to waste a moment. They try to tackle more than one thing at a time, and anything that holds them up—waiting in line, being stuck in traffic, listening to a rambling speaker—is apt to make them impatient and angry.

In contrast, Type B's are low-keyed, relaxed, contemplative. They tend to accomplish things slowly and methodically, to be less concerned with the quantity than with the quality of their output, and to be content with doing a few things really well. Although Type B's are apt to work fewer hours than Type A's, they seem to win just as many promotions and often are highly successful precisely because they don't waste energy worrying about traffic jams and petty details and because their composure inspires confidence. Yet, the notion persists that Type B's are too laid back and that Type A's are more likely to succeed.

Early studies of Type A's suggested that they have heart attacks more frequently and at a younger age than the general population. Their risk of coronary heart disease was believed to be high because their behavior led them frequently into stressful situations, such as arguments and competitive, high-performance jobs. In those situations they were likely to react explosively, setting off the stress response that includes surges in blood pressure and stress hormones (epinephrine, the "fear hormone," and norepinephrine, the "anger hormone"). Such surges can cause damage to the lining of the blood vessels and a buildup of plaque in the veins and arteries, putting the individual at risk for a heart attack or stroke (as discussed in detail in Chapter 15).

Recent evidence suggests that only particular characteristics of the global Type A pattern—specifically, anger and hostility—may increase the risk of heart disease. Studies have shown that heart attacks are more frequent among people who are characterized as hostile and who have a cynical mistrust of others. Other characteristics of the Type A personality, such as competitiveness, drive, and the tendency to be in a hurry, don't seem to be associated with heart disease. It seems, then, that people who habitually respond to life's stresses and challenges

Psychoneuroimmunology   The study of the interactions between the mind and the nervous and immune systems.

Life Events and Disease: Is There a Link?

Some people believe that stressful events predispose a person to illness, whether a cold, mononucleosis, or cancer. Where did this idea originate, and what basis does it have in fact? In 1967 Drs. Thomas Holmes and Richard Rahe published the Social Readjustment Rating Scale (SRRS) in the *Journal of Psychosomatic Research*. The premise of their work was that the more "social readjustments" a person has to make within a certain period of time, the more likely the person is to become sick. Social readjustments are events in a person's life that require change or accommodation—a divorce, a move, the birth of a child, and so on. Holmes and Rahe arrived at their list of social readjustments by examining the life charts of 5,000 patients, noting the events that clustered at times of disease onset, and distilling out a list of 43 life events, both positive and negative, that seemed to be associated with illness. They also weighted the various events, which they referred to as life change units (LCUs), and used the weights to create the SRRS.

Since the development of this assessment instrument, many researchers have investigated the question of whether individuals with high scores are at a greater risk of disease as a result of having to make more readjustments in life. Preliminary studies seemed to confirm the hypothesis. In contrast to control groups, patients with manifestations of disease, such as heart attacks, reported experiencing a greater number of life events and had higher LCU scores. But more recent studies have cast doubt on the hypothesis. These studies have been *prospective*—following healthy people over a period of years to see who becomes ill—as opposed to the earlier *retrospective* studies, which asked people who were already ill to look back and report on past life events. Some of these studies have failed to find a relationship between life events and disease, and others have reported an association weaker than that suggested by earlier studies.

Why the discrepancies among the various studies? One explanation is that in retrospective studies, patients may overreport the number of events they experienced prior to becoming ill. Overreporting would account for the significant associations found in the early studies between life events and illness. However, it would not explain the positive associations reported in some of the prospective studies. A second explanation, and probably the single strongest criticism of life-events studies, is the notion of measuring life events as a single dimension. The SRRS produces one score that encompasses both positive and negative events—marriage as well as divorce, success as well as failure, winning the lottery as well as losing a job. Researchers who have established scores for such other dimensions as "upsettingness," threat, and emotional distress have found that all three of these aspects are independently related to disease.

Finally, some researchers have suggested that the impact of life events on the development of disease may be moderated by personality type. Individuals with certain personality and behavioral

with anger, hostility, and cynicism are at a greater risk of heart disease than people who respond with other emotions and attitudes.

What makes a person a Type A personality? Evidence indicates that some people are born with more explosive, anger-prone personalities. Early childhood experiences, such as rejection or abuse, can also make people hostile and mistrustful. But on the basis of controlled experiments with hundreds of individuals, Dr. Meyer Friedman, the coauthor of *Type A Behavior and Your Heart,* is convinced that Type A's can significantly reduce their risk of heart attacks by modifying their behavior. He claims that his behavior modification program, which is available in do-it-yourself form, has achieved results far superior to those of any other therapy, such as diet, exercise, drugs, or surgery. Through programs like his, Type A's can learn to change their emotional and behavioral responses to stress to promote rather than diminish their cardiovascular health.

If you think you may be a Type A, take the self-assessment quiz in the box entitled, "Are You a Type A or a Type B?" If you are, consider taking some of the suggestions given for derailing your Type A response in the box entitled "Derailing Your Type A Behavior." If you start now to short-circuit your hostile responses, you may be giving yourself the gift of a healthy heart.

Life Events and Disease: Is There a Link? (continued)

characteristics, such as anger and hostility, may be more susceptible to the adverse health effects of life events. Individuals who are more relaxed or more flexible may experience those same events with fewer ill effects.

Although the evidence for life events as a precipitating factor in disease is modest, there does seem to be reason to believe that some life events are potentially disease producing. It may be that only those events that produce emotional distress or increase the possibility of mental illness are risk factors for disease. It may also be that personality and behavioral characteristics moderate the association between life events and disease. Researchers need to pursue this line of study to identify more precisely the life events that carry the highest risk of causing disease.

Early adulthood can be a stressful time, bringing major life changes that require adjustment and accommodation. Listed below, in order of probable severity of effect, are 30 life events that young adults may experience. As explained earlier, we can't say for certain that clusters of events will lead to illness. But we do know that these events increase stress and that stress needs to be managed wisely if the individual is to maintain a healthy equilibrium. If you find that the list includes events that you have experienced recently or expect to experience soon, take the time to develop and cultivate your coping skills—they'll serve you well, both now and in the years to come.

Stressors of Young Adulthood

1. Death of a close family member
2. Death of a close friend
3. Divorce between parents
4. Jail term
5. Major personal injury or illness
6. Marriage
7. Fired from job
8. Failed important course
9. Change in health of a family member
10. Pregnancy
11. Sex problems
12. Serious argument with close friend
13. Change in financial status
14. Change of major
15. Trouble with parents
16. New girl- or boyfriend
17. Increased workload at school
18. Outstanding personal achievement
19. First quarter/semester in college
20. Change in living conditions
21. Serious argument with instructor
22. Lower grades than expected
23. Change in sleeping habits
24. Change in social activities
25. Change in eating habits
26. Chronic car trouble
27. Change in number of family get-togethers
28. Too many missed classes
29. Change of college
30. Minor traffic violations

Stress and Social Support Systems   Is living alone hazardous to your health? Statistics suggest that it may be. Married people live longer than single people and have lower death rates for a wide range of conditions. Married men between the ages of 25 and 64 have a significantly lower death rate from heart disease than do unmarried men. Cancer patients who are married have a 23 percent higher survival rate than single patients do, and people infected with the AIDS virus remain symptom-free for a longer time if they have strong social support systems.

The crucial factor in each case is believed to be the presence of emotional and social supports that connect individuals with others and help them deal with stress. Such support systems seem to have the effect of buffering people from the damaging effects of stress. When such support systems are missing, people are more vulnerable to illness. Social isolation, for example, is now believed to be a major factor in increasing the risk of disease. People who are uninvolved with other people or organizations are especially vulnerable to chronic disease. Individuals with "marginal" social status, such as some homeless or unemployed people, also have increased vulnerability to illness.

To give yourself added protection against stress-related disease, take the time to nourish and maintain your own social support system. It consists of the people with

Are You a Type A or a Type B?

Questionnaires don't provide conclusive assessments of personality types, nor does everyone fall into a neat category. But you can get a general idea of which personality type you more closely resemble by responding to the following statements. Read each statement and circle one of the numbers that follows it, depending on whether the statement is definitely true for you, mostly true, mostly false, or definitely false. Scoring is explained after the questionnaire. If you turn out to be a Type A and would like to relax more, read the tips in the box "Derailing Your Type A Behavior."

	DEFINITELY TRUE	MOSTLY TRUE	MOSTLY FALSE	DEFINITELY FALSE
1. I am more restless and fidgety than most people.	1	2	3	4
2. In comparison with most people I know, I'm not very involved in my work.	1	2	3	4
3. I ordinarily work quickly and energetically.	1	2	3	4
4. I rarely have trouble finishing my work.	1	2	3	4
5. I hate giving up before I'm absolutely sure I'm licked.	1	2	3	4
6. I am rather deliberate in telephone conversations.	1	2	3	4
7. I am often in a hurry.	1	2	3	4
8. I am somewhat relaxed and at ease about my work.	1	2	3	4
9. My achievements are considered to be significantly higher than those of most people I know.	1	2	3	4
10. Tailgating bothers me more than a car in front slowing me up.	1	2	3	4
11. In conversation I often gesture with hands and head.	1	2	3	4
12. I rarely drive a car too fast.	1	2	3	4
13. I prefer work in which I can move around.	1	2	3	4
14. People consider me to be rather quiet.	1	2	3	4
15. Sometimes I think I shouldn't work so hard, but something drives me on.	1	2	3	4
16. I usually speak more softly than most people.	1	2	3	4

	DEFINITELY TRUE	MOSTLY TRUE	MOSTLY FALSE	DEFINITELY FALSE
17. My handwriting is rather fast.	1	2	3	4
18. I often work slowly and deliberately.	1	2	3	4
19. I thrive on challenging situations. The more challenges I have the better.	1	2	3	4
20. I prefer to linger over a meal and enjoy it.	1	2	3	4
21. I like to drive a car rather fast when there is no speed limit.	1	2	3	4
22. I like work that is not too challenging.	1	2	3	4
23. In general I approach my work more seriously than most people I know.	1	2	3	4
24. I talk more slowly than most people.	1	2	3	4
25. I've often been asked to be an officer of some group or groups.	1	2	3	4
26. I often let a problem work itself out by waiting.	1	2	3	4
27. I often try to persuade others to my point of view.	1	2	3	4
28. I generally walk more slowly than most people.	1	2	3	4
29. I eat rapidly even when there is plenty of time.	1	2	3	4
30. I usually work fast.	1	2	3	4
31. I get very impatient when I'm behind a slow driver and can't pass.	1	2	3	4
32. It makes me mad when I see people not living up to their potential.	1	2	3	4

Are You a Type A or a Type B? (continued)

	DEFINITELY TRUE	MOSTLY TRUE	MOSTLY FALSE	DEFINITELY FALSE
33. I enjoy being around children.	1	2	3	4
34. I prefer walking to jogging.	1	2	3	4
35. When I'm in the express line at the supermarket, I count the number of items the person ahead of me has and make a comment if it's over the limit.	1	2	3	4
36. I enjoy reading for pleasure.	1	2	3	4
37. I have high standards for myself and others.	1	2	3	4

	DEFINITELY TRUE	MOSTLY TRUE	MOSTLY FALSE	DEFINITELY FALSE
38. I like hanging around talking to my friends.	1	2	3	4
39. I often feel that others are taking advantage of me or being inconsiderate.	1	2	3	4
40. If someone is in a hurry, I don't mind letting him or her go ahead of me.	1	2	3	4

Scoring

For each statement, two numbers represent Type A answers and two numbers represent Type B answers. Use the scoring sheet to determine how many Type A and Type B answers you gave. For example, if you circled 1, definitely true, for the first statement, you chose a Type A answer. Add up all your Type A answers and give yourself plus 1 point for each of them. Add up all your Type B answers and give yourself minus 1 point for them. Total your score and determine your personality type from the following table:

+20 to +40 = Definite A
 +1 to +19 = Moderate A
  0 to −19 = Moderate B
−20 to −40 = Definite B

1. 1, 2 = A; 3, 4 = B
2. 1, 2 = B; 3, 4 = A
3. 1, 2 = A; 3, 4 = B
4. 1, 2 = B; 3, 4 = A
5. 1, 2 = A; 3, 4 = B
6. 1, 2 = B; 3, 4 = A
7. 1, 2 = A; 3, 4 = B
8. 1, 2 = B; 3, 4 = A
9. 1, 2 = A; 3, 4 = B
10. 1, 2 = B; 3, 4 = A
11. 1, 2 = A; 3, 4 = B
12. 1, 2 = B; 3, 4 = A
13. 1, 2 = A; 3, 4 = B
14. 1, 2 = B; 3, 4 = A
15. 1, 2 = A; 3, 4 = B
16. 1, 2 = B; 3, 4 = A
17. 1, 2 = A; 3, 4 = B
18. 1, 2 = B; 3, 4 = A
19. 1, 2 = A; 3, 4 = B
20. 1, 2 = B; 3, 4 = A

21. 1, 2 = A; 3, 4 = B
22. 1, 2 = B; 3, 4 = A
23. 1, 2 = A; 3, 4 = B
24. 1, 2 = B; 3, 4 = A
25. 1, 2 = A; 3, 4 = B
26. 1, 2 = B; 3, 4 = A
27. 1, 2 = A; 3, 4 = B
28. 1, 2 = B; 3, 4 = A
29. 1, 2 = A; 3, 4 = B
30. 1, 2 = A; 3, 4 = B
31. 1, 2 = A; 3, 4 = B
32. 1, 2 = A; 3, 4 = B
33. 1, 2 = B; 3, 4 = A
34. 1, 2 = B; 3, 4 = A
35. 1, 2 = A; 3, 4 = B
36. 1, 2 = B; 3, 4 = A
37. 1, 2 = A; 3, 4 = B
38. 1, 2 = B; 3, 4 = A
39. 1, 2 = A; 3, 4 = B
40. 1, 2 = B; 3, 4 = A

TACTICS AND TIPS

Derailing Your Type A Behavior

People with Type A personalities tend to be aggressive, ambitious, competitive, restless, and sometimes hostile and distrustful. Hostile Type A's are more vulnerable to heart disease than Type B's, who are more relaxed, laid back, and low-keyed. If you think you are a Type A and would like to be more like a Type B, here are some suggestions from Dr. Meyer Friedman and others to get you started on modifying your behavior.

• Don't wear your watch.
• Drive only in the right lane all day.
• Cancel an errand and go walk in the woods instead.
• Play a game with a child and lose.
• Stop worrying about numbers and how much you get done.
• Ask someone a personal question and listen to the answer.
• Take a long bath.
• Read a novel.

• Ask someone to do you a personal favor.
• Let someone else decide where to go to dinner or what movie to see.
• Become aware of distrustful or hostile thoughts and try to examine them objectively to see if they're really accurate.
• Focus on what's important in your relatively short life and enjoy those things more.

whom you have enduring interpersonal ties, at home, at work, at school, in the community. These are the people you count on to give you emotional support, feedback, and nurturance and with whom you share values and standards. They may be members of your family, or they may be friends and other people with whom you've developed meaningful relationships. Many families don't function very well as support systems for their members, but you can still have a "family" by building emotional ties with others. No matter what kind of stress you're experiencing, it's important to have people with whom you can share your frustrations, complaints, joys, and fears.

The Hardy Personality   You can give yourself another kind of insurance policy against illness by cultivating

Moving is a highly stressful event, but this couple is coping with it wisely. They've taken time out to relax, have a good meal, and replenish their emotional reserves with mutual support.

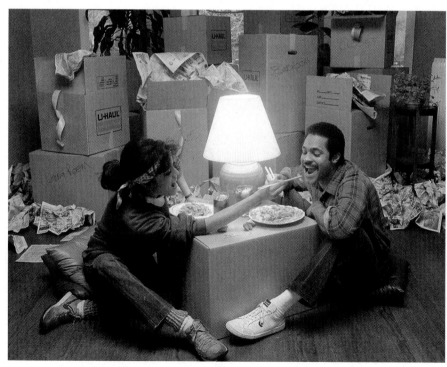

traits associated with what psychologist Suzanne Kobasa calls the "hardy personality." People with this type of personality remain healthy even under extreme stress. Kobasa believes they resist illness because they cultivate what she calls "the three C's of health," challenge, commitment, and control.

■ Exploring Your Emotions

When was the last time you got terribly angry? What did you do? How did you feel afterward? Would you say that you successfully handled this stressful moment? Write down some other ways to deal with stress.

- *Challenge.* People with hardy personalities see change for what it is—a natural, stimulating part of life, not a threat or disruption that has to be avoided at all costs. Hardy people are flexible and open to change, welcoming it as a challenge and an opportunity for growth and learning.
- *Commitment.* These people become deeply involved in their activities, committing themselves to whatever it is they've chosen to do with a strong sense of inner purpose. Their commitment is different from the overcommitted, out-of-control response of Type A's.
- *Control.* Overeating and abusing alcohol and drugs are responses of people who feel at the mercy of life changes. People with hardy personalities act rather than react; they write their own script instead of following one written by someone else. Their control doesn't mean they dominate others, nor does it mean they don't accept things that can't be changed. But they do realize that they have the power to control their lives to a large extent, and their positive attitude helps them deal with adversity when it comes.

Coping with Stress

As you can see, the greatest everyday threats to your health and well-being arise not from wounds or infections but from the effects of stress on your body. When you respond to environmental **stimuli** with excessive amounts of anger, fear, frustration, resentment, or envy, you place a burden on your body that at the very least depletes energy, disrupts your immune system, and im-

pairs cardiovascular health. When you moderate your responses, maintain a strong social support system, and develop healthy ways of coping with stress, you protect yourself from its damaging effects.

There are a number of approaches you can take to coping with stress. Underlying virtually all of them is an awareness of the close connection between your thoughts and feelings and your body's ability to regulate and heal itself. Among the methods described here, try to find and stick with the one that seems most attuned to your needs, tastes, and style. Whether your progress is gradual or swift doesn't matter. What does matter is that you'll be learning to listen to your body. When you recognize the stress response and the emotions and thoughts that accompany it, you'll be in a position to take charge of that crucial moment and handle it in a healthy way.

Time Management   If you're a procrastinator, time management is probably a complete mystery to you. Although occasional postponement of a task may be defensible, chronic procrastination is self-defeating: it creates stress, which then leads to more procrastination, which leads to more stress. Not only does procrastination cause emotional upsets, but it can also sabotage personal relationships, college life, and careers. True, some people refuse to cling to a rigid schedule and work so well under pressure that they can accomplish in a few frantic hours what they couldn't have done as well in a week. But if they gave time management a decent try, even they might find that frenzied last-minute efforts aren't necessarily their key to success.

The reasons for procrastination are as far-ranging and numerous as the excuses made for it (such as "I'll wait until I'm inspired," "What difference will this make in the planetary scheme of things?"). But in general procrastination camouflages self-doubt, an unreasonable desire for perfection, and a reluctance to make changes. The best solution for procrastination is to stop endlessly thinking or talking about what you're going to do and just do it. How can you prod yourself into doing instead of stewing? Here, in abridged form, are some tips from two psychologists who are reformed procrastinators: "Visualize your progress. Optimize your chances. Stick to a time limit. Don't wait until you feel like it. Watch out for your excuses. Focus on one step at a time. Get beyond the first obstacle. Reward yourself after you've made some progress. Be flexible about your goal. It doesn't have to be perfect."

Stimulus (plural stimuli)   Any action, agent, or condition that causes a physiological or psychological response.

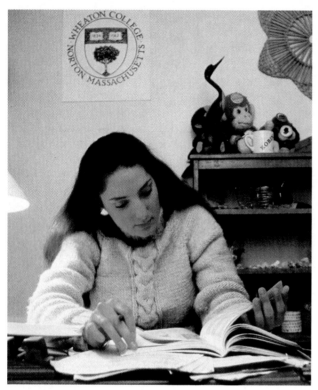

Time management is a critical skill needed to cope with stress. If this young woman allows enough time for studying, sleeping, and recreation, she's well on her way to being in control of her life.

Time pressures can be stressful, though, even if you never procrastinate. Depending on your needs, any or all of the following steps should help you manage your time productively and creatively:

- *Set your priorities.* Split your tasks into three groups: essential, important, trivial. Focus only on the first two; ignore the third.
- *Schedule your tasks for peak efficiency.* Distribute your time not only according to your priorities but also in harmony with your body's natural rhythm. You've undoubtedly noticed that you're most productive at certain times of the day (or night). Schedule your tasks for those hours. Remember, no one can work at top capacity all the time.
- *Aim for realistic goals.* Believable goals will continually spur you on. Strive for the impossible, and you'll almost surely give up.
- *Write down your goals.* First make sure your goals aren't merely wishes. Then fully commit yourself to achieving them.
- *Allow yourself enough time.* It's just wishful thinking to make an unrealistic prediction about how long a project will take. After you've made a reasonable esti-

mate, tack on another 10 or 15 or even 25 percent as a buffer against mistakes or unanticipated problems.
- *Divide your long-term goals into short-term goals.* Instead of waiting for and relying on a large block of time, use snatches of time either to start a project or to keep it moving. Say you have a 50-page report to write and are about to panic. Divide it into three tasks: research, outlining, and writing. Allot enough half-hour or hour time slots to each task. After each hour spent at the library or each few pages written, the progress you've made will make you feel so much better that you'll be stimulated to plow on.
- *Visualize the achievement of your goals.* By mentally rehearsing your performance of a task, you can reach your goal quite smoothly because, after all, you'll have traveled that road before.
- *Sleep on it.* Before you go to sleep, take about five minutes to write down in order of priority the problems you might have the next day. Then ignore them. While you're asleep, your unconscious mind will be hard at work tackling those problems. When you deal with them by rank the next day, you may be surprised at how easily you'll be able to work them out.
- *Delegate responsibility.* If common sense tells you that you need some aid, don't be a martyr. Asking for help isn't a cop-out as long as you don't delegate to others the jobs you know you should do yourself.
- *Say no when necessary.* If the demands made on you don't seem reasonable, just say no—tactfully, but without guilt and endless apologies.
- *Give yourself a break.* Allow time for play—real free time when you ignore the clock and don't compulsively engage in structured activities.

Relaxation Techniques   According to Dr. Herbert Benson of Harvard Medical School, one goal of relaxation techniques is to trigger the relaxation response—a physiological state that is the opposite of the fight-or-flight response. As the body relaxes, the heart rate slows, breathing becomes slower, blood pressure decreases, metabolism and oxygen consumption are reduced, brain waves shift from an alert beta rhythm to a relaxed alpha rhythm, and blood flow to the brain and skin increases, producing a feeling of warmth and quiet mental alertness. Practiced regularly, relaxation techniques can counteract the debilitating effects of chronic stress. They can also be used in stressful situations to help bring the body back to normal levels of functioning.

If you decide to try one of these techniques, practice it every day until it becomes natural to you, and then use it whenever you feel the need. Although you may feel calmer and more refreshed after each session, no matter how inept you are, it may take several weeks for subtle changes to occur. If one technique doesn't seem to work well enough for you after you've given it a good try, have a go at another one. After you've mastered deep relaxation, its effects will carry over into everyday life so that, after a while, you'll probably notice that you have fewer hassles, work more efficiently, and have more free time. None of the techniques takes long to do—for instance, just a few minutes away from the television set should do the trick.

Progressive Relaxation   Here's a technique that, unlike most of the others, doesn't require imagination, willpower, or self-suggestion to master. Progressive relaxation, also known as deep muscle relaxation, helps you become aware of and counteract the tenseness that occurs when you're under stress, by enabling you to identify which muscle groups are involved and relaxing them. Other systems of the body then get the message and ease up on the stress response.

Basically, all you do is tense and then relax each part of your body at least twice, tensing up while inhaling and then relaxing completely while slowly exhaling. As a start, for instance, tense and then relax, in turn, the right fist; right biceps (the large muscle at the front of the upper arm); left fist; left biceps; forehead; eyes; jaw. If you want to relax more quickly, just tense and then relax whole muscle groups at one time (for example, both right and left fists and biceps simultaneously). Once you master this progressive relaxation technique, you can very quickly and effectively relax by simply clenching your fists for a few moments and then fully relaxing them.

Imagery   When you use imagery, or visualization, you can blissfully daydream—without guilt. With this technique, you visualize yourself in a perfectly relaxed state and your body responds to the image as if it were real. You can use imagery not only to help you relax but also as an aid to healing, to changing habits, and to performing well (for example, before taking an exam, playing a sport, writing a paper, or making a public speech).

The next time you're feeling stressed, close your eyes and vividly visualize yourself floating on a cloud, sitting on a mountaintop, or lying in a meadow. Try to involve all five senses (sight, sound, smell, taste, and touch). Or, with eyes closed, imagine your body filled with a deep purple light that you'd like to change to a soothing golden color; then imagine the color changing, and you'll probably feel an easing of your discomfort. If you're worried about doing well at some task, imagine yourself performing it flawlessly.

Meditation   Meditation is a way of politely telling the mind to shut up for a while. The need to periodically stop the incessant mental chatter is so great that, from ancient times, hundreds of forms of meditation have been developed in cultures all over the world. Because medi-

tation has been at the core of many Eastern religions and philosophies, it has acquired an "Eastern" mystique that has caused some people to shy away from it. Yet meditation requires no special knowledge or background. We all know how to meditate; we need only discover that we do and then put our knowledge to use. Whatever philosophical, religious, or emotional reasons may be given for meditation, its power derives from its ability to elicit the relaxation responses.

Meditation helps you tune out the world temporarily, relieving you from both inner and outer stresses. It gives you a chance to transcend past conditioning, fixed expectations, and the trivial pursuits of the psyche; it clears out the mental smog. The "thinker" takes time out to become the "observer": calmly attentive, without analyzing, judging, comparing, or rationalizing. Regular practice of this quiet awareness will subtly carry over into your daily life, encouraging physical and emotional balance no matter what confronts you. For a description of a meditation procedure, see the box entitled, "The Relaxation Response."

Any or all of the relaxation techniques described here should be helpful. Why, then, don't most of them work for long? Because although people might like a certain technique, even become enthusiastic over it, all too often they don't stick with it: after two or three weeks, they slack off, finally abandon it, and resume their seemingly endless search for relief. Most of the methods take time to learn and require a certain amount of discipline, so their appeal tends to fade. Faced with a busy schedule and countless daily hassles, many people find it inconvenient to withdraw, to stop everything while they take time out to practice some form of relaxation. Besides, a few can't seem to relax enough to relax. So let's consider some other possibilities.

Exercise   Exercise is not only beneficial for weight reduction and improving the condition of your cardiovascular system, but it can also make you feel great. Whether your pace is slow or fast, walking just one or two miles can significantly reduce your anxiety level. Exercise also dramatically increases your energy level. After a brisk ten-minute walk, people feel increases in energy and decreases in tension and fatigue for up to two hours. Research has shown that exercise also alleviates depression. In one study, a group of mildly to moderately depressed patients either ran or received short- or long-term psychotherapy. During the first week, the runners reported feeling better, and after only three weeks of running, they were considered "well," with the benefits of their running lasting for at least a year. The exercise group improved as much as the group who received short-term psychotherapy and did even better than patients receiving unlimited long-term therapy.

The Relaxation Response

Relaxation and meditation open the gateway to the relaxation response, which is a set of physiological changes that are scientifically measurable (such as slowed brain waves and decreased heart rate, breathing rate, metabolic rate, and blood pressure). These changes occur as the relaxation response blocks the arousal of the sympathetic nervous system. According to recent experiments, the regular practice of a relaxation-response technique produces special benefits that merely sitting still by oneself does not. By countering the destructive cycle of anxiety, the relaxation response tends to banish inner stresses and exert a healing, calming influence. So it not only helps preserve emotional balance in everyday life, but also enhances therapy for a host of illnesses.

The Procedure

Several years ago, Dr. Herbert Benson developed a simple, practical technique for eliciting the relaxation response. Since then, he has found that combining the technique with the "faith factor" can multiply its benefits. Here is the basic procedure Dr. Benson recommends in *Beyond the Relaxation Response* (1984):

1. Select a word or brief phrase that has a deep meaning for you (such as one that reflects your personal philosophy or religious faith).

2. Take a comfortable position in a quiet environment.

3. Close your eyes.

4. Consciously relax your muscles.

5. Breathe slowly and naturally through your nose, silently repeating your focus word or phrase each time you exhale.

6. Keep your attitude passive—disregard thoughts that drift in.

7. Continue for 10 to 20 minutes, once or twice a day.

Suggestions

If, at least at first, you don't care to combine the technique with the "faith factor," you can pick almost any focus word or phrase, such as "one" or a nonsense word. In Zen meditation, the word *mu* (literally, "absolute nothing") is often used. Some meditators find it helpful to focus on the breath—in, out, in, out—rather than on a word or phrase. Others prefer to focus on an object such as a candle flame. By contrast, in Zen meditation, the eyes are open to discourage a dreamy state but are not focused on anything.

Passively allow relaxation to occur at its own pace, without trying to force it, without making judgments. Whether you think you're doing well or badly, smilingly dismiss the thought. Don't be surprised if your mind refuses to stop its shenanigans for more than a few seconds at a time. It's nothing to get angry about or think about. The more you ignore the intrusions, the easier it will get to do so.

If you want to time your session, peek at a watch or clock occasionally, but don't set a jarring alarm.

Getting to your feet immediately after a session can make you feel slightly dizzy. Sit quietly for a few moments, with eyes closed at first and then open.

The technique works best on an empty stomach—before a meal or about two hours after eating. And avoid those times when you're obviously tired—unless you want to fall asleep.

Although you'll feel refreshed even after the first session, it may take a month or more to get noticeable results. Be patient. Above all, don't harbor expectations or try to aim at a goal. You'll be achieving your goal just by giving the relaxation response a chance—the process itself is the product. Even if you think all you're doing is chasing your mind around and futilely trying to keep it tied down, the relaxation response will be taking place. And long before you assume you know how to elicit the response, its benefits will start showing up in your daily life. Eventually it will become so much a part of you that it will occur spontaneously, or on demand, when you sit quietly for a few moments.

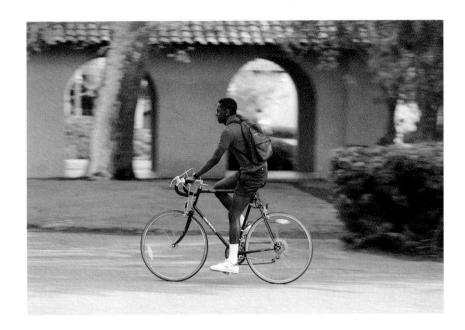

Biking is a particularly effective antidote to stress. It not only provides exercise but helps you avoid all the stresses associated with cars, including getting caught in traffic jams, looking for parking spaces, making insurance payments, and knowing you're producing air pollution.

One way exercise causes changes in mental attitude is through the release of **endorphins,** the body's own opiates. These chemicals are released during the stress of extremely vigorous exercise. Marathon runners often report experiencing euphoria, or a "runner's high" during their long distance workouts. This may be the result of an endorphin release. However, research has shown that even when subjects under stress are given drugs such as naloxone, which block the release of endorphins, they still report feeling less anxiety, depression, tension, anger, and hostility. Endorphins, therefore, aren't the only chemicals working to reduce stress. When neurotransmitters (the chemical messengers of the brain) such as norepinephrine and dopamine are released, we think and react more quickly and feel more motivated and mentally alert. Exercise may increase norepinephrine levels in depressed people and help stabilize their mood.

Whether it's raking leaves, dancing, or running marathons, exercise can be the perfect outlet for reducing your levels of anger and hostility and releasing the physical tension caused by the fight-or-flight syndrome. It is important to remember, however, that strenuous exercise is not necessary for better health. Working small exercises into your daily life can make you feel better, too. Walk to class instead of driving, climb stairs instead of taking the elevator, make a habit of walking with a friend

after dinner. Once you begin incorporating exercise into your life, you may find it harder to live without it.

Nutrition   A sensible diet (see Chapter 12) undeniably helps promote the well-being that enables the body to withstand stress. The basic principles of good nutrition are so easy to learn and to use that their practice can quite rapidly become automatic. The person who is informed and guilt-free about nutrition has an energy bank to draw on whenever stress strikes, as well as a sense of self-control and of self-esteem that is a prime key to managing stress.

Some people react to stress by eating too much, others by eating too little. When you're in deep distress, it may be wise to eat rather lightly, because digestive functions slow or shut down during the stress response (they don't have high priority in the body's attempt to cope).

Although caffeine in small amounts seems to be harmless and definitely provides a mental lift, this stimulant tends to make some persons jittery, irritable, and unable to sleep unless consumed only early in the day. So, when you're under stress, coffee—along with tea, cola, and other soft drinks containing caffeine—may be particularly uncongenial. Eating or drinking chocolate, especially at night, is usually no help either, as it contains a stimulant.

Endorphins   Opiate-like chemical substances, produced in the brain, that help kill pain and produce sedation and euphoria (sense of well-being).

If I Had My Life to Live Over . . .

If I had my life to live over, I'd dare to make more mistakes next time. I'd relax. I'd limber up. I would be sillier than I have been this trip. I would take fewer things seriously. I would take more chances. I would take more trips. I would climb more mountains and swim more rivers. I would eat more ice cream and less beans. I would perhaps have more actual troubles, but I'd have fewer imaginary ones.

You see, I'm one of those people who live sensibly and sanely hour after hour, day after day. Oh, I've had my moments and if I had it to do over again, I'd have more of them. In fact, I'd try to have nothing else. Just moments, one after another, instead of living so many years ahead of each day. I've been one of those persons who never goes anywhere without a thermometer, a hot water bottle, a raincoat and a parachute. If I

had to do it again, I would travel lighter than I have.

If I had my life to live over, I would start barefoot earlier in the spring and stay that way later in the fall. I would go to more dances. I would ride more merry-go-rounds. I would pick more daisies.

Nadine Stair, 85 years old, Louisville, Kentucky. Quoted by Edward A. Charlesworth and Ronald G. Nathan, 1984, in *Stress Management: A Comprehensive Guide to Wellness* (New York: Atheneum), p. 300.

"Stress vitamins"—high-potency formulations that commonly contain vitamins C, E, and B-complex—are worthless in combatting psychological or emotional stress. In fact, because such supplements may contain up to 80 times the U.S. Recommended Dietary Allowance (RDA) for B vitamins and 16 times that for vitamin C, they could even heighten stress through potential side effects.

Humor   Laughter is probably the ultimate stress reliever. A built-in tranquilizer and healer, it is a simple and natural antidote to stress. You can actually alter your mood if you smile, because a smile or a laugh produces changes in the autonomic nervous system.

A genuine belly laugh stimulates the heart and the glandular system and raises both the pulse rate and blood pressure, but afterward the heart rate and blood pressure dip below normal and muscles are more relaxed. In addition, laughter aids digestion and eases pain, apparently by releasing endorphins. Therapeutic humor—which does not include ridiculing, cynical, or sarcastic humor—is an appreciation of life's absurdities and paradoxes. Black humor, which is sometimes so gruesome as to be offensive, is an unconscious means of dealing with fears and anxieties.

Seeing things with humor gives you a break, even if a short one, from the hassles of daily life. It detaches you from both your situation and yourself. Don't allow yourself to be a slave to all the dramas in your life. Develop the ability to laugh at yourself, and you'll always have on hand a stress reliever that is instantly effective.

Changing Your Thinking   Once you get the knack of dealing with stress, you'll probably devise your own special aids. Here, in the meantime, are some suggestions for defusing stress over both the short and the long term.

Worry Constructively   Worrying, someone once said, is like shoveling smoke. Think back to the worries you had last week. How many of them were needless? Worry, if you must, only about things you can control. Try to stand aside from the problem, consider the positive steps you can take to solve it, and then carry them out. You've done what you can; you can quit worrying.

Moderate Expectations   Expectations are exhausting and restricting. The fewer expectations you have, the more you can live spontaneously and joyfully. We assume that people expect a lot from us, just as we do from them. Yet the surest road to failure is to try to please everyone—and that is a road you can choose to bypass. In therapist Fritz Perls's words, "I don't exist to fulfill your expectations, and you don't exist to fulfill mine."

Weed Out Trivia   You can burden your memory with too much information. One of the major sources of stress is trying to remember too many things. Forget the unimportant ones (they will usually be self-evident) and keep your memory free for the essential ones.

Live in the Present   Do you clog your mind with the debris of past events by reliving them? Clinging to experiences and emotions, particularly unpleasant ones, can be a deadly business. Let them go; keep your mind free and clear for what's happening now.

Go with the Flow   A flexible attitude goes a long way toward counteracting the effects of stress. Remember that the branch that bends in the storm doesn't break. Try to flow with your life, accepting the things you can't change.

Be forgiving of faults, your own and others'. Instead of looking forward to being happy at some indefinite point in the future, try to realize that pleasure is integral to being alive and that you can create it every day of your life. Use challenges to help you learn and grow. In this way you can make stress work for you rather than against you, enhancing your overall health.

Summary

Stress-creating situations can be physical or psychological, pleasant or unpleasant. How people respond to stress helps determine their sense of well-being and their feeling of control over their health and their lives.

What Is Stress?

- In Hans Selye's terms, stress is "the body's total biological response to any demand"—including increases in heart rate and blood pressure and the release of stress hormones.
- *Eustress* is pleasant and beneficial; *distress* is unpleasant and can have negative effects.
- Stress is the result of any internal or external disruption of the body's dynamic steady state, or *homeostasis*. The body's response to stress, or general adaptation syndrome (GAS) has three stages: alarm, resistance, and exhaustion. GAS is controlled by the autonomic nervous system; the sympathetic branch puts the body into action, and the parasympathetic branch calms it down.
- The alarm stage of GAS is the fight-or-flight reaction. The hypothalamus stimulates the pituitary gland to release ACTH, which stimulates the adrenal cortex. This event and the stimulation of the adrenal medulla by the sympathetic nerves cause dilation of the bronchi, acceleration of the heart rate, an increase in perspiration, and a release of endorphins.
- The resistance stage of GAS allows the body to readjust; body systems are regulated, and any damage sustained is repaired. Both the alarm and the resistance stages require considerable energy.
- The exhaustion stage occurs only if the body's reserves of energy (including adaptive energy) are depleted in a stress response; the results are distorted perceptions, disorganized thinking, and—in extreme cases—death. Whether the body's reserves of adaptive energy can ever be completely restored after exhaustion is not known.
- Most stresses of modern life can't be handled with a physical response; moreover, many of them continue indefinitely. A person whose body is constantly mobilized against these stresses may become a victim of "diseases of adaptation."

Emotional and Behavioral Responses to Stress

- Stress contributes to the occurrence, course, and deadliness of diseases. Stress-related illness depends not just on the quantity of stressful events in one's life but also on the qualities of events, perception of the events, emotional response to the events, and effectiveness of coping techniques.

The Role of Stress in Disease

- Both emotional and physical stressors lead to a decline in helper T-cells, which control the body's immune response; stress, therefore, affects our ability to fight infection. Ineffective coping techniques make the body even more susceptible because energy is expended fighting stress, not disease.
- The critical factors in a Type A personality (energetic, aggressive, competitive) compared to a Type B personality (relaxed, low-key, contemplative) in terms of risk for heart disease are anger and hostility. Through behavior modification, those with these characteristics can reduce their risk of heart attacks.
- Emotional and social support systems help buffer people from the effects of stress and make illness and disease less likely.
- The "hardy personality" views change as a positive challenge, has a strong sense of inner purpose (commitment), and acts to control health as much as possible.

Coping with Stress

- The greatest everyday threats to health come from the effects of stress on the body. The appropriate responses to stress offer protection against its damaging effects.

- Coping effectively means recognizing the close connections between thoughts and feelings and the body's ability to regulate and heal itself.
- Time management is an effective coping technique for those whose tendency to procrastinate results in the stress of a multitude of tasks, all needing to be done at the last minute. Steps that can be taken include setting priorities, scheduling for peak efficiency, setting realistic goals, writing down goals, allowing enough time, and dividing long-term goals into short-term goals.
- The relaxation response is the opposite of the fight-or-flight response; techniques that trigger it counteract the physiological effects of chronic stress. Characterizing the relaxation response are slower heart and breathing rates, decreased blood pressure, lowered metabolic rate, a relaxed alpha brain rhythm, and increased blood flow to brain and skin.
- Relaxation techniques include progressive relaxation, imagery, and meditation. Progressive relaxation involves tensing and then relaxing parts of the body; practice leads to the ability to quickly relax. The use of imagery or visualization is a form of daydreaming or imagining; it aids not only in relaxing, but also in healing, changing habits, and improving performance. Through meditation, the world with all its stresses can be tuned out.
- Exercise is a coping technique that reduces anxiety and increases energy. Exercise releases endorphins, which are natural opiates; neurotransmitters released during exercise allow quicker thinking and higher levels of alertness.
- Good nutrition helps the body build an energy bank necessary for coping with stress. People who are well-nourished have a sense of well-being that modulates emotional and behavioral responses to stress.
- Laughter promotes physiological responses that lead to a relaxation response; by putting everyday hassles at a distance, it provides a break from stress.
- It's possible to cope with stress through changes in thinking. By eliminating needless worrying, moderating expectations, weeding out trivia, living in the present, and being flexible, people can save energy necessary to deal with unavoidable stress.

Take Action

1. Dr. Edmund Jacobson of the University of Chicago noted that people tense their muscles when they are stressed but don't realize they are doing it. He reasoned that if they can learn to relax, they can lower the stress they experience.

Think about a specific time when you felt anxious or stressed. Now take your pulse rate and record it in your health diary. Learn and practice progression relaxation (see discussion in chapter). Immediately after relaxing the last muscle group, take your pulse rate and record it in your notebook, indicating the time, date, and conditions after which you took it. Was there any difference in your pulse rate? If so and your pulse rate slowed, you may want to incorporate relaxation as a regular technique in your behavioral approach to stress.

2. Think about all the different environments in which you function, including your classrooms, the student union, the dorm, your house. Are some more stressful than others? Make a list of the environments ordered from the most stressful to the least stressful. Indicate next to each environment the reasons you think it is stressful or non-stressful. Now start at the top of your list and record three or more ways to reduce the stressful impact these environments have on you.

3. Turn to the box "Life Events and Disease: Is There a Link?" Using this list as a guide, identify the major events that have occurred in your life in the past six months or are likely to occur in the next six months. Distinguish the events that you can change from those that you cannot change. List the former in your health diary and note how you are going to try to change them.

Behavior Change Strategy

Dealing with Test Anxiety

Are you a person who doesn't perform as well as you should on tests? Do you find that anxiety interferes with your ability to study effectively before the test and to think clearly in the test situation? If so, you may be experiencing test anxiety. People suffering from test anxiety often see tests as threatening, feel inadequate to cope with them, concentrate on the negative consequences of doing poorly, and anticipate failure, which becomes a self-fulfilling prophecy. They often feel so helpless that they can't mobilize their resources to deal with the problem.

Test anxiety can be a serious problem, and it often gets worse rather than better with time. Typically, greater anxiety leads to a poorer performance, which leads to even greater anxiety, and so on. Sometimes the only solution the worried student can think of is to stop taking tests—that is, to drop out of school. Luckily, there are several ways to deal with test anxiety, some of which are also effective ways of dealing with anxiety in other forms, such as phobias and fear of public speaking.

Behavioral approaches to problems like this operate on the assumption that fear and anxiety are learned behaviors and that a person can unlearn them by following appropriate procedures. Test anxiety is seen as an ineffective response to a stressful situation that can be replaced with more effective responses. Two methods that have proven effective in helping people deal with test anxiety are systematic desensitization and success rehearsal. Both can help people interrupt the vicious cycle of fear that prevents them from doing their best in stressful performance situations. If test anxiety is a problem for you, try implementing one of these programs before you take your next exams.

Systematic Desensitization

Systematic desensitization is based on the premise that you can't feel anxiety and be relaxed at the same time. The program described here has three phases—constructing an anxiety hierarchy, learning and practicing deep muscle relaxation, and carrying out the actual steps of the desensitization program.

Constructing an anxiety hierarchy Begin the first phase by thinking of ten or more situations related to your fear, such as hearing the announcement of the test date in class, studying for the test, sitting in the classroom waiting to be handed

an examination booklet, reading the test questions, and so on. Write each situation on an index card, using a brief phrase to describe it on one side of the card and on the other side listing several realistic details that will help you vividly imagine yourself actually experiencing the situation. For example, if the situation is "hearing that 50 percent of the final grade will be based on the two exams," the prompts might include such details as "sitting in the big lecture auditorium in Baily Hall," "taking notes in my blue notebook," "surrounded by many other students," and "listening to Professor Smith's voice."

Next, arrange your cards in order starting with the situation that causes the least anxiety and ending with the situation that causes the most anxiety. Rate each item to reflect the amount of anxiety you feel when you encounter it in the natural environment to make sure your hierarchy is accurate. Assign ratings on a scale of 0 to 100 and make sure that the distances between items are fairly small and approximately equal. When you're sure that your anxiety hierarchy is a true reflection of your feelings, number the cards.

Learning and Practicing Deep Muscle Relaxation The second step of the program involves learning to relax your muscles and to recognize when they are relaxed. A very effective way to do this is through progressive relaxation or deep muscle relaxation, which is described in this chapter. Basically, it consists of alternately tensing and relaxing your muscles, moving from one part of the body to another, while paying attention to the internal activities and sensations you are feeling at the time. Find a quiet, dimly lit setting where you won't be interrupted for 20 or 30 minutes and sit or lie on a comfortable couch or bed. It would be ideal to have instructions recorded on tape—

such as "Make a fist with your left hand. Squeeze it as tightly as you can. (pause) Now relax it completely. Let your hand go limp. Notice how it feels. (pause)"—and listen to the tape the first several times you practice the relaxation procedure. As you became proficient at relaxing, you'll be able to relax without the tape and ultimately to skip steps and go directly to a deeply relaxed state within a few minutes. When you can do this, you're ready to go on to the next phase of the program.

Implementing the Desensitization Program Use the quiet place where you practiced your relaxation exercises. Sit comfortably and place your stack of numbered cards within reach. Take several minutes to relax completely, and then look at the first card, reading both the brief phrase and the descriptive prompts. Close your eyes and imagine yourself in that situation for about 10 seconds. Then put the card down and relax completely for about 30 seconds. Look at the card again, imagine the situation for 10 seconds, and relax again for 30 seconds.

At this point, evaluate your level of anxiety about the situation on the card in terms of the rating scale you devised earlier. If your anxiety level is 5 or below, relax for two minutes and go on to the second card. If it's higher than 5, repeat the routine with the same card until the anxiety decreases. If you have difficulty with a particular item, go back to the previous item and then try it again. If you still can't visualize it without anxiety, try to construct three new items with smaller steps between them and insert them before the troublesome item.

In general, you should be able to move through one to four items per session. Sessions can be conducted anywhere from twice a day to twice a week and should last no more than 20 minutes. Keep track of your progress by recording the names and numbers of the items you imagined successfully during each session, the number of times you imagined each one, and the anxiety rating of each item when you first prepared the hierarchy and after you desensitized yourself to it. It's helpful to graph your progress in a way that has meaning for you.

After you have successfully completed your program, you should be desensitized to the real-life situations that previously elicited anxiety. If you find that you do experience some anxiety in the real situations, take 30 seconds or a minute to relax completely, just as you did when you were practicing. Remember, fear and relaxation are incompatible; you can't experience them both at the same time. You have the ability to choose relaxation over fear.

Success Rehearsal

A variation on desensitization is the approach called success rehearsal. To practice this method, take your hierarchy of anxiety-eliciting situations and vividly imagine yourself successfully dealing with each one. Create a detailed scenario for each situation and use your imagination to experience genuine feelings of confidence. Recognize your negative thoughts ("I'll be so nervous I won't be able to think

straight") and replace them with positive ones ("Anxiety will keep me alert so I can do a good job"). Proceed one step at a time, thinking of strategies for success as you go. These might include the following:

- Before the test, find out everything you can about it—its format, the material to be covered, the criteria used to grade essay answers. Ask the instructor for practice materials.
- Devise a study plan. This might include forming a study group with one or more classmates or outlining what you will study when, where, and for how long.
- Once in the test situation, sit away from possible distractions, listen carefully to instructions, and ask for clarification if you don't understand a direction.
- During the test, answer the easiest questions first. If you don't know an answer and there is no penalty for incorrect answers, guess. If there are several questions you have difficulty answering, review the ones you have already handled. Figure out approximately how much time you have to cover each question or part of the test.
- For math problems, try to estimate the answer before doing the precise calculations.
- For true-false questions, look for qualifiers such as *always* and

never. Such questions are likely to be false.
- For essay questions, look for key words in the question that indicate what the instructor is looking for in the answer. Develop a brief outline of your answer, sketching out roughly what you will cover. Stick to your outline and keep track of the time you're spending on your answer. Don't let yourself get caught with unanswered questions when the time is up.
- Remain calm and focused throughout the test. Don't let negative thoughts rattle you. If you start to become nervous, take some deep breaths and relax your muscles completely for a minute or so.

The best way to counter test anxiety is with successful test-taking experiences. The more times you succeed, the more your test anxiety will recede. If you find that these methods aren't sufficient to get your anxiety under control, you may want to seek professional help with the problem. But whether you use desensitization, success rehearsal, or another approach, it's wise to take action as early as possible to keep test anxiety from significantly interfering with your education plans and career goals.

Selected Bibliography

Benson, Herbert, with William Proctor. 1984. *Beyond the Relaxation Response.* New York: Times Books.

Borysenko, Joan. *Minding the Body, Minding the Mind.* 1987. Menlo Park, Calif.: Addison-Wesley.

Burka, Jane B., and Lenora M. Yuen. 1983. *Procrastination: Why You Do It; What to Do about It.* Reading, Mass.: Addison-Wesley.

Cooper, C. L., and R. Payne. 1988. *Causes, Coping, and Consequences of Stress at Work,* New York: Wiley & Sons.

Friedman, Meyer, and Diane Ulmer. 1984. *Treating Type A Behavior—and Your Heart.* New York: Knopf.

Girdano, Daniel, and George Everly. 1986. *Controlling Stress and Tension: A Holistic Approach,* 2nd ed. Englewood Cliffs, N.J.: Prentice-Hall.

Karasek, Robert, and Tores Theorell. 1990. *Healthy Work: Stress, Productivity, and the Reconstruction of Working Life.* New York: Basic Books.

Kobasa, Suzanne Ouellette. 1982. "The hardy personality: Toward a social psychology of health." In G. S.

Sanders and J. Suls, eds., *Social Psychology of Health and Illness.* Hillsdale, N.J.: Lawrence Erlbaum Associates.

Kobasa, Suzanne Ouellette. 1984 (September). How much stress can you survive? *American Health* 3:64–77.

Martin, Garry, and Joseph Pear. 1983. *Behavior Modification: What It Is and How to Do It,* 2nd ed. Englewood Cliffs, N.J.: Prentice-Hall.

Miller, A., Stress on the job, *Newsweek,* Apr. 25. 1988, pp. 40–45.

Ornstein, Robert, and David Sobel. 1989. *Healthy Pleasures.* Reading, Mass.: Addison-Wesley.

Selye, Hans. 1976. *The Stress of Life,* rev. ed. New York: McGraw-Hill.

Selye, Hans. 1979. Stress: The basis of illness. In Elliot M. Goldwag, ed., *Inner Balance: The Power of Holistic Health.* Englewood Cliffs, N.J.: Prentice-Hall.

Smith, Eleanor. 1987. Meditation goes mainstream. *Washington Post Health,* October 6.

Wechsler, Rob. 1987 (February). A new prescription: Mind over malady. *Discover* 8:51–61.

Recommended Readings

American Health Magazine, Editors of, with Daniel Goleman and Tara Bennett-Goleman. 1986. *The Relaxed Body Book: A High-Energy Anti-tension Program.* Garden City, N.Y.: Doubleday. *Excellent guide to identifying one's stress spiral and creating a program for handling specific problems.*

Brallier, Lynn. 1982. *Transition and Transformation: Successfully Managing Stress.* Los Altos, Calif.: National Nursing Review. *Thoroughly explains how stress arises and then suggests a practical, holistic path to assessing and managing stress.*

Charlesworth, Edward A., and Ronald G. Nathan. 1984. *Stress Management: A Comprehensive Guide to Wellness.* New York: Atheneum. *Offers pointers to identifying areas of stress and describes proven techniques (supported by case examples) for handling stress, overcoming fears, and unleashing creative energy.*

Davis, Martha, Elizabeth Robbins Eshelman, and Matthew McKay. 1982. *The Relaxation & Stress Reduction Workbook,* 2nd ed. Oakland, Calif.: New Harbinger Publications. *Step-by-step instructions for a wealth of techniques, supplemented by questionnaires and personal charts (but skip page 181, which contains misinformation on "stress vitamins" and on hair analysis).*

Hanson, Peter G. 1986. *The Joy of Stress.* Kansas City: Andrews, McMeel & Parker. *Engagingly presented, compact, well-tested advice from a Canadian doctor who shows how to turn stress into an ally rather than an enemy.*

Justice, Blair. 1987. *Who Gets Sick?* Houston: Peak Press. Explores current evidence which suggests that positive attitudes and beliefs can aid in health promotion and disease prevention.

Williams, Redford B. 1989. *The Trusting Heart: Great News about Type A Behavior.* New York: Times Books. Latest research linking hostility and anger to heart disease and how to recognize hostile behavior.

Contents

Making Connections

Your overall health is powerfully influenced by some factors you may not be very aware of—your thoughts and beliefs about yourself, your habitual ways of handling your feelings, the patterns you've developed for interacting with other people. Looking more closely at these components of mental health can give you interesting insights into yourself and lead to unexpected benefits. The scenarios presented on these pages describe situations in which people have to use information, make a decision, or choose a course of action, all related to mental health. As you read them, imagine yourself in each situation and consider what you would do. After you've finished the chapter, read the scenarios again and see if what you've learned has changed how you would think, feel, or act in each situation.

You're intrigued by someone you know slightly at school. She's not particularly attractive, doesn't come from a wealthy or privileged background, and is just an average student. Yet she always seems confident, relaxed, and happy about who she is. It's fun to be around her because she's so energetic and unpretentious. You know a lot of people who have more going for them than she does but are filled with self-doubts. What's her secret, anyway? And how can you get to be as self-assured as she is?

3
Mental Health

Although you basically like your roommate, the two of you have very different ideas and habits and always seem to be at odds. You like to socialize at the student union and study in your room; your roommate prefers to study at the library and socialize in the room. You like to go to bed early; your roommate likes to stay up late listening to music. You're up at 6 and want to hear the news on your radio; your roommate wants to sleep till 8. You joked about it at first, but lately you've been getting on each other's nerves. In fact, you've stopped talking and started slamming doors. You don't want to spend the rest of the year with all this tension in the air. What can you do to improve the situation?

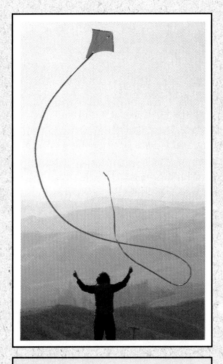

You run into an old friend in a coffee shop and start talking about the "good old days." Things haven't been going too well for her lately, and in the course of the conversation she comments that her life isn't worth much. Then she remarks that people would be better off if she weren't around. When she has to go, you say that you'll see her soon, and she says, "No, you probably won't." You make light of her comments, but later you keep thinking about them. Was she serious? Should you tell anyone or do anything? If so, what?

Things seemed to be going okay for you recently, but last week you had an unpleasant experience you can't understand. You suddenly felt terrified for no reason. You ran back to your room and stayed there until it passed. Now you're worried that it will happen again, and everything seems gray, gloomy, and threatening. You wonder if you're having an allergic reaction to something you ate, or if the medication you're taking for your skin could be causing these feelings. When you mentioned the incident to a friend, she suggested you see someone at the student health services. You're not so sure you want to tell anyone else about it. Should you?

What exactly is *mental* health? Some people justify their lifestyle by claiming that it promotes better mental health than others do, and they may even term those who refuse to accept the lifestyle as "sick" or "crazy." Mental health becomes the focus of battles in legislatures and courts, where expert witnesses contradict each other on whether defendants were mentally healthy enough to have been responsible for their acts or whether people are so mentally ill that they should be treated with medicine or hospitalized involuntarily. When the perpetrator of an especially heinous crime is found "mentally incompetent to stand trial" or "not guilty by reason of insanity," it's not unusual to hear mental illness declared a "myth" promoted by the mental health "establishment."

Is mental health a myth? We don't think so. We think there *is* such a thing as mental health just as there is physical health (and the two are intertwined). Just as your body can work well or poorly, giving you feelings of pleasure or pain, your mind can also work well or poorly, giving you happiness or unhappiness. If you feel pain and unhappiness rather than pleasure and happiness or if you sense that you could be functioning at a higher level, there may be ways you can help yourself, either on your own or with professional help. This chapter will explain how.

What Mental Health Is Not

Mental health is not the same as mental **normality.** Being mentally normal simply means being close to average. You can define your normal body temperature because a few degrees above or below this temperature always means physical sickness. But your ideas and attitudes can vary tremendously without your losing efficiency or feeling emotional distress. And psychological diversity is valuable; living in a society of people with varied ideas and lifestyles makes life interesting. Such a society can respond creatively to unexpected challenges.

Conforming to social demands is not necessarily a mark of mental health. If you don't question what's going on around you, you're not fulfilling your potential as a thinking, questioning human being. For example, our society admires the framers of the U.S. Constitution and the abolitionists who rebelled against injustices. If conformity signified mental health, then political dissent would indicate mental illness by definition (and we have indeed seen that definition used by dictators in this century). Were such a definition valid, Galileo would have been mad for insisting that the earth went around the sun.

Never seeking help for personal problems also does not mean that you are mentally healthy, any more than seeking help proves that you are mentally ill. Unhappy

people may not want to seek professional help because they don't want to reveal their problems to others, may fear what their friends might think, or may not know whom to ask for help. People who are severely disturbed mentally may not even realize they need help, or they may become so suspicious of other people that they can be treated only against their will.

And we cannot say people are "mentally ill" or "mentally healthy" on the basis of symptoms alone. Life constantly presents problems. Time and life inevitably change the environment and change our minds and bodies, and changes present problems. The symptom of anxiety, for example, can help us face a problem and solve it before it gets too big. Someone who shows no anxiety may be refusing to recognize problems or refusing to do anything about them. A person who is anxious for good reason is likely to be judged more mentally healthy in the long run than someone who is inappropriately calm.

Finally, we cannot judge mental health from the way people look. All too often a person who seems to be OK and even happy suddenly takes his (or her) own life. Usually such people lack close friends who might have known of their desperation. We all learn early to conceal and "lie." We may believe that our complaints put unfair demands on others. True, suffering in silence can be a virtue sometimes, but it can also impede help.

What Mental Health Is

It is even harder to say what mental health *is* than what it is *not.* Just as we should think of physical wellness as much more than not being sick, we should view mental health as more than the absence of mental illness.

Mental Health as the Presence of Wellness   Abraham Maslow, an American psychology professor, eloquently described an ideal of mental health in his book *Toward a Psychology of Being.* He was convinced that psychologists were too preoccupied with people who had failed in some way. He also did not like the way psychologists at that time tried to reduce human striving to physiological needs or drives. According to Maslow, there is a *hierarchy of needs,* listed here in order of decreasing urgency: physiological needs, safety, being loved, maintaining self-esteem, and self-actualization. When urgent needs like the need for food are satisfied, less urgent needs take priority. Most of us are well fed and feel reasonably safe, so we are driven by higher motives. Maslow's conclusions were based on his study of a group of visibly successful people who seemed to be living at their fullest. Among them were historical figures such as Abraham Lincoln, Henry David Thoreau, and Ludwig van Beethoven; famous people then living, such as Eleanor

Roosevelt and Albert Einstein; and some of his own friends and acquaintances. He called these people **self-actualized**; he thought they had fulfilled a good measure of their human potential and suggested that such people all share certain qualities:

- They are able to deal with the world as it is and don't demand that it should be otherwise.
- They are able to largely accept themselves, others, and nature.
- They experience profound interpersonal relations.
- They have a continuing fresh appreciation for what goes on around them.
- They are able to direct themselves, rather independently of culture and environment.
- They trust their own senses and feelings.
- They are creative.
- They are democratic in their attitudes.

Let's look at these qualities in a little more detail, using the ideas of Maslow and other theorists.

■ Exploring Your Emotions

When you were a child, how were you taught to handle difficult feelings like anger, fear, and sadness? Do you still use the same methods? How are they working now?

First, mentally healthy people are realistic. If you are realistic, you know the difference between what is and what you want. You also know what you can change and what you cannot. Unrealistic people often get stuck on their idea of what should be. This habit makes them unable to accept what is, so they spend a great deal of energy trying to force the world and other people into their ideal picture. Realistic people accept evidence that contradicts what they want to believe, and if it is important evidence, they modify their beliefs.

A key factor in your mental wellness is self-concept. Mentally healthy people like themselves; in psychological terms, they have a positive self-concept or self-image, or appropriately high self-esteem. They have positive but realistic mental images and positive good feelings about themselves, about what they are capable of, and about what roles they play. People who feel good about themselves are likely to live up to their positive self-image and

enjoy a success that in turn reinforces these good feelings. A good self-concept is based on a realistic view of personal worth. It does not mean being egocentric or "stuck on yourself."

According to Maslow, being free and autonomous is another characteristic of mentally healthy people. Freedom is more than simply not being physically controlled by something or someone outside the self. Many people, for example, shrink from being themselves and from expressing their own feelings because they fear disapproval and rejection. They are unable to act freely and respond only to what they feel as outside pressure. Such behavior is **other-directed.** In contrast, **inner-directed** people find guidance from within, from their own values and feelings. They are not afraid to be themselves. Mentally free people act because they choose to, not because they are driven or pressured.

Mentally healthy people can be comfortable both with silence and with being alone. Maslow believed that mentally healthy people periodically make time for solitude to refresh and renew themselves. Such time seems to help many of these people to welcome the stimulation of company and activity when they return. (In contrast, some people feel they must have a radio or stereo going constantly to drown out the silence, or they do not feel comfortable except in the company of others.)

Being free can give healthy people certain childlike qualities. Very small children have a quality of being "real." They respond in a genuine, spontaneous way to whatever happens. Someone who is genuine needs no pretenses. Being free and genuine means not having to plan words or actions to get approval or to make an impression. It means being unselfconsciously oneself, here and now. This quality is sometimes called **authenticity;** such people are *authentic,* the "real thing."

Mentally healthy people are aware of their own feelings and can express them. One reason why small children often seem so real is that they instantly express how they feel—sometimes to the embarrassment of their parents! Adults and older children have been taught to hide their feelings. Indeed, in most cultures, learning to hide feelings is considered part of growing up. But it would really be healthier for us as individuals to recognize, handle, and express our emotions in appropriate ways. Of course, we must temper emotional self-assertion by considering its effects on others and on ourselves. Expressing anger is not the same as acting it out, for example.

Normality   The mental characteristics attributed to the majority of people in a population at a given time.

Self-actualized   Describes a person who has achieved the highest level of growth in Maslow's hierarchy.

Other-directed   Guided in behavior by the values and expectations of others.

Inner-directed   Guided in behavior by an inner set of rules and values.

Authenticity   Genuineness

Healthy people are capable of physical and **emotional intimacy.** They can expose their senses, feelings, and thoughts to other people. They are open to the pleasure of intimate touching and to the risks and satisfactions of being close to others in a caring, sensitive way. Intimate touching may mean "good sex," but it also means something much more—intense awareness of both your partner and yourself in which contact becomes communication.

Mentally healthy people take responsibility for their own feelings and actions. They do not blame others for what they do or feel. For example, it is both more responsible and more honest to say "I'm feeling rattled" than to say "You're trying to confuse me." A person who no longer says "He made me do it" or "It was all her fault" is moving toward personal responsibility.

Maslow also saw creativity and boldness as characteristic of the group he studied. Mentally healthy people are not necessarily great poets, scientists, or musicians, but they do live their everyday lives in creative ways. "A first-rate soup is more creative than a second-rate painting." Creative people seem to see more and to be open to new experiences; they don't fear the unknown. And they don't need to reduce uncertainty or avoid it, but actually find it attractive.

How did Maslow's group achieve their exemplary mental health, and (more importantly) how can *we* attain it? Maslow does not really answer that question. Undoubtedly it helps to have been treated with respect, love, and understanding as a child, to have experienced stability and been given a sense of mastery. As adults, we probably should concentrate on specific difficulties that block our path to this ideal, as we will discuss later. These difficulties may be ones that almost everyone faces, like achieving healthy and realistic self-esteem or maintaining honest communication, or they may be more specific psychological disorders like **phobias**, depression, or schizophrenia.

Mental Health as the Absence of Sickness

A positive vision of mental health can make you aware of human potential in yourself that you might want to develop. However, many people must struggle with a more limited goal: overcoming troublesome problems in behavior, thinking, or feelings. Wherever you go, you'll find some people who have occasional or permanent psychological problems so severe (or so difficult for others to empathize with) that they cannot function adequately at home, school, or work. Some of these people have specific groups of symptoms (syndromes) that suggest biological disturbances, and we discuss those syndromes later in the chapter.

For these and other reasons, mental health is sometimes defined as the *absence* of mental illness. This definition has the advantage of concentrating attention on the neediest. A broad concept of mental health could lead us to ignore serious mental suffering and to pretend that we or our own loved ones could never have those problems. Or we could use the broad view as an excuse to spend society's resources on the well rather than the sick. In addition, broad definitions like Maslow's ideal can be faulted as being parochial expressions of Western cultural and moral values rather than universally valid scientific facts. Mental illnesses like schizophrenia and depression are reliably identifiable in every culture. On the other hand, a negative definition of mental health can be much too narrow. If we consider everybody mentally healthy who is not severely mentally disturbed, we end up ignoring common psychological problems that can be addressed.

Common Psychological Problems

Two characteristics of mental wellness that Maslow and others emphasize are particularly relevant to how people get along in their everyday lives—(1) having a realistic, positive sense of self and (2) being able to relate well to others, which involves the ability to communicate honestly and openly. These characteristics are not fixed quantities, either completely present or completely absent in people. Different individuals have different levels of self-esteem and different degrees of communication skill. Since self-concept and the ability to communicate are largely the result of learning, they can be changed through relearning.

Achieving Realistic Self-Esteem

Ideally, as children grow up they develop positive feelings about themselves based on their experiences within the family and outside it. They develop a sense of being loved and of being able to give love and to accomplish their goals—in other words, a positive self-concept, or high self-esteem. Sometimes, however, less favorable experiences produce a less positive self-concept. If children feel rejected or neglected by their parents, for example, they may fail to develop feelings of self-worth. They may grow to have a negative concept of themselves.

Another quality of the self-concept is its integration.

Emotional intimacy   A closeness between people that includes a mutual awareness and influence of feelings.

Phobias   Unfounded fears of specific things.

Defenses   Mental mechanisms for controlling anxiety.

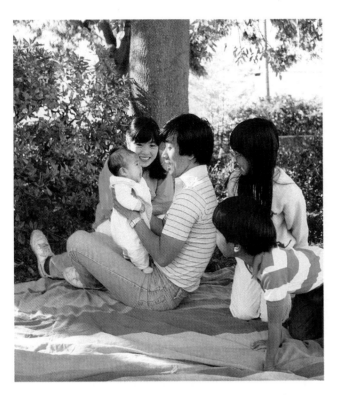

A positive self-concept begins in infancy. Knowing that she's loved and valued by her family gives this 3-month-old a solid basis for life-long mental health.

An integrated self-concept is one that a person has made his or her own—it doesn't feel like someone else's mask or costume that doesn't quite fit. Important building blocks for the self-concept are personality characteristics and mannerisms of the parents, which children can take in uncritically without knowing they have done so. Later, they are surprised when they catch themselves acting like one of their parents, especially if they always objected to such behavior in that parent. Eventually, such building blocks should be reshaped and integrated into a new individual personality.

A further quality of the self-concept is its stability. Stability depends on the integration of the self and its freedom from contradictions. People who have received mixed messages about themselves from parents and friends may have contradictory self-images, which defy integration and which make them open to startling shifts of self-esteem. At times they regard themselves as entirely good, capable, and lovable—an ideal self—and at other times they see themselves as entirely bad, incompetent, and unworthy of love. While at the first pole, they may develop such an inflated ego that they totally ignore other people's needs and see others only as instruments for fulfilling their own desires. At the other pole, they may feel so small and weak that they run for protection to someone who seems powerful and caring. At neither extreme do such people see themselves or others realisti-

cally, and their personal relationships with other people are filled with misunderstandings and ultimately with conflict. The concepts people have about themselves and others are an important part of their personalities; all the qualities of the self-concept profoundly influence interpersonal relations.

As an adult, you sometimes run into situations that challenge your self-concept: people you care about may tell you they don't love you or feel loved by you, or your attempts to accomplish a goal may end in failure. You can react to such challenges in several ways. The best approach is to acknowledge that something has gone wrong and try again, adjusting your goals to your abilities without radically revising your self-concept. A less useful reaction is to deny that anything went wrong or to blame someone else. These psychological **defenses** preserve a good self-concept temporarily, but in the long run they keep you from mastering the challenge. The worst reaction is to develop a lasting negative self-concept in which you feel bad, unloved, and ineffective—in other words, become demoralized. Instead of coping, the demoralized person gives up, reinforcing the negative self-concept and setting in motion a vicious circle of bad self-concept and failure. In people who are biologically predisposed to depressions, demoralization can progress to additional symptoms, discussed later in the chapter.

One method for fighting demoralization is to recognize and test your negative thoughts and assumptions about yourself and others. The first step is to note exactly when an unpleasant emotion—feeling worthless, wanting to give up, feeling depressed—occurs or gets worse, to identify the events or daydreams that trigger that emotion, and to observe whatever thoughts come into your head just before or during the emotion. It is helpful to keep a systematic daily record of such events.

Let's consider the example of Jennifer, a student who went to the college counseling center because she had been feeling "down" lately. Her social life had not been going well, and she had begun to think that it never would—that she was basically just an unattractive person. Asked to keep a daily record, she wrote in it that she felt let down and discouraged when a boyfriend who promised to meet her at 7:30 in the evening was 15 minutes late. The kind of thoughts that occurred to her were "He's not going to come. It's my fault. He has more important things to do. Maybe he's with another girl. He doesn't like me. Nobody likes me because I'm not pretty. What if he got in a car accident?"

People who are demoralized tend to use all-or-nothing thinking: things are either black or white, but never in between. They overgeneralize from negative events. They selectively see the negative and overlook the positive. They jump to negative conclusions. They minimize their own successes and magnify the successes of others. They take responsibility for unfortunate situations that are not

The ability to communicate feelings honestly and clearly is a crucial component of healthy interpersonal relationships. Listening attentively, as the woman on the left has learned to do, is an equally important skill.

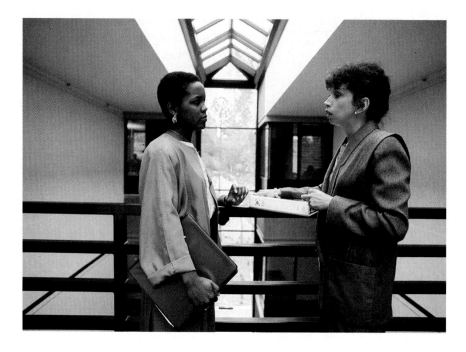

their fault. Jennifer realized that the minute her boyfriend was late she jumped to the conclusion he was not coming. She immediately blamed herself. Then she jumped to more negative conclusions and more unfounded overgeneralizations.

Jennifer needs to develop more rational responses. For Jennifer, more rational thinking could be "He's a little late so I'll have time to reread the study questions." If he had not come after 30 minutes, she might have called him to see if something was holding him up, without jumping to any conclusions about the meaning of his lateness.

In your own fight against demoralization, it may be hard to figure out a rational response until hours or days after the event that upsets you, but once you get used to the way your mind works, you may be able to catch yourself thinking negatively and change it while it's happening.

This approach is not the same as positive thinking—substituting a positive thought for a negative one. Instead, you simply try to make your thoughts as logical and accurate as possible. If Jennifer continues to think she's unattractive, she should try to collect evidence to prove or disprove that. If she has exaggerated her cosmetic defects, as do many demoralized people, her investigations may prove her wrong. For example, she

might ask her friends their candid opinions about her appearance, or she can observe if any men come up to talk to her at parties. She might harbor the false assumption that if she's pretty, everyone must find her pretty. Following this assumption, if she could find one person who did not treat her as if she was attractive, she could continue to believe she isn't pretty. Demoralized people can be so tenacious about their negative beliefs that they make them come true in a self-fulfilling prophesy. Jennifer might conclude that since she is so unattractive no one will like her anyway, so she need not bother to comb her hair carefully or to keep her clothes clean. This behavior could help her negative belief become reality.

Maintaining Honest Communication   A second important area of psychological functioning is relating to others and communicating honestly with them. It can be very frustrating for us and for people around us if we cannot communicate what we want and feel. Others can hardly respond to our needs if they don't know what those needs are. The first step is for us to realize what we want to communicate and then to express it clearly. For example, how do you feel about going to the party instead of to the movie? Do you care if your roommate types a paper late into the night? Some people know what they want others to do, but don't state it clearly because

---

Assertiveness   Expressing wishes forcefully, but not necessarily hostilely.

Psychotic   A mentally disturbed person who has lost contact with reality.

Hallucination   False perception.

Delusion   Firmly held false belief not shared by other members of a person's social group.

Neurotic   A person who is in touch with reality but who has irrational thoughts and feelings.

Tips for Clearer Communication

- When you want to communicate with someone, state your case as clearly as you can. Use "I messages." Ask for what you want directly, instead of hoping that the other person will read your mind. Say what you feel, and what you want to have happen.
- Be specific about the particular behaviors that you like or don't like. Avoid generalizations such as, "You always . . ." and "You never . . ." Avoid blaming, accusing, and belittling. Even if you are 100 percent right, you

have little to gain by putting the other person down. Studies have shown that when people feel criticized or attacked, they became less able to think rationally or solve problems correctly.
- As a listener, don't make assumptions about what the other person is saying. Ask for clarifications. Don't play "fill in the blanks." Develop the skill of reflective listening. Don't judge, blame, or evaluate. Remember, the person may just need to have you there in order to sort

out feelings. By jumping in right away to "fix" the problem, you may actually be cutting off communication. Also, when you listen, be sure you are *really* listening, not off somewhere rehearsing your reply! Try to tune in to the other person's feelings and check them out as well. Do let the other person know that you value what he or she is saying and want to understand. Respect for the other person is the cornerstone of clear communication.

they are afraid that the request or they themselves will be rejected. Such people might benefit from **assertiveness** training. They need to learn to insist on their rights and to bargain for what they want. Assertiveness includes being able to say no or yes depending on the situation.

■ Exploring Your Emotions

The college years are a time when we begin to redefine our relationship with our parents. Are your feelings and attitudes toward your parents changing? Does one or the other still treat you like a child? Do you react to them with childlike behavior? How can you get them to treat you more like an adult?

Because expressing feelings has become so central to pop psychology, many misconceptions have arisen. Neither "sharing" feelings with everyone on every occasion, nor letting feelings alone guide important decisions, are legitimate mental health goals. The word *feel* has at least two fairly distinct meanings in English. Compare "I feel sad" and "I feel that I should stay home tonight." The first sentence expresses an emotion; the second, a politely worded intention, or an intuition of need or duty. To tell people you are sad can imply various things and have various effects: They may feel closer to you and express an intimacy of their own, they may feel guilty because they may feel you are implying that they have caused your sadness, or they may feel angry because they feel forced to help cheer you up. Depending on your intention and prediction of how your statement will be taken,

you may or may not want to make it. To say that you feel like staying home can also have a variety of implications according to the context. You may be politely saying, "Don't bother me," opening a negotiation about what you will do with someone that evening, or expressing your demoralization. Good communication means saying things clearly when you intend to do so. You don't need any special psychological jargon to communicate clearly (see the box "Tips for Clearer Communication").

Psychological Disorders

Some psychological problems are deeper and more disabling than problems of low self-esteem or poor communication. In these cases they are considered psychological disorders. Traditionally, specific psychological disorders have been classified by psychologists and psychiatrists as either psychotic or neurotic. According to these classifications, **psychotics** are so mentally disturbed that they are unable to test their perceptions and beliefs against reality. **Hallucinations** and **delusions** are hallmarks of psychosis. **Neurotics** recognize reality but act irrationally or have irrational thoughts or feelings, which they themselves recognize as irrational but cannot easily correct. Some examples of neurosis are having persistent fears or depression without good reason, having obsessive thoughts, or performing compulsive rituals such as repeatedly checking whether the oven has been turned off or becoming blind or paralyzed without a neurological reason. In its widest sense, any self-defeating behavior or irrational feeling is neurotic. So if we are honest, each of us must admit to being a little neurotic.

■ Exploring Your Emotions

When you see people talking to themselves or acting strangely on the street, how do you feel? What do you do? Do you wonder what's going on in their mind? Do you label them as "sick?" What do you think causes them to act so strangely?

Classifying people or behaviors as psychotic, neurotic, and normal has been criticized as too vague. All people, patients or nonpatients, show a mixture of these behaviors. The latest diagnostic manual of the American Psychiatric Association has dropped the terms **neurotic** and **psychotic** in favor of a classification based on specific symptom patterns, or syndromes. An abbreviated list is shown in Table 3-1. In the manual, detailed criteria for each diagnosis are given. To qualify as a *disorder,* the symptoms must be severe enough to interfere with daily living. Although this diagnostic system is extensive, it is not designed to encompass all human psychological problems and barriers to positive mental health. Diagnoses alone tell little about a person compared to one of Freud's case histories or to a well-written biography.

Some of these disorders are discussed elsewhere in this book—Alzheimer's disease in Chapter 19, disorders associated with psychoactive substances in Chapters 10 and 11, sexual disorders in Chapter 4, and eating disorders in Chapter 13. Here, we focus on schizophrenia, mood disorders, and anxiety disorders.

Schizophrenia   Schizophrenia comes in many forms. It can be severe and debilitating, or it can be quite mild and hardly noticeable. Although people are capable of diagnosing their own depression, they usually don't diagnose their own schizophrenia, because schizophrenics often can't see that anything is wrong. The disorder is not rare; in fact, one out of 100 people has a schizophrenic episode sometime in his or her lifetime. However, because people who are directly and indirectly af-

---

Table 3-1 Diagnostic Classification of Mental Disorders

Disorders usually first evident in infancy, childhood, or adolescence These include *developmental disorders* like mental retardation and autism, *disruptive behavior disorders* like attention-deficit hyperactivity, *tic disorders* like Tourette's disorder, and *eating disorders* like anorexia and bulimia.

Organic mental disorders Disturbances in memory, perception, and mood caused by known bodily diseases; for example, Alzheimer's disease, senile dementia, stroke, intoxication with or withdrawal from alcohol or other psychoactive substances.

Psychoactive substance use disorders A pattern of dependence on or abuse of substances like alcohol, opium-like drugs, barbiturates and other sedatives, amphetamines, marijuana, cocaine, and hallucinogens.

Schizophrenia A disorder in which deteriorating social and work functioning is accompanied by some of the following symptoms: hallucinations, disorganized thoughts, and inappropriate emotions.

Mood disorders Disorders with episodes of depression or mania including *depressive disorders* (one or more depressive episodes) and *bipolar disorders* (one or more manic episodes and often depressive episodes).

Anxiety disorders Disorders characterized by anxiety and avoidant behavior including *simple phobia* (fear of specific objects or situations), *social phobia* (general fear of doing things in front of others, such as speaking or eating), *panic disorder* (panic attacks, diffuse anxiety, and sometimes place phobias), *obsessive compulsive disorder* (obsessions and/or compulsions),

post-traumatic stress disorder (repeated reexperiencing of a severe trauma such as rape or injury-causing accidents in dreams and intrusive memories, often accompanied by anxiety and depression), and *generalized anxiety disorder* (frequent unjustified anxiety and worry).

Somatoform disorders Characterized by the experiencing of bodily symptoms that have no medical basis.

Dissociative disorders States of amnesia, multiple personality, or depersonalization.

Sexual disorders These include *paraphilias* (sexual urges involving nonhuman objects or children or nonconsenting persons) and *sexual dysfunctions* (for example, premature ejaculation or orgasmic dysfunction).

Sleep disorders These include insomnia, hypersomnia, sleep walking, and night terrors.

Personality disorders Inflexible and maladaptive personality patterns such as *paranoid* (actions of people interpreted as deliberately demeaning or theatening), *schizoid* (indifference to social relationships and emotional restriction), *antisocial* (nonconformity to social norms, aggressiveness, absence of guilt or remorse), *borderline* (unstable interpersonal relationships and moods), *histrionic* (excessive but shallow emotionality, attention-seeking), *narcissistic* (grandiosity, lack of empathy, hypersensitivity to criticism), *avoidant* (pervasive social discomfort and timidity), and *passive aggressive* (passive resistance to demands for adequate social and occupational performance).

(from the *Diagnostic and Statistical Manual of Mental Disorders,* American Psychiatric Association, 1987

fected do not like to talk about schizophrenia, its rate of incidence is not generally recognized. In addition, schizophrenics tend to withdraw from society when they are ill, another factor making it seem less common than it is.

Schizophrenia has so many forms that the official psychiatric classification refers to **schizophrenic disorders** rather than "schizophrenia." Some general characteristics of these disorders follow:

- *Disorganized thoughts.* Sometimes a schizophrenic expresses thoughts with unusual words, or mixes words together in a way that is hard for the listener to follow.
- *Inappropriate emotions.* Sometimes all emotion (affect) seems to be absent, and at other times emotions are strong but inappropriate.
- *Delusions.* People with delusions—firmly held false beliefs—may think that their minds are controlled by outside forces, that people can read their minds, that they are great personages like Jesus Christ or the President of the United States, or that they are being persecuted by a group such as the CIA.
- *Auditory hallucinations.* Schizophrenics with auditory hallucinations hear people talking about them and to them when no one is present.
- *Deteriorating social and work functioning.* Social withdrawal and increasingly poor performance at school or work may be so gradual that they are hardly noticed at first.

None of these characteristics is invariably present in schizophrenia. Some schizophrenic people seem to think quite logically except on the subject of their delusions. Others show disorganized thoughts or a lack of thoughts but no delusions or hallucinations.

A schizophrenic person needs help from a mental health professional. Schizophrenia may or may not be accompanied by some form of depression, but in either case suicide is a definite risk. People suffering from schizophrenia may kill themselves to escape from anxiety, confusion, and failure, or to obey inner voices. Expert treatment can reduce the risk of suicide and can minimize the social consequences by shortening the period when symptoms are active.

Treating milder cases of schizophrenia does not require hospitalization. The keystone of successful treatment is medication, taken regularly. These medications are called antipsychotic drugs (or sometimes major tranquilizers) and come in a dozen or so varieties, most of which have

the specific action of blocking a brain chemical called dopamine. Medication is useful at the onset of the disease and whenever thoughts and emotions become unbearably frightening. At such times, medication for schizophrenia is like insulin for diabetes—it makes the difference between being able to function and not. When schizophrenic symptoms get out of control, hospitalization is helpful to find the proper dose and type of medication quickly, to prevent self-destructive acts, and to relieve family and friends from responsibility for restraining the erratic behavior. In some cases, for reasons still unknown, schizophrenia takes a downward course to a point where sustained independent living cannot be maintained. Such people must then be found halfway houses and institutional settings in which they can live.

Mood Disorders   An episode of depression is the most common expression of a mood disorder. Depression comes in many kinds and degrees. Demoralization is usually part of depression, but it's not the whole story. The following description of severe depression, or what psychiatrists call a "major depressive episode," shows what depression can include:

- A feeling of sadness, hopelessness, and sometimes also irritability
- A loss of interest or pleasure in usual activities and pastimes
- Poor appetite and weight loss
- Insomnia, especially early morning awakening
- Restlessness or, alternatively, slowing down in movement and speech (lethargy)
- Loss of sexual drive
- Fatigue
- Thoughts of worthlessness and guilt, sometimes to a delusional degree
- Inability to think or concentrate
- Thoughts of death and suicide

Not all these features are present in every depressive episode. Sometimes instead of poor appetite and insomnia, the opposite occurs—eating too much and sleeping too long. Amazingly, people can suffer the majority of symptoms of depression without feeling sad or hopeless or in a depressed mood, although they usually do experience a loss of interest or pleasure in things (see the box titled Beck Depression Inventory). In some cases, depression is a clear-cut reaction to specific events, such as the loss of loved ones and failing in school or work, while in other cases no trigger event is obvious.

Schizophrenic disorders   Mental disorders that involve a disturbance in thinking and in perceiving reality.

For Some People, Depression Is a Seasonal Disorder

During the winter months, when days are short and nights are long, do you feel lethargic, depressed or crave carbohydrate-rich foods? If so, you may be one of many people who suffer from a condition called seasonal affective disorder (SAD). SAD, one of several types of depressive illnesses, is an extreme form of the winter "blahs." Those who are afflicted by this disorder experience a seasonal pattern of their depressive symptoms.

No one knows exactly what causes SAD. But many experts believe that the condition may result from prolonged secretion or increased levels of melatonin, a hormone that your brain produces during darkness.

In recent years, many SAD patients have benefited from phototherapy—early-morning exposure to special full-spectrum lights. If you think that you suffer from this seasonal condition, see a psychiatrist or psychologist experienced in treating patients with SAD. The most common months for SAD to strike in the northern hemisphere: October through mid-April.

From *Mayo Clinic Health Letter*, February 1989, p. 6.

One of the principal dangers of severe depression is suicide. Although suicide can happen unpredictably and even in the absence of depression, the chances of its happening are greater if the symptoms are numerous and severe. Additional danger signals are

- Expressing the wish to be dead, or revealing contemplated methods
- Increasing social withdrawal and isolation
- A sudden, inexplicable lightening of mood (which can mean the person has finally decided to commit suicide)

Risk factors increase the likelihood of suicide. Some risk factors are

- A history of previous attempts
- A suicide by a family member or friend
- Readily available means such as guns or pills
- Addiction to alcohol or drugs
- Serious medical problems

If you are severely depressed or know someone who is, expert help from a mental health professional is essential. Don't try to do it all yourself. If you suspect one of your friends is suicidally depressed, try to get him or her to see a professional.

Don't be afraid to discuss the possibility of suicide with people you fear are suicidal. You won't give them an idea they haven't already thought of (see the box titled "Myths about Suicide"). If your friend refuses help, you might try to contact your friend's relatives and tell them that you are worried. If the depressed person is a college student, you may need to let someone in your health service or college administration know your concerns. Finally, most communities have emergency help available, often as a suicide prevention agency that has a hot-line telephone counseling service (check the yellow pages).

Treatment for depression depends on its severity and on whether the depressed person is suicidal. The basic treatment is usually some kind of psychotherapy, which may be combined with drug therapy especially if the depression is severe enough to disturb sleep or appetite. "Uppers" such as amphetamines are not good antidepressants. More effective are special drugs that work over a period of two or more weeks. Therefore, when suicidal impulses are too strong, hospitalization for a week or so may be necessary. Electroconvulsive treatment is an effective therapy for severe depression when other approaches have failed.

Manic episodes are less common features of mood disorders, but are often more disturbing to other people than depressive episodes. Superficially, those who suffer from **mania** seem like the opposite of depressed persons. They typically experience exalted moods with unrealistically high self-esteem and boundless energy, stopping to sleep only a few hours a night. Severely manic people might devote themselves to fantastic projects, go on unrestrained buying sprees, or commit sexual indiscretions. Rapid and pressured speech, restlessness, and distractibility are also part of the manic picture. Manic happiness,

Mania   An elated or irritable, hyperactive state of mind.

Beck Depression Inventory

This questionnaire contains groups of statements. Please read each group of statements carefully. Then pick out the *one* statement in each group that best describes the way you have been feeling the *past week, including today*. Circle the number beside the statement you picked. If several statements in the group seem to apply equally, circle the highest number. *Be sure to read all the statements in each group before making your choice.*

1. 0 I do not feel sad.
    1 I feel sad.
    2 I am sad all the time and I can't snap out of it.
    3 I am so sad or unhappy that I can't stand it.

2. 0 I am not particularly discouraged about the future.
    1 I feel discouraged about the future.
    2 I feel I have nothing to look forward to.
    3 I feel that the future is hopeless and that things cannot improve.

3. 0 I do not feel like a failure.
    1 I feel I have failed more than the average person.
    2 As I look back on my life, all I can see is a lot of failures.
    3 I feel I am a complete failure as a person.

4. 0 I get as much satisfaction out of things as I used to.
    1 I don't enjoy things the way I used to.
    2 I don't get real satisfaction out of anything anymore.
    3 I am dissatisfied or bored with everything.

5. 0 I don't feel particularly guilty.
    1 I feel guilty a good part of the time.
    2 I feel quite guilty most of the time.
    3 I feel guilty all the time.

6. 0 I don't feel I am being punished.
    1 I feel I may be punished.
    2 I expect to be punished.
    3 I feel I am being punished.

7. 0 I don't feel disappointed in myself.
    1 I am disappointed in myself.
    2 I am disgusted with myself.
    3 I hate myself.

8. 0 I don't feel I am any worse than anybody else.
    1 I am critical of myself for my weaknesses or mistakes.
    2 I blame myself all the time for my faults.
    3 I blame myself for everything bad that happens.

9. 0 I don't have any thoughts of killing myself.
    1 I have thoughts of killing myself, but I would not carry them out.
    2 I would like to kill myself.
    3 I would kill myself if I had the chance.

10. 0 I don't cry any more than usual.
    1 I cry more now than I used to.
    2 I cry all the time now.
    3 I used to be able to cry, but now I can't cry even though I want to.

11. 0 I am no more irritated now than I ever was.
    1 I get annoyed or irritated more easily than I used to.
    2 I feel irritated all the time now.
    3 I don't get irritated at all by the things that used to irritate me.

12. 0 I have not lost interest in other people.
    1 I am less interested in other people than I used to be.
    2 I have lost most of my interest in other people.
    3 I have lost all my interest in other people.

13. 0 I make decisions as well as I ever could.
    1 I put off making decisions more than I used to.
    2 I have greater difficulty in making decisions than before.
    3 I can't make decisions at all anymore.

Beck Depression Inventory (continued)

14. 0 I don't feel I look any worse than I used to.
    1 I am worried that I am looking old or unattractive.
    2 I feel that there are permanent changes in my appearance that make me look unattractive.
    3 I believe that I look ugly.

15. 0 I can work about as well as before.
    1 It takes an extra effort to get started at doing something.
    2 I have to push myself very hard to do anything.
    3 I can't do any work at all.

16. 0 I can sleep as well as usual.
    1 I don't sleep as well as I used to.
    2 I wake up 2–3 hours earlier than usual and find it hard to get back to sleep.
    3 I wake up several hours earlier than I used to and cannot get back to sleep.

17. 0 I don't get more tired than usual.
    1 I get tired more easily than I used to.
    2 I get tired from doing almost anything.
    3 I am too tired to do anything.

18. 0 My appetite is no worse than usual.
    1 My appetite is not as good as it used to be.
    2 My appetite is much worse now.
    3 I have no appetite at all anymore.

19. 0 I haven't lost much weight, if any, lately.
    1 I have lost more than 5 pounds.
    2 I have lost more than 10 pounds.
    3 I have lost more than 15 pounds.
    I am purposely trying to lose weight by eating less
    _____ yes _____ no

20. 0 I am no more worried about my health than usual.
    1 I am worried about physical problems such as aches and pains; or upset stomach; or constipation.
    2 I am very worried about physical problems, and it's hard to think about anything else.
    3 I am so worried about my physical problems that I cannot think about anything else.

21. 0 I have not noticed any recent change in my interest in sex.
    1 I am less interested in sex than I used to be.
    2 I am much less interested in sex now.
    3 I have lost interest in sex completely.

Add the numbers of the separate items selected. Do not score weight lost on purpose (Item 19). A score of 0–9 would be considered in the normal range, 10–15 would suggest mild depression, 16–23 would be consistent with moderate depression, and a score of 24 or more suggests marked depression.

Anyone who scores between 10 and 23 should repeat the test in two weeks. If the score is still between 10 and 23, and particularly if it has risen, a doctor should be consulted for an evaluation. If the score is greater than 23, a prompt evaluation is certainly indicated. If the score is less than 10 but other indications of depression exist, evaluation is also wise.

It is important not to depend too heavily on any one measure of depression. The subjective experience of depression is highly variable. Some people with normal scores on a depression questionnaire are severely depressed and respond dramatically to treatment.

Source: Aaron T. Beck, 1972.

however, is fragile. When manic people meet opposition to their plans and wishes, their elation gives way to irritability and anger. Even during the greatest elation, doubts and depressive thoughts might make a transitory appearance. Worst of all, over a period of days or months, the mania may fade entirely and be replaced by a depressive episode. Certain people suffer an alternation of manic and depressive episodes; this syndrome is called

Myths about Suicide

Many popular statements made about suicide are false or only true in some cases. These statements may be false generalizations from a few atypical cases, wishful thinking, or just ignorance. People often conceal details about suicides, which promotes false assumptions such as the following.

Myth   People who really intend to kill themselves do not let anyone know about it.

Fact   This belief is a convenient excuse for doing nothing when someone says he or she might commit suicide. In fact, most people who eventually commit suicide *have* talked about doing it.

Myth   People who made a suicide attempt but survived did not really intend to die.

Fact   This may be true for certain people, but people who seriously want to end their life may fail because they misjudge what it takes. Even a pharmacist may misjudge the lethal dose of a drug.

Myth   People who succeed in suicide really wanted to die.

Fact   We cannot be sure of that either. Some people were trying only to make a dramatic gesture or plea for help but miscalculated.

Myth   People who really want to kill themselves will do it regardless of any attempts to prevent them.

Fact   Few people are single-minded about suicide even at the moment of attempting it. People who are quite determined to take their lives today may change their minds completely tomorrow.

Myth   Suicide is proof of mental illness.

Fact   Many suicides are committed by people who do not meet ordinary criteria for mental illness, although people with depression, schizophrenia, and other mental illnesses have a much higher than average suicide rate.

Myth   Certain groups of the population are immune to suicide: alcoholics because they have alcohol as a crutch, elderly men because they have achieved a stable life adjustment, and black teenagers because they are not achievement oriented.

Fact   Certain groups do have low suicide rates, but not these—the first two groups mentioned have much higher than average suicide rates, and the suicide rate for black 15- to 24-year-olds is about the same as for whites of the same age.

Myth   People inherit suicidal tendencies.

Fact   Certain kinds of depression that lead to suicide can be inherited. But many examples of suicide running in a family can be explained by factors such as psychologically identifying with a family member who committed suicide, often a parent.

Myth   All suicides are irrational.

Fact   Maybe by some standards all suicides are "irrational." But many people find it at least understandable that someone might want to commit suicide, for example, when approaching the end of a terminal illness or when facing a long prison term.

---

bipolar disorder because of the two opposite poles of mood. Major tranquilizers are used to treat individual manic episodes, while special drugs like the salt *lithium carbonate* taken daily can prevent future manic and depressive episodes.

Anxiety Disorders   Fear is a basic and useful emotion. Its value for evolutionary survival in prehistoric times cannot be overestimated; for modern humans it provides motivation for self-protection and learning to cope with new or potentially dangerous situations. Only when fear is out of proportion to real danger can it be considered a problem. Anxiety is another word for fear, referring especially to a feeling of fear that is not directed toward any definite threat. Only when anxiety is experienced almost daily or in life situations that recur and cannot be avoided, does it qualify anyone for a diagnosis of anxiety disorder.

The broad concept of anxiety disorders covers a variety of human problems. Here are the main types.

- *Simple phobia* is probably the most common and most understandable anxiety disorder since many of us have a few specific fears—for example, fears of animals or certain locations. Typically feared animals are dogs, snakes, insects, and mice. Frightening locations are

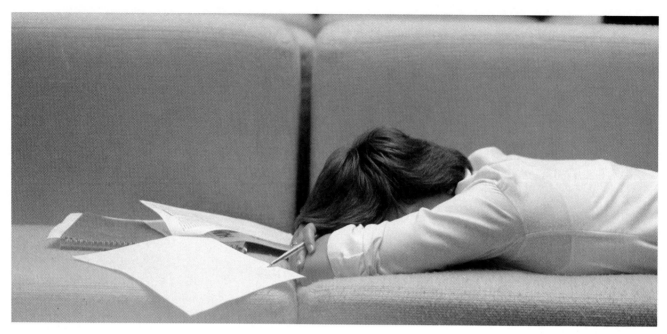

Stressed out from studying—or seriously depressed? Everyone feels dejected or defeated at times, but pervasive feelings of hopelessness, meaninglessness, or guilt signal deeper emotional problems. A person troubled by these feelings can often benefit from professional help.

high places, closed places, and air travel. Sometimes these fears originate in bad experiences with the feared objects, but often there is no such explanation. People who are afraid of witnessing blood or tissue injury are usually those who tend to faint in such situations.

- *Social phobias* are akin to simple phobias, but occur in interpersonal contexts. Those with social phobias fear humiliation or embarrassment while being watched by others. Perhaps the most common social phobia is fear of speaking in public. People also fear choking on food when eating in front of strangers or being unable to urinate in a public lavatory. Some people's social fears are much less specific; extremely shy people, for instance, are afraid in most social situations.

TACTICS AND TIPS

Getting a Grip on Flying Jitters: Tips for Nervous Travelers

More than 25 million Americans experience some level of anxiety about air travel, particularly after news of a plane crash, the Phobia Society of America reports. The most common worries: "Once the plane takes off, I'm powerless" and "Should there be an accident, I'll surely die." To deal with flying jitters, the group recommends that reluctant travelers do the following:

- Avoid caffeine and sugar before and during a flight.
- On takeoff, lean back and let your muscles go limp. Imagine you are a rag doll.
- If you begin to feel anxious, rate your anxiety level on a scale of 1 to 10. Think about different things and note how the level changes when you focus on positive thoughts.
- To curb anxiety, take deep breaths, close your eyes and imagine comforting scenes vividly.
- Stretch, shake your arms and legs to ward off tension.

For information on coping with fears and phobias, write: The Phobia Society of America, P.O. Box 42514, Washington, D.C. 20015-0514.

Adapted from *Washington Post Health*, Aug. 22, 1989, p. 20.

Feeling Shy: The Discomfort of Social Anxiety

Shyness is a form of social anxiety, a fear of what others will think of our appearance or behavior. The accompanying feelings of self-consciousness, embarrassment, and unworthiness can be overwhelming. The distressing telltale symptoms include increased perspiration, clammy hands, trembling hands and legs, butterflies in the stomach, pounding heart, dry mouth, and blushing. The shy person may avoid social gatherings, be unable to make eye contact with another person, and never volunteer or speak up in a public situation.

Research on shyness has boomed in the past few years, as experts try to pin down the cause of shyness. Three major theories have emerged from various studies: Shyness is an inherited personality trait; shyness results when effective social skills are not learned; and shyness is the result of social programming. Evidence suggests that all three premises may be true.

At Harvard University a study being conducted by Jerome Kagan indicates that when faced with the unknown, shy infants and toddlers withdraw. They become reserved and silent, and their heart rate pattern alters. Infants and toddlers who are not shy do not grow wary when presented with unfamiliar stimuli, nor does their heart rate pattern change. By the time the children in this study had entered kindergarten, none of the nonshy children had become shy. About a third of the shy ones

had become less shy; and these, interestingly, were mostly boys. The two-thirds who remained shy still responded to mild stress with apprehension as well as with the increased heart rate they had demonstrated four years earlier. Apparently, the no-longer-shy had been encouraged by their parents to become more assertive and more confident, qualities valued in our society. And those who remained shy probably will always be so. Kagan states, "You begin to get significant predictive correlations to adult behavior around age 5 or 6. Beginning at that time, a boy who is, say, one of the most aggressive in a group of 100 children is likely to be one of the more aggressive adults in that group."

Most shy adults probably were not shy infants. When a schoolchild's self-esteem is battered by family or peers, the child becomes shy. It doesn't take much to make a young person shy, and that shyness emerges in adulthood whenever related situations arise. Adults are shy if they learned early to be uncertain about their looks, say, or their intelligence. They may also become shy when confronted by social groups of a higher or lower class than they were raised in. Also, being surrounded by better-educated people or working alongside more skillful people can bring back shyness.

To define shyness as a fear of social rejection is correct, but it isn't enough. Shyness also in-

cludes an exaggerated sense of self, a concern with one's outward behavior, physiological symptoms, and feelings of self-consciousness. Shy people tend to be self-conscious, self-absorbed, and anxious about how others will view them. They may believe that others are confident in all situations even though very few adults have confidence in their attractiveness to others *and* their social skills *and* their job competence *and* their knowledge *and* their grace and dexterity *and* their techniques in bed. Most people experience the discomfort of shyness in certain situations. While the social scientists continue their research, shy people are taking a pragmatic approach. Some of them are fed up with shortchanging themselves and are reaching out to community center shyness classes, assertiveness training groups, and public speaking clinics. They receive training in social and cognitive skills, assertiveness, and changing negative behavior. These programs are described in greater detail in the Behavior Change Strategy at the end of the chapter.

Shy people may always be shy, but with professional help they can learn behavior that benefits their personal and work lives. And they can learn to tolerate and to modify their physiological symptoms. Many are doing just that. The rest are still sweating it out.

Source: L. F. Jacobson, 1985 (July), The social disease called shyness, *Healthline.*

- *Panic disorder* is characterized by sudden unexpected surges in anxiety, accompanied by symptoms such as rapid and strong heartbeats, shortness of breath, loss of physical equilibrium, and a feeling of losing mental control. Such attacks—the hallmark of **panic disorder**—usually begin in the early twenties and can lead to fear of being in crowds or closed places or of driving or flying. Sufferers fear that a panic attack will occur in a situation from which escape is difficult (as in an elevator), where the attack could be incapacitating and result in dangerous loss of control (as in driving a car), or where no help was available if needed (as when a person is alone). People with this kind of phobia can often do what they would ordinarily avoid if a spouse or trusted companion accompanies them.

- *Obsessive-compulsive disorder* applies to people with obsessions or compulsions or both. **Obsessions** are recurrent, unwanted thoughts or impulses. For example, a parent may have impulses to kill a beloved child; a person may brood over whether he or she contracted AIDS during a handshake; or a person may persistently wonder if he or she has done something unacceptable, such as having hit a pedestrian while driving. **Compulsions** are repetitive, difficult-to-resist actions associated with obsessions. A common compulsion is hand washing, associated with an obsessive fear of contamination by dirt. Others compulsions are counting or repeatedly checking if something has been done—for example, if a door has been locked or a stove turned off. Although obsessive-compulsive disorder is classified as an anxiety disorder, anxiety is not a central symptom and may be absent. Obsessive or compulsive people are sometimes similar to phobics in their avoidances. For example, people who are obsessed with dirt may avoid public lavatories, where they fear contamination.

- *Post-traumatic stress disorder* is a reaction to severely traumatic events (events that produce a sense of terror and helplessness) such as physical violence to oneself or loved ones. Such traumas occur in personal assaults like rape or military combat, natural disasters like floods or earthquakes, and accidental disasters like fires, airplane crashes, and automobile accidents. Symptoms include repeated reexperiencing of the trauma in dreams and intrusive memories, efforts to avoid anything that is associated with the trauma, and a numbing of feelings. Sleep disturbances and other symptoms of anxiety and depression are also often present.

- *Generalized anxiety disorder* is characterized by excessive anxiety and worry about concerns of everyday life. Finances or one's performance at work are typical topics for these worries. As with other anxiety disorders, mental anxiety is often accompanied by bodily expressions of anxiety such as muscle tension, shortness of breath, or rapid heart rate. Ability to fall or stay asleep is often reduced. People with generalized anxiety disorder are often depressed.

Treatment of anxiety disorders is much more controversial than is treatment of schizophrenia or depression. Therapies range from medication to psychological interventions that concentrate on a person's conscious or unconscious thoughts or on overt behavior. The controversy comes from the fact that there are very different models of human nature and each propounds its own idea of the causes and appropriate treatments of psychological disorders. We turn now to a discussion of these models.

Models of Human Nature and Therapeutic Change

How and what people see is shaped largely by the model—the picture—of reality they carry in their minds. Many models of human nature have been suggested, but we will consider only these four: the biological, behavioral, cognitive, and psychoanalytic models. Each model suggests its own kinds of therapy. Although their protagonists may present them as exclusive, the therapies that different models inspire often work best when applied together.

To understand these models it's useful to have a specific example in mind. Let's consider the case of Paul, a college student who finds himself so anxious whenever he's about to contribute to a class discussion that he can barely utter a word in class. In one month all students in this class are expected to make a brief oral presentation on a special topic. Paul's instructor is beginning to believe that Paul is either uninterested, not doing the assigned reading, or not bright enough for college. Paul has always been a shy person, but until recently he's been able to speak in public situations if he really tries. However, a few weeks ago when he began to answer a question in class, he suddenly felt so nervous he couldn't continue. He started to sweat, lost his breath, and could feel his heart pounding in an alarming way. It was terribly embarrassing to have to stop speaking before he could com-

---

Panic disorder A syndrome of severe anxiety attacks accompanied by physical symptoms.

Obsession Recurrent irrational, unwanted thoughts.

Compulsion Irrational, repetitive, forced action, usually associated with an obsession.

plete his answer. Now he gets anxious just going into the classroom. All of this depresses him and makes him think about dropping out of school. Paul's mother was a school teacher until she died of heart disease a year ago. She was a strict person and often critical of her son. Paul's father is still living. He's an easygoing man who tends to drink a bit too much in the evenings and on weekends. We will now present the four principal models, their views on psychological problems, and how they might approach Paul's case.

The Biological Model   The biological model emphasizes that human beings, like other animals, have an evolutionary history that has shaped not only our anatomy and physiology but also our behavior and emotions. The mind's activity depends completely on an organic structure, the brain, whose composition is determined by genes. This structure can be damaged by infectious agents such as viruses or bacteria, or by physical trauma such as that which sometimes accompanies birth. Such damage can produce mental abnormalities. Chemical compounds introduced into the body can induce abnormal mental states that are similar to certain natural mental diseases; chemicals can also partially reverse such mental symptoms.

Certain differences among people in abilities and personality, just as in hair color, may stem from genetic differences present at birth. Evidence shows a link between genes and certain kinds of schizophrenia and depression. Studies of identical and fraternal twins, especially when they have been raised apart, have contributed to that evidence.

Genetic explanations of behavior, however, do not mean that the environment has no influence. Almost half of schizophrenic identical twins have a sibling who is not schizophrenic, although identical twins have exactly the same genes. Genes vary in what is called *penetrance,* the likelihood that their potential will actually be expressed in the individual. Environmental influences include events happening before birth, such as viral infections in the mother; events at the time of birth; and stresses in childhood, adolescence, and adulthood. Stress can produce changes in brain chemistry that result in abnormal thinking, attention, mood, sleep, and other mental functions, just as it may cause the arteries supplying your heart to become clogged.

The biological model is used less in the mental health context than in the mental illness context. Schizophrenia and mood disorders have been of particular interest to biological psychiatrists. Chemists working for pharmaceutical firms have developed dozens of new antipsychotic and antidepressant drugs; those that have shown effectiveness in patients without causing dangerous side effects receive Food and Drug Administration approval, which allows them to be prescribed by psychiatrists and other physicians. Recent investigations on panic disorder show that both antianxiety drugs (minor tranquilizers) and antidepressant drugs can sometimes block panic attacks.

What can a biological model say about our student Paul? He is a shy person, a personality trait that usually begins in early childhood and has a basis in genetic differences. Taking an antianxiety drug before going to class might help him overcome his speech inhibitions, but the dose would have to be low or he might get sleepy and have trouble organizing his thoughts. He would have to be careful not to become dependent on such medicines since his father has tendencies toward alcoholism. If Paul inherited this tendency, he might be prone to addiction to tranquilizers. Since Paul had something like a panic attack when he unsuccessfully tried to answer a question, he might be suffering from a form of panic disorder, in which case certain antidepressants might be advisable.

Although the evidence available today does not firmly prove the correctness of biological models for any mental health problem, such models have been useful in many ways. Some people feel consoled by believing that they have a biological rather than a psychological problem. Somehow that idea relieves them of the tendency to blame themselves or their parents. Biological models have motivated scientists to develop new drugs for treating symptoms. These drugs have been immensely helpful, but it is important not to forget that all drugs have side effects, some of which can harm the patient. Thinking that is too narrowly focused on biology can result in the overprescribing of drugs. Opponents of their use in treating anxiety point out that anxiety can stimulate people to learn better and more mature coping skills. Although antianxiety drugs are seldom physically addicting, they can become a psychologically addictive substitute for more effective ways of dealing with anxiety.

Biological models can also be misused in other ways. Some people promote treatment of mental disease with special diets or vitamins without any scientific evidence that these treatments work. Others try to achieve mental health through drugs such as LSD or mescaline even though any insights attained may prove to be empty when normal consciousness returns and even though fear and paranoia could result. Finally, biological models (like the other models discussed) may be falsely used to excuse people for antisocial acts or to deprive them of their civil rights.

The Behavioral Model   The behavioral model focuses on what people do—on their overt behavior—rather than on brain structures and brain chemistry. Russian physiologist Ivan Pavlov laid the groundwork for the behavioral model in the late nineteenth century when he found that he could train (condition) dogs to salivate in response to various signals. Later, about sixty years ago, in his book *Psychological Care of Infant and Child* (1928), the American psychologist John Watson argued that human psychology also should focus on behavior: "The time has come when psychology must discard all reference to consciousness. . . . [Psychology's] sole task is the prediction and control of behavior."

The behavioral model regards psychological problems as "maladaptive behavior"—bad habits. When and how a person learned bad behavior in the past is less important than what makes it continue in the present. Behaviorists have built their treatment methods on studies of how animals learn and have verified the effectiveness of these methods in studies of humans. They analyze learning in terms of **stimulus, response,** and **reinforcement.**

One (of two) kinds of learning takes place when a stimulus becomes associated with a response. For example, when Paul had his episode of extreme nervousness a few weeks ago, it was perhaps because he was poorly prepared and had good reason to fear criticism; since then his anxiety response may have become conditioned to stimuli that preceded it, such as being in that classroom, looking at notes prepared for speaking, or seeing a classroom of students waiting to hear the speech. That would explain why he is nervous each new time he encounters those stimuli even when he is well prepared.

The second kind of learning explains why a person may repeat a response or not. If a certain response, such as standing up and giving a speech, is followed by a reward (positive reinforcement) like a good grade or compliments, it's more likely that the student will repeat the response in a classroom or in another context. However, if punishment follows the response—in this case, fear or negative feedback about a poor performance—the response is less likely to be repeated. Omission of an expected punishment is also a reward, while omission of an expected reward is a punishment. Paul will be encouraged to repeat his performance if anticipated criticism does not materialize, but discouraged if those he thought would praise him remain silent.

Behavior therapy consists of teaching new adaptive responses and unlearning old maladaptive responses. A wide variety of problems have been treated with behavioral therapy—difficulties in performing tasks, unhealthful habits and addictions, interpersonal conflicts, and irrational fears. The essence of behavior therapy is to analyze the undesirable behavior in terms of the reinforcements that keep it going and then try to alter those reinforcements. Clients are asked to keep a daily behavior diary to monitor the target behavior and events that precede and follow it. Chapter 1 uses overeating as an example, and applies behavioral principles to overcoming it.

Paul might start a behavioral therapy program by writing down each time he makes a contribution to a class-room discussion and how many seconds he actually speaks. He should then develop concrete but realistic goals for increasing this amount each week and contract with himself to reward his successes by spending more time in activities he finds enjoyable. For example, his goals might first be to briefly contribute to class discussions, then to make longer statements, then to volunteer to lead discussions, and finally to give a formal presentation. He can arrange for circumstances that make him more likely to speak—such as adequate preclass preparation or looking at a friendly classmate while speaking—to happen more frequently. Chapter 1 explains other useful measures such as developing social support for change and using role models.

Specific behavioral techniques have been developed for overcoming fears. People might be able to unlearn their irrational fears if they routinely return to feared situations, but often they simply avoid them. Behavioral therapies put people back in feared situations long enough and often enough to extinguish the fear. Two important methods are **desensitization** and **exposure.** Desensitization is useful for phobias of specific objects—for example, snakes or spiders. A person who has a phobia of snakes is first taught to relax and then to begin imagining a small, harmless snake in a secure container some distance away. When the person can imagine this without fear, he or she goes on to imagine more frightening snakes while remaining relaxed. Therapy thus progresses to a point where the person can handle live snakes calmly. A model of a desensitization program is given in the Behavior Change Strategy for Chapter 2.

Exposure therapy is especially useful for phobias of places and activities. It goes beyond relaxation or imagined situations by encouraging people to expose themselves to real places or activities they fear. The treatment program suggested for Paul contained the essential ingredients of exposure—practice in speaking in the classroom arranged in assignments of gradually increasing difficulty. Further elements include staying in a feared situation until the fear has abated somewhat. Leaving when fear is still high causes immediate relief, which acts as a reinforcement of avoidance and escape. Exposure has proved particularly effective in treating people who have become afraid of going shopping because of panic attacks. The sequence of assignments might be (1) going into small stores with a friend, (2) going into small stores alone, (3) going into larger stores with a friend, (4) going into larger stores alone when they are not crowded, and finally (5) going into crowded stores alone. Therapists can have various roles: they help set up the assignments, accompany patients on their assignments, and organize groups of patients to do their assignments together.

Behavioral models can also be useful in taking care of institutionalized people. A mentally retarded person or severe schizophrenic may not respond to verbal requests

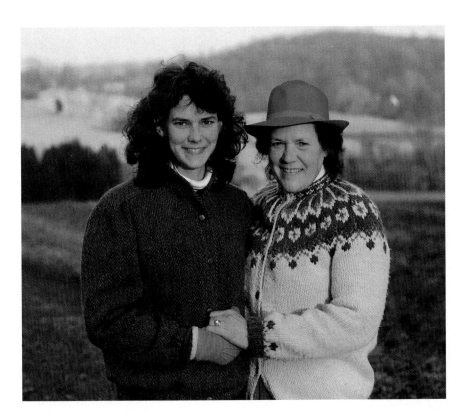

Developing a realistic view of one's parents is an important part of becoming a mentally healthy adult. This mother and daughter have worked out an accepting and loving relationship with one another.

or instructions. Analyzing their behavior in terms of response and reinforcement can give the institution staff ideas for promoting cleanliness, appropriate eating behavior, nonaggressive social interactions, and simple work assignments. First the desired behavior is defined very concretely, and a system of reward and nonreward is set up. For example, washing hands before meals might be rewarded by dessert; doing assigned work might carry the reward of going for a walk outside. Whether it is ever right to use punishments such as electric shocks to change behavior has raised sharp ethical controversy.

The Cognitive Model   The cognitive model emphasizes the effect of ideas on behavior and feelings. Human beings differ from other animals in thinking and expressing themselves in complex ways. In humans (according to the cognitive therapists) behavior results from complicated attitudes, expectations, and motives rather than from simple, immediate reinforcements. When behavioral therapies such as desensitization or exposure work, it is because they change the way a person thinks about the feared situation and his or her ability to cope with

it. Perhaps we should talk about cognitive models, *plural,* because cognitive theorists disagree about the relationship between ideas and other aspects of behavior and about how to change behavior by changing ideas.

One theory says that automatically recurring false ideas produce feelings such as anxiety and depression. Thus identifying and exposing these ideas as false should relieve these painful emotions. When people are anxious, the idea behind the anxiety is "Something bad is going to happen and I won't be able to handle it." Of course, each anxious person has his or her own versions of this basic idea. The therapist challenges such ideas in three ways: (1) showing that there isn't enough evidence for the idea, (2) suggesting different ways of looking at the situation, and (3) showing that no disaster is going to occur. The therapist does not just *state* his or her position, but encourages clients to examine the logic of their own ideas and then to test the truth of the ideas. "Of course, sometimes bad things do happen, and sometimes you can't handle them, at least alone. Life is not simple, and some fear is realistic."

Our student (Paul) who was afraid to speak up in class

Stimulus   Anything that causes an organism to respond.

Response   An organism's reaction to a stimulus.

Reinforcement   Increasing the future probability of a response by following it with rewards.

Desensitization   A therapeutic technique for treating phobias in which a phobic stimulus is vividly imagined while relaxation is maintained.

Exposure   A therapeutic technique for treating fears in which the subject learns to come into direct contact with a feared situation.

probably harbored ideas such as "If I begin to speak, I'll say something stupid; if I say something stupid, the teacher and my classmates will lose respect for me; and then I will get a low grade, my classmates will avoid me, and life will be hell. My heart's pounding; I could die at any minute of heart disease like my mother." In cognitive therapy, Paul would be taught to examine these ideas critically. If he prepares for the presentation, how likely is it that he will sound stupid? Does Paul actually believe that everything he is going to say will be stupid, or is he really aiming for an impossible perfection, every sentence exactly correct and beautifully delivered? Will people's opinion of Paul be completely transformed by how he does in one presentation? Do his classmates even care that much about how well he does? And why does *he* care so much about what *they* think? Paul will be taught to notice thoughts that automatically attack him in feared situations and to substitute more realistic ideas for them. The therapist will advise him to speak in front of the class again and to test his assumptions.

The Psychoanalytic Model   The psychoanalytic model, like the cognitive model, emphasizes thoughts, but it says that false ideas cannot be fought directly because they are fed by other ideas that are **unconscious**. Sigmund Freud, a Viennese neurologist, developed these revolutionary theories around 1900. He discovered that certain paralyses that had no apparent physical basis and certain losses of sensory function (such as some cases of blindness) were better understood in terms of the patients' hidden (unconscious) wishes than in terms of nerve pathways. The ideas that were disturbing behavior were at first hidden from both patient and therapist, but gradually surfaced in dreams, slips of the tongue, and the patient's behavior toward the therapist. Freud removed the moral stigma from such behavior by saying that patients had no conscious intention to deceive. In fact, such behavior was a medical disorder appropriately studied and treated by physicians. Freud also refused to make any sharp distinction between the mentally healthy and the mentally ill. We all have irrational ideas, which may emerge suddenly and demonstrate convincingly that we can't consciously control all of our own acts.

Therapies based on Freud's ideas do not take symptoms as isolated pieces of behavior but as results of a complex system of secret wishes, emotions, and fantasies hidden by active defenses that keep them unconscious. Freud divided the functions of the mind into three parts—the *id, ego,* and *superego.* The id comprises primitive sexual and aggressive drives. The superego is conscience, based on the child's experiences and fantasies of parental approval and disapproval. The ego is the "I" or control center that tries to find satisfactory compromises between the demands of the id and superego and the constraints of external reality. All of the workings of the id and many of the workings of the ego and superego are unconscious. For example, defenses are a part of ego that operates unconsciously to conceal the truth so that people can both lie to themselves and conceal from themselves that they have lied. The concealed truth turns out to derive from id impulses unacceptable to society as well as to the individual's superego.

The master defense is **repression,** which allows us to push down or forget what we don't want to remember. What was once conscious now becomes unconscious— but not inactive or without influence. In the defense of **projection,** we conveniently attribute our unacceptable impulses to others: "I am a gentle, loving person, but X is a real pig, and I'm afraid of him." In **reaction formation,** we conceal unconscious destructive impulses behind exaggerated concern for another person's well-being. And **displacement** shifts our impulses to safer but unsatisfying substitutes, as if a person were to say, "If I cannot be angry at my mother, I'll be angry at my sister instead."

The psychoanalytic model is often criticized nowadays for being unscientific and therapeutically ineffective. Yet its basic ideas persist in the practice of therapists who totally disavow its theoretical structure. One of those ideas is that people will become more mentally healthy if they get to know themselves better, but that self-honesty can be painful. Another idea is that disclosure of one's fears and secrets to a person or a group of people who can be trusted has therapeutic value. Both of these ideas are central in encounter groups and in other group and individual therapies. The psychoanalytic model prescribed that therapists should allow their clients to express themselves as freely as possible in therapy. The therapist is nondirective and tries not to impose his or her own values or ideas about morality or human nature

---

Unconscious   Whatever is in the mind but out of the awareness.

Repression   A psychological defense by which unacceptable thoughts or wishes are excluded from consciousness.

Projection   A psychological defense by which unacceptable thoughts or impulses are attributed to others.

Reaction formation   A psychological defense by which unacceptable feelings or impulses are turned into their opposites.

Displacement   A psychological defense by which unacceptable feelings are transferred from one event or person to a less threatening one.

on a client. Some therapists are influenced by the existential philosophers, who believe that humans are free to decide what they will be. Such therapists often adopt ideals of positive mental health, in contrast to ideas that define mental health as the absence of illness. The earlier section of this chapter entitled "Achieving Realistic Self-Esteem" was based in part on recent psychoanalytic ideas about how people form basic concepts about themselves and others.

If Paul received therapy inspired by this model, he would find a therapist interested not only in his problems in speaking but also in the totality of his personality—his most intimate wishes, hopes, and fears. Paul might learn some new and important things about himself. He would realize that his anxiety in speaking was part of a more general problem of shyness and low self-esteem. Standing up in front of others and letting them see him might make him feel as if he were under attack. For example, he might fear others will notice unpleasant traits he thinks he had. Finally, Paul might recall childhood experiences related to his current difficulties, such as being ridiculed by a parent for a stammer he had as a young child and might understand the impact of his critical mother and her recent death. In doing so he might learn to distance himself from childish ways of thinking and reacting, such as a panicky avoidance of all public speaking.

Implications of the Four Models   The people who believe in the four models we've just described argue out their disagreements. Behaviorists accuse supporters of the biological model of getting stuck in medical ways of thinking and thus of endangering their patients with drug side effects and dependence. Professional rivalries fuel this accusation because behavioral therapists are usually not licensed to prescribe drugs. Behaviorists attack psychoanalytic and other nondirective psychotherapists for making a patient pay for endless, ineffective therapy. Psychoanalytic therapists accuse behaviorists of simplistic thinking, of regarding human beings as behavior machines, with no human rights or responsibilities.

■ **Exploring Your Emotions**

If you were feeling depressed or anxious or were having trouble in your marriage, would you be tempted to see a counselor or therapist? If so, how would you choose among the various therapeutic types? What do you think is the basis for your choice?

The fact is that each model represents certain truths about human beings. Each model can help people dealing with specific types of human problems. When two ther-

apies compete to solve the same problem, scientific studies should be conducted to measure rival claims. At present, strong evidence suggests that therapy is better than no therapy. Showing effectiveness is hardest for therapies that do not focus on specific problems or symptoms, because measuring the changes that occur is difficult, and differences in the therapists' skills may make the difference. There are important practical considerations too. Some people and some problems cannot wait long enough for slowly acting treatments to work.

Getting Help

Self-Help   If you have a personal problem that you would like to solve, an intelligent way to begin is to find out what you can do on your own. Some problems are specifically addressed in this book. Behavioral and some cognitive approaches are especially useful for helping yourself. All of these involve becoming more aware of self-defeating actions and ideas and combatting them in some way: being more assertive when you find yourself backing down; taking the risk of communicating honestly; improving your self-esteem by counteracting thoughts, people, and actions that undermine it; and confronting things you're afraid of rather than avoiding what you fear. Get more information about solving personal problems by seeing what books are available in the psychology or self-help sections of the library or bookstore. Be selective, however—watch out for self-help books making fantastic claims that deviate from the mainstreams of psychological thinking.

Talking to friends (and even parents!) is important too. Just being able to confess what's troubling you to an accepting, empathetic person can bring relief. Comparing notes with people who have problems similar to yours can give you new ideas about coping. Many self-help groups work on the principle of bringing together people with similar problems to share their experiences and support each other. Some support groups are for the families of people with problems; Al-Anon, for the families of alcoholics, is an example.

Professional Help   Sometimes self-help or talking to nonprofessionals is not enough. More objective, more expert, or more discreet help is needed. Many people have trouble accepting the need for professional help to handle personal problems, and often the people who most need help are the most unwilling to get it. You may find yourself someday having to overcome your own reluctance toward seeking help or the reluctance of a friend for whom you want to get help.

David: A True Story

When a person begins to act strangely in public or when with friends or family, others rarely reach an immediate consensus about what this behavior means. Different observers form different opinions. These opinions do not just represent different levels of education or sophistication, because conflicts also occur between the best educated and most knowledgeable. Conflicts between models of mental health are not just theoretical but have practical results, as this true case history illustrates. Only his name and a few details have been changed to protect those involved.

David was a twenty-year-old junior at a large and competitive university, majoring in humanities. He had been the best all-around student in his high school class. The principal of the high school remembered him as brilliant and caring. David had maintained his outstanding academic record. Students in his dorm said he was cheerful, outgoing, and "laid back." For six months he had been attending meditation classes, had become a vegetarian, and had started to jog daily. He avoided all drugs including alcohol. Shortly before spring vacation, he told a friend he had been hearing voices and seeing "real" visions. He was convinced that the end of the world—the "Last Judgment"—was coming. He talked of taking his own life because he felt unworthy and said that his death would help humanity. In contrast to his usual personality, he became withdrawn and isolated. The worried friend called David's father, who lived far away from the university. The father talked to

his son several times on the telephone and arranged to fly up to see him in a week. The day before they were to meet, David jumped off a high bridge and drowned.

How did different people make sense of what happened? In his father's opinion, David's suicide was a result of spiritual striving—a deep interest in Eastern religions—combined with a drive for perfection in everything he attempted. According to his father, David was totally committed in life and in death. The problem his son had faced was trying to live simultaneously in a world of reality and in a world devoted to spirituality.

His friend took a medical point of view. He thought David's visions and voices sounded schizophrenic. The father agreed only partially. From his telephone conversations, he felt that something had temporarily snapped in David's mind. Perhaps a biochemical change had altered his mental state. But during the last telephone call, the day before the suicide, his son seemed to have become completely lucid and calm again. David assured him that he was OK now and that his father could stop worrying. They would see each other soon and be able to hold and love each other. His father found consolation in the thought that his son had found a kind of peace at the end. Yet to many who knew David, the story was only a tragedy—a talented, kind young person with most of his life in front of him died before the seriousness of his problems was recognized and treatment could be begun.

There is a strong temptation to

lay blame here. Was his father spiritualizing a schizophrenic disorder? Of all people, the father, who had known his son for all of his twenty years, should have recognized that something was wrong. But his father lived far away, and was merely empathetically supporting his son's spiritual quest. Religious impulses and spiritual crises are usually not crazy; they can have positive outcomes. And why did his friend not intervene more actively? He could have contacted a dean, faculty member, or someone at the student health service and insisted that someone in authority should step in. Perhaps his respect and admiration for David made him hesitate. David might have felt betrayed if he had been hospitalized. And what kind of university was it, that a student could become so troubled and so few people noticed it? But many large universities do not watch students very closely, because they believe students should be treated as grown-ups, with rights to privacy and to living under a minimum of rules and social requirements. Troubled students often keep to themselves; it would be enforcing conformity not to allow them to do so.

Thus, we cannot convincingly lay blame, but we can hope that in the future better informed students, parents, and college administrators will be more sensitive to serious danger signs such as the ones in this case: hearing voices and seeing visions, a major and sudden change in personality, suicidal thoughts, and the ominous false calm that can follow a firm decision to commit suicide.

Coping with Insomnia

To a sound sleeper, not being able to fall asleep may sound like a minor problem. But to an insomniac, twisting and turning and dreading exhaustion the next day, sleep is a precious necessity that some unexplainable power keeps snatching out of reach. Shakespeare's King Henry IV expresses the torment of insomnia when he says, "O sleep, O gentle sleep, / Nature's soft nurse, how have I frighted thee, / That thou wilt no more weigh my eyelids down / And steep my senses in forgetfulness?"

If you are a poor sleeper, here are some commonsense steps that can help you get a good night's sleep.

First, do you get up at the same time every day and avoid naps during the day? A regular 24-hour rhythm of being awake and asleep promotes alertness during the day and sleepiness at night. Getting up at a regular time is more powerful in setting up that rhythm than going to bed at a regular time. Some insomniacs fall into a cycle of sleeping during the day to make up for lack of sleep at night. Even after a sleepless night, it is important to keep busy and carry on with your normal activities.

Second, are you preparing for sleep properly? Avoid caffeine-containing beverages and alcohol for several hours before bedtime.

Alcohol may push a person into sleep, but such sleep is not normal in quality or duration. Exercise or exciting discussions before bedtime can delay sleep. Relax an hour or so before going to bed by reading, listening to music, or taking a warm bath.

Third, has bed become a place for worry instead of sleep? Some insomniacs spend a lot of their time in bed worrying—often about not sleeping. If you are not sleepy, stay up a little longer. If you go to bed and cannot fall asleep after half an hour, get up and read for a while. In this way, you begin to associate bed with sleep instead of with worried wakefulness.

In some cases, professional help is optimal. Some people are interested in improving their mental health in a general way by going into individual or group therapy to learn more about themselves and how to interact with others. Certain therapies teach people how to adjust the effect of what they say and do on people around them. Clearly, seeking professional help for these reasons is a matter of individual choice. Interpersonal friction among family members or between partners often falls in the middle between necessary and optional. Successful help with such problems can mean the difference between painful divorce and a satisfying relationship.

Following are some strong indications that you or someone else needs professional help:

- If depression, anxiety, or other emotional problems begin to interfere seriously with performance at school, work, or in getting along with other people
- If suicide is attempted or is seriously considered (refer to the danger signals listed in this chapter)
- If symptoms such as hallucinations, delusions, incoherent speech, or loss of memory occur
- If alcohol or drugs are used to the extent that they impair normal functioning during much of the week, if finding or taking drugs occupies much of the week, or if reducing their dose leads to psychological or physiological withdrawal symptoms

Mental health workers belong to several professions. *Psychiatrists* are medical doctors with a full five years of medical training after college, followed by three years of training in psychiatry. *Clinical psychologists* have usually completed a Ph.D. degree requiring at least five years of graduate work after college. *Social workers* typically have master's degrees requiring at least two years of graduate study. The requirements for licensed *counselors* varies from state to state. Some clergymen have special training in *pastoral counseling* in addition to their religious studies.

■ **Exploring Your Emotions**

How do you react when you hear that someone is seeing a psychiatrist or is in therapy? Does it make a difference in how you feel about the person?

These professional groups differ somewhat in their roles. Only psychiatrists prescribe medications. They are experts in deciding whether a medical disease lies behind psychological symptoms. Psychiatrists are usually involved if hospitalization is required. All mental health professionals are trained to practice some kind of psychological therapy, but most restrict themselves to only one or two of the approaches described in this chapter. Psychologists have been important in developing behav-

Group therapy is just one of many different approaches to psychological counseling. If you have concerns you would like to discuss with a mental health professional, shop around to find the approach that works for you.

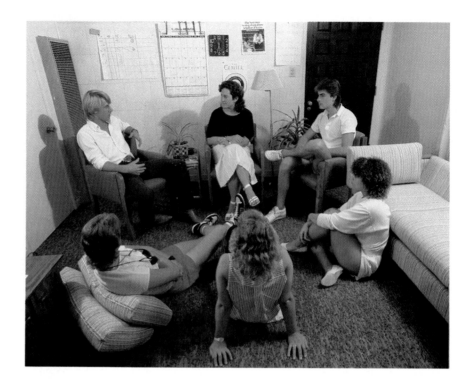

ioral and cognitive therapies and are often expert in these therapies or in psychoanalytically inspired therapies. Social workers have much experience in finding community support for the seriously ill. In hospitals and clinics, various mental health professionals join together in treatment teams. Psychiatric nurses often are important members of these teams.

Where do you actually find these professionals when you need them? College students are usually in a good position to find inexpensive mental health care. Larger colleges have both health services that employ psychiatrists and psychologists and counseling centers staffed by professionals and students (peer counselors). For less severe problems, psychology departments and education departments may offer student counselors. Student newspapers sometimes announce "sensitivity training groups" or other self-awareness groups sponsored by student organizations. Remember, though, that peer counselors are not professionals, and for problems of the kind listed earlier in this section it is better to go to someone with more training and experience. Self-awareness groups are also not really suitable for people who are in a crisis or not functioning.

Community mental health resources may include a school of medicine or teaching hospital with outpatient psychiatric clinics that offer psychological testing, diagnostic screening, and the ongoing services of psychiatrists, psychologists and social workers. If you go first to an interdisciplinary team, you will find out whether your problems have physical origins, you will have access to

professionals qualified to prescribe medication, and you will reap the benefits of several heads. Psychologists, counselors, or psychiatrists working in the community are listed in the local telephone book. Rather than choosing a name at random, get recommendations from a family physician, clergy, friends who have been in therapy, or community agencies.

Financial considerations are important in a country without national health insurance. Be sure to check what kind of mental health benefits your personal health insurance or prepaid medical plan provides. At the time of this writing treatment by a psychiatrist in a private practice setting could cost $100 for a 45-minute session. Therapists in private practice charge more than those affiliated with centers or large institutions, and psychiatrists usually charge more than psychologists, who charge more than social workers or counselors. Group therapy is generally cheaper than individual therapy. Some therapists have a sliding fee scale based on the client's income. If you are not adequately covered by a health plan, don't let that stop you from getting help; investigate low-cost alternatives. City, county, and state governments often support mental health clinics for those who can afford to pay little or nothing for treatment.

It will take a personal meeting to decide whether a therapist is right for you. Besides checking out a therapist's basic professional qualifications, you will need to know whether you feel comfortable with his or her personality, values and belief system, and psychological orientation. Does the therapist seem like a warm, intelligent person who would be able and interested in helping you? Is the therapist willing to talk about the techniques she or he uses? Does the therapist make sense to you? If the first therapist you see seems all right, there is no need to look further; but if you feel at all uncomfortable, it's worthwhile setting up one-shot consultations with one or two others before you make up your mind. If you're not in need of emergency care, be prepared to spend as much time shopping for a therapist as you would for anything else that important. Of course, if you can afford only free or low-cost treatment, your options may be limited.

The number and frequency of sessions depends on the type of therapy. Psychological therapies focusing on specific problems may require eight or ten sessions at weekly intervals. Therapies aiming for psychological awareness and personality change can last months or years with one to four sessions per week. Treatment with medication usually starts with weekly sessions; after the best medication and optimal dose is found, the frequency of sessions is reduced. For schizophrenia or bipolar disorder, medication may have to be continued for years.

Whomever you choose to help you, respect your own judgment as to whether you are actually being helped. Although too much "shopping around" may be a way of avoiding the resolution of problems, you certainly have the right to change therapists if therapy is not helpful after a reasonable period of time. First, ask yourself whether you are displeased because your therapy is raising difficult, painful issues you don't want to deal with. Then express your dissatisfaction to your therapist and deal with it in your session. Finally, if you are convinced that your therapy isn't working or is harmful, find another therapist.

Summary

What Mental Health is Not

- Mental health encompasses more than normality. Psychological diversity is valuable; conformity is not necessarily admirable.
- Getting professional help does not necessarily indicate mental illness. Neither symptoms nor appearances are reliable indicators of mental health.

What Mental Health Is

- Mental health is more than the absence of mental illness.
- Maslow's definition of mental health centered on self-actualization, the highest level of his hierarchy of needs. His ideas and those of others provide a good basis for a definition of mental health.
- Mentally healthy people are realistic and have high self-esteem, or a positive sense of self-worth.
- Being inner-directed is a sign of mental health; it signifies finding guidance from one's own values and feelings. A related quality is authenticity—being genuine and unselfconsciously oneself.
- Mentally healthy people are capable of emotional intimacy, interacting with others in ways that ensure good communication; a strong sense of self allows understanding of others.
- Creativity and boldness are qualities that show an ability to deal with uncertainty and the unknown.
- A definition of mental health as the absence of mental illness allows common psychological problems to be addressed. Although this negative definition can be too narrow, it can provide a balance to the broad concept of mental wellness that can be faulted as more an expression of Western cultural values than a reflection of scientific facts.

Common Psychological Problems

- Self-esteem and the ability to communicate are present in varying degrees in different individuals; both characteristics of mental health can be strengthened through learning.
- A sense of self-esteem develops during childhood as a result of giving and receiving love and learning to accomplish goals. Someone with an unstable self-concept is unable to maintain consistency in relationships.
- Self-concept is challenged every day; healthy people adjust their goals to their abilities if they fail, but unhealthy people rely too much on defenses or become demoralized.
- Fighting demoralization requires recognizing and testing negative thoughts; keeping a daily record can help. Once unpleasant emotions and thoughts have been identified, it's possible to develop rational responses through practice in logical thinking.
- As a facet of mental health, honest communication requires recognition of what needs to be said and the ability to say it clearly. Assertiveness allows people to insist on their rights and to participate in the give-and-take of good communication.
- When people choose to express their feelings, they need to consider their intention and the way their statements will be taken.

Psychological Disorders

- The classification system of neurotic and psychotic disorders has been replaced by a classification system based on specific symptom patterns, or syndromes. People who suffer from disorders have symptoms severe enough to interfere with daily living.
- Schizophrenic disorders are characterized by disorganized thoughts, inappropriate emotions, delusions, auditory hallucinations, and deteriorating social and work performance. Schizophrenia may be accompanied by depression, and suicide is a possibility. Treatment for schizophrenia includes antipsychotic drugs and sometimes hospitalization.
- Depression, a common mood disorder, often includes demoralization as well as feelings of helplessness, loss of pleasure, poor appetite, insomnia, restlessness or lethargy, loss of sexual drive, fatigue, thoughts of worthlessness, inability to concentrate, and thoughts of death or suicide. Loss of interest or pleasure in things seems to be the most universal symptom.
- Severe depression carries a high risk of suicide. Danger signals include expressing the wish to die, social withdrawal and isolation, an inexplicable lightening of mood. Risk factors include previous attempts, suicide by a family member or friend, readily available means, addiction to alcohol or drugs, and serious medical problems. Suicidally depressed people need professional help. Treatment for depression is usually a combination of drug therapy and psychotherapy; when suicidal impulses are strong, hospitalization might be necessary.
- Manic episodes are less common but more disturbing than depression. Symptoms include exalted moods with unrealistically high self-esteem, a need for little sleep, rapid and pressured speech, restlessness, and distractability. Elation usually gives way to irritability and anger and to depression in bipolar disorders. Major tranquilizers are used to treat individual episodes, and special drugs can prevent recurrence.
- Anxiety refers to a fear that is not directed toward any definite threat; when it is experienced daily or in recurrent situations, it becomes a disorder. Anxiety disorders include simple phobias, social phobias, panic disorder, obsessive-compulsive disorder, post-traumatic stress disorder, and generalized anxiety disorder. Treatment of anxiety disorders ranges from giving medication to various forms of therapy.

Models of Human Nature and Therapeutic Change

- Theorists have attempted to understand and explain psychological development and problems by proposing different models of human nature. The biological, behavioral, cognitive, and psychoanalytic models all suggest their own forms of therapy.
- The behavioral model focuses on overt behavior and treats psychological problems as bad habits. The cause of behavior is less important than what makes it continue. Behaviorists analyze learning in terms of stimulus, response, and reinforcement and teach new adaptive responses, partly by analyzing undesirable behavior in terms of the reinforcements that keep it going.
- Behavior self-management techniques are based on the behavioral model. Behavioral therapy uses the techniques of desensitization and exposure for phobias as two important methods.
- The cognitive model considers how ideas affect behavior and feelings; behavior results from complicated attitudes, expectations, and motives—not just from simple reinforcements. Treatment focuses on changing the way a person thinks about situations and abilities.
- The psychoanalytic model asserts that false ideas are fed by unconscious ideas and cannot be attacked directly. Psychological symptoms result from complex—and usually unconscious—interactions between the id, ego, and superego. Although many of this model's original tenets may have been repudiated, its basic ideas persist in many therapeutic practices.
- Each model represents certain truths about human behavior, and the most appropriate therapy depends upon the situation.

Getting Help

- Knowing when self-help or professional help is required for mental health problems is usually not so difficult as knowing how to start or which professional to choose.
- Behavioral and cognitive approaches are useful in self-help. Books are available for guidance; talking to friends or relatives and joining self-help groups are ways to start treatment.
- Professional help is necessary if problems interfere with performance or interpersonal relationships; if suicide is considered or attempted; if hallucinations, delusions, memory loss, or other severe symptoms occur; or if alcohol or drug abuse impairs normal functioning.
- Mental health workers have various forms of training and play different roles in treatment. Several problems can probably be treated best by an interdisciplinary team. It helps to take time choosing a therapist and to continually review the benefits of therapy, changing therapists if necessary.

Take Action

1. Do you remember incidents or moments from childhood that stand out as wonderful or horrible? Write a short essay about two such incidents, including what your feelings were and what you think you learned from them. Then describe what you would do now in the same situations and why.

2. Think about a person you admire. Describe that person in writing, listing the qualities that you admire in him or her. Do you have any of those qualities? What does your list say about the kind of person you want to be?

3. Investigate the mental health services provided on your campus and in your community. What services are available? Consider what ones you would feel comfortable using either for yourself or someone else, should the need ever arise.

4. Many colleges and communities have peer counseling programs, hot-line services (for both general problems and specific issues such as rape, suicide, drug abuse, parental stress, and so on), and other kinds of emergency counseling services. Some of these programs are staffed by volunteers trained in listening, helping, and providing information. Investigate such programs in your school (through the health clinic or student services) or community (look in the yellow pages), and consider volunteering for one. The training and experience can give you invaluable assistance in understanding both yourself and others.

5. Being assertive rather than passive or aggressive is a valuable skill that everyone can learn. To improve your ability to assert yourself appropriately, sign up for a workshop or class in assertiveness training on your campus or in your community.

Behavior Change Strategy

Dealing with Social Anxiety

Everyone is lonely at times, but some people have a harder time meeting new people, initiating friendships, and establishing relationships with members of the opposite sex than others do. In some cases, the problem is social anxiety—also known as shyness, social inhibition, heterosexual anxiety, or interpersonal anxiety. Shyness is discussed in detail in a box in this chapter. This Behavior Change Strategy describes some of the ways the problem of social anxiety is approached in various programs.

Many programs focus on the variety of subtle social skills that are needed to initiate and sustain interpersonal relationships. These skills include appropriate eye contact, sense of humor, reflection, facial expression, initiating topics in conversation, maintaining the flow of conversation by asking questions, and so on. One general plan of treatment assumes a *skills-deficit perspective,* and it teaches college students how to use interpersonal skills to greater personal advantage by means of videotape feedback and modeling (practice exercises). Practice-dating programs in which both partners know that their interaction has been scheduled for practice and self-improvement help extend modeling well beyond the clinic into "real world" social settings.

A slightly different approach stems from the belief that people know well enough what to do to make and keep friends—the problem of social inhibition comes from the anxiety that reduces a person's ability to perform key social skills. Reduced performance produces even greater self-doubt and anxiety, which only interferes further with later performance to produce a vicious circle of damaging experiences. With this approach, people for whom anxiety plays a key role receive special training in relaxation skills and other stress management strategies—perhaps in conjunction with the more complex and time-consuming anxiety-reduction procedure known as *systematic desensitization.*

In most cases shyness and loneliness are not easily diagnosed as being only a problem of skills or only a problem of anxiety. Most programs assume that *both* skills and anxiety play a role, and these programs provide a comprehensive treatment that includes modeling, structural practice, and stress management components.

Programs usually begin with a self-monitoring phase in which all facets of a person's daily routine are noted in a diary format. The Social Activity Diary shows how a coding scheme (noted in the key) can be used to help keep track of the pattern of social contacts, the amount of time spent in effective studying, and the amount of time wasted each day. These patterns are monitored for at least one week so that general trends can be identified.

Depending on the particular program, the shy person is then told to make better use of "wasted

Social Activity Diary

	DATE: 11/16		DATE:		DATE:	
	AM	PM	AM	PM	AM	PM
12		I, I, W				
1		A, W				
2		S				
3		S				
4		S				
5		I, I				
6		W				
7		W				
8		S				
9		S P, P				
10	I, I, S	S				
11	S	W				

KEY
P = Social phone call
I = Social interaction (at least 5 minutes)
A = Social activity
S = Study time
W = Wasted time

time" and to begin to practice some of the skills he or she has learned in the class or clinic in the least troublesome (anxiety-producing) situations. This tactic might be translated into an assignment (and behavioral contract) to initiate brief, nonthreatening conversations with same-sex classmates on an academic topic (the upcoming midterm or the homework assignment, for example). Once these conversations are successfully accomplished, then the next phase of the program could encourage practice of discussions that involve more personal subjects (personal opinions about nonacademic topics). Later assignments might involve members of the opposite sex. The individual steps would form a type of hierarchy, incorporating topics, people, and places, from least to most difficult.

The person would accomplish these steps by using a consistent theme of practice, modeling, and stress management skills while moving up the hierarchy. Using these techniques the person increases social skills and confidence levels, at the same time decreasing anxiety and feelings of insecurity, until social interactions can be sustained with comfort and enjoyment.

To evaluate your own level of social anxiety, examine the following list of statements made by college students identified as lonely in a study conducted at Stanford University. These students said that it was difficult for them to:

- Make friends in a simple, natural way
- Introduce themselves to others at parties
- Make phone calls to others to initiate social activity
- Participate in groups
- Get pleasure out of a party
- Get into the swing of a party
- Relax on a date and enjoy themselves
- Be friendly and sociable with others
- Participate in playing games with others
- Get buddy-buddy with others

These statements suggest a level of social anxiety and inhibition that interferes with dating and making friends. If they describe you, consider looking into a shyness clinic or treatment program on your campus. You have nothing to lose and everything to gain.

Selected Bibliography

American Psychiatric Association. 1987. *Diagnostic and Statistical Manual of Mental Disorders* (DSM-III-R), 3rd ed. revised. Washington, D.C.: American Psychiatric Association Press.

Beck, A. T., A. J. Rush, B. F. Shaw, and G. Emery. 1979. *Cognitive Therapy of Depression: A Treatment Manual.* New York: Guilford.

Berger, P. A., and H. K. H. Brodie,

(eds.). 1986. *American Handbook of Psychiatry.* Vol. 8: *Biological Psychiatry.* New York: Basic Books.

Hatton, C. L., and S. M. Valente, (eds.). 1984. *Suicide: Assessment and*

Intervention. 2nd ed. Norwalk, Conn.: Appleton-Century-Crofts.

Hauri, P. J., and M. J. Sateia. 1985. Nonpharmacological treatment of sleep disorders. Chapter 29 in R. E. Hales and A. J. Frances (eds.), *Psychiatry Update: American Psychiatric Association Annual Review* 4:361–78 (published by the American Psychiatric Press, Washington, D.C.)

Hersen, M., and A. S. Bellack, (eds.). 1985. *Handbook of Clinical Behavior Therapy with Adults.* New York: Plenum Press.

Kohut, H. 1971. *The Psychology of the Self.* New York: International Universities Press.

Lazare, A. 1973. Hidden conceptual models in clinical psychiatry. *New England Journal of Medicine* 288:345–51.

Maslow, A. H. 1968. *Toward a Psychology of Being.* 2nd ed. Princeton, N.J.: Van Nostrand-Reinhold.

Regier, D. A., J. K. Myers, M. Kramer, L. N. Robins, D. G. Blazer, R. L. Hough, W. W. Eaton, and B. Z. Locke, 1984. The NIMH Epidemiologic Catchment Area Surveys. *Archives of General Psychiatry* 41:934–42. (Also see other articles on pp. 942–78 of the same volume.)

Recommended Readings

Agras, S. 1985. *Panic: Facing Fears, Phobias, and Anxiety.* San Francisco: Freeman. *This popular book explains the nature of fears and phobias and how to overcome them.*

Andreasen, N. C. 1984. *The Broken Brain: The Biological Revolution in Psychiatry.* New York: Harper & Row. *Here is a clear, simple presentation of the biology of mental illness.*

Beck, A. T. 1988. *Love is Never Enough.* New York: Harper and Row. *Subtitled "How couples can overcome misunderstandings, resolve conflicts, and solve relationship problems," this book was written by a pioneer in the field of cognitive psychotherapy for couples trying to maintain long-term relationships.*

Emery, G. 1988. *Getting Un-depressed: How a Woman Can Change Her Life through Cognitive Therapy.* New York: Simon and Schuster. *Emery, a student of Beck, has written a self-help book specifically for depressed women.*

Papolos, D. F., and J. Papolos. 1987. *Overcoming Depression.* New York: Harper and Row. *Its subtitle explains its contents: "For the millions who suffer depression and manic depression and for the families affected by these recurring disorders." The book's biological orientation is particularly appropriate for severe mood disorders.*

Patterson, C. H. 1986. *Theories of Counseling and Psychotherapy.* 4th ed. New York: Harper and Row. *This book summarizes the basic principles of a variety of psychological treatments.*

Sarason, I. G., and B. R. Sarason. 1987. *Abnormal Psychology: The Problem of Maladaptive Behavior,* 5th ed. Englewood Cliffs, N.J.: Prentice-Hall. *This up-to-date textbook is a good place to look for more detailed discussions of topics in this chapter.*

Torrey, E. F. 1988. *Surviving Schizophrenia. A Family Manual.* Revised edition. New York: Harper and Row. *This book is a detailed and intelligent account of what schizophrenia is and how to cope with it.*

Zimbardo, P. G. 1977. *Shyness—What It Is. What to Do about It.* Reading, Mass.: Addison-Wesley. *Students and their interpersonal problems are the focus of the research and therapy techniques reported in this book.*

Contents

Making Connections

Humans are sexual beings from birth, but they don't become sexually active until adolescence or adulthood. Most college students—in fact, most adults—are still learning about their sexuality and trying to link what they've heard and read with their own experiences. The scenarios on these pages describe situations involving sex in which people have to use information, make a decision, or choose a course of action. As you read them, imagine yourself in each situation and consider what you would do. After you finish the chapter, read the scenarios again and see if what you've learned about sex has changed how you would think, feel, or act.

An old friend recently called to tell you she's pregnant. She had been trying to conceive ever since she was married a year ago. She says she got pregnant after her husband stopped wearing jockey briefs and started wearing boxer shorts. Is she putting you on?

Periodically, your sister has times when she becomes short-tempered and emotionally excitable, bursting into tears at the slightest upset. She usually craves chocolate and other sweets during these times, but she feels worse after eating them. She knows her symptoms are related to her period, but she doesn't seem to know what to do about it. Recently, you read something about PMS and it really made you think of her. Could that be what's causing her distress? Are there any suggestions you can make to her about it?

Sex and Your Body

Although you've heard a lot about female orgasm, you have yet to experience it yourself. You've been in an intimate relationship for a year now, and you're beginning to wonder if you'll ever have an orgasm. Your partner doesn't seem to know how to help. You're thinking of going to talk to a doctor or therapist at the student health services, but you feel very awkward about discussing it. Do you or don't you have a problem, and if you do, what should you do about it?

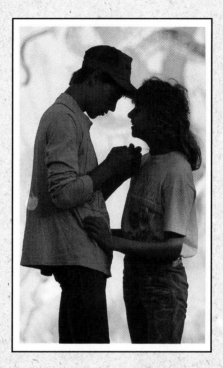

Everyone you know is circumcised, but one of your teammates on the soccer team isn't. He's from another country, and he says most males aren't circumcised there. In fact, he tells you that circumcision is commonly performed only in the United States and a few other countries. Most of the male population of the world isn't circumcised, he says. You find this hard to believe. He assures you it's true. "There aren't any medical reasons to do it," he says. "It's just a custom." Is he right?

After being married for three years, you and your wife have decided that it's time to have a child, even though you have mixed feelings about the responsibilities of becoming a parent. On the night you stop using contraceptives, you have an experience you've never had before—you're unable to sustain an erection long enough to make love. Is something wrong with you? What's going on?

Human beings have a compelling interest in sex. It's the source of our most intense physical pleasures, a central ingredient in many of our intimate emotional relationships, and, of course, the key to the reproduction of our species. These three areas—pleasure, intimacy, and reproduction—are related; in fact, we could say that if sex weren't so pleasurable, so satisfying a part of love relationships, human beings might not be around to enjoy it.

Because of the intensity of the feelings it arouses, communication about sex is often highly emotionally charged. And because of its basic role in human life, sexual expression is usually regulated by society with restrictions and taboos—written and unwritten laws specifying which functions and behaviors are acceptable and "normal" and which are unacceptable and "abnormal." Young people growing up in our society are bombarded with messages about sex from every side, many of them conflicting. The media—television, movies, magazines, popular music—suggest that the average person is a sexual athlete who continually jumps in and out of bed without using contraception, engendering offspring, or contracting disease. Parents, educators, and other responsible adults give a more balanced picture but often convey their own hidden messages as well. More than a few young people get the feeling that sexuality is something to be repulsed by or feared.

In the confusion created by all of these powerful communications, the need for basic information and knowledge can be obscured—information about the body, about sexual functioning, about common sexual problems and ways to solve them. Yet this information is vital to healthy adult life. Once we understand the facts, we have a better basis for evaluating all the messages we get and for making informed, responsible choices about our sexual behavior. If you have questions about aspects of your physical sexuality, this chapter will provide you with some answers. The next chapter will address sexual behavior and intimate relationships.

Sex and Gender: Defining Who You Are

The word *sex* means many things to many people. Strictly speaking, **sex** refers only to the quality of being biologically male or female. In everyday speech, though, the word is sometimes used more loosely, as a kind of shorthand for sexual intercourse, the physical act of making love. It is also used to refer to the masculine and feminine behaviors that people take on, but this is more generally what is meant by **gender**. Your **gender role** is everything you do in your daily life to indicate your maleness or femaleness to others. Your **gender identity** is your personal, inner sense of gender role as a male or female.

Gender role and gender identity are usually in agreement, although some individuals feel ambivalent about their gender and experience a conflict between gender role and gender identity.

■ Exploring Your Emotions

Do you ever wonder if you're sexually "normal"? Do you worry about the size, shape, or appearance of your genitals, about whether your sexual functioning is the same as other people's, or about the acceptability of the thoughts or fantasies that you find erotically exciting? Do you think it would be helpful to know how other people feel about the same things?

The word *sexuality* is the most inclusive of all these terms. It refers to gender, sexual functioning and behaviors, sexual anatomy and physiology, and social and sexual interactions with the same or the opposite sex. Your sense of identity is powerfully influenced by your **sexuality**—you think of yourself in very fundamental ways as male or female, as heterosexual or homosexual, as single, attached, married, divorced. Your sexuality is thus a complex configuration of inborn, biological characteristics and acquired behaviors you learn in the course of growing up in a particular family, community, and society. Although we can discuss the different aspects of sexuality separately—sexual anatomy, patterns of sexual response, sex hormones, intimate relationships, and so on—in practice, none can really be sorted out from the others. They all work together to make people complex sexual beings, defined in many ways by their gender but capable of making choices about how they express their sexuality.

Sexual Anatomy

In spite of their different appearance, the sexual organs of men and women arise from the same structures and fulfill similar functions. Each person has a pair of **gonads**: ovaries are the female gonads, testes are the male gonads. The gonads produce **germ cells** and **sex hormones**. The female germ cells are ova (eggs); the male germ cells are sperm. Ova and sperm are the basic units of reproduction; their union can lead to the creation of a new life.

Female Sex Organs　The external sex organs, or genitals, of the female are called the vulva ("covering") and are illustrated in Figure 4-1a. The mons pubis, a rounded mass of fatty tissue over the pubic bone, becomes covered with hair during puberty. Below it are two paired folds

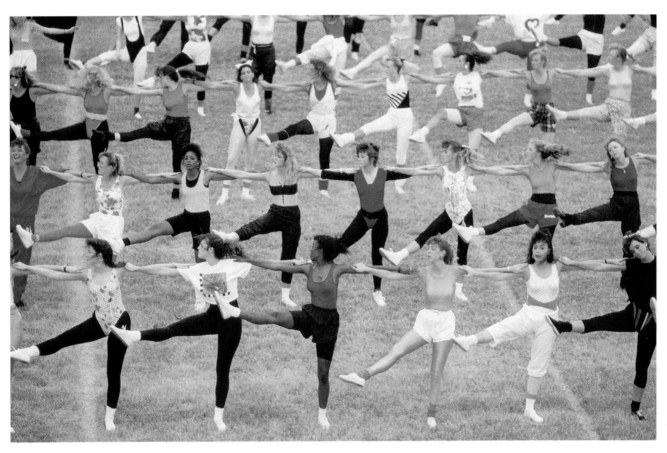

Bodies come in millions of unique sizes and shapes, despite the images promoted in our society. People don't have to conform to any particular physical standards to experience and enjoy their sexuality.

of skin called the labia majora (major lips) and the labia minora (minor lips). Enclosed within are the **clitoris** and its **prepuce** (foreskin), the opening of the urethra, and the opening of the vagina. The clitoris is highly sensitive to touch and plays an important role in female sexual arousal. The clitoris, like the penis, consists of a shaft, glans, prepuce (also called the clitoral hood), and spongy tissue that fills with blood during sexual excitement. The glans is the most sensitive part of the clitoris and is covered by the clitoral hood, which is formed from the upper portion of the labia minora.

The female's urethra leads directly from the urinary bladder to its opening between the clitoris and the opening of the vagina; it conducts urine from the bladder to the outside of the body. Unlike the male's urethra, it is independent of the genitals.

The vaginal opening is partially covered by the hymen. This membrane can be stretched or torn during athletic activities or when a woman has sexual intercourse for the first time. The idea that an intact hymen is the sign of a virgin is a myth.

The vagina is the passage that leads to the internal

Sex   Biological femaleness or maleness.

Gender   Includes not only one's biological sex, but also those psychosocial components that characterize one as a male or female.

Gender role   The different behaviors and attitudes our society expects of women and men.

Gender identity   A person's personal, internal sense of maleness or femaleness.

Sexuality   A dimension of personality shaped by biological, psychosocial, and cultural forces and concerning all aspects of sexual behaviors.

Gonads   Ovaries and testes; primary reproductive organs that produce germ cells and sex hormones.

Germ cells   Sperm and ova.

Sex hormones   Chemical substances that stimulate and promote the development of sexual characteristics.

Clitoris   Highly sensitive, erectile female genital structure.

Prepuce   Foreskin of the penis or clitoris.

Figure 4-1   Female sex organs.

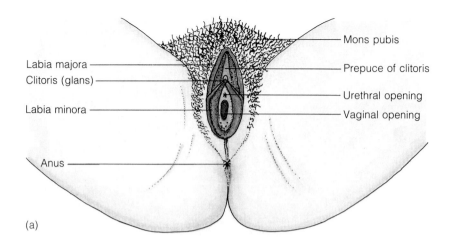

Labia majora
Clitoris (glans)
Labia minora

Mons pubis
Prepuce of clitoris
Urethral opening
Vaginal opening

Anus

(a)

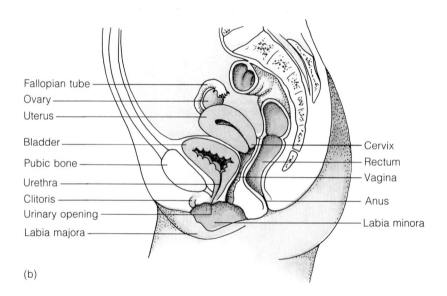

Fallopian tube
Ovary
Uterus

Bladder
Pubic bone
Urethra
Clitoris
Urinary opening
Labia majora

Cervix
Rectum
Vagina
Anus
Labia minora

(b)

reproductive organs (see Figure 4-1b). It is the female organ for sexual intercourse and serves as the birth canal during childbirth. Its soft, flexible walls are normally in contact with each other. A cylinder of muscles surrounds the vagina. During sexual excitement, the tension in these muscles increases and the walls of the vagina swell with blood.

Projecting into the upper part of the vagina is the neck of the uterus, called the cervix. It is inside the pear-shaped uterus, which slants forward above the bladder, that the fertilized egg implants itself and grows into a fetus.

The pair of Fallopian tubes (or oviducts) leads out from the top of the uterus. The fringed end of each tube surrounds an ovary and guides the mature ovum down into the uterus after the ovum bursts from its follicle on the surface of the ovary.

Male Sex Organs   A man's external sexual organs, or genitals, are the penis and the **scrotum** (see Figure 4-2a and 4-2b). The penis consists of spongy tissue that becomes engorged with blood during sexual excitement, causing the organ to enlarge and become erect. The scrotum is a pouch that contains a pair of testes. The purpose

Figure 4-2 Male sex organs.

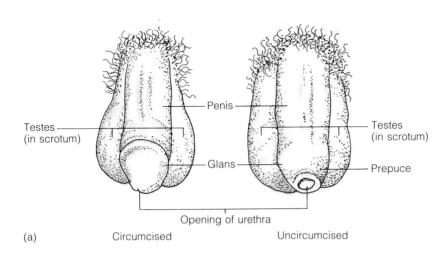

Testes
(in scrotum)

Penis

Testes
(in scrotum)

Glans

Prepuce

Opening of urethra

(a)   Circumcised   Uncircumcised

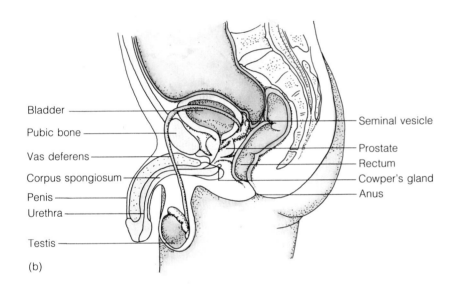

Bladder

Pubic bone

Vas deferens

Corpus spongiosum

Penis

Urethra

Testis

Seminal vesicle

Prostate

Rectum

Cowper's gland

Anus

(b)

of the scrotum is to maintain the testes at a temperature approximately 5° F below that of the rest of the body—that is, at about 93.6° F. The process of sperm production is extremely heat sensitive. In hot temperatures the muscles in the scrotum relax, and the testes move away from the heat of the body. Conversely, in cold temperatures the muscles of the scrotum contract, and the testes move upward toward the body, where they can maintain their 5-degree temperature difference. Even the increase in temperature caused by wearing tight "jockey type" underwear in the summer can interfere with normal sperm production.

The smooth, rounded tip of the penis is the **glans** penis. It is a sensitive part of the penis and an important source of sexual arousal. It is partially covered by the foreskin, or prepuce, a retractable fold of skin that is removed by circumcision in 80 to 85 percent of newborn males in the United States. Circumcision is performed for religious and for hygienic reasons, although the routine practice of circumcision is questioned by some parents and physicians. (See the nearby box entitled "Circumcision: Controversy and Choice.")

Through the entire length of the penis runs a passage called the urethra, which can carry both urine and semen

---

Scrotum The loose sac of skin and muscle fibers that contains the testes.

Glans Rounded head of the penis or of the clitoris.

Circumcision: Controversy and Choice

In 1971 the American Academy of Pediatrics stated that circumcision—the surgical removal of the foreskin of the penis—is an unnecessary medical procedure, and several insurance companies stopped paying for routine circumcision. But in 1988 the group decided to reconsider its position in light of new medical findings. Now the Academy takes a neutral position, stating that circumcision does have some medical advantages but also carries some risks. What are the benefits and risks of this five-minute procedure that is performed on approximately 1.5 million boys born in the United States every year? Who is circumcised, and why? And why do some people oppose it?

As a practice, circumcision can be traced back at least 8,000 years to ancient Middle Eastern civilizations. There are many speculations about why groups began to circumcise their males—as a hygienic procedure, a way to change the appearance of the penis, a "rite of passage" into adulthood, a means of reducing sex drive, a means of increasing sex drive, a means of increasing fertility, and a "mark of purity." The first written account of circumcision appears in the Bible, when Abraham made a "covenant" with God to have all his male descendants circumcised. From that time forward, circumcision took on a religious as well as a cultural significance. Today in the United States, almost all circumcisions of newborns are done for hygienic, cosmetic, and/or religious reasons (Jews being the major group who circumcise for religious reasons, followed by Moslems).

Groups who circumcise their males have always been in the minority. It is estimated that only 15 percent of the world's population practices circumcision. But in the United States, more than 80 percent of all newborn males are circumcised, usually before they leave the hospital. Aside from religious reasons, why are so many American boys circumcised? Dr. Jeffrey Brown, chairman of the Department of Pediatrics at United Hospital in Port Chester, New York, states, "In our patient population, the majority of parents make their decision to circumcise primarily for social or cultural reasons. Some fathers make their decision simply because they want their son to look like them." Concern about the emotional impact of "being different" from peers and the male parent apparently outweigh any concerns about the discomfort or pain of the procedure itself. Rarely is the medical necessity or the cost of the circumcision ($100 to $300) ever mentioned as an issue.

Why is circumcision controversial? Critics of routine newborn circumcision point to its medical disadvantages, which include pain to the infant, the possibility of irritation of the penis, and the risk of complications and surgical errors. They assert that circumcision is "America's leading unnecessary surgery," performed simply as a matter of course in U.S. hospitals.

Proponents of circumcision advocate it for several reasons, the most notable being cleanliness. Bacteria and secretions can be trapped under the foreskin, and uncircumcised boys have to be taught good hygiene to prevent infection. Circumcision removes this potential source of trouble. Circumcised males are also less likely to develop cancer of the penis, a rare disease that occurs almost exclusively in uncircumcised men. In the United States, uncircumcised men have a lifetime risk of one in 600 of getting penile cancer. In parts of the world where circumcision is not practiced and hygiene is poor, the penile cancer rate is higher. Men who develop infection or inflammation of the penis sometimes have to be circumcised later in life, when the operation is more difficult.

It was previously thought that the female sexual partners of uncircumcised men had a higher risk of developing cervical cancer, but new findings indicate that the incidence of cervical cancer depends on many factors. There is some evidence, however, that circumcision may help reduce the spread of sexually transmitted diseases, including AIDS. Finally, recent studies found that urinary tract infections are much more common in uncircumcised infants and can lead to very serious complications of the kidneys. These findings led the American Academy of Pediatrics to adopt its current neutral position on routine circumcision.

Many parents don't hesitate to have their sons circumcised, whether for religious, social, personal, or health reasons. For others, it's a "painful dilemma," in the words of the author of a book about circumcision. Parents who feel the procedure is unwarranted often decide against circumcision (and should be sure to teach their son appropriate hygienic practices). Although circumcision is currently the majority practice in the United States, either decision may be the right one for particular families in particular circumstances.

to the opening at the tip of the glans. Although urine and semen share a common passage, they are prevented from mixing together by muscular sphincters that control their entry into the urethra.

The testes contain tightly packed seminiferous ("sperm-bearing") tubules within which sperm are produced. These tubules end in a maze of ducts that flow into a single storage tube called the epididymis, on the surface of each testis. This tube leads to the vasa deferentia (singular: vas deferens), two tubes that rise into the abdominal cavity and, inside the prostate gland, join the ducts of the two seminal vesicles, whose secretions provide nutrients to semen. The prostate gland produces some of the fluid in semen that nourishes and transports sperm. The tubes of the seminal vesicle and the vas deferens on each side lead to the ejaculatory duct, which joins the urethra. The Cowper's glands (bulbourethral glands) are two small structures flanking the urethra. During sexual arousal, these glands secrete a clear, mucuslike fluid that appears at the tip of the penis. The purpose of this preejaculatory fluid is not known, but it may contain a few sperm in some men. Withdrawal of the penis before ejaculation is therefore not a reliable form of birth control.

Sexual Physiology

As you can see, any description of sexual anatomy alone, no matter how detailed, gives a very incomplete view of human sexuality. The next topic we discuss is sexual physiology—how the sex organs function. This discussion too adds just another piece to the total picture, because sexual functions don't occur in isolation; they are integrated parts of the whole body's operation. Sexual responses involve not just the genitals but the entire body—and the mind as well.

Sexual Stimulation   Sexual activity consists of a stimulus and a response. Erotic stimulation leads to sexual arousal (excitement), which may culminate in the intensely pleasurable experience of **orgasm**. Excitement can come from many sources, both physical and psychological. Although physical stimuli have an obvious and direct effect, some people believe psychological stimuli—thoughts, fantasies, desires, perceptions—are even more powerfully erotic. Regardless of the source of erotic stimuli, all stimulation has a physical basis, which is given meaning by the brain.

Physical Stimulation   Physical stimulation comes through the senses: People are aroused by things they see, hear, taste, smell, and feel. It has even been suggested that they may be attracted and aroused by molecules of specific chemicals, called **pheromones**, that are produced by other people's bodies to create sexual excitement. (See the box entitled "Pheromones and Human Sexuality.") Most often, sexual triggers come from other people, but they may come from books, photographs, paintings, songs, films, or other sources.

The most obvious and effective physical stimulation involves touching. Even though culturally defined practices vary and individual people have different preferences, most sexual encounters eventually involve some form of touching with hands, lips, and body surfaces. Kissing, caressing, fondling, and hugging are as much a part of sexual encounters as they are of expressing affection.

The most intense form of stimulation by touching involves the genitals. The clitoris and glans penis are particularly sensitive to such stimulation. Other highly responsive areas are the vaginal opening, the nipples, the breasts, the insides of the thighs, the buttocks, the anal region, the scrotum, the lips, and the earlobes.

Such sexually sensitive areas, or **erogenous zones**, are especially susceptible to sexual arousal for most people, most of the time. Often, though, it's not *what* is touched but how, for how long, and by whom that determines the response. Under the right circumstances, touching any part of the body can arouse someone sexually.

Psychological Stimulation   Sexual arousal also has an important psychological component, regardless of the nature of the physical stimulation. Fantasies, ideas, memories of past experiences, general "mood"—all can generate excitement. Erotic thoughts may be linked to an imagined person or situation or to a sexual experience from the past. Fantasies often involve activities a person doesn't actually wish to experience in reality, usually because they're dangerous, frightening, or forbidden.

Arousal is also powerfully influenced by emotions. How you feel about a person and how the person feels about you matters tremendously in how sexually responsive you are likely to be. Even the most direct forms of physical stimulation carry emotional overtones. Kissing, caressing, and fondling express affection and caring. The emotional charge they give to a sexual interaction is at least as significant to sexual arousal as the purely physical stimulation achieved by touching. (These issues are discussed further in Chapter 5.)

Orgasm   Discharge of accumulated sexual tension with characteristic genital and bodily manifestation and a subjective sensation of intense pleasure.

Pheromones   Chemical substances produced by animals that are released into the environment and stimulate other animals of the same species; presence in humans is uncertain.

Erogenous zones   Regions of the body highly responsive to sexual stimulation.

Pheromones and Human Sexuality

Various manufacturers of perfumes and colognes claim to sell fragrances that will attract members of the opposite sex. The substance in the fragrance that does the "attracting" is called a pheromone. The word *pheromone* comes from Greek words that literally mean to "transfer excitement." Advertisements for these pheromone-containing fragrances claim that if you use the product, members of the opposite sex will be attracted to you, even from across a crowded room.

Do pheromones really exist? Can we attract members of the opposite sex to us by wearing these substances? Before tackling these questions, let's consider first what scientists know about pheromones from nonhuman research. Biologists use the term *pheromone* to refer to chemical substances secreted by one member of the species that influence the biology and/or behavior of another member of the same species. These substances are released to the environment, make contact with a member of the same species, and produce an effect. For example, female silk moths release a sex attractant pheromone that drifts on the wind and attracts males. Males will fly to the substance even in the absence of females.

There is no doubt that pheromones exist in insects, but do they exist in humans? One more non-

human research study will help us answer this question. In the rhesus monkey, the female vaginal secretions contain a very potent pheromone that attracts males. The pheromone is abundant during the middle of the female monkey's menstrual cycle (monkeys have menstrual cycles like human females), when she is ovulating. Because the male is most attracted to the female just at that time, the chance that copulation will result in fertilization of the ovum is increased.

Human females who are not using oral contraceptives produce the same chemical message identified as the male-attracting pheromone in the rhesus monkey. It is also produced during the middle of the menstrual cycle! Does it attract males? In a very clever study designed to answer this question, researchers prepared a "synthetic" mixture of this potential pheromone and recruited sixty-two young married couples to participate. Each couple received a set of coded treatments packaged in one-dose containers and consecutively numbered. One container held a mixture of the potential pheromone in alcohol, another held only alcohol, another contained plain water, and the fourth held an inexpensive perfume in an alcohol solution.

It was predicted that, if the potential pheromone really worked,

a husband would be more sexually attracted to his wife when she was "wearing" the potential pheromone, and sexual activities would be increased at this time. Each wife was told to rub the contents of an individual container between her breasts at bedtime (neither the wife nor the husband knew the contents of the individual containers). Results: the potential pheromones had no apparent effect on sexual arousal or activity, a conclusion supported by other studies.

A phenomenon that *has* been substantiated in a number of studies is menstrual synchrony, a decrease in time differences between the beginning of menstrual periods among women who live together or spend a lot of time together. A pheromone is thought to be involved in this process. Experiments have shown that exposure to perspiration from the underarms of certain "donor" women produced menstrual synchrony in other women. In this situation the women did not know or ever see the "donor"; these studies seem to argue for the existence of a human pheromone that can in fact change the biological functioning of other individuals.

Source: Adapted from David Quadagno. 1987. Pheromones and human sexuality. *Medical Aspects of Human Sexuality* 21:149–154.

Historically, there have always been people interested in enhancing sexual stimulation through aphrodisiacs—substances believed to increase sexual desire, prolong sexual activity, intensify sexual sensations and responses, or improve sexual performance. Few, if any, substances have ever been shown to have these effects, a fact that

underscores the important role played by psychological and emotional factors in arousal. Despite the lack of evidence for their effectiveness, aphrodisiacs are sought by some people in our society in drugs and alcohol. A list of drugs and their supposed and actual effects on sexual functioning is given in Table 4-1.

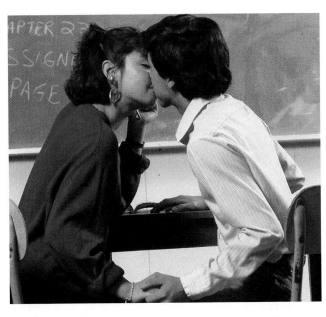

Kissing and touching are among the most common and enjoyable forms of physical stimulation.

Table 4-1 Supposed and Actual Effects of Drugs on Sexual Functioning

Substance	Supposed Effect	Actual Effect
Alcohol	Stimulates sexual desire and sexual activity.	In small amounts, reduces inhibitions and increases sexual desire; with increased consumption, decreases sexual response and sensations from the genitals.
Cocaine ("coke")	Enhances sexual desire and performance.	During early use, some people report enhancement of sexual activities, others poor sexual performance. Chronic abuse frequently leads to diminished sexual desire.
Marijuana ("pot")	Increases sexual desire and performance.	Reduces inhibitions. Actual influence varies from decreased to improved desire and performance.
LSD and other hallucinogens such as mescaline and psilocybin	Increase sexual desire and heighten sexual response.	No physiological effect on reproductive system, but subjective experience of sexual desire and response may be enhanced or diminished.
Cantharidin ("Spanish fly")	Increases desire for sexual activities.	Acts as a powerful irritant; burns lining of bladder and urethra, mimicking sexual stimulation of genitals (causes erection in male, vasocongestion of clitoris, labia, and vagina in female).
Amyl nitrate ("snappers" or "poppers")	Increase pleasure of orgasm.	Dilate (open) blood vessels in genital area and may enhance sensations or perceptions of orgasm. Can produce fainting, headaches, or dizziness.
Amphetamines ("uppers")	Increase sexual desire.	Small doses may enhance sexual desire and response; larger doses lead to sexual dysfunctions.
Barbiturates ("downers")	Increase sexual desire and performance.	In low doses, reduce inhibitions; in larger doses, inhibit sexual arousal and functioning.
Antihypertensives (blood pressure medication)	Control high blood pressure.	Can negatively affect sexual function in men and women, partly because of inhibition of sympathetic nerves of genital region and psychological effects of being treated for high blood pressure.

C. Byer et al. 1988. *Dimensions of Human Sexuality*. (Dubuque: Wm. C. Brown); J. Cocores and M. Gold 1989, Substance abuse and sexual dysfunction. *Medical Aspects of Human Sexuality* 23:22–31.

Sexual Response   In response to effective sexual stimulation, the body shows a predictable set of reactions (see Figure 4-3). Physiologically, these reactions are the same regardless of the nature of the erotic stimulus—whether they are brought about by fantasy, masturbation, sexual intercourse, or some other form of sexual activity. But these experiences may feel quite different subjectively.

Two physiological mechanisms explain most genital and bodily reactions of men and women during sexual arousal and orgasm. These mechanisms are **vasocongestion** and **myotonia**. Vasocongestion is the engorgement of tissues that results when more blood flows into an organ than is flowing out. Thus, the penis becomes erect on the same principle that makes a garden hose become stiff when the water is turned on. Myotonia is increased muscular tension, which culminates in rhythmical muscular contractions during orgasm.

Four stages characterize the sexual response cycle. In the **excitement phase**, the penis becomes erect as its tissues become congested with blood. The testes expand and are pulled upward within the scrotum. In women, the clitoris and the labia are similarly congested with blood, and the vaginal walls become moist with lubricant fluid.

The **plateau phase** is an extension of the excitement stage. Reactions become more marked: in men, the penis becomes harder, and the testes larger. In women, the lower part of the vagina swells, while its upper end expands and vaginal lubrication increases.

In the **orgasmic phase**, rhythmical contractions occur along the man's penis, urethra, prostate gland, seminal vesicles, and muscles in the pelvic and anal regions. These involuntary muscular contractions lead to ejaculation of semen, which consists of sperm cells from the testes and secretions from the prostate gland and seminal vesicles. In women, contractions occur in the lower part of the vagina and in the uterus, as well as in the pelvic region and the anus.

In the **resolution phase**, all the changes initiated during the excitement phase are reversed. Excess blood drains from tissues, the muscles in the region relax, and the genital structures return to their unstimulated state.

More general bodily reactions accompany the changes in the genital organs in both sexes. Beginning with the excitement phase, the nipples of both sexes become erect, the woman's breasts begin to swell, and in both sexes the skin of the chest becomes flushed; all these changes are more marked among women. The heart rate doubles by the plateau phase, and respiration becomes faster. During orgasm, breathing becomes irregular and the person may moan or cry out. A feeling of warmth leads to increased sweating during the resolution phase. Deep relaxation and a sense of well-being pervade the body and the mind.

Male and female reactions during the sexual response cycle differ somewhat. Generally, the male pattern is more uniform, whereas the female pattern is more varied. For instance, the female excitement phase may lead directly to orgasm, or orgasmic and plateau phases may be fused.

Male orgasm is marked by the ejaculation of semen. After ejaculation, men enter a **refractory period** during which they cannot be restimulated to orgasm. Women do not have a refractory period; immediate restimulation is possible.

Sexual stimulation relies on the same set of sensory nerves that transmit other impulses from the body's surface. No special nerves are set aside for conveying sexual sensations. However, specialized nerve centers in the lower portions of the spinal cord regulate the mechanisms of erection and ejaculation. Their actions are **reflexive**; they do not need to be learned (although learned responses may inhibit them).

The ultimate control of sexual functions rests in the brain. As in the lower spinal centers, specific regions in the **limbic system** of the brain control sexual arousal and orgasm. We understand even less how the brain regulates the subjective experience of sexual arousal and the state of altered consciousness experienced during orgasm.

Sex Hormones

Hormones are chemical messages that are secreted directly into the bloodstream by **endocrine glands**. The sex hormones produced by the ovaries and testes greatly influence the development and functions of the reproductive system.

Vasocongestion   Accumulation of blood in tissues and organs.

Myotonia   Increased muscular tension.

Excitement phase   First stage of sexual response cycle, characterized by vasocongestion and myotonia.

Plateau phase   Second stage of the sexual response cycle, characterized by a high and sustained level of excitement.

Orgasmic phase   Third stage of the sexual response cycle, during which myotonia culminates in orgasm.

Resolution phase   Fourth and last stage of the sexual response cycle, during which vasocongestion and myotonia subside.

Refractory period   The period following orgasm during which the male cannot be restimulated.

Reflexive   Involving an involuntary response elicited by a specific stimulus.

Limbic system   A set of structures in the brain regulating motivational-emotional behaviors, including some aspects of sexual activity.

Endocrine glands   Glands that produce hormones.

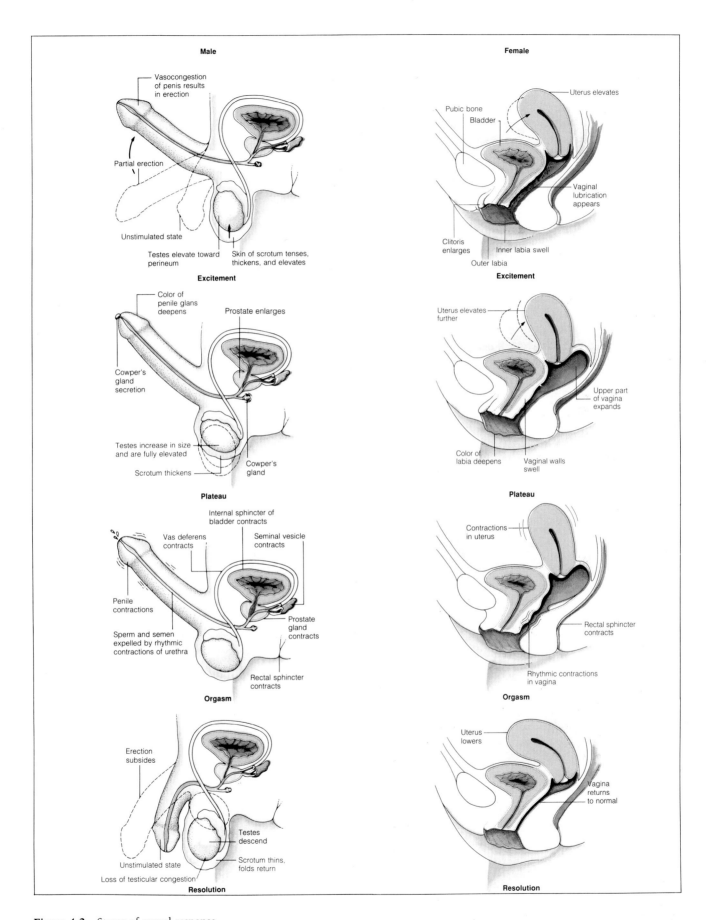

Male

Vasocongestion of penis results in erection

Partial erection

Unstimulated state

Testes elevate toward perineum

Skin of scrotum tenses, thickens, and elevates

Excitement

Female

Pubic bone

Bladder

Uterus elevates

Vaginal lubrication appears

Clitoris enlarges

Inner labia swell

Outer labia

Excitement

Color of penile glans deepens

Prostate enlarges

Cowper's gland secretion

Testes increase in size and are fully elevated

Scrotum thickens

Cowper's gland

Plateau

Uterus elevates further

Upper part of vagina expands

Color of labia deepens

Vaginal walls swell

Plateau

Internal sphincter of bladder contracts

Vas deferens contracts

Seminal vesicle contracts

Penile contractions

Sperm and semen expelled by rhythmic contractions of urethra

Prostate gland contracts

Rectal sphincter contracts

Orgasm

Contractions in uterus

Rectal sphincter contracts

Rhythmic contractions in vagina

Orgasm

Erection subsides

Testes descend

Unstimulated state

Scrotum thins, folds return

Loss of testicular congestion

Resolution

Uterus lowers

Vagina returns to normal

Resolution

Figure 4-3 Stages of sexual response.

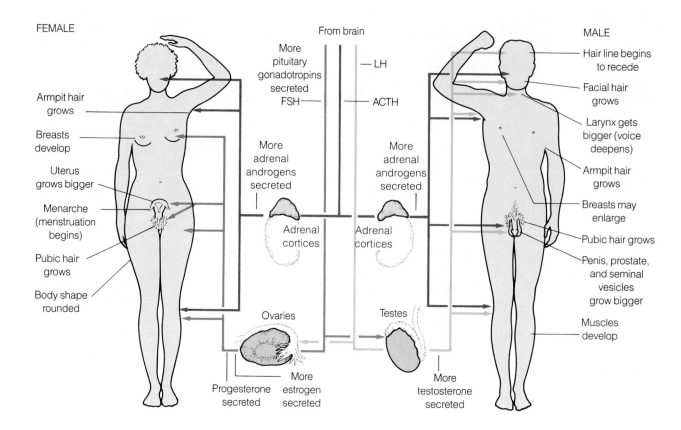

Figure 4-4 Effects of hormones on physical development and sexual maturation at puberty.

The sex hormones made by the testes are called **androgens** (the most important of which is testosterone); the female sex hormones, produced by the ovaries, belong to two groups—**estrogens** and **progestins** (the most important of which is progesterone). In addition to the estrogens and progestins produced by the ovary and testosterone from the testes, the cortex of the **adrenal glands** (located at the top of the kidneys) also produces androgens in both sexes. In fact, ovaries produce small quantities of androgens, and the testes small amounts of estrogens and progestins. Thus, in both males and females, the hormones of the opposite sex are present in small quantities.

The hormones produced by the testes, the ovaries, and the adrenal glands are regulated by the hormones of the **pituitary gland**, located at the base of the brain. This gland in turn is controlled by hormones produced by the **hypothalamus** in the brain (see Figure 4-4).

Developmental Effects of Hormones Hormones from the ovaries and testes exert their primary developmental influences first in the embryo and later during adolescence.

Differentiation of the Embryo The sex of the individual, as male or female, is determined by the fertilizing sperm at the time of conception. All human cells normally contain twenty-three pairs of **chromosomes**, including a pair of **sex chromosomes**. In twenty-two of the pairs, the two partner chromosomes match, but in the twenty-third, the sex chromosomes, two configurations are possible. Individuals with two matching X chromosomes are females, whereas individuals with one X and one Y chromosome—a much shorter chromosome carrying specialized genes—are males. Germ cells (sperm and ova) differ from all other body cells in carrying 23 *single*, not paired, chromosomes—the result of a special kind of cell division in which only one of each chromosome pair is transferred to the new cell. In females, with their XX configuration, all the resulting germ cells will contain an X chromosome. In males, with their XY configuration, some germ cells will contain an X chromosome and some will contain a Y. When the ovum and sperm unite, the two sets of 23 single chromosomes re-form the 23 pairs. If the sperm carries an X chromosome, the baby will be a girl; if it carries a Y chromosome, the baby will be a boy.

The specialized genes on the Y chromosome initiate

the process of sexual differentiation of the reproductive system. Until the sixth week of embryonic life, the reproductive system is undifferentiated. Both sexes have a set of gonads, two sets of tubes, and other related structures. If the undifferentiated reproductive system continued to develop without the influence of sex hormones, it would develop into the normal female system. The gonads would become ovaries and the other structures would become the corresponding female genitals, regardless of the fetus's genetic sex. The specialized genes on the Y chromosome, however, intervene to change this course of events. They influence the undifferentiated gonads to develop instead into testes.

The embryonic testes in turn produce two hormones. The first hormone, testosterone, leads to the further development of male reproductive organs. The second hormone prevents the rest of the undifferentiated structures from developing into female organs. The end result is a normal set of male genital organs.

The common embryonic origin of male and female systems means that every structure in one sex has its developmental counterpart in the other. Thus, the penis corresponds to the clitoris and the scrotal sac to the labia major; all the other male parts have their female counterparts and vice versa.

Reproductive Maturation at Puberty   Although human beings are sexually fully differentiated at birth, the differences between males and females are accentuated at **puberty.** The reproductive system matures, secondary sexual characteristics (such as pubic hair) develop, and the bodies of male and female come to appear more distinctive (see Figure 4-4).

The changes of puberty are initiated by the gonadotropin-releasing hormone (GnRH) of the hypothalamus, under whose influence the anterior pituitary gland increases the production of its two **gonadotropic hormones.** These are the **follicle-stimulating hormone (FSH)** and the **luteinizing hormone (LH)**, which stimulate the ovaries and testes.

■ **Exploring Your Emotions**

Think back to early adolescence and try to recall your feelings about sex as you went through puberty. Many adolescents feel overwhelmed by changes in their bodies and a variety of emotions—worry, guilt, excitement, elation—about their sexuality. Do you have any of the same feelings about sex that you had then? Are you satisfied with the adjustment to sexuality that you've made so far in your life?

The first menstrual period, or menarche, occurs at the average age of 12.8 years in the United States, but it may also normally start several years earlier or later. Until recently, the age of first **menstruation** had been steadily going down, but it has stabilized over the past several decades.

The first sign of female puberty is breast development, followed by a rounding of the hips and buttocks. As the breasts develop, hair appears in the pubic region and later in the underarms. Shortly after the onset of breast development, girls show an increase in growth rate. Generally speaking, breast development begins at about age 8 to 13, and the time of rapid body growth occurs between 9 and 15 years of age. Estrogens and progestins as well as androgens from the adrenal glands are responsible for the physical changes that occur in the female at puberty.

In the female, FSH stimulates the immature ovarian follicles to mature. The follicles are the site of egg pro-

---

Androgens   Male sex hormones produced by the testes in males and by the adrenal glands in both sexes.

Estrogens   A class of female sex hormones, produced by the ovaries, that bring about sexual maturation at puberty and maintain reproductive functions.

Progestins   A class of female sex hormones, produced by the ovaries, that sustain reproductive functions.

Adrenal glands   Endocrine glands, located over the kidneys, that produce androgens (among other hormones).

Pituitary gland   An endocrine gland at the base of the brain that produces gonadotropic (FSH and LH) and other hormones.

Hypothalamus   A region of the brain above the pituitary gland whose hormones control the secretions of the pituitary and that is also involved in the nervous control of sexual functions.

Chromosomes   The threadlike bodies into which the genetic material within the cell nucleus is organized.

Sex chromosomes   The X and Y chromosomes, which determine the sex of the individual.

Puberty   The period of biological maturation during adolescence.

Gonadotropic hormones   Follicle-stimulating hormone (FSH) and luteinizing hormone (LH), produced by the pituitary gland in both sexes.

Follicle-stimulating hormone (FSH)   The pituitary hormone that stimulates maturation of the ovum in the female and sperm production in the male.

Luteinizing hormone (LH)   The pituitary hormone that causes ovulation and stimulates the production of progestins in the female and androgens in the male.

Menstruation   The normal bleeding phase of the menstrual cycle of women, characteristic of primates (humans, apes, and monkeys); a woman's "period."

Understanding the Menstrual Cycle

The menstrual ("monthly") cycle is one of the key physiological functions of the female body. An ovarian, or estrus, cycle is characteristic of all female mammals but menstruation, periodic uterine bleeding that accompanies the ovarian cycle, occurs only in women, in female apes, and some monkeys.

The average length of the menstrual cycle is 28 days, although somewhat longer and shorter cycles are also quite common and normal. Because the onset of bleeding is easier to note than its gradual cessation, the day that bleeding starts is counted as the first day of a given cycle.

The menstrual cycle is controlled by mechanisms involving hormones released by the hypothalamus, the pituitary, and the ovaries. The cycle has four stages, as illustrated in the diagram—the menstrual phase, the preovulatory phase, the ovulation phase, and the postovulatory phase. The diagram shows the events occurring in the uterus and the ovaries and the hormone output by the anterior pituitary and ovaries over the course of the cycle.

The preovulatory phase starts as soon as menstrual bleeding from the previous cycle has ended. The anterior pituitary produces large amounts of follicle-stimulating hormone (FSH) and a small amount of luteinizing hormone (LH). Under the influence of FSH, an ovarian follicle begins to mature and produces in turn increasingly higher level of estrogens. In response to estrogen stimulation, the uterine lining thickens with increased numbers of blood vessels and uterine glands.

In the ovulation phase at mid-cycle, the ovum is released as LH production surges and FSH output decreases. Gonadotropic hormones that control the output of ovarian hormones are in turn regulated by the level of ovarian hormones, through a negative feedback mechanism. Thus, the increased level of estrogens de-presses FSH production. Following ovulation, the follicle transforms into the corpus luteum ("yellow body"), which produces progesterone.

In the post-ovulatory phase, the secretion of progesterone begins to rise. Under the combined influence of estrogens and progesterone, the endometrium continues to develop and the uterine glands secrete nutrient materials. The endometrium is now ready to receive and sustain the fertilized ovum if fertilization has occurred. The levels of ovarian hormones then remain high and the uterine lining is maintained intact through pregnancy. If pregnancy doesn't occur, the high levels of estrogens and progesterone gradually fall.

Below a certain level of hormonal support, the uterine lining can no longer be maintained and begins to slough off, initiating the final menstrual phase of the cycle. As levels of ovarian hormones drop, their inhibiting effect on the pituitary gonadotropins is lifted. FSH

---

duction. The cells of the maturing follicle in turn produce estrogens. Under the effect of LH, the egg is released from the follicle (this process is called ovulation). The remains of the follicular cell become the **corpus luteum** (literally "yellow body"), which is stimulated by LH to produce progestins. These two hormones, FSH and LH, are responsible for the **menstrual cycle**. (See the box entitled "Understanding the Menstrual Cycle.")

Reproductive maturation of boys lags about two years behind that of girls and usually begins at about 10 or 11 years of age. Enlargement of the testes, development of pubic hair, growth of the penis, the onset of ejaculation (usually at about age 11 or 12), deepening of the voice, the appearance of facial hair, and a period of rapid growth complete the process.

The hormonal basis for physical changes in the male at puberty is quite similar to that of the female. Hypothalamic hormones trigger the anterior pituitary to pro-

---

Corpus luteum   The part of the ovarian follicle left after ovulation, which secretes hormones during the second half of the menstrual cycle.

Menstrual cycle   The monthly ovarian cycle in the female that leads to menstruation in the absence of pregnancy.

Menopause   Cessation of menstruation in middle-aged women.

Understanding the Menstrual Cycle (continued)

and LH production now begins to rise, and a new cycle starts.

When pregnancy occurs, the hormone human chorionic gonadotropin (HCG) sustains the corpus luteum in maintaining high levels of estrogens and progestins. Hence, the uterine lining (which now houses the embryo) does not slough off and the pregnant woman misses her period.

Birth control pills (see Chapter 6) consist of synthetic estrogens and progestins. Because the pills maintain high blood levels of these hormones, gonadotropin production is suppressed by negative feedback. Ovulation does not occur, and the woman cannot get pregnant. A reliable way of predicting the most fertile time in the menstrual cycle (when ovulation has occurred) is to subtract 14 days from the onset of the menstrual flow. This time—14 days plus or minus 2 days—is the interval between ovulation and menstruation. This information about the approximate date of

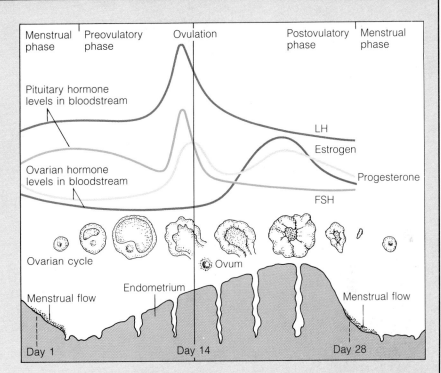

ovulation can be used in fertility treatment, when a woman wants to become pregnant, and in the natural family planning method of birth control, when she wants to avoid pregnancy (see Chapter 6).

duce gonadotropins. FSH promotes the maturation of sperm; LH stimulates testicular cells to produce testosterone, which brings about most of the male changes of puberty.

Aging and Human Sexuality   As a woman approaches 50, her ovaries gradually cease to function and she enters the **menopause** (cessation of menstruation). The associated drop in hormone production causes a set of symptoms that are troublesome for some women.

Among the most common physical symptoms of menopause are hot flashes (or flushes), experienced by three out of four women. They consist of a sensation of warmth rising to the face from the upper chest with or without perspiration and chills. Other symptoms include headaches, dizziness, palpitations, and joint pains. Osteopo-

rosis can develop (that is, the bones can become more porous), making older women more liable to suffer fractures (see Chapter 12). Some menopausal women become moody, even markedly depressed. They also complain of tiredness, irritability, and forgetfulness. Estrogen replacement significantly improves most of these symptoms. As a result of the decrease in estrogen production, the vaginal walls thin and the lubricatory response to sexual arousal diminishes. As a result, sexual intercourse may become painful. Hormonal treatment or the use of lubricants during intercourse eliminates these problems.

Some women have a difficult time making the psychological adjustment to this stage of life, associating it with a loss of youth and sexual attractiveness. Others welcome it as a time of increased personal freedom, when the responsibilities of child rearing are over and sexuality can

Although sexual physiology changes as people get older, many men and women readily adjust to these alterations. Sexual activity can continue throughout life for individuals like this healthy and vigorous couple in their mid-60s.

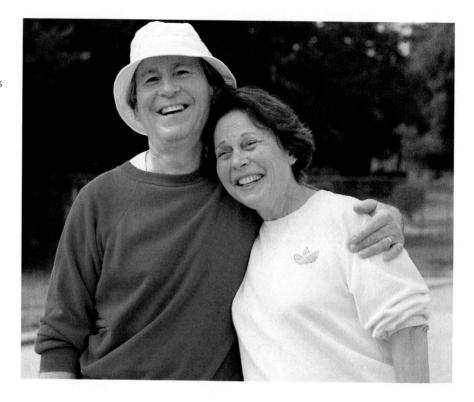

be enjoyed without fear of pregnancy. Today, with longer life expectancies, many women are rejecting the view that the childbearing years are the central period of female life, flanked by youth and old age. Instead, they see three equally important periods characterized by particular biological and psychological concerns—a time of growing and learning, a time of childbearing and nurturing (or creative expression), and a time of inner growth and repose. Menopause is seen as signaling the end of one phase of life and the beginning of another, equally meaningful one.

■ Exploring Your Emotions

Many people in their sixties, seventies, and eighties continue to enjoy sex as a vital part of their lives. What are your attitudes toward older people and sex? How would you feel if your grandmother were to describe her sexual experiences to you?

Men do not experience a drop in hormone production in midlife comparable to that experienced by women, although testosterone levels gradually decline with age. Nonetheless, the pattern of male sexual responses definitely changes. As they get older, men depend more on direct physical stimulation for sexual arousal. They take longer to get an erection and find it more difficult to maintain. Orgasmic contractions are less intense.

At the same time, many men go through a period of reassessment and readjustment in middle age (sometimes popularly referred to as "midlife crisis"), which may have repercussions for their sexuality. As with women, sexual activity can continue to be a source of pleasure and satisfaction for men as they grow older. When problems do arise, they are more often due to psychological reactions to bodily changes than to the physical changes themselves.

Hormones and Behavior   Hormones clearly affect our development, but how do they affect our sexual behaviors? Their role isn't completely clear. Experiments have shown that hormones have a direct effect on behavior in animals. Male rats, for example, are typically more aggressive than female rats and less likely to show nurturing behavior to newborn rat pups. Testosterone seems to be a crucial factor in determining these behaviors. Female rats exposed to testosterone prior to birth are more aggressive and less nurturing than normal females, and male rats deprived of testosterone prior to birth are less aggressive and more nurturing than normal males.

In humans the situation is much more complicated because of the enormous influence of cultural learning on behavior. If we see boys being aggressive or girls being nurturant, for example, we really can't tell how much of their behavior is genetically or hormonally influenced and how much of it they've learned through interactions with their environment—parents, peers, the media, and so on. It's probably safe to say that some genetic or hormonal "sexualization" occurs before birth in humans but that environmental influences can modify or override any biological inclinations.

The effect of hormones on sexual interest and activity is a bit clearer, as suggested by the upsurge of sexual interest at puberty. As sex hormones flood the body, young teenagers find themselves experiencing powerful sexual impulses and attractions. After puberty, hormones seem to play a role in maintaining sexual functions, at least in men. When men experience a significant decline in testosterone production, their sex drive and their ability to have erections and orgasms suffer over a period of time. When they're treated with testosterone, their sexual functions improve.

In women, on the other hand, fluctuations in hormones don't seem to affect sexual interest or ability to reach orgasm. Women who take estrogens and progestins in birth control pills, for example, don't necessarily have increased interest in sex, and women whose hormonal levels have dropped at menopause don't have less interest. Concentrations of sex hormones fluctuate during the menstrual cycle, but sex drive doesn't seem to change consistently with these phases. It's possible that the hormones responsible for female sexual function are actually androgens, which continue to be produced by the adrenal cortex throughout a woman's life.

Whatever the effects of sex hormones on behavior, it's clear that both gender identity and sexual behavior in humans are largely shaped by cultural factors. Children learn to act "like girls" or "like boys" by absorbing countless subtle messages every day about gender-appropriate behavior. Older children and adults receive equally powerful messages about socially acceptable behavior. Thus, although hormones make it possible for us to act sexually and may predispose us to act one way or another, how (and whether) we engage in sexual behavior is greatly influenced by our culture and our sexual upbringing.

Sexual Health: Disorders and Dysfunctions

Both psychological and physical problems can interfere with normal sexual functioning. If you are not in good physical health, for example, or if you are experiencing high levels of stress or anxiety, your sexual functioning might very well be negatively affected. Sexual problems

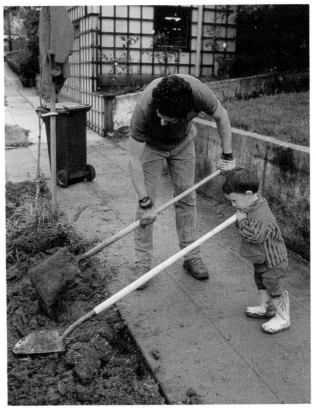
Hormones affect what we do in some ways, but our sense of gender identity and many of our behaviors are overwhelmingly influenced by cultural factors. This little boy is learning "male" behaviors by imitating his dad.

caused mainly by biological or physical conditions are referred to as **sexual disorders**; problems of psychological origin are called **sexual dysfunctions**.

Common Sexual Disorders   Sexual disorders may be physiological in origin, but they may also be the result of infections, which can be prevented.

* *Vaginitis* is inflammation of the vagina and can be caused by a variety of organisms, including *Candida* (yeast infection), *Trichomonas* (trichomoniasis), and *Gardnerella* (nonspecific vaginitis). The symptoms include a vaginal discharge and some irritation. Vaginitis is easily treated with various medications. In the case of trichomoniasis, both partners must be treated, as the organism can also be harbored in the male genital tract. (See Chapter 17 for a more detailed discussion of trichomoniasis.)

Sexual disorders   Disturbances in sexual desire, performance, or satisfaction having physical origins.

Sexual dysfunction   Disturbances in sexual desire, performance, or satisfaction having psychological origins.

Premenstrual Syndrome: Still a Mystery

A week or two of tension, mood swings, fatigue, and depression every month is the lot of millions of women who have premenstrual syndrome (PMS). The physical and emotional symptoms that precede menstruation may dominate a woman's life, leading her to plan her activities around the days or weeks she knows she'll be experiencing them. Despite decades of study, researchers still don't understand exactly what causes PMS or why some women are more vulnerable to it than others.

PMS seems to affect some 5 to 7 percent of menstruating women seriously enough to interfere with their work or lifestyle, according to a report issued in 1989 by the American College of Obstetricians and Gynecologists. But many more women—20 to 40 percent, by some estimates—may suffer less severe premenstrual symptoms in the few days before their periods. PMS usually occurs in women between 25 and 45 years of age, but it never occurs in pregnant women. The most frequently reported symptoms are tension, anxiety, and fluid retention in the 7 to 10 days preceding menstruation, although the spectrum of symptoms can be much broader. Some women experience sleep

disturbances, irritability, migraine headaches, a craving for carbohydrates, constipation, and hot flashes. Others experience psychological symptoms including feelings of fatigue, sadness, and, in the most severe cases, depression that may require drug treatment and psychotherapy.

Years ago, physicians thought PMS was a purely psychological problem, but today we know this isn't true. As medical researchers measure with ever-increasing precision the various chemicals in the body, particularly brain chemicals, PMS provides an intriguing example of the frontier between biology and behavior. PMS is now classified as a biobehavioral problem—the latest medical catchword for problems that can have both physical and psychological components.

Although researchers don't know exactly what causes PMS, they do know that symptoms are somehow linked to the monthly fluctuations of a variety of substances in the body. In the normal, 28-day menstrual cycle, there are two phases: a follicular phase, when the egg develops, and a luteal phase, when the egg is discharged and can be fertilized. These two phases are controlled by the brain

through chemical signals sent from the brain to the pituitary gland and the ovaries.

Researchers had speculated that women who suffer from PMS might have some kind of imbalance of the hormone progesterone during the luteal phase of the cycle. But that theory is being revised, thanks to the use of sophisticated medical technologies that allow much more precise measurement of many substances involved in the menstrual cycle, including estrogen, progesterone, estradiol, and the naturally occurring opiate known as beta-endorphin. For example, when researchers used experimental drugs to alter the menstrual cycle, speeding or delaying onset of bleeding, PMS symptoms still occurred in about half the women. This leads researchers to speculate that PMS might be triggered by something other than changes in progesterone levels.

Another theory suggests that some women with PMS may be experiencing withdrawal from their own levels of beta-endorphin. Researchers have found that blood levels of beta-endorphin dropped sharply in the majority of women with PMS during the week preceding their periods. Women

---

- *Endometriosis* is the growth of endometrial tissue (tissue normally found lining the uterus) outside of the uterus. It occurs most often in women of childbearing age, and pain in the lower abdomen and pelvis is the most common symptom. Endometriosis can cause serious problems if left untreated because the endometrial tissue can scar and partially or completely block the oviducts, causing infertility (difficulty in conceiving) or sterility (inability to conceive). Endometriosis is treated with hormone therapy and/or surgery.
- *Pelvic inflammatory disease* (PID) is an infection of the uterus, oviducts, or ovaries and is caused when micro-

organisms spread to these areas from the vagina. Approximately 50 to 75 percent of PID is caused by sexually transmitted organisms associated with diseases such as gonorrhea and *Chlamydia* infections. PID can cause scarring of the oviducts, resulting in infertility or sterility. Symptoms include pain in the abdomen and pelvis and fever. The treatment involves bed rest and antibiotic therapy. Prompt treatment lessens the chances of infertility and sterility. (Sexually transmitted diseases are discussed in detail in Chapter 17.)
- *Menstruation* is a normal biological process, but it may cause distressing physical or psychological symptoms

Premenstrual Syndrome: Still a Mystery (continued)

without PMS symptoms were found to maintain consistently high levels of beta-endorphin. When the drug naloxone was given to the women with PMS, beta-endorphin levels remained high in 70 percent of the subjects. Help for other women may come from a variety of other treatments under investigation: oral contraceptives; light therapy (exposing women to fluorescent lights for several hours each day prior to menstruation); antidepressants; anti-anxiety agents; and other drugs that improve mood and diminish appetite.

What seems clear is that most over-the-counter medications do not help. Many nonprescription drugs contain antihistamines (a throwback to the days when PMS was thought to be some kind of allergy), diuretics (to compensate for bloating and water retention), and painkillers such as acetaminophen (the active ingredient in Tylenol). Unfortunately, no scientific evidence confirms that any of these measures work. PMS is under intensive study by the National Institute of Mental Health (NIMH) and many other agencies and research centers, so it may be just a matter of time before the mystery of this syndrome is unrav-

Who's Affected: Primarily 25-to-45-year-old women.

When it Occurs: For the 7 to 10 days before menstruation. PMS symptoms generally end when the period begins.

How Common: 20 to 40 percent of the menstruating women report some symptoms from time to time, but only 5 to 7 percent of women need medical treatment for severe problems.

Symptoms: Breast tenderness, craving for sweet or salty foods, headache, anxiety, fatigue, depression, water retention.

Cause: Unknown.

Treatment: No proven therapies. Researchers are studying a wide range of experimental treatments, including progesterone supplements, light therapy, naloxone and antidepressants.

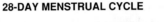

28-DAY MENSTRUAL CYCLE

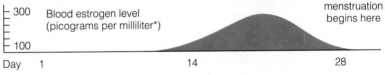

Blood estrogen level (picograms per milliliter*)

menstruation begins here

Day   1   14   28

*a picogram equals one millionth of a gram

–The Washington Post

eled and effective treatments are made available.

In the meantime, women can take a few behavioral steps to treat the symptoms of PMS: eat a nutrient-rich diet; decrease alcohol, caffeine, nicotine, and salt use to lessen nervousness, depression,

and bloating; and increase exercise to stimulate relaxation. This approach is sensible and safe and may relieve the discomfort of PMS.

Adapted from Balancing between behavior and biology, *Washington Post Health* (October 10, 1989), p. 11.

in some women. Two common problems are dysmenorrhea and premenstrual tension. Dysmenorrhea (the word means "painful menstruation") is characterized by cramps in the lower abdomen, backache, a bloated feeling, nausea, vomiting, diarrhea, and loss of appetite. Some of these symptoms can be attributed to uterine muscular contractions called spasms, which are caused by prostaglandins, (chemicals released from the uterine lining as it is shed during menstruation). Any drug such as aspirin or ibuprofen that blocks the effects of prostaglandins will usually be effective in alleviating some of the symptoms of dysmenorrhea.

Premenstrual tension involves negative mood changes and physical symptoms associated with the time before the onset of the menstrual flow (hence the name "premenstrual"). A more serious condition, premenstrual syndrome (PMS), is experienced by a smaller number of women before the menstrual flow. PMS is considered to be a severe form of premenstrual tension by many physicians. (The box entitled "Premenstrual Syndrome: Still a Mystery" describes some research on this problem.)

Sexual Dysfunctions   Sexual dysfunction encompasses disturbances in sexual desire, performance, or satisfaction. Although a wide variety of physical conditions and drugs may interfere with sexual functions (for instance, diabetes may interfere with the blood and nerve supply to sex organs), sexual dysfunctions more often result from psychological causes and problems in intimate relationships. The same two mechanisms—vasocongestion and myotonia—that form the bases of the sexual response cycle are also at the root of the main forms of sexual disturbance: inability to become aroused and problems with orgasm.

■ Exploring Your Emotions

Do you remember things you were told about sex as a child, such as that touching your genitals was "bad"? When you think about such messages from your current point of view, are some of them positive and helpful and some negative and not so helpful? Might any of them be affecting your sexual functioning today?

Common sexual dysfunctions in men include **erectile dysfunction** (previously called impotence), which is the inability to have or maintain an erection that is sufficient for sexual intercourse; **premature ejaculation**, which is ejaculation before or just on penetration of the vagina; and **retarded ejaculation**, the inability to ejaculate once an erection is achieved. Many men will experience occasional difficulty in achieving an erection or ejaculating because of excessive alcohol consumption, fatigue, or stress. In fact, it is estimated that 50 percent of all men in the United States experience occasional bouts of erectile dysfunction and retarded ejaculation. Usually, the dysfunction disappears when the interfering factor is removed. Because of the powerful effect of psychological factors on sexual behavior, especially anxiety about performance, an understanding attitude on the part of the sexual partner is an important component in restoring sexual functioning.

Two sexual dysfunctions in women are **vaginismus**, in which the woman experiences painful involuntary muscular spasms when sexual intercourse is attempted, and **orgasmic dysfunction**, which is the inability to experience orgasm. Vaginismus is a conditioned reflex probably related to fear of intercourse. Orgasmic dys-

function has been the subject of a great deal of discussion over the years as people debated the nature of the female orgasm and what constitutes dysfunction in women. Many women experience orgasm but not during intercourse, or they experience orgasm during intercourse only if the clitoris is directly stimulated at the same time. Do these patterns of response reflect normal female sexual functioning, or are they forms of orgasmic dysfunction? In general, the inability to experience orgasm under certain circumstances is a problem only if the woman considers it a problem. If a woman does believe that she has a problem—for example, if she has never experienced orgasm under any circumstances—then she is considered to have orgasmic dysfunction.

Treating Sexual Dysfunction   Most forms of sexual dysfunction can be treated. The first step is to treat any underlying medical condition. Approximately 10 to 20 percent of all sexual dysfunctions stem from disease. Diabetes and heart disease, for example, may cause erectile dysfunction. Medications and drugs, especially depressants such as alcohol, may also inhibit sexual responses. Anyone experiencing sexual difficulties should have a thorough physical examination.

If no physical problem is found, the problem may be psychosocial in origin. Psychosocial causes of dysfunction include troubled relationships, lack of sexual skills, irrational attitudes and beliefs, anxiety, and psychosexual trauma, such as sexual abuse or rape. Many sexual myths, including some of those listed in the box entitled "Myths about Human Sexuality," can interfere with the sexual performance or satisfaction of people who believe them. Through their difficulties, their partners are affected as well. Like other skills, sexual competence is learned. We learn what makes us and others feel good by talking with them about sex, reading about it, watching films, and experimenting. Many people, however, do not acquire sexual skills because they lack the opportunity to experiment or because their cultural background causes even the thought of sexual behavior to create overwhelming anxiety for them.

Many of these problems can be addressed by **sex therapy** methods that seek to modify the behavior patterns that are interfering with satisfactory sexual relationships. The behavioral treatment of sexual dysfunction concentrates on reducing performance anxiety, changing self-defeating expectations, and learning sexual skills. Many

---

Sex therapy   Treatment of sexual dysfunction.
Erectile dysfunction   Inability to have or maintain an erection.

Premature ejaculation   Involuntary orgasm before or shortly after the penis enters the vagina; ejaculation that takes place sooner than desired.

Retarded ejaculation   Inability to ejaculate when one wishes to during intercourse.

Myths about Human Sexuality

Myth: The bigger the man, the bigger the penis; the larger the nose, the larger the penis; men with bigger penises are more virile and make better lovers.

Fact: There is no known correlation between the size of the penis and body build, nor does the size of the penis determine the capacity to enjoy or provide sexual pleasure.

Myth: Ancient cultures had secret potions to enhance the sexual drive.

Fact: So they believed, as many cultures still do, but there is no evidence that sexual stimulants (aphrodisiacs) work other than by suggestion.

Myth: A woman who does not reach orgasm does not get pregnant.

Fact: Female orgasm is not necessary for pregnancy.

Myth: If you have sexual intercourse often when you are young, you will "run out of steam" when you get older.

Fact: On the contrary, men and women who are sexually active as young adults are more likely to remain so in their older years.

Myth: Sexual relations interfere with athletic performance.

Fact: Not so. Baseball manager Casey Stengel may have said it best when he told his players, "Going to bed with a woman never hurt a ballplayer. It's staying up all night looking for them that does you in."

Myth: Masturbation is an unnatural, immature act that can cause blindness, insanity, and numerous other ailments.

Fact: Masturbation is a natural function. People in most cultures masturbate, many of them throughout their lives. Many sexually active people with available partners masturbate as an additional gratification. There is no evidence that masturbation impairs physical or mental health.

Myth: The uncircumcised male has more control over the timing of ejaculation than does the circumcised male.

Fact: Masters and Johnson found no difference between uncircumcised men and circumcised men in sensitivity of the penis or in ability to control ejaculation.

Myth: The hymen is always stretched or torn on the occasion of first intercourse, and therefore a woman without an intact hymen cannot be a virgin.

Fact: The hymen can be torn by many kinds of nonsexual activities such as horseback riding and riding a bicycle and therefore is not a reliable indicator of virginity or its absence.

Myth: Women's intellectual and perceptual-motor performance varies with the phase of the menstrual cycle.

Fact: Although some women report feeling that they perform less well at various intellectual and perceptual-motor tasks during the premenstrual and menstrual phases of the cycle, no controlled study to date has found any clear relationship between phases of the cycle and any type of performance.

Myth: Women experience two types of orgasm, "clitoral" and "vaginal."

Fact: All orgasms in women are physiologically identical.

Myth: Heterosexual individuals respond differently to sexual stimulation than do homosexuals.

Fact: Heterosexual and homosexual men and women respond in exactly the same biological manner to psychological or physical sexual stimulation. In all cases, there is vasocongestion and the development of muscle tension regardless of sexual orientation or source of sexual stimulation.

Human sexuality is not just a matter of bodies responding to each other. This young couple's physical experiences together will be powerfully affected by their emotions, ideas, and values and how they choose to express them.

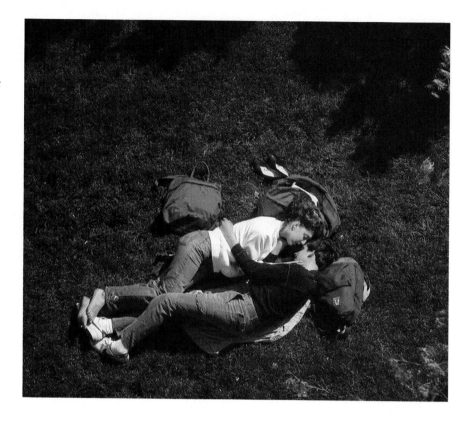

sex therapists use techniques pioneered by William Masters and Virginia Johnson in the 1960s. The therapy program usually includes "bibliotherapy" (reading self-help sex manuals) and learning new patterns of sexual behavior.

For example, a man experiencing erectile dysfunction learns to relax and receive sexual stimulation. He and his sexual partner first massage each other without touching the genitals, using verbal instructions and guiding each other's hands to communicate. Genital touching follows after a few sessions. The partners follow a gradual series of sexual activities that alleviates performance anxiety and ultimately ends in intercourse. Masters and Johnson report that erectile dysfunction has been reversed in 72 percent of the couples they have treated with this method. Premature ejaculation, another common problem, is often treated by the "squeeze technique," in which the tip of the penis is squeezed when the man feels he is about to ejaculate. This technique is reported to be effective in 90 percent of the men treated.

Women who seek treatment for orgasmic dysfunction often have not had the chance to learn through trial and error what types of stimulation will excite them and bring them to orgasm. Most sex therapists prefer to treat this problem with masturbation. Women are taught about their own anatomy and sexual responses and then are encouraged to experiment with masturbation until they experience orgasm. Once they can masturbate to orgasm, they may need additional treatment to transfer this learning to sexual intercourse with a partner.

Although sex therapy techniques may seem to focus narrowly on physiological responses, they actually highlight the fact that sex is not merely a mechanical body response. Sexual problems are closely tied in with emotional and psychological concerns and with a person's thoughts, perceptions, beliefs, values, and relationships with others. The same can be said for all sexual functioning. This chapter has focused on the physical aspects of sex. The next chapter addresses sexuality in the broader context of sexual behavior and intimate relationships. Together, the two chapters reflect the complexity and wholeness of human sexuality.

Vaginismus Painful, involuntary muscular contractions in the vagina that occur when sexual intercourse is attempted.

Orgasmic dysfunction The inability to experience orgasm.

Summary

- The conflicting messages and information people receive about sex can be confusing, but knowledge about the body's sexual functioning and sexual problems and ways to solve them is vital to a healthy life.

Sex and Gender: Defining Who You Are

- The word *sex* refers to biological identity as male or female, but in ordinary usage it has wider meanings. Gender roles and gender identity describe actions and feelings related to maleness and femaleness.
- Sexuality is a complicated concept involving sexual anatomy, sexual response, sex hormones, and intimate relationships; sexuality develops from both inborn, biological characteristics and acquired behavior.

Sexual Anatomy

- The sexual organs of men and women arise from the same structures and fulfill similar functions. Gonads in both sexes produce germ cells and sex hormones.
- Female external sex organs are called the vulva; the clitoris plays an important role in sexual arousal. The vagina leads to the internal sex organs; it is the female organ for sexual intercourse and serves as the birth canal.
- Male external sex organs are the penis and the scrotum; the glans penis is an important source of sexual arousal. The prepuce partly covers the glans; its removal in circumcision continues to be a common—but controversial—procedure in the United States. The scrotum maintains the temperature of the testes 5° lower than that of the rest of the body.

Sexual Physiology

- Sexual functions are integrated parts of the whole body's operations.
- Sexual activity consists of a stimulus and a response. Stimulation may be physical or psychological.
- Physical stimulation comes from the senses—from seeing, hearing, tasting, smelling, feeling, touching.
- Sexual arousal also has a psychological aspect. Fantasies and memories can generate excitement, and emotions also have a powerful effect on stimulation.
- Vasocongestion (engorgement of tissues) and myotonia (increased muscular tension culminating in muscular contractions) are the primary physiological mechanisms of sexual response.
- The sexual response cycle has four stages: excitement, plateau, orgasmic, and resolution. Specific genital changes accompany each stage, as do more general body reactions.

- The brain controls sexual functions; specific regions in the limbic system of the brain control arousal and orgasm.

Sex Hormones

- Hormones are chemical substances secreted directly into the bloodstream by endocrine glands.
- The testes produce androgens (especially testosterones); the ovaries produce estrogens and progestins (especially progesterone). The adrenal glands produce androgens in both sexes.
- Hormones from ovaries and testes exert influence first in the embryo, then in adolescence.
- The fertilizing sperm determines the sex of the individual. Some male germ cells contain an X chromosome; some contain a Y chromosome. The sperm cell unites with an ovum (always an X chromosome), forming XX or XY pairs. XY pairs lead to development of a male embryo.
- The specialized genes on the Y chromosome initiate the process of sexual differentiation in the embryo. The common embryonic origin of male and female systems means that every structure in one sex has a developmental counterpart in the other.
- The reproductive system matures at puberty. The hypothalamus influences the anterior pituitary gland to increase production of follicle-stimulating hormone (FSH) and the luteinizing hormone (LH), which stimulate the ovaries and testes.
- Breast development is the first sign of puberty in the female, followed by rapid body growth. FSH and LH stimulate maturation of ovarian follicles and release of eggs—ovulation. The first menstruation occurs during this period.
- The reproductive system of boys matures later than that of girls. FSH promotes the maturation of sperm. LH stimulates testicular cells to produce testosterone, which brings most of the male changes of puberty.
- Ovaries cease to function as women approach 50, and they enter menopause. Some symptoms may be troublesome; estrogen replacement therapy can help. Many women see menopause as the beginning of an important new life phase.
- Men do not experience a drop in hormone production in midlife, though testosterone production gradually decreases. The pattern of male sexual responses changes with age. Many men do go through a period of readjustment and reassessment (a "midlife crisis").
- The role hormones play in sexual behavior is not clear. Although in animals testosterone clearly causes aggressiveness and its absence promotes nurturance, in hu-

mans, the influence of cultural learning complicates the equation.

• The effect of hormones on sexual interest and activity is clear in teenagers. As males age, hormones seem to play a role in maintaining sexual functions. In women, fluctuations in hormones don't seem to affect sexual interest or the ability to reach orgasm.

Sexual Health: Disorders and Dysfunctions

• Physical and psychological problems can both interfere with sexual functioning. Sexual disorders are caused by physical conditions; sexual dysfunctions have psychological origins.

• Common sexual disorders may be physiological or may be the result of infection. They include vaginitis, endometriosis, pelvic inflammatory disease, dysmenorrhea, and premenstrual tension.

• Problems with vasocongestion and myotonia are at the root of the main forms of sexual dysfunction—inability to become aroused and problems with orgasm.

• In men, dysfunctions include erectile dysfunction, premature ejaculation, and retarded ejaculation. Occasional episodes of erectile dysfunction and retarded ejaculation can be due to excessive alcohol consumptions, fatigue, or stress. Dysfunction in women includes vaginismus and orgasmic dysfunction. Inability to experience orgasm under certain circumstances is a problem only if the woman considers it so.

• Treatment for sexual dysfunction first of all addresses any underlying medical conditions such as diabetes and heart disease or causes like drugs and alcohol. Problems can be psychosocial in origin—coming from troubled relationships, lack of sexual skills, misinformation. Sexual competence is learned; sex therapy can help teach new patterns of sexual behavior.

Take Action

1. Sexual myths and misconceptions abound in our culture. Create a list of myths you've heard. Find out the facts by consulting books and pamphlets mentioned here or available through your school health center.

2. There are many reputable self-help books about sexual functioning available in libraries and bookstores. If you're not satisfied with your level of knowledge and understanding, consider doing some reading.

3. If you think you may have PMS, keep a diary of your moods, time of day they occur, foods you eat, and when your period occurs. If there seems to be a cyclical character to your moods, consider taking some of the steps suggested in the box on PMS.

4. Interview an older person to find out what sexual attitudes were when he/she was your age. In what ways are things different today? In what ways are they the same?

Selected Bibliography

Cole, E., and E. Rothblum. 1989. *Women and Sex Therapy*. Binghamton, N.Y.: Haworth Press.

Cocores, J., and M. Gold. 1989. Substance abuse and sexual dysfunction. *Medical Aspects of Human Sexuality* 23:22–31.

Kelly, K. 1987. *Females, Males and Sexuality*. Albany: State University of New York Press.

Leiblum, S., and R. Rosen. 1989. *Sexual Desire Disorders*. New York: Guilford.

Rosen, R., and Gayle Beck. 1989. *Patterns of Sexual Arousal*. New York: Guilford.

Wells, J. 1989. Sexual language usage in different interpersonal contexts: A comparison of gender and sexual orientation. *Archives of Sexual Behavior*, 18:127–143.

Recommended Readings

Boston Women's Health Collective. 1984. *The New Our Bodies, Ourselves*. New York. Simon and Schuster. *A very readable book concerned with all aspects of female sexuality.*

Denney, N., and D. Quadagno. 1988. *Human Sexuality*. St. Louis. Times-Mirror Mosby. *A human sexuality textbook with a complete discussion of all of the biological aspects of human sexuality that are presented in this chapter.*

The Diagram Group. 1977. *Man's Body*. New York: Bantam Books. *While this book is relatively old it is still an excellent source of information about male sexuality. No newer book like this exists.*

Leiblum, S., and R. Rosen. 1989. *Principles and Practice of Sex Therapy*. New York: Guilford. *Timely, up-to-date information on the treatment of sexual dysfunctions.*

Olds, S. 1985. *The Eternal Garden: Seasons of Our Sexuality.* New York: Times Books. *A very readable book that presents an overview of our sexuality from birth to old age.*

Spencer, S. and A. Zeiss. 1987. Sex roles and sexual dysfunction in college students. *Journal of Sex Research* 23:338–347. *An article of interest to college-aged individuals dealing with the nature and prevalence of sexual dysfunction in this age group.*

Spence, A. 1989. *Biology of Human Aging.* Englewood Cliffs, N.J.: Prentice-Hall. *An excellent account of how the reproductive structures change with age and the impact of these changes on sexual functioning.*

Contents

Making Connections

I ntimate relationships, with or without a sexual component, are an important part of wellness—people need to feel connected with others in order to function at their highest level. But intimacy and successful relationships are elusive for many people, as current divorce rates testify. The scenarios presented on these pages describe situations in which people have to use information, make a decision, or choose a course of action, all related to intimate relationships. As you read them, imagine yourself in each situation and consider what you would do. After you've finished the chapter, read the scenarios again and see if what you've learned has changed how you would think, feel, or act in each situation.

Two months after you got to college, your parents informed you that they were separating. They said they'd been unhappy for years and were just waiting for all the children to leave home to get a divorce. They obviously think that this is no one's business but their own and that you and your brothers are old enough to take it all in stride. But you've been feeling disoriented, angry, and anxious ever since they gave you the news. Is there anything you can do about your feelings, or will they pass in time?

You've become seriously involved with someone who comes from a different ethnic, religious, and socioeconomic background than you do. The two of you are intrigued by the differences in how you were brought up, how you express your feelings, and what you want to accomplish in life. Even though you both identify strongly with your own backgrounds, it seems to be a case of opposites attracting. Your parents, however, are concerned that the two of you have too many differences. Successful relationships and happy marriages, they say, are based on common backgrounds and interests. They want you to date other people, preferably people more like yourself. Are they being unreasonable, or do they have a point?

5
Sexual Behavior and Intimate Relationships

A lot of men in your dorm are eager to be involved in sexual relationships and make it seem as if sleeping with different women is a required part of growing up. You were brought up to believe that sex was an important part of love and marriage, not something you did casually. But sometimes when you hear your friends talking about how great a sexual experience was, you think you ought to take the plunge. Are you hopelessly old-fashioned, or is it okay to want to wait? Should you be guided by the beliefs you were brought up with, or should you reconsider in light of what others are telling you?

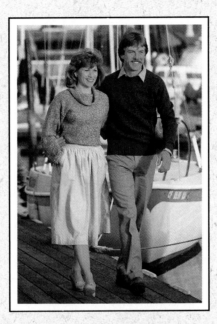

You've been dating a man seriously for several months and are thinking of moving in with him. The only thing is, you wonder if you'll become too isolated living with him. He likes spending all his free time with you and objects to your spending time with other friends. He's asked you to quit your part-time job at the library so you'll have more time for him, and now he wants you to drop out of the drama club as well. He says he loves you and wants to be with you all the time. You love him too and want to pursue the relationship, but you feel a little uncomfortable with his demands. Is he being unreasonable? Or are you being too sensitive? What should you do?

You recently had a troubling experience that you can't stop thinking about. You accepted a date with an attractive man from one of your classes. He took you to dinner at a fancy restaurant, ordered expensive food and wine, and charmed you with his sophisticated conversation. Afterwards you went back to his apartment and had some more wine. Then he began to make sexual advances, persisting even though you told him you weren't ready to go that far with him. The more you resisted, the more forceful he became, finally succeeding in having sex with you. Afterwards he said you led him on by going out to dinner with him and then back to his apartment. He said any man would have interpreted your actions the way he did. You're not sure why you went to his apartment, but you do know that you feel confused, guilty, and violated. Was what happened your fault? How can you make sure it doesn't happen again?

Human beings need social relationships; people cannot survive as solitary creatures. Nor could the human species survive if adults didn't cherish and support each other, if they didn't form strong mutual attachments with their infants, and if they didn't create families in which to care for children. People need other people in the same way they need food to eat and air to breathe.

The most characteristic basis for human relationships appears to be love, although it is often mixed with other emotions. Fear, anger, hatred, compassion, nurturance, and other intense feelings, needs, and desires also hold people together in relationships. But love in its many forms—parental, filial, platonic, romantic—is the wellspring from which much of life's meaning and delight flows. People devote tremendous energy to keeping up friendships, seeking mates, nurturing intimate relationships, maintaining marriages—all for the pleasure of loving and being loved.

The role of love in passionate attachments between adults in our society is obscured by a fairly recent development. In the beginning of this century, Sigmund Freud proposed a theory of psychological development that placed sexuality at the heart of the human experience. Freud's notion of sexuality as the predominant and overriding human **drive** has saturated our whole culture. There is no doubt that sexual behavior—all activities that lead to sexual arousal—is a natural and highly significant element that pervades and even defines many relationships. But whether it is the overriding human drive is questionable. In very few past societies has sexual fulfillment been elevated to such preeminence in the list of human aspirations as it is in ours.

Whether it is the primary drive or not, sexuality is so pervasive a motivator of behaviors that no discussion of intimacy and human relationships can proceed without considering its effects. Optimal health includes understanding and accepting the role of sexuality and sexual relationships in one's life. In this chapter we first consider the thread of sexuality in human relationships, and then we turn to a broader view of intimate relationships in general.

Sexuality in Human Relationships

Aspects of Sexual Behavior   Many behaviors stem from sexual impulses, and sexual expression takes a variety of forms. Probably the most basic aspect of sexuality is reproduction, the process of producing offspring. Sexual behaviors related to reproduction include sexual intercourse, contraception, pregnancy, childbirth, and breast-feeding. As important as reproduction is, the intention of creating a child accounts for only a small measure of sexual activity; most people have sex for other rea-

sons, as well, very often hoping that it *won't* result in pregnancy.

■ **Exploring Your Emotions**

Is sexuality an important part of relationships for you? Do you think you could have a friendship with a member of the opposite sex without its becoming a sexual relationship?

Sexual excitement and satisfaction are nonreproductive aspects of sexual behavior. The intensely pleasurable sensations of arousal and orgasm are probably the strongest motivators for human sexual behavior. People are infinitely creative in the ways they seek to experience erotic pleasure; common expressions of nonreproductive sexuality are kissing and fondling, intercourse in any number of different positions, and oral-genital stimulation.

Another, perhaps more complex aspect of sexuality is the expression of love, affection, and emotional intimacy. Although love can be expressed through sexual behaviors, people who don't love each other can enjoy sex and have a passionate relationship, and people who do love each other can sometimes have impersonal sex. Sexual activity can be mechanical and hurried whether or not two people are in love with each other. A love relationship marked by caring and respect protects both partners against the risk of being used sexually.

■ **Exploring Your Emotions**

What are your expectations of love? How much are your expectations shaped by movies and magazines, by what your friends expect, by what you've observed of your parents' relationship and of the relationships of other adults? Are there any contradictions among these views? If so, can you reconcile them?

Love relationships without a sexual component—relationships between parents and children, siblings, friends, and companions—are far more common than those with it. Even partners in an intimate relationship sometimes agree to abstain from physical intimacies because of religious or moral values, a lack of sexual desire, or the wish to avoid the complications of a sexual relationship. Today, with attitudes toward sex becoming somewhat more conservative, fewer relationships have a sexual component than was true even a few years ago. (See the box entitled "Three Couples.")

The most profound but least noticed expressions of sexuality are gender identity—the very basic sense a person has of being male or female—and gender role—the characteristics and behaviors that go along with that self-perception. Some gender characteristics are determined

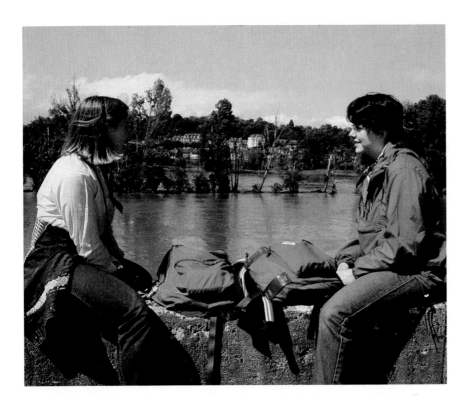

Close relationships without a sexual component are more common than those with sex. Friendship satisfies the human needs for affection, affirmation, sharing, and companionship.

biologically, such as the genitals a person is born with and the secondary sex characteristics that develop at puberty. Others are defined by society and learned in the course of growing up. These characteristics vary from one society to another and from one time to another. In the United States today, for example, many women shave their legs and wear make-up; in Muslim countries, women wear robes and veils that conceal their faces and bodies. Each set of behaviors expresses some learned aspect of the female gender role in that society, and each set would be inappropriate in the other society.

Roots and Development of Sexual Behavior   Why do most of us have a deep impulse to act sexually? Are we born programmed to behave sexually, or do we learn sexual behaviors, or both?

Innate or Learned?   Various theories attempt to account for human sexual behavior on the basis of a sexual **instinct** or drive. They suggest that an innate force (called "libido" in psychoanalytic theory) impels us to seek sexual satisfaction even against considerable obstacles. This concept of a sexual instinct presupposes that some be-

haviors—mating, "nesting," and "mothering" impulses, for example—are programmed into us from conception. Just as our cells carry blueprint instructions for determining our physical appearance, our master program instructs us to perform certain acts. Students of animal social behavior assume that the patterns of human sexual behavior are predetermined by evolution and that differences in human responses to these instinctive urges are the result of the influence of society.

Behavioral scientists place much greater emphasis on the role of learning than they do on instinct. They assume that various forms of **conditioning** and **social learning** shape our sexual behaviors. One model of social learning is embodied in the concept of **sexual scripts.** Such scripts are learned during development and function like a blueprint, influencing why, with whom, how, and under what circumstances a person has sexual relations.

A more integrative approach explains sexual behavior as the outcome of interacting biological and psychosocial factors. In this view the interactions between the nervous system and the endocrine systems (the glands and other structures that secrete hormones into the bloodstream) maintain the sexual machinery, and biological factors

---

Drive   Innate behavioral force that moves one to act.

Instinct   Unlearned, goal-directed motivational force.

Conditioning   A basic form of learning that establishes acquired responses.

Social learning   Acquiring personal and social behavior through learning.

Sexual scripts   Socially learned patterns of sexual behavior.

Three Couples

Couples on today's college campuses show a wide range of attitudes toward love and sex. For some, love alone is not a sufficient justification for sexual intercourse; the more permanent commitment of marriage is a necessary prerequisite. For others, sex is considered permissible if a man and woman love each other; in this view, sex is an expression of love and caring. For still others, sex is acceptable even without love; sex is considered an enjoyable activity to be valued for its own sake. The following couples represent each of the three types.

A Sexually Traditional Couple: Paul and Peggy

Peggy believes that intercourse before marriage is wrong. She explained that "even if I were engaged, I wouldn't feel right about having sex." Many of Peggy's girlfriends are having sexual affairs, which Peggy accepts "for them." It's not right for Peggy, however, and she believes that Paul respects her views. For his part, Paul indicated that he would like to have intercourse with Peggy, but he added that intercourse "just isn't all that important for me."

A Sexually Moderate Couple: Tom and Sandy

Three weeks after their first date, Tom told Sandy that he loved her. She was in love, too, and their relationship grew quickly. In a few months they were spending weekends together at one of their dorms. They slept in the same bed but did not have intercourse. Although Tom was very attracted to Sandy, he was slow to initiate intercourse. "I didn't want to push it on her," he said. "I felt that we shouldn't have sex until our relationship reached a certain point. [Sex] is something I just can't imagine on a first date." Tom and Sandy first had intercourse with each other just before becoming engaged. For Tom, "Sex added another dimension to our relationship; it's a landmark of sorts."

A Sexually Liberal Couple: Jennifer and Michael

Jennifer and Michael had been dating for about two weeks when they returned to Jennifer's apartment after a movie one Saturday night. They began kissing in front of the TV, and then Jennifer asked Michael if he wanted to spend the night. She told him she was very attracted to him, and he said he was attracted to her too. That night was the beginning of their sexual relationship. For Jennifer and Michael, having sex was part of getting to know each other. It added a closeness to their relationship that both of them wanted and enjoyed.

The central distinction between these three orientations concerns the links between sexual intimacy and emotional intimacy. For traditionalists, emotional intimacy develops in the context of limited sexual activity; sexual intercourse is tied not only to love but to a permanent commitment as well. For moderates, emotional intimacy sets the pace for sexual intimacy. As feelings of closeness and love increase, greater sexual exploration is possible. For liberals, sexual intimacy and emotional intimacy need not be related. Sex can be enjoyed in its own right, or sexual intimacy can be a route to developing emotional intimacy.

Adapted from Rubin/McNeil 1985 *The Psychology of Being Human* (New York: Harper & Row), p. 532.

---

predispose a person to act certain ways. These predispositions are then further elaborated and given meaning by cultural forces. Our actual behavior is shaped by the interplay of our predispositions and our learning experiences throughout life.

Social Learning   From birth children are influenced to act as female or male. Social learning processes encourage traits and behaviors traditionally deemed appropriate for one sex or the other. Children begin to conceptualize the world as consisting of males and females, and they try to act like their own sex. Parents usually give children gender-specific names, clothes, and toys. In conversations they are far more likely to tell a boy why the car is accelerating, and a girl why the cookies aren't chewy. Family and friends create an environment that teaches the child whether to become a woman or a man and how to act appropriately. Teachers, television, books, and even strangers model these gender roles.

Historically, gender roles have tended to highlight and emphasize the differences between males and females, but new gender roles are emerging in our society that reflect more of a mix of male and female characteristics and behaviors. This tendency toward **androgyny** greatly broadens the range of experiences available to both males and females. Many educators, parents, and others have attempted to erase the lines between stereotypically masculine and feminine behaviors for children in hopes of freeing them from the constraints of inflexible gender roles.

Androgynous adults are less stereotyped in their thinking, in how they look, dress, and act, in how they divide work in the home, in how they think about jobs and careers, and in how they express themselves sexually. Women today are able and even expected to be much more assertive, competitive, ambitious, and powerful than they were allowed to be in the past, and men are able to be more sensitive, articulate, nurturing, and emotionally expressive. Children who are exposed to androgynous models are likely to have more choices when they grow up, although many learned gender role behaviors are so subtle that it's virtually impossible to escape them.

Childhood Sexual Behavior   The capacity to respond sexually is present at birth. Ultrasound studies suggest that boys experience erections in the uterus. After birth, both sexes have the capacity for orgasm, though many babies may not experience it. As people grow, many discover this capacity through self-exploration. Sexual behaviors gradually emerge in childhood in the form of self-stimulating play. Self-exploration and touching the genitals are common forms of play, observed among infants as young as 6 months. They gradually lead to more deliberate forms of **masturbation** with or without orgasm.

Children often engage in sexual play with playmates by exploring each others' genitals. These activities are often part of games like "playing house" or "playing doctor." By age 12, 40 percent of boys have engaged in sex play; the peak exploration age for girls is age 9, by which time 14 percent have had such experiences. Although parents and teachers actively teach and socialize children, in our culture they largely avoid the task of sexual education or carry it out indirectly.

Adolescent Sexuality   A person who has experienced puberty is biologically an adult. But in psychological and social terms, human beings need five to ten more years to attain full adult status. This discrepancy between biological and social maturity creates considerable confusion over what constitutes appropriate sexual behavior during adolescence.

Sexual fantasies and dreams become more common and explicit in adolescence than at earlier ages, often as an accompaniment to masturbation. Most teenage boys and somewhat fewer girls masturbate more or less regularly. Once puberty is reached, orgasm among boys is accompanied by ejaculation. Teenage boys also experience **nocturnal emissions** ("wet dreams"). Some girls also have orgasmic dreams. In general, masturbation does not carry the social stigma and imagined perils of former times, but adolescents—and many adults as well—are often still embarrassed by it.

Sexual interaction in adolescence usually takes place between peers in the context of dating, which fulfills a variety of other social functions as well. Sexual intimacy is usually expressed in such relationships through petting and necking, which may involve kissing, caressing, and stimulating the breasts and the genitals. These activities lead to sexual arousal but may or may not culminate in orgasm.

Many American teenagers now also engage in **premarital sexual relations**, although the threat of AIDS is probably causing a decrease in casual sexual activity. About 55 percent of unmarried people have had **sexual intercourse** by the age of 18 and 75 percent by the age of 20. Rates for premarital sex vary considerably from one group to another, however, based on ethnic, educational, religious, geographic, and other factors. Engaging in **coitus** for the first time is affected by these same factors plus psychological readiness, fear of consequences, being in love, going steady, peer pressures, and the need to act like an adult, gain popularity, or rebel, among other factors. Some people thoughtfully weigh decisions and others plunge recklessly. Teenagers who engage in sexual intercourse or are close to doing so generally value personal independence, have loosened family ties in favor of more reliance on friends, and are more apt to experiment with drugs or alcohol and to engage in political activism than their contemporaries.

Adolescent sexual behaviors are not confined to **heterosexual** relationships. Beginning in childhood, sex play involves members of one's own sex as well as of the opposite sex. **Homosexual** attractions, with or without sexual encounters, are likewise common in adolescence.

Androgyny   A blending of male and female characteristics and roles, especially a lack of sex-typing with respect to roles.

Masturbation   Self-stimulation to obtain sexual arousal and orgasm.

Nocturnal emissions   Orgasm and ejaculation (wet dream) during sleep.

Premarital sexual relations   Coitus before marriage.

Sexual intercourse   Sexual relations involving genital union; coitus; also called "making love."

Coitus   Sexual intercourse.

Heterosexual   Sexual orientation toward and preference for the opposite sex.

Homosexual   Sexual orientation toward and preference for the same sex.

The Roots of Sexual Orientation

Why is it that some people are heterosexual and others homosexual? A short answer is that we don't know. Despite much study and speculation, when, how, and why we develop our sexual orientation is still unclear.

Studying the roots of sexual orientation would be the most appropriate way to understand the choice between heterosexuality and homosexuality. Yet research in this area usually has been aimed at discovering the causes of homosexuality because it is atypical in the general population and scientists often investigate what is unusual.

Because exclusive homosexuality precludes reproduction, it is biologically maladaptive for human societies as a whole, although not necessarily for individuals. But the same concern with reproduction does not apply to bisexuality. In fact, one wonders why we aren't sexually attracted equally to men and women. After all, we love members of both sexes, and love and sexuality often go together.

It has long been argued that homosexuality is "unnatural," but if by "natural" we mean what exists in nature, that position is not tenable. Same-sex interactions can be observed among many different species of animals. Whether homosexuality is socially acceptable or not, homosexual behavior is certainly not a modern human invention.

Much research about biological determinants of homosexuality has focused on genetic and hormonal factors. Studies have found that the brothers of gay men are more likely to be homosexuals than the brothers of heterosexual men, especially if they are twins. But in such studies, genetics, heredity, and common patterns of upbringing cannot readily be sorted out.

Investigators have also noted differences between physical structures, blood chemistry, and metabolic processes of homosexuals and heterosexuals. Yet inconsistencies in methodology and outcomes make these studies inconclusive.

The search for psychosocial determinants likewise has failed to reveal consistent patterns. Psychoanalysts have pointed to parental relationships as a basis for growing up to be gay. Typically, gay men report having detached and hostile fathers and seductive and domineering mothers. Social learning theorists have pointed to poor peer relationships, atypical sexual experiences, and homosexual seduction in childhood as factors in homosexuality. A prime learning mechanism in social learning theory—imitation—can't be used to explain homosexuality, because homosexuals come almost entirely from heterosexual families. One can find cases to fit any theory, but none can be generalized as a sole cause of homosexuality.

Nonetheless, some interesting patterns in sexual development cast some light on this matter. By the time boys and girls reach adolescence, their sexual preferences are already largely set. Romantic attraction to the same sex is present several years before any homosexual activity takes place. Adolescents who become gay are not particularly lacking in heterosexual experience—they just don't find such experiences as gratifying. Gender nonconformity—effeminate boys and tomboyish girls—is strongly linked to the development of homosexuality.

These findings indicate once again the futility of trying to understand sexual orientation and behavior outside of the broader context of gender identity and personality development. Sexual orientation has to be considered an integral part of life.

Adapted from A. P. Bell, et al. 1981. *Sexual Preferences: Its Development in Men and Women* (Bloomington: Indiana University Press).

For many these are youthful experiments and don't mean that participants will ultimately be homosexual. For a minority they may be a factor in adult **sexual orientation** (see the box entitled "The Roots of Sexual Orientation"). Most adult gay men and women trace their preferences to their early years.

Adult Sexuality   Early adulthood is a time when people make important life choices, a time of increasing responsibility in terms of interpersonal relations and family life. In recent years, both in the United States and abroad, there has been a definite trend toward marriage at a later age than in past decades. And before marriage, more

Sexual orientation   Preference for opposite sex, same sex, or both as sexual partners.

young adults are driven by an internal need to become sexually knowledgeable. Today more people in their twenties believe that becoming sexually experienced rather than preserving virginity is an important prelude for selecting a mate. According to psychologist Erik Erikson, developing the capacity for intimacy is a central task for the young adult.

Adult sexuality can include any of the sexual behaviors and practices described in this chapter. In mature love relationships, people ideally are able to integrate all the aspects of intimacy—physical, sexual, emotional—so that sexuality is a deeply meaningful part of how they express love. People can continue to enjoy sexual activities throughout their entire lives, varying and expanding the scope of their experiences as they gain more understanding of their own and their partners' needs and desires.

Sexual Orientation

Homosexuality   About 5 to 7 percent of our population, approximately 12 million people, is estimated to be exclusively homosexual, sexually and romantically attracted to and satisfied only by members of their own sex. A larger number of bisexuals are sexually attracted, to various degrees, to both men and women. Currently, most homosexual men prefer to be called gay, and women lesbian. The "gay liberation" movement of the 1970s and 1980s helped to dispel some of the historical prejudice against them, but homosexuality still has not received widespread societal approval.

■ Exploring Your Emotions

What are your feelings about homosexuality? Do your attitudes differ from those of others in your family or of your friends? Could a difference of opinion about homosexuality seriously affect a friendship or family relationship?

The sexual practices of gay men and women resemble those of their heterosexual counterparts except for coitus. In addition to kissing and fondling, gay sex relies more heavily on oral-genital stimulation as a means of attaining orgasm, and gay men engage more frequently in anal intercourse. About a quarter of all lesbians and a tenth of all gay men form close and stable ties with one partner. Before the AIDS epidemic, many gay men interacted with numerous sexual partners whom they would meet in gay bars, baths, and other designated meeting places. AIDS has led many gay men to curtail and change their patterns of sexual behavior drastically—cutting out sex with anonymous partners, for instance, and using condoms during all sexual contact that involve potential exchange of body fluids. Much of the gay lifestyle depends on whether individuals are overt or covert homosexuals. Those who feel forced to be secretive abut their sexual preference may lead double lives, one public and one

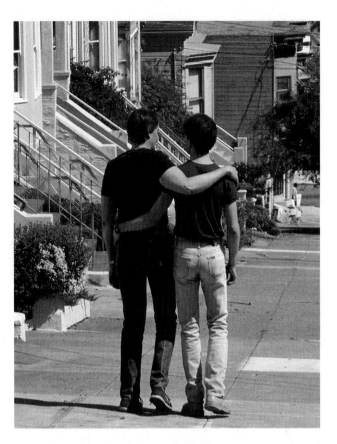

Greater openness has made gay men and lesbians more visible than they used to be, although they still constitute a minority of the population and have not received widespread societal approval.

private. Those who have "come out" participate more actively in the gay subculture.

Heterosexuality   The great majority of people—more than 80 percent and perhaps above 90 percent—are heterosexual, sexually attracted to and satisfied by members of the opposite sex. The origins of heterosexuality aren't understood any better than the origins of homosexuality, although Freud's theory of the Oedipus complex is a well-known attempt to explain sexual orientation. According to this theory, children are romantically and sexually attracted to the parent of the opposite sex during the stage of psychosexual development that occurs between the ages of 3 and 5, but fear of punishment leads the child to renounce the attraction and identify with the parent of the same sex. This identification results in a heterosexual orientation in adolescence and adulthood (and failure to resolve the Oedipal issues, according to Freud, results in a homosexual orientation). Although many psychologists accept the role of Oedipal relationships in personality development, they question their role in the development of sexual orientation.

■ **Exploring Your Emotions**

Are there some actions and activities you feel are appropriate only for men or only for women? How do you feel about women asking men out on dates or making sexual advances? How about wives taking the initiative sexually with their husbands?

The heterosexual lifestyle usually includes all the behavior and relationship patterns that are described in this chapter, such as dating, engagement and/or living together, and marriage. Legally recognized and binding marriage is available in our society only to heterosexual couples, so gay couples cannot legally marry. (Some religious organizations do solemnize gay unions.) As mentioned earlier, heterosexuals and homosexuals practice basically the same sexual behaviors except for coitus, but the heterosexual path is the more common and sanctioned one in our society.

Varieties of Human Sexual Behavior   Most people express their sexuality in a variety of ways. Some sexual behaviors are **autoerotic**—aimed at self-stimulation only, such as masturbation—while **sociosexual** practices involve interaction with others in behaviors such as kissing and coitus. Some people choose not to express sexuality and practice celibacy instead.

Celibacy   Continuous abstention from sexual activities with others is the practice of **celibacy.** Celibacy can be a conscious and deliberate choice or it can be necessitated by circumstances. Health considerations—concerns about recurring vaginal infections, sexually transmitted diseases, and particularly the spread of AIDS—may contribute to a decision to practice celibacy. Religious and moral beliefs may lead some people to celibacy, particularly until marriage or until an acceptable partner appears. Some people get no pleasure from sexual intimacy, and some find the energy and time spent seeking it a distraction from other more creative endeavors. Still others simply don't have access to a partner.

Sexual abstention can be practiced temporarily or on a periodic basis, often for years, and sometimes for a lifetime. Some celibates masturbate; others engage in no sexual activities at all. A disadvantage of the celibate life is that it may lack physical contact and affection.

Autoeroticism and Masturbation   The most common autoerotic sexual activity is **erotic fantasy**, mental experiences that arise in the imagination and range from fleeting thoughts to elaborate scenarios. Fantasies may be replays of past sexual experiences, or they may be fabrications based on unfulfilled wishes or drawn from books, drawings, or photographs. As mentioned in Chapter 4, people often don't want to act out their fantasies and wouldn't even if they had the chance.

■ **Exploring Your Emotions**

How aware are you of your own sexual wishes and preferences? Do you feel that your sexual impulses are healthy and acceptable, or do they make you feel uncomfortable? Do you feel safe with your sexual fantasies and confident that you can control your sexual behavior?

Masturbation typically involves manually stimulating the genitals, rubbing them against objects (such as a pillow), or using stimulating devices such as vibrators. Although commonly associated with adolescence, for many masturbation remains a sexual outlet throughout adult life. It may be used as a substitute for coitus and other sociosexual behaviors or as part of sexual activity with a partner. Masturbation gives a person control over the pace, time, and method of sexual release and pleasure. Most men and women masturbate. On average, two of three college students masturbate a few times a week, others do it more or less frequently, and some don't do it at all.

Touching and Foreplay   Tactile stimulation—touching—is integral to sexual experiences, whether in the form of massage, kissing, fondling, or holding. The entire body surface is a sensory organ, and touching almost anywhere can enhance intimacy and sexual arousal. Some body areas, known as erogenous zones, are much more sensitive to touch as a sexual stimulus than others; lips, genitals, and nipples in particular are generously endowed with sensory nerve endings. Touching can convey a variety of messages, including affection, comfort, and a desire for further sexual contact.

■ **Exploring Your Emotions**

What sexual practices are acceptable to you and what ones are unacceptable? What influences your feelings about them? Are there sexual practices that you object to but find arousing anyway? Remember, there's a big difference between what you think and what you do.

During arousal many men and women manually and orally stimulate each other by touching, stroking, and caressing their partner's genitals. Men and women vary greatly in their preferences for the type, pacing, and vigor of such **foreplay**. Working out the details to accommodate each other's pleasure is a key to enjoying these activities. Direct communication about preferences can enhance sexual pleasure and protect both partners from physical and psychological discomfort.

Oral-Genital Stimulation   **Cunnilingus** (the stimulation of the female genitals with the lips and tongue) and **fellatio** (the stimulation of the penis with the mouth) are quite common practices. A survey of several thousand college students in sexuality classes spanning 15 years revealed that approximately 89 percent of women and 82 percent of men had both administered and received oral-genital stimulation (although prevalence varies in different populations). Oral sex may be practiced either as part of arousal and foreplay or as a sex act culminating in orgasm. Like all acts of sexual expression between two people, oral sex requires the cooperation and consent of both partners. If they disagree about its acceptability, they need to discuss their feelings and try to reach a mutually pleasing solution.

Anal Intercourse   Another practice, less common but well known, is anal stimulation and penetration by the penis or a finger. About 10 percent of heterosexuals and 50 percent of homosexual males regularly practice anal intercourse. The receiver does not usually reach orgasm from anal intercourse, though men usually experience orgasm while penetrating. Many people have strongly negative attitudes toward anal sex because they consider it unclean, unnatural, or unappealing. Because the anus is composed of delicate tissues that tear easily under such pressure, anal intercourse is one of the riskiest of sexual behaviors associated with transmission of the AIDS virus, gonorrhea bacterium, and syphilis organism. Routine use of condoms is recommended for anyone engaging in anal sex. Special care and precaution should be exercised if anal sex is practiced—cleanliness, lubrication, and gentle entry at the very least. Anything that is inserted into the anus should not subsequently be put into the vagina unless it has been thoroughly washed. Bacteria naturally present in the anus can cause vaginal infections.

Sexual Intercourse   For most adults, most of the time, sexual intercourse is the ultimate sexual experience. Men and women engage in coitus—make love—to fulfill both sexual and psychological needs. The most common practice involves the man placing his erect penis into the woman's dilated and lubricated vagina after sufficient arousal.

Much has been written on how to enhance pleasure through various coital techniques, positions, and practices. For a woman the key factor in physical readiness for coitus is adequate vaginal lubrication, and psychologically to be aroused and receptive. For a man, conditions and the partner must arouse him to attain and maintain erection. Personal preferences vary, but most people prefer a safe, private setting. Candlelight and music, for example, can enhance the mood of the occasion. Psychological factors and the quality of the relationship are more important to overall sexual satisfaction than sophisticated or exotic sexual techniques.

Sexual activities give rise to intensely pleasurable human experiences and emotions, and at the same time can produce one of the most precious—and expensive and needy—of human products, a child. Along with the pleasure comes the responsibility of practicing safe, sane, and considerate sex. This responsibility is dramatically apparent today in light of both our staggering population increase and the AIDS epidemic, which brings the possibility of death through reckless sexual pursuit. Contraception has long been necessary in light of the heavy price attached to having a child. (Contraception is discussed in Chapter 6.) For the small amount of effort necessary to practice safe sex, the benefit is life-enhancing. Safe sex practices are discussed in detail in Chapter 17.

Problematic Sexual Behaviors   Atypical sexual behaviors are by definition less common types of sexual expression, and they are usually considered undesirable by others. Atypical here refers to adult behaviors such as exhibiting one's genitals in public, peeping uninvited into strangers' homes, child abuse, incest, and rape. The people who repeatedly and persistently prefer certain unusual behaviors to legitimate outlets for sexual gratification are classified as **sex offenders** if their sexual activity violates moral and legal codes, offends the public sense of decency, or threatens others. While some unwilling recipients of less intrusive variant sexual expressions, such as peeping or exposing, may be psychologically traumatized, many recipients are not. Because of this and the fact that many of these behaviors do not generally

---

Autoerotic behavior   Activities aimed at sexual self-stimulation.

Sociosexual behavior   Sexual activities involving other people.

Celibacy   Continuous abstention from sexual activities.

Erotic fantasy   Sexually arousing thoughts and daydreams.

Foreplay   The kissing, touching, and other oral-genital contact that stimulates people toward intercourse.

Cunnilingus   Oral stimulation of the female genitals.

Fellatio   Oral stimulation of the penis.

Sex offender   One who engages in sexual behaviors prohibited by law.

involve physical or sexual contact with another, some behaviors are viewed as minor sex offenses. Other more severe forms of sexual victimization are major offenses. Almost all sex offenders are men, though occasionally a woman is cited for sexual harassment in the office or female day care workers are charged with sexual abuse of children.

The search for genetic and hormonal causes for these deviant behaviors has been inconclusive. Psychoanalytic theory explains them as unresolved immature sexual impulses from childhood. Other theorists explain these behaviors as products of social learning.

Some atypical sexual behaviors can be partially explained by the concept of a **paraphilia**, a condition in which a person's sexual arousal and gratification depend on an unusual object or act. From a mental health perspective, however different, odd, or unusual a sexual behavior may be, even if it appears to be paraphilial, it is not considered pathological so long as it injures no one and involves only consenting adults. But because paraphilias are often accompanied by a thinly veiled hostile element, they become vehicles for more aggressive aspects of sexuality, male sexuality in particular. The most common paraphilias are listed below.

Voyeurism is the practice of watching others engage in sexual activities, usually without their knowledge or consent.

Exhibitionism, also known as exposing or "flashing," involves exhibiting the genitals to an involuntary observer. Usually the exhibitionist masturbates during or after the act, drawing sexual pleasure from the observer's shocked reaction.

Fetishism involves becoming sexually aroused by an inanimate object or a part of the human body, such as hair, feet, or a pair of pantyhose or underpants.

Pedophilia is sexual attraction to children.

Transvestism, or cross-dressing, involves repeatedly wearing the clothes of the opposite gender for the purpose of sexual arousal. **Transsexualism,** a gender disorder, is to be distinguished from transvestism: a transsexual wishes to be a member of the opposite sex and to have an anatomical gender change. Transsexuals also cross-dress, not for sexual arousal but for a sense of emotional completeness.

Bestiality, or zoophilia, involves sexual contact with animals.

Sexual sadism involves sexual gratification through inflicting psychological and physical suffering on another person. **Masochism** is the erotic enjoyment of one's own suffering. Sadomasochism clearly demonstrates that dominance and aggression can play a role in sexual arousal.

Coercive Sex   The use of force and coercion in sexual relationships is one of the most serious problems in human interactions. Its most extreme manifestation is rape, but **sexual coercion** commonly occurs in many subtler forms. Coercion—forcing a person to submit to another's sexual desires—is often used to intimidate younger, more naive people, as in cases of incest and pedophilia.

Child Molestation and Incest   Sexual interactions forced on a child by an adult are known as molestation or sexual abuse. Molesters are often pedophiliacs, usually male, and typically interested in prepubescent girls or boys, although many victims are younger. In most cases the pedophile is a relative, family friend, or someone known to the child. Sexual contacts are typically brief and consist of genital manipulation; genital intercourse is rarely attempted. However, the potential for violent abuse exists, and evidence suggests that some child molesters may progress to more violent sexual offenses, such as rape. Child abusers usually have poor interpersonal and sexual relations with other adults, and they may feel socially inadequate and inferior. The problem is subtle because offenders often strongly deny the harm of their deeds, and children, who may have strong affection and fear for the adult offender, may support the offender and turn against accusors. The degree of trauma for the victim can be very serious, but varies with the encounters, their frequency, and the parents' response. Children must be protected from being molested again.

Incest is sexual activity of any kind between members of the same family, including grandparents, adopted children, stepparents, and in-laws. It is not so rare in our society as most people believe—estimates suggest that perhaps 50,000 children are abused sexually by their parents or guardians each year. It is far more frequent between brothers and sisters and between fathers and daughters than between mothers and sons. Adults who abuse children in their families may be pedophiliacs, but very often they are simply sexual opportunists or people with poor impulse control and emotional problems. Incest is usually an intensely damaging psychological experience that contributes to persistent sexual difficulties. Today incest is forbidden in virtually every society, with punishments varying from social disapproval to jail sentences.

Many studies have shown that people who were involved in incest as children never tell anyone about it and retain feelings of guilt, shame, resentment, anger, or low self-esteem as a result of the experience. Very often they have difficulty in establishing intimate relationships in adulthood as a result of the incest. If you were involved in incest or sexual abuse as a child and feel it may be interfering with your functioning today, you may want to address the problem. A variety of approaches may help, such as joining a support group of people who had

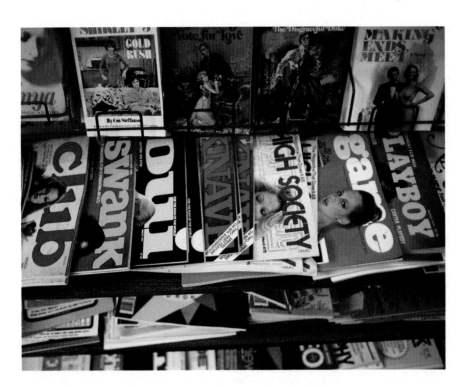

Erotic magazines tend to depict sexuality in an unrealistic and distorted way. By depersonalizing women and glamorizing male forcefulness, they may promote some of the attitudes that lie behind sexual harassment and sexual assault.

similar experiences, confiding in a partner or friend, or seeking professional help. Some people have experienced tremendous relief by confronting the person who abused them years earlier, but the possible consequences of this course of action have to be carefully considered, preferably with the help of a counselor or therapist.

Sexual Harassment Widespread wishful thinking probably underlies the commonly held notion that women say no to sex even when they mean yes. As a result, some men consider **sexual pressuring** legitimate even when women are clearly refusing sex. Women are becoming less willing to put up with such unwelcome advances, and perpetrators are becoming more aware of victims' feelings. When sexual pressuring involves someone in a vulnerable position—such as an employee pressured by the boss or a student by a professor—it constitutes **sex-**

ual harassment and takes on the form of blackmail: either you give me sex or I will fire (fail) you. Men are usually, but not always, the offenders, partly because they are more often in positions of power. Abuse of power for sexual gain is fairly widespread. A recent survey of 17,000 federal employees found that 42 percent of women and 15 percent of men had been sexually harassed.

If you have been the victim of sexual harassment, you can take action to stop it. If it's emotionally possible for you, confront your harasser either in writing, over the telephone, or in person, informing him or her that the situation is unacceptable to you and you want the harassment to stop. If that doesn't work, begin to assemble a file of memos documenting the harassment, noting times, places, and circumstances of each incident, along with any witnesses who may be able to support your

---

Paraphilia Variant choice of sexually arousing activities or partners.

Voyeurism Secretly watching others undress or engage in sexual activities for one's own sexual pleasure.

Exhibitionism Exhibiting one's genitals to unwilling observers to derive sexual pleasure; "flashing."

Fetishism Sexual attachment to inanimate objects or body parts.

Pedophilia Coercive sexual interactions between adults and children.

Transvestism Repeatedly dressing in clothes of the opposite gender for sexual pleasure; cross-dressing.

Transsexualism Rejecting one's assigned gender and feeling trapped in a wrong-sex body.

Bestiality (zoophilia) Sexual interactions between humans and animals.

Sexual sadism Inflicting psychosocial and physical pain to obtain sexual arousal.

Masochism Suffering pain to obtain sexual enjoyment.

Sexual coercion Use of physical or psychological force or intimidation to force a person to submit to sexual demands.

Incest Sexual activity between close relatives, such as siblings or parents and their children.

Sexual pressuring Persistently making unwanted sexual advances.

Sexual harassment Sexual pressuring of someone in a vulnerable or dependent position, such as a youth, student, naive person, or employee.

claims. You may discover others who have been harassed by the same person, which will strengthen your case. Then file a grievance with the harasser's supervisor or employer, such as someone in the dean's office if you are a student or someone in the personnel office if you are an employee.

If your attempts to deal with the harassment internally aren't successful, you can file an official complaint with your city or state Human Rights Commission or Fair Employment Practices Agency or with the federal Equal Employment Opportunity Commission. You may also wish to pursue legal action under the Civil Rights Act or under local laws prohibiting employment discrimination. Very often the threat of a lawsuit is enough to stop the harasser.

Sexual Assault: Rape   Sexual coercion that relies on the threat and use of physical force or takes advantage of circumstances that render a person incapable of giving consent (such as when drunk) constitutes **sexual assault** or **rape.** When the victim is younger than the legally defined "age of consent," the act constitutes **statutory rape,** whether or not coercion is involved. Any woman—or man—can be a rape victim. It is conservatively estimated that at least 3.5 million females are raped annually in the United States. Some men are raped by other men, perhaps 10,000 annually—and not all of these rapes are committed in prison.

Rape victims suffer both physical and psychological injury. For most, physical wounds are not severe and heal within a few weeks. Psychological pain may endure and be substantial. Even the most physically and mentally strong are likely to experience shock, anxiety, depression, shame, and a host of psychosomatic symptoms after being victimized. These psychological reactions following rape are called rape trauma syndrome, which is characterized by fear, nightmares, fatigue, crying spells, and digestive upset. Self-blame is very likely; society has contributed to this tendency by perpetrating the myths that women can actually defend themselves and that no one can be raped if she doesn't want to. Fortunately, these false beliefs are dissolving in the face of evidence to the contrary.

Men who commit forcible rape may come from any social class and be any age. About half of all rapists are exploiters in the sense that they rape on the spur of the moment and mainly want immediate sexual gratification. About a fourth of them attempt to compensate for feelings of sexual inadequacy and inability to obtain satisfaction otherwise. A fifth of rapists are more hostile and sadistic and are not primarily interested in sex but in hurting and humiliating a particular woman or women in general.

Sometimes husbands rape wives. Strong evidence suggests that one of every seven American women who have ever married has been raped by her husband or ex-husband. One study found that 60 percent of 430 battered women had been raped by their husbands. There is little evidence that mates rape because wives have refused reasonable sexual requests. Rather it appears that the husbands liked violent sex and used physical force to intimidate and control the wives. In some cases the situation grows out of a relationship characterized by poor communication and verbal and sometimes physical violence. A charge of mate rape can now be taken to court in over half the states.

The role of **pornography** in rape and other acts of violence against women has been investigated in recent years. Many educators, social scientists, and feminists distinguish between "soft porn" or **erotica**—the explicit or implicit depiction of sexual activities in which mutual empathy and enjoyment are reflected—and "hard porn"—the explicit depiction of sexual activities involving violence, exploitation, and degradation of victims. People use soft porn to learn about different sexual behaviors and to become sexually aroused; heavy exposure to it seems to lead to satiation and boredom rather than to changes in sexual behavior. Hard porn, on the other hand, with its focus on violence and dominance, is associated with aggressive feelings and antisocial attitudes, especially toward women. But it appears to be the violence itself, not the sexual content of pornography, that stimulates aggression. Furthermore, there is no reliable evidence that pornography by itself causes men to rape women.

Date Rape   Most college women are in much less danger of being raped by a stranger than of being sexually assaulted by a man they date. Surveys suggest that as many as one woman in four has had experiences in which the man she was dating persisted in trying to force sex on her despite her pleading, crying, screaming, or resisting.

Sexual assault   Use of force to gain sexual access to someone.

Rape   Coercing a person into sexual relations by threats or use of force.

Statutory rape   Sexual interaction with someone below the legal age of consent.

Pornography   Explicit depiction of sexual activities; made to sell.

Erotica   Sensual depictions of adults engaging in sexual activities.

Monogamous   Referring to the condition of being married to only one person at a time.

One of every 6 to 15 women has been raped by a man she knew or was dating. Most cases of date rape are never reported to the police, partly because of the subtlety of the crime. Usually no weapons are involved and direct verbal threats may not have been made. Rather than being terrorized, the victim usually is attracted to the man at first. Victims of date rape tend to shoulder much of the responsibility for the incident, questioning their own judgment and behavior rather than blaming the aggressor. Many college women are especially vulnerable to date rape because of their relative inexperience and lack of sophistication about men.

One factor in date rape appears to be the double standard about appropriate sexual behavior for men and women. Although the general status of women in society has improved, it is still a commonly held cultural belief that nice women don't say yes to sex (even when they want to) and that real men don't take no for an answer. The scenario in which a woman puts up token resistance but then willingly yields to a man's forceful sexual advances is a common one in books and films. The message is not lost on millions of men who want to "score" sexually.

There are also widespread differences between men and women in how they perceive romantic encounters and signals. In one study, researchers found that men tend to interpret women's actions on dates, such as smiling or talking in a low voice, as indicating an interest in having sex, while the women interpreted the same actions as just being "friendly." Men's thinking about forceful sex also tends to be unclear. One psychologist reports that men find "forcing a woman to have sex against her will" more acceptable than "raping a woman," even though the former description is the definition of rape.

Aside from the double standard and unclear perceptions and thinking about sex, men who rape their dates tend to have certain attributes, including hostility toward women, a belief that dominance alone is a valid motive for sex, and an acceptance of sexual violence. They may feel that force is justified in certain circumstances, such as if they are sexually involved with a woman and she refuses to "go all the way," if the woman is known to have slept with other men, or if the woman shows up at a party where people are drinking and taking drugs. The man often primes himself to force himself sexually on his date by drinking, which lowers his ordinary social inhibitions. Many college men who have committed date rape tried to seduce their dates by plying them with alcohol and marijuana first.

Date rape is largely a result of sexual socialization in which the man develops an exaggerated sexual impulse and puts a premium on sexual conquests. Sex and violence are linked in our society, and coercion is accepted by some adolescents as an appropriate form of sexual

expression. Both males and females can take actions that will reduce the incidence of date rape in our society; see the box entitled "Dealing with Rape" for specific guidelines and suggestions.

Intimate Relationships

Sexual attraction is an important bond that holds people together in intimate relationships, but it isn't the only bond, nor even the most important one. Many human needs are satisfied in intimate relationships—needs for approval and affirmation, for companionship, for meaningful ties and a sense of belonging, for a partner with whom to face life's challenges. Truly satisfying and lasting intimate relationships go well beyond sexual behavior.

The early stages of many intimate relationships are often exhilarating, filled with romance, passion, emotional excitement. Lovers are preoccupied with each other, idealizing virtues and ignoring faults. They live in a tumultuous state of "being in love," prey to their wildly fluctuating feelings of joy—when love is reciprocated—and despair—when uncertainty takes over or rejection seems possible. Researchers are now investigating the neurological and hormonal changes that produce these symptoms in the "lovesick." Some partners work successfully to maintain emotional excitement in their relationship; others lose the shine with age.

Love has other faces and deeper roots than those found in relationships built solely on either the erotic or the romantic aspects. The need to love and to be loved may be the most powerful motivating force in human behavior. Loving another person is an alternative to selfishness. Relationships built on altruism, caring, nurturing, and mutually fulfilling needs enhance and enlarge the partners and bring out their generous, giving capabilities. These feelings are the basis for friendship and companionship, regardless of other aspects of a relationship—whether sexual, parental, brotherly, or other. Many relationships initially based on sexual and spiritual attraction develop from wild passion to a deep, affectionate, long-lasting attachment to another person over the course of time. As an intimate relationship grows, it provides the partners with feelings of closeness, contentment, and joy. It supplies the security and support that helps them grow in both inner and outer ways and to function well in the world. It also provides the most solid foundation for raising children.

Most people seek intimacy in long-term, **monogamous** relationships, especially marriage. Over 90 percent of all Americans marry at least once in their lifetime. In 1987, 63 percent of the adult population (18 years and older) were married, 22 percent were single (primarily in the

Dealing With Rape

To reduce the risk of being raped, try not to let yourself get into vulnerable situations; specifically

- Avoid dark, lonely city streets or parks.
- Stay aware of your surroundings and notice if anyone is following you.
- Have your keys out in your hand as you approach your car or house so you can get inside quickly, and lock the door behind you.
- Avoid showing that you are alone in a house or apartment.
- Find out with certainty who is at the door before opening it.
- Try to look confident, strong, and purposeful when you're out by yourself.
- Try to remain as cool as possible in all situations.
- Think out in advance what you would do if you were threatened with rape.

When asked what to tell women who found themselves facing a rapist, an experienced counselor responded:

Please be very careful about giving specific advice on what to do. There is great disagreement on the subject. Some rapists say that if a woman had screamed or resisted loudly, they'd have run; others report they'd have killed her. Self-defense training is valuable in that it helps a woman feel and act more assertively, but it is risky in that none of us really knows how we would use it when scared to death—and badly or ineffectively used active self-defense could get us killed. Some say it is best to seem to give in quietly so as to avoid being injured or killed, and to try to calm the rapist, to win time, so that escape is more likely should the opportunity arise. The trouble with telling a woman she *should* resist and yell is that she adds to her already large burden of guilt if she does not do so, and it plays into the hands of prosecutors and those who insist (against the law) that a woman isn't really raped unless she is beaten up or shows signs of struggle. I think it is best to give various options and then say that each woman and each rapist and each situation are unique, and the woman should respond in whatever way she thinks best.

If you are threatened by a rapist and decide to fight back, here is what Women Organized Against Rape (WOAR) recommends:

- *USE YOUR VOICE!* Yell and keep yelling. (This may sound obvious but you would be surprised how few people have ever really yelled. It takes practice and you should do it today.) Yelling will clear your head and start your adrenalin going. It may scare your attacker and also bring help.
- If you just throw your hands out for striking, they can be grabbed by an attacker and used to get you down.
- If an attacker grabs you from behind, use your *elbows* for striking the neck or his sides, or even his stomach to take him by surprise.
- Don't forget that a rapist also feels pain and is also afraid of pain, plus he is afraid of getting caught. Try to use this weakness to get away.
- Your legs are the strongest part of your body—they have been carrying you around all of your life. Your kick is longer than his reach and a series of hard, fast kicks should keep him away from you. Always kick with your rear foot and with the toe of your shoe. Aim low to avoid losing your balance.
- His most vulnerable spot is his *knee;* it's low, difficult to protect, and easily knocked out of place. The most effective kick is a glancing one across his kneecap.
- Don't try to kick a rapist in the crotch. He has been protecting this area all of his life. In addition, he may grab your foot, knocking you off balance.
- Trust your gut feelings. If you feel you are in danger, don't hestitate to run and scream. It is better to feel foolish than to be raped. In any situation, screaming and a general uproar are strongly recommended.
- Remember that ordinary rules of behavior don't apply. It's OK to vomit, act "crazy," or claim to have a sexually transmissible disease.
- When you do decide to fight, always accompany it with a strong bellowing war cry.
- Don't ever expect a single blow to end the fight. Don't give up, keep fighting. Your objective is to get away, and to get away as soon as you can.
- If a rapist is carrying a weapon, you shouldn't fight unless absolutely necessary.

Dealing With Rape (continued)

If you are raped, WOAR gives the following advice:

- Tell what happened to the first friendly person you meet.
- Call the police. Use the emergency number. Give your location and tell them you were raped.
- Try to remember as many facts as you can about your attacker: clothes, height, weight, age, skin color, etc. Try to remember his car, license number, the direction in which he went, etc. Write all this down right away.
- *Don't* wash or douche before the medical exam, or you destroy important evidence. *Don't* change your clothes, but bring a new set with you if you can.
- At the hospital you will have a complete exam, including a pelvic exam. Show the doctor any bruises, scratches, etc.
- Tell the police simply but exactly what happened. Try not to get flustered. Have a friend or relative accompany you if possible. Be honest and stick to your story.
- If you do not want to report the rape to the police, see a doctor as soon as possible. Make sure you are checked for pregnancy and venereal disease.
- Contact an organization with skilled counselors so you can talk about the experience. Look in the telephone directory under "Rape" or "Rape Crisis Center" for a hotline number to call or a local chapter of WOAR.

To avoid date rape:

- Believe in your right to control what you do. Set limits and communicate these limits clearly, firmly, and early. Say "no" when you mean "no."
- Be assertive with someone who is sexually pressuring you. Often men interpret passivity as permission.
- Remember that some men assume sexy dress and a flirtatious manner mean a desire for sex.
- Remember that alcohol and drugs interfere with clear communication about sex.
- Use the statement that has proven most effective in stopping date rape: "This is rape and I'm calling the cops."

Guidelines for men:

- Be aware of social pressure. It's OK not to "score."
- Understand that "no" means "no." Don't continue making advances when your date resists or tells you she wants to stop. Remember that she has the right to refuse sex.
- Don't assume sexy dress and a flirtatious manner are invitations to sex, that previous permission for sex applies to the current situation, or that your date's relationships with other men constitute sexual permission for you.
- Remember that alcohol and drugs interfere with clear communication about sex.

Adapted from Daniel Goleman, When the rapist is not a stranger, *New York Times,* August 29, 1989, pp. B1 and B11, and M. S. Calderone and E. W. Johnson, *The Family Book about Sexuality.* (New York: Harper and Row, 1989), pp. 176–7.

youngest age groups), and 15 percent were widowed or divorced. One of the clearest benefits of intimate relationships can be seen in health statistics: married people enjoy better health and have lower death rates than single, widowed, or divorced people for a wide range of conditions, including heart disease.

Although intimacy is clearly an important and desirable component of a healthy life, it can be elusive. Many relationships founder on the rocks of poor communication, lack of understanding, or personal psychological problems. What are the characteristics of successful relationships, and how can people work toward them?

Characteristics of Relationships That Work   Constructive partnerships—in which both parties grow and realize their potential—share some characteristics. Ideally, an intimate relationship evolves through the sharing of private, inner feelings. Its strength derives from mutual affection, trust, acceptance, respect, understanding, and a willingness to make oneself emotionally available. A central tenet in human relationship building is affirmation—the art of giving and receiving support. People who successfully affirm themselves and others believe both in their own capability of actively, adequately, and creatively nurturing others and in unlimited potential growth, strength, and beauty in the people they nurture. Each partner is an emotional resource for the other.

Worthwhile relationships carry both rights and responsibilities. Partners have the right to be themselves and to be valued for what they are. They also have the right to the freedom to grow—even to grow apart. If one person demands that the other change—or stay the same—in order to preserve the relationship, it may already be doomed. Both partners have the right to the private time and space they need to pursue their own interests, tap their own resources, and sort out their thoughts and feelings. They have the right to expect honesty and to be able to trust the other.

At the same time, if the partners want a relationship to work, they have to accept responsibilities. Primary among these is commitment—to each other and to the relationship. A relationship represents an investment of time, energy, and effort, and without them, it will quickly diminish and lose its value. Partners also have to take responsibility for themselves as individuals, for their own emotions and personal lives.

Passive or dependent partners pose burdens on a relationship by relinquishing decisions and responsibilities, often complaining or blaming the partner for things that go wrong. On the other hand, a partner who assumes a strong take-charge posture may encourage passivity by undermining the other's resolve to actively assume responsibility. Such a lop-sided partnership has the qualities of a parent-child relationship rather than those of a strong give-and-take peer relationship.

Healthiest relationships evolve between people who take responsibility for themselves financially, spiritually (they create sufficient excitement and passion from things they do for themselves) and emotionally (they develop a support group). The strongest foundation for a primary relationship is self-knowledge, a strong sense of personal worth, and a continuing pursuit of personal interests, friendships, and inner truths.

A critical component of any satisfying relationship is the ability to communicate. Relationships that survive are usually those in which the partners verbally share their expectations and limitations with each other. Successful communication begins with active listening—sending back and acknowledging the partner's message rather than conveying one's own message. In all relationships, including those between parents and children, attempts to communicate can be cut off by a variety of counterproductive responses, such as preaching, advising, agreeing, disagreeing, analyzing, giving logical arguments, sympathizing, probing, and humoring (see the box entitled "Conflict Management: Learning to Fight"). The first requirement for true communication is that the message simply be heard and understood. Sometimes a person just needs to talk or unburden him- or herself, and it may be enough to listen and reflect back what is said.

At other times, a reaction or opinion may be desired, and the partner has to expose his or her own thoughts and feelings. Some subjects are harder to discuss than others, such as specific emotional and sexual needs and desires. Since no one can read minds, partners may have

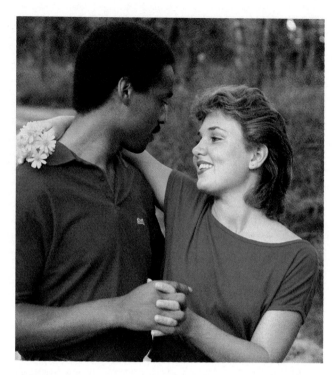

Most people choose a partner from a fairly small pool of candidates very much like themselves. Interracial couples face certain obstacles in their relationship, but they can overcome them if they are compatible, tolerant of differences, and good at communicating with each other.

to make clear statements and requests in order to be understood: "I don't like it when you . . .", "I would like you to . . ." The partner of whom the request is made has to retain the option of refusing if giving appears to be at his or her emotional expense. People have to say no even to reasonable requests when they don't have the patience, psychological energy, or time to comply. Good communication doesn't mean that people always reach agreement, but it does mean that they talk about their concerns, no matter how uncomfortable or unpleasant the issue may be.

These are some of the characteristics that have been observed of relationships that provide lasting satisfaction for the partners—mutual respect, trust, and affection; commitment; respect for one's own and the other's rights; acceptance of responsibility for oneself in the relationship; and open communication. Successful relationships also depend on the characteristics of the partners and how they interact. What are the important qualities a person should look for in a compatible intimate?

Selecting a Compatible Partner   There aren't any set rules for choosing partners in intimate relationships, but the process is neither random nor mysterious. Most men and women select partners for stable relationships quite carefully and through a fairly predictable process. Although the pool of potential candidates appears huge,

Conflict Management: Learning to Fight

Conflicts in intimate relationships may result from differences in emotional and sexual needs, in tastes in music or political views, or even in degrees of neatness. Frustration and anger in intimate relationships cannot be entirely avoided. This is not something to feel guilty about, but rather an indication that strong feelings of dissatisfaction need to be worked out. Expressing dissatisfaction usually does not mean you do not care for your partner. (If lack of caring is the real message, actions will show it and arguing won't help.)

Women, in particular, have been taught to deny their aggressive feelings. But now many therapists are recognizing the value of expressing anger and conflict. They are training clients in conflict management, a skill everyone needs. This does not mean that you are entitled to have a temper tantrum at any time over any issue. To be constructive, the anger must be kept within reasonable bounds. Physical violence is always completely unacceptable.

The point of a fruitful argument is not to insult or demean your partner but to discuss or explain whatever is bothering you, to give the other person an opportunity to explain and make amends, thereby clearing the air and improving your mutual understanding. The aim is not victory for one and defeat for the other, but some reasonable compromise. Here are some suggestions for managing conflict:

1. Try not to start an argument unless you know what you are angry about. If you are jealous, don't pretend your anger is about the choice of restaurant. And don't argue just to get attention.

2. Try to determine whether your feelings and their intensity are appropriate to the issue. Don't dramatize.

3. Know what you want to accomplish. Are you just letting off steam? Making a point? Will you insist on behavior change? Settle for compromise? State your complaint and your desires simply and clearly. Then wait for a response.

4. Allow enough time. Avoid jumping into an argument five minutes before you are scheduled to go out for a night on the town or if you are expecting company. Pick a time and place where you can both be open without embarrassing each other. That will give you time to cool off and to think through the problem.

5. Try not to lay on the guilt. Relating what you feel—anger, hurt—is more effective than blaming and accusing. And don't leave in the middle of an argument.

6. Do not let the situation overwhelm you. If you feel overpowered by the other person, say so and ask for the courtesy of speaking your mind without interruption. If you feel intimated, say so. Remember, you are supposed to be equals.

7. Listen. See if your partner has acceptable reasons for her or his actions. Laziness, greediness, and selfishness are not good reasons. If you are the defendant, acknowledge what you hear by repeating the accusation to make sure you heard it clearly.

8. Try corresponding by mail. Personal feelings can sometimes be more easily influenced by logic and rational thought with some emotional distance.

9. If you are the one confronted, do not immediately try to defend yourself or feel righteously indignant. Let the other person vent his or her wrath. Don't crumble in guilt or defensiveness. Don't close yourself off angrily. Don't deny the conflict.

10. So far as possible, focus on the particular issue at hand. Deal with one problem at a time. Criticize your partner's behavior but do not attack his or her personality. Stick to concrete actions and avoid abstractions.

---

most people pair with someone who lives in the same geographical area and who is similar in racial, ethnic, and socioeconomic background; educational level; lifestyle; physical attractiveness; and other traits. In simple terms, people select partners like themselves.

First attraction is based on easily observable characteristics—looks, dress, social status, and reciprocated interest. Although people may fall in love and be tempo-rarily swept away by their feelings, wildly romantic love is not really a good basis for a successful relationship. The idealization and euphoria of romantic love cloud people's perceptions and judgments, preventing them from seeing each other as they really are. An episode of being in love may last a week or two or go on for many years. The turmoil usually winds down gradually as one or both partners gain a more realistic view of the other.

At this point, personality traits and private behaviors become more significant factors in how the partners view each other. They begin to get a better idea of each other's capacity for closeness and readiness to form an intimate relationship. Through sharing and revealing their inner feelings and thoughts, they gradually gain a deeper understanding of each other. The emphasis shifts to basic values, such as religious beliefs, political persuasion, sexual attitudes, and future aspirations regarding career, family, and children. At some point, they decide whether the relationship feels viable and is worthy of their continued commitment. If they are compatible, people who were once "in love" with each other gradually shift into more enduring forms of love, affection, and deep attachment.

When people choose compatible intimates, they can't assess "applicants" the way employers do, but they can use some standards to evaluate possible partners. Perhaps the most important question they can ask themselves is, How much do we have in common? Although differences add interest to a relationship, especially at first, similarities in education, socioeconomic background, values, tastes, and interests increase the chances of a relationship's success.

If there are major differences between the partners, such as in educational level, religion, or ethnic background, partners should ask, first, How tolerant of differences are we? And second, How well do we communicate? Tolerance and good communication skills go a long way toward making a relationship work, no matter how different the partners. Several specific issues that arise in relationships are addressed in the compatibility quiz presented in the box "How Compatible Are You and Your Prospective Partner?" Try answering these questions to clarify your thinking on some important issues and to assess your compatibility with a partner, either current or future.

Living Together: A Growing Trend   In Western societies, courtship during a period of **engagement** has traditionally provided a socially approved means for individuals to get to know each other. Dating and going steady usually precede engagement or substitute for it. Intimate relationships that last long enough are usually formalized around a living arrangement. In our culture, this arrangement has typically taken the form of marriage, but a growing number of couples are choosing **cohabitation** (living together without legal recognition) instead of marriage or as a prelude to it. They are usually interested in establishing a relationship based more on

companionship and emotional commitment than on formal ties.

Currently, over 2 million couples (about 4 percent of single adults) live together without being married. This figure represents a 47 percent increase since 1980, a rise that clearly reflects changing social norms about the acceptance of premarital sex. Several other factors are involved in this change as well, including increased availability of contraceptives, the trend for people to wait longer before getting married, and a larger pool of divorced people who have the option of living with someone.

Cohabitation is more popular among younger people than older, although a significant number of older couples live together without marrying because they would lose a source of income, such as Social Security benefits, if they were to marry. According to the U.S. Bureau of the Census, 22 percent of unmarried people who lived together in 1987 were under 25 years of age, 61 percent were between 25 and 44, 11 percent were between 45 and 64, and 6 percent were 65 and older. Over 30 percent of the couples had children younger than 15 living in their households. For many younger couples, cohabitation is either temporary or the prelude to marriage. Only a minority of these couples find cohabitation a satisfactory long-term alternative to marriage.

Whatever the reasons for choosing cohabitation, living together provides many of the benefits of marriage—companionship, a setting for an enjoyable and meaningful relationship, the opportunity to develop greater intimacy through learning, compromising, and sharing. It also provides the opportunity for more frequent and varied sexual experiences than dating does and the development of a more trusting and satisfying sex life.

For those who choose it, living together also has certain advantages over marriage. For one thing, it can give the partners a greater sense of autonomy. They don't feel bound by the social rules and expectations that are part of the institution of marriage. They may find it easier to keep their identity and more of their independence, and they don't incur the same obligations that marriage brings. If things don't work out, they may find it easier and less complicated to leave a relationship that hasn't been legally sanctioned.

But living together has its liabilities, too. In most cases, the legal protections of marriage are absent, such as health insurance benefits and property and inheritance rights. These considerations can be particularly serious if the couple has children, from either former or current relationships. Since social acceptance of cohabitation is

---

Engagement   Provisional agreement to marry.

Cohabitation   To live together in a sexual relationship when not legally married.

How Compatible Are You and Your Prospective Partner?

Are you and your prospective mate compatible? To find out, take this quiz and let your partner do the same. Then compare your answers.

According to psychologist Karen Shanor of Washington, D.C., who helped put this quiz together, the more areas of agreement here, the less possible conflict in marriage.

However, she says, it's no fun to be married to a clone, so it's OK to have some disagreement—provided that you're able to compromise or, at least, agree to disagree.

This quiz is not meant to be a valid scientific measure of your compatibility. It was put together as an exercise to get you thinking about situations that can be difficult and cause stress in a relationship.

The issues were chosen because they have specifically been mentioned by various couples who have sought counseling from Shanor.

1. How many of the 10 items on this list do you have in common with your prospective mate: religion, career, same home town or neighborhood, friends, education level, income level, cultural pastimes, sports/recreation activities, travel, physical attraction?
a. Almost everything on the list.
b. Quite a few.
c. A few.
d. Almost none.

2. Would you prefer a relationship that is
a. Male-dominated.
b. Female-dominated.
c. A partnership.

3. What banking arrangement sounds best after marriage?
a. Separate account.
b. Joint account.
c. Joint account, but some cash for each of you to spend as you please with no accounting.

4. If you share an account, whose responsibility should it be to balance the checkbook and pay bills?
a. The man in the family.
b. The woman in the family.
c. Whoever is better at math and details.

5. If you inherited $10,000, would you prefer it to be:
a. Saved toward a major purchase.
b. Spent on something you could enjoy together such as a vacation.
c. Spent on luxury items you could enjoy individually, such as a fur coat or golf clubs.

6. Where do you think you should spend major holidays?
a. With his family.
b. With her family.
c. Alternating with his and her family.
d. At your place and inviting the relatives.
e. Just the two of you at home, or with friends, or off on vacation.

7. How frequently do you want to see your in-laws if they live in the same town?
a. Only on special occasions and holidays.
b. Twice a month.
c. At least once a week.

8. How frequently do you enjoy talking with your own parents?
a. Every day.
b. Once a week.
c. Once a month or less.

9. If you both have careers, what will be your priority?
a. Marriage before career.
b. Marriage equally important to career.
c. Career before marriage; my spouse is going to have to be understanding.

10. If you are offered a career promotion with a hefty raise making your income much more than your spouse's but involving a move out of state, would you
a. Expect your mate to be agreeable to relocation.
b. Try a commuter marriage; only seeing each other weekends or occasionally.
c. Say no rather than move; money isn't everything.

11. If your new spouse sets aside one evening a week to go out with a friend or friends of his or her same sex would you feel
a. Jealous of the time away from you.
b. Happy that he or she has friends.
c. This should not go on; let your feelings be known.

12. If you've had a bad day at the office and come home feeling moody, would you prefer that your mate
a. Back off, get out of the way.
b. Act sympathetic, be a good listener.
c. Discuss the events that led to your mood, perhaps offering some alternative suggestions for dealing with the people or problems that made you unhappy.

How Compatible Are You and Your Prospective Partner? (continued)

13. If your mate does something that makes you extremely angry, are you most likely to
a. Forgive and forget it.
b. Hurl insults.
c. Mention you are angry at an appropriate time, preferably when the anger is first felt and explain why without making derogatory accusations.

14. If you can't stand his or her friends and he or she can't stand yours, how will you deal with this after marriage? (You may choose more than one.)
a. Cultivate new friends that you both can enjoy.
b. See your friends by yourself and let him or her do the same.
c. Phase out the friends you knew before marriage; expect your partner to do the same.

15. If you and your spouse-to-be are different religions, would you expect to
a. Convert before marriage.
b. Have him or her convert before marriage.
c. Take turns attending each other's place of worship.
d. Observe religious days separately.
e. Not worry about it; religion is not an issue in your relationship.

16. When do you want to start a family?
a. As soon as possible.
b. After you have spent a few years enjoying your relationship as a couple.
c. As soon as careers are firmly established.
d. Never.

17. What is your attitude about housework? (You may check more than one.)
a. It is unmasculine for a man to do it. A woman should do all of it even if she chooses to have a career.
b. It is fine for a man to help, but only with certain tasks, such as mowing the lawn or taking out the trash.
c. If a woman works outside the home, cleaning should be shared.
d. Even if a woman does not work outside the home, cleaning should be shared.
e. Hire a maid; regardless if it fits the family budget.

18. Before marriage, you go out as a couple several times a week. A few months after marriage, you realize that you are going out a lot less. Would you consider this
a. OK. The pace was exhausting.
b. Dull. You worry that you are being taken for granted.
c. Not OK. You and your mate should make plans for some evenings out or evenings at home with friends.

19. You need to buy a new suit. Your spouse wants to come along. Would you see this as a sign of
a. Interest in spending time with you.
b. Crowding your relationship.
c. Watch-dogging your taste or pocketbook.

20. How would you prefer to spend your annual vacation? (Check as many as apply.)
a. On a trip by yourself.
b. On a trip with your mate.

c. On a trip with your mate and another couple.
d. Visiting your relatives or in-laws at their homes.
e. At a beach relaxing.
f. Engaged in an active sport such as skiing, tennis camp, or hiking/camping.
g. Traveling to another city for sightseeing/shopping.
h. At home catching up on repairs, appointments, books, visits with friends.
i. I would rather take a vacation less frequently than once a year and spend this money on rent or mortgage, enabling us to live in a more convenient or prestigious neighborhood.

21. If you were hunting for a place to live, would you prefer being in
a. The country.
b. The suburbs.
c. The city.

22. If your spouse-to-be had many loves before he or she met you, would you prefer that he or she
a. Keep the details to himself or herself.
b. Tell you everything.
c. Answer truthfully, but only the questions you ask, such as what broke up each relationship.

23. If your new spouse is in a romantic mood and you are not, how would you be most likely to respond?
a. Communicate your mood; suggest another time.
b. Pretend you are feeling romantic.
c. Invent an excuse rather than communicate your mood.

How Compatible Are You and Your Prospective Partner? (continued)

Psychologist Karen Shanor Explains

1. The more you have in common, the more of your life you can share and enjoy together.

2. Research and experiences of many couples have shown that the equal relationship is most successful.

3 and 4. There is no one right answer. Decide what works best for you and creates the least tension in your relationship.

5. We've all learned early in life to spend our limited money in certain ways. For some, it's on clothes; for others, it's on home or travel. Unless we understand our priorities and communicate them to our partner, we can find ourselves in great financial conflict and tension.

6. Very often we expect others to celebrate holidays as we do and give them the same sense of importance as the family in which we grew up. This isn't always so. Be able to compromise on this one.

7 and 8. Some are happy going for years at a time without seeing relatives. Others intentionally buy the house next door and want to drop in every day. Most important here is to let your spouse know that he or she comes first before parents and in-laws.

9. Talk about career and marriage priorities. Can you be accepting of your spouse's choice if he or she considers time spent on work more important right now than time spent with you?

10. There is no one right answer. Decide what works best for you and creates the least tension in your relationship.

11. It's healthy to have friends. You can't realistically expect your mate to spend 24 hours around the clock with you. If you or your mate go off for a time with friends, it wouldn't be too mushy to kiss, hug, or otherwise reassure your mate by words or actions that he or she is still first in your life. A spouse needs to hear this.

12. There are times when answer A would be best; other occasions call for B or C. Be sensitive to your mate's mood. If you are the one in the bad mood, don't expect your mate to read your mind as to whether you need space, sympathy or discussion. Clue him or her in.

13. Answer C is best. Somewhere along the way, people have to learn how to express anger constructively.

14. Be careful here. If you make his or her old friends feel left out or unimportant, they could work on your prospective mate to break up your relationship.

15. If you have major differences on this one, you may want to consider terminating the relationship instead of committing to marriage.

16. It's impossible to have half a child. Compromise won't work on this one, so it is best to speak your mind before marriage.

17. The most successful marriages are the ones in which men and women do not limit themselves in the traditional masculine-feminine roles. The sharing of responsibility heightens a sense of trust, caring and cooperation.

18. Sometimes the pace during dating is frantic. It is nice to calm down, but not nice to settle down to the point that each of you is taking the other for granted. Marriage requires continual work if you are going to keep adventure and interest in the relationship.

19. Whether you see it as interest, crowding, or distrust, communicate your feelings to your mate. If you'd rather shop alone, let that be known too.

20. Agree upon your needs in advance of the annual vacation, or what should be a time of relaxation away from the daily grind will turn into a source of tension and arguments. There is nothing wrong with separate vacations if one of you wants to fish on the lake and the other enjoys sightseeing.

21. If you are set on a particular style of living and not willing to change it after marriage, speak up before you say, "I do."

22. In general, it is not a good idea to go into great detail about past relationships because they are not totally relevant to your current one. However, trust and honesty are very important. If your partner asks a question, answer honestly but think very carefully. If you are the one doing the questioning, ask yourself, "Do I really want to hear this?"

23. There are times in your relationship when you may not want to go along with your spouse's romantic feelings, but it is generally best to communicate in a nice way without making him or her feel rejected or unloved that you simply are not in the mood. Do suggest another time.

not universal, couples may feel pressure from family members or others to marry or otherwise change their living arrangement, especially if they have young children.

Although many people choose cohabitation as a kind of trial marriage, there is little evidence as yet that people who live together before getting married have happier or longer-lasting marriages. It may just be that whatever patterns are going to develop in the relationship, whether deeper intimacy or disillusionment, develop earlier than if the couple had not lived together before marriage.

Marriage: Formalizing an Intimate Relationship   So much conflict seems to be involved in marriage, and so many marriages break up, that it's fair to ask why so many people marry in the first place. The answer is simple: Marriage fulfills a number of basic needs, and its long history has made it an integral part of our culture. There are many important social, moral, economic, political, and other aspects of marriage, although these have changed over the years. In the past, people married mainly for practical economic and social purposes, such as raising children and rendering services to each other and society. Today, people marry more for personal, emotional reasons. This shift in emphasis places a greater burden on marriage to fulfill needs and expectations, sometimes unreasonably high ones. Let's look more closely at some personal aspects of marriage.

Benefits of Marriage   The primary functions and benefits of marriage are those of any intimate relationship: affection, personal affirmation, companionship, sexual fulfillment, emotional growth. Marriage also provides a nurturing setting in which to care for and socialize children, although a growing number of couples choose to remain childless. Raising children places enormous additional demands on a couple's time, energy, and financial resources, especially since society delegates to parents the primary responsibility for their children's physical, emotional, social, and moral well-being and development.

■ **Exploring Your Emotions**

What are your expectations of marriage? Do you think it should last forever? What influences your views of marriage?

Marriage is also important for its provision for the future. By committing themselves to remain together through good times and bad, men and women provide themselves with lifelong companions with whom to share the joys and sorrows of life. They also provide themselves with some insurance for their later years, when they may be ill or have other problems. Many couples arrive at a new appreciation of the benefits of marriage in their later years, when they can again enjoy the affection and com-

panionship that brought them together at the beginning of their marriage.

The opportunity to have a regular sex life is one of the chief benefits of marriage, and marital happiness is linked with satisfying sexual relations. But couples vary tremendously in their sexual desires, tastes, and needs. Some couples have intercourse every day or several times a day; others would find this frequency exhausting and unpleasant. If the partners agree and are satisfied, nearly any kind of sex life can be part of a happy marriage.

The Intimate Relationship over the Life Cycle of the Marriage   A marriage relationship isn't static, even though we've been led to believe that the prince and princess simply live happily ever after. Sometimes relationships lose their vitality, becoming meaningless and frustrating. Sometimes they grow more vital, becoming profoundly satisfying and meaningful. Whatever the overall pattern, relationships continually fluctuate and change as the partners grow, change, and enter new stages of life.

At first two different individuals must make many marital adjustments as they learn to live with one another. They have to adjust to each other's personal habits, learn to give and receive affection and love, work out their preferred modes of sexual expression, decide on a division of labor, adjust their social relationships with friends and family, develop ways of making decisions, and address many other tasks of marriage. Parenthood brings a new set of adjustments—shifting the focus of family emotions and activities, learning to care for a child, working out child care arrangements, making career decisions.

Partners must adjust further to each change in the family constellation or life cycle, whether it's the birth of another child, the beginning or the end of the school years, middle age, divorce, the death of a spouse, the birth of grandchildren, old age. Many studies and surveys show that all these changes affect marital happiness and satisfaction in generally consistent and predictable ways. In general, marital satisfaction is high at the beginning of marriage, drops during the child-rearing years when demands are greatest, and rises again after the last child has left home. Contrary to popular thinking, both men and women seem to be happier later in life than they were when they were younger.

Changing Roles in Marriage   Because marriage and family are such important institutions in our society, powerful roles are associated with them. Historically, men have been the providers and breadwinners in our society, and this is still their key role today. Men derive much of their self-esteem, personal satisfaction, and social status from their work, but they also have to contend with job-related stress, especially if they bear all the financial responsibility for supporting a family. Men suffer many more stress-related illnesses and health problems than women, although women are catching up. The time men have to

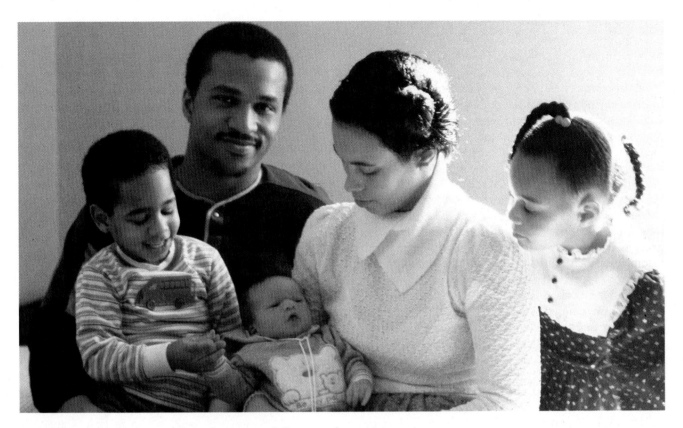

Every change in the family constellation brings new challenges to the marriage relationship. This couple will need flexibility, commitment, and continuing good will to adjust to their new roles as parents of three.

spend with their children is also limited, which means that both they and their children are deprived of important parent-child interactions.

The role of women has fluctuated more over time than that of men. In some periods, women have been mainly homemakers and caregivers, and in other periods, particularly during wars, they have been an important part of the labor force. Current social and economic trends seem to have produced a more or less permanent change in women's roles. Today, over 50 percent of married women are in the labor force, including women with babies under 1 year of age. Among women whose youngest child is in elementary or high school, almost 75 percent are working. Another significant change is that women currently head one-third of all families in the United States.

Even though social and economic patterns have changed, family roles have not kept up, and many married women who work full-time also continue to take most responsibility for the home and children. Most husbands have not taken on major housekeeping roles, even though they pay lip service to the fairness of sharing roles. The result is that working mothers put in a "second shift" after they come home from work, cooking, cleaning, and caring for the children. This pattern means that women are exhausted, men are still missing chances for

learning and growth, and children have less attention paid to their personal and social needs. This is just one of the marriage-related issues that people will be facing in the years ahead.

■ **Exploring Your Emotions**

What do you think are appropriate roles and activities for husbands and wives? If both husband and wife work full-time, do you think they should share housework and child care equally? What influences your view?

Marriage is a high-gain, high-risk proposition. Despite many changes and problems, it still offers a reasonable framework in which to work out the ups and downs of life for most couples. The vast majority of people seek to fulfill their intimacy needs through marriage—at least once. But as everyone knows, many marriages fail, ending in disillusionment and divorce. Handling the breakup of an important relationship is one of the most difficult experiences human beings can face.

Ending a Relationship Even when they begin with the best of intentions, intimate relationships may not last. Sometimes a couple is mismatched to begin with, or the association doesn't evolve and thrive over time. Although it's tempting to see relationships that fail as mistakes, some relationships simply outlive their usefulness as partners grow in unexpected and divergent ways.

Sexual intimacy is one of the earliest casualties of a faltering relationship. On the other hand, sexual incompatibilities can contribute to other problems in a relationship, creating additional strain. If a couple is unhappy, partners may lose interest and seek intimacy elsewhere. Extramarital affairs are common among both men and women in unhappy marriages. Most but not all such involvements further disrupt the relationship.

Some relationships prove unworkable because couples expect too much of them—no one can satisfy all the needs of another person—or because their aspirations are incompatible. The partners may lack the ability to solve problems and make compromises. They may lose the motivation and commitment to save the marriage. Even if they learn communication skills and resolve some problems through counseling, the relationship will fail if the partners are no longer willing to put energy into it.

Divorce—A Modern Cure-All?   Currently, over half of all marriages in the United States end in divorce. The divorce rate—the number of divorces per 1,000 people in the population—peaked in 1979 and then leveled off and even declined a little. The main reason for this trend is probably that the oldest members of the "baby boom" generation (people born between 1945 and 1960) reached prime divorcing age in the late 1970s. Although the trend is toward fewer divorces, the United States has one of the highest divorce rates in the world.

Very few couples decide to divorce without agonizing over it for months or even years. Even when they are very unhappy, have no loving feelings for their partner, believe it would be better to be out of the marriage than in it, or are having an extramarital affair, there may be other factors they have to weigh. These include financial considerations, religious beliefs or moral values, social or family pressure to stay married, the potential effect on children, and the likelihood of finding a new partner. If the decision is for divorce, the partners usually have to go through a painful adjustment (although in particularly unhappy or abusive marriages, the divorce may be a welcome relief). Divorce is typically an emotionally traumatic experience for everyone involved, often accompanied by shock, fear, anger, loneliness, despair, physical symptoms such as insomnia and diminished memory, and behavioral changes such as increased drinking or smoking. Children are especially vulnerable to the trauma of divorce, and sometimes counseling is appropriate to help them adjust to the changes in their lives.

About 75 to 80 percent of all people who divorce re-

marry, often within three to five years. One result of the high divorce and remarriage rates is a growing number of "blended" families, those made up of new spouses and their children from previous marriages. These families have many complicated relationships to work out and many adjustments to make, although there is no evidence that they are inherently less successful than first marriages.

Breaking Up   Although ending an important intimate relationship of shorter duration isn't as painful as ending a marriage, it can still be difficult and traumatic. Both partners often feel attacked and abandoned, but feelings of distress are likely to be more acute for the person who doesn't initiate the breakup. If you are involved in a breakup, following a few simple guidelines can make the ending easier for both partners.

- Give the relationship the best chance you can before breaking up. If it still isn't working, you'll know that you weren't able to make it succeed even with your best efforts. You'll feel less guilt and regret and have fewer doubts that you did the right thing.
- Be fair and honest. If you are the one initiating the breakup, don't try to make your partner feel responsible. You owe it to both of you to learn something from the experience so you'll have a better chance of avoiding the same mistakes in another relationship.
- Be tactful and compassionate. You can leave the relationship without putting your partner down or deliberately damaging his or her self-esteem. Rather than dwelling on your partner's shortcomings, emphasize your mutual lack of fit and admit your own contributions to the problem.
- If you are the rejected person, give yourself time to resolve the bitterness you may feel. Then be forgiving. If the relationship was important to you, you will need to go through a process of mourning. You may feel disbelief at first ("This can't be happening to me!"), then anger, sadness, and finally acceptance. Despite all the romantic talk about your "one and only," there are actually many potential candidates with whom you can establish intimate relationships.
- Find the value in the experience. Ending a close relationship can teach you valuable lessons about your needs, preferences, strengths, and weaknesses. Try to use your insights to make changes in yourself and to increase your chances of success the next time around.

Singlehood   Despite the prevalence and popularity of marriage, and despite the fact that less than 10 percent of the population never marries, a significant proportion of adults in our society are single. In 1987, about 22 percent of whites 18 years and older were single; for blacks, the figure was 34 percent, and for Hispanics, 26 percent. Included in the category "singles" are young people who have not married yet but plan to in the future, people who are living together, and people of all ages who would like to marry but haven't found a suitable mate. In other words, the category includes people of all ages who are single both by choice and by chance.

Being single doesn't mean that people don't have close relationships, however. They may date, enjoy active and fulfilling social lives, and have a variety of sexual experiences and relationships. When social psychologist Jonathan Freedman asked single and married people what made them happy, single men and women both listed friends and social life and being in love as very important factors. Unlike married people, singles are free to pursue and enjoy friendships with a variety of people of both sexes.

■ **Exploring Your Emotions**

How do you feel about single people? Do you think they're anxious to get married, or do you think they're happy to be single? What are the sources of your feelings about singlehood?

Other advantages of being single include economic self-sufficiency, more opportunities for personal and career development without concern for family obligations, greater variety in sexual partners, and more freedom and control in making life choices. Single people don't have to answer to a partner about how they live, take someone else's wishes into account, or compromise on what they want to do. On the other hand, loneliness and lack of companionship are significant disadvantages of being single, along with economic hardships (mainly for single women) and being deprived of the benefits of intimacy. Single people, both male and female, experience some discrimination and often are pressured to get married.

Nearly everyone has at least one episode of being single in adult life, whether it's prior to marriage, between marriages, following divorce or the death of a spouse, or for the entire adult life span. How enjoyable and valuable this single time is depends on several factors, including how deliberately the person has chosen it, how satisfied the person is with social relationships, standard of living, and job, how comfortable the person feels when alone, and how resourceful and energetic the person is about creating an interesting and fulfilling life. But a fulfilling life nearly always involves other people. No one can be happy completely isolated or deprived of human companionship. Single or married, young or old, people continue to need meaningful relationships throughout life.

Summary

- Even if not the overriding drive that Freud deemed it, sexuality is so powerful a motivator in human affairs that understanding and accepting its role in one's life is necessary to optimal health.

Sexuality in Human Relationships

- The most basic aspect of sexuality is reproduction. Nonreproductive aspects are sexual excitement and satisfaction.
- Love relationships without a sexual component are far more common than those with it.
- Gender identity and gender role are also aspects of sexuality. Some gender characteristics are determined biologically and others are defined by society.

Roots and Development of Sexual Behavior

- Many theories of sexual behavior are based on the concept of a sexual instinct or drive. Behavioral scientists assume that conditioning and social learning shape sexual behaviors. An integrative approach to sexual be-

havior explains it as the outcome of interacting biological and psychosocial factors.
- Social learning processes encourage traits and behaviors traditionally deemed appropriate for one sex or the other. Today gender roles are emerging that reflect an androgynous mix of male and female characteristics and behaviors.
- The ability to respond sexually is present at birth. Sexual behaviors emerging in childhood include self-exploration, perhaps leading to masturbation.
- Although puberty indicates biological adulthood, people need five to ten additional years to reach social maturity. Sexual fantasies and dreams and nocturnal emissions are characteristic of adolescence; most sexual interaction takes place in the context of dating.
- Developing the capacity for intimacy and becoming sexually experienced now seem to be important tasks of young adults.
- Although prejudice against homosexuals is not so great as it once was, homosexuality still has not received widespread societal approval. Sexual practices resemble

those of heterosexuals, except for coitus. AIDS has led many gay men to curtail and change their patterns of sexual behavior.

- Most people are heterosexual; Freud's Oedipus theory attempts to explain heterosexual orientation, but most psychologists don't accept his explanation.
- Celibacy is continuous abstention from sexual activities with others; it may be a conscious choice or may be necessitated by other factors.
- Autoerotic activity includes fantasy and masturbation. Fantasies are imaginary experiences or replays of past sexual experiences. Masturbation may be a substitute for coitus or a part of sexual activity with a partner.
- Touching is integral to sexual experience; the erogenous zones are more sensitive to touch than are the other body areas. People vary in their preferences for foreplay and need to communicate their wishes.
- Cunnilingus and fellatio may be part of arousal and foreplay or sex acts culminating in orgasm. Anal intercourse is less common and can be risky because of the threat of AIDS.
- Intercourse is the ultimate sexual experience for most adults. The key factor for a woman is adequate vaginal lubrication and psychological arousal; a man needs to be aroused enough by conditions and his partner to attain and maintain an erection.
- The pleasure of sexual activities must be accompanied by the responsibilities of contraception and safe sex.
- People are considered sex offenders if their sexual activity violates moral and legal codes, offends the public sense of decency, or threatens others.
- Some deviant sexual behaviors can be explained by the concept of a paraphilia, a condition in which a person's sexual arousal and gratification depend on an unusual object or act.
- Coercive sex is a serious problem in human relationships. Rape is the most extreme manifestation.
- Child molestation often results in serious trauma for the victim; often the pedophile is a relative, friend, or someone known to the victim. Incest contributes to persistent sexual difficulties.
- Sexual harassment is sexual pressuring of someone in a vulnerable position—an employee or student, for example.
- Rape victims suffer both physical and psychological pain. Society has contributed to the tendency for self-blame by perpetrating the myth that women can actually defend themselves and can't be raped if they don't want to be. Rape can happen within marriage.
- Erotica is distinguished from "hard" pornography, which depicts sexual activities involving violence, exploitation, and degradation of victims. The violence of pornography, not the sexual content, stimulates aggression.

- Date rape occurs in part because of the double standard about appropriate sexual behavior for men and women.

Intimate Relationships

- "Being in love" often means passion and emotional excitement, but in a long-term relationship it usually develops into a deep, affectionate attachment that supplies security and support.
- Many people seek intimacy in long-term monogamous relationships, especially marriage; a clear benefit is better health and lower death rates.
- Constructive intimate partnerships are based on affirmation, the art of giving and receiving support. Responsibilities in a relationship include commitment to the other and a commitment to the self.
- The ability to communicate is crucial to any relationship. Successful communication begins with listening and avoids counterproductive responses.
- Most people select partners carefully and through a predictable process. How much a couple has in common is of special importance; similarities increase the chances of a relationship's success.
- Cohabitation provides many of the benefits of marriage and may give partners a greater sense of autonomy.
- Marriage fulfills basic human needs and is an integral part of our culture. Today personal emotional reasons supersede economic and social reasons for marriage.
- Relationships change in marriages as partners enter new stages of life. Children always necessitate adjustments. Marital satisfaction is high at the beginning of marriage, drops during child-rearing years, and rises when the last child has left home.
- Men and women have always had specific roles associated with marriage and the family. Women's roles have changed more than men's have, and yet they seem to have retained most responsibility for tasks at home while entering the labor force.
- More than half of all marriages in the United States end in divorce. The decision is rarely made easily and is often delayed because of financial considerations, religious beliefs or moral values, and effects on children.
- Most divorced people remarry, leading to "blended" families with complicated relationships.
- Ending any relationship can be difficult. It helps to give the relationship the best chance possible; to be honest, tactful, and compassionate; to resolve the bitterness; and to find value in the experience.
- In any given year, a significant proportion of adults are single, by choice or by chance. Advantages of singlehood include economic self-sufficiency, opportunity for career and personal development, and more freedom and control in making life choices. Loneliness and lack of companionship are significant disadvantages.

Take Action

1. List in your health diary the characteristics and behaviors that you associate with being male or female. Where do you think you learned your ideas? When you examine them closely, are there any you'd like to change?

2. What approach do you take when it comes to communicating your feelings and needs to the people with whom you live or have important relationships? Think of a particular issue that has been bothering you and write down the statements you would make if you were discussing it with the appropriate person. Examine your statements to see if unrelated feelings or issues are coming through in them. Devise a strategy for dealing with the issue, using the guidelines in the box on conflict management.

3. If you have an intimate sexual relationship with a regular partner, think honestly about what is satisfying about it and what you would like to change. Is there anything you want to try but have been afraid to ask for? Take a chance and bring it up with your partner.

4. What are you looking for in a partner? Make a list of desirable qualities (such as a good sense of humor, generosity, and so on). Are they qualities you think you have? How realistic are your ideals?

Selected Bibliography

Crooks, Robert and Karla Baur. 1987. *Our Sexuality,* 3rd ed. Menlo Park, Calif.: Benjamin/Cummings.

Dorn, Lois. 1983. *Peace in the Family.* New York: Pantheon Books.

Haas, Kurt, and Adelaide Hass. 1987. *Understanding Sexuality,* St. Louis: Times Mirror/Mosby.

Masters, William H., Virginia E. Johnson, and Robert C. Kolodny. 1988. *Human Sexuality,* 3rd ed. Boston: Scott, Foresman.

Rice, F. P. 1990. *Intimate Relationships, Marriages, and Families.* Mountain View, Calif.: Mayfield.

Recommended Readings

Calderone, Mary S., and Eric W. Johnson. 1989. *The Family Book About Sexuality,* rev. ed. New York: Harper and Row. *A comprehensive guide to the development of sexuality throughout life, appropriate for a family reference book. The authors present both sides of controversial issues and stress the importance of sex education. This edition sensitively addresses teenage sex, pregnancy, homosexuality, and sexuality in the elder years.*

Davis-Kasl, Charlotte. 1989 (August). Women, sex and addiction. *East West* 19:34–9. *An insightful analysis of the codependent personality and how it functions in sexual relationships, using sex to buy love while staving off fears of abandonment, trying to fuse to another because it does not know its own boundaries. The author deduces the traits and behaviors requisite for successful relationships.*

Gaylin, Willard, and Ethel Person. 1988. *Passionate Attachments: Thinking about Love.* New York: The Free Press. *A fresh and compelling collection of essays in which humanists and scientists explore the nature and complexities of love, relating it to sexual behaviors, personality development, mythology, mental health, and the essence of humanity.*

Weinrich, James D. 1987. *Sexual Landscapes.* New York: Scribner. *A provocative tour of our sexual taboos and discomforts, wherein the author challenges our assumptions. Weinrich presents the results of fascinating research and controversial new theories on why we love and lust.*

Contents

Making Connections

Probably no single behavior has more potential for upsetting a young person's life plans than unprotected sexual activity, yet many people leave contraception up to chance. More than a million unplanned teenage pregnancies in the U.S. every year testify to the confusion and ambivalence surrounding contraceptive use in our country. The scenarios presented on these pages describe situations in which people have to use information, make a decision, or choose a course of action, all involving choices in contraception. As you read them, imagine yourself in each situation and consider what you would do. After you've finished the chapter, read the scenarios again and see if what you've learned has changed how you would think, feel, or act in each situation.

When you went home for Thanksgiving, you accidentally left your birth control pills at school. You missed three days, but started taking them again as soon as you got back, five days ago. Are your birth control pills providing you with effective contraception right now?

After a romantic evening with a man you've been dating for a few months, you and he go back to his room with the intention of having sex. Once you get there, you find he doesn't have any condoms. He assumed you had a diaphragm or took the pill. In fact, he says, "It's your responsibility—you're the one who could get pregnant." Is he right? Who *is* responsible? Is it up to you to get some contraceptives for future occasions?

6

Contraception

You call an old friend to see if you can get together and are shocked to discover he's had to drop out of college to support his wife and their new baby. You can't hide your dismay, because you knew he had plans to graduate and go on to law school. When he explains that he and his wife were relying on withdrawal as a contraceptive method, you're even more upset, since that's what *you* rely on. He says he was sure he withdrew in time, but she got pregnant anyway. Does this mean that you're not using a safe method? Is there anything you can do to make it safer, or should you start using contraceptives?

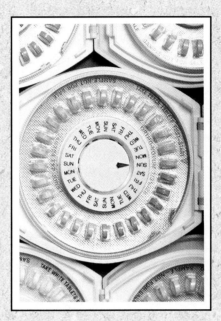

Even though you're seriously involved with your boyfriend, you're hoping to go to medical school after college and get established in your profession before you even think about getting married and starting a family. A career is very important to you, but children are too. You've thought quite a lot about abortion and come to the conclusion that you could never have one. All of this means that not getting pregnant by accident is a very high priority for you. What contraceptive method is the best choice for you?

You want to use vaseline to lubricate your condom before you make love, but your girlfriend says it's too risky. She claims that oil makes latex condoms break. You've never heard that and in fact often use vaseline or an oil-based hand lotion as lubrication. Is she wrong, or are you taking a big chance?

In her lifetime, the ovaries of an average woman produce over 400 eggs, one a month for about three and a half decades. Each is capable of developing into a human being if fertilized by one of the millions of sperm a man produces in every ejaculate. Furthermore, unlike most other mammals, human beings are capable of sexual activity at any time of the month or year. These facts help explain why people have always had a compelling interest in controlling fertility and in preventing unwanted pregnancies. Historical writings dating back to the fourth century B.C. mention the use of douches, sponges, and crude methods of abortion. Other materials mentioned as potential contraceptives include lemon juice, parsley, seaweed, olive oil, camphor, and opium. The underlying principle of these trial-and-error methods, although not clearly understood at the time, was basically the same as that of the **contraceptives** used today: the female's ovum (egg) was blocked from uniting with the male's sperm (**conception**), thereby preventing pregnancy.

Fortunately, modern contraceptive methods are much more predictable and effective than those used in the past. Today, people have many choices when they're making decisions about sexual and contraceptive behavior. And because the prevention of unintended pregnancies and **sexually transmissible diseases (STDs)** is such a crucial element in lifelong health and well-being, these decisions are among the most significant young people can make. However, because these decisions are also emotional, complex and difficult, they are often avoided or dealt with in ineffective ways.

While biological, social, and media pressures often encourage sexual activity at ever younger ages, few forces in the United States support a factual, realistic discussion of the importance of either postponing sexual intercourse or using contraception when intercourse is chosen. Our present superficial approaches to education are clearly ineffective: The United States has one of the highest teen pregnancy rates of all developed nations. Because many of women's changing roles are hampered severely by unplanned child rearing and the option of turning to abortion is becoming more restricted, the problem is even worse than the numbers show.

This chapter provides a basic framework of information on the various contraceptive methods, along with their advantages and disadvantages for different individuals. We hope that the issues we raise will provoke and clarify personal questions for you and encourage open discussion with others. The most critical decisions for you, however, will involve the time and type of sexual involvement best for you and the commitment to always protect yourself against unwanted pregnancy and STDs.

Principles of Contraception

A variety of approaches has proven effective in preventing conception; these approaches are based on different principles of birth control. Barrier methods work by physically blocking the sperm from reaching the egg. Diaphragms, condoms, and several other methods are based on this principle. Hormonal methods alter the biochemistry of the woman's body, preventing ovulation and producing changes that make it more difficult for the sperm to reach the egg if ovulation does occur. Birth control pills operate on this principle. A variety of so-called natural methods of contraception are based on the fact that egg and sperm have to be present at the same time if fertilization is to occur. Finally, surgical methods—female and male sterilization—more or less permanently prevent transport of the sperm or eggs to the site of potential conception.

All the contraceptive methods have advantages and disadvantages that make them appropriate for some people but not for others or at some periods of life but not at others. Factors that affect the choice of method include effectiveness, convenience, cost, reversibility, side effects and risk factors, and protection against STDs. Later in this chapter, we help you sort through these factors to decide on the method that's best for you if you are sexually active.

■ **Exploring Your Emotions**

Did your parents tell you anything about contraception? Are your ideas and needs different from their expectations for you?

Contraceptive   Any agent that can prevent conception. Condoms, diaphragms, intrauterine devices, and oral contraceptives are examples.

Conception   The fusion of ovum and sperm, resulting in a zygote (fertilized egg).

Sexually transmissible diseases (STD)   Any of several contagious diseases such as syphilis and gonorrhea contracted through intimate sexual contact.

Theoretical effectiveness   The failure rate of a contraceptive when it is used "exactly as directed." It cannot be accurately measured, but it is inferred from studying the most successful users.

Use effectiveness   The failure rate of a contraceptive when used under average conditions by average people.

Continuation rate   The percentage of women who continue to use a particular contraceptive after a specified period of time.

Myths about Contraception

Myth Taking borrowed birth control pills for a few days before having sexual relations gives reliable protection against pregnancy.

Fact Instructions for taking birth control pills must be followed carefully to provide effective contraception. With most pills, this means starting them with a menstrual period and then taking one every day.

Myth Pregnancy never occurs when unprotected intercourse takes place just before or just after a menstrual period.

Fact Menstrual cycles may be irregular, and ovulation may occur at unpredictable times.

Myth During sexual relations, sperm enter the vagina only during ejaculation and never before.

Fact The small amounts of fluid secreted before ejaculation may contain sperm.

Myth If semen is deposited just outside the vaginal entrance, pregnancy cannot occur.

Fact Sperm can live up to six or seven days within the woman's body and are capable of traveling through the vagina and up into the uterus and tubes.

Myth Douching immediately after sexual relations can prevent sperm from reaching and fertilizing an egg.

Fact During ejaculation (within the vagina), some sperm begin to enter the cervix and uterus. Since they are no longer in the vagina, it is impossible to remove them by douching after sexual relations.

Myth If a woman doesn't have an orgasm, pregnancy is unlikely to occur.

Fact The sperm and the egg can travel and unite to begin a pregnancy with or without female orgasm.

Myth A woman who is breast-feeding does not have to use any contraceptive method to prevent pregnancy.

Fact Frequent and regular breastfeeding may at times prevent ovulation, but does not do so in a consistent, reliable fashion.

Myth Women can't become pregnant the first time they have intercourse.

Fact *Any time* intercourse without protection takes place, sperm may unite with an egg to begin a pregnancy. There is nothing unique about first intercourse to prevent this.

Myth A pill is readily available as postcoital contraception.

Fact "Morning after pills" are not available in most U.S. clinics, as they have not been approved by the Food and Drug Administration.

The category *effectiveness* requires further explanation. Physicians and research scientists distinguish two kinds of effectiveness for contraceptive methods. **Theoretical effectiveness** is the failure rate of a contraceptive when it is "used exactly as directed." This rate cannot be accurately measured, but it can be inferred from studying the most successful users. **Use effectiveness** is the failure rate of a contraceptive when used under average conditions by average people. A third measure of effectiveness is provided by the **continuation rate**—the percentage of people who continue to use the method after a specified period of time. This measure is important because many unintended pregnancies occur when a method is stopped and not immediately replaced with another. Thus, a contraceptive with a high continuation rate would be more effective at preventing pregnancy than one with a low continuation rate.

We turn now to a description of the various contraceptive methods, discussing first those that are reversible and then those that are permanent.

Reversible Contraceptives

Reversibility is an extremely important consideration for young adults when they choose a contraceptive method, since most people either plan to have children or at least want to keep their options open until they're older. In this section we discuss the reversible contraceptives, be-

To be effective, contraceptives should be used in exactly the right way. A careful explanation by a health care professional helps this young woman understand the importance of taking birth control pills according to instructions.

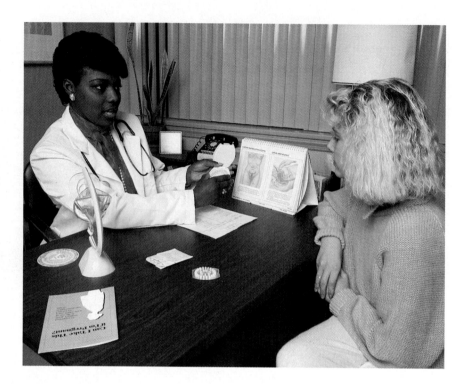

ginning with the hormonal methods, then moving to the barrier methods, and finally covering the natural methods.

Oral Contraceptives—The Pill   A century ago or more, a researcher made a key observation: **ovulation** does not occur during pregnancy. Further research showed that ovulation is controlled by the **corpus luteum**, a gland that in nonpregnant women appears and disappears with each new menstrual cycle. It forms in the ovary after ovulation and then degenerates at the end of the cycle and is absorbed into the system. In pregnant women, however, the corpus luteum remains and continues to secrete a hormone called **progesterone.**

To test the theory that progesterone prevents ovulation, extracts of progesterone were given to animals that were not pregnant. Ovulation did not occur in most cycles. Researchers later found that when **estrogen**, a hormone produced in the ovaries, was given along with progesterone, ovulation was prevented more consistently. Estrogen, progesterone, and certain closely related laboratory-made compounds are the active ingredients in **oral contraceptives** (OCs), or birth control pills.

In addition to preventing ovulation, the birth control pill also has other backup contraceptive effects. It hampers the movement of sperm by thickening the cervical mucus, alters the rate of ovum transport by means of its hormonal effects on the oviducts, and may inhibit implantation by changing the lining of the uterus, in the unlikely event that a fertilized ovum reaches that area.

Today, the birth control pill is the most widely used form of contraception among unmarried women and is second only to sterilization among married women. The most common type of pill is the combination pill. Each one-month packet contains three weeks of pills that combine varying types and amounts of estrogen and progesterone. Most packets also include one week of inactive pills to be taken following the hormone pills; others instruct the woman to simply take no pills at all for one week before starting the next cycle. During the week in which no hormones are taken, a light menstrual period occurs. Because many different types of combination pills are available today, if minor problems occur with one brand, women can switch to another. The overall trend has been toward lower-dose pills (those with 50 micrograms or less of estrogen), which offer the same high effectiveness rate with fewer unwanted side effects.

A second, much less common, type of OC is the "minipill," a small dose of a synthetic progesterone taken every day of the month. Because the minipill contains no estrogen, it has fewer side effects and health risks, but it also carries a higher risk of pregnancy and irregular bleeding.

Users must start the first cycle of the birth control pill with a menstrual period (the first day, the fifth day, or the following Sunday, depending on the instructions given with each specific pill); this procedure eliminates the possibility of beginning pills during an unsuspected pregnancy and will most effectively prevent ovulation the first month of use. Thereafter, users must take each cycle completely and according to instructions. A few pills taken before sexual relations will not prevent pregnancy.

During the first cycle or two when hormonal adjustment is occurring in the body, slight bleeding may occur between periods. This spotting is considered normal, and users should continue the daily intake of one pill. During the first month, when maximal levels of hormones have not yet been reached, full effectiveness cannot be guaranteed and using an additional backup method, such as foam and/or condoms, is recommended. Similarly, if users forget any pills, effectiveness decreases and backup contraception should be used for the rest of that particular cycle. Pregnancy is practically impossible if a pill has been taken every day according to instructions. Women who did not take a pill every day and then miss a period, and those who skip periods more than once, should consult their physician.

Pill use in the United States reached an all-time high in the mid-1970s and then declined rather rapidly between 1975 and 1977, following intense publicity regarding possible increased risks of heart attacks and strokes. In recent years, however, many of those risks have been reduced by using lower-dosage pills and by clarifying the personal factors that place a specific woman in a high-risk category. Currently, the pill is again the birth control method of choice for many American women, especially those in the younger age groups. A marked decline in pill use has occurred among women who have been married more than ten years, with the main replacement method being surgical sterilization. Among couples in whom neither partner has been sterilized, however, no other birth control method comes close to the birth control pill in popularity.

Advantages   The main advantage of the oral contraceptive is its high degree of effectiveness in preventing pregnancy. Nearly all unplanned pregnancies result because the user did not take the pill as directed. The pill is relatively simple to use and does not require any interruptions that could hinder sexual spontaneity. Most women also enjoy the predictable regularity of periods, as well as the decrease in cramps and other premenstrual symptoms. For young women, its reversibility is especially important; **fertility** (ability to reproduce) returns

after the pill is discontinued, although not always immediately. The medical advantages include a decreased incidence of the following conditions: benign breast disease, iron-deficiency anemia, pelvic inflammatory disease (PID), ectopic pregnancy, endometrial cancer (of the lining of the uterus) and ovarian cancer. Women who have never used the pill are twice as likely to develop endometrial or ovarian cancer as users who have taken it for at least 12 months.

Disadvantages   The hormones in birth control pills influence all tissues of the body, and they can lead to a variety of minor disturbances, and for some women, to serious side effects. Symptoms of early pregnancy—morning nausea, weight gain, and swollen breasts, for example—may appear during the first few months of oral contraception. They usually disappear by the fourth cycle. Other complaints include depression, nervousness, changes in the sex drive, dizziness, generalized headaches, migraine headaches, bleeding between periods, and changes in the lining of the walls of the vagina, with an increase in clear or white discharge from the vagina. Chloasma, or "mask of pregnancy," sometimes occurs, causing brown "giant freckles" to appear on the face. Acne may develop or worsen, but in most women, using the pill causes acne to clear up, and it is sometimes prescribed for young women for that purpose.

Yeast fungus infections are more common among women who are taking the pill. These infections are not serious, but the itchiness and increased discharge in the vagina that accompany them are often extremely uncomfortable. Medical treatment, usually in the form of vaginal creams, gives prompt relief most of the time.

Serious side effects of pill use have been reported in a small number of women. These include blood clots, stroke, heart attack, concentrated mostly in cigarette smokers, and benign tumors of the liver that may bleed and rupture. Pill users also show a slight increase in the incidence of high blood pressure, which is usually quickly reversed on discontinuation of the pill, and of gall bladder disease.

Many investigations regarding oral contraceptive use and breast cancer have shown no increased risk among users. Some recent reports, however, have suggested that certain subgroups of women may be at higher risk. These

---

Ovulation   The release of the egg (ovum) from the ovaries.

Corpus luteum   A gland in the ovary that forms after ovulation; secrets progesterone. If the ovum is not fertilized, the corpus luteum degenerates each month (menstruation).

Progesterone   A hormone produced by the corpus luteum and, during pregnancy, by the placenta. Used in oral contraceptives to prevent ovulation.

Estrogen   A hormone produced by the ovaries. An active ingredient in birth control pills.

Oral contraceptive (OC)   Any of various hormone compounds in pill form taken by mouth. Oral contraceptives prevent conception by preventing ovulation.

Fertility   Ability to reproduce.

Risk Factors for Oral Contraceptives

Use of oral contraceptives is not recommended for women who have or have had any of the following conditions:

Blood clots

Heart disease or stroke

Any form of cancer or liver tumor

Vaginal bleeding from unknown causes

Use of oral contraceptives is questionable and ongoing medical evaluation is recommended for women who have any of the following conditions:

Severe headaches, especially migraines

High blood pressure

Diabetes or strong family history of diabetes

Gallbladder, kidney, or liver disease or acute mononucleosis

Sickle cell disease

Major surgery planned in next four weeks, especially surgery requiring immobilization, or major injury to lower leg

Being 35 years of age or older and currently a heavy smoker

Use of oral contraceptives is probably OK but ongoing medical observation is important for women with any of the following conditions:

Family history of death from heart attack before age 50, especially in a mother or sister

Family history of high blood levels of cholesterol

Depression, asthma, epilepsy, or varicose veins

Based on R. A. Hatcher et al. 1988. *Contraceptive Technology, 1988–89* (New York: Irvington), pp. 209–210.

---

include women who started the pill early in life (under the age of 25) or before their first full-term pregnancy, or those who had used the pill for five or more years. In January 1989, a special advisory committee to the Food and Drug Administration reviewed the studies conducted to date and concluded that the evidence was too weak to warrant a change in pill use or a new warning label. However, young women who have been on the pill for some time may want to consider another method when lifestyle permits.

Similarly, although many earlier studies showed no causal relationship between pill use and cervical cancer, some recent investigations have indicated an increased risk that rises with increased duration of OC use. In addition to pill use, other behavioral characteristics, such as sexual relationships at an earlier age and with a greater number of partners and smoking are also related to cervical cancer. Regular Pap smears for the detection of earlier cervical changes are especially important in pill users. Also, because other temporary cervical changes found in some women on OCs may contribute to an increased susceptibility to the STDs chlamydia and gonorrhea, regular screening for those diseases is also recommended.

In trying to decide whether to use oral contraception, each woman needs to weigh the benefits against the risks.

For most women, the known, directly associated risk of death from use of the pill is much lower than the risk of death from pregnancy. This is especially true as newer, low-dose combinations become available. Although many long-term effects are still not completely understood, thereby complicating the decision-making process, there are many important actions that the potential user can take to make the most informed decision possible. She can discuss and evaluate with a health care professional the risk variables that are known and that apply to her; request a low-dosage pill; stop smoking; carefully and consistently follow the pill-taking instructions; be alert to preliminary danger signals (severe headaches, problems with vision, severe pain in the abdomen, chest, or legs); have regular checkups of her blood pressure, weight, and urine, and an annual examination of the thyroid, breasts, abdomen, and pelvis. By following these measures, women can better evaluate and actively affect the benefit-risk ratio of pill use. Conditions that indicate a woman should not take oral contraceptives (or should take them with ongoing medical supervision) are listed in the box "Risk Factors for Oral Contraceptive Use."

Effectiveness   As explained earlier, theoretical effectiveness is the failure rate of a contraceptive when it is "used exactly as directed." For the combination pill, the theoretical effectiveness is 1 pregnancy per 1,000 women (or 0.1 pregnancy per 100 women) during one year of use. Use effectiveness, the failure rate of a contraceptive when it is used under average conditions by average people, includes pregnancies that result from erratic pill taking, as well as those that occur when a woman stops taking pills and fails to use another method of contraception. This figure will differ markedly, as it depends on numerous patient variables. A typical first-year failure rate is 3 percent. Again, it's critical that the woman become thoroughly informed in regard to all aspects of pill use and that she follow all guidelines carefully. The continuation rate for OCs has also varied considerably from one group of users to another, with the range being 50 to 75 percent after one year.

The "Morning After" or Postcoital Pill   Another hormonal method of contraception, but a much less commonly used one, is the "morning after" pill. One type contains large doses of **diethylstilbestrol (DES)**, a synthetic preparation of estrogen, and was approved by the FDA in the mid-1970s as a postcoital contraceptive. In recent years, however, DES has been used infrequently, because it has been linked to cervical and vaginal cancers in daughters of women who had taken the drug to avoid miscarriage (a common practice from 1945 to 1960). If a pregnancy does result after DES use, a therapeutic abortion should be considered because of possible damage to the fetus.

Another "morning after" pill, a combination of estrogen and progesterone, was recently approved in western Europe for emergency situations. This same pill, although approved by the FDA for other uses in the United States, has not been approved specifically for postcoital purposes and probably will not be in the near future because of opposition to its acting as an **abortifacient** in some cases. It is not actually one pill but a series that must be started within 72 hours (preferably within 12–24 hours) after unprotected sexual intercourse. No serious side effects have been observed with this medication when taken under medical supervision.

The Intrauterine Device (IUD)   Placing objects inside the uterus is one of the oldest methods of birth control. Over two thousand years ago, Hippocrates, the Greek physician, described various devices, including one that was inserted into the uterus through a piece of lead tubing. The possibility of intrauterine methods of birth control was almost ignored in modern times until E. Grafenberg, a German physician, reported his use of an intrauterine ring of silkworm gut and silver in 1930. Grafenberg's ring did not work because of flaws in design and insertion techniques. Improvements in materials, design, and insertion techniques greatly increased the acceptability of the **intrauterine device (IUD)**, and in the United States there was a sharp increase in its use between 1965 and 1973.

By 1976, however, there was a slight decline, which was probably related to the publicity about the increased risk of serious infections with the widely used Dalkon Shield and its withdrawal from the market. An even greater decline in IUD use resulted from the 1985–1986 decisions to discontinue U.S. marketing of the Lippes Loop, the Copper 7, and the Copper T, the IUDs used by most women. The companies manufacturing these IUDs decided to stop U.S. distribution, not because of new findings of increased medical risk, but due to the financial risk of ongoing lawsuits. In 1987, only about 3 percent of all women who used contraception had IUDs. Only one IUD, the hormone-releasing Progestasert, remained available to women in the United States until 1989, when another type, the T-380A, also known as the ParaGard, was approved for use. The T-380A offers the advantage of a four-year life span, as compared to the Progestasert's one-year replacement requirement and may lead to a resurgence in IUD use.

No one knows exactly how IUDs work. They may cause biochemical changes in the uterus, such as the production of specific cells that destroy the egg and/or sperm; they may immobilize sperm in the uterus or shorten the normal travel time of the egg in the Fallopian tube; or they may interfere with the implantation of eggs in the uterus. Progestasert acts primarily by slowly releasing the hormone progesterone, which makes the uterine lining unsuitable for implantation. The amount of progesterone released is very small and does not change hormone levels in the bloodstream. In the T-380A, a small amount of copper surrounding its T-shaped arms and leg seems to facilitate the contraceptive biochemical changes in the uterus. Again, the effects of the copper seem to be localized to the uterus.

Before an IUD is inserted, a medical history and a gynecological examination should be completed to rule out the presence of pregnancy, infection, anatomical abnormalities, or other potentially complicating conditions. If none of these complications exists, the IUD is threaded into a sterile inserter, which is then introduced through

---

Diethylstilbestrol (DES)   A synthetic hormone that produces the effects of natural estrogen. DES is not considered safe.

Abortifacient   Agent or substance that induces abortion.

Intrauterine device (IUD)   A plastic device inserted into the uterus as a contraceptive.

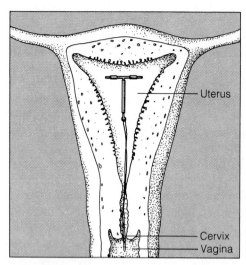

Figure 6-1   An IUD (Progestasert) properly positioned in the uterus. The attached threads that protrude from the cervix into the upper vagina allow the woman to check to make sure that the IUD is in place.

the cervix until it reaches the lowermost portion of the uterus. The plunger pushes the IUD into the uterus, and the inserter is withdrawn. The threads protruding from the cervix are trimmed so that only 1 to 1½ inches remain in the upper vagina. These are not noticeable during coitus. (See Figure 6-1.) An IUD can be inserted any time during the menstrual cycle, as long as pregnancy has been ruled out.

IUDs with nylon threads can usually be removed by pulling on the threads. Only a trained professional should undertake this process, however, because the cervix might have to be expanded, or dilated. Timing of removal can be crucial; some unwanted pregnancies have resulted when sperm have survived from intercourse that took place a couple of days before the IUD was removed.

Advantages   Intrauterine devices are highly reliable (second only to the pill) and are simple and convenient to use, requiring no attention except for a periodic check of the string position. They do not require the user to anticipate or interrupt sexual activity. Usually IUDs have only localized side effects, and in the absence of complications, such as infection, their effects are considered fully reversible. In most cases fertility resumes as soon as the IUD is removed. While the initial cost of IUD insertion may be substantial, the long-term expense is low.

Disadvantages   Most side effects of IUD use are limited to the genital tract. By far the most common complaint is abnormal menstrual bleeding. The menstrual flow tends to appear sooner, last longer, and become heavier after insertion of an IUD. Bleeding and spotting between

periods may also occur. Another common complaint is pain, particularly uterine cramps and backache, side effects that seem to occur most often in women who have never been pregnant. Uterine cramps that accompany insertion usually disappear after a few days, but in some cases they are severe enough to require the removal of the device.

Spontaneous expulsion of the IUD happens in 5 to 10 percent of all users within the first year after insertion. If a woman does not notice that she has lost it, an unwanted pregnancy may result. Most expulsions occur during the first months after insertion, usually but not always during the menstrual period, so checking tampons or menstrual pads for the device is a wise precaution. It is also a good idea to check occasionally that the device is in place by locating the threads, particularly prior to sexual activity. Expulsion after the first year is uncommon. If one IUD is expelled, the risk of expelling another IUD becomes two to three times greater, although about one-half of all women who experience a first expulsion eventually retain the device. The older the woman is and the more children she has had, the less likely she is to expel the device.

A serious complication sometimes associated with IUD use is **pelvic inflammatory disease (PID)**. Most pelvic infections among IUD users are relatively mild and can be treated successfully with antibiotics. However, early and adequate treatment is critical, for a smoldering infection can lead to tubal scarring and subsequent infertility. Recent studies on IUDs have been encouraging, showing that any risk of infection is largely limited to the first four months after IUD insertion and to women exposed to STDs. Evidence suggests that infection risk may be reduced if women take an antibiotic when the IUD is inserted, the time when vaginal bacteria is most likely to be transmitted into the uterus. It also appears that there is virtually no increased risk of infection and infertility when a woman has a mutually faithful sexual relationship with only one partner, a situation in which exposure to the leading causes of PID, chlamydia and gonorrhea, is unlikely.

In about one of 2,000 insertions, the IUD punctures the wall of the uterus and migrates into the abdominal cavity. No evidence has been found that IUDs cause cancer in women, but the long-term effects are not well known.

Most doctors advise against the use of IUDs by young women who have never been pregnant because of the increased incidence of side effects in this subgroup and the risk of infection with the possibility of subsequent infertility. The IUD is not recommended for women of any age who have a history of pelvic infection, suspected pregnancy, large tumors of the uterus or other anatomical abnormalities, irregular or unexplained bleeding, history of ectopic pregnancy, rheumatic heart disease, or diabetes.

Early IUD danger signals that the user should be alert for are abdominal pain, fever, chills, foul vaginal discharge, irregular menstrual period, and other unusual vaginal bleeding. An annual checkup is important and should include a Pap smear and a blood check for anemia if menstrual flow has increased. (And in the case of Progestasert use, the IUD must be replaced every twelve months.)

Effectiveness   The use effectiveness rate of IUDs is about 6 pregnancies per 100 women during the first year of use. Many of these pregnancies are due to undetected partial or complete expulsion of the device. For all types the failure rate tends to decline rapidly after the first year. Because most pregnancies occur in the first few months after IUD insertion, some doctors advise using an additional method of contraception during that time. Regular checking of the cervix to verify the presence of thread and absence of the IUD stem is also recommended.

Pregnancy may occur with the device in place. If the patient wishes to maintain the pregnancy, the IUD should be removed. Following removal, there is a slightly increased incidence of a **spontaneous abortion** (miscarriage). Birth defects are no more common among babies born of such pregnancies than among other babies. Pregnancies with an IUD left in place may lead to fatal infection or bleeding, and they have a 50 percent chance of ending in miscarriage.

The continuation rate of IUDs is 70 to 85 percent after one year of use.

Condoms   In the sixteenth century, the Italian anatomist Fallopius described the use of linen sheaths worn over the penis as a protection against disease. By the eighteenth century the contraceptive function of the **condom** had been recognized, and the French and English used condoms made of sheep gut or the amniotic membrane of newborn lambs. Sheaths of animal skin were too expensive for most people, but the vulcanization of rubber in 1844 made a less expensive condom possible. Since the early 1900s, "rubbers" have, by and large, replaced animal skin condoms.

The condom is still one of the most popular contraceptives in North America. In recent years, its sales have increased dramatically, partly due to fear of STDs, particularly AIDS and herpes. Of all condoms purchased, at least one-third are bought by women (see the box "Condoms—Growing in Popularity"). This figure will no doubt increase, as more women become aware of the serious risks associated with STDs. Currently, condom use is relied on more than any of the other **barrier methods** and is the third most popular of all birth control methods used in the United States, exceeded only by the pill and sterilization.

■ **Exploring Your Emotions**

How do you feel about buying contraceptives at the drugstore? About asking for a prescription contraceptive at your health clinic or from your physician? What is the basis for your feelings? Have they changed as you've gotten older?

The user or his partner must put the condom on the penis before it is inserted into the vagina, because the small amounts of fluid that may be secreted unnoticed prior to **ejaculation** often contain sperm capable of causing pregnancy. The rolled-up condom is placed over the head of the erect penis and unrolled down to the base of the penis, leaving a half-inch space (without air) at the tip to collect semen. If the user has not been **circumcised**, he must first pull back the foreskin of the penis. He and his partner must be careful not to damage the condom with fingernails, rings, or other rough objects.

Some condoms are sold already lubricated. If the users wish, they can lubricate their own condoms with contraceptive foam, creams, or jelly or water-based preparations such as KY Jelly. All products that contain mineral oil—including baby oil, Vaseline Intensive Care lotion, Nivea hand lotion, and regular Vaseline petroleum jelly—should never be used; studies have shown that they cause latex condoms to begin to disintegrate within 60 seconds, thereby markedly increasing their chances of breaking. Vegetable-based cooking oils—including Mazola and Wesson oils, as well as olive oil, Crisco, and butter—are also damaging.

When the male loses his erection after ejaculating, the condom loses its tight fit. To avoid spilling semen, the condom must be held around the base of the penis as the penis is withdrawn. If any semen is spilled on the vulva, the sperm may find their way to the uterus.

Pelvic inflammatory disease (PID)   An infection that progresses from the vagina and cervix and eventually moves into the pelvic cavity.

Spontaneous abortion   A miscarriage; the premature expulsion of a nonliving fetus.

Condom   A sheath, usually made of thin rubber, designed to cover the penis during sexual intercourse. Used for contraception and to prevent disease.

Barrier method   A contraceptive that acts as a physical barrier, blocking the sperm from uniting with the egg.

Ejaculation   An abrupt discharge of semen from the penis after sexual stimulation.

Circumcise   To remove the foreskin of the penis.

Spermicide   An agent that kills sperm.

Condoms—Growing in Popularity

Embrace Her, Plan Ahead, and Play Safe aren't suggestions for lovers, and Duke, Mentor, and Nightrider aren't TV heroes—they're all condoms, the contraceptive that's rapidly becoming the method of choice for millions of people. Condoms are an old standby as a method of preventing pregnancy, but recently they've achieved new status as a method of protection against STDs, including AIDS. Even people who have been sterilized are using condoms to protect themselves from disease.

Worldwide, 40 million couples use condoms for contraception. Two-thirds of them live in developed countries, with Japan accounting for about 25 percent of all condom sales. About $350 million worth of condoms were sold in the United States in 1988, with women purchasing about 40 percent of them. Unfortunately, many teenagers continue to view the use of condoms as a contrived mechanical process that identifies their sexual activity as planned and removes the sense of spontaneity. The attitude that intercourse must be spontaneous to be an expression of love needs to be replaced with more practical and realistic ideas.

Condoms are recommended because they

- Are relatively inexpensive compared with the pill, the IUD, and the diaphragm.
- Are readily accessible—they can be purchased without a prescription in drugstores, convenience stores, campus dormitories, student unions, hotels, and so on.
- Are moderately effective when used correctly as a contraceptive, especially in conjunction with vaginal foam.
- Require a couple's shared responsibility.
- Help prevent the transmission of the AIDS virus and other STDs, such as herpes, venereal warts, gonorrhea, trichomoniasis, and hepatitis B, especially if they're lubricated with nonoxynol-9 (latex condoms only).
- May slow or reduce the development of cervical abnormalities that could lead to cancer.

Condoms don't have to interfere with sexual arousal or pleasure. They come in an array of styles, shapes, colors, thicknesses, and textures and their use can be integrated into sexual activities before intercourse. Although

they're not 100 percent effective either as a contraceptive or as protection from disease, they improve your chances on both counts. Use them properly by following these guidelines:

- Buy latex. If you're allergic to rubber, try wearing a lambskin condom under a latex one.
- Buy fresh. Patronize a busy, reputable pharmacy where there's likely to be a high turnover. Don't remove the condom from its individual sealed wrapper until you're ready to use it. Don't use it if it looks dried out or discolored.
- Buy a water-based lubricant, preferably one that contains nonoxynol-9.
- Buy a good design, preferably one with a reservoir tip at the end.
- Wear it right, rolling it down over the penis as soon as it's erect and before you continue foreplay. Remove it after ejaculation before the penis becomes flaccid. Use a new condom every time you have intercourse.

Adapted from Bernard Goldstein. 1989. Condoms—On a roll! *Healthline*, August.

Prelubricated condoms are now available containing nonoxynol-9, the same spermicidal agent found in many of the contraceptive foams and creams that women use. Since the **spermicide** kills many of the sperm soon after ejaculation, its addition may significantly decrease contraceptive failure associated with breakage and the spilling of semen.

Advantages Condoms are easy to purchase and are available without prescription or medical supervision. They are simple to use and allow increased male participation in contraception. Condoms do not require daily use during intervals of sexual inactivity, and their effects are immediately and completely reversible. In addition to being free of medical side effects (other than occasional allergic reactions), condoms made of rubber (not the lambskin type) help to protect against STDs, which in turn may diminish the likelihood of cervical cancer in some women.

Disadvantages The two most nearly universal complaints about condoms are that they diminish sensation and interfere with spontaneity. Although some people find these drawbacks serious, others consider them only mi-

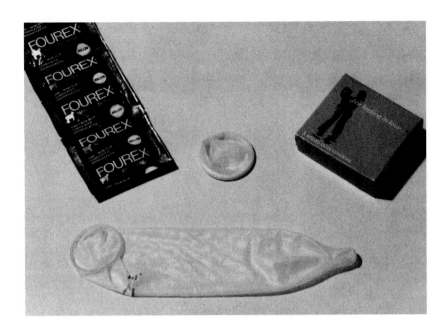

Condoms are a very popular, moderately effective form of contraception. They are more effective if used together with spermicidal foam. The elongated tip on the unrolled condom is a reservoir to collect semen.

nor disadvantages. It is hard to think of a human activity in which losing sensation and spontaneity would be less welcome than in coitus. Many couples, however, learn to creatively integrate condom use into their sexual activities. Indeed, it can be a way to improve communication and add shared responsibility to the relationship.

Effectiveness Condoms, when used exactly as directed during each act of intercourse, have a theoretical effectiveness of 3 pregnancies per 100 women during one year of use. In actual use, however, the failure rate varies considerably. First-year rates among typical users average about 12 percent. At least some of these pregnancies happen because the condom is carelessly removed after ejaulation. Some may also happen because of a break or a tear, which is estimated to occur once in every 150 to 200 instances. Since heat destroys rubber, condoms should not be stored for long periods in a wallet or in the glove compartment of a car. Some consumer advocates have suggested that if kept away from heat and light, condoms will remain safe from three to five years. Manufacturers of condoms in the United States recently agreed to put expiration dates on their products and are in the process of determining what a safe "shelf life" would be.

If a condom breaks or is carelessly removed, the risk of pregnancy can be reduced somewhat by the immediate use of a vaginal spermicide. The use effectiveness of the condom can be greatly improved and approaches that of the pill if a spermicidal foam is also inserted just *before* intercourse.

The most common cause of pregnancy with condom users is "taking a chance"— that is, not using a condom

at all—or waiting to use it until after preejaculate fluid (which may contain some sperm) has already entered the vagina.

Female Condoms Female condoms are currently undergoing extensive studies in Europe and the United States and should soon be available for public marketing. The new device called Femshield in England is known only as WPC-333 thus far in the United States. The female condom is a disposable device that comes in one size and consists of a soft, loose-fitting polyurethane sheath with two flexible rings (see Figure 6-2). The ring at the closed end is inserted into the vagina and placed at the cervix much like a diaphragm, while the ring at the open end remains outside the vagina. The walls of the condom protect the inside of the vagina. It can be

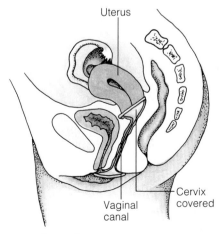

Figure 6-2 Female condom.

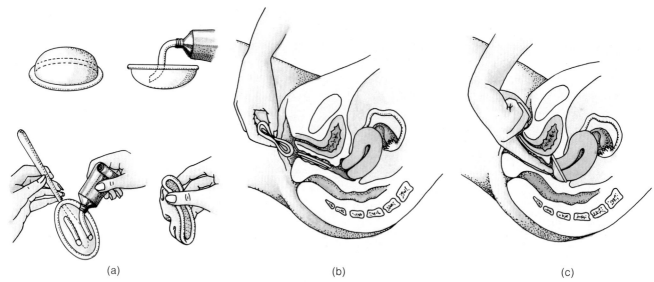

(a)   (b)   (c)

Figure 6-3 Use of the diaphragm: (a) spermicidal jelly is placed in the concave side of
the diaphragm, and the diaphragm is pressed firmly between the thumb and forefinger;
(b) diaphragm is inserted in the vagina; (c) diaphragm is checked for correct position
against the cervix.

inserted well before intercourse, and should be used with a water-based lubricant to prevent penile irritation.

Advantages For many women, the greatest advantage of the female condom will be the control it allows them. Along with serving as a contraceptive, it also offers the couple improved protection against STDs because it allows less skin-to-skin contact than the male condom.

Disadvantages As with the traditional condom, decreased sensation and interference with spontaneity are likely to be common complaints.

Effectiveness Exact effectiveness rates have not been established, but the stronger polyurethane appears less likely to tear than the latex in male condoms and thus may offer greater reliability.

The Diaphragm and Jelly Before oral contraceptives were introduced, about one-fourth of all American couples who used any form of contraception relied on the **diaphragm.** Many former diaphragm users have been won over to the pill or to IUDs, but the diaphragm continues to offer advantages that are important to certain couples. About 4 percent of all women who use contraception use diaphragms.

Wilhelm Mensinga, a German physician, invented a rubber diaphragm in the late 1800s, and there have been few changes in design since. The diaphragm is a dome-shaped cup of thin rubber stretched over a collapsible metal ring. When correctly used with spermicidal cream or jelly, the diaphragm covers the mouth of the cervix, blocking sperm from entering the uterus.

Diaphragms can be obtained only by prescription. Because of individual differences in women, a diaphragm must be carefully fitted to ensure that it will be both effective and comfortable, and only a trained person can make these adjustments. The fitting should be checked with each routine annual medical examination, as well as after childbirth, abortion, or a weight change of more than 10 pounds.

Before inserting the diaphragm, the woman should spread about a tablespoon of spermicidal jelly or cream over the surface of the dome that will be against the cervix. The diaphragm is easiest to insert if the user squats, lies down, or stands with one foot raised. The user squeezes the diaphragm into a long narrow shape with one hand. She holds the labia apart with the other hand and pushes the diaphragm up along the back wall of the vagina as far as it will go, keeping it behind the cervix. She then tucks the front rim up behind the pubic bone. (See Figure 6-3.) Because the vagina tilts backward, a user who inserts the diaphragm while she is standing up must insert it almost horizontally.

After the diaphragm is inserted, its position should be checked. The cervix should be located and felt through the dome of the diaphragm to make sure that it is completely covered and that the front rim of the diaphragm is pushed up behind the pubic bone.

The diaphragm must not be inserted more than six hours before intercourse. If the time between insertion and coitus is longer than six hours, an applicatorful of spermicide should be inserted into the vagina, or the diaphragm should be taken out and spermicide freshly applied before it is reinserted. Additional cream or jelly should also be inserted into the vagina before any additional act of coitus. The diaphragm must be left in place for at least six hours after the last act of coitus to give the spermicide enough time to kill all the sperm.

To remove the diaphragm, the user simply hooks the front rim down from the pubic bone with one finger and pulls it out. After the diaphragm is removed, it should be washed with mild soap and water, rinsed, and patted dry. It should then be examined for holes or cracks. Defects are mostly likely to develop near the rim, and they can usually be spotted by looking at the diaphragm in front of a bright light. After the diaphragm is inspected, it can be dusted with cornstarch (*not* talcum powder, which may damage the diaphragm and irritate the vagina) and stored in its case.

Advantages   Diaphragm use is less intrusive than condom use because a diaphragm can be inserted up to six hours before intercourse. Its use can be limited to times of sexual activity only, and it allows for immediate and total reversibility. The diaphragm is free of medical side effects (other than rare allergic reactions). When used along with spermicidal jelly or cream, it may offer limited protection against certain STDs, but should never be used for full protection as a substitute for condoms.

Disadvantages   Diaphragms must always be used with a spermicide, and therefore a user must keep both of these somewhat bulky supplies with her whenever she anticipates sexual activity. Diaphragms require extra attention, since they must be cleaned and stored with care to preserve their effectiveness. Some women cannot wear a diaphragm because of their vaginal anatomy. In other women, diaphragm use can cause an increase in bladder infections. It has also been associated with a slightly increased risk of **toxic shock syndrome (TSS)**, an occasionally fatal disease related to tampon use. To diminish the risk of TSS, women should wash their hands carefully with soap and water before inserting or removing the diaphragm, should not use the diaphragm during menstruation or whenever there is an abnormal discharge,

and should never leave the device in place for more than 24 hours.

Effectiveness   When used consistently, the diaphragm has a theoretical effectiveness of 2 to 3 pregnancies per 100 women during one year. In actual practice, women rarely use the diaphragm correctly every time they have intercourse. Typical use effectiveness of the diaphragm varies from 14 to 18 pregnancies per 100 women during the first year of use. The main causes of failures are inaccurate fitting and incorrect insertion. Sometimes, too, the vaginal walls expand during sexual stimulation, allowing the diaphragm to be dislodged. This displacement seems to happen most commonly with the woman-on-top position.

The Cervical Cap   The **cervical cap** is another barrier device. It consists of a thimble-shaped rubber or plastic cup that fits snugly over the cervix and is held in place by suction. It is used in a manner similar to the diaphragm, a small amount of spermicide being placed in the cup before each insertion. Use of the cervical cap in the United States has been limited, because it was only recently approved for marketing. Wider distribution is now underway.

Advantages   Advantages of the cervical cap are similar to those associated with diaphragm use. In addition, it can be used as an alternative for women who have anatomical features that preclude diaphragm use, such as very lax vaginal tone, pressure discomfort, or recurrent urinary infections with diaphragm use. It may be left in place for up to 48 hours, compared with 24 hours for the diaphragm; and because the cap fits tightly, it does not require reintroduction of spermicide with repeated intercourse.

Disadvantages   Along with most of the disadvantages associated with the diaphragm, difficulty with insertion and removal is a more common problem for cervical cap users. In addition, tests have shown that women who use the cap rather than the diaphragm initially have a higher rate of abnormal Pap smears. In most cases these result from inflammation or infections of the cervix, conditions that are easily treatable. As a safety precaution, the FDA

Diaphragm   A contraceptive device consisting of a flexible, dome-shaped cup that covers the cervix. The diaphragm prevents sperm from entering the uterus.

Toxic shock syndrome (TSS)   A disease whose major symptoms include high fever, vomiting, diarrhea, headache, sore throat, and rash. Although primarily associated with menstruating women who use tampons, the disease has also been reported in men. It is usually caused by the bacterium *Staphylococcus aureus*. Mortality rate has decreased from 10–15 percent to 3 percent or less due to earlier recognition and treatment.

Cervical cap   A thimble-shaped cup that fits over the cervix, to be used with spermicide.

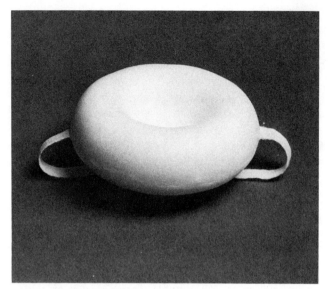

The contraceptive sponge is inexpensive and can be purchased without a prescription. In actual use, it is less effective than a condom and about as effective as a diaphragm used with spermical jelly.

has stated that the cap should be prescribed only for women with normal Pap smears and that a repeat test should be done after three months of use to confirm that no changes have occurred.

Effectiveness   Studies completed thus far indicate that cervical cap effectiveness is about 17 percent, similar to that of the diaphragm.

The Sponge   The **sponge**, a more recent addition to the barrier methods, is a round, absorbent device about 2 inches in diameter with a polyester loop on one side (for removal) and a concave dimple on the other side, which helps it fit snugly over the cervix. Most sponges are made of polyurethane and are presaturated with the same spermicide that is used in contraceptive creams and foams. The spermicide is activated when moistened with a small amount of water just before insertion. The sponge, which can be used only once, acts as a barrier, as a spermicide, and as a seminal fluid absorbent.

Advantages   The sponge offers advantages similar to those of the diaphragm and cervical cap. In addition, sponges can be obtained without a professional fitting, and they may be safely left in place for twenty-four hours without the addition of spermicide for repeated intercourse.

Disadvantages   Reported disadvantages include difficulty with removal and an unpleasant odor if left in place for more than eighteen hours. Allergic reactions, such as irritation of the labia, are more common with the sponge than with other spermicide products, probably because the overall dose contained in each sponge is significantly higher than that used with the other methods. (It contains 1 gram of spermicide compared to the 60–100 mg present in one application of other spermicidal products.) Because the sponge has also been associated with toxic shock syndrome, the same precautions must be taken as described for diaphragm use. A sponge user should be especially alert for symptoms of TSS when the sponge has been difficult to remove or was not removed intact. We do not know how much spermicide is absorbed through the vaginal walls with this device, or what possible effects are caused by recurring, extended exposure.

Effectiveness   The use effectiveness of the sponge is similar to that of the diaphragm (16 pregnancies for 100 women during one year) for women who have never experienced childbirth. For women who have had a child, however, sponge effectiveness is significantly lower than diaphragm effectiveness. One possible explanation is that the one size now marketed may be insufficient to adequately cover the cervix after childbirth. To ensure effectiveness, the user should carefully check the expiration date on each sponge, as shelf life is limited.

Vaginal Spermicides   In recent years spermicidal compounds developed for use with a diaphragm have been adapted for use without a diaphragm by combining them with a bulky base. Foams, creams, jellies, and vaginal suppositories are all available. Foam is sold in an aerosol bottle or a metal container with an applicator that fits on the nozzle. Creams and jellies are sold in tubes with an applicator that can be screwed onto the opening of the tube. (See Figure 6-4.)

Foams, creams, and jellies must be placed deep in the vagina near the cervical entrance and must not be inserted more than one-half hour before intercourse. After an hour, their effectiveness is drastically reduced, and a new applicatorful must be inserted. Another application is also required before each repeated act of coitus. If the woman wants to **douche**, she should wait for at least eight hours after the last coitus to make sure that there has been time for the spermicide to kill all the sperm.

In recent years the spermicidal suppository has become widely marketed and publicized in the United States. It is small and easily inserted like a tampon. Because body

---

Sponge   A contraceptive device about 2 inches in diameter that fits over the cervix and acts as a barrier, spermicide, and seminal fluid absorbent.

Douche   To apply a stream of water or other solutions to a body part or cavity such as the vagina; not a contraceptive technique.

Figure 6-4   Application of spermicide.

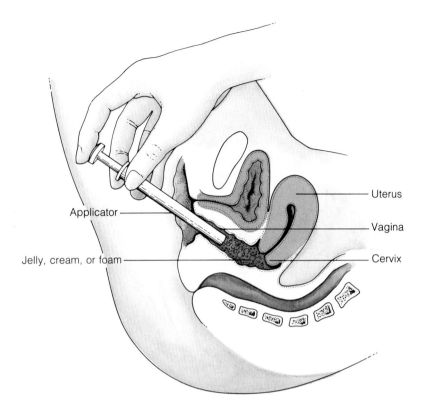

Applicator

Jelly, cream, or foam

Uterus

Vagina

Cervix

heat is needed to dissolve and activate the suppository, it is important to wait at least ten minutes after insertion before having intercourse. The suppository's spermicidal effects are limited in time, and coitus should take place within one hour of insertion. An additional suppository is required for each additional act of intercourse.

The latest addition to the vaginal spermicides is the vaginal contraceptive film (V.C.F.) a paper thin 2-inch square of film that incorporates the same spermicide as the methods already discussed. It is folded over one or two fingers and placed high in the vagina, as close to the cervix as possible. In about ten minutes the film dissolves into a gel that exerts a contraceptive effect against sperm for about 1½ hours. An additional film must be inserted each time intercourse is repeated.

Advantages   The use of vaginal spermicides is relatively simple and can be limited to times of sexual activity. They are readily available in most drugstores and do not require a prescription or a pelvic examination. Spermicides allow for complete and immediate reversibility; the only known medical side effects are occasional allergic reactions. Vaginal spermicides may offer limited protection against some STDs, but should never be used instead of condoms for reliable protection.

Disadvantages   All vaginal spermicides when used alone must be inserted shortly before intercourse, so their use may be seen as an annoying disruption. Some women find the slight increase in vaginal fluids after spermicide use unpleasant, but for most this effect is negligible.

Some studies have indicated that spermicide use around the time of conception may be associated with a higher rate of miscarriage, low birth weight, and certain birth defects. Other investigations have not found any such relationship, and no definitive conclusion can be made at this time. Similarly, the effects on the user herself of extended exposure to spermicide are unknown at present.

Effectiveness   The reported effectiveness rates of vaginal spermicides cover a wide range, again depending partly on how consistently and carefully instructions are followed. The average use effectiveness is about 21 pregnancies per 100 women during the first year of use. Of the various type of spermicides, foam is probably the most effective, because its effervescent mass forms a more dense and evenly distributed barrier to the cervical opening. Creams and jellies give only minimal protection unless used with diaphragms or cervical caps. Vaginal spermicides are used by many couples in combination with condoms or as a backup with other birth control methods.

Abstinence, Fertility Awareness, and Withdrawal
Millions of people throughout the world do not use any of the methods we have described. Either they will not because of religious conviction or cultural prohibitions

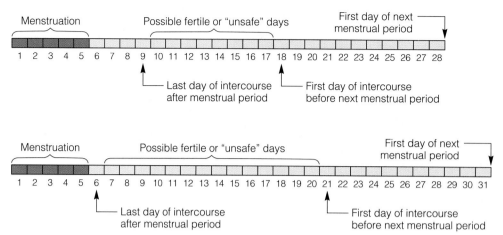

Figure 6-5   The Fertility Awareness Method of contraception, showing the safe and unsafe days for a woman with a regular 28-day cycle (top), and a woman with an irregular cycle, ranging from 25 to 31 days (bottom).

or they cannot because of poverty or lack of information and supplies. If they use any method at all, they are likely to use one of the following relatively "natural" methods of attempting to prevent conception.

Abstinence   **Abstinence**, the decision not to engage in sexual intercourse for a chosen period of time, has been followed by human beings throughout history for a variety of reasons. Until relatively recently, many people abstained because they had no other birth control measures. Today, with other methods available, about 5 percent of all American women who use birth control rely on periodic abstinence as a birth control method. To some of them, all other methods simply seem unsuitable. Concern regarding possible side effects, STDs, and unwanted pregnancy may be factors. Or intercourse may be temporarily avoided because of medical reasons such as recent illness or surgery. In other cases, abstinence may be seen as the wisest choice in terms of personal emotional needs. A period of abstinence may be chosen as a time to focus energies on other aspects of interpersonal or personal growth. Religious and cultural beliefs are sometimes motivating factors. For a variety of reasons, what may seem "right" and highly desirable for one person may be unacceptable for another. External pressure alone, either from individuals or from society at large, is being recognized as an unsatisfactory reason to engage in intercourse.

Many couples who do choose to abstain from sexual intercourse in the traditional sense turn to other mutually satisfying alternatives. When open communication be-

tween partners exists, many new avenues may be explored. These may include dancing, massage, hugging, kissing, petting, mutual masturbation, and oral-genital sex. Sexual feelings and intimacy may be expressed and satisfied through a wide range of activities.

Fertility Awareness Method (FAM)   **FAM** is based on avoiding coitus during the fertile phase of a woman's menstrual cycle. Ordinarily only one egg is released by the ovaries per month, and it lives about twenty-four hours unless it is fertilized. Sperm deposited in the vagina are apparently on the average capable of fertilizing an egg for about six to seven days; so conception theoretically can only occur during eight days of any cycle. Predicting *which* eight days these are is difficult. It is done either by the calendar method or by the temperature method. Information on cyclical changes of the cervical mucus has also been helpful in determining the time of ovulation.

The *calendar method* is based on the knowledge that the average woman releases an egg fourteen to sixteen days before her next period begins. Few women menstruate with complete regularity, so a record of the menstrual cycle must be kept for twelve months, during which time some other method of birth control must be used. The first day of each period is counted as Day 1. To determine the first fertile, or "unsafe" day of the cycle, subtract 18 from the number of days in the shortest cycle. To determine the last unsafe day of the cycle, subtract 11 from the number of days in the longest cycle. The calendar method is illustrated in Figure 6-5.

The *temperature method* is based on the knowledge that a woman's body temperature drops slightly just before ovulation and rises slightly after ovulation. A woman using the temperature method records her basal, or resting, body temperature (BBT) every morning before getting out of bed and before eating or drinking anything as the activities may alter the results. Once the temperature pattern can be seen (usually after about three months), the period unsafe for coitus can be calculated as the interval from Day 5 (Day 1 is the first day of the period) until three days after the rise in BBT. To arrive at a shorter unsafe period, some women combine the calendar and the temperature methods, calculating the first unsafe day from the shortest cycle of the calendar chart and the last unsafe day as the third day after a rise in the BBT.

The *mucus method* is based on changes in the cervical secretions throughout the menstrual cycle. During the preovulatory phase, cervical mucus increases and is clear and slippery. At the time of ovulation some women can detect a slight change in the texture of the mucus and find that it is more likely to form an elastic thread when stretched between thumb and finger. After ovulation these secretions become cloudy and sticky and decrease in quantity. Infertile, safe days are likely to occur during the relatively dry days just before and after menstruation. (See Figure 6-6.) This is also called the **Billings method.** These additional clues have been found helpful by some couples who rely on the Fertility Awareness Method. One possible problem that may interfere with this method is that vaginal infections or vaginal products or medication can also change cervical mucus.

FAM is not recommended for women who have very irregular cycles—about 15 percent of all menstruating women. Any woman for whom pregnancy would be a serious problem should not rely on the FAM alone, because the failure rate is high—approximately 20 percent among typical users during the first year of use.

Withdrawal Probably the oldest known method of contraception, and also the least effective, is **withdrawal.** In this method (or "nonmethod," as some call it), the male removes his penis from the vagina just before he ejaculates. Withdrawal has three advantages: it is free, it requires no preparation, and it is always available. For many people, these advantages are far outweighed by the disadvantages: the male has to overcome a powerful bio-

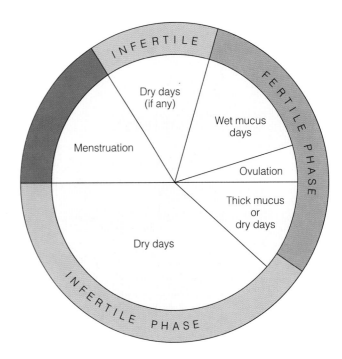

Figure 6-6 The Billings method relies solely on the presence and quality of cervical mucus to indicate fertile and infertile periods of the menstrual cycle. The beginning of the fertile period is indicated by the onset of mucus flow. The day of the "peak mucus symptom" is the last day of wet, slippery mucus, after which mucus thickens and disappears. The fertile period is presumed to last until four days after the peak symptom.

logical urge. The fear that withdrawal may be too late can detract from sexual pleasure for both partners. Also, since in many societies a woman takes longer than a male does to reach orgasm, withdrawal before the woman's orgasm is likely and can leave the couple frustrated if she relies on coitus for satisfaction. And most important, the failure rate for withdrawal is high: 20 to 25 pregnancies per 100 women during one year. One key factor in this high failure rate is the degree of self-control necessary. In addition, preejaculatory fluid, which may contain viable sperm, is commonly secreted unnoticed before actual ejaculation occurs.

Figure 6-7 summarizes the use effectiveness of eight reversible contraceptive methods.

Abstinence Avoidance of sexual intercourse. This is one method of birth control.

Fertility Awareness Method (FAM) A method of preventing conception based on avoiding coitus during the fertile phase of a woman's cycle.

Billings method A method of predicting the fertile period in a woman's cycle by means of the texture, color, and amount of cervical mucus.

Withdrawal Sexual intercourse purposely interrupted by withdrawing the penis before ejaculation (to avoid conception).

Contraceptive Method
(during the first year of actual use)

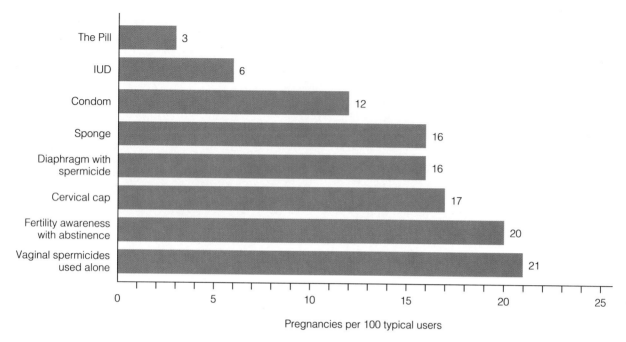

Pregnancies per 100 typical users

Figure 6-7 Use effectiveness of light reversible contraceptive methods.

Permanent Contraception—Sterilization

Surgical attempts to control human fertility have a long history. Most were mutilating, dangerous, and ineffective until aseptic surgery (surgery without the danger of infection) and anesthetics became available in the late nineteenth century.

Sterilization is permanent, and it provides complete protection, with no further action needed at any time. For these reasons, it is becoming an increasingly popular method of birth control. At present it is the most commonly used method in the United States. It is especially popular among couples who have been married ten or more years, as well as among couples who have had all the children they intend.

An important consideration in choosing sterilization is that, in most cases, it cannot be reversed. Although the chances of restoring fertility are being increased by modern surgical techniques, such operations are costly and pregnancy can never be guaranteed. Some couples choosing male sterilization are using sperm banks as a way of extending the option of childbearing. Some recent studies have indicated that male sterilization is preferable to female sterilization in a variety of ways. The overall cost of a female procedure is about four times that of a male procedure, and women are much more likely than men to experience both minor and major complications following the operation. Furthermore, regret seems to be somewhat higher in women than in men after sterilization.

Although some doctors will perform surgery for sterilization on request, most require a thorough discussion with both partners before the operation. Most doctors also recommend that people who have religious conflicts, psychiatric problems related to sex, or unstable marriages not be sterilized. Young couples with one or two children, who might later change their minds and want more, are also frequently advised not to undergo sterilization.

Male Sterilization or Vasectomy **Vasectomy** involves severing the **vasa deferentia,** two tiny ducts that transport sperm from the testicles to the seminal vesicles. The testicles continue to produce sperm, but the sperm are absorbed into the body. Since the testicles contribute only about one-tenth of the total seminal fluid, the actual quantity of ejaculate is only slightly reduced. Hormone output from the testicles apparently continues with very little change and secondary sex characteristics are not altered.

Vasectomy is ordinarily done in the doctor's office and takes about 30 minutes. The patient is instructed to present himself with all pubic hair shaved. After the scrotal region is washed with a surgical cleanser, a local anesthetic is injected into the skin of the scrotum and near the vasa. Small incisions are made at the upper end of the scrotum where it joins the body, and the vas deferens on each side is exposed, severed, and tied off or coagulated with electrocautery. The incisions are then closed with sutures, and a small dressing is applied. (See Figure 6-8.)

As the local anesthetic wears off, the patient feels a dull ache in the surgical area and often in the lower abdomen. Pain and swelling are usually slight and can be relieved with an ice bag, aspirin, and use of a scrotal support. Bleeding and infection occasionally develop but are in most cases easily treated. Most men are ready to return to work in two days.

Men can have sex again as soon as they feel no further discomfort; for most men this means after about a week. Another method of contraception must be used for the first few weeks after vasectomy, however, because sperm produced before the operation may still be present in the semen. To make sure that sperm are no longer in the ejaculate and that another method of contraception is no longer necessary, a semen specimen should be examined under a microscope.

Recent investigations do not support an earlier hypothesis that a vasectomy may accelerate atherosclerosis (the formation of fat deposits that clog arteries). In fact, one very large-scale study found no long-range complications of any type following vasectomy and actually found lower death rates from cancer and heart disease among vasectomized men when comparing them to matched controls who had not been sterilized. The researchers concluded that perhaps the vasectomized men were healthier to start with in some way.

In about 1 percent of vasectomies, a severed vas rejoins itself, and sperm can again travel up through the duct and be ejaculated in the semen. Because of this possibility, some doctors advise that a semen specimen be examined yearly.

Although some surgeons report pregnancy rates of about 80 percent for partners of men who have their vasectomies reversed within ten years of the original procedure, most studies report considerably lower rates. In

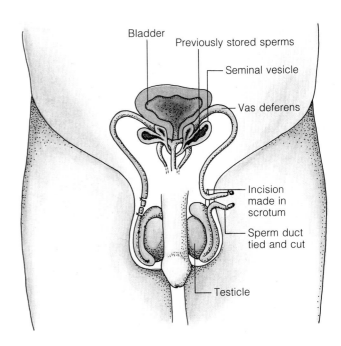

Figure 6-8   Vasectomy is a comparatively simple surgical procedure.

at least 50 percent of vasectomized men the process of absorbing sperm (instead of ejaculating it) results in antisperm antibodies that may interfere with later fertility. Other factors, such as length of time between the vasectomy and the reversal surgery, may also be important predictors of reversal success.

Female Sterilization   The most common method of female sterilization involves severing or in some manner blocking the oviducts, thereby preventing the egg from reaching the uterus and the sperm from entering the tubes. Ovulation and menstruation continue, but the unfertilized eggs are released into the abdominal cavity and absorbed. Hormone production by the ovaries and secondary characteristics are not affected.

One method of **tubal sterilization** is accomplished by making a small incision in the abdominal wall, locating each oviduct, bringing it into view, severing it, removing a small section, and tying or stapling shut the two ends. (See Figure 6-9.) Another method involves making the

---

Sterilization   Surgically altering the reproductive system to prevent pregnancy. Vasectomy is the procedure in males, tubal sterilization or hysterectomy in females.

Vasectomy   Surgical severing of the ducts that carry sperm to the ejaculatory duct.

Vasa deferentia   (*Vas deferens,* singular form) The two ducts that carry sperm to the ejaculatory duct.

Tubal sterilization   Severing or in some manner blocking the oviducts. This prevents ova (eggs) from reaching the uterus.

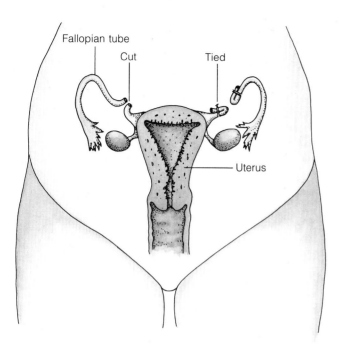

Fallopian tube
Cut
Tied
Uterus

Figure 6-9   Tubal sterilization is more complex than vasectomy.

incision through the vaginal wall, an approach that leaves no visible scar but is associated with a higher complication rate. Also, some conditions such as obesity or recent pregnancy make this method difficult or impossible. Either a regional or a general anesthetic can be used with these two types of tubal sterilization, and the operation takes about thirty minutes. If no complications occur, many hospitals allow the patient to return to her home the same day. The operation can be performed shortly after a normal delivery, or in the case of cesarean section immediately after the incision in the uterus is repaired.

Female sterilization by the standard abdominal or vaginal procedure is riskier than male sterilization. About 7 percent of the patients experience problems after the operation. Such problems arise mainly from the wound, infection, or bleeding. Serious complications are rare, and the death rate is low—especially when regional rather than general anesthesia is used.

An increasing number of tubal sterilizations are being done by a method called **laparoscopy.** A laparoscope, which is a tube containing a small light, is inserted through a small abdominal incision, and the surgeon looks through it to locate the oviducts. Instruments are passed either through the laparoscope or through a sec-

ond small incision, and the two oviducts are cauterized (sealed off) by electrocautery. Either a regional or general anesthetic can be used, but a general anesthetic is more common. The operation takes 15 minutes and can be done without overnight hospitalization. Most women leave the hospital two to four hours after surgery. Complications, such as bowel injury and hemorrhage, occur in 0.1 to 7 percent of laparoscopic sterilizations. This figure varies widely depending on the experience of the surgeon and type of equipment available. The mortality rate is low.

Laparoscopy has approximately the same failure rate as standard tubal ligations: about 3 out of every 1,000 cases. Reversibility rates are 50–70 percent for all methods.

Complaints of long-term abdominal discomfort and menstrual irregularity have been reported following female sterilization, but these have been difficult to interpret. Most women are satisfied. The number of women who feel regret varies in follow-up studies, and this fact, too, is difficult to interpret. Regret, when it does appear, seems to be related to previous difficulties, initial doubts and reservations, feelings of being pressured by the spouse, or changes in marital and family circumstances.

Hysterectomy, removal of the uterus, is the preferred method of sterilization for only a small number of women, usually women with preexisting menstrual problems. Because of the risks involved, hysterectomy is not recommended unless the patient has serious gynecologic problems such as disease or damage of the uterus and future surgery appears inevitable.

New Methods of Contraception

Even with all the improvements of recent years, the best of the present methods of contraception have drawbacks. The search still continues for the ideal method, the one that will be more effective, safer, cheaper, easier to use, more readily available, easily reversible, and acceptable to more people.

Many people place a high priority specifically on an increase in the male contraceptive alternatives. Throughout history, the responsibility for birth control has been assumed predominantly by women, partly because women have greater personal investment in preventing pregnancy with its many risks and childbearing with the many demands that fall mostly on women. Some women

---

Laparoscopy   Examining the internal organs by inserting a tube containing a small light through an abdominal incision.

Hysterectomy   Total or partial surgical removal of the uterus.

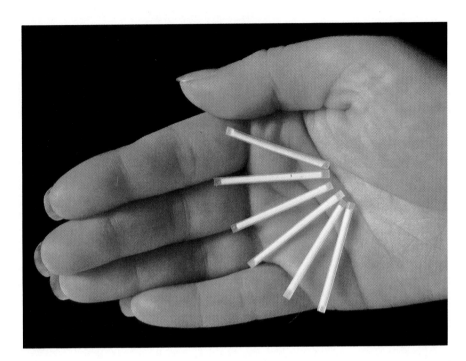

Contraceptive implants, filled with synthetic hormones and inserted under the skin on the arm or leg, can provide five years of protection against pregnancy.

in some settings see complete control as crucial. More birth control options have been available for female use, because there are more ways to intervene in the female reproductive system. Another factor may be the continuing underrepresentation of women in medicine, scientific research, pharmaceutical management, the FDA, and other political forces. Participation by women and an emphasis on their needs regarding birth control has been limited in these areas.

Some new methods are currently considered very promising. Two methods, injection and implant, have actually been approved and made available for public use in several countries around the world. However, it appears unlikely that U.S. manufacturers will introduce any new methods in the near future, partly because preclinical safety testing is so expensive and because the number of liability claims against these firms is skyrocketing. Some of the newest methods being studied are listed below.

• *Long-acting injectables.* Injections of progestin, a laboratory-made progesterone, every ninety days are almost 100 percent effective in preventing pregnancy. Progestins have several contraceptive effects: cervical mucus becomes thick and hampers the movement of sperm; transport of the egg through the tubes may be slowed down; changes in the uterine lining may prevent implantation; and subtle hormonal shifts may result in the inhibition of ovulation. This method still has disadvantages, however, including irregular menstrual bleeding patterns in the uterus and long delays (twelve

to twenty-one months) in the return of ovulatory cycles after injections are stopped. Less frequent injections of higher doses are also being tested.

• *Implants.* In this method, two to six capsules that are 1 inch long and spaghetti-width are filled with progestin and inserted under the skin of the inner arm or thigh. They can provide protection for up to five years. Side effects are similar to those of long-acting injectable progestins. Fertility quickly returns, however, on implant removal. One type of implant, called Norplant, is already approved in several countries, including the United States.

• *Vaginal ring.* The vaginal ring resembles the rim of a diaphragm and is molded with a mixture of progestin and estrogen. The woman inserts the ring herself and wears it for three weeks, during which time the hormones are absorbed into her bloodstream, preventing ovulation. Menstruation follows removal, and then a new ring is inserted.

• *Chemical contraceptives for men.* Male and female hormones can interfere with sperm development in the male in a way similar to ovulation suppression in the female. However, effectiveness of these hormones is often unpredictable and side effects may include both the loss of libido (sex drive) and the development of female secondary sex characteristics—for example, enlarged breasts.

Gossypol, a derivative of cottonseed oil used for several years in China, also results in very low sperm counts. Reported side effects include disturbances in potassium metabolism and general weakness. Also, animal studies in the United States indicate that it may be carcinogenic.

- *Contraceptive immunization.* Immunity to fertility has—rarely—occurred because a man has been (nonexperimentally) sensitized to his own sperm cells. He then produces antibodies that inactivate sperm as if they were a disease. In theory, a woman could be purposely sensitized against her own egg cells or against her partner's sperm cells. Experimentally, at least, the theory works, but widespread human testing cannot begin until several questions have been answered. How long the immunity would last and how to control it are not yet known, and serious allergic reactions could be a life-threatening problem.

- *Reversible sterilization.* Present methods of sterilization of both men and women are reversible 50–70 percent of the time. Several new techniques of sterilization are being studied in the hope that restoring fertility can be made easier and more predicable.

    Female sterilization has been attempted by injecting liquid silicone into the Fallopian tubes, where it solidifies and forms a plug. In animal experiments, however, such plugs have been readily dislodged by normal muscle activity, so this method is not likely to be very effective.

    In men, totally blocking sperm flow with removable clips and with various plugs has been tried, but both clips and plugs damaged the vasa, making restoration of fertility less likely. Recanalization of the vas, a phenomenon in which the sperm make a new path around the plug, has also occurred with plugs. Some of the plugs tested contain a tiny valve that can be opened manually or magnetically.

    Even when tissue damage and recanalization can be prevented, researchers face another problem: some vasectomized men develop antibodies to their sperm, which may persist after vasectomy reversal.

- *Prostaglandins.* A new and promising use of **prostaglandins** is their application to tampons, which are inserted to bring on menstruation shortly after a period is missed. Prostaglandins tampons used regularly at the end of each cycle could induce menstruation each time whether or not the cycle had been fertile.

- *Luteinizing Hormone-Releasing Hormone (LHRH).* LHRH, a naturally occurring compound in both men and women, acts on the pituitary gland, triggering the release of its hormones, which in turn play an essential role in sperm formation and ovulation. Synthetic analogs of LHRH, which are over 100 times as powerful as natural LHRH, are currently available. After these analogs are administered, the levels of pituitary hormones rise sharply, followed by a drop to subnormal levels, probably because the pituitary gland is overstimulated and exhausted. Once the low levels are established, it appears that in women (on whom most of the studies thus far have been completed) the pituitary-ovary cycle is effectively disrupted, and ovulation and menstruation stop temporarily. No immediate side effects have been detected. However, many questions regarding this complex interaction and its long-term effects remain, and any possible clinical application is undoubtedly several years away.

Issues in Contraception

The subject of contraception is closely tied to several issues that are currently receiving much attention in the United States—issues like premarital sexual relations, gender differences, and sex education for teenagers.

When Is It OK to Begin Having Sexual Relations?
One issue that strongly affects a society's approach to contraception is the question of when to begin having sexual relations. Opinions on this issue will largely determine one's views on sex education and contraception accessibility. A wide range of responses to this question can be found in the United States: only after marriage, when 18 years or older, when in a loving, stable relationship, when the partners have completed their education and/or could support a child, and whenever both partners feel ready and are using protection against pregnancy and STDs.

Opinions on sexual behavior shift from one decade to another. Although attitudes toward sexual relations became more liberal through the 1960s and 1970s, people started holding more restrictive views as the 1980s passed. For example, between 1985 and 1987, according to one recent poll, the proportion of people in the United States who opposed all sexual relations before marriage increased seven percentage points, the first reversal since 1969 (see the box entitled "Public Opinion on Premarital Sex"). Although public opinion in 1987 was almost evenly divided, with 46 percent of Americans thinking premarital sex was wrong, 48 percent finding it accept-

Prostaglandins   Naturally occurring chemicals, two of which induce abortion of the embryo or fetus when injected into the amniotic sac or inserted into the uterus.

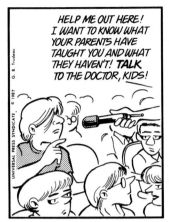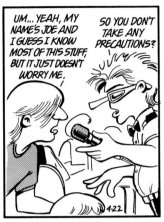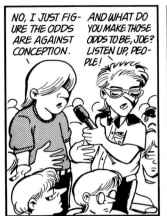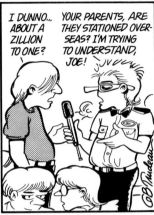

Doonesbury Copyright 1989 G. B. Trudeau. Reprinted with permission of Universal Press Syndicate. All rights reserved.

able, and 6 percent with no opinion, women and older adults were more inclined than men and younger adults to disapprove. The most common reasons given by individuals for their disapproval were moral or religious beliefs (83 percent); risk of STDs (20 percent); and risk of pregnancy (13 percent).

Closely related to the issue of beginning sexual relations is the more personal question: What would you consider the ideal amount of previous sexual experience for you and your spouse at the time of your marriage? Again, the views on this vary, especially in terms of what is desirable for men and for women. While chastity is still more commonly deemed desirable for women, being "sexually experienced" is often valued more highly for men.

As more women consider careers for themselves and therefore often delay childbearing and even marriage, the likelihood of sexual activity and the critical need for pregnancy prevention only increase. As a result, making decisions about sexual activity and contraception becomes even more important to those starting college or a career. Unfortunately, however, many individuals in this age group, even those who protect their health in all other areas of their life, do end up taking high risks in their sexual behavior. Ambivalence and lack of communication about who will "take charge" is common and is partly due to the denial and hypocrisy regarding sexual behavior in our society.

Contraception and Gender Differences   A second issue, one all couples must confront, is the differing significance of contraception to women and men; the consequences of not using contraception are markedly different for men and women. In past years, women have accepted the primary responsibility of contraception, along with related side effects and health risks, partly because of the wider spectrum of birth control methods

available to them. Men still have very few contraceptive options, with condoms being the only nonpermanent method. Recently, however, their participation has become critical, since condom use is central to "safer sex," even when OCs or other female methods are being used.

■ **Exploring Your Emotions**

What are your ideas about responsibility for contraception? Where did you get them? Are they tied to other ideas you have about male and female gender roles?

Although dependent primarily on cooperation of the man, condom use and the prevention of STDs has potentially greater consequences for the woman. While men may suffer only local and short-term effects from the most common diseases (not including AIDS), women face an increased risk of serious long-term effects, such as cervical cancer and/or pelvic infection with associated infertility, from these same prevalent STDs. In other words, although dependent on the male, condom use is clearly a more important issue for women. Future availability of a female condom may offer a helpful alternative.

Similarly, the experience of an unintended pregnancy is very different for the two involved partners. While men do suffer emotional stress from such an unexpected occurrence (and share financial and/or custodial responsibilities), women are much more intimately affected, simply by the natural, biological processes of the pregnancy and the outcome, whether abortion, adoption, or parenting. In addition, our societal attitudes are more severely punitive toward the woman and place much greater responsibility and blame on her when an unintended pregnancy occurs; the focus is almost entirely on the "girl who got into trouble" or the "unwed mother," with no mention of the "unwed father."

Public Opinion on Premarital Sex

Gallup polls indicate that Americans have adopted a more conservative stance toward premarital sex in recent years. The first poll shown here gives the percentages of people who said premarital sex was wrong or not wrong in 1969, 1973, 1985, and 1987. The second poll characterizes the respondents who said it was wrong by sex, age, religion, education, and geographic region. The third characterizes them by reasons given for believing that premarital sex is wrong.

Premarital Sex			
	Wrong	Not wrong	No opinion
1987	46%	48%	6%
1985	39	52	9
1973	48	43	9
1969	68	21	11

Premarital Sex			
(Percent Saying "Wrong")			
	1987	1985	1969
National	46%	39%	68%
Men	39	32	62
Women	53	44	74
18–29 years	27	18	49
30–49 years	41	35	67
50 & older	65	56	80
Protestants	52	46	70
Catholics	39	33	72
College education	40	31	56
High school	42	40	69
Grade school	60	60	77
East	37	40	65
Midwest	42	36	69
South	61	48	78
West	40	24	55

Why Premarital Sex Is Wrong						
	Moral, Religious Reasons	Risk of Disease	Risk of Pregnancy	Should Be Virgins	Other	No Opinion
National	83%	20%	13%	9%	5%	3%
Men	85	18	11	6	4	3
Women	82	21	14	10	6	3
College graduates	89	22	11	7	6	2
College incomplete	81	18	17	6	8	4
High school graduates	84	21	9	7	3	3
Not high school graduates	81	19	14	13	4	3
Protestants	88	12	18	8	4	3
Catholics	78	13	20	9	6	3
18–29 years	75	27	17	17	6	2
30–49 years	80	27	15	7	4	4
50 & older	88	13	9	7	5	5

Note: Totals exceed 100 percent because of multiple mentions.

Source: G. Gallup. 1987. More today than in 1985 say premarital sex is wrong. The Gallup Report 263: 20.

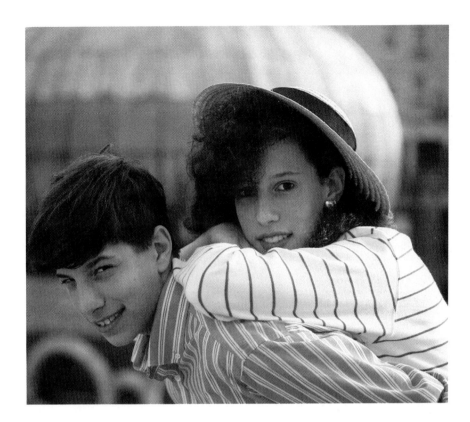

How old should people be when they become sexually active? The answer to this question depends on the personal values, beliefs, and experiences of the individuals involved.

Fortunately, there is a growing interest in the roles and responsibilities of men in family planning. For example, an American Public Health Association (APHA) Task Force on Men in Family Planning and Reproductive Health recently completed a review of available resources in this area. This group concluded that there is a serious lack of both educational materials and clinical programs that focus on male contraception and reproductive health. They emphasized that better printed material and audiovisual supplies, as well as specific training, are needed by health care workers in order to provide more balanced services. Especially needed is a greater emphasis on gender differences and couple communication.

Sex and Contraceptive Education for Teenagers   A third controversial question focuses on the best approach for sex education and pregnancy prevention programs for teenagers. Again, opinion in the United States is sharply divided. Certain religious groups express concern that more sex education, and especially the availability of contraceptives, will lead to more sexual activity and promiscuity. They maintain that greater access to improved contraception was a key factor contributing to the "sexual revolution" in the 1960s and that the ensuing liberal sexual attitudes have been generally more destructive than helpful. They point to an increase in divorces, a dramatic rise in STDs, and a general breakdown in morality as related negative effects.

■ **Exploring Your Emotions**

What are your feelings about sex education for children? Do you think it promotes responsibility or promiscuity or neither? Are you satisfied with what you were taught? What effect did it have on your sexual behavior?

Many in this group urge that educational responsibility be emphasized in the home, where parents can instill moral values, including premarital abstinence. According to some in this group, young people should primarily be taught and assisted to "just say no." They see most public education about contraception, and especially facilities that make supplies available, as only increasing the problem.

Other groups in the United States argue that encouraging public availability of contraceptive information and supplies does not necessarily result in an increase in promiscuous sexual behavior and point to the fact that many young teens are already pregnant when they first visit a health care facility. These groups assert that parents today aren't dealing effectively with the issue of sexuality and related problems and that a broader, coordinated approach involving public institutions, such as the school, are needed along with parental input. These groups encourage attempts by community facilities to help young individuals better understand their own sex-

Planned Parenthood

"Every child a wanted child": since its stormy beginnings over sixty years ago, Planned Parenthood Federation of America has sought to end compulsory parenthood by making birth control devices accessible to all who want them. Taking up their cause in local communities and courtrooms throughout the nation, Planned Parenthood has committed itself to making all Americans aware of the problems caused by unrestrained population growth, both here and abroad.

Planned Parenthood's educational goals are equally far-reaching. In the offices of all of its affiliates, basic birth control information is provided through films, group discussions, and individual counseling sessions. In addition, many affiliates offer special discussion groups for young people, where participants can talk about their anxieties, ask their questions, and share their problems in a supportive environment.

All the agency's affiliates also provide educational services within the community. Its trainers prepare teachers, social workers, nurses, and clergy to educate others in matters related to human sexuality and birth control.

Since Margaret Sanger, the agency's founder, began her courageous fight for voluntary parenthood, Planned Parenthood has actively opposed state and federal laws that interfere with parenthood by choice. In 1969, the agency published the nation's first county-by-county study of birth control needs and services among low-income women. This study was probably the single most important piece of research leading to the Family Planning Services and Population Research Act of 1970. With the passage of this act, the federal government for the first time authorized funds ($225 million) for birth control research, expanded family planning services, and the creation of the Office of

Population Affairs within the Department of Health, Education, and Welfare.

Planned Parenthood's activities literally span the globe. The International Planned Parenthood Federation (IPPF) is the world's largest voluntary family planning organization. Dedicated to the formation and support of national family planning associations throughout the world, it assists in developing programs to educate people about the personal, social, and economic benefits of family planning. IPPF also provides technical information to several agencies of the United Nations and gives national associations financial support and technical assistance.

To contact Planned Parenthood, write:

Planned Parenthood Federation
of America
810 Seventh Ave.
New York, NY 10019

uality and to utilize contraception when needed. Increased availability of contraceptive information and the methods themselves is seen as a necessary and realistic part of this approach.

While sexual and contraceptive education in public facilities remains a volatile issue, there is overall growing support for such programs. Many studies do seem to show that sexually active students who receive sex education are more likely to use contraceptives and that those who are not sexually active are not encouraged to initiate such behavior. However, these programs are receiving increasing support mainly because of the prevalent fear of AIDS and other STDs. In fact, in some cases the focus of "sex ed" is almost exclusively on disease prevention, with little attention given to pregnancy prevention. Although not as deadly as the AIDS epidemic, the more than 1 million teen pregnancies that occur each year in the United States is a serous public health prob-

lem and warrants much greater national attention than it has received in the past.

Which Contraceptive Method Is Right for You?

If you are sexually active, you need to use the contraceptive method that will work the best for you. The process of choosing and using a contraceptive method can be complex and varies greatly from one couple to another. Each individual must consider many variables in deciding which method is most acceptable and appropriate for her or him. Some important considerations are:

1. *Individual health risks of each method in terms of personal and family medical history.* IUDs are not recommended

for any young women without children, because of an increased risk of pelvic infection and subsequent infertility. Oral contraceptives should be used only after a clinical evaluation of one's medical history. Other methods have only minor and local side effects.

2. *Implications of unwanted pregnancy and therefore the importance of effectiveness.* Oral contraceptives, when taken correctly, offer by far the best protection against pregnancy. Condoms, diaphragms, and cervical caps should be combined with a spermicide and used with every intercourse. Neither FAM nor withdrawal is very effective and should never be relied upon when pregnancy prevention is important. (The box "Improving the Effectiveness of Your Contraception Method" gives further details.)

3. *Possible risks of sexually transmissible diseases.* Condom use, preferably with foam, is of critical importance whenever any risk of STD is present. This is especially true when you are not in an exclusive, long-term relationship or when you are taking the pill, because cervical changes occurring during hormone use may lead to increased vulnerability to certain diseases. Abstinence or outercourse (pleasure-giving activities that don't involve intercourse or any other exchange of body fluids) can be a satisfactory alternative for some individuals and couples.

4. *Convenience and comfort of the method as viewed by each partner.* The oral contraceptive is generally ranked high in this category unless there are negative side effects and health risks or if forgetting to take the pill is a problem. Some users think condom use disrupts spontaneity and lowers penile sensitivity. (Creative approaches to condom use and the improved quality of new models can decrease these complaints.) The diaphragm, cap, sponge, and spermicides can be inserted before intercourse begins, but are still considered a significant bother by some.

5. *Type of relationship.* The barrier methods require more motivation and a sense of responsibility from *each* partner than pill taking does. When the method depends on the cooperation of one's partner, assertiveness is necessary, no matter how difficult. This is especially true in new relationships, when condom use is most important. When sexual activity is infrequent, a barrier method may make more sense than the daily OC.

6. *Ease and cost of obtaining and maintaining each method.* With OC use, an annual pelvic exam and periodic clinic checks are required and important. In addition, the cost of the pills themselves tends to be higher than barrier supplies for most couples, although insurance plans will sometimes cover pill expense. Diaphragms also require an initial exam and fitting.

7. *The method's acceptability in terms of religious or other philosophical beliefs.* According to the religious beliefs of some individuals, abstinence is the only acceptable form of sexual behavior in all premarital relationships. Even after marriage, the Catholic Church holds that all artificial birth control is wrong and the FAM is the only permissible contraceptive method.

Whatever your needs, circumstances, or beliefs, do make a choice about contraception—not choosing anything is the one method known *not* to work. This is an area in which taking charge of your health has immediate and profound implications for your future. The method you choose today won't necessarily be the one you'll want to use your whole life or even next year. But it should be one that works for you right now. Contraception is something you can't afford to leave to chance.

■ **Exploring Your Emotions**

What are the relevant factors that you need to consider in choosing a contraceptive method? Which one would be best for you? Why?

Summary

- Because preventing unintended pregnancy and sexually transmissible diseases is so crucial to optimal health, decisions about sexual behavior and contraception—although emotional, complex, and difficult—are crucial.

Principles of Contraception

- The barrier method of contraception physically prevents the sperm from reaching the egg; hormonal methods are designed to prevent ovulation, fertilization, and/or implantation; and surgical methods permanently block the movement of sperm or eggs to the site of potential conception.

- Choice of contraceptive method depends on effectiveness, convenience, cost, reversibility, side effects and risk factors, and protection against STDs. The concept of effectiveness includes theoretical effectiveness, use effectiveness, and continuation rate.

Improving the Effectiveness
of Your Contraceptive Method

Combination oral contraceptive	Follow pill-taking instructions carefully and consistently. Use a backup method such as foam or condoms during the first month.
IUD	Have IUD inserted by experienced clinician.
	Frequently check for IUD's position during the first few months. (User should feel thread in cervical opening but not the stem of the IUD.)
	Use a backup method such as foam or condoms during the first three months and, if desired, at mid-cycle thereafter.
Condom	Use with every act of intercourse.
	Put condom on erect penis before *any* penis-vagina contact.
	Leave space in tip of condom for semen.
	Remove carefully to avoid spillage.
	Avoid damage to condom; handle carefully.
	Avoid heat and Vaseline or any products containing mineral or vegetable oils.
	Do not use after two years.
	Buy a good brand (ask your pharmacist).
	Use foam along with condom.
Diaphragm and jelly	Use with every act of intercourse.
	Ask for thorough instruction with initial fitting.
	Have diaphragm and its fit checked every one to two years by an experienced clinician. Replace if necessary. Also have fit checked after a weight change of more than 10 pounds.
	Always use ample amounts of jelly or cream; add as necessary.
	Check position after insertion. Front rim must be behind pubic bone, and dome must cover cervix.
	Inspect regularly for defects or holes.
	Avoid use of Vaseline or any products containing mineral or vegetable oils or perfumed powders, including talcum powder, as they can damage the latex and irritate the vagina.
Vaginal spermicides	Use with every act of intercourse.
	Follow instructions regarding time limits of effectiveness.
	Use ample amounts.
	When using foam, shake vigorously before use.
	Use condoms along with spermicide.
FAM	Combine calendar, temperature, and mucus methods.
Withdrawal	Avoid penis-vagina contact during secretion of preejaculatory lubricating fluid (very difficult to detect).
	Use foam along with coitus interruptus.

Whenever you discontinue one method, immediately replace it with another. Many unplanned pregnancies occur when couples "take a chance" between methods.

Reversible Contraceptives

- Reversibility in contraceptives is especially important to those who have not yet had children or might want more.
- In oral contraceptives (OCs), a combination of estrogen and progesterone prevents ovulation, hinders the movement of sperm, and affects the uterine lining so that implantation is inhibited.
- OC users take estrogen/progesterone pills for three weeks and inactive pills (or no pills) for one week. A variation of the OC, the minipill, contains no estrogen.
- Advantages of OCs include its high degree of effectiveness, simplicity of use, freedom from interruption during foreplay and intercourse, and reversibility. In addition to minor disadvantages, possible serious side effects include blood clots, stroke, and heart attacks.
- Pill effectiveness, theoretically 1 pregnancy in 1,000, is about 3 in 100 in first-year users. It is the most effective reversible method.
- One "morning after" pill, diethylstilbestrol (DES), is used infrequently because it has been linked to cancers in daughters of women who took the drug. Another pill, with fewer health risks than DES, has been approved for "morning after" use in Europe. In this country it is available to physicians and clinics for other purposes but does not have FDA approval for postcoital use.
- How intrauterine devices work is not clear; they may cause biochemical changes in the uterus, immobilize sperm in the uterus, shorten the travel time of the egg in the oviduct, or interfere with the implantation of the egg in the uterus.
- Advantages of IUDs include reliability, simplicity of use, freedom from interruption during coitus, and—in the absence of complications—reversibility. Spontaneous expulsion is a possibility.
- Pelvic inflammatory disease (PID), a serious complication possible with IUD use, can lead to infertility if not treated with antibiotics. An annual checkup helps reduce all risks and complications.
- Condoms are the most popular barrier method, and their use has increased dramatically, partly because of their effectiveness against STDs.
- The condom must be put on the penis before it is inserted into the vagina so that sperm-containing pre-ejaculatory fluids don't cause pregnancy. Lubricants containing mineral or vegetable oil will cause the condom to disintegrate and cannot be used.
- Advantages of condoms include availability and ease of purchase, simplicity of use, immediate reversibility, protection against STDs, and freedom from side effects.
- Although theoretical effectiveness is 3 percent pregnancies, use effectiveness averages 12 percent during the first year.

- Female condoms, not yet available in the United States, are made of a polyurethane sheath with two flexible rings; they can be inserted well before intercourse.
- When used correctly, with spermicidal cream or jelly, the diaphragm covers the mouth of the uterus and blocks sperm from entering. Diaphragms require a prescription, and a careful fitting is necessary.
- A diaphragm must be inserted within six hours of intercourse and must be kept in place for six hours afterward. Although theoretical effectiveness is 2–3 percent pregnancies, use effectiveness is 14–18 percent.
- The cervical cap is a rubber or plastic cup that adheres to the cervix through suction. It is available for women who have anatomical features that preclude diaphragm use; it can be kept in place for 48 hours. Effectiveness is similar to that of the diaphragm.
- The sponge is a round absorbent device with a concave dimple on one side that helps it fit snugly over the cervix. It is made of polyurethane and saturated with spermicide. Sponges act as barriers, spermicides, and absorbers of seminal fluid. Use effectiveness is 16 percent pregnancies in women who have not yet had children.
- Vaginal spermicides come in the form of foams, creams, jellies, and suppositories. They must be inserted less than one-half hour before intercourse.
- Because of religion, culture, poverty, or lack of information, many people use no contraception at all or use "natural" methods. Abstinence may be chosen out of fear of STDs or because of personal needs.
- The Fertility Awareness Method (FAM) is based on avoiding coitus during the fertile phase of a woman's menstrual cycle. The one egg released per month lives about twenty-four hours and sperm can fertilize an egg for six to seven days, so fertilization is possible during eight days of each cycle. A calendar method, a basal body temperature method, and a mucus method may be used to determine the fertile period. FAM is not recommended if menstrual cycles are irregular or if pregnancy would be a problem; the failure rate is around 20 percent during the first year.
- When withdrawal is used, the male must remove his penis from the vagina just before he ejaculates. The failure rate is 20–25 percent in the first year.

Permanent Contraception—Sterilization

- Sterilization is permanent, and no further contraceptive action is needed. Reversibility can never be guaranteed. Male sterilization may be preferable to female sterilization because of costs, complications, and feelings of regret.
- Vasectomy—male sterilization—involves severing the vasa deferentia. No long-term complications have been

discovered. The failure rate is about 1 percent. Reversibility has been reported as high as 80 percent but is probably lower.

- Female sterilization involves severing or blocking the oviducts so that the egg cannot reach the uterus. The abdominal, vaginal, and laparoscopic methods are all done in the hospital or an outpatient surgery center, and the woman usually returns home the same day. Laparoscopy has the fewest complications. The failure rate is about 3 in 1,000; reversibility is 50–70 percent.

- Hysterectomy is not recommended except for women with serious gynecologic problems.

New Methods of Contraception

- The ideal contraceptive in terms of effectiveness, safety, and reversibility has yet to be found.

- Long-lasting (90-day) injections of progestin are nearly 100 percent effective. Implants of progestin can protect for up to five years. The vaginal ring is molded with hormones and worn for three weeks, preventing ovulation.

- Chemical contraceptives for men are unpredictable and can cause loss of sex drive and development of female secondary characteristics. Theoretically, a woman could be immunized against her own eggs or her partner's sperm. Methods of reversible sterilization have not been very successful and, in men, are complicated by the development of antibodies to sperm. Other hormonal methods are still being studied.

Issues in Contraception

- Opinions on when to begin having sexual relations are tied to views on sex education and contraception accessibility. Because women today frequently delay childbearing, decisions about sexual activity and contraception are essential for optimal health.

- Although condom use depends on male cooperation, the implications of not using them are greater for women, both in terms of pregnancy and the consequences of STDs.

- Opinion in the United States is divided on the issues of sex education and availability of contraceptives for teenagers; increasing support for such programs is probably due to fear of AIDS, although the issue of teen pregnancy needs more attention.

Which Contraceptive Method Is Right for You?

- Issues to be considered in choosing a contraceptive include (1) individual health risks of each method, (2) importance of effectiveness in terms of implications of unwanted pregnancy, (3) possible risk of sexually transmissible diseases, (4) convenience and comfort of the method as viewed by each partner, (5) type of relationship, (6) cost and ease of maintaining each method, (7) acceptability in terms of religious or philosophical beliefs.

Take Action

1. Consider the different methods of contraception described in this chapter. In your health diary, rank the methods according to how they suit your particular lifestyle. Take into account such considerations as how often you have sexual intercourse, convenience, and cost.

2. Consider what health risks you or your partner takes (or would take) by using a particular contraceptive method. For example, if you smoke and take birth control pills, you increase your risk of heart attack or stroke. In your health diary, make a list of the different methods and any additional risks associated with them for you or your partner. Don't forget to include the risk of pregnancy. Compare this list with your list for item 1.

3. In your health diary, list the positive behaviors and attitudes that help you adhere to your beliefs about contraception (for example, not drinking alcohol or drinking only in moderation makes it unlikely that you would make an unwise choice because you had had too much to drink). Are there ways you can strengthen these behaviors? Then list behaviors and attitudes that might interfere with your effective use of contraception. Can you do anything to change or improve any of these?

Selected Bibliography

Djerassi, Carl. 1989 (July 28). The bitter pill. *Science.* 245:356–361.

Forrest, Katherine A., Janice M. Swanson and Douglas E. Beckstein. 1989. The availability of educational and training materials on men's reproductive health. *Family Planning Perspectives,* 21(3):120–122.

IUDs—A new look. 1988. Population information program—The Johns Hopkins University. *Population Reports,* Series B, No. 5, pp. 1–31.

Johnson, Jeanette H. 1989. Weighing the evidence on the pill and breast cancer. *Family Planning Perspectives* 21(2):89–92.

Kjersgaard, Anne G., Ingrid Thranov, Ole Vedel Rasmussen, and Jens Hertz. 1989. Male or female sterilization: A comparative study. *Fertility and Sterility* 51(3):439–443.

Lee, Nancy C., George L. Rubin, and Robert Borucki. 1988. The intrauterine device and pelvic inflammatory disease revisited: New results from the women's health study. *Obstetrics and Gynecology.* 72(1):1–6.

Louv, William C., Harland Austin, Jeffrey Perlman, and W. James Alexander. 1989. Oral contraceptive use and the risk of chlamydial and gonococcal infections." *American Journal of Obstetrics and Gynecology* 160(2):396–402.

Mishell, Daniel R. 1989. Contraception. *New England Journal of Medicine* 320(12):777–787.

Murray, Pamela P., Bruce V. Stadel, and James J. Schlesselman. 1989. Contraceptive use in women with a family history of breast cancer." *Obstetrics and Gynecology* 73(6):977–983.

Oral contraceptives and breast cancer. *International Planned Parenthood Federation Medical Bulletin* 23(4): August 1989, p. 3.

Rosoff, Jeannie I. 1989. Sex education in the schools: Policies and practice. *Family Planning Perspectives* 21(2):52, 64.

Thomas, Patricia. 1988. Contraceptives. *Medical World News* 29(5):49–68.

Voeller, Bruce, Anne H. Coulson, Gerald S. Bernstein, and Robert M. Nakamura. 1989. Mineral oil lubricants cause rapid deterioration of latex condoms. *Contraception* 39(1):95–102.

Recommended Readings

Boston Women's Health Book Collective. 1984. *The New Our Bodies, Ourselves.* New York: Simon and Schuster. *Comprehensive paperback, written from a woman's viewpoint. Broad coverage of many women's health concerns, with an emphasis on psychological, as well as physical factors. A favorite for many years. Periodically updated.*

Family Planning Perspectives (journal published bimonthly). New York: Alan Guttmacher Institute. *An excellent journal focused entirely on family planning issues. A good source for latest research findings. Some articles are quite technical (science based and statistics oriented), but all are very readable.*

Hatcher, R. A., F. J. Guest, F. H. Stewart, G. K. Stewart, J. Trussell, S. Cerel, and W. Cates. 1988. *Contraceptive Technology 1988–89.* New York: Irvington. *A compact, reliable source of up-to-date information on contraception, with a focus on the technological aspects, rather than the psychological. The information is somewhat geared toward health care providers, but suitable for all readers. Many references and sources of information are included. Updated every two years.*

Contents

Making Connections

Whether your connection with the abortion issue is political, social, or personal, it's likely that your life will be touched by this complex and emotional issue in the 1990s. The scenarios presented on these pages describe situations in which people have to use information, make a decision, or choose a course of action, all relating to abortion. As you read them, imagine yourself in each situation and consider what you would do. After you've finished the chapter, read the scenarios again and see if what you've learned has changed how you would think, feel, or act in each situation.

Your friends are talking about a film they saw that claims to show the reactions of a 12-week-old fetus in the process of being aborted. They say you can see the fetus thrashing around in fear and even "screaming." You find it hard to believe that a fetus at that stage of development could have such a response. Your friends say that if you don't believe it, you should see the film. Could seeing the film prove your opinions to be correct or incorrect? Is there another way to get answers to your questions?

You and your boyfriend took a chance on having sex without contraception a while ago, and now you've missed your period. You haven't been able to think very clearly about what that might mean or focus on any kind of decisive action. Your boyfriend is pushing you to see a doctor or get a pregnancy test. He says that if you're going to want an abortion, the earlier you have it, the better. You want to wait a little longer and see if you get your next period. Which would be the better course of action?

7
Abortion

As the oldest of eight brothers and sisters, you've been around young children and babies your whole life. That's why you don't think you can end your accidental pregnancy with an abortion. It's also why you don't want to have a large family yourself or begin having children at 20. You're leaning toward giving the baby up for adoption, but you're worried that it won't be loved as much as you would love it or have a good home. Are your concerns justified? Is there any way you can ensure your child's well-being? How can you get the information you need to make your decision?

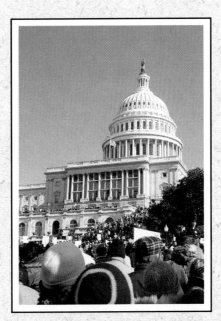

Your roommate had an abortion several months ago. You expected her to be depressed afterwards, but instead she was euphoric. She said she was so relieved that she felt she'd gotten a whole new lease on life. She talked about how blue the spring sky was and how sweet the air smelled. But lately she's been unusually quiet and subdued, avoiding social occasions and spending a lot of time by herself. Could she still be reacting to the abortion? If so, is there anything you can do to help?

You agree to drive a friend to a women's health center in a nearby metropolitan area for an abortion. When you get there, you find a demonstration going on outside the clinic. While you're waiting to drive your friend home, you go outside and listen to an argument between two opposing demonstrators. One of the things the "pro-life" demonstrator says is that many abortions are performed on fetuses that could survive outside the womb if given the chance. The pro-choice advocate responds that most abortions are performed in the first eight weeks of pregnancy, long before the fetus could survive outside the womb. The pro-life advocate says that in any event conception marks the beginning of life and that fetuses are human beings with civil rights. The pro-choice advocate responds, "What about the woman's rights? We're not pro-abortion—we're pro-choice." Although you've thought about the abortion issue, you don't really know where you stand. Are some of these claims true and others false? What information do you need to form your own opinion about abortion?

In the United States today, few issues are as complex and emotion-filled as abortion. While most public attention has focused on legal definitions and restrictions, the most difficult aspects of abortion actually take place at a much more personal level. Because the majority of women having abortions are young, many college students have had some type of direct exposure to these more personal experiences of abortion. This gives them an inside perspective on the dilemma.

On campuses today, as in our society at large, many powerful forces (including the great emphasis on sexuality and on the "good times" that follow alcohol consumption) contribute to the high rate of unintended pregnancy and abortion. At all school levels and in the general public, there is simultaneously great resistance to confronting these related issues openly and honestly—resulting in a lack of programs to deal with the problem at a preventive level.

With their inside vantage point, college students are in a key position to understand and to address the contributing factors, as well as the broad effects of unintended pregnancies and abortion. Instead of simply attempting to legislate certain behaviors, they can choose to grapple with the complex human factors that go into the prevention as well as the "treatment" of unintended pregnancy. This chapter will provide basic information on abortion, including the current focuses of controversy. We hope it will act as a springboard for you to form your own views and, more importantly, personal plans for constructive action.

The Abortion Issue

The following discussion presents various perspectives on abortion. The word **abortion**, by official or strict definition means the expulsion of a fetus from the uterus before it is sufficiently developed to survive. As commonly used, however, *abortion* refers only to those expulsions that are artificially induced by mechanical means or drugs, and *miscarriage* is the word generally used for a spontaneous abortion, one that occurs naturally with no causal intervention. In this chapter, the word *abortion* will be used to mean a deliberately induced abortion.

History of Abortion in the United States   For more than two centuries, abortion policy in the United States followed English common law, which made the practice a crime only when performed after "quickening" (fetal

movement that begins at about twenty weeks). There was little public objection to this policy until the early 1800s when an anti-abortion movement began, led primarily by physicians who questioned the doctrine of quickening and who objected to the growing practice of abortion by untrained persons (in part because it weakened their control of medical services).

■ **Exploring Your Emotions**

Modern medical technology makes it possible to identify fetuses with some genetic, chromosomal, and other defects before birth. Do you think these fetuses should be aborted? Why or why not?

This anti-abortion drive gained minimal attention until the mid-1800s, when newspaper advertisements for abortion preparations became common and concern grew that women were using abortion as a means of birth control (and perhaps to cover up extramarital activity). There was much discussion about the corruption of morality among women in the United States, and by the 1900s, virtually all states had anti-abortion laws. These laws stayed in effect until the 1960s, when courts began to invalidate them on the grounds of constitutional vagueness and violation of right to privacy.

Current Legal Status   In 1973, the abortion issue was thrust to the center of legal debate when the U.S. Supreme Court made abortion legal in the landmark case of *Roe vs. Wade.* To replace the restrictions most states still imposed at that time, the justices devised new standards to govern abortion decisions. They divided pregnancy into three parts or trimesters, giving a pregnant woman less choice about abortion as she advances toward full term. In the first trimester, the abortion decision must be left to the judgment of the pregnant woman and her physician. During the second trimester, similar rights remain but a state may regulate factors that protect the health of the woman, such as type of facility where an abortion may be performed. In the third trimester, when the fetus is viable (capable of survival outside of the uterus), a state may regulate and even bar all abortions except those considered necessary to preserve the mother's life or health.

After 1973, various campaigns were waged to overturn the Supreme Court decision and to ban abortions by amending the U.S. Constitution. In addition, many other

---

Abortion   The premature expulsion or removal of an embryo or fetus from the uterus.

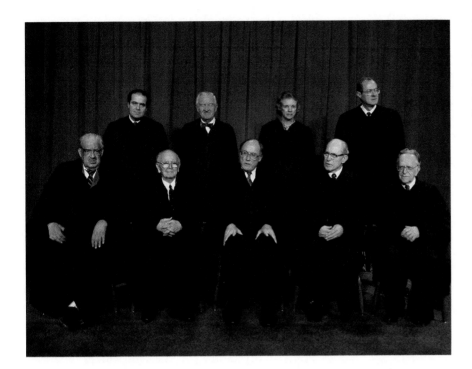

In 1989 the U.S. Supreme Court upheld the legality of abortion but ruled that the states could impose restrictions on it. These Supreme Court justices will be responsible for handing down further decisions and setting legal policy on abortion in the 1990s.

forms of increased abortion regulation were introduced into legislative bodies at the local, state, and national levels, although most were rejected. The U.S. Supreme Court, which heard arguments on abortion cases nearly every year, continued to uphold its 1973 decision. However, with the presidential appointments of conservative justices in the mid-1980s, the Court's vote in favor of abortion rights, originally seven to two in 1973, dwindled to an unpredictable five-four lineup.

In July 1989, another legal milestone was reached, when the Supreme Court handed down its decision in *Webster vs. Reproductive Health Services*. The Court did not overturn *Roe*, but did let stand several key restrictions on abortions enacted by the Missouri legislature in 1986. The two most severe restrictions forbid the use of all public facilities, resources, and employees for abortion services and require costly and time-consuming tests to determine fetal viability whenever the doctor estimates the fetus to be 20 weeks or older. The majority of justices also rejected *Roe's* framework of trimesters, a structure that attempted to balance women's rights against fetal rights and did not replace it with any other standard for weighing those rights. In addition, the justices declined to specifically address the preamble of the Missouri law that stated, "the life of each human being begins at conception," saying that it was only a "value judgment" and that it did not "regulate abortion."

Since the Webster decision gave few guidelines (other than that further state restrictions will probably be upheld), chaos can be expected at the state levels. Great

disparities in the availability of legal abortion are likely to exist from one area of the country to another, causing a checkerboard effect (see Figure 7-1). States where abortion laws had been liberalized prior to the 1973 *Roe* decision, mostly in the West, the Northeast, and the Middle Atlantic regions, will probably not change their laws significantly. Other states, mainly those where fundamentalist or Mormon influence is strong, will probably decide to bar all abortions, except those necessary to save the woman's life or perhaps in cases of rape and incest. Those states in between are likely to add other regulations, such as those that would require waiting periods, parental or spousal consent, detailed descriptive information, and very strict licensing of all abortion facilities.

■ Exploring Your Emotions

Some people believe that teenagers should have their parents' permission before they can have an abortion and married women should have their husbands' permission before they can have an abortion. How do you feel about these restrictions?

While not banning abortion outright, the addition of these various regulations will seriously restrict accessibility to abortion for many women, especially those with limited resources. For example, the indigent and the young will be most affected by any prohibitions placed

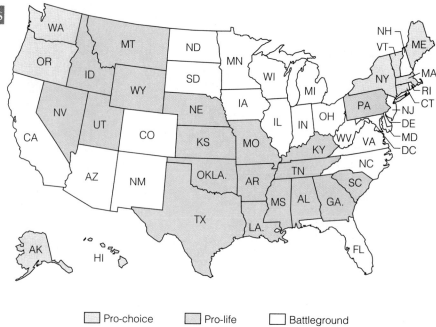

Figure 7-1 Disparities in attitude toward legal abortion in the 50 states.

Pro-choice   Pro-life   Battleground

on public facilities and funding. These are the same women who will be most affected by legal changes necessitating travel for a legal abortion and laws requiring additional tests in the case of late abortion (since they make up the bulk of those having late abortion). Concerns have been expressed that the new regulations may result in a two-tiered health care system, one for women with means and another for those without. (Table 7-1 lists the average cost of an abortion in the United States.)

The complete overturning of *Roe vs. Wade* by the Supreme Court may well occur as numerous new test cases are brought for its consideration. Such a reversal would permit, but not require, states to prohibit all abortion. In the absence of federal legislation, differences in availability, cost, and timing of abortion would continue to exist from one state to another, depending on each one's laws and court interpretations. Both pro-choice and prolife groups would most likely move to the national level, seeking federal legislation, the former to ensure abortion rights and the latter to make abortion a federal crime. However, legal experts are divided as to what constitutional authority the U.S. Congress may have to pass either pro- or anti-abortion legislation. Prolonged confusion and even more heated debate are likely to follow.

Moral Considerations   Along with the legal debates has come ongoing arguments between "pro-life" and "pro-choice" groups regarding the ethics of abortion, what is right and what is wrong in a moral sense (see the box

entitled "The Opposing Views"). Central to the pro-life position is the belief that the fertilized egg must be valued as a human being from the moment of conception, and abortion at any time is equivalent to murder. This group holds that any woman who has sexual intercourse knows that pregnancy is a possibility, and should she willingly have intercourse and get pregnant she is morally obligated to carry the pregnancy through. Pro-life followers encourage adoption for women who feel they are unable to raise the child and point out how many couples are seeking babies for adoption. Pro-lifers do not see the availability of legal abortion as essential to women's well-being, but view it instead as having an overall destructive effect on our traditional morals and values.

Table 7-1 The cost of an abortion U.S. National Average Price in 1989	
Gestation period	**Cost**
First 12 weeks of pregnancy	$210
12 to 16 weeks	$400–600
17 to 20 weeks	$600–900
20 to 22 weeks	$900+
Source: National Abortion Foundation.	

The Opposing Views

Restrictions Mean Suffering, Death

by Kate Michelman

Nineteen eighty-nine was a pivotal year in the battle to protect the right to choose abortion. The Supreme Court ruling in *Webster vs. Reproductive Health Services* in July and the nationwide political mobilization in the fall made abortion a dominant issue in the United States. The 1990s are shaping up as the decade of choice in America. In the coming years, state legislatures, the Congress, courts, and the electorate itself will have to address abortion and the related issues of birth control and sex education.

Abortion is a complex issue for everyone. It involves the most fundamental questions about religion, ethics, morality, and the role of government in decisions involving family planning. It touches all Americans, from policy makers to individual voters. But most importantly, it affects women with unwanted pregnancies and their families. The central question in the debate is simple: Who decides? Who should resolve these difficult issues? Should it be politicians? Should it be those who call themselves "pro-life"? Or should it be the women and families directly involved?

Those of us who support abortion rights believe that women and families must make these decisions for themselves and that the choice in each case is an individual one. We are pro-choice, not "pro-abortion." Abortion is an issue about which there are deep and honest differences of opinion. We respect those differences. As diffi-

cult as it is morally for some people to accept abortion, we feel there is a greater wrong in forcing a woman to undergo the demanding, intimate, and at times, life-threatening experiences of pregnancy and childbirth. For some women, the pain and suffering of being denied the choice to end a pregnancy is so extreme that they have risked and lost their lives in order to avoid it. We defend the right of women to choose whether or not to have an abortion. We also work to prevent any parent, spouse, doctor, or politician from ever forcing an abortion on any woman who does not want one.

A small, extremist minority cannot be allowed to impose its views and take away our most fundamental liberty: the right to choose. This right establishes that an outsider cannot determine when or whether an individual may have a family. The anti-choice minority claims that human life begins at conception. In fact, there is no consensus about when human life begins. Certainly, women recognize that a fetus has the potential for human life. But "when human life begins" is a moral, religious, ethical, and philosophical question. Only the woman involved can weigh the moral issues. No government can possibly legislate these wrenching decisions.

For seventeen years *Roe vs. Wade*, the landmark decision legalizing abortion in all fifty states, has been the law of the land. It provided that abortion in the first

three months of pregnancy, defined as the first trimester, be free from government interference and established some limits on abortion in the second and third trimesters. Many politicians have placated anti-choice forces by stating their personal opposition to abortion, but have not had the power to act on it. In its 1989 decision in *Webster vs. Reproductive Health Services*, the Supreme Court ruled that states could enact legislation that severely restricts abortion. The political aspect of the abortion issue has taken on a new complexity.

In some areas, anti-choice forces are asking politicians to translate their personal ambivalence toward abortion into public policy by enacting onerous restrictions on abortion. On the other hand, the pro-choice majority will be scrutinizing the actions of elected officials as they deal with this issue. Pro-choice voters are making clear to politicians who restrict abortion that, as a consequence, pregnant women will be forced either to bear unwanted children or to suffer the pain and degradation of illegal abortions. Many women will die.

Consider, also, what happens to children who are born unwanted. For women facing crisis pregnancies, adoption can be an option. But it is the worst kind of deceit to claim that there is a loving family waiting to adopt the child of every woman—from teenage welfare mothers to drug addicts.

Part of our work is directed to

The Opposing Views (continued)

prevent pregnancies and to reduce the need for abortion. We support sex education and safe, accessible contraception. We work to assure that every child is fed, housed, and educated.

The decision to have an abortion is not an easy one. We would all like to see fewer women facing crisis pregnancies and the wrenching decisions they involve. But, in reality, whether or not to have an abortion is often a choice women face. The world is not perfect; there will always be a need for abortion services. Women are entitled to make these decisions themselves, in consultation with families, trusted friends, religious counselors, and doctors, if they so wish. The option of whether or not to have an abortion is a fundamental right. Politicians, extremists, and clinic protesters have no right to interfere with this right.

A woman's right to choose safe, legal, and accessible abortion should not be restricted by anti-choice politicians. As a nation we must trust women to use their personal judgment in making thoughtful, conscientious decisions regarding procreation. Sometimes those decisions involve terminating a pregnancy. The National Abortion Rights Action League (NARAL) is committed to defending the right of all women to make these personal decisions and to ensuring that abortion is accessible to all women who choose it.

Kate Michelman is the Executive Director of NARAL.

The Opposing Views

The Fetus Is Life Itself

J. C. Willke, M.D.

In looking at abortion, the first question to ask is: What is this that grows within the woman? Is this human life? Or, when will it be? If it's not human life, then a case can be made to permit abortion. If, however, this being is fully human, sexed, alive, complete, and intact from the first-cell stage, then a second human life exists and we have a collision of the rights of two humans.

So, first, let's ask: Is this human life? The answer lies in books on biology, embryology, and fetology. In these sciences there is no disagreement on the facts of when human life begins. At the union of sperm and ovum there exists a living, single-celled, complete human organism. It is already male or female, is alive and growing, and is human, as the forty-six human chromosomes in the cell's nucleus mark this microscopic being as a member of the human family. This is arguably the most complicated cell in the entire world; it contains more information than could be contained in all of NASA's computers. As this single-celled human organism divides and subdivides, each cell in turn contains progressively less information, is more specialized.

At one week of life, this embryonic human attaches to the nutrient lining of the woman's womb and soon sends into her body a hormonal message that stops her period. About four days after the time when the woman's period

The Opposing Views (continued)

would have begun, the embryo's heart begins to beat. At forty days brain waves can be recorded. By ten weeks the structure of the body is completely formed. By three months all organ systems are functioning. To deny that fully human life begins at fertilization is to deny the known facts of fetal development and biological science.

Some argue that life existed in the sperm and ovum and will exist in the future. True, but we are not asking about generic life, but rather about this one unique individual's human life, which begins at fertilization and ends at death.

Some would measure the beginning of human life with a theologic yardstick, speaking of soul, God, and creation. In a secular state, however, we cannot use a theologic belief to define when human life begins for the purpose of making laws that either protect or allow the destruction of that life.

Others use various philosophic definitions of when the fullness of humanness exists, such as when cognition and self-consciousness are possible, when love is exchanged, when a being is declared to be "humanized" or "socialized," or when certain biologic mileposts are reached. Though these definitions are arrived at by intellectual processes, they cannot be scientifically proven. Open to diametric disagreement among people of good will, these definitions are also beliefs. We should not impose either religious or philosophic beliefs upon others in our culture. If one defines human life from the facts of natural science, human life, complete and intact, begins at

fertilization. That is a fact that we must face and work with.

Because this is human life from the very moment of conception, the issues touching that life are civil rights and human rights and the laws protecting those rights.

Now, let us ask a second question: Should there be equal protection under the law for all living humans? Or, should the law discriminate fatally against entire classes of humans, in this case against those still living in the womb?

Interestingly enough, our nation faced a similar situation once before—slavery. In 1857 the Supreme Court ruled in the Dred Scott case that black people were not legal persons before the law. They were the property of the slave owner, who could buy, sell, or even kill them. Abolitionists' protests were countered: "Now look, you find slavery morally offensive? Well, you don't have to own a slave. But don't force your morality on the owner, for he has the constitutional right to choose to own a slave." In 1973 the Court did it again. In *Roe vs. Wade*, also by a 7 to 2 margin, it ruled that unborn people were not legal persons. They were the property of the owner (the mother), who could keep or kill. Pro-lifers objected, to hear the same response. "Look, you find abortion morally offensive. Well, you don't have to have one. But don't force your morality on the owner (the woman) for she now has the constitutional right to choose, to kill."

The Dred Scott decision discriminated by skin color; *Roe vs. Wade* discriminates by place of

residence: still living in the womb. Each is a civil rights outrage.

A woman has a right to her own body, but to say that the little passenger residing within her is part of her body is to utter a biologic absurdity.

But she does not want this child? Since when does anyone's right to live depend upon someone else wanting them? Killing the unwanted is a monstrous evil.

A woman's issue? Did you know that women make up the overwhelming majority in the pro-life movement and that opinion polls consistently show more opposition to abortion from females than from males?

So, should a woman have the right to choose? I have a right to free speech, but not to shout "fire" in a theater. A person's right to anything stops when it injures or kills another living human.

No one should minimize the problems of pregnant women. With adequate counseling, informed consent, involvement of parents, husbands, and friends, we can help solve most of their problems, but sadly, never all of them. The pivotal question is, Should any civilized nation give to one citizen the absolute legal right to kill another to solve that first person's personal problem? I think not. We must give women far more help, both privately and publicly than is available today. But, we simply cannot continue to solve their personal problems by allowing the ghastly violence of killing tiny, innocent humans.

Dr. Willke is President of the National Right To Life Committee, Inc., in Washington, D.C.

"Pro-life" groups oppose abortion on the basis of their belief that life begins at the moment of conception.

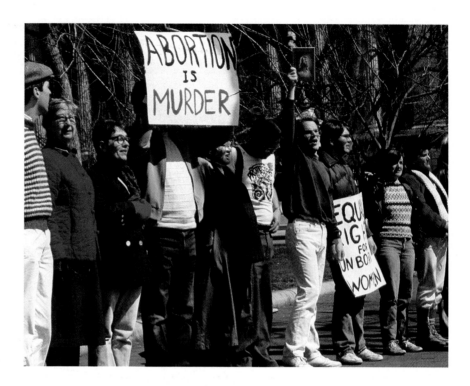

By contrast, the pro-choice viewpoint holds that distinctions must be made between the stages of fetal development and that preserving the fetus of early gestation is not always the ultimate moral concern. Members of this group maintain that women must have the freedom to decide whether and when to have children; they argue that pregnancy can result from contraceptive failure or other factors out of a woman's control. When pregnancy does occur, pro-choice individuals believe that the most moral decision possible must be determined according to each individual situation, and that in some cases greater injustice would result if abortion were not an option. If legal abortions were not available, some pro-choice supporters say, "back-alley shops" and do-it-yourself techniques with their many health risks, as well as the births of unplanned children, would again grow in number. Others argue that discrimination in health care would result, since wealthy women could more easily make the travel arrangements necessary for a legal abortion elsewhere. Still others emphasize that some physicians, because of their strong personal convictions regarding abortion rights, would feel forced into becoming law-breakers.

■ **Exploring Your Emotions**

The women most affected by abortion regulation are those who are young and poor. How do you feel about this inequity?

Some individuals strongly identify exclusively with either the pro-life or the pro-choice stance, but many people have moral beliefs that are blurred, less defined, and in some cases a mixture of the two. A common assumption is that all religious organizations and individuals adhere to the pro-life position. This notion can be misleading. Although some generalizations can be made, moral positions regarding abortion can vary widely among religious believers just as they can differ markedly among individuals who consider themselves nonreligious.

Public Opinion   In general, U.S. public opinion on abortion is somewhat flexible and seems to change depending on the specific situation. Many individuals approve of legal abortion as an option when destructive health or welfare consequences could result from continuing pregnancy, but they do not advocate abortion as a simple way out of an inconvenient situation. Overall, most adults in the United States continue to approve of legal abortion and are opposed to overturning the basic right to abortion established in *Roe vs. Wade* (see the public opinion polls in this chapter). But the amount of public support will vary considerably, depending on the circumstances surrounding the abortion request (see Figure 7-2). Most people see many areas of ambiguity in the abortion issue.

For example, people who feel that abortion should be available in early pregnancy often question at which stage in later pregnancy the fetus's rights should take prece-

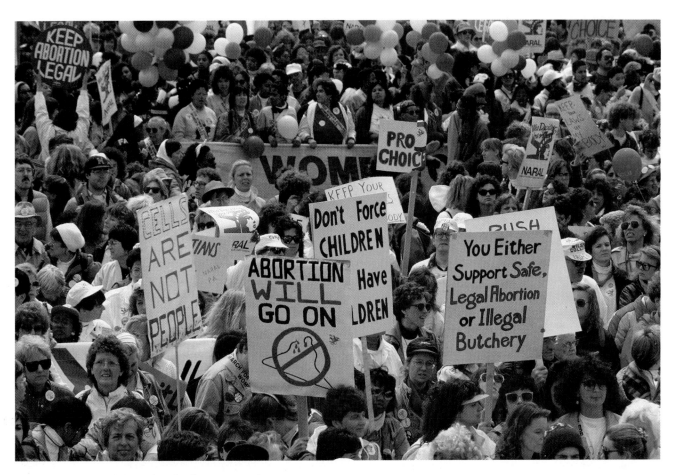

"Pro-choice" groups believe that the decision to end or continue a pregnancy is a personal matter that should be left up to the individual.

dence over the woman's rights. The 1973 U.S. Supreme Court decision considered viability the key criterion in establishing the point beyond which a woman's right to choose abortion becomes markedly restricted. In 1973, viability was generally considered to be about twenty-six to twenty-eight weeks. Today it is about twenty-four weeks, with isolated cases of survival at twenty-three weeks. Although neonatal intensive care units continue to advance technologically, most experts feel that viability cannot ever be expected beyond this limit.

Other individuals associate fetal rights not with viability but with earlier developmental characteristics such as onset of heartbeat, brain size, and nervous system maturity. *The Silent Scream,* a widely shown film that used computer-enhanced ultrasound images, purports to depict a twelve-week-old fetus "screaming in pain" during an abortion procedure, attributing a fully human response to the fetus. Critics contend that the film was manipulated, with portions of the footage being sped up to project the illusion of a fetus thrashing in terror. Experts in fetal medicine have refuted the film's medical premises, stating that at twelve weeks fetal responses are

simply reflex activity and that brain and nervous systems are insufficiently developed to feel pain. In fact researchers have recently described evidence that minimal nervous system connections necessary for brain function don't develop until after the fifth month of pregnancy.

■ **Exploring Your Emotions**

How do you define life? When do you think it begins? How does your answer affect your position on abortion?

Still other individuals argue that the embryo becomes a human being at the point of individuation or twinning, which occurs two to three weeks after conception. (Before that time, the embryo has not yet differentiated into either a single or an identical twin pregnancy.) Others believe that the moment of conception is the only critical point to consider. For them, all other developmental stages are irrelevant to the abortion debate. As can be seen from such wide variation of opinion, objective

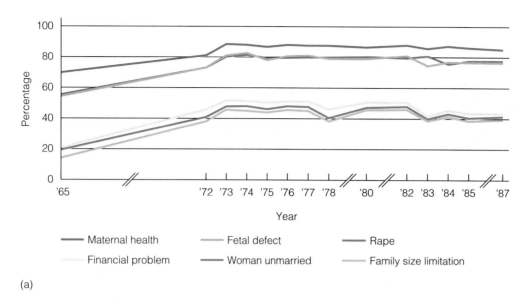

(a)

VITAL STATISTICS

Figure 7-2   (a) Percentage of public approving of abortion under various circumstances, by survey year, 1965–1987. (b) The reasons women choose abortions (respondents could give more than one answer).

measures of humanness and clear-cut guidelines regarding fetal rights are elusive, and decisions ambiguous.

Although opinions vary as to whether, or when, in pregnancy, abortion rights should be tightly regulated by law, most people agree that abortions done later in pregnancy present more difficulties in personal, medical, philosophical, and social terms. Who are the women who have late abortions? Of all abortions done after the twenty-first week of gestation, 44 percent are performed on teenagers. Possible explanations include teenagers' ignorance, denial, fear, and lack of supportive family or friends. Other typical recipients of late abortions include poor women who may have more difficulty finding suitable facilities as well as necessary funds, and premenopausal women who fail to recognize a delayed period as pregnancy. Another small group of women who may seek late abortion are those who have learned through **amniocentesis** (the withdrawal and analysis of amniotic fluid) that the fetus is suffering from a specific abnormality, such as Down's syndrome. Because the results of this test are not available until the nineteenth or twentieth week of pregnancy, abortion, if chosen, is necessarily delayed. (Chorionic villus-sampling, a genetic diagnosis technique that can be performed in the first trimester, is becoming more available. However, this technique does not diagnose neural tube defects and also carries slightly more risk for the fetus.)

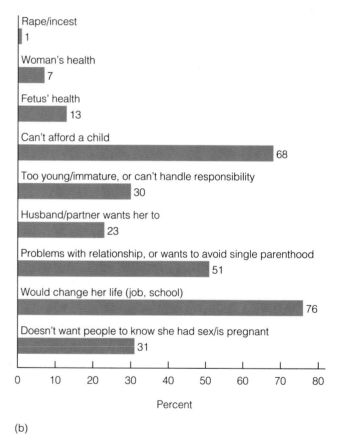

(b)

Personal Considerations   For the pregnant woman who is considering abortion, the usual legal and moral arguments may sound quite meaningless as she attempts to weigh the many short- and long-term ramifications for

Amniocentesis   Withdrawal of fluid from the amniotic sac.

Public Opinion on Abortion

A majority of Americans believe that women should retain the right to abortion as established in *Roe vs. Wade* in 1973. The first poll shown here indicates that in December 1988, all groups except those who did not graduate from high school and those who said that religion is very important opposed the overturning of this law. (Even so, a majority of both Catholics and Protestants opposed the overturning of the law.)

The second set of polls, conducted in July 1989 immediately following the Supreme Court decision in *Webster vs. Reproductive Health Services*, showed that a majority still did not want *Roe vs. Wade* overturned and disapproved of the court's decision to allow the states to restrict women's right to abortion.

The third poll, conducted just before the *Webster* decision, shows that voters disapprove of candidates who want to restrict the right to abortion more than they disapprove of candidates who favor abortion. It also indicates that many Americans favor certain kinds of restrictions on abortion.

December 1988 Gallup Poll

OVERTURN RIGHT TO ABORTION			
	Favor	Oppose	No opinion
NATIONWIDE	37%	58%	5%
Men	36	57	7
Women	37	59	4
18-29	30	69	1
30-49	37	57	6
50 and older	41	51	8
College graduates	29	66	5
Some college	33	62	5
High school grads	34	59	7
Not high school graduates	54	41	5
Protestants	39	56	5
Catholics	39	54	7

Importance of Religion:

	Favor	Oppose	No opinion
Very important	49	45	6
Fairly important	24	72	4
Not very important	19	77	4
Republicans	41	54	5
Democrats	36	58	6
Region East	35	60	5
Midwest	34	59	7
South	44	51	5
West	31	64	5

"Do you ever wonder whether your own position on abortion is the right one or not?"

EVER QUESTION OWN OPINION?	
	Dec. 1988
Yes	33%
No	60
Not sure	7

Public Opinion on Abortion (continued)

Do you agree:	Yes
I would never vote for any candidate who favors abortion.	24%
I would never vote for any candidate who would restrict women's right to have an abortion.	32

Do you favor or oppose restrictions in your state that would:	Favor	Oppose
Require parental consent before a teenager has an abortion?	72%	25%
Require testing for fetus viability outside the womb?	48	38
Require doctors to inform parents about alternatives?	81	16
Prohibit public spending on abortion?	37	57

From a telephone poll of 504 adult Americans taken for *Time/CNN* on July 6 (1989) by Yankelovich Clancy Shulman. Sampling error is ±4.5 percent.

Time, July 17, 1989.

July 1989 Gallup Poll

■ Do you approve or disapprove of the Supreme Court decision allowing states to pass laws that restrict abortion (*Webster vs. Reproductive Health Services*, July 1989)?

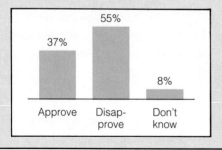

■ In 1973, the Supreme Court ruled that states cannot place restrictions on a woman's right to an abortion during the first three months of pregnancy. Would you like to see this ruling overturned or not?

	July 1989
Overturn	34%
Not overturn	58
Don't know	8

all lives directly concerned. If she chooses abortion, can she accept that decision in terms of her own religious and moral beliefs? What are her long-range feelings likely to be regarding this decision? What are her partner's feelings regarding abortion, and how will she deal with his responses? Does she have a supportive relative or friend who will help her through this time of emotional adjustment? Which medical facility offering abortions would be most suitable for her? What about transportation and costs? (See Figure 7-3 for a profile of women who choose abortion.)

■ **Exploring Your Emotions**

How would you feel if you discovered that a fetus you were carrying (or your partner was carrying) had a serious genetic defect? Would you be likely to choose abortion? How much would the nature of the defect and its consequences for the baby and you affect your decision?

For the woman who decides against abortion and chooses instead to continue the pregnancy, there are other questions. If she decides to raise the child herself,

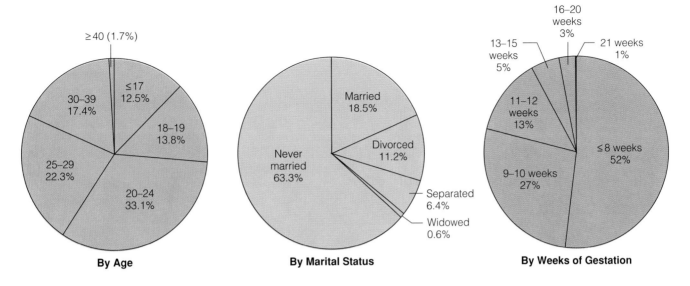

By Age By Marital Status By Weeks of Gestation

VITAL STATISTICS

Figure 7-3 Who has abortions? Percentage distribution of all women who had abortions in 1987.

will she have the critical resources to do it well? Is a supportive, lasting relationship with her partner likely? If not, how does she feel about being a single parent? Are family members available to help with the many demands of child rearing? If she is young, what will the effects be on her own growth? Will she be able to continue with her educational and other personal goals? What about the ongoing financial responsibilities?

■ **Exploring Your Emotions**

Some men feel strongly that they should have a say when their partner is considering abortion. Others feel it's up to the woman. How do you feel about men's roles and rights in decisions about abortion?

If the pregnant woman considers adoption, she will have to try to predict what her emotional responses will be throughout the full-term pregnancy and the adoption process. What are her long-range feelings likely to be? What is the best setting for her during her pregnancy? How can she best maintain continuity with the rest of her life and her long-term goals? Which adoption facility is likely to make the most suitable arrangements for her and her baby? A public or a private agency? Is anonymity between the adoptive parents and herself desirable or not? Does she have someone she trusts to help her with these difficult decisions? (The box entitled "Adoption: How Viable an Alternative?" addresses some of these questions.)

Current Trends Clearly, all responses to unintended pregnancy can be difficult, including abortion and especially late abortion. Fortunately, with the increased accessibility to legalized abortion following the mid-1970s, the rate of late abortions dropped steadily, until fewer than 1 percent of all abortions were performed at more than twenty weeks and fewer than 9 percent at more than twelve weeks by the mid-1980s. Also, the overall abortion rate, which rose during most of the 1970s and leveled off around 1980 fell significantly between 1982 and 1985 (see Figures 7-4 and 7-5).

The effects of the 1989 *Webster* decision and related restrictions are hard to predict. While some foresee a sharp decrease in the number of abortions in the United States, others argue that the overall total will change very little. Women seeking abortions usually do so with very strong motivation and determination and are not likely to be deterred easily. With the current availability of interstate transportation, many women may be able to travel whatever distances are necessary for a legal abortion. Others might well turn to more accessible, but illegal, nonmedical practitioners. Still others may find local physicians who feel strongly about abortion rights and who therefore continue to perform abortions even under illegal circumstances, finding reassurance from those legal scholars who predict that many juries would not be willing to convict either the woman or the doctor of criminal activity. Although even women living in highly restricted areas may continue to obtain abortions, they are likely in most cases to face significant increases in expense and time delays (see the box entitled "Facts about Abortion").

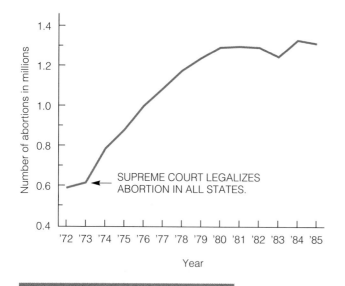

VITAL STATISTICS

Figure 7-4   Legal abortions in the United States.

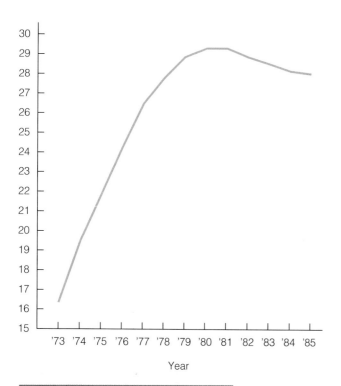

VITAL STATISTICS

Figure 7-5   Rate of abortions per 1,000 women aged 15–44.

There is also growing speculation regarding the possible impact of the new "abortion pill," RU-486, now approved for use in France and China (see discussion later in this chapter). Although unlikely to be approved soon in the United States, this pill may become widely available through illegal channels, according to experts who point to the many other illicit drugs prevalent in our society. Other groups are suggesting that menstrual extraction kits, packaged with use instructions for lay individuals, may offer a self-help option for abortion seekers. Although both of these measures, along with the numerous other do-it-yourself techniques that are likely to surface, carry serious health risks, they would undoubtedly be sought out by a certain number of women. Of great concern is the fact that "home remedies" may simply damage the fetus instead of causing an abortion.

Unless coupled with attention to the prevention of unwanted pregnancy, especially among the young and single women who make up the majority of those seeking abortions, legal changes alone will probably not decrease the number of abortions dramatically. (Figure 7-6 lists abortion rates for seventeen countries.)

■ **Exploring Your Emotions**

If you were pregnant (or if your partner were pregnant), what do you think you would do? Would you be more likely to favor marriage, single parenthood, adoption, or abortion? Would your decision depend on the circumstances, or do you have strong opinions and beliefs that would guide you under any conditions? If so, what are the sources of your opinions and beliefs?

We hope the recent surge of public interest in sexual behavior (largely due to fear of sexually transmitted diseases) will lead to more open discussion regarding sexuality and the wide variety of human responses to this basic drive. With more communication and broader understanding of personal needs (including needs for intimacy and closeness), individuals and couples could perhaps choose more wisely the social and sexual behavior that would meet those needs most positively, both in the short and the long run. For those who choose to include sexual intercourse as part of their relationships, birth control should be made readily available and effectively used (see Chapter 6). Other measures that might help to decrease the demand for abortion include the following economic and social reforms: increased options for working women; more dual parenting; maternal/paternal leaves; improved child care facilities; and quality pre- and postnatal care available for all economic levels.

Adoption: How Viable an Alternative?

Many people on the "pro-life" side have encouraged women to deal with unwanted pregnancies through adoption rather than abortion. But only a small percentage of pregnant women are taking this advice. Of the estimated 3 million unwanted pregnancies in the United States each year, about half are terminated by abortion. Of the 1.5 million babies born each year following unwanted pregnancy, only about 2 percent are placed for adoption—about 25,000 babies.

At the same time, an estimated 1 to 2 million qualified couples in the United States would like to adopt a baby, which means there are at least forty potential families for each baby currently placed for adoption. There are also un-counted thousands of babies and children living with biological parents who are unable to provide even minimal care for them. Why are these three parties—couples seeking children to adopt, parents unable to care for their children, and the children themselves— having such a hard time making connections with each other? Why is adoption not a more attractive or viable alternative to marriage, single parenthood, or abortion?

One reason seems to be that there is much less social stigma attached to unmarried pregnancy than there was twenty or twenty-five years ago. At that time, about 50 percent of white single women under 25 routinely gave up their babies for adoption. Today, young women, especially teenagers, are under pressure from friends and family to keep their babies. Single parenthood is a choice commonly made by young mothers today, despite the disruption of their

lives and the problems both they and their children face.

Another reason is the prevailing assumption that children are better off with their biological parents under almost any circumstances. Federal child welfare-reform legis-lation passed in 1980 made the reuniting of families the highest priority when children are removed from their homes. Legislation also provides financial incentives to help keep biological families to-gether, which effectively discour-ages adoption. Women who want to keep their babies are eligible for Aid to Families with Dependent Children, food stamps, food sup-plements, and other government assistance, worth perhaps $8,000 a year. Women who want to place their babies for adoption, at least through most public and private agencies, have no such financial incentive.

Another factor working against adoption is the assumption on the part of many social workers that pregnant women want to keep their babies—otherwise, they would have had abortions. But this assumption may not be true. Critics of the nations' 2,500 public and private adoption agencies claim that few of them offer coun-seling that really helps women consider their options and assess their abilities to be parents.

All these factors work together to produce a small pool of babies placed for adoption each year— at least the babies most in demand, who are healthy white newborns. Many more babies and children are in need of homes but are unlikely to be adopted, including babies born to drug-addicted mothers, babies with AIDS, and older children with or without

physical, mental, emotional, or behavioral problems. Minority children's chances of being adopted are lowered by the common policy of discouraging cross-racial adop-tions. Since there are many more white couples who want to adopt a baby than black, the number of potential matches shrinks even further.

If most adoption agencies are unsuccessful both in recruiting single pregnant women who will give up their babies and in finding babies for adoptive parents, where are people turning? Many adop-tions are being arranged through private adoption lawyers and agencies that aggressively reach out to pregnant women through advertising and publicity. One controversial agency in Chicago arranges 300 adoptions per year (in contrast to the typical agency's 12), finding healthy white infants for wealthy white parents—at a cost of $20,000 each.

Many couples have turned in recent years to so-called inde-pendent or private adoptions, those undertaken without the supervision of licensed agencies. Such adoptions are legal in all but six states (Connecticut, Delaware, Massachusetts, Michigan, Minne-sota, and North Dakota) and may account for 60 percent of all infant adoptions today. In this kind of adoption, the would-be parents put personal ads in newspapers and send resumes and letters to lawyers, obstetricians, and clergy across the nation in the hope of finding a pregnant woman willing to relinquish her baby. They usually pay the mother's medical expenses and sometimes her living expenses before and after the baby is born. The biological mother

Adoption: How Viable an Alternative? (continued)

has the opportunity to choose the adoptive family and in many cases to keep in touch with them and her child, and the adoptive parents have the chance to control at least part of the baby's prenatal life. Like expensive agency adoptions, independent adoptions run the risk of being construed as cases of "baby selling" in which lawyers, brokers, or mothers sell babies to the highest bidders.

Recently, some private groups, including evangelical churches, have been taking steps to encourage adoption by opening a kind of institution that was common in American cities until about 1970— the unwed mother's home. Pregnant single women are invited

to live in these dormitories until they give birth, and then their babies are placed for adoption. One institution that has served as a model for the new wave of maternity homes is the Edna Gladney Foundation in Fort Worth, Texas, which serves about 280 pregnant women each year.

With the Supreme Court decision of July 1989 in place, many states have begun to search for alternatives to abortion. Some states already have much higher rates of adoption than others (Utah, Idaho, South Dakota, Oregon, and Alaska are in the lead). If abortion becomes more restricted in coming years, adoption may become more common. Even if

abortions were completely illegal, of course, women would continue to have them as they have in the past, when undeterred by cost, difficulty, or social pressure. Carrying a baby to term and putting it up for adoption can be a traumatic and even impossible alternative for some women, accompanied by intense feelings of loss, grief, and regret. For other women, however, it may be the best of all possible solutions.

Based on "Abortion and the adoption option," *Washington Post Health*, Aug. 15, 1989, pp. 6–7; "Where have all the babies gone?" *Money*, Dec. 1988, pp. 164–176; and "The adoption option," *American Demographics*, Oct. 1989, p. 11.

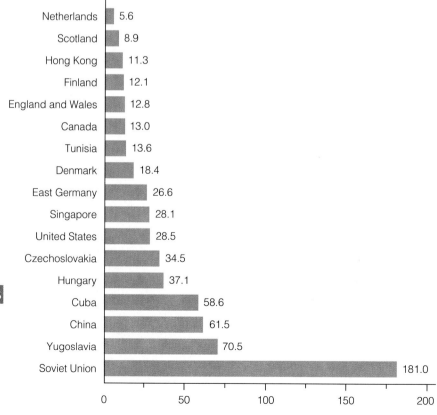

VITAL STATISTICS

Figure 7-6 National abortion rates— number of abortions per 1,000 women age 15–44. Figures are for 1984 except for Canada and Soviet Union (1982), China and Singapore (1983), and Tunisia (1985).

Number of abortions per 1,000 women ages 15 to 44

Netherlands	5.6
Scotland	8.9
Hong Kong	11.3
Finland	12.1
England and Wales	12.8
Canada	13.0
Tunisia	13.6
Denmark	18.4
East Germany	26.6
Singapore	28.1
United States	28.5
Czechoslovakia	34.5
Hungary	37.1
Cuba	58.6
China	61.5
Yugoslavia	70.5
Soviet Union	181.0

Facts about Abortion

Incidence of Abortion

- More than 50 percent of the pregnancies among American women are unintended—one-half of these are terminated by abortion.
- In 1985, there were about 1.5 million abortions in the United States. From 1973 through 1988, more than 22 million legal abortions took place in the United States. Since 1967, when many states began liberalizing their abortion laws, almost 24 million legal abortions have been performed.
- Each year nearly 3 out of 100 women aged 15–44 have an abortion—40 percent have had at least one previous abortion and 45 percent have had a previous birth.
- The abortion rate—the number of abortions per 1,000 women aged 15–44—in 1975 was 22; in 1980, 29; and in 1985, 28.
- The United States has one of the higher abortion rates among developed countries; U.S. rates of abortion and unintended pregnancy are about five times those of the Netherlands. But some other countries, notably China and the Soviet Union, have much higher rates than the United States.

Who Has Abortions?

- The majority of women obtaining abortions are young: 61 percent are under age 26, including about 26 percent who are teenagers (age 11–19); only 18 percent are over 30.
- 18–19-year-old women have the highest abortion rate—63 per 1,000 women.
- The proportion of pregnancies terminated by abortion is higher among unmarried women (61 percent), women aged 40 and older (49 percent), and teenagers (42 percent) than among all women (30 percent).
- Poor women are about three times more likely than women who are financially better off to have abortions. Nevertheless, 11 percent of abortions are obtained by women whose household incomes are $50,000 or more.
- Women who report no religious affiliation have a higher rate of abortion than women who report some affiliation. Catholic women are about as likely to obtain an abortion as are all women nationally, and Protestants and Jews are less likely. Catholic women are 30 percent more likely than Protestants to have abortions.
- One in six abortion patients in 1987 described herself as a born-again or evangelical Christian; they are half as likely as other women to obtain an abortion.
- 70 percent of women having an abortion say that they intend to have children in the future.
- Most women who have an abortion after 15 weeks of pregnancy have had problems detecting their pregnancy, and almost one-half are delayed because of problems, usually financial, in arranging an abortion.
- Women using contraceptives account for 43 percent or 1.5 million of unintended pregnancies a year; 57 percent or 1.9 million are among those not using contraceptives.

Abortion and Teenagers

- Among teenagers, 82 percent of pregnancies are unintended.
- Of the 1.6 million abortions obtained by U.S. women in 1985, 416,000 were obtained by teenagers.
- 42 percent of women who become pregnant as teenagers choose abortion, while 58 percent continue their pregnancies to term (excluding those who miscarry).
- Of teenagers having abortions, three-fourths say they cannot afford to have a baby, and two-thirds think they are not mature enough.
- More than one-fourth of unmarried teenagers under age 18 who get abortions have never used birth control. Of those who have, most have often used one of the less effective ones, such as the condom or withdrawal.
- Teenagers are more likely than older women to have abortions during the second three months of pregnancy, when health risks associated with abortion increase significantly.
- 55 percent of teenagers under age 18 who obtain an abortion do so with their parents' knowledge—the younger the teenager, the more likely that her parents know.

From *Facts in Brief: Abortion in the United States.* (New York: The Alan Guttmacher Institute), Nov. 1, 1989.

Methods of Abortion

"Morning after" pills (see Chapter 6) and IUDs inserted immediately after unprotected sexual relations are generally not considered **abortifacients** (agents that produce abortion) from a medical viewpoint, because they act before implantation of the fertilized egg, should one be present. Therefore, these topics are not discussed here.

RU-486   Initially RU-486 (trade name Mifepristone) was incorrectly referred to as a "morning after" pill; it is now known as a menses inducer or more commonly as an abortion pill. RU-486, which must be taken by the forty-ninth day following the last menstrual period, blocks uterine absorption of progesterone, thereby causing the uterine lining and any fertilized egg to shed. When given in combination with another drug and under medical supervision, RU-486 results in fewer health risks than surgical abortion and has a 95 percent success rate. Although currently marketed in China and France, legal availability of RU-486 is unlikely in the United States in the near future due to the strong anti-abortion lobby. Use of RU-486 as a once-monthly "contraceptive" (given just before an expected menstrual period) has also been studied, but because of possible problems with timing its administration and concerns about its being an abortifacient, this mode of use appears limited as well.

Menstrual Extraction   Developed in the early 1970s, **menstrual extraction** is the vacuum aspiration of uterine contents shortly after a missed period. It was originally defined as a procedure to be done up to the forty-second day after the last menstrual period and before the absence or presence of a pregnancy was confirmed. Initially, menstrual extraction was seen as safe, cost effective, and as especially suitable for those women uncomfortable with the notion of abortion. Complication rates, including incomplete evacuation, infection, and continuing pregnancy, were higher than expected, however, and menstrual extraction is now rarely performed in the United States.

With the likelihood of increased restrictions on abortion, however, interest in menstrual extraction has again emerged in certain groups as a possible self-help option. Physicians warn that such procedures can be dangerous; complications include, missing the fertilized egg, lacerating the cervix, perforating the uterus, and spreading bacterial infection.

Vacuum Aspiration   First developed in China in 1958, **vacuum aspiration** (also called suction curettage) has rapidly become the preferred method for abortions up to the twelfth week of pregnancy. It can be done quickly, and the risk of hemorrhage or other complications is small. It is usually done on an outpatient basis.

A sedative may be given, along with a **local anesthetic.** A speculum, a device used to open the vaginal entrance, is inserted into the vagina, and the cervix is cleansed with a surgical solution. The cervix is dilated and a suction curette—a specially designed hollow tube—is then inserted into the uterus. The curette is attached to the rubber tubing of an electric pump, and suction is applied (see Figure 7-7). In about 20 to 30 seconds the uterus is emptied. Moderate cramping is common during evacuation. To ensure that no fragments of tissue are left in the uterus, the doctor usually scrapes the uterine lining with a metal curette, an instrument with a spoonlike tip. The entire operation takes only five to ten minutes.

After a few hours in a recovering area, the woman can return home. She is usually instructed not to douche, have coitus, or use tampons for the first week or two after the abortion and to return for a two-week post-abortion examination. This examination is important to verify that the abortion was complete and that no signs of infection are present.

Dilation and Curettage   In **dilation and curettage** (commonly called **D & C**) the embryo and placenta are removed by surgical instruments rather than by suction.

Abortifacient   Agent or substance that produces abortion.

Menstrual extraction   The vacuum aspiration of uterine contents shortly after a missed period.

Vacuum aspiration   Also called *suction curettage,* this procedure involves removal of the embryo or fetus by means of suction.

Local anesthesia   (also called **regional anesthesia**) Use of agents that block the nerves carrying pain signals to the brain; in abortion and childbirth the nerves running from the pelvic area to the brain are affected while leaving the woman awake and alert.

Dilation and curettage (D & C)   Dilation of the cervix and scraping of the uterus to remove the embryo or fetus or for other medical conditions of the uterus.

Dilation and evacuation (D & E)   The method of abortion most commonly used between 13 and 15 weeks of pregnancy. Following dilation of the cervix, both vacuum aspiration and instruments are used as needed.

General anesthesia   Use of agents that usually produce unconsciousness to relieve pain.

Amniotic sac/Amniotic fluid   The bag of watery fluid lining the uterus, which envelops and protects the fetus.

Hysterotomy   A modified cesarean section in which the fetus is removed.

Cesarean section   A surgical incision through the abdominal wall and uterus; performed when vaginal delivery of a baby is not advisable.

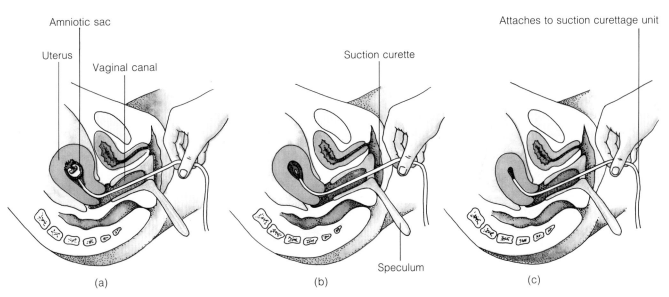

Amniotic sac

Uterus

Vaginal canal

Suction curette

Attaches to suction curettage unit

Speculum

(a)   (b)   (c)

Figure 7-7   Vacuum aspiration takes only five to ten minutes and can be performed up to the twelfth week of pregnancy.

After the cervix is dilated, a curette is used to scrape the tissues from the wall of the uterus; an ovum forceps, a long grasping instrument, is also used. Because a D & C takes longer, causes a greater loss of blood, and requires a longer recovery period, it has been largely replaced by vacuum aspiration.

Dilation and Evacuation   The method most commonly used between thirteen and fifteen weeks of pregnancy and now preferred by some physicians up to and past twenty weeks is **dilation and evacuation** (often referred to as D & E). This procedure combines and extends both vacuum aspiration and D & C, using greater cervical dilation, larger suction curettes, and heavier forceps as required. Intravenous fluid that includes a medication to increase uterine contractions and thus limit blood loss is often given during or after the procedure. Either local or **general anesthesia** is used. Both the time required for the D & E and the recovery time are slightly longer than for vacuum aspiration.

Medical Methods   After the fifteenth week of pregnancy, one of the following medical methods is used in many centers because suction becomes more difficult. With saline instillation, the oldest of these methods, a local anesthetic is given, and a long needle is inserted through the abdominal and uterine walls into the **amniotic sac. Amniotic fluid** is drained from the sac and replaced with an equal amount of 20 percent salt solution. The injection must be made slowly and with great care to avoid introducing the solution into the woman's

circulation. The woman must be fully awake to report pain or other symptoms.

The death of the fetus, which occurs immediately due to the disruption in chemical balances essential to life, is followed by labor and delivery within a day or two. The uterus is scraped to reduce chances of infection or hemorrhage. The recovery period is slightly longer than for suction (vacuum) curettage, and complications are more frequent.

Prostaglandins, a group of naturally occurring chemicals, also bring on abortion, apparently by stimulating contractions of the uterus. They can be injected into the amniotic sac or inserted through the cervical canal into the uterus. Their major shortcoming is their effect on the muscles of the digestive tract, which produces nausea, vomiting, and diarrhea. Refined prostaglandins have fewer side effects than natural ones. Another chemical, urea, is often used in combination with prostaglandins to facilitate labor.

Hysterotomy   Abortion by **hysterotomy** is a major surgical procedure (a modified **cesarean section**) usually performed under a general anesthetic, although a spinal anesthetic may be effective. Incisions are made in the walls of the abdomen and the uterus and the fetus and placenta are removed. Some doctors insist that caesarean section be used for all subsequent deliveries to avoid the risk that the uterus will rupture during labor contractions although this practice is decreasing. The saline and prostaglandin methods have largely replaced hysterotomy.

Abortion Complications

Along with questions regarding the actual procedure of abortion, many individuals have concerns regarding possible aftereffects. Over the past years, several detailed and long-term studies have focused on both physical and psychological concerns; slowly, more information is being gathered on this important subject.

Possible Physical Effects   The incidence of immediate problems following abortion (infection, bleeding, trauma to the cervix or uterus, and incomplete abortion requiring repeat curettage) varies widely. The overall incidence is significantly reduced with good patient health, early timing of abortion, use of the suction method and local anesthesia, performance by a well-trained clinician, and availability and use of prompt follow-up care.

Problems related specifically to infection can be decreased through pre-abortion testing and treatment of asymptomatic gonorrhea and other infections. Also, some clinicians routinely give antibiotics after abortion, while others treat only those patients who have a history of or current symptoms of pelvic infection. All patients should thoroughly understand the postabortion danger signs (see Table 7-2) and should not hesitate to report any concerns.

Excessive bleeding during or after abortion is rare with early vacuum aspiration. In later pregnancies, the use of uterus-contracting medications reduces the risk significantly. Again, early reporting and treatment of any heavy bleeding are very important.

Cervical trauma or laceration and uterus perforation are uncommon as well, especially in early abortion with a well-trained clinician. In more advanced pregnancies, slow and careful dilation of the cervix before abortion can diminish these risks.

Incomplete abortion means that some pregnancy tissue has remained in the uterus. With this condition, or when blood clots form in the uterus shortly after abortion, severe cramping and signs of infection often occur and a repeat vacuum aspiration is usually needed. On rare occasions, a pregnancy may continue after incomplete abortion. The recommended two-week postabortion exam is important to establish that the abortion was complete.

Studies on long-term complications (subsequent infertility, spontaneous second abortions, premature delivery,

and low-birth-weight babies) have not been conclusive. The risk of postabortion infertility seems to be very low, especially when any signs of infection are reported and treated promptly.

Also, there is apparently no effect on outcome of future pregnancies when an early vacuum aspiration is performed with minimal cervical dilation; with later abortions and with repeated or multiple abortions, there is only a slight risk, if any. One recent study suggests that "neither single nor multiple induced abortions as now performed are likely to increase the risk of miscarriage in subsequent pregnancies." The same study indicated that when two or more abortions were performed *before* 1973, the odd ratio for subsequent miscarriage rose to 2.6. The authors concluded that after the legalization of abortion in 1973, improved techniques have resulted in decreased cervical trauma and thereby greatly diminished any risk of future miscarriages. For Rh-negative women, dangerous sensitization (the buildup of antibodies) can be minimized by an injection of Rh-**immune globulin** given within seventy-two hours of the procedure.

Table 7-2 Danger signs after abortion

- Fever (temperature 100.4°F or more)
- Abdominal pain or cramps (severe or increasing)
- Abdominal tenderness with pressure, walking, coughing
- Bleeding that is heavy or lasts longer than 3 weeks
- Foul-smelling vaginal discharge
- Rash, hives, asthma (possible medication reaction)
- Normal menstrual period has not begun within 6 weeks

Source: R. A. Hatcher et al. 1988. *Contraceptive Technology 1988–1989.* (New York: Irvington), p. 396.

■ **Exploring Your Emotions**

How would you feel if you discovered that your mother had had an abortion? What does your reaction to this question tell you about your feelings on the abortion issue?

Immune globulin   A sterile solution of specific proteins that carry many antibodies normally present in human blood; a passive immunizing agent derived from adult human blood. One type of immune globulin carries antibodies to the Rh factor in the blood.

The risk of mortality associated with childbirth is about 11 times as high as that associated with abortion. The risk of death associated with abortion increases with the length of pregnancy, from 1 death for every 500,000 abortions at eight weeks or less to 1 per 30,000 at sixteen to twenty weeks and 1 per 8,000 at twenty-one or more weeks. The risk of death associated with abortion decreased more than fivefold from 1973 to 1985, with 3.4 deaths per 100,000 legal abortions in 1973 declining to 0.4 in 1985.

Possible Psychological Effects   Psychological side effects of abortion are less clearly defined. Responses vary and depend on the individual woman's psychological makeup, family background, current personal and social relationships, surrounding cultural attitudes, and many other factors. A woman who has specific goals with a somewhat structured life pattern may incorporate her decision to abort as the unequivocally "best" and acceptable decision more easily than a woman who feels uncertain about her future.

Although some women experience great relief after abortion, and virtually no negative feelings, most go through a period of ambivalence. Along with relief, they often feel a mixture of other responses, such as guilt, regret, loss, sadness, and/or anger. When a woman feels she was pressured into sexual intercourse or into the abortion, she may feel bitter. If she has strongly believed abortion to be immoral, she may wonder if she is still a good person. Many of these feelings are strongest immediately after abortion, when hormonal shifts are occurring; such feelings often pass quite rapidly. Others take time and fade only slowly. It is important for a woman to realize that such a mixture of feelings is natural, enabling her to accept all her reactions and to share them with others (see the box entitled "Personal Decisions about Abortion").

For a woman who does experience painful feelings, talking freely with a close friend or family member who is understanding and trustworthy can be very helpful. Supportive people can help her feel positive about herself and her decision. Although a legal and common procedure in the United States, abortion is still treated very secretively in most of our society, so it is easy for a woman to feel unique, isolated, and alone. Some women may specifically seek out other women who have had an abortion. Many clinical centers that offer abortions make such peer counseling available. Other women find they can identify with case histories in books written on abortion, which can help them deal with their own reactions. In a few cases, unresolved emotions may persist, and a woman may need more professional counseling, and should seek it.

Decision Making and Unintended Pregnancy

When faced with an unintended pregnancy, women differ greatly in their approach to decision making. Unprotected sexual intercourse may be followed immediately by a vague sense of anxiety. When symptoms of pregnancy appear, some women (especially young women) respond with denial, ascribing the delayed menstruation and other signs to other causes. Several days or weeks may elapse before the woman finally has the pregnancy confirmed (a major cause of late abortions). After a positive test, women often feel a mixture of anxiety, depression, guilt, and anger, sometimes tinged with some anticipation and delight. The actual decision making can vary widely. Some women calmly and resolutely make a choice within a very short time, while others, feeling panic and chaos, wrestle with the decision for several weeks. For some women, it is the first time in their lives that they feel unable to find a "right" answer, and instead must settle for a "best" but difficult solution.

The response of a woman's partner can have a significant influence on how she experiences an unintended pregnancy. Men's emotional reactions can vary considerably. Some withdraw and choose to remain completely detached; others simply press for the most expedient solution (abortion). Still others feel very emotionally involved and wish to play an active role in decision making. Partners can be very helpful, both in weighing important considerations and in actually helping with the chosen course of action. Some couples find that an abortion experience draws them closer together; for others, it's the last straw in an already unstable relationship. When one or both partners decide the relationship is at a dead end, they have to give it up and move on.

Parents can also be helpful. However, when there are marked disagreements, a stressful situation can become even more difficult. According to most state laws, the woman, who is the one most directly affected by unintended pregnancy, has the final rights in the decision. Pressure is growing, however, to require spousal and/or parental consent in an increasing number of states.

■ **Exploring Your Emotions**

Abortion is a complex issue that can't be resolved on the basis of facts alone; it ultimately involves personal beliefs and feelings. Do you have a position on this issue? If so, is it the same as or different from that of others in your family? Have you been influenced by friends, classmates, or the media? Do you think your position reflects your most deeply held personal beliefs?

Personal Decisions about Abortion

When unintended pregnancy occurs, decisions regarding the best possible solution will vary according to each personal and social situation. The following examples show how some women in a variety of circumstances responded.

Stephanie

Stephanie hadn't been careless—the contraceptive device she'd used had failed. "I want a baby in what I think is a healthy circumstance," she said. "I don't have a husband. I don't have a man who really wants this child. Russ will see me through an abortion, but he's walking out of my life when it's over."

After the abortion: "I felt abandoned. I wanted a lot of hugging and to know that somebody cared." The father had offered to accompany her to the clinic where she had her abortion and to spend the weekend with her, but he didn't behave lovingly. "Russ couldn't deal with the experience and was quite cruel, really. I suppose he was frightened, but that didn't make it any easier for me. He stayed with me, but when I wanted to be held, he said, 'Don't hug me; we're just friends.' Considering I'd just gone through an abortion in order not to have this person's child, I thought that was a ludicrous thing to say."

Maggie

Maggie said she felt like a "bad girl" when she found out she was pregnant and didn't know which of two men was the father. "I guess my religious background came through. I felt I was being punished for having sex even though I didn't rationally believe my behavior was wrong. The guilt was pretty bad, and I really needed someone to tell me I was all right."

Maggie's closest girlfriend went to the clinic and stayed with her after the abortion. Like all women who have had abortions, Maggie was in need of comforting. "Eventually that 'bad girl' feeling wears off, but it takes time."

Karen

Karen chose not to have an abortion, but to give her baby up for adoption. When the Bakerfields arrived at the hospital and walked down the corridor, Karen held out her baby to them. The baby was wearing a T-shirt with the inscription, "I love my Mommy and Daddy!" Then the Bakerfields and Karen prayed together, and Karen formally relinquished her child to their care.

"I was so happy to give life to someone else to start a family," Karen said. "That excited me. It still excites me." Karen has told her story to a number of high school audiences, and generally they are puzzled about her decision. What Karen tries to communicate is that love motivated her.

"I never had a father, really, growing up," she said. "By giving my baby to the Bakerfields, I gave her a father. She needed that."

Laura

After eight pregnancy tests and eight personal denials, my father confronted me by asking if I was pregnant. I answered, scared, "yes."

"My father gave me an ultimatum: to have an abortion or leave the family. I chose to leave.

Knowing I had to leave the house I went to the crisis pregnancy center. They took care of me.

I am currently at home again with my three-month-old boy. I am now engaged and looking forward to having my own family soon."

Laurie

"At first, Mark didn't want to talk about my pregnancy. Finally he said 'It's totally up to you. If you want to have the baby, I'll stay with you, and if you want to get married, I'll probably marry you. I don't really care, but it's not going to be any different from the way it is now. I won't turn into the president of IBM. You have to decide.'"

Mark is not financially secure; Laurie is a freelance writer with a fluctuating income. She chose not to have the child, "because parenthood would have been entirely my responsibility—Mark wouldn't have supported us—and I don't have the resources to cope with that. It was the first time I'd been pregnant and maybe my last chance. At thirty-nine, how many more opportunities are you going to have?"

Susan

Susan was a freshman in college and was very caught up in her new academic and social activities. Bill (another student) and she had been dating for about three months, when one evening she decided to "take a chance" since she had just finished her menstrual

---

Personal Decisions about Abortion (continued)

period. When her next period was two weeks overdue, she had a pregnancy test. It was positive.

When Bill first learned of the pregnancy, he became distant, but he did agree to help pay for an abortion. Soon, however, he withdrew completely and had no further contact with Susan. The hardest time for Susan was before the abortion when she found herself crying frequently. She talked a lot with her close girlfriends, who comforted her. After the abortion, she felt very strongly

that she had made the best decision, but she did occasionally wonder how she would feel in future years. After meeting a new boyfriend with whom she could talk openly, Susan felt more certain than ever that she had made the right choice.

Helen

Helen was attending a junior college along with working part-time when she found out she was pregnant. Both Mike and she came

from very religious backgrounds, and, for them, marriage was the only acceptable solution. They had met just a couple of months before the pregnancy, and it was only after marriage that they got to know each other well. Now, twelve years later, they have two children and a reasonably stable life together. Although both feel that their relationship lacks closeness, deriving little joy or satisfaction from their times together, they are certain that the decision they made was the best one for them.

No matter which of the available options to unintended pregnancy is chosen, a series of questions is likely to arise that must be addressed (see the section on personal considerations). Although a prompt decision carries critical advantages, careful consideration is important. If there are strong feelings of uncertainty or ambivalence, hasty action should be avoided.

Having a supportive confidant, such as a male partner, other close friend, or family member, can be very important in sorting out complex feelings. Along with listening and offering understanding and perspective, supportive people can help find suitable medical personnel and plan financial arrangements. Once a course of action has been chosen, a sense of moving ahead usually follows and the next step toward resolution can occur.

■ **Exploring Your Emotions**

Women choose abortion for a wide variety of reasons: the pregnancy threatens their health; having a child would interfere with their educational or career plans; the pregnancy resulted from rape or incest; they can't afford to have a child; they don't want to be single parents; the child has a birth defect; and so on. Under what circumstances (if any) do you think abortion is justified?

Summary

Most people in our society resist confronting the interrelated issues of sexuality, unintended pregnancy, and abortion; as a result, pregnancy prevention programs are limited in number and scope.

The Abortion Issue

• The common use of the word *abortion* refers only to artificially induced expulsion of the fetus (using drugs or mechanical means).

• Until the mid-1800s abortion in the United States was legal if it took place before the twentieth week; more restrictive laws passed by the various states remained in effect until they began to be invalidated by courts in the 1960s.

• The 1973 *Roe vs. Wade* Supreme Court case devised new standards to govern abortion decisions; it was based on the trimesters of pregnancy and limited a woman's choices as she advanced through pregnancy.

- Although the Supreme Court continued to uphold its 1973 decision, challenges were made to it nearly every year; in 1989 in *Webster vs. Reproductive Health Services,* the Court let stand restrictions imposed by Missouri and rejected the trimester framework. *Webster* did not overturn Roe and gave few guidelines, leaving room for further restrictions to be enacted by the states.
- Among the results of *Webster* will probably be great differences in laws between the states and perhaps discrimination in health care because wealthier women will be able to travel to get legal abortions. The confusion and debate that have ensued from Webster will probably last throughout the 1990s.
- The controversy between pro-life and pro-choice movements centers on the issue of when life begins. Pro-life groups believe that a fertilized egg is a human life from the moment of conception and that any abortion is a murder. Pro-choice groups distinguish between stages of fetal development and argue that a woman's right to live her life as she chooses can supersede the rights of the fetus in early stages of development.
- Overall public opinion in the United States supports legal abortion and opposes overturning *Roe vs. Wade.* Opinion changes according to individual situations, and fetal viability outside the uterus is usually the criterion for deciding when the fetus's rights supersede the woman's. Today viability is considered to be twenty-four weeks.
- Most people agree that abortions done late in pregnancy present personal, medical, philosophical, and social problems. Almost half of these are done on teenagers, but other recipients include poor women, women nearing menopause, and women who have waited for the results of amniocentesis.
- The woman considering abortion needs to consider her own religious and moral beliefs, her long-range feelings, support from others, availability, and cost. The woman who decides against abortion needs to make decisions about keeping the child, perhaps being a single parent, or choosing adoption.
- Although the overall abortion rate rose during the 1970s, it leveled off around 1980 and fell significantly between 1982 and 1985.

Methods of Abortion

- RU-486, an abortion pill, blocks uterine absorption of progesterone, which causes the uterine lining and any fertilized egg to shed. Under medical supervision, it is safer than surgical methods and has a 95 percent success rate. It is not available in the United States.
- Menstrual extraction is the vacuum aspiration of uterine contents shortly after a missed period; complication rates are high, and it is rarely used in the United States, though some fear that it will become a self-help method if restrictive abortion laws are passed.

- Vacuum aspiration, the preferred method of abortion until the twelfth week of pregnancy, uses an electric pump to remove the uterine contents; the physician also scrapes the uterine lining with a metal curette. The operation takes only five to ten minutes and is done on an outpatient basis.
- Dilation and curettage (D & C) uses surgical instruments rather than suction to remove the uterine contents. Dilation and evacuation (D & E) combines and extends vacuum aspiration and D & C and is the most commonly used method between thirteen and fifteen weeks.
- Saline instillation or prostaglandins are used for abortions after the fifteenth week of pregnancy; the saline solution causes fetal death, and prostaglandins stimulate uterine contractions. Hysterotomy, a major surgical procedure, has been replaced by prostaglandins and saline instillation.

Abortion Complications

- Physical complications following abortion can be reduced with good patient health, early timing, use of the suction method and local anesthesia, a well-trained physician, and follow-up care. Infections can be reduced through pre-abortion testing and use of antibiotics. A two-week postabortion exam can establish that the abortion was complete.
- The risk of postabortion infertility is very low, and miscarriage rates following abortion have fallen greatly since abortion became legal, probably because techniques have improved.
- Psychological side effects of abortion vary with the individual. Most women go through a period of ambivalence; the strongest feelings usually occur immediately after the abortion. Having a supportive partner, friend, and family can be helpful.

Decision Making and Unintended Pregnancy

- Women who face unintended pregnancy differ in the way they make decisions; some make their choice calmly and quickly, while others struggle for weeks. It is often a matter of finding the "best," not necessarily the "right" solution.
- The woman's partner can positively influence her experience of an unintended pregnancy—giving support and helping with the decision. On the other hand, unintended pregnancies often mean the end of an unstable or unsatisfactory relationship.
- Parents can be helpful, unless disagreements lead to more stress; in most states today, the woman has the final say in the matter, though new legal changes in several states may change that.

Take Action

1. Now that you have information about abortion, reevaluate your contraceptive practices. If they aren't adequate to prevent unintended pregnancy, make any changes that you consider necessary to protect yourself.

2. Describe in writing the feelings you would have if you were faced with a decision about abortion right now. Decide on a course of action, and then project the consequences of your decision into the future. Describe how your decision might affect the course of your life and how you might feel about it a month from now, a year from now, ten years from now, and twenty years from now.

3. Write a one-page essay presenting your personal opinion on the abortion issue. Include arguments to refute the points typically made by the opposing side. Then write an essay presenting a convincing case for the opposite position. Make sure your arguments are clearly stated and that you can defend them, where appropriate, with facts.

4. Interview someone who has had an abortion or the partner of someone who has had an abortion. What can you learn from his or her experience? Does it offer insights into the issue or influence your position? Write an essay describing the person's experience, your reaction to it, and how you think the experience would have been different if abortion had been illegal at the time (or legal at the time, if it was an illegal abortion).

Selected Bibliography

Abortion surveillance: preliminary analysis—United States, 1984, 1985. *Journal of the American Medical Association* 260(23):Dec. 16, 1988, pp. 3410, 3412.

The American Psychiatric Association testifies on abortion before Koop. *Psychiatric News*, Apr. 1, 1988, pp. 1, 6, and 14.

The battle over abortion (several cover stories). *Newsweek*, July 17, 1989, pp. 14–27.

Hennessey, Patricia. 1989. Supreme Court puts women at risk. *Conscience*, 10(4):1–5.

Holt, V. L., et al. 1989. Induced abortion and the risk of subsequent ectopic pregnancy. *American Journal of Public Health* 79(9):1234–1238.

Kaplan, John. 1988 (Fall). What if the Supreme Court changed its mind? *Stanford Lawyer*, pp. 11–13 and 52–54.

Koop, C. Everett. 1989. A measured response: Koop on abortion. *Family Planning Perspectives* 21(1):31–32.

Rhoads, George G., et al. 1989. The safety and efficacy of chorionic villus sampling for early prenatal diagnosis of cytogenetic abnormalities. *New England Journal of Medicine* 320(10):609–617.

Rossi, Alice S., and Bhavani Sitaraman. 1988. Abortion in context: Historical trends and future changes. *Family Planning Perspectives* 20(6):273–281.

Want a baby? (several cover stories on adoption). *Time*, Oct. 9, 1989, pp. 86–95.

Recommended Readings

Mohr, J. C. 1978. *Abortion in America: The Origins and Evolution of National Policy, 1800–1900.* New York: Oxford University Press. *A historical perspective of views on abortion within American society. Includes a discussion of the powerful role that physicians played in the formation of public opinion and related legal decisions.*

Rubin, Eva R. 1987. *Abortion, Politics, and the Courts: Roe v. Wade and Its Aftermath.* Westport, Conn: Greenwood Press. *A thoroughly researched account of recent history on the abortion controversy in the United States. Gives a brief overview of the nineteenth-century views and the reform movements of the 1950s and 1960s. Primary focus is on* Roe v. Wade *and its aftermath.*

Stewart, Felicia, et al. 1987. *Understanding Your Body: Every Woman's Guide to Gynecology and Health.* New York: Bantam Books. *A comprehensive guide to women's gynecological health. Describes various treatment options for common problems. Includes up-to-date information on contraception and abortion.*

Contents

Making Connections

Some people have a child when they're in their teens or twenties, others wait until they hear their "biological clock" ticking in their mid- or late thirties, and still others never have children at all. Whatever your choice, it's critical for your health and happiness that you take control of your own fertility and make the decisions that are right for you. The scenarios presented on these pages describe situations in which people have to use information, make a decision, or choose a course of action, all related to pregnancy, childbirth, and becoming a parent. As you read them, imagine yourself in each situation and consider what you would do. After you've finished the chapter, read the scenarios again and see if what you've learned has changed how you would think, feel, or act in each situation.

You've been jogging regularly for a few years and plan to continue right through your pregnancy. But your mother thinks you're increasing your risk of miscarriage by being too active. She had three miscarriages herself and says you were born only because she spent so much time in bed while she was pregnant with you. Is she being overcautious on your account, or are you taking a chance?

You and your wife are taking prepared childbirth classes, and some of the other parents-to-be have some very clear expectations and opinions about birth and child rearing. They make it sound as if any woman who takes pain-relieving drugs during birth, has a cesarean delivery, or doesn't breastfeed is a failure, or worse. You find it hard to believe there's only one "right" way to have a baby and care for it. You're afraid your wife will be setting herself up for disappointment and guilt if she adopts the same attitudes. Is it true that all births are "natural" these days? Should every woman breastfeed her baby? What can you say to balance what you hear from others?

8

Becoming a Parent: Pregnancy and Childbirth

Although you haven't had much contact with children, you've always assumed you would be a father some day. Now that you've been married three years, you'd like to start a family. Your wife, who is an artist, says she just isn't ready to give up all her activities for a child. In fact she says she's not sure she'll ever be ready. You don't think a child will interfere that much with her activities or your lifestyle together. Babies spend most of their time sleeping, you tell her. And how much can something that only weighs 8 pounds change your life? She's not convinced. Is she right to hesitate, or should you both just take the plunge?

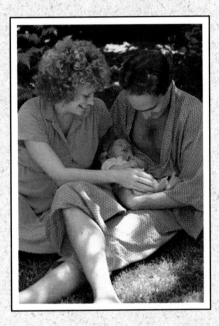

You have a friend who is six months pregnant and hasn't yet seen a physician or had any prenatal care. She says she's young and healthy and doesn't need any medical supervision to know how to have a baby. Now she's talking about having a home birth and wants you to be present, although she hasn't found a midwife or other attendant. Is it true that women without health problems have no need of medical attention during pregnancy? Is there any advice you can give her about prenatal care or home birth?

Now that you're six weeks pregnant, you've started thinking about the kind of birth experience you want to have. Some good friends of yours had a home birth last year with a midwife attending, and although the birth went fine, some complications afterward sent them rushing to the hospital. Because of their experience, your husband thinks home birth is too risky, and you feel too that you might never be able to forgive yourself if anything went wrong. On the other hand, you hate the idea of having such an important and personal experience as childbirth in a sterile hospital environment, where you're afraid you won't have any say in what happens. Do you have to accept a routine hospital birth? Should you plan to have a home birth and be ready to get to the hospital if necessary? Is there a compromise between the two?

Deciding whether to become a parent is one of the most important decisions you will ever make. Having a child changes your life forever; deciding not to have children has equally far-reaching implications. Yet many people approach this momentous decision with only the vaguest notion of what is involved in pregnancy, childbirth, and parenting. An estimated half of the 3.6 million babies born every year in the United States are from unintentional pregnancies, and many of the other half are conceived without any preplanning.

Exploring Your Emotions

If you decide not to have children, how do you think you will feel about your decision ten, twenty, or thirty years from now? What factors will influence your decision and your subsequent feelings?

Today, with changing cultural expectations and increasingly sophisticated contraceptive technology, you have more choice about becoming a parent than people have ever had before. Until recently it was expected that virtually every married couple would have children. Now you can choose whether, when, and how you want to have a child; you can also make choices that minimize the risks and maximize the benefits for yourself, your partner, and your children. This chapter presents information that you can use both now and later in your life to make the decisions about children and parenting that are right for you.

Preparation for Parenthood

Before you decide whether or when to become a parent, you'll want to consider your suitability and readiness to parent; once you (and your partner) are expecting a baby, you'll want to decide who will help deliver your child and where, what prenatal tests you'll need, and what feeding method you'll use. If you're lucky, you won't have to consider issues of infertility, but you should be aware that infertility problems increase with a woman's age.

Deciding to Become a Parent   Many factors have to be taken into account when you are considering parenthood. The following are some questions you should ask yourself and some issues you should consider when making this decision. Some issues are relevant to both men and women; others apply only to women.

- Your physical health and your age. Are you in reasonably good health? If not, can you improve your health by changing your lifestyle by modifying your diet or giving up cigarettes or drugs? Do you have physical conditions, such as overweight or diabetes, that will require extra care and medical attention during pregnancy? Do you or your partner have a family history of genetic problems that a baby might inherit? If you both have a history of the same genetic problem, chances are greater that a baby would inherit it.
- Pregnant teenagers have special health concerns. They have to eat well enough to supply the needs of their own growing bodies as well as the baby's. Many teenagers have poor eating and health habits, and often they can't afford adequate prenatal care. Becoming a mother after 35 has risks too; women under 20 and over 35 have babies with a higher incidence of Down's syndrome. After 30 women risk greater infertility and may find it harder to become pregnant.

Exploring Your Emotions

How do you feel about the prospect of having a baby being completely dependent on you for food, shelter, clothing, attention, and love for several years of your life? Can you support a child emotionally?

- Your financial circumstances. Can you afford a child? Will your health insurance cover the costs of pregnancy, prenatal tests, delivery, and medical attention for mother and baby before and after the birth, including physicians' fees and hospital costs? Supplies for the baby are expensive too—diapers, bedding, cribs, strollers, car seats, clothing, food and medical supplies, and child care. The first few years of raising a baby can easily cost $10,000, and if the mother has quit her job or is on maternity leave, the family must live on one income. Costs increase as the child grows. Some families find they need a bigger apartment or house or a bigger or safer car. For the latest figures on the cost of raising a child, see the box "How Much Does a Child Cost?"
- Your relationship with your partner. Are you in a stable relationship, and do both of you want a child? Are your views compatible on such issues as child-rearing goals, the distribution of responsibility for the child, and work and housework?
- Your educational, career, and child care plans. Have you completed as much of your education as you want right now? Have you sufficiently established yourself in a career, if that is something you want to do? Have you investigated maternity leave and company-sponsored child care? Do you and your partner agree on child care arrangements, and does such child care exist in your community? Many child development experts

How Much Does A Child Cost?

Although the number of babies born in the early 1990s is expected to rival the number born in the late 1950s and early 1960s—the peak of the baby boom—there's no comparison between the two eras when it comes to expense. Babies cost about twice as much as they did thirty years ago, even adjusting for inflation. Back then, a baby's first year cost parents about $800, equivalent to $2,892 in today's goods and services. Today, the nationwide figure is $5,774.

What costs so much more? Day care. Few families needed day care thirty years ago. Today, more than half of first-time mothers are back at work before their children celebrate a first birthday. Day care costs parents across the United States an average of $2,184 during the first year, assuming a new mother takes a three-month ma-

ternity leave. In some states, the figure is much higher, up to well over $4,000. That puts the total cost at over $7,800.

But day care isn't the only new expense. Car seats, disposable diapers, formula, and sophisticated photographic equipment also add to the expense facing first-time parents. Some new baby items are legally required (car seats), recommended by pediatricians (formula, rather than cow's milk), or demanded by harried parents (disposable diapers).

Thirty years ago, a "car seat" was just an expanse of vinyl or car upholstery next to mom or dad. Today, babies are strapped into expensive, form-fitted chairs that protect them in case of an accident. Parents may need two car seats during the first year—one for the newborn and another for the older infant. The cost: about $100.

Other high-tech tools include portable cribs ($65), safety gates ($30), umbrella strollers ($35), and sling seats that parents use to carry the baby next to their bodies ($35).

In the 1950s, a baby had about 50 cloth diapers that its stay-at-home mother had time to launder. Now parents spend $570 in the first year on 3,000 disposable diapers, which may be convenient for the household but cause a problem for the nation's landfills. And few parents used to have expensive photographic equipment. Today, about 16 percent of parents with babies own a video camera, and the number is rising. Most parents own 35-mm camera equipment.

Is the expense of the first year a warning of 17 costly years to come? Research confirms that it is. The total cost of raising a child from birth to age 18 is about $100,000, according to the U.S. Department of Agriculture. And that doesn't include the cost of college. Some grown children even return to their parents' home for a period of time after college because they find it too expensive to live on their own. Perhaps the only consolation for today's struggling parents is that it's cheaper to have a child now than it will be 30 years from now!

$5,774

THAT'S HOW MUCH A BABY COSTS IN ITS FIRST YEAR OF LIFE...

That's a national figure, one that includes material goods and some services, but excludes such additional costs as trips to the pediatrician for illnesses.

Food	$855
Diapers	$570
Clothes	$352
Furniture	$995
Bedding	$223
Medicine*	$396
Toys	$199
Day care	$2,184

* Vitamins, personal care products
Sources: U.S. Bureau of the Census, National Center for Health Statistics, U.S. Department of Agriculture, American Baby

Adapted from Blayne Cutler. Ringing up baby. *San Jose Mercury News*, February 25, 1990, p. 1L.

advise against full time child care for babies under 1 year of age because it can disrupt their attachment to their parents. The child care issue, which some people consider the most difficult one in parenting, requires a great deal of thought.

- Your emotional readiness for parenthood. Are you prepared to have a helpless being completely dependent on you twenty-four hours a day? Do you have the emotional reserves to care for and nurture an infant? Are you willing to change your lifestyle to provide the best conditions for a baby's development, both before and after birth?
- Your social support system. Do you have a network of family and friends who will help you with the baby? Are there community resources that you can call on for additional assistance? A family's social support system is one of the most important factors affecting their ability to adjust to a baby and cope with new responsibilities.
- Your personal qualities, attitudes toward children, and aptitude for parenting. Do you like children? Do you think time with children is time well spent? Do you feel good enough about yourself to love and respect others? Do you have safe ways of handling anger, frustration, and impatience?

■ **Exploring Your Emotions**

Do you want to have children? What is the basis for your feelings and desires? Can you distinguish personal reasons from cultural expectations? Would people think of you as selfish if you decided not to have children?

- Your philosophical beliefs. Some people question the value of bringing more people into an already overcrowded world. Many countries have yet to stabilize their populations, the United States among them; worldwide population is expected to soar from 5 billion in 1990 to 9 billion in 2030. Given these figures, some people feel that human beings have already fulfilled the biblical directive to be fruitful and multiply, and they choose to remain childless.

Preparing for Pregnancy and Childbirth   Once a pregnancy begins, there are many decisions and choices to consider. Some important decisions involve the type of practitioners and environment the parents want for their birth. Many hospitals and physicians no longer follow rigid routines, offering instead a variety of options to parents. Parents should inquire about the use of anesthesia and fetal monitoring, the practices of inducing labor and using forceps for delivery, and the criteria for performing **cesarean sections**. They should know whether the father will be allowed in the delivery room, whether the baby will be able to stay with the mother after birth (a practice known as rooming-in), and whether other children in the family will be allowed to visit.

■ **Exploring Your Emotions**

Would you take advantage of a prenatal diagnostic tool like amniocentesis to find out ahead of time if your child had a genetic abnormality? If such an abnormality was discovered, would you choose to terminate the pregnancy? What criteria would you use to make your decision? From whom would you seek advice and with whom would you discuss the dilemma?

Many families are choosing alternative settings and methods of childbirth, both at home and in alternative birth centers. In some states, trained and certified nurse-midwives can attend women with low-risk pregnancies in home births, give prenatal and postnatal care and treatment and perform the delivery. Despite precautions, home births are not without risks. Many hospitals have introduced alternative birth centers in response to the criticisms of traditional hospital routines. The centers are alternatives to home births, where emergencies may not be adequately handled, and to traditional hospital births, where procedures sometimes seem too rigid and impersonal. Alternative birth centers provide a comfortable, emotionally supportive environment in close proximity to up-to-date medical equipment. A 1989 study of alternative birth centers concluded that the properly administered ones are as safe as hospitals for most births.

Prospective parents also have the option of obtaining information about their baby before it's born—including its sex and whether it has certain genetic abnormalities or birth defects—through prenatal testing. The most common tests now used are ultrasound, amniocentesis, and chorionic villus sampling. Ultrasound provides a visual image of the fetus in the uterus, showing its position, size and gestational age, and the presence of certain anatomical problems, such as cleft palate. Amniocentesis involves the extraction of amniotic fluid from the uterus and the genetic analysis of the fetal cells it contains. This analysis can reveal a variety of abnormalities, including Down's syndrome and sickle-cell anemia.

Cesarean section   A surgical incision through the abdominal walls and uterus, performed to extract a fetus.

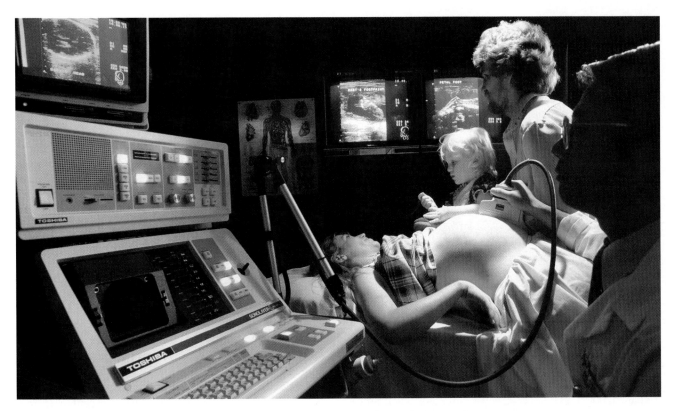

Ultrasound provides information about the position, size, and physical condition of a fetus in the uterus. This couple and their first child can see the baby move and perhaps tell its sex by watching it on the screen.

Many hospitals routinely advise all mothers over the age of 35 to have amniocentesis because of their higher risk of passing on a genetic disorder.

The newest technique, chorionic villus sampling, involves the extraction of a sample of chorionic tissue (part of the fetal support system in the uterus) and its analysis for genetic abnormalities. Chorionic villus sampling can be done much earlier than amniocentesis, so that if parents choose to abort a fetus, they can do so sooner and more safely. Genetic counselors explain the results of the tests so that parents can understand their implications.

Parents-to-be also have to decide whether to breastfeed or bottlefeed their child. In general, breastfeeding is preferred to bottlefeeding because human milk is perfectly suited to the baby's nutritional needs and digestive capacities and because it supplies the baby with antibodies that protect it against diseases. Breastfeeding is also beneficial to the mother, because it stimulates contractions that help the uterus return to normal more rapidly. On the other hand, breastfeeding can be confining for women planning to return to work. Because drugs taken by the mother show up in breast milk, including antacids, laxatives, and hormones, she has to avoid medications as long as she nurses her baby.

Although health care practitioners recommend breastfeeding for a number of practical reasons, the decision about how to feed the baby is ultimately up to the parents. Both methods of feeding can be part of loving, secure mother-child relationships. In many cases, personal, social, and cultural values or considerations take precedence over professional advice.

These are just a few of the decisions and issues prospective parents have to face before their child is born. The greater range and variety of choices available to parents have brought greater responsibility for making informed decisions. Some people have responded to this increased freedom and responsibility by adopting attitudes that are just as narrow and rigid as hospital practices used to be. They become vocal advocates of the new childbirth practices without taking unexpected circumstances or personal preferences into account. Such attitudes tend to restrict people's choices rather than broaden them.

■ **Exploring Your Emotions**

If you are a woman and want to have a child, what kind of birth experience do you want to have? If you are a man, do you want to participate and have a role in your partner's birth experience, or would you rather just leave it to her?

Actually, a variety of birth situations and child-rearing practices can have positive physical and psychological outcomes, especially if parents are encouraged to choose what feels comfortable to them. The important thing is that people give sufficient thought to the issues to make the right choices. Having a child is one of the most arduous, important, and rewarding enterprises that human beings undertake. The more you know about it—about conception and pregnancy, fetal development and prenatal care, birth and parenting—the more capable you will be of making intelligent, informed decisions about it.

Understanding Fertility   That anyone ever gets pregnant is a miracle; that we can now prevent pregnancy because we understand the female fertility cycle is a miracle of quite a different sort. Conceiving is a highly complex process, and although many couples conceive readily, others can testify to the difficulties that can be encountered.

Conception   Every month during a woman's fertile years, her body prepares itself for **conception** and childbearing. In one of her **ovaries** an egg ripens and is released, bursting from its **follicle.** The egg is then drawn into an **oviduct** (or **Fallopian tube**) through which it travels to the **uterus.** The journey takes three to four days. The lining of the uterus has already puffed out to assist the implanting of a **fertilized egg,** or zygote. An unfertilized egg lives about twenty-four hours and then disintegrates. It is expelled along with the uterine lining during menstruation. Each egg is about the size of a pinpoint, 1/250 inch in diameter, and about a half million eggs are in a girl's ovaries at birth. Only about 400 to 500 of them will ripen and be released during her lifetime.

Sperm cells are much smaller than eggs (1/8,000 inch in diameter). They are also much more plentiful; an average ejaculation contains about 400 million. During ejaculation, sperm cells travel from the testicles, where they develop, through two ducts (vasa deferentia) and the

seminal vesicles, pouches where they are temporarily stored. At the prostate gland, they enter the urethra, through which orgasm propels them with great force into the woman's vagina.

A sperm cell—unless it fertilizes an egg—lives only about a week. Many sperm cells do not survive the acidic environment of the vagina. Those that do quickly migrate to the cervix, the "neck" of the uterus, where secretions are more alkaline and thus more hospitable. Once through the cervix and into the uterus, many sperm cells are diverted to the wrong oviduct or get stuck along the way. Those that enter the tube that harbors the traveling egg face one more obstacle: tough skin that encases the egg. However, each sperm cell that touches the egg deposits an enzyme that dissolves parts of the membrane. The first sperm cell that bumps into a bare spot on the egg cell can swim into the cell to merge with the nucleus, and **fertilization** occurs. The sperm's tail, its means of locomotion, gets stuck in the outer membrane and drops off, leaving the sperm head inside the egg. Now no more sperm can enter the egg, possibly because once it has been fertilized it releases a chemical that makes it impregnable.

The ovum (egg) carries the hereditary characteristics of the mother and her ancestors; sperm cells carry the hereditary characteristics of the father and his ancestors. Together they contain the **genetic code,** a set of instructions for development. Each parent cell—egg or sperm—contains 23 chromosomes, and each of these chromosomes in turn contains at least 1,000 genes, so small that they cannot be seen through a microscope. These genes are packages of chemical instructions for designing every part of a new baby. They specify that the infant will be human; what its sex will be; whether it will tend to be (depending also on its environment) short, tall, thin, fat, healthy or sickly; how intelligent it can be; and hundreds of other characteristics. Together, they provide the blueprint for a new and unique person.

Conception   The formation of a zygote (fertilized egg), the cell resulting from the fusion of ovum and sperm, and in normal conditions capable of survival and maturation in the uterus.

Ovary   One of the two female reproductive glands in which ova (eggs) and hormones are formed.

Follicles   The thousands of protecting, enclosing spherical bubbles in the ovaries in which ova mature. Each follicle contains a liquid supplied with estrogen.

Oviducts (Fallopian tubes)   The two passages through which ova travel from the ovaries to the uterus; "normal" place for fertilization.

Uterus   The hollow, thick-walled, muscular organ in which the egg develops into a child; located directly above the vagina; the source of menstrual flow; the womb.

Fertilized egg   The egg after it has been penetrated by a sperm; a zygote.

Sperm cell   A mature male germ cell that serves to impregnate the ovum.

Fertilization   The initiation of biological reproduction, as, for example, when the sperm and ovum unite to form a zygote (fertilized egg).

Genetic code   Master blueprint message directing the body's growth and cell differentiation, contained in genetic material.

Human chorionic gonadotropin (HCG)   A hormone found only in pregnant women; its presence is the basis for pregnancy testing.

Infertility   Inability to reproduce.

Artificial insemination   The act of placing semen in the vagina or uterus by means other than sexual intercourse.

In vitro fertilization   Combining ovum and sperm in a laboratory dish for the purpose of fertilization.

Pregnancy Tests   Some women wish to know immediately whether or not they are indeed pregnant. They can test for pregnancy with home testing kits sold over the counter in drugstores. These kits detect a hormone found only in pregnant women, called **human chorionic gonadotropin** (HCG). Home test kits come equipped with a small sample of red blood cells coated with HCG antibodies, to which the user can add a small amount of her own urine. If the concentration of HCG is great enough, it will clump together with the HCG antibodies, indicating that the user is pregnant.

These home tests are 85–95 percent reliable. If used too early in the pregnancy, the HCG concentrate is not great enough to clump. Other conditions that also produce a false negative include an unclean test tube, vaginal or urinary infection, presence of some drugs or oral contraceptives, and moving the test while it's working. False positives can occur when the user is near menopause, has uterine cancer, has been recently pregnant, or waits too long to read the results. Blood tests administered and analyzed by a medical laboratory give more accurate results.

Problems of Infertility   Although the main concern for many women and men, especially if they are young and single, is how *not* to get pregnant, the reverse is true for millions of couples who have difficulty conceiving. Perhaps 15 to 20 percent of all couples in the United States are unable to have the children they want. Treatment for **infertility** enables about half of the couples who seek help to have a child, but in many other cases nothing helps.

■ **Exploring Your Emotions**

If you were thirty-five and it didn't seem likely that you were going to have a child, would you consider extraordinary measures—such as single parenthood via adoption or artificial insemination—to do so? What do you think would be the difficulties involved in such a course of action, and what would be the rewards?

A variety of conditions may cause infertility. Women may fail to ovulate or they may have menstrual cycle irregularities, endometriosis (a condition in which abnormal tissue in the pelvic cavity prevents conception), hormonal imbalances, or scar tissue in the oviducts. Some women have physical abnormalities, such as an unusually shaped uterus, that make it more difficult for them to carry a pregnancy to term. Other women develop an allergic response that kills their partner's sperm.

In men, infertility is caused mainly by low sperm counts or sperm with poor motility (ability to move). These problems can often be traced to injury of the testicles, infection (especially from mumps during adulthood), radiation, gland disorders, birth defects, or subjecting the testicles to high temperatures, such as those produced by hot baths or tight-fitting underwear. Semen quality appears to improve with regular sexual activity rather than following abstinence.

Some kinds of infertility can be treated; others cannot. Surgery can sometimes repair oviducts, clear up endometriosis, and correct anatomical problems. Fertility drugs can help a woman ovulate, although they carry the risk of causing multiple births. Surgery can sometimes reverse a vasectomy.

If these procedures don't work, more advanced techniques may help. Male infertility can sometimes be overcome by collecting and concentrating the man's sperm and introducing it mechanically into the woman's vagina or uterus, a procedure known as **artificial insemination**. Some kinds of female infertility can be by-passed with **in vitro fertilization**. In this procedure, eggs are removed from the woman's ovary and fertilized in a laboratory dish by her partner's sperm. One or more of the resulting embryos is implanted in the woman's uterus. Embryos that aren't used are often frozen and stored for the couple to use later. If one partner is infertile, a donor can supply the sperm or egg.

Some aspects of in vitro fertilization have sparked intense moral and legal debate. A recent court case involved the status of frozen embryos after the parents divorced. The court ruled in favor of the wife, who planned to use the embryos to have children, and against the husband, who no longer wanted to father a child with his ex-wife and asked that the embryos be destroyed. Another case involved the legal status of frozen embryos as heirs to the estate of their parents, who were both killed in a plane crash before the embryos could be implanted.

The most controversial of all approaches to infertility is surrogate motherhood. This practice involves a contract between a fertile woman who agrees to carry a fetus and a couple who wishes to have a child but cannot because the woman is infertile. The surrogate mother agrees to be artificially inseminated by the husband's sperm, carry the baby to term, and give it to the couple at birth. In return, the couple pays her for her services. Some people question the morality of paying a woman to carry a baby. They see surrogate motherhood as an arrangement essentially to sell a baby, and they worry about the psychological consequences for children who learn their biological mothers "sold" them. Experience has shown, too, that some surrogate mothers have a very difficult time giving up the baby they have carried and are unwilling to fulfill the contract after the birth, causing emotional trauma for themselves and the couple.

All these treatments for infertility are expensive and

Six Ways to Start a Family

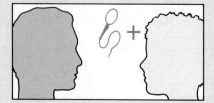

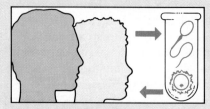

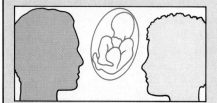

Traditional

1. Couple conceives a child.

2. The child stays with the couple, who are its genetic and legal parents.

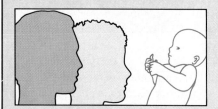

Adoptive

1. Couple is unable to conceive or chooses not to.

2. An adoption agency matches the couple with child to be adopted.

3. Adoption papers are signed. Couple accepts parental responsibilities but has no genetic link to the child.

Donor Sperm

1. Couple is unable to conceive because male is infertile.

2. Sperm purchased from a sperm bank is used to impregnate the woman by artificial insemination.

3. The child is genetically linked to the mother but not the father. The sperm donor—the biological father—has no legal link to the child.

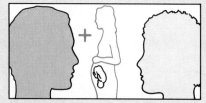

Surrogate Mother

1. Couple is unable to conceive because the female is infertile or pregnancy would be too risky.

2. A second woman is selected to be inseminated with the father's sperm. She signs a contract agreeing to bear the child and give it up after birth, usually for a sum of money.

3. Shortly after birth, the child is given to the couple. The child is genetically linked to the father but not to the mother. Whether the woman who bore the child—the biological mother—has the right to change her mind and keep the child is still open to question.

In Vitro Fertilization

1. Although male and female produce sperm and eggs, the couple is unable to conceive.

2. Sperm and egg are combined in a laboratory.

3. The fertilized egg is implanted back into the woman.

4. The child stays with the couple, who are its genetic and legal parents.

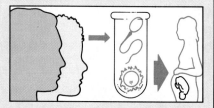

Host Uterus

1. Although male and female produce sperm and eggs, they are unable or unwilling to have a pregnancy.

2. Sperm from the male and egg from the female are combined in a laboratory.

3. The fertilized egg is implanted into a second woman, who agrees to bear the child and give it up, usually for a sum of money.

4. Shortly after birth, the child is given to the couple. Although brought to term in the uterus of another woman, the child's genes all come from the couple.

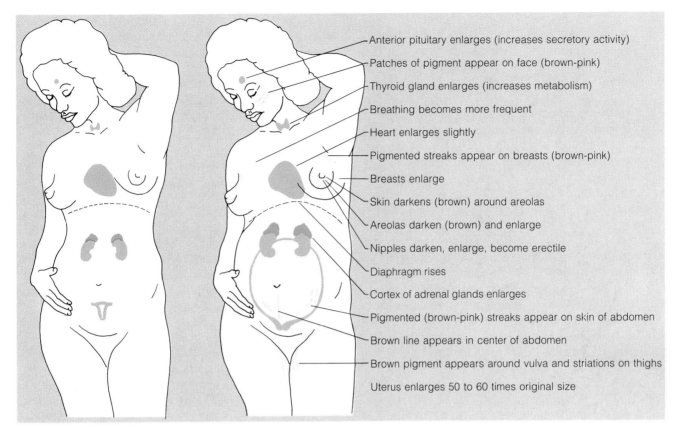

Anterior pituitary enlarges (increases secretory activity)
Patches of pigment appear on face (brown-pink)
Thyroid gland enlarges (increases metabolism)
Breathing becomes more frequent
Heart enlarges slightly
Pigmented streaks appear on breasts (brown-pink)
Breasts enlarge
Skin darkens (brown) around areolas
Areolas darken (brown) and enlarge
Nipples darken, enlarge, become erectile
Diaphragm rises
Cortex of adrenal glands enlarges
Pigmented (brown-pink) streaks appear on skin of abdomen
Brown line appears in center of abdomen
Brown pigment appears around vulva and striations on thighs
Uterus enlarges 50 to 60 times original size

Figure 8-1   Physiological changes during pregnancy: *(left)* the female body at the time of conception; *(right)* development after 30 weeks of pregnancy.

emotionally draining, and their success is uncertain. Couples undergoing fertility treatment may lose perspective on the rest of their lives and seek solutions that seem radical to outsiders, if they can afford them. Others remain childless or turn to adoption, which can also be difficult and expensive. Support groups for infertile couples can provide help in this difficult situation, but there are few easy answers to infertility. One measure that you can take now to avoid infertility is to protect yourself against STDs and to treat promptly and completely any diseases you do contract.

Pregnancy

Pregnancy is usually discussed in terms of **trimesters**— three periods of three months (or thirteen weeks) each, based mainly on fetal development. During the first trimester, the mother experiences relatively few bodily changes and some fairly common symptoms. During the

second trimester, often the most peaceful time of pregnancy, the mother gains weight, looks noticeably pregnant, and may experience a general sense of well-being if she is happy about having a child. The third trimester is the hardest for the mother. She must breathe, digest, excrete, and circulate blood for two people. The weight of the fetus, the pressure of its body on her organs, and its increased demands on her system cause discomfort and fatigue. As a result, the mother may become increasingly lethargic and impatient to give birth.

Changes in the Woman's Body   Hormonal changes begin as soon as the egg is fertilized, and for the next nine months the woman's body continually prepares the way for the fetus. Her ribs flare out long before the uterus needs room to expand, for example, and her uterus expands long before the fetus needs room to grow. Her overall body metabolism becomes more efficient to provide a positive nutritional balance for herself and the fetus. Let's take a closer look at the changes of early, middle, and late pregnancy (see Figure 8-1).

Trimester   One of the three thirteen-week periods of pregnancy.

Early Signs and Symptoms Early recognition of pregnancy is important, especially for women with physical problems and nutritional deficiencies. The pregnancy symptoms described here are not absolute indications of pregnancy, but they are reasons to visit a gynecologist.

- Missed menstrual period. If an egg has been fertilized and implanted in the uterine wall, the uterine lining is retained to nourish the embryo. A woman who misses a period after having unprotected intercourse may be two weeks pregnant. After missing a second period, she should visit a gynecologist.
- Slight bleeding. During early pregnancy, slight bleeding may follow the implanting of the fertilized egg in the uterine wall. Because it happens about when a period is expected, the bleeding is sometimes mistaken for menstrual flow. It usually lasts only a few days.
- Nausea. About two-thirds of pregnant women feel nauseated, probably as a reaction to increased levels of progesterone and other hormones. The nausea is often called morning sickness, but some women have it all day long. It frequently disappears by the twelfth week.
- Sleepiness, fatigue, and emotional upset. These symptoms result from hormonal changes.

Miscarriage and Ectopic Pregnancy Complications may prevent full-term development of the fetus. Sometimes genetic or physical defects in a fetus will cause **spontaneous abortion**—also known as **miscarriage**—to occur, terminating the pregnancy. Although the exact frequency of spontaneous abortion is unknown, it is estimated that 10–40 percent of pregnancies end this way, some without the woman's awareness that she was pregnant. Most of these miscarriages occur within the first trimester.

Earlier miscarriages may appear as a heavier than usual menstrual flow; later ones may involve uncomfortable cramping and profuse bleeding. One miscarriage doesn't mean that later pregnancies will be unsuccessful. Of women who have three or more miscarriages, the cause in about 40 percent is an abnormal uterus or ovaries that do not produce enough progesterone. Recently, a third significant cause of repeated miscarriage has been identified as an inappropriate maternal immune response to the type of fetal cell that contacts the mother's tissues. These women can now be immunized with cells from the father or from the placenta.

Sometimes the developing embryo attaches itself to the wall of an oviduct instead of making its way to the uterus. These **ectopic pregnancies** are dangerous because the embryo can grow only so much before the tube bursts. If the embryo isn't removed surgically, the mother can die of internal bleeding. An early prenatal exam can reveal whether the embryo is growing properly in the uterus.

Continuing Changes in the Woman's Body The most obvious changes during pregnancy occur in the reproductive organs. During the first three months, the uterus enlarges to about three times its nonpregnant size, but it still cannot be felt in the abdomen. By the fourth month, it is large enough to make the abdomen protrude. By the seventh or eighth month, the uterus pushes up into the rib cage, which makes breathing slightly more difficult. The breasts enlarge and are sensitive by the eighth week and may tingle or throb. The pigmented area around the nipple, the areola, darkens and broadens. After the tenth week, **colostrum**, a thin milky fluid, may be squeezed from the mother's nipples, but actual secretion of milk is prevented by high levels of estrogen and progesterone.

Other changes are going on as well. Early in pregnancy, the muscles and ligaments attached to bones begin to soften and stretch. The joints between the pelvic bones loosen and spread, making it easier to have a baby but harder to walk. The circulatory system becomes more efficient to accommodate the blood volume, which increases by 50 percent, and the heart pumps it more rapidly. Much of the increased blood flow goes to the uterus and placenta. The mother's lungs also become more efficient, and her rib cage widens to permit her to inhale up to 40 percent more air. Again, much of the oxygen goes to the fetus. The kidneys become highly efficient, removing waste products from fetal circulation and producing prodigious amounts of urine by midpregnancy.

How much weight should a woman gain during pregnancy? Women of normal weight gain an average of 18 to 25 percent of their initial weight: 20 to 28 pounds for a woman weighing 110; 23 to 32 pounds for a woman weighing 128 pounds. Reducing diets during pregnancy can deprive the fetus of needed nutrients and they are discouraged even among overweight mothers. About 60 percent of weight gained relates directly to the baby—about 7.5 pounds for the baby and 8.5 pounds for the

---

Spontaneous abortion Termination of pregnancy when the uterine contents are expelled; causes vary, but can include an abnormal uterus, insufficient hormones, and genetic or physical fetal defects.

Ectopic pregnancy A life-threatening situation where a fertilized egg implants itself into an oviduct instead of the uterus; the embryo must be surgically removed.

Colostrum The thin, milky fluid secreted by the mammary glands around the time of childbirth until milk comes in, about the third day.

False labor Preliminary uterine contractions that occur throughout pregnancy and that do not progress to labor.

Lightening A labor process in which the uterus sinks downward about 2 inches because the baby's head, or other body part, settles far down into the pelvic area.

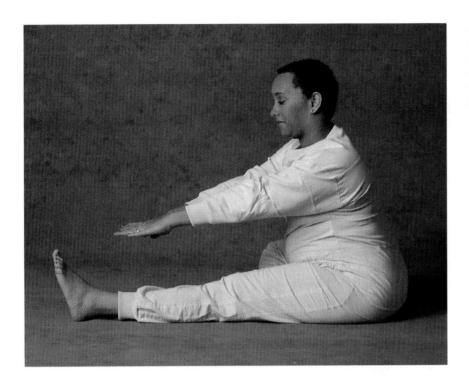

A woman's body changes drastically during pregnancy to accommodate and nourish the growing fetus. Prenatal exercise helps this woman stay healthy while her body works to sustain two lives.

placenta, amniotic fluid, heavier breasts and uterus—and 40 percent accumulates over the mother's entire body as fluid (blood, about 4 pounds) and fat (4 to 8 pounds). But gains in total pregnancy pounds vary strikingly, and similarities in total weight gain appear to conceal large differences in components of gain. As the woman's skin stretches, small breaks may occur in the elastic fibers of the lower layer of skin, producing "stretch marks" on her abdomen, hips, breasts, or thighs. Increased pigment production darkens the skin in 90 percent of pregnant women, especially in places that have stretched.

Sexual activity often changes during pregnancy. Varying hormone levels and increased sensitivity in the genital area cause some women to become more interested in sexual intercourse and others less interested. Both responses are common and are influenced by the woman's and her partner's attitudes toward sexuality during pregnancy. Intercourse is possible throughout pregnancy, but physical awkwardness in later months may interfere with comfort. Open communication between the partners is essential to a satisfying sexual relationship during pregnancy.

Rapid changes in hormone levels can cause a pregnant woman to experience unpredictable emotions and general "weepiness." A great part of pregnancy is beyond the woman's control—her changing appearance, her energy level, her variable moods—and some women need extra support and reassurance to keep on an even keel. Hormonal changes can also make women feel exhilarated and

euphoric, although for some women such moods are temporary.

Changes and Complications of Later Stages of Pregnancy By the end of the sixth month, the increased needs of the fetus place a burden on the mother's lungs, heart, and kidneys. Her back may ache from the pressure of the baby's weight and from having to throw her shoulders back to keep her balance while standing (see Figure 8-2). Her body retains more water, perhaps up to three extra quarts of fluid. Her legs, hands, ankles, or feet may swell, and she may be bothered by leg cramps, heartburn, or constipation. Despite discomfort, both her digestion and her metabolism are working at top efficiency.

The uterus prepares for childbirth throughout pregnancy with preliminary contractions, or **false labor** pains. Unlike true labor pains, these contractions are usually short, irregular, and painless. The mother may only be aware that at times her abdomen is hard to the touch. These contractions become more frequent and intense as the delivery date approaches.

In the ninth month, the baby settles into the pelvic bones, usually head down, fitting snugly. This process, called **lightening**, allows the uterus to sink down about two inches, producing a visible change in the mother's profile. Pelvic pressure increases and pressure on the diaphragm lightens. Breathing becomes easier; urination becomes more frequent. Sometimes, after a first pregnancy,

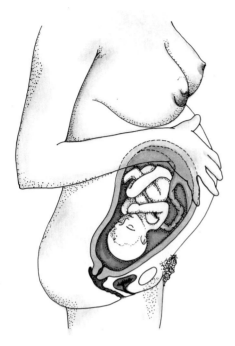

Figure 8-2   Position of the uterus and fetus after 32 weeks of pregnancy.

the baby doesn't settle down into the pelvis until **labor** begins.

A potentially serious condition that occasionally develops in the later months of pregnancy (usually not before the twenty-fourth week) is **preeclampsia, or toxemia of pregnancy**. Blood pressure rises, the face and legs swell, and excess protein appears in the urine. In later stages, vision blurs and the head aches continually, leading eventually to convulsions, coma, and even death. A woman who notices facial edema (swelling) should see her physician immediately. Changes in blood pressure are normally noticed and tracked by the physician or midwife during routine prenatal examinations.

Fetal Development   Now that we've seen what happens to the mother's body during pregnancy, let's consider the

development of the fetus. By the end of the first trimester, the baby's anatomy is almost completely formed; further refinements are made during the second trimester; and needed fat and pounds are added during the third trimester (see Figure 8-3).

First trimester   About 30 hours after the egg is fertilized, the cell reproduces itself by dividing in half. The process of cell division repeats many times. As the cluster of cells drifts down the oviduct, several different kinds of cells emerge. The entire genetic code is passed to every cell, but each cell follows only a segment of the code; if this were not the case, there would be no different organs or body parts. For example, all cells carry genes for hair color and eye color, but only the cells of the hair follicles and irises respond to that information.

On about the fourth day after fertilization, the cluster, now about thirty-six cells and hollow, arrives in the uterus. In this form it is known as a **blastocyst**. On the sixth or seventh day, the blastocyst burrows into the uterine lining, usually along the upper curve (see Figure 8-4). One week after conception the cells number over 100, and the cluster is now considered an **embryo**. It begins to draw nourishment from the **endometrium**, the uterine lining.

Soon, the spherical cluster collapses in on itself, and the inner cells now transform themselves by separating into three layers. One layer composes inner body parts, the digestive and respiratory systems; another layer becomes the skin, hair, and nervous tissue; and the middle layer becomes muscle, bone, marrow, blood, kidneys, and sex glands.

The outermost shell of blastocyst cells becomes the **placenta**, umbilical cord, and **amniotic sac**. A network of roots called **chorionic villi** sprouts from the blastocyst and eventually forms the placenta. Tapping the small blood vessels in the endometrium, the villi firmly implant the cell cluster and draw nourishment from the mother's blood through a thick, spongy layer into the embryo's blood. They remove waste products by the same route.

By the end of the first month the embryo is a finely

Labor   The act or process of birthing a child, expelling it with the placenta from the mother's body by means of uterine contractions.

Preeclampsia (toxemia of pregnancy)   A series of metabolic disturbances characterized at first by a rise in blood pressure, excess albumin in the urine, and fluid retention. More severe symptoms follow in the second stage and, without appropriate medical attention, can cause death.

Blastocyst   A stage of human development, lasting only from about Day 6 to Day 14, during which the cell cluster divides into the embryo and the placenta.

Embryo   The developing cluster of cells from the end of the first week to the end of the eighth week following conception.

Endometrium   The mucus membrane that forms the inner lining of the cavity of the uterus.

Placenta   The organ through which the fetus receives nourishment and empties waste via the mother's circulatory system; after birth, the placenta is expelled from the uterus.

Amniotic sac   The bag of watery fluid that lines the uterus and surrounds and protects the fetus.

Chorionic villi   Threadlike blood vessels that sprout from the blastocyst into the mother's vessels to draw out blood and nourishment.

Fetus   Developmental stage of a human from the ninth week after conception to the moment of birth.

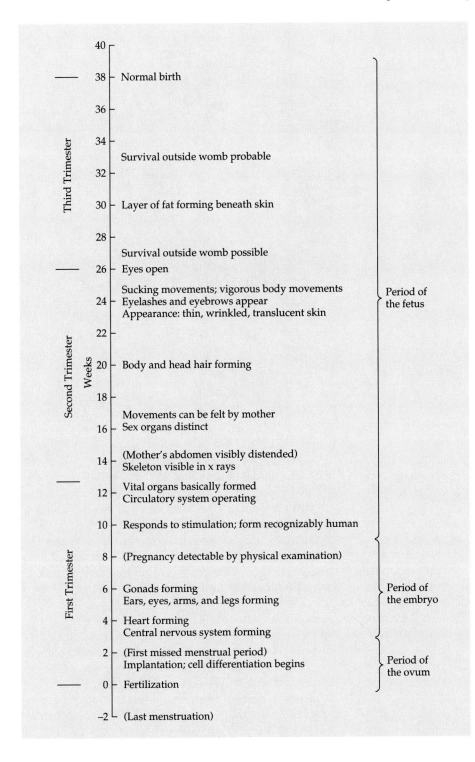

Figure 8-3 Chronology of milestones in prenatal development.

structured although incomplete body. By the end of the second month, the brain sends out impulses that coordinate the functioning of other organs. The embryo is now considered a **fetus**, and all further bodily changes will be in size and refinements of working parts. In the third month the fetus begins to be quite active. By the end of the first trimester, the fetus is about four inches long and weighs 1 ounce.

Second Trimester To achieve its growth during the second trimester—to about 14 inches and 2 pounds—the fetus must have large amounts of food, oxygen, and water, which come from the mother through the placenta. The placental system is so efficient that within an hour or two the fetus receives any substance entering the mother's bloodstream. All body systems are operating, and the fetal heartbeat can be heard with a stethoscope.

Figure 8-4 A cross section of the uterus in pregnancy.

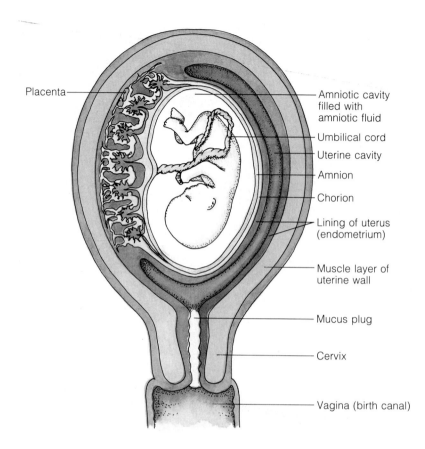

Placenta

Amniotic cavity filled with amniotic fluid

Umbilical cord

Uterine cavity

Amnion

Chorion

Lining of uterus (endometrium)

Muscle layer of uterine wall

Mucus plug

Cervix

Vagina (birth canal)

Fetal movements can be felt by the mother beginning in the fourth or fifth month. Against great odds, a fetus born prematurely at the end of the second trimester might survive.

Third Trimester The fetus gains most of its birth weight during the last three months. Some of the weight is fatty tissue under the skin that insulates the fetus, supplies food, and gives a baby its characteristic chubbiness. The fetus must obtain large amounts of calcium, iron, and nitrogen from the food the mother eats. Some 85 percent of the calcium and iron she consumes goes into the fetal bloodstream.

Although the fetus may live if it is born during the seventh month, it needs the fat layer acquired in the eighth month and time for the organs, especially the respiratory and digestive organs, to develop. It also needs the immunities that the mother's blood supplies in the last three months. Her blood protects the fetus against all the diseases to which she has acquired immunity. These immunities wear off within six months after birth, but they can be replenished by the mother's milk if the baby is breast fed.

The Importance of Prenatal Care Adequate prenatal care—appropriate diet, exercise, and rest, avoidance of drugs, and regular medical evaluation—is essential to the health of both mother and baby. The pregnant woman cannot help but be responsible for the condition of the baby she carries. Everything she eats, drinks, and does affects the fetus to one degree or another. The baby gets its nutrients and oxygen from the mother's bloodstream and has its wastes removed the same way. Many harmful substances can also be passed on to the baby via the placenta and umbilical cord. For these reasons, taking care of her health during pregnancy is a lifelong investment in her child's health.

Regular Checkups In the woman's first visit to her obstetrician, she will be asked for a detailed medical history of herself and her family. The physician or midwife will note especially any hereditary conditions that may assume increased significance during pregnancy. The tendency to develop gestational diabetes (diabetes during pregnancy only), for example, can be inherited. Appropriate treatment during pregnancy reduces the risk of serious harm from the condition, if it does develop.

The woman is given a complete physical exam and is informed about appropriate diet. She returns for regular checkups throughout the pregnancy, during which her blood pressure and weight gain are measured and tracked and the size and position of the fetus are monitored, among other things. Regular prenatal visits also give the mother a chance to discuss her concerns and to assure herself that everything is proceeding normally. Early advice from physicians, midwives, health educators, and

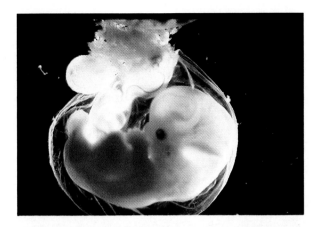

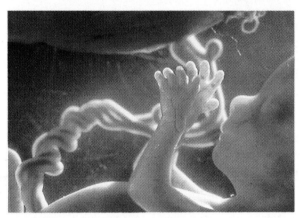

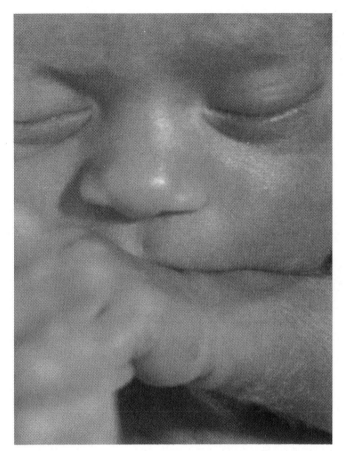

A six-week-old (top left) embryo has simple internal organs, including a beating heart, and is about 1 inch long. By the end of the first trimester, all the major body structures are formed, and some systems are functioning. By the fourth month, the fetus (bottom left) is growing rapidly and is about 10 inches long. Weighing about 6 ounces, it moves vigorously in the uterus and can suck, frown, and turn its head. At seven months, the fetus (right) weighs about 3 pounds and has grown to about 15 inches. Although it can now survive if born prematurely, it needs two more months in the womb to gain weight and acquire a layer of fat.

teachers of childbirth classes provides the mother with invaluable information.

■ Exploring Your Emotions

When you imagine having a baby, do you ever consider the possibility of having a child with a mental or physical disability, such as Down's syndrome or deafness? What do you think your reactions would be? Do you consider the possibility of having to have a cesarean delivery?

Blood Tests   A blood sample is taken during the initial prenatal visit to reveal blood type, anemia, and Rh incompatibilities. The Rh factor is a protein found in the blood. If an Rh-positive father and an Rh-negative mother conceive an Rh-positive baby, the baby's blood will be incompatible with the mother's. If some of the baby's blood enters the mother's bloodstream during delivery, she will develop antibodies to it just as she would toward

a virus. If she has subsequent Rh-positive babies, the antibodies in the mother's blood, passing through the placenta, will destroy the fetus's red blood cells, possibly leading to jaundice, anemia, mental retardation, or death. This condition is completely treatable with a serum called Rh immune globulin, which destroys Rh-positive cells as they enter the mother's body and prevents her from forming antibodies to them. (Blood tests can also reveal the presence of some sexually transmissible diseases, discussed later in the chapter.)

Prenatal Nutrition   An appropriate diet throughout pregnancy is essential for both the baby and the mother. Not only does the baby get all its nutrients from the mother, it also competes with her for nutrients not sufficiently available to meet both their needs. When a woman's diet is low in iron or calcium, the baby receives most of it and the mother may become deficient in it. To meet the increased nutritional demands of her body, a pregnant woman shouldn't just eat more; she should make sure that her diet is adequate in all the basic nutritional categories. In the second and third trimesters, requirements increase for kcalories and most nutrients, including protein, calcium, the B vitamins, vitamins A, C, D, and E, iodine, iron, magnesium, and zinc. With the possible exception of iron, for which some authorities recommend a supplement, all these nutrients can be obtained from a sensible, varied diet designed for a healthy pregnancy. Table 8-1 provides nutritional guidelines for pregnancy.

Avoiding Drugs   In addition to the food the mother eats, the drugs she takes and the chemicals she is exposed to affect the fetus. Some experts believe that everything the mother ingests eventually reaches the fetus. Some drugs—such as cold medicine or cough syrup—harm the fetus but not the mother because the fetus is in the process of developing and because the proper dose for the mother represents a massive dose for the fetus.

During the first trimester, when basic body structures are rapidly forming, the fetus is extremely vulnerable to environmental factors such as viral infections, radiation, drugs, and other **teratogens**, any of which can cause **congenital malformations** (birth defects). The most susceptible body parts are those growing most rapidly at the time of exposure. The rubella (German measles) virus, for example, can cause a congenital malformation of a delicate system such as the eyes or ears, leading to blindness or deafness if exposure occurs during the first trimester, but does no damage later in the pregnancy. Similarly, the tranquilizer thalidomide taken early in pregnancy prevented the formation of arms and legs in fetuses, but taken later, when limbs were already formed, it caused no damage. Other drugs can cause damage throughout prenatal development.

Currently, there is an alarming increase in the number of babies born who were exposed during the prenatal period to damaging psychoactive drugs, most notably cocaine. Babies exposed to cocaine are likely to be born prematurely and to have malformed hearts and skulls. They tend to be extremely irritable, ultrasensitive to noise and touch, difficult to comfort or console, and unable to respond normally to the people who care for them. Because these early problems affect every area of functioning, including social, emotional, language, and intellectual development, only time will tell how extensive the damage from prenatal exposure to cocaine will be.

An even more prevalent problem is prenatal exposure to alcohol, another teratogen. High levels of alcohol con-

sumption during pregnancy are associated with mental retardation, low birth weight, abnormal smallness of the head, and distinctive facial features. Babies with this pattern of characteristics suffer from fetal alcohol syndrome (FAS). Although occasional or moderate drinking was earlier thought to have no negative effects on the fetus, researchers now doubt that any level of alcohol consumption is safe, and they recommend total abstinence during pregnancy.

Cigarette smoking is associated with several adverse conditions in newborns, including low birth weight. Researchers have observed that fetal breathing and movement become more rapid and agitated when the level of nicotine in the mother's bloodstream is high. A direct cause-and-effect relationship is difficult to establish between cigarette smoking and problems at birth, but infants whose parents smoke are unusually susceptible to pneumonia and bronchitis during their first year. Since no benefits for either the mother or the fetus come from smoking, many mothers stop smoking during pregnancy. Other agents and conditions known to affect prenatal development are shown in Table 8-2.

Infections are another serious problem for the fetus, contracted either during or before birth. The four most serious infections are the sexually transmissible diseases syphilis, gonorrhea, herpes simplex, and AIDS. Syphilis can infect and kill a fetus; if the baby is born alive, it will have syphilis. Penicillin given to the mother during pregnancy cures syphilis in both mother and fetus. Gonorrhea can infect the baby during delivery and cause blindness. In many states, newborns' eyes are routinely treated with silver nitrate or another antibiotic to destroy gonorrheal bacteria. Herpes simplex can also be transmitted to the baby during delivery if the mother's infection is in the active phase. If this is the case, the baby is delivered by cesarean section. Herpes can damage the baby's eyes and brain, and no cure has yet been discovered for it.

Currently, the most serious infection a newborn can contract is AIDS, when the AIDS virus crosses the placenta from an infected mother. The babies most at risk for this fatal disease are those whose mothers are intravenous (IV) drug abusers or the sexual partners of IV drug abusers. There is no cure, and the baby usually dies before the age of 2. Physicians now recommend that all women at risk for AIDS have a blood test before becoming pregnant.

Prenatal Activity and Exercise   Physical activity during pregnancy contributes to mental and physical well-being.

Congenital malformation   A physical defect existing at the time of birth, either inherited or caused during gestation.

Teratogen   An agent or influence that causes physical defects in a developing embryo.

Table 8-1 Nutritional guidelines for pregnancy

Food Group	Nutrients Provided	Daily Requirements	Sources and Equivalents
Milk and milk products	Calcium, protein, vitamins, minerals, kcalories	4 servings	1 serving = 1 C milk, yogurt, custard, or milk pudding 1½ oz. cheddar-type cheese 1½ C cottage cheese
Meat and other protein sources	Protein, minerals, vitamins, kcalories	3 servings, 2–3 oz. each	1 3 oz. serving = 1 chicken leg ½ chicken breast 1 lean hamburger 1 medium pork chop 1 small fish fillet ½ serving = 3 T peanut butter 2 oz. cheddar-type cheese ¾ C cooked dried beans, chickpeas, or lentils ¾ C cottage cheese 1 C tofu 4 T sunflower seeds 1½ C yogurt 2 eggs
Fruit and vegetables	Vitamins C and A, other vitamins and minerals, fiber, kcalories	1 serving vitamin C source every day, 1 serving vitamin A source every other day + 2–3 additional servings (4 servings total)	Vitamin C sources: broccoli, brussel sprouts, cabbage, cantaloupe, cauliflower, citrus fruits, bell pepper, spinach, strawberries, potatoes, tomatoes Vitamin A sources: dried apricots, cantaloupe, carrots, squash, sweet potatoes, leafy green vegetables, broccoli, cabbage, pumpkin
Enriched or whole-grain breads and cereals	Protein, iron, B vitamins, other vitamins and minerals, kcalories	4–5 servings	1 serving = 1 slice bread ½ bagel or English muffin 1 biscuit or dinner roll ½ C cooked cereal ½– ¾ C dry cereal 5–7 crackers ½ C cooked macaroni, noodles, or spaghetti 1 tortilla 1 pancake ½ C cooked rice
Fats and sweets	kcalories	No specific recommendations beyond nonpregnant requirement of 1 T polyunsaturated fat per day	These fat sources all have about 45 kcalories: 1 t butter or margarine 1 slice bacon 2 T half and half 1½ T sour cream 1 T cream cheese 1 t salad oil 1 t mayonnaise 1 T French dressing ⅛ avocado 6 small nuts

Sources: Ellen Satter. 1986. *Child of Mine* (Palo Alto, Calif.: Bull Publishing); Mike Samuels and Nancy Samuels. 1979. *The Well Baby Book* (New York: Summit Books); Laurel Robertson, Carol Flinders, and Bronwen Godfrey. 1976. *Laurel's Kitchen* (Petaluma, Calif.: Nilgiri Press).

Table 8-2 Environment Factors Associated with Impairments during Prenatal Development

Agent or Condition	Effects
Rubella (German measles)	Blindness; deafness; heart abnormalities stillbirth
Cytomegalovirus (CMV)	Microcephaly (smaller than normal head); motor disabilities; hearing loss
Syphilis	Mental retardation; physical deformities; in utero death and miscarriage
AIDS virus	Death, often within two years of birth
Addictive drugs	Low birthweight; possible addiction of infant to the drug; hypersensitivity to stimuli; higher risk for stroke and respiratory distress
Smoking	Prematurity; low birthweight and length
Alcohol	Mental retardation; growth retardation; increased spontaneous abortion rate; microcephaly; structural abnormalities in the face; lowered IQ
Irradiation	Physical deformities; mental retardation
Inadequate diet	Reduction in brain growth; smaller than average birthweight; decrease in birth length; rickets
Tetracycline	Discoloration of teeth
Streptomycin	Eighth cranial nerve damage (hearing loss)
Quinine	Deafness
Barbiturates	Congenital malformations
DES (diethylstilbestrol)	Increased incidence of vaginal cancer in adolescent female offspring; impaired reproductive performance in same population
Valium	Cleft lip and palate
Accutane (13-cis-retinoic acid, a new drug used to treat acne)	Small or absent ears; small jaws; hydrocephaly; heart defects
Endocrine disorders	Cretinism; microcephaly
Maternal age under 18	Prematurity; stillbirth; increased incidence of Down's syndrome
Maternal age over 35	Increased incidence of Down's syndrome
Malnutrition	Lower birthweight; abnormal reflexes and irritability; altered brain growth
Environmental chemicals (e.g., benzene, formaldehyde, PCBs, etc.)	Chromosome damage; spontaneous abortions; low birthweight

Source: Judith Schickedanz, Karen Hansen, and Peggy Forsyth. 1990, *Understanding Children*. (Mountain View, Calif.: Mayfield), p. 100.

Many women continue working at their jobs until late in their pregnancies, provided the work isn't so physically demanding that it jeopardizes their health. At the same time, pregnant women need more rest and sleep. They become fatigued more easily because the energy demands on their bodies are so great. They need adequate rest and sleep to maintain their own and the fetus's well-being.

The prospective mother can and should continue all reasonable exercising that she is accustomed to, such as tennis, swimming, low-impact aerobics, gardening, or dancing, unless or until her pregnancy inhibits movement. The amniotic sac protects the fetus so that normal activities will not harm it. More strenuous activities that could result in a fall, such as skiing, skating, or horseback riding, are best delayed until after the birth. A pregnant woman who hasn't been exercising and wants to start should first consult with her physician.

Prenatal exercise classes are valuable because they teach exercises that tone the body muscles involved in birth, especially those of the abdomen, back, and legs. Toned-up muscles aid delivery and help the body regain its nonpregnant shape afterward. A program of prenatal exercises is illustrated in the box "Exercises for Pregnancy and Birth."

Preparing for Birth   As hospital childbirth practices have been increasingly challenged over the last 20 years, many women have chosen to learn techniques in childbirth preparation classes that help them deal with the discomfort of labor and delivery without pain-relieving drugs. One method of **prepared childbirth** was developed by Dr. Grantly Dick-Read, an English physician. Dick-Read believed that the pain experienced by women during birth results from learned fears that interfere, through tension, with the birth process.

To dispel these fears, childbirth educators teach parents the details of the birth process as well as relaxation techniques to use during labor and birth. Several similar methods of childbirth training are used now, including the Bradley method and the Lamaze method, all designed to ease birth through knowledge, relaxation, and physical conditioning. Most hospitals and childbirth educators tend to instruct parents in a combination of Lamaze and other relaxation techniques.

Childbirth classes are almost a routine part of the prenatal experience for both mothers and fathers these days. The mother learns and practices a variety of techniques so she can choose what works best for her during labor.

The father typically acts as a coach, supporting the mother emotionally and helping her with her breathing and relaxing. He remains with the mother throughout labor and delivery, even when a cesarean section is performed. It can be an important and fulfilling time for the parents to be together.

Childbirth

By the end of the ninth month of pregnancy, most women are tired of being pregnant; both mother and father are impatient to start a new phase of their lives. Because prepared childbirth classes are now so widespread, most couples find the actual process of birth to be an exciting and positive experience.

Labor and Delivery   The birth process occurs in three stages (see Figure 8-5). Labor starts when hormonal changes in both the mother and the baby cause strong, rhythmic uterine **contractions** to begin. These contractions exert pressure on the cervix, the neck of the uterus, causing it gradually to pull back and open, or dilate (a process known as effacement). The contractions also pressure the baby to descend into the mother's pelvis, if it hasn't already.

This first stage of labor averages about 13 hours for a first birth, although there is wide variation among women. Contractions usually last about 30 seconds and come every 15 to 20 minutes at first, more often later. The prepared mother relaxes as much as possible during these contractions to allow labor to proceed without being blocked by tension. In some women, the amniotic sac ruptures and the fluid rushes out. This speeds up labor and usually indicates that the second stage is about to begin. If the sac doesn't rupture, the attendant often ruptures it to shorten labor.

When the cervix is completely dilated, the second stage of birth, referred to as expulsion, begins. The baby is slowly pushed down, through the bones of the pelvic ring, past the cervix, and into the vagina, which it stretches open. The mother bears down with the contractions to help push the baby down and out. The baby's back bends, the head turns to fit through the narrowest parts of the passageway, and the soft bones of the baby's skull actually move together and overlap as it's squeezed

---

Prepared childbirth   Preparation for birth that includes physical conditioning, instruction in the process of birth and what to expect, and psychological and emotional conditioning so that fear and anxiety are kept to a minimum, making childbirth as pain-free as possible. It can include but does not require labor and delivery without drugs.

Contraction   (uterine) A shortening of the uterus that reduces its size and eventually expels the fetus.

Exercises for Pregnancy and Birth

The following series of twelve exercises takes about fifteen to twenty minutes to perform. You can do them daily, if you wish.

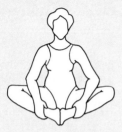

1. Groin stretch (helps make the delivery position more comfortable)

Start by holding your ankles with the soles of your feet touching each other. Lean forward and press your knees down with your elbows, feeling a gentle stretch in your groin and inner thighs. Hold the position for ten to thirty seconds. Repeat three times.

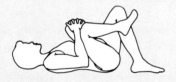

2. Single knee tuck (stretches lower back to help prevent or reduce back pain)

Start on your back with knees bent and the soles of your feet flat. Bring one knee to your chest, feeling a gentle stretch of the lower back. Relax the lower back as you hold for ten seconds. Switch knees and repeat the entire cycle three times.

3. Double knee tuck (stretches lower back to help reduce low-back pain)

See illustration for single knee tuck, above. Start on your back with knees bent and soles flat. Grip both knees and bring your knees to your chest. Keep the back relaxed as you hold the gentle stretch for three to ten seconds. Repeat three times.

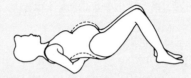

4. Pelvic tilting on back (to strengthen the abdominal muscles)

Start on your back with knees bent. Place one hand in the hollow of your back, the other on the rim of the hip. Slowly tighten the abdominal and buttock muscles by pushing down on your hand with the small of your back. Rock the baby back into the pelvic cradle as you roll your hips back gently. Breathe out as you contract the abdominal muscles. Hold the contraction for three to six seconds and then relax as you breathe in. Keep your back flat throughout. Repeat three to five times.

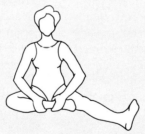

5. Hamstring stretch (to stretch the hamstring muscles)

Start with one leg straight, the other tucked in. Reach for the ankle of the extended leg, feeling the gentle stretch of the muscles in the back of the thigh. Hold the stretch for ten to thirty seconds. Switch legs and repeat the entire cycle three times.

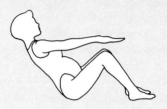

6. Sit-back (for abdominal strength and endurance)

Start in an upright sitting position. Reach forward with your arms and sit back to a 45° angle. Hold the V-like position for three to six seconds. Repeat three times.

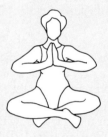

7. Chest push (for strength and endurance of the chest muscles)

Start with your elbows bent and palms together. Press your palms firmly together so that you can feel the tightening of the pectoral muscles under the breasts. Hold the press for three to six seconds. Repeat three times.

Exercises for Pregnancy and Birth (continued)

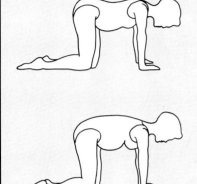

8. Pelvic tilting on all fours (to strengthen abdominal muscles)
Start in a kneeling position with your arms extended for support. Pull your back and pelvis up into a catlike position. Hold for three to six seconds and relax to the starting position, but never let your spine sag. Repeat three times.

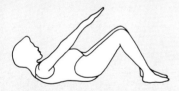

9. Modified sit-up (to strengthen abdominal muscles)
Start flat on your back with knees bent. Tilt your pelvis up, flattening your back. Extend your arms and slowly curl up. Tuck your chin in and come up one vertebra at a time as you lift your head first and then your shoulders. Stop when you can see your heels and hold for three to six seconds before returning to the starting position. Repeat three times.
Don't do this exercise if your abdominal muscles have separated (come to a point).

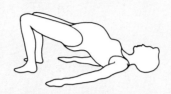

10. Back arch (to strengthen lower back muscles)
Start on your back with knees bent and arms flat alongside. Do a pelvic tilt and then lift your tailbone, buttocks, and lower back from the floor. Hold this position for three to six seconds with your weight resting on your feet, arms, and shoulders. Return to starting position and repeat three times.

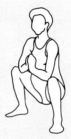

11. Squat (to strengthen thigh and hip muscles)
If you have no knee problems, start with your feet flat on the floor, squatting halfway down. Hold for three to six seconds, then stand up. Eventually go into full squat. If necessary, have a partner hold your hands to assist with balance. Repeat three times. If you have knee problems, limit movement to half squat.

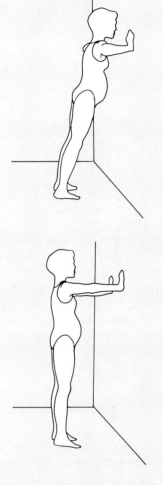

12. Wall push-away (for strength and endurance of the arms and shoulders and for flexibility of the Achilles tendon)
Start supporting yourself with your arms extended against the wall. Bend your arms, allowing your head and upper body to slowly come toward the wall. Hold this position for ten seconds so that you can feel the stretch of your calves and Achilles tendon. Push away slowly to starting position. Repeat three times.

Source: Ivan Kusinitz and Morton Fine, 1987. *Your Guide to Getting Fit* (Mountain View, Calif.: Mayfield), pp. 209–212.

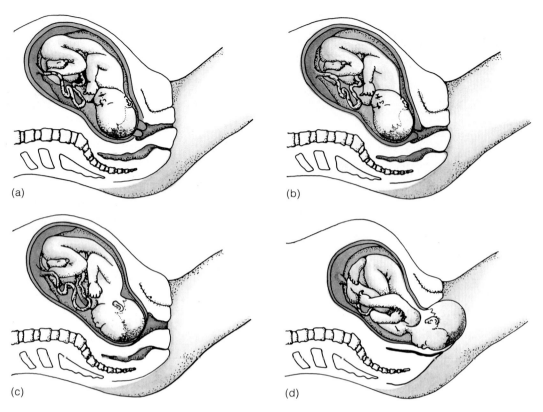

Figure 8-5 The birth process: (a) full-term fetus before labor begins; (b) early stages of labor; cervix begins to dilate; (c) second stage of labor; cervix completely dilated; baby's head begins turning toward mother's back; (d) late stage of labor; baby's head is completely turned; head begins to emerge.

Table 8-3 The Apgar Scale

Criterion	Score		
	0	1	2
Color	Blue, pale	Body pink; extremities blue	All pink
Heart rate	Absent	Less than 100	Greater than 100
Respiration	Absent	Irregular, slow	Breathing and crying
Reflex irritability	No response	Weak (grimace)	Vigorous (sneeze, cough)
Muscle tone	Completely flaccid	Limp, some flexion of extremities	Active, resilient

through the pelvis. When the top of the head appears at the vaginal opening, the baby is said to be crowning. The baby's head emerges and then, with the next push, the body. Many attendants now routinely place the baby on the mother's abdomen immediately following birth. A variety of conditions can lead to birth by cesarean section, the delivery of the baby through an incision in the mother's abdominal wall. This procedure is discussed in the box entitled "Cesarean Births—Why Are They Increasing?"

The third stage of labor, known as afterbirth, is the delivery of the placenta. This usually occurs within 10 to 20 minutes of the baby's birth and is accomplished with a few strong uterine contractions. In the meantime, the attendant ties and cuts the umbilical cord, and the baby takes its first breath and cries. This first breath

Cesarean Births—Why Are They Increasing?

The number of cesarean deliveries performed in the United States has risen dramatically in recent years, causing concern among parents and medical personnel alike. What are the facts behind the controversy? Why are babies delivered by cesarean section, and why is the number of such operations increasing?

Cesarean sections are performed when a baby can't be delivered vaginally. Sometimes a mother's pelvis isn't big enough for the baby's head to pass through during birth. Sometimes the baby is in a feet-down or buttocks-down position in the uterus rather than in the usual head-down position, or even lying sideways across the uterus, all of which make vaginal birth difficult. Mothers with diabetes, high blood pressure, kidney or heart disease, or toxemia often deliver their babies by cesarean section to reduce the stress on their bodies.

Sometimes a woman is unable to sustain labor. Contractions slow down or stop, and the cervix shows no progressing dilation. After 24 hours, physicians usually perform a cesarean section. This reduces the risk of infection to the newborn, which can be high once the protective membranes have ruptured. In the past, cesareans were also performed when women had previously had cesarean births. Physicians believed that the pressure of labor and vaginal delivery on the uterine wall would rupture the old incision. This has not proven to be true, and many women now have vaginal births after cesarean births.

Cesarean sections are major surgery and carry some risk themselves, although much less than 15 or 20 years ago. Better antibiotics and refined understanding and use of anesthesia make the procedure relatively safe. Women now are often given a local anesthetic and remain conscious during the whole operation. The father can be in the operating room if the mother is given a local anesthetic.

Between 1965 and 1980 cesarean deliveries increased from 5 percent to 15 percent of all births in the United States. By 1987 the nationwide cesarean rate was reported to be 24 percent, with even higher rates in some states. The hospitals with very high cesarean rates are usually university hospitals, where many more high-risk pregnancies are handled than in the average community hospital.

One reason for higher cesarean rates is that hospitals now have more sophisticated techniques for detecting fetal distress. Fetal monitoring, for example, can reveal a slowed fetal heart rate due to inadequate oxygen during labor, possibly leading to a decision for cesarean section. Advocates of increased reliance on cesareans claim that the procedure makes birth safer for mothers and babies in a situation where prolonged, stressful labor is the alternative. They point to reduced maternal and neonatal mortality rates and the better health of newborns (fewer babies are born with brain damage from labor and delivery trauma).

Critics of the increased reliance on cesarean deliveries, including many physicians and surgeons, believe that cesareans are often performed unnecessarily and that labor isn't well managed by medical personnel in this country. They claim that not all relevant staff members, for example, can accurately interpret signs of fetal distress. They suggest that cesarean sections are frequently performed more for the convenience of the physician than for the mother's or baby's health. Until physicians can document the need for a cesarean in each and every case, and until the public becomes more aware of the benefits of this procedure for some mothers and babies, this debate is likely to continue.

Adapted from Judith Schickedanz, Karen Hansen, and Peggy Forsyth. 1990. *Understanding Children* (Mountain View, Calif.: Mayfield), p. 85.

requires five times as much effort as an ordinary breath because thousands of tiny uninflated air sacs in the lungs must be expanded.

The attendant cleans the baby, weighs it, and assesses its general condition, usually with the **Apgar scale** (see Table 8-3). The baby is scored 0, 1, or 2 for skin color,

Apgar scale   A method for assessing the general condition of the newborn soon after birth.

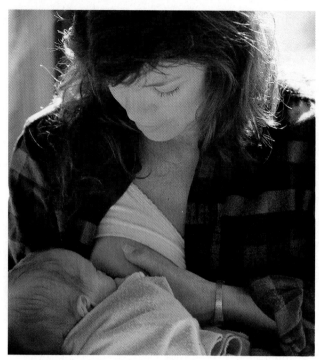

Breastfeeding is an ideal method of feeding an infant because the mother's milk contains antibodies against disease and is perfectly suited to the baby's nutritional needs. But women who choose bottlefeeding can still experience the physical contact and emotional closeness that are such an important part of the parent-child relationship.

heart rate, respiration, reflex irritability, and muscle tone. A total score of 10 indicates that a baby is in the best possible physical condition. The baby is then usually wrapped tightly in a blanket and returned to the mother, who may begin to nurse the baby right away.

The Puerperium　The **puerperium** is the time after childbirth during which the mother's reproductive organs slowly return to the nonpregnant state, usually over the course of six or eight weeks. Following a vaginal delivery, mothers usually leave the hospital within one to three days; following a cesarean section, they usually stay longer. Many women experience fluctuating emotions during the puerperium as hormone levels change. A few experience some **postpartum depression**, and of these, a small number experience depression serious enough to warrant hospitalization. Postpartum depression can be treated successfully.

When a mother doesn't nurse, menstrual periods usually return within about ten weeks. Breastfeeding can prevent the return of menstruation for as long as six months. The hormone prolactin, which aids milk production, suppresses hormones vital to the development of mature eggs. However, ovulation—and pregnancy—can occur before menstruation returns, so breastfeeding is not a contraceptive method. If the mother becomes pregnant while still nursing, she should stop nursing to ensure good nutrition for the unborn child.

Parenting

A great deal of time, energy, and effort is put into educating parents-to-be about prenatal care and childbirth these days, but comparatively little is spent directly educating parents about caring for their children after birth and over the long term. Many parents leave the hospital knowing only how to feed and diaper their baby, if that. They learn nearly everything else on the job, usually by trial and error. Most parents use their own parents as models of how to raise children, unless they make a conscious effort to do otherwise.

■ Exploring Your Emotions

Did your parents enjoy having children? What did they do in bringing you up that you liked and would repeat with your own children? What did you not like? If you think they made mistakes, what would you do differently?

This chapter can't begin to address the complex issues involved in parenting, but a few points can be made. Besides providing a safe and healthy physical environment for the child, the parents' mission is to help the child develop into an independent, responsible, competent human being. Parents have to teach and show by example the values and qualities that they want their children to have as they grow into adults. They do this best by treating them with love and respect, by disciplining—that is, teaching—them appropriately, by communicating honestly with them, and by giving them their time and attention. All these actions and attitudes create feelings of positive self-worth in the child.

Puerperium　The period of about six to eight weeks after labor during which the mother's reproductive organs, particularly the uterus, return to the nonpregnant state.

Postpartum depression　An emotional low experienced by the mother following childbirth; infrequently intensifies until medical attention is necessary.

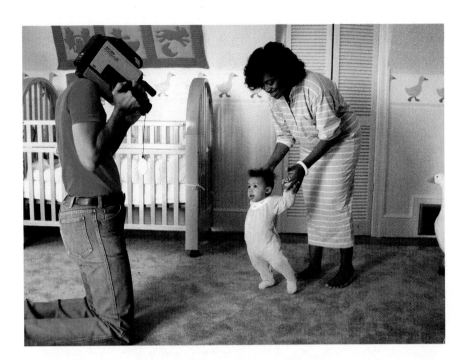

Good parenting isn't automatic; people have to work at it. New parents like this couple learn how to nurture their baby by observing friends, reading, taking classes, and just trying things out to see if they work.

A crucial factor in the early parent-child relationship is attachment—the strong emotional tie that develops between the baby and the adult who cares for the baby, usually the mother. Research in child development has demonstrated that a secure early attachment relationship helps the child to develop and function well socially, emotionally, and intellectually. An insecure or anxious attachment relationship is consistently associated with later problems, including aggressive, hostile, or harassing behavior, withdrawal or fearfulness, and low self-esteem.

Parents foster secure attachment relationships in the earliest weeks and months by responding sensitively to the baby's true needs. Parents who respond appropriately to the baby's signals of gazing, looking away, smiling, and crying establish feelings of trust and effectiveness in their child. They feed the baby when it's hungry, for example; respond when it cries; interact with it when it gazes, smiles, or babbles; and stop stimulating it when it frowns or looks away. Parents of anxiously attached babies tend to misread or ignore their babies' signals, responding inappropriately or not at all. In cases where the attachment relationship is severely disrupted, the result may be child abuse. (The box entitled "Child Abuse" gives more information on causes and possible solutions to this problem.)

■ **Exploring Your Emotions**

Have you thought about how your life would change if or when you have a baby? What would you be willing or unwilling to give up? What do you think the gains would be?

Parents can learn to respond sensitively to their babies, and they can learn other good parenting techniques as well. Parenting well doesn't come automatically; good parents work at it and evolve. They learn what to expect from their children and themselves by observing other children and parents, comparing ideas and experiences with other parents, reading about child development and behavior, and taking classes on parenting.

Parents at home with young babies may socialize informally or in classes (such as "baby gym" classes) with other parents and babies. Later, they may observe their children at day care or preschool and gain insights into parenting by talking with experienced teachers (see the box entitled "Choosing the Best Child Care"). Sometimes pediatricians can solve puzzles or provide just the right advice. Parents may be motivated to examine their own backgrounds and childhoods to discover what they liked and want to repeat and what they disliked and want to discard. If they feel they need more help than they're getting with parenting, they may join support groups or seek counseling or family therapy.

Education and information about pregnancy and childbirth reduce pain and increase satisfaction with those important events. The same is true of parenting, except that parenting goes on for years and is continually evolving. Parents no sooner learn how to cope with a toddler than they have a preschooler, no sooner understand their child than they have an adolescent or a young adult. Perhaps the best qualification for parenting in the long run is the willingness to change, to adapt, to learn, and most of all to accept the person the child turns out to be.

Child Abuse

Statistics suggest that about 1 million children, most of them under the age of 3, are maltreated by their parents or other caregiving adults every year. Most fatalities occur in the newborn to 1-year-old age group. What causes adults to physically, emotionally, or sexually abuse their children or neglect them to the point of harm? Studies show that most child battering is done by apparently "normal" people in a critical period. Generally, abusive parents, overwhelmed by life circumstances, strike out because of rage, resentment, or sheer ignorance.

Multiple factors may be at work. Some parents begin abusing their children as a reaction to stress and strain caused by family troubles such as marital discord, financial hardship, or mental illness. Where there is violence within the family, the typical pattern shows the husband hitting the wife and the wife hitting a child. When there is abuse in a family with a number of children, it is likely to be centered on one child. Some children pose more stress to parents and are more vulnerable to beatings or other abuse: premature or low-birth-weight babies, children who are colicky, those who are more difficult to toilet train, and physically handicapped or mentally retarded children.

Incidents of abuse and neglect often happen in families that are socially isolated, without continuing relationships with friends or sympathetic relatives. There are also parents who lack understanding of a child's physical, emotional, and psychological needs, who ignore a child's crying, or who react with impatience. Maltreatment has also been traced to compulsive disciplinarians who live by the dictum "spare the rod and spoil the child." Many abusive parents were themselves beaten as children and they repeat the cycle. Some child advocates find an entrenched pattern of violent child-rearing in our country. And abuse begets abuse.

What can be done to help abused children and abusive parents? Child welfare experts estimate that four out of five abusive families can be helped with proper treatment. Two kinds of treatment are important. One is the telephone hotline, providing support, reassurance, and information twenty-four hours a day, seven days a week, for parents who have reached the end of their rope. The other is long-term therapy, which can help parents come to terms with their own histories and learn how to love and care for their children. Abused children may be removed from the home and placed in foster care while both they and their parents receive therapy, but in most cases the goal is to reunify the family.

What can you do if you suspect that a family you know is abusive? The best approach is to contact a community agency by looking in the yellow pages of the telephone book. Look under "Family Services," "Family Stress Center," or "Parental Stress Hotline." Explain your concerns and ask for advice. If you would like more information about child abuse, you can contact one of the following agencies:

- The American Humane Association is a national federation of individuals and agencies working toward prevention of abuse and exploitation of children. For information, write American Humane Association, Child Protection, 9725 E. Hampden, Denver, Colorado 80231.
- The Child Welfare League of America is the national standard-setting organization for public and voluntary child welfare agencies in the United States and Canada. Their address is 67 Irvine Place, New York, New York 10003.
- The National Center on Child Abuse and Neglect (NCCAN) serves as the focal point for federal activities related to child abuse and neglect. For information, including the resource center in your area, write to: National Center on Child Abuse and Neglect, P.O. Box 1182, Washington, D.C. 20013.
- The National Committee for Prevention of Child Abuse is a volunteer network dedicated to involving citizens in actively preventing child abuse. For information, write to The National Committee for Prevention of Child Abuse, 332 S. Michigan Avenue, Suite 1250, Chicago, Illinois 60604.
- Parents Anonymous is a nationwide organization with local chapters where groups of parents meet with the aim of changing their behavior by understanding and rechanneling destructive attitudes and actions. For information, write Parents Anonymous, 22330 Hawthorne Blvd., Suite 208, Torrance, California 90505.

Adapted from "To Combat and Prevent Child Abuse and Neglect," Theodore Irwin, Public Affairs Pamphlet #588. Copyright © 1980 by the Public Affairs Committee, Inc. Used by permission.

Choosing the Best Child Care

With the number of working mothers and two-career families on the rise, finding acceptable child care is rapidly becoming the most difficult and worrisome aspect of child rearing in the United States today. The U.S. Census Bureau estimated in 1987 that 26.5 million children aged 14 and under (out of 52 million such children) were cared for during some part of the day by adults other than their parents. The youngest children—infants, toddlers, and preschoolers— present the biggest problem for parents. What are the best choices for them, and what criteria can they use to evaluate facilities and caregivers?

The best choice, but also the most expensive, is having a qualified person come into the home— a nanny. Being cared for in the home means less disruption for the child and more control for the parent, who can screen candidates, get references, and select a person who interacts well with the child. Additionally, if the child is sick, the parent can still go to work. The next best option is a neighborhood day care home in which a well-trained and credentialed individual takes in three or four children. When considering this option, parents should inquire why the woman takes children into her home (often it's so she can be at home with her own child), observe how she deals with the children, and evaluate the home (see the list of guidelines).

The third and most common option, and the one over which parents have the least control, is the day care center. Before enrolling their child in a day care center, parents should assure themselves that it provides a safe, healthy, nurturing environment that supports play and fosters learning. The following are guidelines they can use in their evaluation:

Safety is a prime consideration for infant and toddler facilities. Does this day care center provide a safe environment? For example,

- Are electrical outlets covered?
- Are heaters out of reach?
- Are drapery cords removed or tied up?
- Is furniture stable, in good repair, and in compliance with consumer protection safety standards?
- Are all medicines and cleaning supplies well out of reach of children?
- Is there a fire evacuation plan? Are fire extinguishers and first aid equipment available?
- Do the personnel know infant CPR and first aid?
- Are children well supervised?

Health is also a prime consideration. Does this day care center provide a healthy environment? For example,

- Is the facility clean?
- Do caregivers wash their hands frequently, using dispenser soap and paper towels, especially before preparing food and after changing diapers?
- Do they wash the children's hands regularly, especially before eating?
- Are toys cleaned daily?
- Is the diapering area cleaned after each change?
- Is food prepared properly and dishes washed with hot water?
- Are the children well, or are sick children present?

- Are all children up to date on their immunizations?

Learning and playing are what children do. Does this day care facility provide a stimulating, challenging environment that promotes exploration and allows hands-on experiences? For example,

- Is there a variety of toys and materials from which the children can choose? Are toys age-appropriate?
- Is there open space that encourages movement and private space where children can be alone?
- Is there a lot of color?
- Are there cubbies for children's personal belongings and comfortable areas for relaxing and resting?
- Are there large, low windows (made of safety glass)?
- Are toys and furniture the right size for children?
- Is the environment fairly orderly, and can the noise level be controlled when necessary (for example, when some children are sleeping)?
- Are there places for sand and water play?
- Outdoors, are there areas with grass and sand? Is there a place to play on riding toys? Is equipment safe and age-appropriate?

The **qualities of the caregivers** themselves are of prime importance. Do they provide nurturing care and support for children's social, emotional, and intellectual development? For example,

- Is there one adult for every three or four babies under 1 year of age?

Choosing the Best Child Care (continued)

- Is there one adult for every four or five toddlers?
- Are caregivers well trained?
- Do they respect children, no matter how young?
- Do they support positive self-images for all the children? Do they encourage cultural identification?
- Do they treat boys and girls the same?
- Do they demonstrate good judgment, humor, and a commitment to children?
- Can they communicate with parents and regard them as partners? Do they listen?

- Do they demonstrate an understanding of appropriate behavior at different stages of child development?
- What is their approach to resolving problems? Are there a lot of rules, or are children helped to work things out themselves?
- What is the daily schedule like? Do the children have free time to spend as they wish?

A careful inspection and evaluation of the day care center, both indoors and out, and an interview with the people who will actually be caring

for the child are essential if parents are going to be satisfied with their choice. Finding the best affordable child care goes a long way toward resolving the conflict working parents inevitably feel. It also helps them relax and enjoy their children when they're with them, knowing they're well cared for the rest of the time.

Sources: Janet Gonzalez-Mena and Dianne Widmeyer Eyer. 1989. *Infants, Toddlers, and Caregivers* (Mountain View, Calif.: Mayfield); Eleanor Reynolds. 1990. *Guiding Young Children* (Mountain View, Calif.: Mayfield).

Summary

- Today it's possible to choose whether, when, and how to have a child; it's also possible to make choices in young adulthood that will help keep all options open for the day one is ready to have a child.

Preparation for Parenthood

- Factors to consider when deciding if and when to have a child include (1) physical health and age, (2) financial circumstances, (3) relationship with partner, (4) educational, career, and child care plans, (5) emotional readiness for parenthood, (6) social support system, (7) personal qualities, attitudes toward children, and aptitude for parenting, and (8) philosophical beliefs.
- Risks are high for teenagers, who are still growing themselves and often can't afford prenatal care, and for women over 35, who have a higher incidence of babies with Down's syndrome.
- Once a woman is pregnant, she and her partner need to decide on a health practitioner and environment for birth.
- Prenatal tests, including amniocentesis, ultrasound, and chorionic villus sampling, provide information about sex, size, and genetic abnormalities.

- Breastfeeding provides a food suited to the baby's nutritional needs and digestive capacities; human milk supplies the baby with antibodies against diseases. Bottlefeeding can also be a part of a loving parent-child relationship.
- The wider variety of choices available to prospective parents has ironically sometimes led to adoption of rigid, narrow viewpoints, where new childbirth practices are advocated to the exclusion of all others. Positive outcomes are most likely if the parents choose what feels comfortable to them.
- Fertilization is a complex process culminating when *one* sperm (out of the millions released in one ejaculation) penetrates the membrane of the one egg released in a month.
- Home pregnancy tests detect the presence of human chorionic gonadotropin in urine; their 85–95 percent reliability rate is not as good as that of tests analyzed in a medical laboratory.
- Infertility probably affects 15–20 percent of all couples in the United States. Surgery and drugs can cure some problems, and more advanced techniques include in vitro fertilization and artificial insemination.

- One way to avoid some forms of infertility is to protect oneself against STDs and to get treatment for any diseases contracted.

Pregnancy

- Pregnancy is usually divided into trimesters based on fetal development; the third trimester is most difficult for the mother because of increased demands on her system.
- Early signs and symptoms include a missed menstrual period; slight bleeding at the time a period is expected; nausea; and sleepiness, fatigue, and emotional upset.
- Spontaneous abortion can be caused by genetic or physical fetal defects, an abnormal uterus, insufficient progesterone production in the ovaries, or inappropriate maternal immune response to fetal cells.
- An ectopic pregnancy occurs when a fertilized egg attaches itself to the wall of an oviduct instead of the uterus; if the embryo isn't removed, the tube can burst and the mother can die of internal bleeding.
- In pregnancy the uterus enlarges until it pushes up into the rib cage, the breasts enlarge and secrete colostrum, the muscles and ligaments soften and stretch, and the circulatory system and lungs become more efficient, as do the kidneys.
- Women usually gain an average of 24 to 28 pounds in pregnancy, with the baby accounting for about 7.5 pounds.
- Pregnancy sometimes leads to either increased or decreased interest in sexual activity; intercourse throughout pregnancy is possible but often awkward and uncomfortable in later stages. Mood changes are also common throughout pregnancy.
- Preeclampsia is a potentially fatal complication that may develop in later stages; high blood pressure, facial swelling, and protein in the urine are early symptoms of this dangerous condition.
- The fetal anatomy is almost completely formed in the first trimester and is refined in the second; needed fats and pounds are added during the third trimester.
- One week after conception, the cells that have developed from the fertilized egg implant in the uterine wall and become an embryo. Its inner cells immediately develop into three layers, which form body systems, structures, and tissues. Its outer cells become the placenta, umbilical cord, and amniotic sac. By the end of the second month the embryo is a fetus, and its brain coordinates the functioning of other organs.
- In the second trimester all body systems are operating, and the fetal heartbeat can be heard through a stethoscope; the mother feels movement beginning in the fourth or fifth month.
- In the third trimester the fetus gains most of its weight, and the respiratory and digestive systems complete development. The mother's blood supplies immunities to the baby, which last for about six months after birth.
- Medical care during pregnancy involves a complete history and physical at the beginning and regular checkups for blood pressure, weight gain, and size and position of the fetus.
- Blood tests reveal blood type, anemia, STDs, and Rh incompatibilities. If mother and child are Rh incompatible, serum immune globulin is given after birth of the first child to protect later children.
- A pregnant woman needs to make sure her diet is adequate in all basic nutritional categories since she needs sufficient nutrients for the baby and herself. Requirements for kcalories and most nutrients increase in the second and third trimester.
- The drugs a mother takes and chemicals she is exposed to can cause congenital malformations, as can radiation and viral infections. Prenatal exposure to cocaine and alcohol are especially serious problems; all the effects of such exposure are not yet known. Cigarette smoking is associated with low birth weight and respiratory infections during the first year.
- STDs, especially syphilis, gonorrhea, herpes simplex, and AIDS, are dangerous to the fetus. The AIDS virus crosses the placenta, and infected babies usually die before age 2.
- Physical activity during pregnancy contributes to physical and mental well-being; although adequate rest is necessary, the pregnant woman should continue all reasonable exercise, discontinuing only those that could result in a fall.
- In prepared childbirth the parents learn the details of the birth process as well as relaxation techniques; the idea is that by reducing fear and tension, the mother will have less pain and will deal with it better.

Childbirth

- The first stage of labor begins with contractions that exert pressure on the cervix, causing it to pull back and dilate. The baby descends into the mother's pelvis; the amniotic sac ruptures.
- The second stage of labor begins when the cervix is completely dilated. The baby is pushed down into the vagina, and the mother bears down until the baby emerges. Certain conditions can lead to cesarean section, where the baby is delivered through an incision in the mother's abdominal wall.
- The third stage of labor is delivery of the placenta. The umbilical cord is cut, and the baby takes its first breath.
- The puerperium is the time after childbirth when the mother's reproductive system returns to normal; changing hormone levels make postpartum depression a possibility.

Parenting

- Although childbirth education is more and more prevalent, few new parents are educated in how to raise a child.
- The parents' goal is not only to provide a safe and healthy physical environment but also to help a child develop into an independent and responsible person. Teaching by example and creating a feeling of self-worth are essential.
- Attachment between parent and child is crucial to the child's social, emotional, and intellectual development. Paying attention to an infant's needs helps establish feelings of trust and effectiveness.
- It's possible to learn how to be a good parent through observation, discussion, reading, and classes. What's necessary is adaptability, openness, and tolerance.

Take Action

1. Research your family tree to see if there are any genetic diseases that run in your family or ethnic or racial group (such as Tay-Sachs disease or sickle-cell anemia). If you turn up any problems, use the library to discover the latest medical thinking on possible treatments.

2. Interview your parents to find out what your birth was like. What were the cultural conditions like at the time, and what were their personal preferences? Find out as much as you can about hospital procedures, use of anesthesia, length of hospital stay, and so on. Did your father have a role in your birth?

If possible, interview your grandparents or someone of their generation. How was their experience different from your parents'?

3. Investigate the childbirth facilities in your community. If possible, visit the maternity wing of a hospital and an alternative birth center. What do you like about them, and what do you not like?

Selected Bibliography

Eisenberg, Arlene, Heidi Eisenberg Murkoff, and Sandee Eisenberg Hathaway. 1984. *What to Expect When You're Expecting.* New York: Workman.

Feinbloom, Richard I., and Betty Yetta Forman. 1985. *Pregnancy, Birth, and the Early Months.* Menlo Park, Calif.: Addison-Wesley.

Hayes, Cheryl D., ed. 1987. National Research Council: Panel on Adolescent Pregnancy and Childbearing. *Risking the Future: Adolescent Sexuality, Pregnancy, and Childbearing,* Vol. I. Washington, D.C.: National Academy Press.

Scher, Jonathan, and Carol Dix. 1983. *Will My Baby Be Normal: How to Make Sure.* New York: Dial.

Schickedanz, Judith, Karen Hansen, and Peggy Forsyth. 1990. *Understanding Children.* Mountain View, Calif.: Mayfield.

Shapiro, Howard I. 1983. *The Pregnancy Book for Today's Women.* New York: Harper and Row.

Sussman, John R., and B. Blake Levitt. 1988. *Before You Conceive: the Complete Prepregnancy Guide.* New York: Bantam.

Warschaw, Tessa Albert, and Victoria Secunda. 1988. *Winning with Kids: How to Negotiate with Your Baby Bully, Kid Tyrant, Loner, Saint, Underdog or Winner So They Love Themselves and You, Too.* New York: Bantam.

White, Burton L. 1980. *A Parent's Guide to the First Three Years.* Englewood Cliffs, N.J.: Prentice-Hall. A mine of carefully researched advice on child rearing.

Recommended Readings

Bundy, Darcie. 1985. *The Affordable Baby: A complete Consumer Guide to Costs and Comparisons for Parents-To-Be.* New York: Harper and Row.

Gonzalez-Mena, Janet, and Dianne Widmeyer Eyer. 1989. *Infants, Toddlers, and Caregivers.* Mountain View, Calif.: Mayfield. *A practical guide to caring for infants and toddlers, with emphasis on how to provide the best conditions for children's physical, emotional, social, and intellectual development.*

Main, Frank. 1986. *Perfect Parenting and Other Myths.* Minnesota: CompCare Publications. *Realistic guidance in lowering expectations and dealing with the confusion and complexities of family life.*

Reynolds, Eleanor. 1990. *Guiding Young Children.* Mountain View, Calif.:

Mayfield. *A child-centered approach to caring for preschool children, based on a problem-solving philosophy of freedom with responsibility and full of practical techniques and examples.*

Sears, William, M.D. 1982. *Creative Parenting.* New York: Everest House. *From conception through birth to early adolescence, this book deals with all aspects of practical child care.*

Silverman, Marvin, and David A. Lustig. 1987. *Parent Survival Training: A Complete Guide to Modern Parenting.* N. Hollywood, Calif.: Wilshire. *A behavior therapy guide to taking charge of your relationship with your children and to creating a home environment consisting of love, warmth, respect, and minimal conflict.*

Contents

Making Connections

Smoking is hazardous to everyone's health, smoker and nonsmoker alike. This is part of the reason that the tobacco issue is likely to remain a battleground for conflicting rights and opposing interests throughout the 1990s. The scenarios presented on these pages describe situations involving tobacco use in which people have to use information, make a decision, or choose a course of action. As you read them, imagine yourself in each situation and consider what you would do. After you've finished the chapter, read the scenarios again and see if what you've learned has changed how you would think, feel, or act in each situation.

Since coming to college you've been smoking a few cigarettes a day, sometimes getting them from friends and sometimes buying a pack yourself. Now you're away for a ski weekend at your parents' cabin and are surprised to discover how much you want a cigarette. In fact, you can't stop thinking about where you can go to buy a pack. Is it the circumstances, or are you hooked?

While you're waiting for a bus in a crowded terminal, the person sitting next to you lights up a cigarette. You ask her if she would mind not smoking, since you don't want to breathe in the smoke. She replies that she *would* mind and suggests that you find another seat. "You nonsmoking fanatics make me mad with all your talk about the right to breathe clean air," she says. "What about *my* rights? I've been smoking for 30 years, and I've got a right to smoke if I want to." Does she have a point? What should you do?

9
Toward a Tobacco-free Society

A good friend of yours is a pack-a-day smoker and has no interest in quitting. Here's why: Her grandmother, age 90, has been smoking for 50 years and has no sign of heart disease, lung cancer, or any other smoking-related illness. "All she has is a smoker's cough," your friend says. "Otherwise, she's perfectly healthy. If nothing's happened to her, why should anything happen to me?" Are there any flaws in your friend's reasoning?

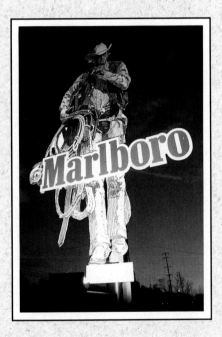

During Christmas vacation you discover that your 15-year-old sister has started smoking cigarettes. When you ask her why, she says she and some of her friends are smoking because they heard it was a good way to keep their weight under control. You point out that smoking is a health hazard, but she says that you have to smoke for years before you damage your lungs. She's just going to enjoy it while she's young and stop smoking before it affects her health. Besides, she tells you, she can quit any time she wants. How much of what she says is true? What advice can you give her?

A friend offers you some chewing tobacco, saying it will give you a pleasant lift. He tells you it's not dangerous to your health because you don't smoke it. You're skeptical, but he points out that a lot of professional athletes not only use it but also endorse it in ads. "Would they do that if it was dangerous?" he asks. You're tempted because you really enjoyed cigarettes when you used to smoke. Should you give it a try?

"The air nimbly and sweetly recommends itself unto our gentle senses," wrote William Shakespeare as he expressed how exhilarating it feels to take in sweet, clean air. But taking a deep breath isn't so pleasant for smokers. Their inhalation is likely to be interrupted by a racking, brittle "smoker's cough." The smoke from their cigarettes makes the air less sweet for others, too. In fact, it's now known that cigarette smoking poses a health threat to nonsmokers as well as smokers. Smoking causes more ill health than any other single behavior or combination of behaviors affecting health. And according to the Surgeon General of the United States, smoking remains the leading preventable cause of illness and death in the United States (see Table 9-1). These facts have been documented by thousands of carefully executed studies.

Why, then, with this kind of documented evidence would people continue to smoke or take it up in the first place? People continue to smoke despite the evidence that it is harmful primarily because they have become addicted to a powerful drug found in tobacco—**nicotine.** Like alcoholics and heroin addicts, smokers who try to stop experience strong withdrawal symptoms. Drinking alcohol and coffee enhances these symptoms. While it is unclear how long the transition from experimental to regular smoking takes, results from several recent studies suggest that teenagers become addicted more quickly than was previously believed. (See the box "Nicotine Dependence: Are You Hooked?" for some symptoms of addiction.)

Tobacco has some adverse effects on health in whatever form it is used. Although low-tar or low-nicotine cigarettes may reduce risks, some smokers who switch to low-tar or low-nicotine brands will probably smoke more cigarettes to match their previous absorption levels of nicotine. Researchers warn there is no such thing as a "safe" cigarette. Many smokers have switched from cigarettes to other forms of tobacco such as cigars, pipes, clove cigarettes, and smokeless tobacco. However, each of these alternatives is far from safe.

Why People Use Tobacco

Just like all other addictions, the problem of nicotine needs to be addressed not just in terms of cure but also in terms of prevention. What personal and societal forces induce people to start smoking, and what forces encourage them to continue? This section examines nicotine addiction in more detail and tries to answer the question of why people use tobacco.

Nicotine Addiction Regular tobacco use and especially cigarette smoking is not just a psychological habit but a classic case of addiction, or physical dependence on nicotine. Addicted tobacco users must keep a continuous

	VITAL STATISTICS

Table 9-1 Estimated Risks of Various Activities

Activity or Cause	Annual Fatalities per 1 Million Exposed Persons
Active smoking	7,000
Alcohol	541
Accident	275
Disease	266
Motor vehicles	187
Alcohol-involved	95
Non-alcohol-involved	92
Work	113
Swimming	22
All other air pollutants	6
Football	6
Electrocution	2
Lightning	0.5
DES in cattlefeed	0.3
Bee sting	0.2
Basketball	0.02

Source: Active smoking, CPS-II; NHISs 1965, 1985; U.S. Bureau of the Census (1974, 1986).

amount of nicotine circulating in the blood and going to the brain. If that amount falls below a certain level or if they stop using tobacco, they experience withdrawal symptoms. In one experiment, subjects were given cigarettes that tasted and looked exactly the same but varied in the amount of nicotine they contained. Although they didn't know how much nicotine they were getting, the subjects automatically adjusted their rate of smoking and depth of inhalation to ensure that they absorbed their usual amount of nicotine. In other studies, heavy smokers were given nicotine without knowing it—and they cut down on their smoking without a conscious effort.

■ **Exploring Your Emotions**

Did people in your family smoke when you were growing up? Do you think it's affected your feelings and attitudes about smoking today? If so, how?

These unconscious adjustments made by many smokers may explain why low-nicotine cigarettes are as harmful as high-nicotine ones. Using these cigarettes, many smokers merely puff more frequently, inhale more

Nicotine Dependence: Are You Hooked?

You may be dependent on nicotine if you have used tobacco for at least one month and experience one or more of the following characteristics:

- You have made a serious, but unsuccessful, attempt to stop using tobacco or permanently reduce the amount you use.
- Your attempts to stop smoking have led to physical withdrawal symptoms (including a craving for tobacco, anxiety, irritability, restlessness, difficulty in concentrating, headaches, drowsiness and stomach upset).
- You continue to use tobacco even when you have a serious physical problem (such as cardiovascular or respiratory disease) that you know is worsened by tobacco.
- You develop a "tolerance" to tobacco. A certain dose of the drug (in this case, a particular number of cigarettes that you smoke during the day) produces less effect over time; increasing doses are necessary to achieve a desired sensation.

In all these criteria, the central element of addiction is that the substance controls your behavior by producing temporary alterations in your mood when it is not in your system.

From *Mayo Clinic Health Letter*, May 1989, p. 6.

---

deeply, smoke down to a short butt, or continue smoking, thus exposing themselves and those around them to a greater total amount of smoke.

Like other drug addicts, the chronic tobacco user or smoker who stops suddenly is likely to experience physiological withdrawal symptoms. Sudden abstinence can change brain waves, heart rate, and blood pressure. People who quit "cold turkey" are often irritable, complain of insomnia, muscular pains, headache, nausea, and other discomforts. They are easily distracted and perform poorly on objective tests that require sustained attention. Most heavy smokers continue their addiction not for pleasure but because they are unwilling to go through the uncomfortable withdrawal process.

Secondary Reinforcers   Why do smokers have such a hard time quitting even when they want to? Social and psychological forces combine with physiological addiction to maintain the tobacco habit (see the box entitled "For Smokers Only: Why Do You Smoke?"). Many people, for example, have established habits of smoking while doing something else—while talking, while working, while drinking, and so on. It's difficult for these people to quit smoking because the activities they associate with it continue to trigger their urge for a cigarette. Psychologists call such activities **secondary reinforcers;**

they act together with the physiological addiction to keep the smoker dependent on tobacco.

Why Start in the First Place?   Most people start smoking as teenagers or young adults. Research studies have identified certain behavioral patterns in these people. Smoking at an early age is often linked to curiosity, low self-esteem, and status seeking. The urge to imitate close friends, older siblings, and parents is an important factor. Most teenage smokers report that their best friends and parents are smokers. For many teenagers, the choice to smoke or not revolves around their desire to conform to a particular group. Older teenagers tend to report their smoking behavior in more personal terms—stimulation, pleasure, or relief from unpleasant moods such as anxiety or depression. Despite their keen awareness of the health hazards of smoking, they often defend their behavior with rationalizations like "my grandmother smoked and lived to be 80" or "you can get killed just by crossing the street."

Who Uses Tobacco?   Different people smoke for different reasons but underlying psychological or physiological processes may be associated with all drug addiction or dependence. People who smoke, for example, are also more likely to drink coffee and alcohol and use other

---

Nicotine   A poisonous substance found in tobacco and responsible for many of the effects of tobacco.

Secondary reinforcers   Stimuli that are not necessarily pleasurable in themselves, but have been associated with other stimuli that are pleasurable.

For Smokers Only: Why Do You Smoke?

Although smoking cigarettes is physiologically addicting, people also smoke for reasons other than nicotine craving. They differ in the way they use smoking in their lives, the purpose it serves for them, and the circumstances in which they're likely to smoke more or less. Knowing what your motivations and satisfactions are can ultimately help you quit.

What kind of smoker are you? What do you get out of smoking? This test is designed to provide you with a score on each of six factors that describe many people's smoking. Your scores will help you identify what you use smoking for and what kind of satisfactions it gives you. With this information in hand, you're in a better position

to tackle the behavior change strategy described at the end of the chapter.

Here are some statements made by people to describe what they get out of smoking cigarettes. How *often* do you feel this way when smoking them? Circle one number for each statement. Be sure you answer every question.

		ALWAYS	FREQUENTLY	OCCASIONALLY	SELDOM	NEVER
A.	I smoke cigarettes in order to keep myself from slowing down.	5	4	3	2	1
B.	Handling a cigarette is part of the enjoyment of smoking it.	5	4	3	2	1
C.	Smoking cigarettes is pleasant and relaxing.	5	4	3	2	1
D.	I light up a cigarette when I feel angry about something.	5	4	3	2	1
E.	When I have run out of cigarettes I find it almost unbearable until I can get them.	5	4	3	2	1
F.	I smoke cigarettes automatically without even being aware of it.	5	4	3	2	1
G.	I smoke cigarettes to stimulate me, to perk myself up.	5	4	3	2	1
H.	Part of the enjoyment of smoking a cigarette comes from the steps I take to light up.	5	4	3	2	1
I.	I find cigarettes pleasurable.	5	4	3	2	1
J.	When I feel uncomfortable or upset about something, I light up a cigarette.	5	4	3	2	1
K.	I am very much aware of the fact when I am not smoking a cigarette.	5	4	3	2	1
L.	I light up a cigarette without realizing I still have one burning in the ashtray.	5	4	3	2	1
M.	I smoke cigarettes to give me a "lift."	5	4	3	2	1
N.	When I smoke a cigarette, part of the enjoyment is watching the smoke as I exhale it.	5	4	3	2	1
O.	I want a cigarette most when I am comfortable and relaxed.	5	4	3	2	1
P.	When I feel "blue" or want to take my mind off cares and worries, I smoke cigarettes.	5	4	3	2	1
Q.	I get a real gnawing hunger for a cigarette when I haven't smoked for a while.	5	4	3	2	1
R.	I've found a cigarette in my mouth and didn't remember putting it there.	5	4	3	2	1

For Smokers Only: Why Do You Smoke (continued)

How to Score

1. Enter the numbers you have circled to the smoking questions in the spaces below, putting the number you have circled to question A over line A, to question B over line B, and so on.

2. Total the 3 scores on each line to get your totals. For example, the sum of your scores over lines A, G, and M gives you your score on *Stimulation*—lines B, H, and N give the score on *Handling*, etc.

Scores can vary from 3 to 15. Any score 11 and above is *high*; any score 7 and below is *low*.

What Your Scores Mean

The six factors measured by this test describe one or another way of experiencing or managing certain kinds of feelings. Three of these feeling-states represent the *positive* feelings people get from smoking: (1) a sense of increased energy or *stimulation*, (2) the satisfaction of *handling* or manipulating things, and (3) the enhancing of *pleasur-*

able feelings accompanying a state of well-being. The fourth is the *decreasing of negative feelings* by reducing a state of tension or feelings of anxiety, anger, shame, etc. The fifth is craving for a cigarette, representing a strong physiological or psychological *addiction* to cigarettes. The sixth is *habit* smoking, which takes place in an absence of feeling and is purely automatic smoking.

A score of 11 or above on any factor indicates that this factor is an important source of satisfaction for you. The higher your score (15 is the highest), the more important a particular factor is in your smoking and the more useful the discussion of that factor can be in your attempt to quit.

Stimulation   If you score high or fairly high on this factor, it means that you are one of those smokers who is stimulated by the cigarette—you feel that it helps wake you up, organize your energies, and keep you going. If you try to give up smoking, you may want a safe substitute, a *brisk walk* or moderate exercise, for example,

whenever you feel the urge to smoke.

Handling   Handling things can be satisfying, but there are many ways to keep your hands busy without lighting up or playing with a cigarette. Try doodling or toying with a pen, pencil, or other small object.

Accentuation of Pleasure—Pleasurable Relaxation   It is not always easy to find out whether you use the cigarette to feel *good*, that is, get real, honest pleasure out of smoking, or to keep from feeling so *bad*. About two-thirds of smokers score high or fairly high on *accentuation of pleasure*, and about half of those also score as high or higher on *reduction of negative feelings*.

Those who do get real pleasure out of smoking often find that an honest consideration of the harmful effects of their habit is enough to help them quit. They substitute social or physical activities and find they do not seriously miss their cigarettes.

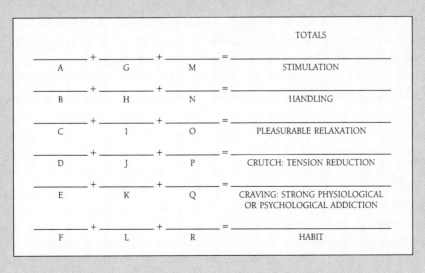

For Smokers Only: Why Do You Smoke? (continued)

Reduction of Negative Feelings, or "Crutch"   Many smokers use the cigarette as a kind of crutch in moments of stress or discomfort, and on occasion it may work; the cigarette is sometimes used as a tranquilizer. But heavy smokers, those who try to handle severe personal problems by smoking many times a day, are apt to discover that cigarettes do not help them deal with their problems effectively.

When it comes to quitting, this kind of smoker may find it easy to stop when everything is going well but may be tempted to start again in a time of crisis. Again, physical exertion or social activity may serve as useful substitutes for cigarettes, even in times of tension. The choice of a substitute depends on what will achieve the same effect without having any appreciable risk.

Craving or Strong Addiction   Quitting smoking is difficult for people who score high on this factor. For them, the craving for the next cigarette begins to build up the moment they put one out, so tapering off is not likely to work. They must go "cold turkey." It may be helpful for them to smoke more than usual for a day or two, so that the taste for ciga-

rettes is spoiled, and then isolate themselves completely from cigarettes until the craving is gone. Giving up cigarettes may be so difficult and cause so much discomfort that once they do quit, they will find it easy to resist the temptation to go back to smoking because they remember how agonizing it was to quit once.

Habit   These smokers are no longer getting much satisfaction from cigarettes. They just light them frequently without even realizing it. They may find it easy to quit and stay off if they can break the habit patterns they have built up. Cutting down gradually may be quite effective if there is a change in the way the cigarettes are smoked and the conditions under which they are smoked. The key to success is becoming *aware* of each cigarette when it's smoked. This can be done by asking, "Do I really want this cigarette?" Habitual smokers may be surprised at how many they don't want.

Summary

If you don't score high on any of the six factors, chances are that you don't smoke very much or haven't been smoking for very

many years. If so, giving up smoking—and staying off—should be easy. If you score high on several categories, you apparently get several kinds of satisfaction from smoking and will have to find several solutions. Certain combinations of scores may indicate that giving up smoking will be especially difficult. Those who score high on both *reduction of negative feelings* and *craving*, may have a particularly hard time in going off smoking and in staying off. However, there are ways to do it; many smokers represented by this combination have been able to quit.

Quitting smoking isn't easy. It usually means giving up something pleasurable that has a definite place in your life. In the end, of course, it's worth it, because you repay yourself with pleasures of a more solid kind. Now that you have some ideas about why you smoke, read the Behavior Change Strategy at the end of the chapter for a plan that will help you quit.

Adapted from Daniel Horn and Associates. 1983 (October). *A Self-Test for Smokers* (Test 3), DHEW Publication No. (CDC) 75-8716 (Washington, D.C.: U.S. Department of Health and Human Services).

psychoactive drugs. Some studies have found that over 90 percent of heroin addicts and 80 percent of alcoholics are heavy cigarette smokers. Both coffee and alcohol are synergistic with smoking—that is, coffee and alcohol both enhance the unpleasant symptoms of withdrawal and so encourage the smoker to light up.

Nevertheless, no single factor has yet been found to predict who will smoke and who will quit. No personality measures can successfully identify which people will re-

spond to stop-smoking programs. Some demographic variables are correlated with smoking. Wealthier, more educated people are less likely to start smoking and are more successful in their efforts to quit. Since the U.S. Surgeon General's initial report on the health hazards of smoking, physicians and other health professionals have stopped smoking at a higher rate than have most other professionals. However such statistics aren't very useful in predicting individual behavior.

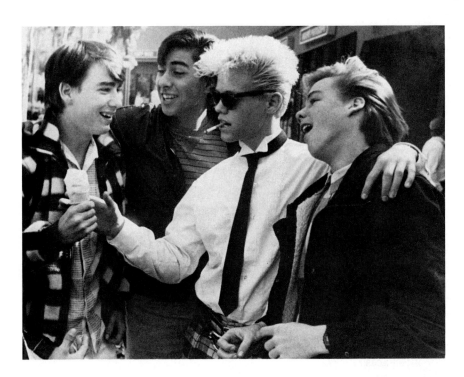

Most smokers start smoking as teenagers and have an expensive cigarette habit by the time they're young adults. Like these teens, they imagine that smoking gives them an air of worldly sophistication—just as the tobacco companies would have them believe.

■ **Exploring Your Emotions**

How do you think you would feel if you found your 12-year-old child smoking? Would your feelings depend on whether you yourself were a smoker or a nonsmoker?

Cigarette smoking has declined substantially among all men in the United States and slightly among all women in the United States but hardly at all among people without a high school diploma. From 1965 to 1987, smoking among men 20 years of age and older decreased from 50.2 to 31.2 percent (see Table 9-2). Among women, smoking decreased from 31.9 to 26.5 percent. Smoking among whites fell steadily. Among blacks, the prevalence of smoking changed little until 1974 when the prevalence began to decline at a rate similar to that of whites. Smoking has consistently been higher among blue-collar workers than among white-collar workers. Of all adults who smoked at any time during the year 1985–1986, 70 percent had made at least one serious attempt to quit during their lifetime. The prevalence of smoking among high school seniors decreased from 29 percent in 1976 to 21 percent in 1980, after which it leveled off at 18 to 21 percent. The best sociodemographic predictor of smoking patterns appears to be level of educational attainment.

Between 1964 and 1987, use of smokeless tobacco (snuff and chewing tobacco) declined among men and women 21 years of age and older. However, among males aged 17 to 19, snuff use increased fifteenfold, and use of chewing tobacco increased more than fourfold from 1970 to 1987 (see Table 9-3, and the box entitled "Smokeless

VITAL STATISTICS			
Table 9-2 Percentage of Adults Who Smoke Cigarettes, by Sex and Age—United States, 1987			
Age (yrs)	Men	Women	Total
18–24	28.1	26.1	27.1
25–44	35.6	30.8	33.2
45–64	33.5	28.6	30.9
65–74	20.2	18.0	19.0
75 or older	11.3	7.5	8.9
Total	**31.2**	**26.5**	**28.8**

From Centers for Disease Control. 1989. *Morbidity and Mortality Weekly Report.* 38(40):685-686.

Tobacco: An Unsafe Alternative"). From 1964 to 1987, the prevalence of pipe and cigar smoking declined by 80 percent among men.

Health Hazards

It's hard to believe that anyone in the United States doesn't know about the harmful effects of tobacco on the heart and lungs. In fact, tobacco adversely affects nearly every part of the body—including brain, stomach, and mouth.

VITAL STATISTICS

Table 9-3 Percentage of Men Who Use Non-cigarette Tobacco,* by Age and Form of Smokeless Tobacco or Alternative Smoking Method—United States, 1987

Age (yrs)	Smokeless Tobacco Form		Alternative Smoking Method	
	Chewing Tobacco	Snuff	Pipes	Cigars
18–24	5.5	6.4	0.8	1.6
25–44	3.2	3.1	2.9	5.8
45–64	3.9	1.6	5.1	7.0
65–74	5.0	1.9	5.0	5.2
75 or older	6.1	2.7	4.1	3.9
Total	**4.0**	**3.1**	**3.4**	**5.3**

Prevalence of use among women was 0.5% or less.

From Centers for Disease Control. 1989. *Morbidity and Mortality Weekly Report.* 38(40):685–686.

Tobacco Smoke: A Poisonous Mix   Tobacco smoke contains hundreds of damaging chemical substances. Smoke from a typical unfiltered cigarette contains about 5 billion particles per cubic millimeter—50,000 times as many as are found in an equal volume of polluted urban atmosphere. The particles in tobacco smoke are made up of several hundred different chemicals, many of them toxic. These particles, when condensed, form the brown, sticky mass called **cigarette tar.**

Some chemicals in tobacco are **carcinogenic;** that is, they cause cancer (see Table 9-4). Other chemicals in tobacco tar are **cocarcinogens;** they do not themselves cause cancer but combine with other chemicals to stimulate the growth of certain cancers, at least in laboratory animals. The phenols present in tar, for example, although not particularly carcinogenic themselves, greatly increase the carcinogenic power of benzopyrene, a substance also contained in tar. Still other compounds, which may not directly cause cancer, irritate the tissues of the respiratory system and damage the respiratory cilia, which operate to keep the air passages free of mucus and dust.

Smoking interferes with the functioning of the respiratory system and often leads rapidly to the conditions called smoker's throat, smoker's cough, and smoker's bronchitis, as well as shortness of breath. Besides respiratory problems, common physical complaints of smokers include loss of appetite, diarrhea, fatigue, hoarseness,

weight loss, stomach pains, and insomnia. These conditions usually disappear in people who stop smoking.

Nicotine is the predominant **psychoactive drug** in tobacco. When a person inhales smoke, the nicotine in it passes through the membrane of the lung tissue and rapidly enters the bloodstream. The heart pumps about 15 percent of the nicotine directly to the brain, which absorbs all of it. This process takes about 7 seconds. When the nicotine hits the brain, it produces several effects, including the release of hormones called **catecholamines.** Both blood pressure and heart rate go up. The change in the body's metabolism is the "lift" that smokers crave. For every puff, the smoker gets a "shot" or "fix" of nicotine. Throughout the day, smokers automatically and unknowingly maintain the nicotine level in their brains by varying the number of cigarettes they smoke and by the way they inhale. In this way, they sustain the "lift" effect without inducing the unpleasant side effects of smoking, such as becoming dizzy and nauseated.

Cigarette smoke also contains carbon monoxide, the deadly gas in automobile exhaust, in concentrations 400 times greater than is considered safe in industrial workplaces. Not surprisingly, smokers often complain of breathlessness when they require a burst of energy to run across campus for their next class. Carbon monoxide displaces oxygen in red blood cells, depleting the body's supply of life-giving oxygen for extra work. Carbon monoxide also impairs visual acuity, especially at night.

Cigarette tar   Brown sticky mass caused when the chemical particles in tobacco smoke condense.

Cocarcinogen   A substance that works with a carcinogen to produce a cancer.

Carcinogenic   Cancer causing.

Psychoactive drug   A drug that affects the brain or nervous system.

Catecholamines   Hormones secreted by the adrenal glands, especially during stress.

Smokeless Tobacco: An Unsafe Alternative

In February 1986, Congress passed the Comprehensive Smokeless Tobacco Health Education Act, which requires manufacturers of chewing tobacco and snuff to include health warning labels on packages. The warnings, which will be emphasized by arrows and circles, are shown in Table 9-5.

Chewing tobacco and snuff contain tobacco leaf and a variety of sweeteners, other flavorings, and scents. In chewing tobacco, the leaf may be shredded (loose-leaf), pressed into bricks or cakes (plugs), or dried and twisted into ropelike strands (twists). A portion is either chewed or held in place in the cheek or between the lower lip and the gum. The two categories of snuff, dry and moist, are made from powdered or finely cut tobacco leaves. In some countries, dry snuff is sniffed through the nose, but in the United States both dry and moist snuff are "dipped" by tucking a small amount (pinch) between the lip or cheek and the gum. Nicotine from the tobacco is absorbed into the bloodstream and produces mental effects described by users as relaxing or stimulating.

In 1985 an expert panel assembled by the National Institutes of Health concluded that despite their hazards, smokeless tobacco products have been gaining rapidly in popularity—especially among teenagers. The panel estimated that at least 10 million Americans had used smokeless tobacco products within the previous year, with 3 million users under the age of 21. Another national study found that 16 percent of male youths 12 to 17 years old had used some form of smokeless tobacco during the previous year, while a local study found that tobacco chewing and snuff dipping had tripled between 1976 and 1982 among boys ages 12 to 14.

The rise in popularity is obviously related to advertising that associates chewing and dipping with "macho" images and athletic prowess. Ads for smokeless tobacco have appeared mainly in male-oriented outdoor publications such as *Field and Stream, Outdoor Life,* and *Sporting News.* U.S. Tobacco Company's Skoal has been a major sponsor of Atlanta Braves baseball telecasts. The company also promotes its products through scholarship offers to rodeo riders. Race car driver A. J. Foyt, four-time winner of the Indianapolis 500, races automobiles bearing bold logos for Copenhagen Snuff. Prominent baseball and football players have appeared in testimonial ads.

Rep. Henry Waxman (D-Calif.), who played a major role in passage of the new law, hopes the warning labels will make it obvious to children that "smokeless tobacco products are not bubblegum." The law also bans radio and television advertising of the products and requires manufacturers to reveal to the U.S. Department of Health and Human Services what additives and flavorings they contain.

Chemical analysis of various smokeless products has found three types of chemicals known to produce cancer: polycyclic aromatic amines, nitrosamines, and polonium 210, which is radioactive. Dr. Gregory Connolly, director of the dental division of the Massachusetts Department of Public Health, calls smokeless tobacco use "a chemical time bomb ticking in the mouths of hundreds of thousands of boys in this country."

The risk is not confined to oral cancer. Smokeless tobacco can cause tooth decay, gingivitis (inflammation) and recession of the gums, especially where the tobacco is habitually placed. Epidemiological data on the incidence of heart disease in smokeless tobacco users have not yet been collected. But it is known that chewing and dipping produce blood levels of nicotine similar to those in cigarette smokers that elevate blood pressure, heart rate, and blood levels of certain fats. Other chemicals in smokeless tobacco are believed to pose risks to developing babies in pregnant female users.

Because of its nicotine content, smokeless tobacco is also highly addicting. Some users even keep it in their mouth while sleeping. Psychologist Elbert Glover of East Carolina University has reported that only one out of 14 participants at recent quit-smokeless-tobacco clinics was able to stop for more than four hours.

Source: Stephen Barrett, 1986. Smokeless tobacco is dangerous, *Healthline,* December.

Table 9-4 Risks of Smoking and Benefits of Quitting

Risks of Smoking	Benefits of Quitting
Shortened life expectancy. 25-year-old 2-pack-a-day smokers have life expectancy 8.3 years shorter than nonsmoking contemporaries. Other smoking levels: proportional risk.	**Reduces risk of premature death** cumulatively. After 10–15 years, ex-smokers' risk approaches that of those who have never smoked.
Lung cancer. Smoking cigarettes is a major cause.	Gradual decrease in risk. **After 10–15 years, risk approaches that of those who have never smoked.**
Larynx cancer. 2.9 to 17.7 times that of nonsmokers. Risk is in all smokers (including pipe and cigar).	**Gradual reduction of risk** after smoking cessation. **Reaches normal after 10 years.**
Mouth cancer. Cigarette smokers have 3 to 10 times as many oral cancers as nonsmokers. Pipes, cigars, chewing tobacco also major risk factors. Alcohol seems synergistic carcinogen with smoking.	Reducing or eliminating smoking/drinking reduces risk in first few years; **risk drops to level of nonsmokers in 10–15 years.**
Cancer of esophagus. Cigarettes, pipes, and cigars increase risk of dying of esophageal cancer about 2 to 9 times. Synergistic relationship between smoking and alcohol.	Since risks are dose related, reducing or eliminating smoking/drinking **should have risk-reducing effect.**
Cancer of bladder. Cigarette smokers have 7 to 10 times risk of bladder cancer as nonsmokers. Also synergistic with certain exposed occupations: dyestuffs, etc.	**Risk decreases gradually to that of nonsmokers over 7 years.**
Cancer of pancreas. Cigarette smokers have 2 to 5 times risk of dying of pancreatic cancer as nonsmokers.	Since there is evidence of dose-related risk, reducing or eliminating smoking should have risk-reducing effect.
Coronary heart disease. Cigarette smoking is major factor; responsible for 120,000 excess U.S. deaths from coronary heart disease each year.	**Sharply decreases risk after one year.** After 10 years ex-smokers' risk is same as that of those who have never smoked.
Chronic bronchitis and pulmonary emphysema (COLD). Cigarette smokers have 4–25 times risk of death from these diseases as nonsmokers. Damage seen in lungs of even young smokers.	**Cough and sputum disappear** during first few weeks. **Lung function may improve** and rate of deterioration slow down.
Stillbirth and low birth weight. Smoking mothers have more stillbirths and babies of low birth weight—more vulnerable to disease and death.	Women who stop smoking before fourth month of pregnancy **eliminate risk of stillbirth and low birth weight** caused by smoking.
Children of smoking mothers are smaller, underdeveloped physically and socially, seven years after birth.	Since children of nonsmoking mothers are bigger and more advanced socially, inference is that **not smoking during pregnancy might avoid such underdeveloped children.**
Peptic ulcer. Cigarette smokers get more peptic ulcers and die more often of them; cure is more difficult in smokers.	Ex-smokers get ulcers but these are **more likely to heal rapidly and completely** than those of smokers.
Allergy and impairment of immune system.	Since these are direct, immediate effects of smoking, they are obviously **avoidable by not smoking.**
Alters pharmacologic effects of many medicines and diagnostic tests and greatly increases risk of thrombosis with oral contraceptives.	**Majority of blood components elevated by smoking return to normal after cessation.** Nonsmokers on oral contraceptives have much lower risks of thrombosis.

Source: Adapted from American Cancer Society, *Dangers of Smoking, Benefits of Quitting and Relative Risks of Reduced Exposure,* rev. ed., pp. 8–9.

Immediate Effects of Tobacco Use   The beginning smoker often has symptoms of mild *nicotine poisoning:* dizziness; faintness; rapid pulse; cold, clammy skin; and sometimes nausea, vomiting, and diarrhea. The seasoned smoker occasionally suffers these effects of nicotine poisoning, particularly after quitting and returning to a previous level of consumption. The effects of nicotine on smokers vary, depending greatly on the size of the nicotine dose and how much tolerance previous smoking has built up. Nicotine can either excite or tranquilize the nervous system, depending on dosage. Generally the smoker feels stimulated first. This stimulation gives way to feeling tranquil and then depressed.

Nicotine has many other effects. It stimulates the part of the brain called the **cerebral cortex.** It also stimulates the adrenal glands to discharge adrenalin. And it inhibits the formation of urine, constricts the blood vessels, especially in the skin, increases the heart rate, and elevates blood pressure. Higher blood pressure, faster heart rate, and constricted blood vessels require the heart to pump more blood. In healthy people, the heart can usually meet this demand, but in people whose coronary arteries are damaged enough to interfere with the flow of blood, the heart muscle may be strained.

People who smoke often do not feel as hungry as people who do not. Smoking depresses hunger contractions and causes the liver to release glycogen, which slightly raises the level of sugar in the blood. Smoking also dulls taste buds so that food does not taste as good. People who quit smoking usually notice how much better food tastes. Figure 9-1 summarizes these immediate effects.

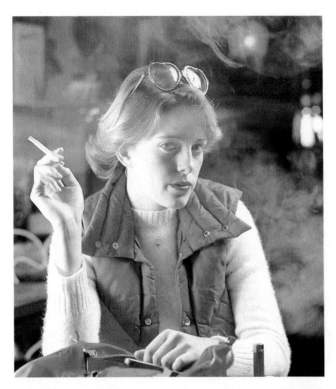

Cigarette smoke contains many toxic and carcinogenic chemicals that affect both the person smoking and the people breathing the second-hand smoke. A growing body of evidence links second-hand smoke not only with lung cancer and other respiratory diseases but also with cardiovascular disease.

All smokers absorb some gases, tars, and nicotine from cigarette smoke, but smokers who inhale bring most of these substances into their bodies and keep them there. In one year, a typical one-pack-per-day smoker takes in 50,000 to 70,000 puffs. Smoke from a cigarette, pipe, or cigar directly assaults mouth, throat, and respiratory tract; the nose—which normally filters about 75 percent of foreign matter in the air we breathe—is completely bypassed.

In a cigarette, the unburned tobacco itself acts as a filter. As a cigarette burns down, there is less and less filter. Thus, more chemicals are absorbed into the body during the last third of a cigarette than during the first. A smoker can therefore cut down on absorption of harmful chemicals by not smoking cigarettes down to short butts. Any gains, of course, will be offset by smoking more cigarettes, inhaling deeper, or puffing more frequently.

Long-Term Effects of Tobacco Use   Beginning in 1964, the U.S. Surgeon General's office issued a number of reports evaluating three major types of evidence linking smoking with disease. The first type of evidence was based on animal studies: nicotine and other chemicals in tobacco smoke were given to animals, and damage to their tissues was measured. The second type of evidence was gathered from clinical and autopsy studies of tissue damage occurring most often in smokers. The third type of evidence came from two kinds of population studies: (1) past smoking habits of people with a particular disease and (2) studies that followed groups of smokers and nonsmokers over a period of years to record the occurrence and progress of certain diseases, including chronic cough and sputum production—sure signs of bronchitis. These studies also compared death rates and causes of death for the two groups.

Cerebral cortex   The outer layer of the brain, which controls the complex behavior and mental activity of human beings.

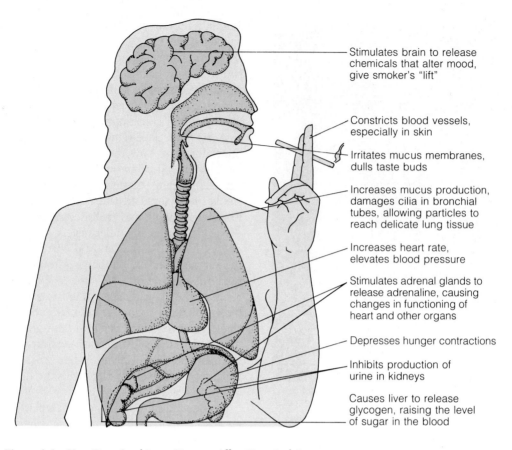

Stimulates brain to release
chemicals that alter mood,
give smoker's "lift"

Constricts blood vessels,
especially in skin

Irritates mucus membranes,
dulls taste buds

Increases mucus production,
damages cilia in bronchial
tubes, allowing particles to
reach delicate lung tissue

Increases heart rate,
elevates blood pressure

Stimulates adrenal glands to
release adrenaline, causing
changes in functioning of
heart and other organs

Depresses hunger contractions

Inhibits production of
urine in kidneys

Causes liver to release
glycogen, raising the level
of sugar in the blood

Figure 9-1   How Does Smoking a Cigarette Affect Your Body?

A great deal of scientific evidence now indicates that the total amount of tobacco smoke inhaled is a key factor contributing to disease. People who smoke more cigarettes per day, inhale deeply, puff frequently, smoke cigarettes down to the butts, or begin smoking at an early age run a greater risk of disease than do those who behave more moderately or who do not smoke at all. Many diseases have already been linked to smoking; and as more research is done, even more diseases associated with smoking are being uncovered. The most costly ones, to society as well as to the individual, are cardiovascular diseases, respiratory diseases such as emphysema and lung cancer, and other cancers. Although cancer tends to receive the most publicity, **coronary heart disease (CHD)** is actually the most widespread single cause of death for cigarette smokers.

Coronary Heart Disease   Cigarette smoking is strongly related to various cardiovascular disorders that involve the heart and blood vessels. CHD is one type and often results from a disease called **atherosclerosis**, in which fatty deposits called **plaques** form on the inner walls of heart arteries, causing them to narrow and stiffen. The crushing chest pain of **angina pectoris**, a primary symp-

tom of CHD, results when the heart muscle or **myocardium** does not get enough oxygen. Sometimes a plaque forms at a narrow point in a main coronary artery. If the plaque completely blocks the flow of blood to a portion of the heart, that portion may die. This type of heart attack is called a **myocardial infarction.** CHD can also interfere with the normal electrical activity of the heart, resulting in disturbances of the normal heartbeat rhythm. Sudden and unexpected death is a common result of CHD, particularly among smokers. (See Chapter 15 for a more extensive discussion of cardiovascular disease.) Deaths from CHD associated with cigarette smoking are most common in people 40 to 50 years old. This age bracket is almost twenty years younger than the age at which people are most likely to die from lung cancer caused by smoking. Cigar and pipe smokers run a lower risk than do cigarette smokers.

We do not completely understand how cigarette smoking increases the risk of CHD. Researchers, however, are beginning to shed light on the process. Smoking reduces the amount of **HDL** cholesterol (**high-density lipoprotein**, the "good" cholesterol) and thus promotes plaque formation and speeds blood clotting. Smoking may also increase tension in the heart muscle walls, speed up the rate of muscular contraction, and increase the heart rate. The workload of the heart thus increases, as does its need for oxygen and other nutrients. Carbon monoxide produced by cigarette smoking combines with hemoglobin in the red blood cells, displacing oxygen and thus providing less oxygen to the heart.

As suggested earlier, the risks of CHD decrease rapidly when the person stops smoking, particularly for younger smokers whose coronary arteries haven't yet been extensively damaged. Cigarette smoking has also been linked to other cardiovascular diseases, including:

1. **Stroke,** a sudden interference with the circulation of blood in a part of the brain.
2. **Aortic aneurysm,** a bulge in the aorta caused by weakening in its walls.
3. **Pulmonary heart disease,** a disorder of the right side of the heart, caused by changes in the blood vessels of the lungs.

Lung Cancer   Cigarette smoking is the primary cause of lung cancer. The dramatic rise in lung cancer among women clearly parallels the increase of smoking in this group; lung cancer now exceeds breast cancer as the leading cause of cancer deaths among women. The risk of developing lung cancer increases with the number of cigarettes smoked each day, the number of years smoking, and the age at which the person started smoking.

While cigar and pipe smokers run a higher risk for lung cancer than nonsmokers do, the risk is lower than for cigarette smokers. Smoking filter-tipped cigarettes slightly reduces health hazards, unless the smoker compensates by smoking more, as is often the case.

The evidence suggests that after a year without smoking the risk of lung cancer decreases substantially. After ten years, the incidence of lung cancer among ex-smokers approaches the incidence of those who never smoked. If smoking is stopped before cancer has started, lung tissue tends to repair itself, even if changes leading to cancer are already present.

Research has also linked smoking to cancers of the mouth, pharynx, esophagus, pancreas, bladder, kidney, cervix, and stomach.

Emphysema   Smoking is the primary cause of **emphysema,** a particularly disabling condition. The walls of the air sacs in the lungs lose their elasticity and are gradually destroyed. The lungs' ability to obtain oxygen and remove carbon dioxide is impaired. A person with emphysema becomes breathless, is constantly gasping for air, and has the feeling of drowning. The heart must pump harder and may become enlarged. The person frequently dies from a damaged heart. There is no known way to reverse this disease. In its advanced stage, the victim is bedridden and severely disabled.

Chronic Obstructive Lung Disease   Chronic obstructive lung disease (COLD), also known as chronic obstructive pulmonary disease (COPD), refers to pulmonary emphysema and chronic bronchitis. Chronic bronchitis is a persistent, recurrent inflammation of the bronchial tubes. When the cell lining of the bronchial tubes is irritated, it secretes excess mucus. Bronchial congestion is followed by a chronic cough, which makes breathing more and more difficult. The risk of developing COLD rises with the number of cigarettes smoked and falls when smoking ceases.

Cigarette smokers are up to eighteen times more likely to die from emphysema and chronic bronchitis than are nonsmokers. If smokers have chronic bronchitis, they face a greater risk of lung cancer, no matter how old they are or how many (or few) cigarettes they smoke. Chronic bronchitis seems to be a shortcut to lung cancer.

Even smokers of high school age show impaired respiratory function, compared with nonsmokers of the same age. Although pipe and cigar smokers are more likely to die from COLD than are nonsmokers, they have a smaller risk than do cigarette smokers.

For most people in the United States, cigarette smoking is a more important cause of COLD than air pollution. But exposure to both air pollution and cigarette smoking is more dangerous than exposure to either by itself.

Coronary heart disease (CHD)   Heart disease caused by hardening of the arteries that supply oxygen to the heart muscle.

Atherosclerosis   Heart disease caused by the deposit of fatty substances in the walls of the arteries.

Plaque   A deposit on the inner wall of blood vessels. Blood can coagulate around a plaque and form a clot.

Angina pectoris   Chest pain due to heart disease.

Myocardium   The muscle of the heart.

Myocardial infarction   Heart attack caused by plaque that completely blocks a main coronary artery.

High-density lipoprotein (HDL)   Blood fats that help keep cholesterol in a watery state and thus are protective against heart diseases.

Stroke   An impaired blood supply to some part of the brain, resulting in the destruction of brain cells (also called cerebrovascular accident).

Aortic aneurysm   A blood-filled bulge in the aorta due to a weakening in its walls.

Pulmonary heart disease   A disorder of the right side of the heart caused by changes in the blood vessels of the lungs.

Emphysema   Loss of lung tissue elasticity and breakup of the many small air sacs in the lungs so that fewer, larger, and less elastic air sacs are formed. The progressive accumulation of air causes difficulty in breathing.

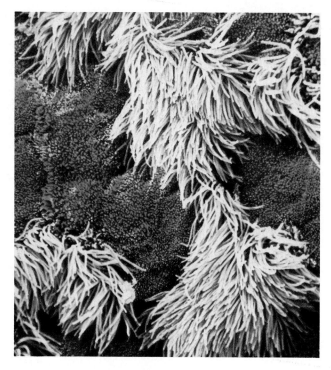

The respiratory tract is kept clean and healthy by cilia (stained yellow in this photomicrograph), which constantly sweep debris up and out of the bronchial tubes, and by goblet cells (orange), which produce mucus to trap dust particles. Cigarette smoke damages and eventually destroys the cilia, robbing the respiratory system of a major defense against injury and disease.

Even when the smoker shows no signs of lung impairment or disease, cigarette smoking damages the respiratory system. Normally the cells lining the bronchial tubes secrete mucus, a sticky fluid that collects particles of soot, dust, and other substances in inhaled air. Mucus is carried up to the mouth by the continuous motion of the cilia, hairlike structures that protrude from the inner surface of the bronchial tubes (see photo). If the cilia are destroyed or don't work or if the pollution of inhaled air is more than the system can remove, the protection provided by cilia is lost.

Cigarette smoke first slows, then stops the action of the cilia. Eventually it destroys them, leaving delicate membranes exposed to injury from substances inhaled in cigarette smoke or from the polluted air in which the person lives or works. Special cells of the body, the

macrophages (literally "big eaters"), also work to remove foreign particles from the respiratory tract by engulfing them. Smoking appears to make macrophages work less efficiently.

Although cigarette smoking can cause many respiratory disorders and diseases, the damage is not always permanent. Once a person stops smoking, steady improvement in overall lung function usually takes place. Chronic coughing subsides, phlegm (mucus) production returns to normal, and breathing becomes easier. The likelihood of lung disease drops sharply. People of all ages, even those who have been smoking for decades, improve after they stop smoking. If given a chance the human body has remarkable powers to restore itself.

Other Health Hazards   Tobacco use is associated with many other health hazards. For example, people who smoke cigarettes are more likely to develop peptic ulcers than nonsmokers and are more likely to die from them, especially ulcers of the stomach. People with ulcers should stop smoking immediately because smoking impairs the ability of the ulcer to heal. Many of the hazards associated with tobacco use have only recently been discovered, so we are not sure if they are causally related or if they merely exist together. Premature skin wrinkling, premature baldness, gum disorders, and allergies have all been associated with cigarette smoking. Recent research also suggests that smoking may harm the immune system. Further research may link tobacco use to still other disorders.

Cumulative Effects   Statistical data can illustrate the cumulative effects of tobacco use. These effects fall into two general categories. The first category is reduced life expectancy. A male who takes up smoking before age 15 and continues to smoke is only half as likely to live to age 75 as is a male who never smokes. If he inhales deeply, he risks losing one minute of life for every minute of smoking. Females who have similar smoking habits also have a reduced life expectancy.

The second category involves quality of life. A national health survey begun in 1964 shows that smokers spend one-third more time away from their jobs because of illness than do nonsmokers. Female smokers spend 17 percent more days sick in bed than do female nonsmokers (this includes women who work both inside and out-

---

Macrophages   Large cells in the body that absorb dead tissue and dead cells.

Mainstream smoke   Smoke that is inhaled by a smoker and then exhaled into the atmosphere.

Sidestream smoke   "Second-hand smoke" that comes from the burning end of a cigarette, cigar, or pipe.

Carboxyhemoglobin   A compound formed when carbon monoxide displaces oxygen from red blood cells; it seriously limits the body's ability to use oxygen.

side the home). Lost work days associated with cigarette smoking number in the millions.

Both men and women smokers show a greater rate of acute and chronic disease than do those who have never smoked. The U.S. Public Health Service estimates that if all people had the same rate of disease as those who never smoked there would be 1 million fewer cases of chronic bronchitis, 1.8 million fewer cases of sinusitis, and 1 million fewer cases of peptic ulcers in the country every year.

The Effects of Smoking on the Nonsmoker

The movement to protect people from tobacco smoke is gaining strength. Nonsmokers are insisting on the right to breathe clean air. FAA regulations now prohibit smoking on all flights in the continental limits of the United States of six hours or less, which effectively prohibits smoking on all domestic flights.

Sidestream Smoke   Also called second-hand smoke, **sidestream smoke** enters the atmosphere from the burning end of the cigarette, cigar, or pipe. Smoke that the smoker inhales and then exhales is referred to as **mainstream smoke.** Studies have shown that sidestream smoke has (1) twice as much tar and nicotine as does mainstream smoke; (2) three times as much benzopyrene, a cancer-causing agent; (3) almost three times as much carbon monoxide, which robs the blood of vital oxygen; and (4) three times as much ammonia. Nearly 85 percent of the smoke in a room where someone is smoking comes from sidestream smoke. Of course, sidestream smoke is diffused through the air, so nonsmokers don't inhale the same concentrations of toxic chemicals that the smoker does. Still, the nonsmoker is at risk from the mainstream smoke exhaled by the smoker as well as from the sidestream smoke polluting the environment.

One of the main ingredients of tobacco smoke is carbon monoxide, a poisonous, odorless gas that is also spewed forth from automobile exhausts. When inhaled, this gas displaces oxygen from red blood cells and forms **carboxyhemoglobin**, a dangerous compound that seriously limits the body's ability to use oxygen. Studies have shown that in rooms where people are smoking, levels of carbon monoxide can exceed those permitted by the Federal Air Quality Standards for outside air. Nonsmokers can still be affected by the harmful levels of sidestream smoke hours after they have left a smoky environment. Carbon monoxide still lingers in the bloodstream five hours later.

A particularly unpleasant side effect of smoking for nonsmokers is tobacco odor. Have you ever gone to a party with smokers and noted, much later or even the next day, a strong odor of tobacco in your hair and clothes? The human body acts as a magnet to tobacco smoke. Burning tobacco smoke creates a high electrical potential, whereas the water-filled human body has a low one. The smoke in a room gravitates and clings to people in much the same way as iron filings are attracted to a magnet. Aldehydes and ketones (chemicals in tobacco smoke) produce the penetrating odor, and the tars hold them to your skin and your clothes. The smoker may not be sensitive to the odor because smoke destroys the inner lining of the nose. Research has found that smoke contamination is so intense that demands on an air conditioning system can increase to as much as 600 percent to control the smell.

Effects of Passive Smoking on Children   Babies and young children breathe faster than adults, and they therefore inhale more air as well as more of the pollutants in the air. Studies have shown that children inhale three times more pollutants per unit of body weight than do adults. This intake is particularly harmful because young lungs need clean air for optimal development.

Babies of parents who smoke at home have much more pneumonia and bronchitis than do babies of nonsmoking parents, particularly in their first year of life. Studies show that the mother's smoking has the most impact on the child's lung function, probably because the mother is usually the primary caregiver. And since women are smoking more, more children are affected.

Asthma, the most frequent cause of school absenteeism from a chronic condition, can be a serious lung disease. The rise in deaths from asthma may be associated with exposure to the combined effect of cigarette smoke and air pollution. Even among nonasthmatic children, researchers have found that respiratory illnesses occur more than twice as often among children whose parents smoke at home as among those with nonsmoking parents.

■ **Exploring Your Emotions**

How do you feel when you see teenagers smoking? Pregnant women? Older people? Are your feelings related to personal experiences you've had?

One study divided 441 nonsmokers into those with a history of allergies and those without. Of both groups, 70 percent suffered from eye irritations caused by smoke. The allergic group suffered the most symptoms, from breathlessness to headaches, nasal congestion, and cough. Even among the nonallergic group, 30 percent developed headaches and nasal discomfort, while 25 percent developed coughs.

VITAL STATISTICS

Facts about Smoking

According to statistics gathered by the Coalition of Smoking or Health:

- In 1915, most tobacco was used for pipes, cigars, and chewing tobacco, and cigarette smoking was uncommon. Lung cancer was virtually unknown.
- Today, about 30 percent of the adult population smokes cigarettes, and 120,000 people die of lung cancer every year.
- In 1964—the year of the first Surgeon General's Report linking smoking with heart disease—42 percent of adult Americans smoked. Since 1964, the smoking rate in the U.S. has dropped by 20 percent
- 92 percent of all smokers say they would like to quit.
- 90 percent of all smokers began to smoke before the age of 19; 60 percent began before the age of 14.

- 20 percent of all high school seniors smoke. About 40 percent of high school seniors do not believe there is a great health risk in smoking.
- 350,000 Americans die every year from diseases caused by cigarette smoking, representing one in seven deaths.
- 1,000 people quit smoking every day—by dying. That is equivalent to two fully loaded jumbo jets crashing every day, with no survivors.
- The tobacco industry spends $2.5 billion per year on advertising and promotion to reach smokers. That is approximately $40 for every smoker—or $10 for every man, woman, and child.
- The tobacco industry is the largest advertiser in print media and outdoor (billboard) advertising. The top four advertisers in

these media are cigarette companies.
- In 1985, per capita consumption of cigarettes in the United States was 3,384 cigarettes per person—representing $35 billion spent by consumers for cigarettes. In 1986, 600 million cigarettes were sold in the United States.
- It costs the American economy approximately $65 billion a year to cover cigarette-related health care costs and loss of worker productivity.
- According to recent polls, 30 percent of the American public is unaware that smoking causes heart disease. Nearly 50 percent of women polled did not know that smoking during pregnancy increases the risk of stillbirths and miscarriage.

From *Healthline*, February 1988.

Smoking and Pregnancy   Smoking during pregnancy can seriously harm both the mother and the unborn baby. It is especially harmful for mothers who are very young or older, or who are poorly nourished, anemic, or have other health problems. These harmful effects include increased risk of spontaneous abortion and stillbirths. If the baby is born alive, it runs an increased risk of congenital abnormalities and premature birth, and its birth weight is likely to be lower than normal. Low birth weights are associated with increased mortality and a variety of diseases, especially infections.

In addition, evidence suggests that infants born to smoking mothers are more likely to die from sudden infant death syndrome (SIDS), also known as crib death, and are more likely to show long-term impairments in physical growth and intellectual development. Moreover, as if these problems weren't enough, animal research evidence indicates that certain cancers are more common in animals that were exposed as fetuses to cigarette smoke.

What Can Be Done?

There are probably no safe levels of tobacco smoke inhalation. Researchers have found an increased risk of lung cancer in nonsmoking women married to men who smoke. This is not surprising, because we know that ingredients in tobacco smoke cause lung cancer at a higher rate among smokers. Given these findings, nonsmokers should not hesitate to assert their right to breathe clean air, free from harmful and irritating tobacco smoke (see Figure 9-2 for a nonsmoker's Bill of Rights). This right supersedes the right to smoke when the two conflict. Nonsmokers have the right to express—firmly but politely—their adverse reactions to tobacco smoke. They have the right to voice their objections when smokers light up. Nonsmokers have the right to act through legislative channels, social pressures, or any other legitimate means—as individuals or in groups—to prevent or

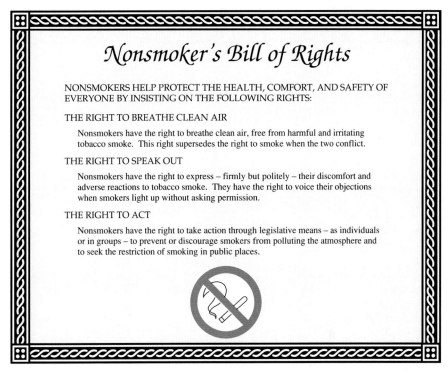

Figure 9-2   Nonsmoker's Bill of Rights.

discourage smokers from polluting the environment and to seek the restrictions of smoking in public places. Refer to the box titled "What Can Nonsmokers Do?" for ideas on a few things you can do.

Action at the Federal Level   The Comprehensive Smoking Act was signed into law in 1984. One of the act's major provisions replaced the old health warning on cigarette packages ("The U.S. Surgeon General has determined that cigarette smoking is dangerous to your health") with the new warnings shown in Table 9-5. The act also requires that cigarette companies disclose to the U.S. Department of Health and Human Services a complete list of all chemicals and other ingredients added to cigarettes during the manufacturing process.

■ **Exploring Your Emotions**

How do you feel when someone near you lights up a cigarette? What knowledge or experience influences your feelings? If it bothers you but you have difficulty asserting yourself, what feelings are making you uncomfortable? Can you think of ways to deal with them?

Also at the federal level, Congress permanently extended the 16 cents excise tax on cigarettes in 1986. Tax

bills introduced in 1985 removed the tax deduction for cigarette advertising and promotion activities, such as sponsorship of sports events and music festivals. In addition, one federal court and three federal agencies have now held that sensitive nonsmokers are "handicapped persons" and can take legal action to require employers to provide a "reasonable accommodation" to the handicap.

Politics, Tobacco, and Tobacco Interests   More and more restrictions are being placed on smoking in public buildings and in other public places. After a long, hard-fought battle with the powerful Tobacco Institute, Congress banned smoking on all domestic airline flights within the continental limits of the United States. These efforts have been somewhat successful in reducing cigarette smoking in some age groups, but they are opposed by an impressive concentration of economic, social, and political power. Tobacco interests wield enough power to keep the U.S. government subsidizing them with millions of dollars each year despite the fact that the government is supporting an aggressive antitobacco campaign.

As smoking has declined among better-educated, wealthier segments of the American population, tobacco companies have redirected their marketing efforts toward

Table 9-5 Health Warnings Required on Tobacco Packages and Advertisements in the United States

CIGARETTES

Warning(s)	Effective Dates	Packages	Advertisements, Including Outdoor Billboards
CAUTION: Cigarette Smoking May Be Hazardous to Your Health.	January 1, 1966–October 31, 1970	X	
WARNING: The Surgeon General Has Determined That Cigarette Smoking Is Dangerous to Your Health.	November 1, 1970–October 11, 1985	X	
	1972–October 11, 1985		X
SURGEON GENERAL'S WARNING: Smoking Causes Lung Cancer, Heart Disease, Emphysema, and May Complicate Pregnancy. SURGEON GENERAL'S WARNING: Quitting Smoking Now Greatly Reduces Serious Risks to Your Health. SURGEON GENERAL'S WARNING: Smoking by Pregnant Women May Result in Fetal Injury, Premature Birth, and Low Birth Weight. SURGEON GENERAL'S WARNING: Cigarette Smoke Contains Carbon Monoxide.	October 12, 1985–present	X	X

SMOKELESS TOBACCO

Warnings	Effective Dates	Packages	Advertisements, Not Including Outdoor Billboards
WARNING: This product may cause mouth cancer. WARNING: This product may cause gum disease and tooth loss. WARNING: This product is not a safe alternative to cigarettes.	February 27, 1987–present	X	X

WARNING:

This product is not a safe alternative to cigarettes

Smokeless tobacco warnings must be in circle-and-arrow format.

Source: Surgeon General's Report, 1988.

What Can Nonsmokers Do?

- Tell family, friends, co-workers, students, and strangers that you mind if they smoke.
- Put stickers and signs in your home, car, classroom, and office. Request seating in nonsmoking sections when you travel. Wear buttons.

- Ask your doctor and dentist or health professional to restrict smoking in their waiting rooms and to establish no-smoking regulations in all health care facilities, including hospitals.

- Contact the American Lung Association, the American Cancer Society, or the American Heart Association to discuss ways to protect nonsmokers.

minorities, the poor, and young women, populations among whom smoking rates are still high. The practice of targeting specific segments of the smoking market has become extremely controversial, especially when the segment has unusually high risks for the fatal diseases caused by smoking. Recently, the R. J. Reynolds Tobacco Company canceled its plans to market Uptown, a brand of cigarettes designed to appeal to blacks, after the U.S.

Secretary of Health and Human Services accused the company of "promoting a culture of cancer." The American Cancer Society saw the Uptown campaign as an escalation in the exploitation of blacks, who are more likely to smoke than whites and who suffer the health effects of smoking in numbers far greater than their proportion in the population.

Tobacco marketers have been trying to appeal specif-

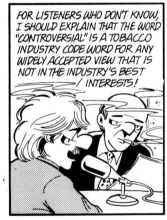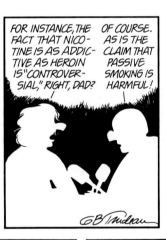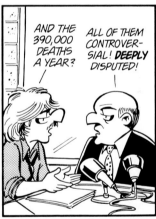
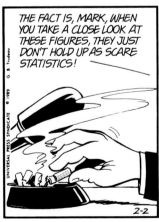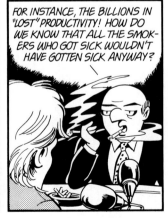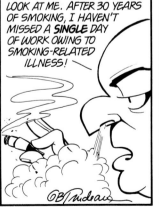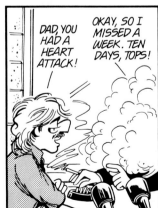

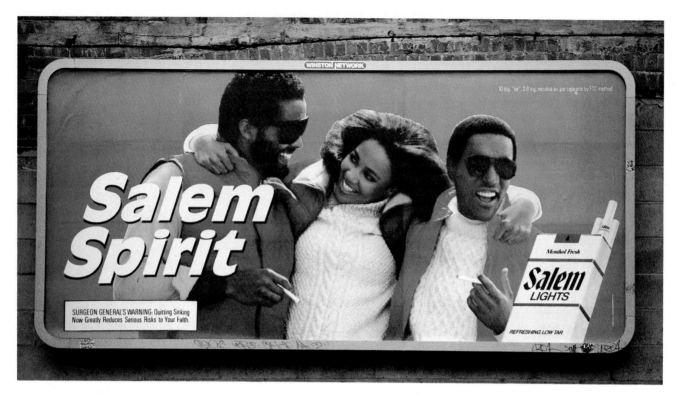

With business shrinking, tobacco companies are targeting narrower segments of the market and mounting aggressive advertising campaigns to lure smokers away from competing brands. Half to two-thirds of all black smokers smoke menthol cigarettes, so ads for the three leading menthol brands are often aimed at this population.

ically to women for years, usually by connecting smoking with thinness (the dominant women's brand is Virginia Slims). The Reynolds company recently targeted a certain segment of the women's market with their brand Dakota, aimed at 18- to 20-year-old women—the only group of Americans whose rate of smoking continues to increase. With their immensely profitable industry shrinking, to-bacco companies are concentrating on appealing to nar-rower and narrower market segments with an ever-increasing array of brands and styles—over 350 in all. As companies compete for customers in the years ahead, more social, ethical, and legal questions are likely to be raised about cigarette manufacture and marketing.

How Can a Tobacco User Quit?

Studies have shown that most ex-smokers quit on their own without participating in a particular program. Yet some programs may be more helpful than others and may vary in their ability to help different kinds of people.

Types of Programs   Most stop-smoking programs em-phasize one of various pharmacological, psychological,

or health education approaches. Some combine more than one approach. The health education programs often assume that if a person learns the facts about smoking he or she will make the rational decision to stop smoking. But human behavior is quite complex and not necessarily rational, and the failure rates of these programs tend to be quite high. One reason is that nicotine's powerful ad-dicting qualities often overwhelm the smoker's conscious desire to quit.

■ **Exploring Your Emotions**

Restrictions on smoking are increasing in our society. Do you think they're fair? Do they infringe on people's rights? Do they go too far or not far enough?

Most smoking programs treat quitting as an event and assume that when the program is over, the smoking problem will also be over. And, in fact, most programs can demonstrate a high quit rate initially, but after one year most people have started smoking again. These pro-grams provide a social environment with psychological supports that no longer function for the smoker when the program ends. The behavioral reinforcers that main-

---

Nicotine Gum: Hope for Smokers

For people who really want to quit smoking but haven't been able to, nicotine gum may offer some hope. For use under medical supervision, nicotine gum is marketed as a prescription product under the brand name Nicorette by Merrell Dow Pharmaceuticals, Inc., a subsidiary of the Dow Chemical Company. A 96-piece package of Nicorette costs about $20. Each piece of gum contains 2 mg of nicotine, which, when the gum is chewed slowly, is absorbed through the lining of the mouth over a 20- to 30-minute period. Chewing one piece of gum per hour produces blood nicotine levels comparable to those obtained with hourly cigarette smoking. Any nicotine that is swallowed has little effect on the body. The gum provides a substitute for oral activity and can prevent nicotine withdrawal symptoms, allowing the smoker to break the behavioral habits of smoking without suffering the discomforts of nicotine withdrawal.

Most users find that 8 to 10 pieces of gum a day are sufficient to control their craving for cigarettes. Side effects are common but mild. Most of them disappear by themselves within a week or can be controlled by chewing more slowly. After a few months,

use of the gum is tapered off and stopped.

An FDA advisory committee that reviewed the evidence concluded that nicotine gum increases the likelihood of smoking cessation when used together with appropriate counseling. The product is most suitable for smokers in whom the addictive component is strongest—those who smoke 30 or more cigarettes per day or those who find that the most difficult cigarette to give up is the first one in the morning.

Nicotine gum is not a "miracle" drug, but it can be very helpful to those who have a strong desire to become nonsmokers for good. Recent studies involving hard-core smokers found that success rates using nicotine gum and counseling were three times as high as with counseling alone or with counseling and placebo gum containing nicotine in nonabsorbable form. Perhaps one day nicotine gum will also be approved for use as a temporary substitute for smoking in situations like airplane trips or meetings, so that smokers can maintain their nicotine levels without disturbing the people around them.

Merrell Dow supplies doctors with detailed information on how to select and prepare patients for

using the gum. Users receive a 24-page booklet and, upon request, two newsletters about smoking cessation and nicotine gum treatment. Doctors are being urged to provide at least one follow-up visit per month over the treatment period (usually three to four months).

If you smoke, there is certainly good reason to stop. No matter how long you have smoked, it is still beneficial to quit. During the first day after quitting, the heart and lungs begin to repair the damage caused by cigarette smoke. Smoker's cough usually disappears within a few weeks, energy and endurance may increase, and taste and smell may return for foods that haven't been enjoyed for years. After ten to fifteen years, the risk of dying from heart and blood vessel disease goes down to the level of nonsmokers. The risk of lung cancer decreases, and so does the incidence of respiratory infections and lung tissue destruction, which are responsible for emphysema. Given these health statistics, smokers should consider using any means necessary—including nicotine gum—to quit.

Source: Stephen Barrett. 1985. Nicotine gum: New hope for smokers. *Healthline*, May.

---

tained abstinence are no longer present. Learning theory suggests that when the reinforcers disappear, so does the behavior. Giving up smoking (or other drug dependencies) is a long-term, intricate process. Heavy smokers who say they've just stopped "cold turkey" aren't revealing the thinking and struggling and other mental processes that contributed to their final conquest over this powerful addiction.

Pharmacological programs often substitute nicotine-containing substances such as chewing gum. Some of

these programs are effective when combined with psychological and social reinforcement. However, success rates are usually lower than 25 percent after a one-year follow-up. Their major drawback is that nicotine addiction remains untreated. When these nicotine-containing substitutes for cigarettes are discontinued, many people begin to smoke again. In addition, many people don't find these substitutes very satisfying and complain about side effects. (See the box "Nicotine Gum: Hope for Smokers" for more details.)

The lengthy process of giving up smoking is influenced by many factors, and none, unfortunately, is highly predictive of success. Stop-smoking programs that combine several approaches have the most promise. These programs, which sometimes operate in industrial settings, may attract people who would not otherwise participate in a smoking clinic. They frequently alter the social environment by setting up demands and expectations that make smoking undesirable. Peer support is often a powerful influence in behavior, as witnessed by the experience of Alcoholics Anonymous. The persistent encouragement of colleagues, family, and friends can be critical in giving up drug dependencies. Providing individual or group incentives can be combined with other techniques. Feedback on cardiac and respiratory status can be a compelling method to help some people stop smoking. And documenting improvement in vital functions after the person has quit smoking can continue to provide positive reinforcement. A behavioral approach to quitting is described at the end of this chapter.

Benefits of Quitting   Studies have shown that when smokers stop, a number of changes occur. Food is absorbed more efficiently, appetite increases, and the senses of taste and smell improve. In some people these changes lead to a slight weight gain—but they are signs of improved health. Cardiovascular changes include improved circulation (in hands and feet especially), reduced heart rate, lowered blood pressure, increased HDL (the good cholesterol), and increased heart efficiency during rest and exercise. Many ex-smokers report more energy, increased alertness, and need for less sleep. Because of increased microcirculation in the skin, some people report improved facial complexion.

■ **Exploring Your Emotions**

If you are a smoker and have tried to quit and failed, how did it make you feel? How did you deal with your feelings?

As one might expect, respiratory changes are often pronounced. An immediate improvement appears in the efficiency of oxygen exchange between the lungs and the circulatory system, maximal breath capacity increases, and breathing rate decreases. Gradually the "smoker's cough" declines and long-term respiratory conditions—such as bronchitis, emphysema, and asthma—improve.

The younger people are when they stop smoking, the more pronounced the health improvements. And these improvements gradually but invariably increase as the period of nonsmoking increases.

Summary

- Smoking is the largest preventable cause of ill health and death in the United States. Nevertheless, addiction to nicotine causes millions to continue smoking.

Why People Use Tobacco

- Regular tobacco use is not just a psychological habit but also a matter of physical dependence on nicotine. This addiction requires keeping a continuous amount of nicotine circulating in the blood and going to the brain. Secondary reinforcers—habits associated with smoking—make quitting even more difficult.
- People who begin smoking are usually imitating others; they may have low self-esteem or may be seeking stimulation or relief from unpleasant moods; despite awareness of risks, they rationalize their behavior.
- Tobacco users often use other psychoactive drugs; coffee and alcohol use enhance withdrawal effects of nicotine. Wealthier, more educated people are less likely to smoke; although cigarette, pipe, and cigar smoking have been decreasing, use of chewing tobacco and snuff increased from 1970 to 1987.

Health Hazards

- Tobacco smoke is made up of particles of several hundred different chemicals, many of which are toxic. When the particles condense, they form tar.
- Some chemicals in tobacco are carcinogenic; others irritate the respiratory system, causing smoker's cough and other symptoms.
- Nicotine, a psychoactive drug, causes a "lift" in body metabolism; it enters the brain through the bloodstream and triggers the release of catecholamines, which cause both the blood pressure and heart rate to go up.
- Carbon monoxide in cigarette smoke displaces oxygen in red blood cells, depleting the body's supply of oxygen.

- Symptoms of nicotine poisoning include dizziness; faintness; rapid pulse; cold, clammy skin; and sometimes nausea, vomiting, and diarrhea. The dosage of nicotine usually determines whether it acts as a stimulant or a tranquilizer.
- Nicotine stimulates the cerebral cortex and the adrenal glands (which discharge adrenalin); by raising blood pressure, increasing the heart rate, and constricting blood vessels, it forces the heart to pump more blood—which can strain the heart muscle if the coronary arteries are already damaged.
- Smoking depresses hunger contractions, causes the liver to release glycogen, and dulls taste buds—all resulting in a decrease in appetite.
- The total amount of tobacco smoke inhaled is a key factor in disease.
- Coronary heart disease is the most widespread cause of death for cigarette smokers. Smoking's reduction of high-density lipoproteins probably promotes plaque formation and speeds blood clotting. The risks of CHD decrease rapidly when smoking is stopped. Cigarette smoking has also been linked to stroke, aortic aneurysm, and pulmonary heart disease.
- Cigarette smoking is the primary cause of lung cancer; the risk increases with amount of tobacco smoked, years spent smoking, and age at which smoking started. Lung tissue repairs itself if smoking is stopped. Smoking is linked to many other cancers as well.
- Smoking is the primary cause of emphysema, a condition in which the walls of the air sacs in the lungs lose their elasticity and are gradually destroyed; as a result, the lungs can't obtain oxygen or remove carbon dioxide. The heart may become enlarged; the disease is not reversible.
- In chronic bronchitis the bronchial tubes are inflamed; the irritated cell lining secretes mucus, which causes congestion and a chronic cough. A high risk of lung cancer is associated with chronic bronchitis. Exposure to air pollution in conjunction with cigarette smoking increases the risk of chronic obstructive lung disease.
- Cigarette smoking also damages the cilia in the bronchial tubes, eventually killing them, and hinders the work of macrophages.
- Damage from smoking is not always permanent, and lung function usually improves when a person quits.
- Cigarette smokers are more likely to develop peptic ulcers and to die from them than are nonsmokers. Also associated with smoking are gum disorders, premature skin wrinkling and baldness, and allergies. Tobacco use leads to lower life expectancy and to a diminished quality of life.

Effects of Smoking on the Nonsmoker

- Sidestream smoke contains more toxic chemicals than mainstream smoke although nonsmokers don't inhale them in as concentrated a form as smokers do. Sidestream smoke is a health hazard for nonsmokers.
- Babies and young children inhale more air than adults do and so take in more pollutants; children whose parents smoke are especially susceptible to respiratory diseases.
- Smoking during pregnancy increases the risk of spontaneous abortion, stillbirth, congenital abnormalities, premature birth, and low birth weight. Crib death and long-term impairments in physical and intellectual development are also risks.

What Can Be Done?

- Because there are probably no safe levels of tobacco smoke inhalation, smokers need to assert their rights to breathe clean air, using legislative channels, social pressures, or other means to discourage smokers from polluting the air.
- In 1984 Congress replaced the warning on cigarette packages with stronger ones. Congress has also extended taxes on cigarettes, removed tax deductions for cigarette companies, and has further restricted smoking on airplanes.
- Federal efforts to reduce cigarette smoking are undermined by the forces of the tobacco industry, which is itself subsidized by the federal government. Recently tobacco companies have aimed marketing programs at narrower segments of the population in which smoking is still popular.

How Can a Tobacco User Quit?

- Although most ex-smokers quit on their own, some smokers benefit from stop-smoking programs. Learning the facts about smoking isn't enough because the addictive powers of nicotine are overwhelming. Giving up smoking is a long-term process that must deal with reinforcers and other mental processes.
- Pharmacological programs don't treat the underlying nicotine addiction; they need to be combined with psychological and social reinforcement. Combination programs usually have the best success.
- Cardiovascular and respiratory functions improve when smoking stops.

Take Action

1. Look through some popular magazines and examine the cigarette ads. What market are they targeting? How do they try to appeal to their audience? How do the advertisers deal with the Surgeon General's warning? Write a short essay describing your findings.

2. Make a tour of the public facilities in your community and on your campus, such as movie theaters, auditoriums, business and school offices, and classrooms. What kinds of restrictions on smoking do these places have? In your opinion, are they appropriate? If you feel more restrictions are in order, write a letter to the editor of your school or local newspaper making your case. Support it with convincing arguments and appropriate facts.

3. Draw up a list of statements you might make to a smoker in various situations. Consider carefully how you can be assertive rather than aggressive or passive, how you can increase the likelihood of compliance by being courteous, and how you can make sure your statements don't threaten the person's dignity. The next time you're in an appropriate situation, use one of your statements. If it doesn't have the desired effect, think about why and modify it for the next time.

Behavior Change Strategy

Quitting Smoking

If you are a smoker and would like to quit, begin by scoring yourself on the statements listed in the box "For Smokers Only: Why Do You Smoke?" Clues and information about the reasons you smoke, the ways you respond to nicotine addiction, and other aspects of your behavior will be helpful as you plan a strategy for quitting. You may also want to review the general discussion of behavior management plans given in Chapter 1. Once you're ready, think of quitting smoking as being divided into three phases: (1) preparing for quitting, (2) quitting, and (3) maintaining nonsmoking behavior.

Preparing for Quitting   Preparation for quitting involves collecting personal smoking information in a detailed smoking diary, as described in Chapter 1. Notice that the diary enables you to collect two major types of information—cigarettes smoked and smoking urges. Part of the job is to identify patterns of smoking that are connected with routine situations (for example, the coffee break smoke, the after-dinner cigarette, the tension reduction cigarette, and so on). Use this information in combination with your self-assessment scores to discover the behavior chains involved in your smoking habit.

The second major task of this preparation phase is to learn how to use nonsmoking relaxation methods. Many smokers find that they use cigarettes to help them unwind in tense situations or to relax at other times. Because smoking performs this function, it will be difficult to eliminate unless you find effective substitutes. Since it takes time to become proficient at using progressive relaxation, initial practice of this procedure is recommended early in the process of preparation. Refer to the more detailed discussion of progressive relaxation found in Chapter 2.

Quitting   Quitting smoking is the first goal most smokers want to reach, but staying off cigarettes is the ultimate objective. Quitting involves establishing a personal quit contract that specifies the day and time when you will stop smoking as well as possible rewards for quitting.

When drawing up a personal contract, smokers are usually torn between quitting abruptly (the so-called cold turkey approach) or through gradual reduction (one step at a time). Research favors the abrupt approach but with enough time set aside to learn and practice effective quitting skills.

Maintaining Nonsmoking   Maintaining nonsmoking over time is the ultimate goal of any stop-smoking program, and it is the third phase of this program. The lingering smoking urges that remain once you have quit are the targets of work and planning because they will cause relapse if left unattended. Just as there are patterns to smoking, there are also patterns to lingering smoking urges. Keep track of these urges in your smoking diary. Patterns are often linked to situations in what seem like simple and innocuous ways. If you always used to sit on the couch every evening to read the paper and have a cigarette, then even after you have quit smoking you may have smoking urges in that situation. By changing something in the situation—sitting in another chair or reading in another room—you may be able to break the strength of past associations. In the same way you will have to practice a new repertoire of non-smoking skills if stress or boredom is a strong smoking-urge "signal" for you. Use relaxation procedures, take a brisk walk, have a stick of gum, or substitute some other activity for smoking.

Cognitions, too, can be a source of considerable trouble during the maintenance phase of becoming an ex-smoker. Testing yourself ("I can prove that I'm strong; I'll put the pack out in front of me to prove my strength") and remembering cigarettes as long-lost friends or part of a better time in your life ("the good old days") can erode your sense of resolve and your skills in resisting lingering smoking urges. Identifying and listing personal prosmoking self-statements ("It's probably not that bad for me—I'm still young" or "I'll just have one and then no more") can be very

helpful in alerting you to how you can unwittingly undermine your own progress.

Finally, keep track of the emerging benefits that come from having quit smoking. Items that might appear on such a list include improved stamina, an increased sense of pride at having kicked a personally troublesome problem, improved sense of taste and smell, no more smoker's cough, and so on. And be sure to reward yourself for every week you stick to your plan. You deserve it for kicking a powerful addiction!

Selected Bibliography

Burros, M. 1988. The smoking law revisited. *New York Times,* October 12.

Cancer Facts and Figures. 1990. New York: American Cancer Society.

Eriksen, M. P., C. A. LeMaistre, and G. R. Newell. 1988. The health hazards of passive smoking. *Annual Review of Public Health* 9:47–70.

Heart Facts. 1990. New York: American Heart Association.

A Lifetime of Freedom from Smoking. 1989. New York: American Lung Association.

U. S. Surgeon General. 1989. *Reducing the Health Consequences of Smoking.* Bethesda, Md.: U.S. Department of Health and Human Services.

Recommended Readings

Boyd, G., and C. M. Darbey, eds. 1990. *Smokeless Tobacco Use in the United States.* NCI Monograph, National Cancer Institute. *A comprehensive examination of the role of smokeless tobacco in causing cancer.*

Journal of the American Medical Association, January 6, 1989. *This issue of JAMA is devoted mostly to smoking and includes the following articles: Trends in cigarette smoking in the United States, the cost-effectiveness of counseling smokers to quit, and many others.*

Leventhal, H., K. Glynn, and R. Fleming. 1987. Is the smoking decision an "informed choice"? Effect of smoking risk factors on smoking beliefs. *Journal of the American Medical Association* 257(24):3373–3376. *A cogent exploration of the kinds of apparent psychological options people have and their willingness to engage in detrimental behaviors.*

Schelling, T. C. 1986. Economics and cigarettes. *Preventive Medicine* 15(5):549–560. *A discussion of how politics and the marketplace drive the consumption of cigarettes.*

Contents

Making Connections

The use of alcohol pervades our culture so thoroughly that no one is immune to its effects. Although personal and social expectations vary, the reality is that virtually everyone, at some point, is faced with a decision about whether, what, or how much to drink. Knowing your options is the best guarantee that you will make the right choice. The scenarios presented on these pages describe alcohol-related situations in which people have to use information, make a decision, or choose a course of action. As you read them, imagine yourself in each situation and consider what you would do. After you've finished the chapter, read the scenarios again and see if what you've learned has changed how you would think, feel, or act in each situation.

Your fraternity is doing its usual planning for the Homecoming weekend party, which includes huge quantities of beer, wine, and hard liquor. During past Homecomings, some outrageous things have been done at your house. This year, you've been asked by your college administration to take measures to control your guests. They've specifically asked you to limit the consumption of alcohol and to serve some nonalcoholic beverages. What can you serve to comply with this request and yet ensure that people have a good time?

You like your uncle Joe a lot when he's not drinking, but he's hard to take when he's under the influence. He's spoiled innumerable Thanksgivings, Christmases, and other family celebrations with his drunken behavior, which is sometimes angry, sometimes weepy, and always loud. You're going home for the holidays and really feel compelled to say or do something about it, for the sake of both your family and your uncle Joe. Your mother has always said that he takes after their father and that there's nothing you can do about it. Is it true that you can't influence him? Should you say something to him, and if so, what?

10
The Responsible Use of Alcohol

You wanted everyone to have a good time at a party you gave in your apartment, so you made sure there was plenty of beer and wine. But now, as your guests are leaving, you realize that one person who is quite drunk has to drive himself and his date home. Other guests are expressing concern about them to you and urging you to insist that they stay overnight. They even say you should take the man's car keys. You're not sure you have the right to do that. After all, he's an adult and freely made the choice to drink as much as he did. What are your responsibilities in this situation? Should you intercede, or should you let them go?

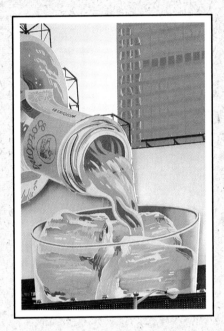

Your sister refrained from drinking any alcohol throughout her pregnancy, but once the baby was born she started drinking beer again, usually one a day. The last time you visited her, you saw that she was sipping a beer while she was nursing the baby. She explained that her doctor told her it would help her relax and "let down" her milk. "So no alcohol goes into the milk?" you ask her. She's not sure about that, but she thinks it probably doesn't or else her doctor wouldn't have recommended it. Does the alcohol she drinks reach her milk, or does it all get metabolized in her body? Is there any information or advice you can give your sister?

You didn't realize it was getting so late and find that you're still feeling slightly drunk when it's time to drive your moped home from a Friday night gathering at a local pub. A friend orders you a cup of strong coffee and urges you to eat a lot of potato chips to speed absorption of the alcohol in your stomach. She says if you take several deep breaths and do a few jumping jacks when you get outside, you'll be just fine. Is she right that these are good activities to help you sober up?

People long ago recognized the power of alcoholic beverages: The "spirit" changed feelings and behavior. Ever since, **alcohol** has had a somewhat contradictory role in human life. It has been associated with good times, cheerfulness, and conviviality, but it is also associated with escape, with blotting out the world, with inch-by-inch suicide, and with general self-destructiveness. Many of our slang expressions for **intoxication** reflect its less positive aspects—"blasted," "smashed," "bombed," "wasted."

Alcohol is probably the oldest drug in the world; we have evidence that beer and berry wine were used at least by 6400 B.C., and probably even earlier. Alcohol has been used in religious ceremonies, in feasts and celebrations, and as a medicine for thousands of years. Beer is a mild intoxicant brewed from a mixture of grains. Wines are made by **fermenting** the juices of grapes or other fruits.

Once the **distillation** process was developed (about A.D. 800), the spirit could be concentrated in a purer and more potent form. It was called *al-kuhl*, an Arabic word meaning "finely divided spirit." Throughout history alcohol has been more popular than any other drug in the Western world in spite of a great variety and number of prohibitions against it. In fact, forbidding the use of alcohol seems only to make it more popular. Even the newer **psychoactive drugs** have not diminished that popularity.

■ **Exploring Your Emotions**

How was alcohol used in your family when you were growing up, and what are your associations with it? Was it used for family celebrations? Was there alcohol abuse in your family? If so, how did you react at the time? How do you feel about it now?

Most of us think of alcohol the way it's portrayed in ads—as part of good times at the beach, social occasions, and elegant gatherings. Used in moderation, alcohol can enhance social occasions by loosening inhibitions and creating a pleasant feeling of relaxation. Among some people, alcohol is an integral part of celebrations and special events. But the use of alcohol can also be an unhealthy adaptation. Like other drugs, alcohol has definite physiological effects on the body that can impair functioning in the short term and cause devastating damage in the long term. For some, alcohol becomes an addiction, leading to a life of recovery or to debilitation and death.

The use of alcohol is a complex issue, one that demands conscious thought and informed decisions. In our society, some people choose to drink in moderation, some choose not to drink at all, and others realize too late that they've made an unwise choice—when they become dependent on alcohol, are involved in an alcohol-related accident, or simply wake up to discover they've done something they regret. This chapter discusses the complexities of alcohol use and provides information that will help you make the choice that's right for you.

The Nature of Alcohol

Have you ever noticed that one of your friends *seems* to be able to drink throughout a party without being noticeably affected, while another friend seems quite drunk after only an hour? Can some people "handle" alcohol better than others? Is it possible to drink a safe amount of alcohol? Many of the misconceptions about alcohol and how it affects people can be clarified by understanding the chemistry of alcohol and how it's metabolized in the body.

The Chemistry of Alcohol   Ethyl alcohol, in various concentrations, is the common psychoactive ingredient in wine, beer, and what are called *hard liquors*. The concentration of alcohol in table wines is about 9 to 14 percent. Other wines such as sherry, port, and Madeira contain about 20 percent alcohol. These types are called *fortified wines* because distilled alcohol has been added to them. The stronger alcoholic beverages, such as gin, whiskey, brandy, and rum and liqueurs, are made by distilling brewed or fermented grains or other products. These beverages contain (usually) from 35 to 50 percent alcohol, a concentration about ten times that of beer. Except for kcalories, these beverages have little or no nutritional value.

Alcohol concentration in a beverage is indicated by the **proof value**, which is two times the percentage concentration. If a beverage is 100 proof, it contains 50 percent

---

Alcohol   The intoxicating ingredient in fermented liquors. A colorless, pungent liquid.

Intoxication   The state of being mentally affected by a chemical.

Fermented   Describes a substance in which complex molecules have been broken down by the action of yeast or bacteria. Fermentation of certain substances produces alcohol.

Distillation   The process of heating a mixture and recondensing the vapor. This process intensifies the mixture's properties and eliminates impurities. Distillation is used in manufacturing whiskey and brandy.

Psychoactive drugs   Drugs that affect the brain or nervous system.

Proof value   Two times of percentage of alcohol.

Blood alcohol concentration (BAC)   The amount of alcohol in the blood in terms of weight per unit volume. Also referred to as blood alcohol level (BAL).

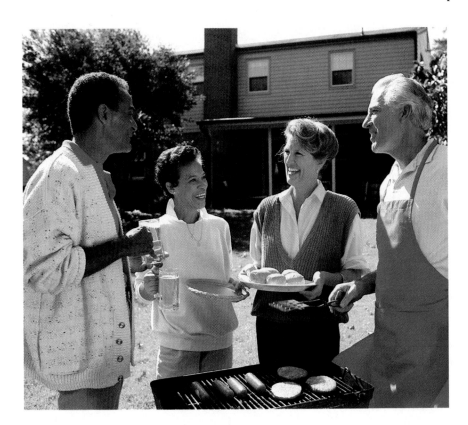

Alcoholic beverages like beer and wine are an integral part of social occasions for many people. A central nervous system depressant, alcohol acts to loosen inhibitions; when used in moderation, it tends to make people feel more relaxed and sociable.

alcohol. Two ounces of 100-proof whiskey contain one ounce of pure alcohol. The proof value of the stronger alcoholic beverages can usually be found on the bottle labels. A convenient way of remembering alcohol concentrations is that the usual 12-ounce bottle of beer, 5-ounce glass of table wine, and cocktail with 1½ ounces of liquor all contain the same amount of alcohol—about 0.6 ounces.

It is important to know that there are different kinds of alcohol. In this chapter the term *alcohol* refers to ethyl alcohol, which is the only kind of alcohol that can be drunk. Other kinds of alcohol such as methanol (wood alcohol) and isopropyl alcohol (rubbing alcohol) are also intoxicating, but they can cause blindness or other serious problems when consumed in even low doses.

Metabolism   How quickly someone becomes intoxicated and the level of intoxication depend not only on the amount of alcohol consumed but also on personal factors like weight and sex and on circumstantial factors like amount of food eaten. These all figure in the process of alcohol metabolism.

Blood Alcohol Concentration   Alcohol is absorbed into the bloodstream from the stomach and small intestine. How long absorption from the stomach takes depends on the amount, type, and proof of the beverage, the time taken to drink it, and whether or not there is food in the stom-

ach. For example, a glass of champagne drunk quickly on an empty stomach will be absorbed at a more rapid rate (and could have greater immediate effects) than a larger amount of sherry sipped slowly after a large meal. Food in the stomach slows the absorption process by acting as a barrier between the alcohol and the stomach wall.

Another factor affecting rate of alcohol absorption in the stomach is whether the drinker is male or female. Recent medical research has shown that women become drunk more quickly than men do because their stomachs are less able to neutralize alcohol. Women have less of the stomach enzyme that metabolizes alcohol, so more of the alcohol goes directly into their bloodstreams through the stomach wall. The effect is even more pronounced among alcoholic women because their stomachs apparently stop digesting alcohol at all. For them, drinking has the same effect as injecting alcohol intravenously.

Alcohol not absorbed in the stomach moves with any other undigested stomach contents into the small intestine. Here, absorption is rapid and complete because the walls of the small intestine have a large surface area and are highly permeable to alcohol. Neither the **blood alcohol concentration (BAC)** nor the presence of food affects absorption from the small intestine. Usually all alcohol is absorbed before it has the chance to reach the colon.

After alcohol is absorbed through the wall of the stom-

Table 10-1 Effects of Alcohol		
Blood Alcohol Concentrations (Percent)	Common Behavioral Effects	Hours Required for Alcohol to Be Metabolized
0.00–0.05	Slight change in feelings—usually relaxation and euphoria. Decreased alertness.	2–3
0.05–0.10	Emotional lability with exaggerated feelings and behavior. Reduced social inhibitions. Impairment of reaction time and fine motor coordination. Increasingly impaired during driving. Legally drunk at 0.08 in several states and .10 in many others.	4–6
0.10–0.15	Unsteadiness in standing and walking. Loss of peripheral vision. Driving is extremely dangerous. Legally drunk at 0.15 in all states.	6–10
0.15–0.30	Staggering gait. Slurred speech. Pain and other sensory perceptions greatly impaired.	10–24
More than 0.30	Stupor or unconsciousness. Anesthesia. Death possible at 0.35 and above.	More than 24

Source: Adapted from U.S. Department of Health and Human Services, 1989.

ach or small intestine, it is distributed via the blood throughout the tissues of the body. In general, less alcohol becomes concentrated in fatty tissues. Since women usually have a higher percentage of fat at any given body weight than men do, more alcohol remains in their bloodstream than is the case for men. This is another factor accounting for higher BACs in women when the same amount of alcohol is consumed.

As the blood circulates through the liver, a certain amount of the alcohol passes into the liver cells, where it is transformed into energy and other products. The rate of this metabolic process stays about the same in each individual. A person who weighs 150 pounds and has normal liver function **metabolizes** on the average about 0.3 ounce of alcohol per hour—about half a bottle of beer.

About 2 to 10 percent of alcohol is not metabolized in the liver, but is excreted unchanged, mostly via the lungs and kidneys. This is the basis of breath and urine analyses for alcohol levels and the reason for the telltale smell of alcohol on a user's breath.

If an individual drinks slightly less alcohol each hour than the amount he or she can metabolize in an hour—about half a bottle of beer or half of an ordinary-size drink—the BAC remains low. People can drink large amounts of alcohol this way over long periods of time without becoming noticeably intoxicated.

If this same individual drinks more than he or she can metabolize, his or her BAC will steadily increase, and he or she will become more and more drunk (see Table 10-1). Despite popular myths, there is no way that people can significantly speed up their metabolism of alcohol. The rate of alcohol metabolism is the same whether the person is asleep or awake (see the box entitled "Myths about Alcohol").

We do not know exactly how alcohol acts to influence individual behavior, but we can measure its effects according to relationships and factors that apply to most drugs. One important factor in the action of alcohol is the **dose-response relationship.** The influence of alcohol on behavior is likely to depend on how much the person takes in. The concentration of alcohol in the blood

---

Metabolize To chemically transform food and other substances in the body into energy and wastes.

Dose-response relationship The relationship between the amount of a drug taken and the intensity or type of drug effect.

Sedate To calm by the use of a drug that quiets the activity of the nerves.

Myths about Alcohol

Myth   You can speed up the metabolism of alcohol by exercising, drinking coffee or taking other central nervous system stimulants, or by breathing fresh air.

Fact   Once alcohol is absorbed, there are no ways of appreciably accelerating its breakdown.

Myth   Alcoholics can "handle their alcohol" better than nonalcoholics.

Fact   In the early stages of alcoholism, this is sometimes true. However, in later stages of alcoholism, tolerance to alcohol often decreases. In some severe alcoholics, tolerance fluctuates from day to day; on one day a liter of wine has little behavioral effect, on another day, one glass of wine causes intoxication.

Myth   When you are under the influence of alcohol, you are so relaxed you are less likely to get hurt in an accident.

Fact   Alcohol slows protective reflexes and impairs coordination. People under the influence of alcohol are at much greater risk of injury (and death) from accidents.

Myth   Most alcoholics are consciously aware of drinking too much.

Fact   Denial—the unconscious psychological process that blocks awareness of reality—is an almost universal characteristic of alcoholics and other drug abusers. There is a clinical adage: "the two hallmarks of alcoholism are drinking too much and denying that you drink too much."

Myth   An alcoholic must want help before he or she will respond to it.

Fact   Many alcoholics respond to coercive intervention—to save their relationships, their careers, or their driver's license—even though they continue to deny their drinking problems.

Myth   Only an alcoholic can understand and help another.

Fact   Recovering alcoholics do have something unique to offer—a positive, encouraging example. But most of us have experienced and can empathize with the feelings

associated with excessive drinking—anxiety, depression, loneliness, remorse.

Myth   An alcoholic must "hit bottom" before he or she is ready to stop drinking.

Fact   Alcoholics do not have to lose all before they are motivated to stop. People vary markedly in what induces them to change their behavior. For some, the first blackout or alcohol-related automobile accident fosters abstinence.

Myth   The first step in the treatment of alcoholism is hospitalization.

Fact   Most alcoholics can be treated on an outpatient basis. Those with medical complications such as delirium tremens or seizures may require hospital care.

Myth   There is only one kind of effective treatment for alcoholism.

Fact   Different treatments work for different people—"different strokes for different folks." Shopping around is often required.

(BAC) is a major determinant of drug effects. Alcohol at low concentrations makes people feel relaxed, jovial, and euphoric, but at higher concentrations people are much more likely to feel angry, **sedated,** or sleepy.

How Much Is Safe?   The effects of alcohol are first recognized at BACs of about 0.03 to 0.05 percent. These effects may include light-headedness, relaxation, and release of inhibitions. When the BAC reaches 0.1 percent, a major reduction in most sensory and motor functioning

occurs. At 0.2 percent, the drinker is totally unable to function, either physically or psychologically. Usually coma accompanies a BAC of 0.35 percent, and any higher level can kill a person. Figure 10-1 shows the results of a study of the relationship between drinking and driving. How much a person drinks (the dose) has an effect on how he or she drives (the response).

The estimated number of drinks is shown on the bottom axis of Figure 10-1. This representation is a rough guide in which one drink can be one cocktail, a 5-ounce

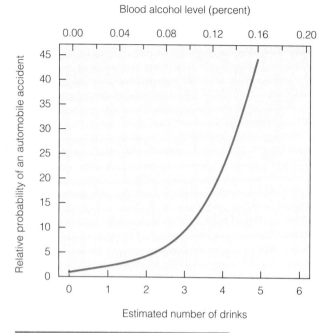

Blood alcohol level (percent)

Figure 10-1 The dose-response relationship of alcohol levels and automobile accidents.

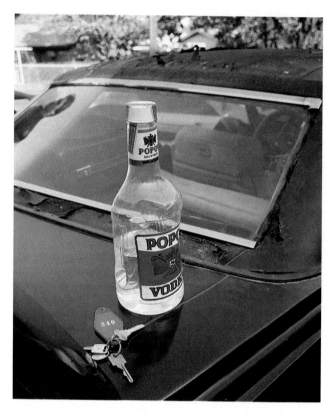

Alcohol interferes with judgment, perception, coordination, and other areas of mental and physical functioning and is a factor in a majority of all fatal automobile accidents. The driver of this car was lucky—a suspicious police officer intervened before an accident occurred.

glass of table wine, or one bottle of beer. The drinker is assumed to be a man of average weight (150 pounds), and the drinking takes place in one hour. It takes more drinks to achieve a given BAC if the person weighs more, if he has eaten recently, or if the drinking is done more slowly. It takes less time for a woman to achieve a given BAC, as explained earlier. The vertical axis represents how likely the drinker is to have an automobile accident compared to a sober driver. In other words, a man driving with a BAC of 0.10 (the legal limit in most states) is about ten times more likely to be involved in an accident that someone with no alcohol in his or her blood. Clearly, low doses of alcohol do not greatly increase risk, but as the dose increases, the risk of an automobile accident increases at a spectacular rate. The number of drinks it takes the average person to reach the legal BAC limit is shown in Figure 10-2. Remember that these amounts are approximate, since BACs vary depending on many factors, including gender. While you can do something about your own drinking, it's harder to protect yourself against someone else; the box titled "Protecting Yourself on the Road" gives some hints.

Alcohol and Health

By now, everyone knows that driving under the influence of alcohol is dangerous to your health, but other health consequences of drinking are less well known. What are the effects of alcohol on your body? Can drinking be part of a lifestyle devoted to wellness?

Immediate Effects of Alcohol Most people are familiar with the usual effects of alcohol on behavior. Low doses of alcohol—a drink or two over the course of the evening can help one relax and feel more at ease. Most drinkers experience mild euphoria and become more sociable. When people drink in social settings, alcohol often seems to act as a **stimulant**, enhancing conviviality or assertiveness. This response probably occurs, however, because alcohol acts on people to make them lose their **inhibitions**, not because it stimulates the nervous system.

With higher doses these pleasant effects tend to be replaced by more negative ones—interference with motor coordination, intellectual functions, and verbal performance. The individual often becomes irritable and may be easily angered or given to crying. Drinkers who take very high doses risk pronounced depression of the **central nervous system**, with **stupor**, unconsciousness, even death.

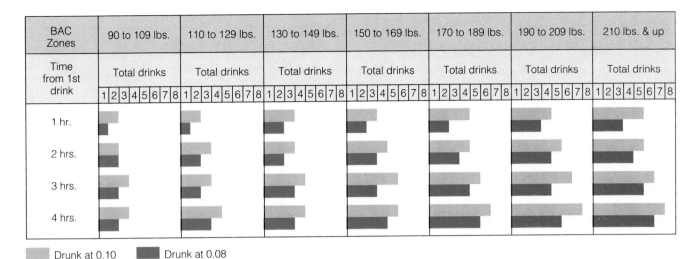

BAC Zones	90 to 109 lbs.								110 to 129 lbs.								130 to 149 lbs.								150 to 169 lbs.								170 to 189 lbs.								190 to 209 lbs.								210 lbs. & up							
Time from 1st drink	Total drinks								Total drinks								Total drinks								Total drinks								Total drinks								Total drinks								Total drinks							
	1	2	3	4	5	6	7	8	1	2	3	4	5	6	7	8	1	2	3	4	5	6	7	8	1	2	3	4	5	6	7	8	1	2	3	4	5	6	7	8	1	2	3	4	5	6	7	8	1	2	3	4	5	6	7	8

Drunk at 0.10   Drunk at 0.08

Figure 10-2   Blood alcohol concentrations and body weight. A BAC of 0.08 is considered legally drunk in four states, and a BAC of 0.10 is considered legally drunk in most other states. This chart illustrates the number of drinks it takes the average person of a specific weight to reach each BAC.

■ Exploring Your Emotions

Have you ever said or done anything while under the influence of alcohol that you regretted later? If so, how did you deal with the consequences? Did you change your behavior so it didn't happen again?

Shakespeare accurately described the effects of alcohol on sexual performance. He said (in *Macbeth*) that "it stirs up desire, but it takes away the performance." Small doses may improve sexual performance for individuals who are especially anxious or self-conscious, but higher doses usually make it worse. Excessive alcohol use on either an acute or chronic basis can result in reduced erection response and reduced vaginal lubrication.

Alcohol causes blood vessels near the skin to dilate, so drinkers often feel warm; their skin flushes, and they may sweat more. Flushing and sweating contribute to loss of heat, and so the internal body temperature falls. High doses of alcohol may impair the body's ability to regulate temperature, causing it to drop sharply, especially if the surrounding temperature is low. Drinking alcoholic beverages to keep warm in cold weather does not work, and it can even be dangerous.

Alcohol, particularly in large amounts, definitely changes sleep patterns. Alcohol may facilitate falling asleep more quickly, but the sleep is often light, punctuated with awakenings, and unrefreshing. Even after the habitual drinker stops drinking, his or her sleep may be altered for weeks or months. Users of alcohol frequently awaken with a "hangover"—headache, nausea, stomach distress, and generalized discomfort.

■ Exploring Your Emotions

How much do you think your mood and behavior change when you drink? How do you feel about such changes? What changes in your mood and behavior do other people see?

Alcohol acts as a depressant on the central nervous system. This fact is the overall reason for the changes that result from drinking. Physiologically, it first depresses a part of the brain that is involved in coordinating various parts of the nervous system. It also interferes with the processes that control inhibitions and depresses the function of nerves, muscles, including the heart muscle, and many other body tissues. We do not know precisely how alcohol exerts these effects.

Stimulant   Something that increases nervous or muscular activity.

Inhibition   The blocking of impulse or inclination.

Central nervous system depressant   Any chemical that affects the brain or spinal cord and decreases nervous or muscular activity.

Stupor   A state of dulled mind and senses in which an individual has little or no appreciation of his or her surroundings.

Protecting Yourself on the Road

Social drinkers and alcoholics alike are a menace behind the wheel. One-half of all traffic fatalities are associated with alcohol use, and one-third of all alcohol-related traffic accidents involve drivers between the ages of 16 and 24. People who drink and drive are unable to drive responsibly because their judgment is impaired, their reaction time is slower, and their coordination is reduced. No one can drive skillfully and safely when under the influence of alcohol.

What can you do to protect yourself from alcohol-related accidents on the road? If you are out of your home and drinking, follow the practice of having a "designated driver," an individual who refrains from drinking in order to provide safe transportation home for others in the group. The responsibility is rotated, so different people take the role of designated drivers on different occasions. In Sweden and the United Kingdom, where the practice originated, designated drivers place their car keys in their empty beverage glasses so they are not served. In the United States, designated drivers sometimes wear a special button to indicate their role for that evening.

Of course, even if you follow safe practices, you may encounter a drunk driver on the road. To reduce your chances of being involved in an accident caused by someone else, learn to be alert to the erratic driving that signals an impaired driver. Warning signs include the following:

- Unusually wide turns
- Straddling the center line or lane marker
- Driving with one's head out of the window or with the window down in cold weather
- Nearly striking an object or another vehicle
- Weaving or swerving
- Driving on other than the designated roadway
- Stopping with no apparent cause
- Following too closely
- Responding slowly to traffic signals
- Abrupt or illegal turns
- Rapid acceleration or deceleration
- Driving with headlights off at night

If you see any of these warning signs, what should you do?

- If the driver is ahead of you, maintain a safe following distance. Do not try to pass, because the driver may swerve into your car.
- If the driver is behind you, turn right at the nearest intersection. Let the driver pass and then return to your route.
- If the driver is approaching your car, move to the shoulder and stop. Avoid a head-on collision by sounding your horn or flashing your lights.
- When approaching an intersection, slow down and expect the unexpected.
- Fasten your seat belt, place children in approved safety seats, and keep your doors locked.
- Report suspected impaired drivers to the nearest law enforcement agency by phone. Give a description of the vehicle, license number, location, and direction the vehicle is headed.

Don't become a statistic. Be alert, don't drink and drive, and use a designated driver to make sure you come home alive and safe.

Adapted from The designated driver: Being a friend, *Healthline*, December 1986.

Effects of Chronic Use Alcohol even in relatively small amounts can alter liver function. With continued use of alcohol, liver cells are damaged and then progressively destroyed. The destroyed cells are often replaced by fibrous scar tissue, a condition known as **cirrhosis of the liver.** As cirrhosis develops, the individual may progressively lose his or her capacity to tolerate alcohol, because there are fewer remaining liver cells to metabolize whatever alcohol is in the bloodstream. Alcohol-precipitated cirrhosis is a major cause of death in the United States. Alcohol can also irritate and inflame the pancreas, causing nausea, vomiting, abnormal digestion, and severe pains in the abdomen. It may harm the kidneys over longer periods of time, but such harm does not happen often.

Alcohol can also affect the cardiovascular system. Again, the dosage and duration of alcohol use are critical considerations. Moderate doses of alcohol—one or two drinks a day—may reduce slightly the chances of heart attack in some people. The reasons for this finding are poorly understood, but may be the result of moderate amounts of alcohol increasing blood levels of certain **high-density lipoproteins (HDLs).** Higher doses of alcohol, however, are associated with cardiovascular problems. In some people, more than two drinks a day will elevate blood pressure, making strokes and heart attacks more likely. Some alcoholics show weakening of the heart muscle, a condition known as **cardiac myopathy.** Cardiac myopathy can be caused by the direct toxic effects of alcohol, or indirectly by the malnutrition and vitamin deficiencies that many alcoholics experience from their poor diets and gastrointestinal disturbances. In summary, although the relationships between alcohol and cardiovascular disease are multiple and complex, the net result is clear—excessive drinking increases the risk of disease. These health risks progressively increase as the amount of excessive drinking increases.

Chronic alcohol use has been linked to certain cancers of the upper digestive and respiratory tracts. It is difficult to get a clear picture of the relationship, however, because most heavy drinkers also smoke cigarettes, a practice that definitely increases the risk of several types of cancer. Alcohol may be the main factor in certain cancers such as those involving the pancreas. It may also increase the risk already present from tobacco use. Some recent studies link heavy alcohol use and breast cancer, but these remain controversial.

Overall, alcohol has a damaging effect on the body, affecting brain cells, bone cells, and many other organs and tissues. Alcohol abusers have life spans that are ten to twelve years shorter than average. Alcohol use is also frequently associated with suicide, homicide, and fatal accidents both on and off the road.

Fetal Alcohol Syndrome Many studies of animals and humans indicate that alcohol ingested during pregnancy can harm the fetus. Women who drink, especially in excessive amounts, are at increased risk of giving birth to children who have a collection of birth defects known as the **fetal alcohol syndrome.** These children are small at birth, are likely to have heart defects, and often have abnormal anatomical features, including small, wide-set eyes. Even with the best of care, their physical and mental growth rate is slower during childhood than normal. In adolescence they sometimes catch up with their age mates in terms of physical size but not usually in mental abilities. Most remain mentally retarded, with IQs in the 40 to 80 range. Other forms of the fetal alcohol syndrome do not involve obvious retardation or anatomical changes, but instead, subtle problems with learning and fine motor coordination.

Although researchers initially thought that fetal alcohol syndrome was caused by poor nutrition associated with the alcoholism of the mother, subsequent research indicates that it results directly from excessive alcohol intake. We should remember that alcohol is very soluble in water and blood is primarily water. Thus, any alcohol ingested rapidly enters the mother's blood and quickly crosses the placenta into the circulation of the fetus; when the mother has a blood alcohol concentration of 0.03, so does her fetus. There is no precise blood alcohol threshold level above which damage occurs and below which there is no danger. Instead the frequency and severity of defects progressively increase as the amount of drinking increases. Exposing the fetus to alcohol or other drugs during the first twelve or thirteen weeks of pregnancy is particularly hazardous because, during this time, the critical formation of the central nervous system, heart, and other organs occurs. As discussed in Chapter 8, the safest course of action is abstinence. Occasionally, newly born babies of alcoholic mothers show withdrawal reactions. These withdrawal problems are similar to those experienced by older individuals.

Any alcohol consumed by a nursing mother quickly enters the breast milk. What impact this has on the child or the mother's milk production is a matter of controversy. Dosage may again be the key issue. Some pediatricians argue that very small amounts of alcohol—half a glass of wine—may provide some useful relaxation to mother and child, but that large amounts are too sedating and may interfere with subsequent child development.

Medical Uses and Possible Health Benefits of Alcohol Alcohol can be effective for some medical purposes. Alcohol sponges are commonly used to reduce fever because alcohol cools the skin by evaporation. In concentrations of 70 percent by weight, alcohol kills bacteria. It is used as an astringent and skin cleanser in treating skin disorders. Contrary to a popular myth, however, alcohol is not a good antiseptic for open wounds. It injures exposed tissues and may form a coagulant that protects rather than destroys bacteria. If no antiseptic is available, it is usually better to just clean the wound with water and soap, and try to keep it clean while seeking medical attention.

People who associate alcohol with dining pleasure may feel hungrier and digest their food better if they take a small amount of alcohol—a bottle of beer, a glass of

---

Cirrhosis A disease of the liver caused by excessive and chronic drinking. Contrary to earlier medical belief, cirrhosis occurs even when nutrition is adequate.

High-density lipoprotein (HDL) Waxy substance in the blood thought to protect against heart disease.

Cardiac myopathy Weakening of the heart muscle through disease.

Fetal alcohol syndrome Birth defects caused by excessive alcohol consumption by the mother.

wine—with their meals. Drinking alcohol has been thought by some to be useful in treating angina pectoris, a painful disorder in which the heart is unable to get enough oxygen. Most physicians feel that there are much more effective drugs for this condition, and any beneficial effect of alcohol is due to sedation rather than improvement in blood circulation.

Relationships between alcohol use and mortality rates are complex. As one would predict, both abstainers and moderate drinkers live longer than heavy drinkers. Some recent studies also suggest that people who regularly drink moderate amounts of alcohol—fewer than three drinks per day—live longer than those who abstain completely. However, these findings are controversial and may reflect unrepresentative sampling techniques.

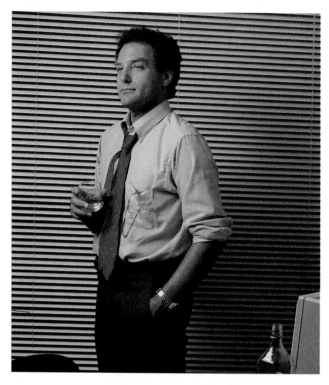

Drinking alone during the day is a sign of alcohol abuse. Although alcohol may seem to provide temporary relief from uncomfortable feelings, it offers no actual solutions to personal problems.

Misuse of Alcohol

Addiction to alcohol—like addiction to tobacco and other psychoactive drugs—affects more than just the user. Alcoholics can wreak havoc within a family, and children are often those most severely affected. But alcohol can be abused even when there's no true addiction; even though the rate is falling, too many victims of traffic accidents are actually victims of weekend drinkers.

Alcohol Abuse   Recent definitions make a distinction between alcohol abuse and alcohol dependence, or alcoholism. According to the third edition (revised) of the *Diagnostic and Statistical Manual of Mental Disorders* (1987) of the American Psychiatric Association, **alcohol abuse** involves either (1) continued use of alcohol despite knowledge of having a persistent or recurrent social, occupational, psychological, or physical problem that is caused by or exacerbated by use of alcohol, or (2) recurrent use of alcohol in situations when use is physically hazardous (such as driving while intoxicated). The term **alcohol dependence**, which is also called **alcoholism**, refers to more extensive problems with alcohol use, usually involving tolerance or withdrawal.

Other authorities use different definitions to describe problems associated with drinking. The important point is that one does not have to be an alcoholic to have problems with alcohol. The person who drinks only once a month, perhaps after an exam, but then drives while intoxicated is an alcohol abuser.

There are different patterns of alcohol abuse. Here are four common patterns:

1. *Regular daily intake of large amounts.* This continuous pattern is the most common adult pattern of excessive consumption in most countries.
2. *Regular heavy drinking limited to weekends.* This continuous pattern is commonly followed by teenagers and college students.
3. *Long periods of sobriety interspersed with binges of daily heavy drinking lasting for weeks or months.* This episodic or "bender" pattern is common in the United States but quite uncommon in France, although the per capita consumption of alcohol is higher in France.
4. *Heavy drinking limited to periods of stress.* This "reactive" pattern is associated with periods of anxiety or depression; for example, examination or other performance fears, interpersonal difficulties, school or work pressures.

Alcohol abuse   The use of alcohol to a degree that causes physical damage, impairs functioning, or results in behavior harmful to others.

Alcohol dependence   Either pathological use of alcohol or impairment in functioning due to alcohol and tolerance or withdrawal; alcoholism.

Alcoholism   Chronic psychological and nutritional disorder from excessive and compulsive drinking; alcohol dependence.

Seven Ways to Drink Less

When You're the Guest

- Let your waistline be your incentive. For the same 215 calories in two seven-ounce gin and tonics, you can have 3 ounces of broiled, trimmed sirloin and get the meat's additional nutrients.
- At a restaurant, order the food first, not a drink. Then if you want a drink you'll probably have time for only one before the meal is served.
- Avoid drinks made with carbonated mixers, especially if you're thirsty. You'll gulp them down.
- Remember that the pressure to have a drink may often be in your imagination. It is becoming more and more acceptable to say "no thanks" to alcohol.

When You're the Host

- Have plenty of nonalcoholic beverages on hand and make sure they are as accessible and as attractive as the alcoholic drinks.
- If it's a dinner party, try to serve dinner on schedule, before there's time for a second drink.
- Experiment with various juices and beverages until you come up with an alcohol-free concoction all your own. Or stick to traditional punches and blends, but leave out the alcohol.

Adapted from *University of California, Berkeley, Wellness Letter*, April 1987.

How can you tell if you are beginning to abuse alcohol or if someone you know is doing so? Look for the following warning signs:

1. Drinking alone or secretively.
2. Using alcohol deliberately and repeatedly to perform or get through difficult situations.
3. Feeling uncomfortable on certain occasions when alcohol is not available.
4. Escalating alcohol consumption beyond an already established drinking pattern.
5. Consuming alcohol heavily in risky situations; for example, before driving.
6. Getting drunk regularly or more frequently than in the past.
7. Drinking in the morning or at other unusual times.

The box titled "Seven Ways to Drink Less" gives some hints to help cut back on drinking.

Alcoholism   People of all social and economic classes use alcohol excessively, not just people who are considered to be skid row bums, who actually account for only a small percentage of the total alcoholic population and usually represent the final stage of a drinking career that began years before. Among white American men, excessive drinking usually begins in the teens or twenties and gradually progresses through the thirties until the person is clearly identified as alcoholic by the time he is in his late thirties or early forties. It is relatively uncommon for alcoholism to begin in men after the age of 45 unless there are also psychiatric problems such as depression.

■ **Exploring Your Emotions**

How do you feel about alcoholism? Do you think of it as a disease, a weakness, an affliction, a choice? What is the basis for your attitude?

The "natural history" of alcoholism in women differs from that of men. Women tend to become alcoholic at a later age and with fewer years of heavy drinking. It is not unusual for women in their forties or fifties to become alcoholic after years of controlled drinking, whereas this pattern occurs infrequently in men. Women alcoholics also develop cirrhosis and other medical complications somewhat more often than men.

There are notable differences in patterns of alcoholic drinking among various racial and ethnic groups. For example, urban black males commonly start excessive drinking at a younger age than do urban white males, develop serious medical and neurological illnesses at an earlier age, and have a higher rate of alcoholism-related suicides. Excessive drinking among Native Americans varies from tribe to tribe and does not follow a consistent pattern. There is a low rate of alcoholism in Asia, and a high rate among many Northern Europeans.

Estimating the prevalence of alcoholism is complicated by disagreement about definition and other methodological problems. Although the figure of 9 or 10 million American alcoholics has often been cited, it is not based on scientific studies. More systematic studies of smaller geographic areas such as counties or states suggest that about 3 percent of all men are alcoholic and perhaps 0.1

to 1 percent of all women. It is somewhat easier to determine the quantity of drinking done by a given population. Studies show that about 20 percent of American men are heavy drinkers, meaning they drink daily and drink six or more drinks several times a month.

We do not know exactly what causes alcoholism. Probably a variety of factors are involved, all of which vary from individual to individual. Recent reliable studies have compared individuals who were adopted when they were young and individuals who lived with their biological parents. These studies showed that people are more likely to be alcoholics if either one or both of their biological parents are alcoholics. Alcoholism in adopted parents, however, does not make individuals either more or less likely to become alcoholics. In other words, there apparently is a genetic contribution to susceptibility to alcoholism. Not all children of alcoholics become alcoholics, however, and it is clear that many other factors are involved. No changes in the brain chemistry of alcoholics or the children of alcoholics have been identified. Personality disorders, being subjected as a child to destructive child-rearing practices, and imitating parents' and other important people's abuse of alcohol may all play a part. People who begin drinking excessively during their teenage years are especially prone to alcoholism later in life. Common psychological features of individuals who excessively use alcohol are denial ("I don't have a problem") and rationalization ("I drink because I need to socialize with my customers.")

Certain social factors have been linked with alcoholism. These include urbanization, disappearance of the extended family, general loosening of kinship ties, increased mobility, and changing religious and philosophical values.

Complications The consequences of alcoholism are well known. Many of these consequences stem from the fact that all people (including nonalcoholics) develop a **tolerance** to alcohol after repeated use. They require greater and greater amounts to produce the same psychological effect, but these larger amounts increase the chances of adverse physical effects.

Tolerance, however, develops at different rates to different effects of alcohol. For example, alcohol-induced depression of the respiratory system develops slowly and only to a small extent. Thus alcoholics are only slightly less susceptible to lethal respiratory depression from overdose than are moderate users. The same is true for users of barbiturates and most other sedating drugs.

When people continue to abuse alcohol for long periods of time, their tolerance may begin to decrease. Some chronic alcoholics have very little tolerance for alcohol, in part because their livers are so damaged that they no longer have adequate amounts of the enzymes necessary to metabolize alcohol.

When alcoholics stop drinking or cut their intake way down, they will have **withdrawal symptoms.** These can vary from merely unpleasant feelings to serious, even life-threatening, disorders. The jitters, or "shakes," are the most common withdrawal symptom and may last as long as two weeks. Seizures are less common, but they are more serious. Still less common is the severe withdrawal reaction known as the **DTs (delirium tremens)**, a dramatic state characterized by disorientation, confusion, and vivid **hallucinations**, often of vermin and small animals.

Since alcohol is water soluble and distributed throughout most of the body, it can harm many different organs and tissues. Damage to the liver in the form of cirrhosis is just one well-known example. Asthma, gout, diabetes, and recurrent infections are more common in heavy drinkers than in people who drink moderately or not at all. Other medical and psychiatric complications are associated with excessive alcohol use. Some of these alcohol-related medical problems are made worse by nutritional deficiencies that often accompany alcohol abuse. Disorders of the liver, stomach, and intestine are especially common, as are diseases of the nervous system, but all vary among users. One individual may primarily have defects of the central nervous system, serious damage to the memory, and no liver or gastrointestinal damage. Another individual, with a similar drinking and nutrition history, may have advanced liver disease and no memory defects.

An alcoholic's medical and psychiatric problems often respond rapidly to hospitalization, tranquilizers, and the elimination of alcohol from the diet. These problems are likely to return, however, if the person starts drinking

---

Tolerance Lower sensitivity to a drug so that a given dose no longer exerts the usual effect and larger doses are needed.

Withdrawal symptoms Unpleasant physical and mental sensations experienced when abstaining from a drug to which one is addicted.

DTs (delirium tremens) A state of confusion brought on by reduction of alcohol intake in a person addicted to alcohol. Other symptoms are sweating, trembling, anxiety, and hallucinations.

Hallucinations False perceptions that do not correspond to external reality. A person who hears voices that are not there or who sees visions is having hallucinations.

Paranoia A mental disorder characterized by false beliefs that one is being persecuted, often beliefs of a grandiose and logically systematic nature. There are no hallucinations, and intelligence is not impaired.

Children of Alcoholics: The Struggle to Recover

One out of eight Americans—about 30 million people—grow up in alcoholic households, according to the Children of Alcoholics Foundation. For these children, life is a struggle to deal with constant stress, anxiety, and embarrassment. Family life centers on the drinking parent, and children's needs are often ignored.

Children in alcoholic households often adapt to their situation by learning patterns of interaction and methods of coping that help them survive childhood but that don't support their own healthy development. They may be victims of violence, abuse, neglect, or incest in the home, all of which contribute to long-lasting emotional scars. When they grow up, children of alcoholics are more likely to become alcoholic and to marry an alcoholic than the general population. They are also more likely to abuse other drugs and develop an eating disorder.

Until recently, children of alcoholics were considered no different from other children with family difficulties and were largely ignored by treatment programs, which tended to focus on the alcoholic parent. But today, professionals recognize the special problems and needs of children of alcoholics, and family-oriented therapy has become a major focus of alcoholism rehabilitation.

If you are the child of an alcoholic, be aware, first, that you are not alone. Millions of people across the country have been through the same problem and have dreamed of having a happy family life in which drinking is not an issue. Realize, too, that other people can understand what you have been through and can help. Find a person you can trust—perhaps a teacher, a friend, a member of the clergy—and confide

in him or her. It may seem safer to keep your feelings secret, but talking about the problem is the first step toward a healthy readjustment. Finally, acknowledge that your parent's alcoholism is not your fault. Many children of alcoholics carry a burden of guilt from early childhood, when they could not understand that they weren't the cause of their parent's behavior. This unexamined assumption causes part of the emotional pain experienced by children of alcoholics.

Several support groups exist for children of alcoholics. To get help for yourself or someone you know, call one of the local Al-Anon or AlaTeen agencies listed in your telephone book. You can also call or write the Children of Alcoholics Foundation at 540 Madison Avenue, New York, NY 10022, (212) 980-5394.

---

again. Some people have what is called **paranoid** personalities. If they use alcohol excessively, they may suffer delusions, jealousy, suspicion, and mistrust—so-called alcoholic paranoia. Other psychiatric problems associated with alcoholism include profound memory gaps (amnesia), which are sometimes filled by conscious or unconscious lying (confabulation).

Alcohol use causes more serious social problems than all other forms of drug abuse combined. The 1983 statistics of the National Council on Alcoholism concluded that 10 million Americans were alcoholic; for each of these, another three to four people were directly affected. In a 1989 Gallup poll, one in five Americans said that drinking had been a cause of trouble in their family (see the box entitled "Children of Alcoholics: The Struggle to Recover").

An estimated 3.3 million 14- to 17-year-olds are showing signs of potential alcohol dependency. These numbers are far greater than those associated with cocaine,

heroin, or marijuana use. The social and psychological consequences of excessive drinking in young people is more difficult to measure than the risks to physical health. One of the consequences is that excessive drinking interferes with learning the interpersonal and work skills that are required for adult life. Excessive drinkers sometimes narrow their circle of friends to other heavy drinkers and thus limit the range of people they can learn from. Perhaps most important is that people who were excessive drinkers in college are more likely to have social, occupational, and health problems when they are studied 20 years later.

■ **Exploring Your Emotions**

What, if any, were your experiences with alcohol in high school, and what were the experiences of your friends and classmates? How do you feel about those experiences now?

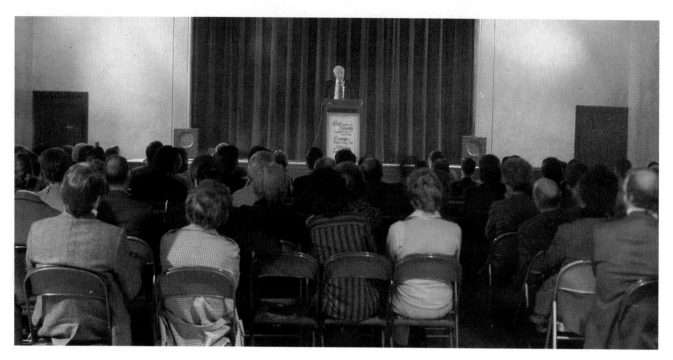

Over 800,000 people in the United States and Canada belong to Alcoholics Anonymous, the oldest and best known recovery program. According to AA, alcoholics must recognize that they are "powerless over alcohol" and seek help from a "higher power" in order to regain control of their lives.

The important point is that despite media attention to cocaine and other chemicals, the U.S. Surgeon General reminds us that alcohol remains our number one drug problem.

Treatment It is important to realize that some alcoholics recover without professional help. It is unknown how often this occurs, but perhaps as many as 25 percent of alcoholics "spontaneously" stop drinking or reduce their drinking to the point where problems do not occur. In a 1981 study of "problem drinkers," 9 percent of American adults were currently experiencing drinking problems. Another 9 percent had had drinking problems in the past but no longer did. One of the great debates in the field is whether "true" alcoholics can become controlled or social drinkers. Studies indicate this may occur, but that many alcoholics must practice total abstinence to avoid an eventual return to problem drinking.

In any event, the majority of alcoholics do not stop their chronic excessive use of alcohol on their own. For these people, treatment is difficult. However, although we do not have satisfactory ways to treat all people who have alcohol problems, cautious optimism has replaced the widely held view of "nothing can be done" that prevailed a few years ago.

Many different kinds of treatment programs exist. Some, such as Alcoholics Anonymous, emphasize group and "buddy" support as well as personal testimonies.

Other programs emphasize making changes in lifestyle and learning specific techniques such as stress management. The best treatment programs often involve a combination of a variety of techniques, such as Alcoholics Anonymous, psychotherapy (individual, group, and especially family or couple), and chemical therapies. None of these has been successful for all patients. As with the treatment of other drug dependencies, one major problem in treating alcoholics is predicting ahead of time which treatment will be most useful for a particular individual. Another major treatment problem has to do with long-term effectiveness. For example, one chemical treatment involves the use of disulfiram (trade name, Antabuse). Disulfiram causes patients to become violently ill whenever they drink. What usually happens is that after taking the drug for a while, the patient declares him or herself to be "cured" and decides that he or she no longer needs the drug. The effect of the drug does not wear off for about four days, so the patient is able to avoid impulse drinking and may even gain enough momentum to stay "cured"—for a time. After weeks or perhaps months of not taking the drug, many patients start drinking again.

Prescribing chemical substitutes such as diazepam (Valium) or chlordiazepoxide (Librium) for alcohol is a controversial treatment. Proponents argue that at least the more toxic alcohol is being replaced by a less toxic drug and thus the health hazard is reduced. Others claim that one drug dependency is merely being exchanged for another and many of the behavioral problems associated with the chemical abuse are unchanged. Like many controversies in the field of alcoholism and drug abuse, this one is unlikely to be resolved, because value judgments are involved.

Helping a friend or relative with an alcohol problem requires skill and tact. One of the first steps is making sure you are not an "enabler" or "co-dependent"—someone who, perhaps unknowingly, allows another to continue excessive use of alcohol. Enabling takes many forms. One of the most common is making excuses or covering up for the alcohol abuser—saying "he has the flu" when it is really a hangover. Whenever you find yourself minimizing or lying about someone's drinking behavior, a warning bell should sound. Often another important step is open, honest labeling—"I think you have a problem with alcohol." Such explicit statements usually elicit emotional rebuttals and may endanger a relationship. In the long run, however, you are seldom most helpful to your friends when you allow them to deny their problems with alcohol or other drugs. Even when problems are acknowledged there is commonly reluctance to obtain help. Your best role might be to obtain information about the available resources and persistently encourage their use.

Drinking Behavior and Responsibility

The responsible use of alcohol means drinking in such a way as to keep your BAC low so that your behavior is always under your control. Sometimes people lose control when they misestimate how much they can drink; other times they set out deliberately to get drunk. When you want to drink responsibly, it's helpful to know, first of all, why you drink. The following are the ten most common reasons given by college students for drinking alcohol:

1. "It increases my feelings of sociability."
2. "It relieves anxiety or tension."
3. "It makes me feel elated or euphoric."
4. "It makes me less inhibited in thinking, saying, or doing certain things."
5. "It enables me to go along with my friends."
6. "It enables me to experience a different state of consciousness."
7. "It makes me less inhibited sexually."
8. "It enables me to stop worrying."
9. "It alleviates depression."
10. "It makes me less self-conscious."

■ **Exploring Your Emotions**

How do you perceive a nondrinker in a social situation where others are drinking? Does it seem like an acceptable choice to you? What is the basis for your attitude?

If you drink, what are your reasons for doing so? Are you attempting to meet underlying needs that could best be addressed by other means? Or is your drinking moderate and responsible? Here are some tips for keeping your drinking under control:

- *Drink slowly.* Learn to sip your drinks rather than gulp them. It helps to develop the habit of deliberately tasting and smelling the nuances of alcoholic beverages so that you can determine their similarities and differences. Learn to compare and contrast the different kinds of wines and beers. Don't drink alcoholic beverages to quench your thirst.
- *Space your drinks.* Learn to drink nonalcoholic drinks at parties—juices or tonic water without the alcohol, for example—or intersperse these with alcoholic drinks. Learn to refuse a round: "I've had enough for right now." Parties are easier for some people if they hold a glass of anything nonalcoholic that has ice and a twist of lime floating in it so that it looks as if they were drinking alcohol. Other people are comfortable in openly requesting "mocktails"—drinks like "virgin screwdrivers" that have all the ingredients of the cocktail except the alcoholic beverage. Such requests provide a healthy model for others.
- *Eat before and while drinking.* Avoid drinking on an empty stomach. Food in your stomach will not prevent the alcohol from eventually being absorbed, but it will slow down the rate somewhat, and thus the peak blood alcohol level will usually be lower.
- *Know your limits and your drinks.* Learn how different blood alcohol concentrations affect you. In a safe setting such as your home, with your roommate or a friend, see how a set amount—say, two drinks an hour—affects you. A good test is walking heel to toe in a straight line with your eyes closed or standing with your feet crossed and trying to touch your finger to your nose with your eyes closed.

However, be aware that in different settings your performance, and especially your ability to judge your behavior, may change. At a given blood alcohol concentration, you will perform less well when surrounded by activity and boisterous companions than you will in a quiet test setting with just one or two other people. This impairment results partially because alcohol reduces your ability to perform when your brain is bombarded by multiple stimuli. It is useful to discover the

Young People Take Action: Students Against Driving Drunk

Students Against Driving Drunk (SADD) was established in 1981 to improve young people's knowledge and attitudes about alcohol and drugs to help save their lives—and the lives of others. The program has three major components:

First, it provides a series of lesson plans to present the facts about drinking and driving, permitting students to make informed decisions.

Second, it mobilizes students to help one another through peer pressure to face up to the potential dangers of mixing driving with alcohol or drugs.

And third, it promotes a frank dialogue between teenagers and their parents through the SADD "Contract." Under this agreement both students and their parents pledge to contact each other should they ever find themselves in a potential DWI (driving while intoxicated) situation.

CONTRACT FOR LIFE

A Contract for Life
Between Parent and Teenager
The SADD Drinking-Driver Contract

Teenager   I agree to call you for advice and/or transportation at any hour, from any place, if I am ever in a situation where I have been drinking or a friend or date who is driving me has been drinking.

_____
Signature

Parent   I agree to come and get you at any hour, any place, no questions asked and no argument at that time, or I will pay for a taxi to bring you home safely. I expect we would discuss this issue at a later time.

I agree to seek safe, sober transportation home if I am ever in a situation where I have had too much to drink or a friend who is driving me has had too much to drink.

_____
Signature

_____
Date

S.A.D.D. does not condone drinking by those below the legal drinking age. S.A.D.D. encourages all young people to obey the laws of their state, including laws relating to the legal drinking age.

Distributed by S.A.D.D., "Students Against Driving Drunk"

---

rate at which you can drink without increasing your BAC. Be able to calculate the approximate amount a given drink will increase your BAC.

• _Cultivate and model responsible attitudes toward alcohol._ Our society teaches us attitudes toward drinking that increase the chances for alcohol-related problems, if not for ourselves, then for others (see the box "A Nation Gets Serious about Sobriety"). Many of us have difficulty expressing disapproval to someone who has drunk too much. We are amused by the antics of the "funny" drunk. We tend to accept the alcohol industry's linkage of drinking with virility or sexuality. And we treat abstainers as odd. These attitudes are not healthy.

■ **Exploring Your Emotions**

How do you feel about alcohol advertising and marketing? Do you think it's ethical to sell a potentially dangerous substance by appealing to people's desires and vulnerabilities? Do you think liquor manufacturers ought to be held responsible for the damage alcohol inflicts on some people?

• _Learn to be a responsible host or hostess regarding alcohol._ In medieval England an important legal precedent, the dramskeeper's principle, was established. This principle put the responsibility for alcohol-related injuries or untoward results of the guest's drunken behavior on

A Nation Gets Serious about Sobriety

Call it raised consciousness. Call it social responsibility. Call it the law. By any name, there is a growing trend in the United States on the part of both consumers and manufacturers to rethink drinking.

"Social change takes a long time. But we are seeing a change," says the spokesperson for Beer Drinkers of America, a responsible-drinking advocacy group with a national membership of about 400,000. "People aren't drinking to excess any more. It is becoming more and more socially unacceptable, especially drinking and driving. You don't hear the jokes about it that you may have heard in the past. People really do take car keys away from people."

National Highway Traffic Safety Administration statistics seem to back that up. They show that the number of people killed in car accidents in the United States in which at least one driver was considered legally intoxicated has declined steadily in recent years: 46 percent in 1982, 41 percent in 1986, 39 percent in 1988. In the same period, more than 400 laws imposing stiffer penalties for drinking and driving have passed in the United States. Four states—Oregon, Utah, Maine, and California—have set .08 percent blood alcohol concentration as the level at which a driver is considered legally drunk. (In most other states, the level is .10 percent.) A person weighing 160 pounds could reach a BAC of .08 percent after consuming as few as two drinks in one hour, according to the California Department of Motor Vehicles.

New laws help keep drunk drivers off the roads, but social consciousness has changed as well. Mothers Against Drunk Driving (MADD) is often credited for first bringing drinking and driving issues to public awareness in the early 1980s. MADD's public awareness campaign was followed by numerous public and private responsible-drinking campaigns, research studies, and health warnings. Bars and restaurants began posting signs suggesting responsible drinking habits, offering rides home, and sending their employees to classes to learn how to determine if a customer has had too much to drink.

The big breweries, wineries, and liquor distillers started changing their advertising strategies as well. Today, most spend a portion of their multimillion-dollar advertising budgets to push responsible drinking. For example, the 1988–89 holiday season's Coors Light jingle, "It's the right time now," was incorporated into a television commercial that pointed out the "right time"—cut to a lively group watching a football game on a living-room TV—and "wrong time"—the picture changes to a man leaving a bar alone, car keys in hand—for beer consumption.

Annual spring college-break events in Florida—many of them sponsored by beer companies—have traditionally revolved around drinking. In the past few years, however, a strong shift has been made away from activities such as beer-chugging contests toward nondrinking events such as concerts, free movies, and volleyball exhibitions.

The printed word is another source of continuing public awareness. In 1989, almost every major newspaper and magazine published a story dealing with alcohol use and abuse, ranging from newsmagazines to *Good Housekeeping* and *TV Guide*. *Discover* magazine ran a story about a study that concluded country music is more likely to lead to alcohol abuse than are pop or rock music. (The slower the tempo, the faster the drinking, according to the story. Songs with 85 beats per minute led to the least drinking, and songs with 60 beats per minute led to excessive drinking.) Several magazines had celebrities (including Drew Barrymore, Tai Babilonia, and John Larroquette) talking about their bouts with alcoholism and how life is better sober. *Car & Driver* magazine editors devoted 10 pages to proving that "drunk driving is as dangerous as smoking crack, running through Tehran with a 'Death to the Ayatollah' sign, or playing marbles in the first turn of the Indy 500."

Are enough people getting the message? Some organizations, such as MADD, the National Commission on Drunk Driving, and the National Highway Traffic Safety Administration, don't think so. They cite the 23,352 alcohol-related deaths in the United States in 1988 and point out that there is no way to measure what those deaths meant to the wives, husbands, mothers, fathers, and children of the people who died. Despite improvements, they say, there is still work to be done. Attitudes and behavior do take a long time to change, especially when it comes to something as popular and complex as drinking, but signs indicate that a start has been made.

Adapted from Toni Mazzacane, 1990. Driven to stop drinking. *San Jose Mercury News*, January 9, p. D1.

the innkeeper or tavern owner. Although the legal force of this principle has been muted over the centuries, it is a useful guide for our obligations to our guests. Acquire the habit of serving nonalcoholic beverages as well as alcohol. Popular nonalcoholic drinks include soft drinks, sparkling water and fruit juice in a variety of flavors (sales of these beverages have increased 600 percent in the last decade), drinks made from mixers without the alcohol, and alcohol-free wine and beer. Always serve food along with alcohol, and stop serving alcohol an hour or more before people will leave. Eliminate one drink more—for the road. Be able to insist that a guest who had too much take a taxi, ride with someone else, or stay at your house rather than drive.

- *Learn about alcohol abuse prevention programs at your school.* What alternatives are being developed to "keg parties" and other events where heavy drinking is fostered? Are programs available for students who are at high risk for alcohol abuse—such as students whose parents abused alcohol? Are counseling or self-help programs such as Alcoholics Anonymous available for students who are having problems with alcohol?
- *Refer to the Behavior Change Strategy at the end of this chapter* for more suggestions on developing responsible drinking habits.

Summary

- Although alcohol has long been a part of human celebrations, it is a drug capable of causing addiction and harmful physiological effects.

The Nature of Alcohol

- Ethyl alcohol is the psychoactive ingredient in alcoholic beverages. The proof value of an alcoholic beverage is two times the percentage concentration.
- How long it takes for alcohol to be absorbed into the bloodstream from the stomach depends on the amount, type, and proof of the beverage, the time taken to drink it, and whether there is food in the stomach.
- Women become intoxicated more quickly than men do because their stomachs have less of the enzyme that metabolizes alcohol.
- After alcohol is absorbed, it is distributed throughout the body via the bloodstream. The liver metabolizes alcohol as the blood circulates through it; the rate of the metabolic process stays about the same for each individual. What is not metabolized is excreted via the lungs and kidneys.
- If people drink less alcohol each hour than the amount they can metabolize in an hour, the blood alcohol content remains low. The BAC increases when people drink more than they can metabolize.
- The influence of alcohol on behavior is likely to depend on how much a person takes in. A major reduction in sensory and motor functioning occurs at a BAC of 0.1 percent.

Alcohol and Health

- Alcohol helps people relax; in social settings it often acts as a stimulant, probably because it helps people lose their inhibitions. At higher doses alcohol interferes with motor coordination, intellectual functions, and

verbal performance. At very high doses, stupor, unconsciousness, and even death are possible.
- Alcohol affects internal body temperature, changes sleep patterns, and has an adverse effect on sexual performance.
- Continued alcohol use causes cirrhosis, in which damaged and destroyed liver cells are replaced by fibrous scar tissue.
- Although moderate doses of alcohol may reduce the chances of heart attack by increasing blood levels of HDL, higher doses are associated with cardiovascular problems, including cardiac myopathy.
- Alcohol has also been related to certain cancers. Abusers have shorter life spans than the average, and alcohol is also associated with suicide, homicide, and fatal accidents.
- Women who drink while pregnant risk giving birth to children with fetal alcohol syndrome. This syndrome can mean physical abnormalities and mental retardation; in less severe forms it still involves learning problems and fine motor coordination. There is no safe level of drinking during pregnancy.
- Alcohol consumed by a nursing mother quickly enters breast milk and can interfere with the child's development.
- Although alcohol has medical benefits when it is used externally to reduce fever and clean the skin, any medical effects that come from drinking alcohol are questionable.

Misuse of Alcohol

- Alcohol abuse involves either (1) continued use of alcohol despite knowledge that it causes recurrent social, occupational, physical, and psychological problems, or (2) recurrent use of alcohol in situations where use is physically hazardous.

- Alcohol dependence, or alcoholism, involves more extensive problems with alcohol abuse, usually involving tolerance or withdrawal.
- Alcohol abuse follows different patterns, such as daily intake of large amounts, heavy weekend drinking, long periods of sobriety interspersed with binges of heavy drinking, or heavy drinking limited to periods of stress.
- Warning signs of alcohol abuse include drinking alone, using alcohol to get through difficult situations, feeling uncomfortable when alcohol is not available, escalating alcohol consumption, heavy use in risky situations, getting drunk regularly, and drinking at unusual times.
- Alcoholism affects people from all social and economic classes; excessive drinking often begins in the teens and twenties for men, though later for women.
- Rates of alcoholism differ among racial and ethnic groups. Perhaps 3 percent of all men and 0.1 to 1 percent of all women are alcoholics.
- There is a genetic contribution to alcoholism, but other factors are involved. Personality disorders, destructive child-rearing practices, and the desire to imitate others are all involved. Social factors involved include urbanization, disappearance of the extended family, increased mobility, and changing values.
- Consequences of alcoholism usually stem from the tolerance that develops after continued use. When greater amounts are needed to produce the same psychological effect, the chances of adverse physical effects increase.
- When alcohol has been used so long and so excessively that liver damage occurs, tolerance begins to decrease.
- Withdrawal symptoms occur when alcoholics stop drinking or drastically reduce their intake. These vary from unpleasant sensations to life-threatening disorders.

- Alcohol damages not only the liver but also the stomach, intestines, kidneys, bronchi, and peripheral nerves; its effects vary with the individual. Medical treatment can help when alcohol is stopped.
- Psychiatric problems involved with alcohol abuse include paranoia and memory loss.
- Alcoholism causes many social problems; it especially affects the children in a family. Furthermore, millions of teenagers show signs of potential alcohol dependency; they risk not only their physical health but also their occupational and social lives.
- Some alcoholics recover without professional help; still a matter of controversy is the question of whether true alcoholics can become controlled drinkers.
- The best treatment programs involve a variety of techniques, such as buddy support, psychotherapy, and chemical therapies. Long-term effectiveness needs to be considered in evaluating any treatment program. The use of chemical substitutes has been challenged as not dealing with underlying problems.
- Helping someone who abuses alcohol means avoiding being an enabler. Open, honest labeling is important; the best way to help might be to obtain information about available resources and persistently encourage their use.

Drinking Behavior and Responsibility

- The responsible use of alcohol means keeping the BAC low and behavior always under control. Ways to do so include drinking slowly and spacing drinks, eating before and while drinking, being a responsible host or hostess, having responsible attitudes toward alcohol, and learning about alcohol abuse prevention programs.

Take Action

1. In your health diary, list the positive behaviors that help you drink responsibly. Consider how you can strengthen these behaviors. Then list the behaviors that interfere with responsible drinking for you. Which ones can you change?

2. Make a list of the statements you might make to a person you cared about who you thought was developing a drinking problem; statements you might make to a person who was planning to drive under the influence of alcohol, both with and without you in the car; and questions you might ask a friend about your own behavior when you drink. Consider using some of these statements when an appropriate situation arises.

3. List and describe what you can do as the responsible host of parties or social gatherings. What nonalcoholic beverages can you serve, and what can you do to keep your guests safe when they leave your home?

4. Some Alcoholics Anonymous groups encourage visitors. If your local chapter does so, attend a meeting to see how the organization functions. What behavioral techniques are used to help people stop drinking? How effective do these techniques seem to be? If there is a local "co-dependent" or Al-Anon group, attend one of their meetings. What themes are emphasized? Do any themes apply to your relationships?

5. Go through your favorite magazines and note advertisements for alcoholic beverages. What psychological techniques are used to sell the products? What are the hidden messages? How much do you think you're responding to such hidden messages when you drink?

Behavior Change Strategy

Developing Responsible Drinking Habits

How much do you drink? Is it the right amount for you? You may know the answer to this question already, or you may not have given it much thought. Many people learn through a single unpleasant experience how alcohol affects their bodies or minds. Others suffer ill effects but choose to ignore or deny them.

To make responsible, informed choices about alcohol, consider, first, whether there is any history of alcohol abuse or alcoholism in your family. Since there does seem to be a genetic component to the problem, this information is important to your decisions about alcohol. If someone in your family is dependent on alcohol, you may have a higher-than-average likelihood of becoming dependent too.

Second, consider whether you are dependent on other substances. Do you smoke, drink strong coffee every day, use other drugs regularly? Does some habit control your life (going out for a pack of cigarettes in the middle of the night, taking risks to get drugs)? Some people have more of a tendency to become addicted than others, and a person with one addiction is often likely to have other addictions as well. If this is the case for you, again, you may need to be more cautious with alcohol.

Keep a Record

Once you have answered these questions, find out more about your alcohol-related behavior by keeping track of your drinking for two weeks in your health diary. Keep a daily alcohol behavior record like the one illustrated in Chapter 1 for eating behavior. For every drink, include

- the time of day
- what the drink was
- how fast you drank it
- where you were
- what else you were doing
- how others influenced you
- what made you want to drink
- your feelings at the time
- your thoughts and concerns at the time
- changes in your feelings while you were drinking and afterwards
- any further consequences of having the drink

Analyze Your Record

Next, analyze your record to detect patterns of feelings and environmental cues. Do you always drink when you're at a certain place or with certain people? Do you sometimes drink just to be sociable, when you don't really want a drink and would be satisfied with a nonalcoholic beverage? Do you drink alcohol when you're thirsty? Refer to the list in this chapter of reasons given by college students for drinking to see if any of your reasons are the same. Also refer to the list of warning signs of alcohol abuse given in the text. Are any of them true for you? For example, do you feel uncomfortable in a social situation if alcohol is *not* available?

Set Goals

Now that you've analyzed your record, think about whether you want to change any of your behaviors. This might be the case if you tend to drink too much, even without driving, because alcohol damages your body. It should definitely be the case if you drink and drive or if you're becoming dependent on alcohol. Decide on goals that will give you the best

health and safety returns, such as a beer or a glass of wine with dinner, one drink per hour at a party, or no alcohol at all.

Devise a Plan

Refer back to your health diary to see what kinds of patterns your drinking falls into and where you can intervene to break the behavior chain. You may be able to change the antecedents of your behavior, for example, by stocking your refrigerator with alternative beverages, such as juices or sparkling water. If you feel self-conscious about ordering a nonalcoholic drink when you're out with a group, try recruiting a friend to do the same. If it's impossible to avoid drinking in some situations, such as at a bar or a beer party, you may decide to avoid those situations for a period of time.

Instead of drinking, you can try other activities that produce the same effect. For example, if you drink to relieve anxiety or tension, try adding 20 or 30 minutes of exercise to your schedule to help you manage stress. Or try doing a relaxation exercise or going for a brisk walk to help reduce anxiety before a party or date. If you drink to relieve depression or to stop worrying, consider finding a trustworthy person (perhaps a professional counselor) to talk to about the problem that's bothering you. If you drink to feel more comfortable sexually, consider ways to improve communication with your partner so you can deal with sexual issues more openly. When these activities are successful, they will reinforce your responsible drinking decisions and make it more likely that you'll make the same decisions again in the future.

For other ways to monitor and control your drinking behavior, see the suggestions given in the box entitled "Seven Ways to Drink Less" and in the section "Drinking Behavior and Responsibility."

Reward Yourself and Monitor Your Progress

If changing your drinking behavior turns out to be unusually difficult, it may be a clue that drinking was becoming a problem for you—all the more reason to get it under control now. Be sure to reward yourself as you learn to drink responsibly (or not at all), using the personal rewards you listed in your health diary at the beginning of this course. You may lose weight, look better, feel better, and have higher self-esteem as a result of limiting your drinking. Keep track of your progress in your health diary and revise your strategy if you start to revert to unhealthy or out-of-control patterns. Stay with your program by recruiting support, using a buddy, looking to a role model, and managing stress with healthy coping techniques. Remember, when you establish sensible drinking habits, you're planning not just for this week or month but for your whole life.

Selected Bibliography

American Psychiatric Association. 1987. *Diagnostic and Statistical Manual of Mental Disorders: Third Edition–Revised*. Washington, D.C.: American Psychiatric Association.

Brown, Stephanie. 1988. *Treating Adult Children of Alcoholics: A Developmental Perspective*. New York: Wiley.

Goodwin, Donald W. 1985. Alcoholism and genetics. The sins of the father. *Archives of General Psychiatry* 42(2):171–74.

Kinney, Jean, and Gwen Leaton. 1987. *Loosening the Grip: A Handbook of Alcohol Information*, 3rd ed. St. Louis: Mosby.

Kissin, Benjamin, and Henri Begleiter. 1983. *The Pathogenesis of Alcoholism: Biological Factors*. Vol. 7: *The Biology of Alcoholism*. New York: Plenum Press.

Kissin, Benjamin, and Henri Begleiter. 1983. *The Pathogenesis of Alcoholism: Psychosocial Factors*. Vol. 8: *The Biology of Alcoholism*. New York: Plenum Press.

Kolata, Gina. 1990. Study tells why alcohol is greater risk to women. *The New York Times*, January 11, p. A1.

Peele, S. 1986. The implications and limitations of genetic models of alcoholism and other addictions. *Journal of Studies of Alcoholism* 47(1):63–73.

Russell, R. 1986. *What Should We Teach About Alcohol?* Piscataway, N.J.: Rutgers Center of Alcohol Studies.

U.S. Public Health Service. 1987. *Alcohol and Health: Sixth Special Report to the U.S. Congress*. Washington, D.C.: U.S. Department of Health and Human Services.

U.S. Public Health Service. 1988. *Women and Alcohol Use: A Review of the Research Literature*. Washington, D.C.: U.S Department of Health and Human Services.

U.S. Public Health Service. 1989. *Surgeon General's Workshop on Drunk Driving: Background Papers*. Washington, D.C.: U.S. Department of Health and Human Services.

Volger, R. E., and W. R. Bartz. 1982. *The Better Way to Drink: The Alternative That Works*. New York: Simon and Schuster.

Recommended Readings

Alcoholics Anonymous, 3rd ed. 1976. New York. Alcoholics Anonymous World Services. *This is the "Big Book," the basic text for AA. It includes the founding tenets of AA and vivid histories of recovering alcoholics.*

Bassini, Richard. 1985. *How to Cut Down on Your Social Drinking*. New York: Putnam's. *More tips for reducing your alcohol intake.*

Dorris, Michael. 1989. *The Broken Cord*. New York. Harper and Row. *A personal story and an up-to-date source of information on the fetal alcohol syndrome.*

Goodwin, Donald. 1981. *Alcoholism: The Facts*. New York: Oxford University Press. *A scholarly, well-written book that critically reviews a great deal of research in alcoholism.*

Kissin, Benjamin, and Henri Begleiter. 1976. *Social Aspects of Alcoholism*. New York: Plenum. *A classic reference text that summarizes social science studies in alcoholism.*

Ray, Oakley, and Charles Ksir. 1987. *Drugs, Society, and Human Behavior*, 4th ed. St. Louis: Mosby. *An entertaining, popular college text that skillfully underscores societal factors that influence alcohol use.*

Steiner, Claude. 1971. *Games Alcoholics Play*. New York: Grove Press. *An interesting, readable book on the common behavioral patterns followed by people with alcohol problems.*

Contents

Making Connections

Some drugs improve people's lives; others destroy them. Drugs are everywhere in our society, and knowing how to handle situations involving them is crucial to maintaining control of your life. The scenarios presented on these pages describe situations in which people have to use information, make a decision, or choose a course of action, all involving the use of drugs. As you read them, imagine yourself in each situation and consider what you would do. After you've finished the chapter, read them again and see if what you've learned has changed how you would think, feel, or act in each situation.

Even though you enjoy drinking a lot of black coffee, you've decided to give it up because you've been feeling pretty nervous and jittery lately. You figured it would help you restore some calm to your life. You didn't have any coffee yesterday or today, and you're surprised to discover how much you want a cup. You also have a splitting headache that isn't responding to aspirin. You know you liked coffee, but this is ridiculous. What's going on?

A friend of yours has been snorting cocaine occasionally for the last six months, and lately he's been jumpy, harried, and distracted a lot of the time. Although he says he's too smart to get hooked, you're starting to wonder just how much he's taking. He's borrowed money from you and hasn't paid you back, and yesterday he told you he ran into some trouble the last time he went to the city. Now he wants to borrow money again. He's a good friend and you'd like to lend it to him, but you're worried that you might just be helping him get into more trouble. Is it likely that your friend has a drug problem? Should you lend him the money, no questions asked? Should you confront him with your concerns? What's the best thing to do in this situation?

11

The Use and Abuse of Psychoactive Drugs

You're at a party with friends where people are dancing, listening to music, and drinking beer. No one seems to make anything of it when someone brings out some marijuana and begins rolling a joint. Pretty soon it's being passed in your direction, although you notice that some people just pass it on without smoking it. You've never had marijuana, and you hesitate to try it. The person next to you says, "Don't you smoke? How come?" Should you take a puff to get out of answering that question? Why did some people not smoke it?

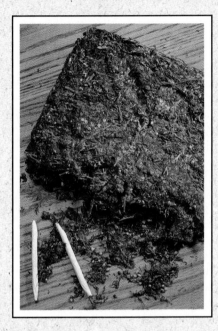

You realized too late that you hadn't allowed enough time for one of your term papers and that you were going to have to stay up all night to finish it. When you mentioned it to a friend, she offered you a Tenuate, a drug she takes as an appetite suppressant. You take it and find yourself soaring through your work. Your topic strikes you as intensely interesting, your ideas seem crystal clear, and words flow effortlessly from your pen. But suddenly at 3 o'clock in the morning it ends; your euphoria vanishes and a black cloud takes its place. All you can think of is putting on your coat and running over to your friend's place to get another pill. What happened? What kind of drug did you take? What are the risks in taking a drug like this?

Your aunt has been taking Valium under her physician's supervision for quite a while, and lately you notice that she's moving around awfully slowly and having trouble speaking clearly. You asked your father about it, and he said she's "addicted to that damn drug she takes." How could she be "addicted" to a prescription drug under a physician's care? Can she get off it, and is she in danger if she doesn't?

The United States and many other countries are drug societies today. The use of drugs for both medical and social purposes is common and widespread. The prevailing attitude among many people is that all problems, no matter how big or small, have chemical solutions. Our expectations about drugs are fed by medical research findings, by advertisements, by social pressures, by our fast-paced, quick-fix life, and by our personal hopes for easy answers to life's difficult questions. Many people have learned to seek immediate relief from even the mildest physical or emotional discomfort by finding a drug to do the trick.

Drugs are defined as chemicals other than food intended to affect the structure or function of the body. They include prescription medicines, such as antibiotics or tranquilizers; over-the-counter remedies, such as aspirin or antihistamines; legal substances, such as alcohol, tobacco, and caffeine products; and illegal substances, such as cocaine, marijuana, and heroin. This chapter focuses primarily on **psychoactive drugs**, chemicals that can alter a person's experiences or consciousness—sensations, feelings, thoughts, or the functions of the nervous system. Although psychoactive drugs are often thought of in terms of illegal substances, many drugs have psychoactive properties, including alcohol, tobacco, and a number of prescription and over-the-counter drugs. Those drugs are discussed in other chapters.

The Drug Tradition

Human beings have been altering consciousness with drugs since prehistoric times. As mentioned in Chapter 10, alcohol has been used for thousands of years, to heal, to celebrate, to intoxicate. All over the world, native populations have known about the psychoactive properties of various local plants, such as the coca plant in South America, the opium poppy in the Middle East and Far East, *Cannabis sativa* (the source of marijuana) in many areas, and various mushrooms and other plants. All of these drugs have been used for religious, medicinal, and personal reasons, usually under controlled circumstances, such as in ceremonies.

In the nineteenth century, chemists were successful in extracting the active elements from medicinal plants, such as morphine from the opium poppy and atropine, a muscle spasm reliever, from belladonna. This was the beginning of *pharmacy*, the art of compounding drugs, and of *pharmacology*, the science and study of drugs.

From this point on, a variety of drugs began to be produced, including cocaine, heroin, and codeine (see Figure 11-1).

At first these drugs were used freely as ingredients in medicines that could be purchased without a prescription. They were even used in nonalcoholic beverages; Coca-Cola originally contained a small amount of cocaine, which accounted for the "lift" it provided. As a result of the heavy use of drugs in medicines and commercial products, by 1900 many people were addicted to them in Europe and the United States. Pure food and drug legislation was passed to protect consumers, and the use of drugs dropped sharply over the course of the next fifty years.

In the 1960s, there was a surge in the recreational use of drugs, such as marijuana, cocaine, amphetamines, LSD, and a variety of other psychoactive drugs synthesized in laboratories. Use continued to rise until the late 1970s, when it stabilized and began to decline slightly, at least for many drugs. The exception is cocaine, whose use and abuse continue to grow in some populations. Today, the drug scene in the United States is dominated by a multibillion dollar criminal drug industry that thrives on the dependencies and recreational habits of large segments of the population.

Use, Abuse, and Dependence

Why do people use drugs today? The answer to this question depends on both the user and the drug. Young people, especially young people from middle-class backgrounds, are frequently drawn to drugs by the allure of the exciting and illicit. They may be curious, rebellious, or vulnerable to peer pressure. They may want to appear to be daring and to be part of the group. They may want to imitate adult models in their lives or in the movies. Most people who have taken illicit drugs have done so on an experimental basis, typically trying the drug one or more times but not continuing beyond that. The main factors in the initial choice of a drug are whether it is available and whether other people around are already using it.

Although some people use drugs because they have a desire to alter their mood or are seeking a spiritual experience, others are primarily motivated by a desire to escape boredom, anxiety, depression, feelings of worthlessness, or other distressing symptoms of psychological problems. They use drugs as a way to cope with the

---

Drugs Chemicals other than food intended to affect the structure or function of the body.

Psychoactive drug Any chemical other than food that when taken into the body can alter the user's consciousness.

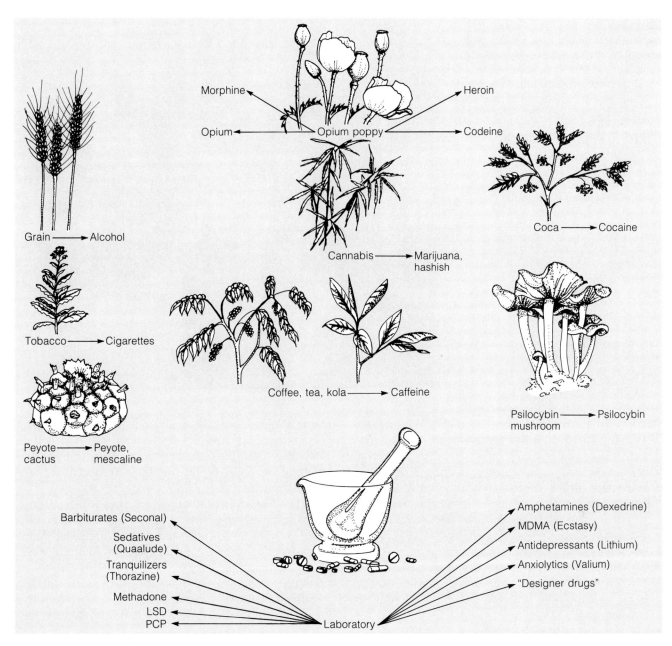

Figure 11-1   Sources of selected psychoactive drugs.

difficulties they are experiencing in life. The common practice in our society of seeking a drug solution to every problem is a factor in the widespread reliance on both illicit drugs and prescription drugs like Valium.

■ **Exploring Your Emotions**

How do you feel about people taking psychoactive drugs? Do you feel differently about people using marijuana, cocaine, or Valium than about people using alcohol? If so, why?

For minorities living in poverty in the inner cities, many of these reasons for using drugs apply in magnified form. The problems are more devastating, the need for escape more compelling. The buying and selling of drugs reflect issues of race, class, and economics more than personal quests or uncertain values. The problems associated with the inner-city drug culture in the United States are discussed in more detail elsewhere in this chapter.

Drug Abuse   What does it mean when we say a drug is abused? All drugs have the potential for misuse and

Many people try drugs out of curiosity and take them for a relatively brief period of time. Like these teenagers, they usually drink beer and smoke marijuana with friends in social situations, using the drugs to change their perceptions and alter their moods.

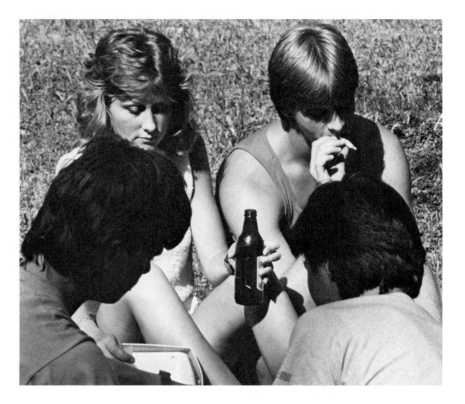

abuse. A drug is misused when it is taken for a purpose or in a way for which it was not intended. For example, if you borrow some of your roommate's antibiotic to treat your ear infection, you are misusing a drug. **Drug abuse** goes beyond misuse. It occurs when a drug is taken to the extent that it causes physical damage to the user; impairment of the user's ability to function in social situations, in school, or on the job; or behavior that is harmful to others. Sometimes the original abuse of a drug came about unexpectedly as a by-product of its medical use, as in the case of cocaine. Many of the drugs discussed here are used or were originally used to treat pain or other symptoms.

Drug Dependence   Drug abuse is different from drug **dependence** (or dependency), formerly called addiction. Two different kinds of dependence are distinguished, physical and psychological, although in practice they are usually intertwined.

A key feature of physical dependence is the presence of **withdrawal** symptoms when the user tries to give up the habit or cut down on the dose. Withdrawal symptoms from opiates may include sweating, running nose, and yawning. If the level of the drug in the bloodstream continues to drop, symptoms get worse and may include weakness, nausea, vomiting, stomach pains, diarrhea, and aches and pains. A dose of the drug puts an imme-

Figure 11-2   "Chipping" versus developing tolerance. When a user allows intervals between doses, tolerance doesn't build up.

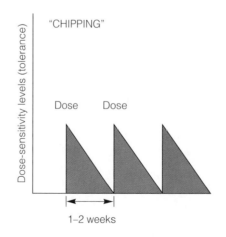

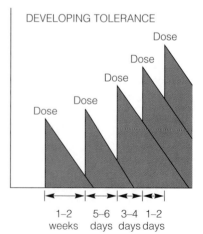

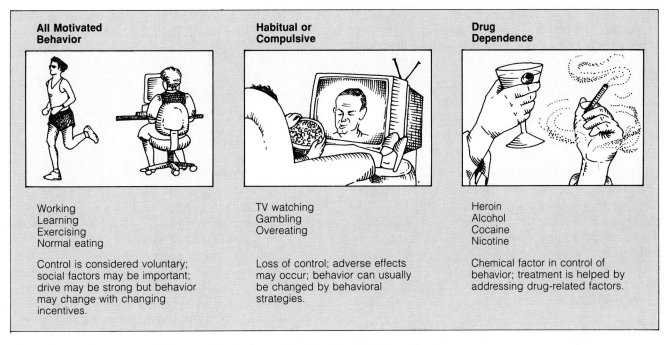

All Motivated Behavior	Habitual or Compulsive	Drug Dependence
Working Learning Exercising Normal eating	TV watching Gambling Overeating	Heroin Alcohol Cocaine Nicotine
Control is considered voluntary; social factors may be important; drive may be strong but behavior may change with changing incentives.	Loss of control; adverse effects may occur; behavior can usually be changed by behavioral strategies.	Chemical factor in control of behavior; treatment is helped by addressing drug-related factors.

Figure 11-3 Behavior control. A progression from normal to dependent behavior occurs in some areas of life for some people. The key feature of this progression is loss of control.

diate end to these unpleasant symptoms.

Physical dependence is often associated with **tolerance**. Users develop a tolerance for the drug and need larger and larger doses to achieve the same effect. Users sometimes try to stay one step ahead of the game by using a technique called "chipping" (see Figure 11-2). They take only infrequent, low doses in a usually futile attempt to avoid getting hooked. But too often the time between doses shortens, the dose gets bigger, and tolerance develops. The usual starting dose of heroin, for example, is about 3 mg, but tolerance can lead within a few months to doses of 1,000 mg.

Psychological dependence involves a strong repetitive need, or craving, for the change in feelings and mood that a particular drug provides. Some drugs induce euphoria, others reduce unpleasant psychological states, and still others just cause a change—in some instances a change that many would deem unpleasant. Psychological dependence is strongly affected by social factors; particular situations, times of day, or people may trigger the compulsive craving for the drug. Personality traits can also play a role in whether a person develops a psycho-

logical dependence on a particular drug. In some ways, people can become psychologically dependent on things other than drugs, too, such as gambling, overeating, or sex (see Figure 11-3).

■ **Exploring Your Emotions**

Most people have things they have to do every day or else they don't feel comfortable or good about themselves— taking a shower, going for a jog, spending some time reading or relaxing. Do you have any of these "good habits" or "positive addictions"? Do you have others? What are they?

The opiates (morphine, heroin, codeine, and so on) are common dependency-producing psychoactive drugs, although the physiological mechanism of dependency is not fully understood. The **central nervous system (CNS)** depressants, including alcohol, and the CNS stimulants, including nicotine, also induce physical dependency to varying degrees. Marijuana in moderate doses and the psychedelics and deliriants do not produce physical dependence. Psychological dependence is a pos-

---

Drug abuse Taking drugs to a degree that causes physical damage, impairs functioning, or results in behavior harmful to others.

Dependence (dependency) A behavior pattern of compulsive drug users. The pattern is characterized by preoccupation with acquiring the drug and using it. It used to be termed *addiction.*

Withdrawal The process of abstaining from a drug on which one has been dependent.

Tolerance Lower sensitivity to a drug so that a given dose no longer exerts the usual effect and larger doses are needed.

Central nervous system (CNS) The brain and spinal cord.

sibility for all drugs and, as mentioned earlier, is often mixed with physical dependence. Getting off drugs for a short time is relatively easy; most drug abusers have done it many times. The hard part is adjusting to life without the drug or finding something to take its place.

How Drugs Affect the Body

Like alcohol and tobacco, the psychoactive drugs discussed in this chapter have effects that are extremely complex and highly variable. The same drug may affect different users differently or the same user in different ways under different circumstances. The effects of a drug depend on three general categories of factors: (1) drug factors—the properties of the drug itself and differences in how it's used, (2) user factors—the physical characteristics of the user, and (3) psychological and social factors.

Drug Factors   When different drugs or dosages produce different effects, the differences are usually caused by one or more of five different drug factors:

- The **pharmacological properties** of the drug are its overall effects on a person's body chemistry, behavior, and psychology. Some drugs are classified according to what kind of effect they have on the body, such as the CNS stimulants and the CNS depressants. Other drugs are classified by their chemical makeup, such as the opiates, which are derived from opium.

    Of all the millions of chemicals known, only a few have pharmacological properties that lead humans to use and abuse them. These voluntarily self-administered chemicals are alcohol, nicotine, and the drug groups discussed in this chapter—opiates; barbiturates and other sedative-hypnotics; tranquilizers; caffeine and amphetamine-like stimulants; cocaine; psychedelics; certain deliriants; and marijuana. With the exception of the psychedelics, all of these drugs are also self-administered by laboratory animals. The pharmacological properties that make them attractive to humans in social settings also make them appealing to animals.

- The **dose-response function** is the relationship between the amount of drug taken and the intensity or type of drug effect. This relationship is not necessarily a direct one in which increasing the dose simply increases or intensifies the effect. Rather, the effect can change with a higher dosage. A familiar example is the person who becomes friendly after one cocktail but belligerent and hostile after four. With some drugs there is a plateau in the dose-response function in which a larger dose has no effect on the response. With LSD, for example, the greatest changes in perception occur at a certain dose, and no further changes in perception take place if higher doses are taken.

- The **time-action function** is the relationship between the time elapsed since a drug was taken and the intensity of its effect. The effects of a drug are greatest when concentrations of the drug in the tissues are changing the fastest, especially if they are increasing. A constant drug level, even a high one, is less likely to change the user's experience or behavior. For example, with alcohol, immediately after a person takes a drink, the alcohol begins to be absorbed in the digestive tract and the level of alcohol in the blood begins to rise rapidly. As the alcohol is metabolized, the blood alcohol level gradually falls, as explained in Chapter 10. Intoxication is usually greater when the level is rising than when it is falling, even though there may actually be somewhat less alcohol in the blood when it is rising.

- The *cumulative effects* of psychoactive drugs may be different from the effects of a single dose, because over time the drugs produce physiological alterations in the body that change their effects. A given amount of alcohol, for example, will generally affect a habitual drinker less than an occasional drinker. Tolerance to some drugs, such as LSD, builds rapidly. To experience the same effect, a user has to abstain from the drug for a period of time before that dosage will again exert its original effects.

- The *method of use* has a direct effect on how strong a response a drug produces. Methods of use include ingestion, inhalation, injection, and absorption through the skin or tissue linings. If a drug is taken by a method that allows the drug to enter the bloodstream and reach the brain rapidly, the effects are usually stronger than when the method involves slower absorption. For ex-

---

Pharmacological properties   The overall effects of a drug on the individual's behavior, psychology, and chemistry. This term also refers to the amount of the drug required to exert various effects, the time course of these effects, and other characteristics of the drug such as its chemical composition.

Dose-response function   The relationship between the amount of a drug taken and the intensity or type of drug effect.

Time-action function   The relationship between the time elapsed since a drug was taken and the intensity of a drug effect.

Biochemical   Describes the branch of chemistry that deals with the life processes of plants and animals.

Set   A person's expectations or preconceptions in a given situation.

Placebo   An inert or innocuous medication that is given in place of an active drug; it is often called a sugar pill.

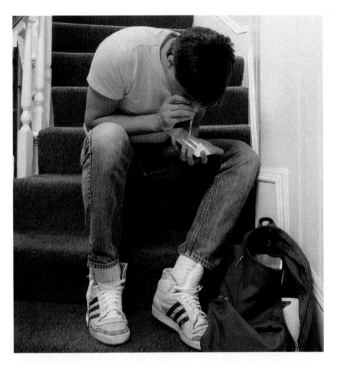

Most middle-class users sniff, or "snort," cocaine, a method of use that produces effects in two to three minutes. With other methods, such as injecting it intravenously, inhaling vapors, or smoking crack, the effects of cocaine are felt within seconds. Method of use is just one variable in the overall effect of a drug on the body.

ample, injecting a drug generally produces stronger effects than swallowing the same drug. Drugs are usually injected one of three ways: intravenously (IV, or mainlining), intramuscularly (IM), or subcutaneously (SQ, or "skin popping"). Inhaling (smoking) marijuana produces about three times the effects of the same dose taken by mouth, at least for people who are used to smoking.

Different methods of drug use are associated with different "costs," or risks. For example, injecting drugs often involves the sharing of needles, which may be contaminated with disease agents from another user's blood. In some groups, the primary route of AIDS infection is through contaminated needles. AIDS and other infections carried in the blood can be avoided by not sharing needles and by sterilizing needles that are shared, although sterilization has to be done carefully because viruses can be transmitted in very small amounts of blood.

User Factors   The second category of factors that determine how a person will respond to a particular drug involves the person's physical characteristics. Body mass is one variable that can make a difference in response. The effects of certain drugs on a 100-pound person will

be twice as great as the effect of the same amount of the drug on a 200-pound person. Other variables include general health and various subtle **biochemical** states, including genetic factors. For example, some people have an inherited ability to rapidly metabolize a cough suppressant called dextromethorphan, which also has psychoactive properties. These people must take a higher than normal dose to get a given cough suppressant effect.

If a person's biochemical state is already altered by another drug, this too can make a difference in the effect of a drug. Some drugs intensify the effects of other drugs, as is the case with alcohol and barbiturates, both CNS depressants. Some drugs block the effects of other drugs, such as when an anxiolytic is used to relieve anxiety caused by cocaine. Interactions between drugs, including many prescription and over-the-counter drugs, can be unpredictable and dangerous.

One physical condition that requires special precautions is pregnancy. It can be risky for a woman to use any drugs at all during pregnancy, including alcohol and common over-the-counter drugs like cough medicine. The risks are greatest during the first trimester of pregnancy when the fetus's body is rapidly forming and even small chemical alterations in the mother's body can have a devastating effect on development. Even later, the fetus is more susceptible than the mother to the adverse effects of any drugs she takes.

Psychological and Social Factors   Sometimes a user's response to a drug is affected strongly by factors other than the pharmacological or the physiological ones. With large doses, the chemical properties of the drug do seem to have the strongest influence on the user's response. But with small doses, psychological and social factors are often more important. These factors are known as the set and the setting.

The **set** is the user's expectations about how he or she is going to respond to the drug. When people strongly believe that a given drug will affect them a certain way, they are likely to experience those effects regardless of the drug's pharmacological properties. The **placebo** effect—when an individual receives an inert substance and yet responds as if it were an active drug—is a well-documented example of set.

■ **Exploring Your Emotions**

What do you think are a woman's responsibilities to her unborn child? Does she have an obligation to avoid drugs and alcohol during pregnancy? What about smoking cigarettes and eating junk food? If she doesn't follow her physician's advice, should she be held legally responsible for the effects on the child?

The **setting** is the physical and social environment surrounding the drug use. If a person uses marijuana at home with trusted friends and pleasant music, the effects are likely to be different from the effects if the same dose is taken in an austere experimental laboratory with an impassive research technician. Similarly, the dose of alcohol that produces mild euphoria and stimulation at a noisy, active cocktail party might induce sleepiness and slight depression when taken at home while alone.

■ Exploring Your Emotions

Do you ever have a vague craving for something and not know what you wanted? Have you ever stared into the refrigerator looking for some food or drink that you think might make you feel better? Have you ever eaten too much candy or ice cream, drunk too much coffee or Coke, or smoked too many cigarettes? If so, do you think your motivations differ from those of a drug user?

Experiments have been conducted in which some subjects smoked small quantities of marijuana while others (unknowingly) smoked a substance that smelled and tasted like marijuana but was not. The intensity of the **"high"** the subjects experienced was not related to whether or not they had actually smoked marijuana. In other studies, subjects who smoked low doses of real marijuana that they believed to be a placebo experienced no effects from the drug. Clearly, the setting and the set had greater effects on the smokers than the drug itself.

Representative Psychoactive Drugs

What are the major psychoactive drugs, and how do they produce their effects? We discuss six different representative groups in this chapter: (1) opiates, (2) CNS depressants, (3) CNS stimulants, (4) psychedelics, (5) marijuana and other cannabis products, and (6) deliriants. As mentioned earlier, some of these drugs are classified according to how they affect the body; others—the opiates and the cannabis products—are classified according to their chemical makeup.

Opiates   The opiates, also called narcotics, are natural or synthetic (laboratory-made) drugs that relieve pain, cause drowsiness, and induce **euphoria**. Opium, morphine, heroin, methadone, codeine, and meperidine are examples of drugs in this class. The opiates tend to reduce anxiety and to produce lethargy, apathy, and an inability to concentrate. Opiate users become less active and less responsive to frustration, hunger, and sexual stimulation. These effects are more pronounced in novice users; with repeated use, many effects diminish.

Although the euphoria associated with opiates is an important factor in their abuse, many individuals experience a feeling of vague uneasiness when they first use these drugs. They may feel nauseated, vomit, or have other unpleasant sensations. As mentioned earlier, the opiates are often dependency-producing. The reasons for this are not entirely clear, but it undoubtedly is due to a combination of pharmacological, psychological, and social factors.

The various opiates have similar effects, but they do differ in dose-response and time-action characteristics. They are sometimes injected under the skin, into the muscles, or directly into the veins. They may also be taken into the body by **absorption** from the stomach and intestine, the nasal membranes, or the lungs. As mentioned earlier, how the drug is taken determines how quickly it enters body tissue. If it is injected intravenously or smoked, the tissue level will change rapidly, and more behavioral changes will result.

A great deal of recent research has been devoted to the study of **endorphins**, opiates that occur naturally in the body. Endorphins appear to control pain and regulate emotional states and sensory input. Some researchers believe they are responsible for the phenomenon known as "runner's high," the feeling of euphoria some runners experience, and other researchers think they may play a role in premenstrual syndrome (PMS). Endorphins and the receptors for them in the brain may play a role in the dependency process that occurs with the opiates.

A relatively recent addition to the group of psychoactive chemicals are the "designer drugs." These are new compounds that are produced in clandestine laboratories by modifying the chemical structure of older, often naturally occurring drugs. Because they are "new" drugs, they aren't illegal until they are specifically outlawed. Designer heroin, or 3-methylfentanyl, also known as "China White," is an example of a synthetic opiate. It was initially touted as a "safe" opiate but was subsequently found to have most of the negative effects of heroin.

Central Nervous System Depressants   Central nervous system **depressants**, or **sedative-hypnotics**, slow down the overall activity of the nervous system. The result ranges from mild sedation to death, depending on the various factors involved—which drug is used, how it's taken, how tolerant the user is, and so on. The most common CNS depressants are alcohol (discussed in Chapter 10), **barbiturates**, antianxiety agents, and various other drugs with similar effects.

Effects   CNS depressants reduce anxiety and produce mood changes, muscular incoordination, slurring of speech, and drowsiness or sleep. Mental and motor functioning are also affected, but the degree varies from person to person and also depends on the kind of task the

---

Signs of Drug Dependence

If you notice changes in behavior and mood in someone you know, they may signal a growing dependence on drugs. Signs that a person's life is beginning to center on drugs include the following:

1. Sudden withdrawal or emotional distance

2. Rebellious or unusually irritable behavior

3. Loss of interest in usual activities or hobbies

4. Decline in school performance

5. Sudden change in group of friends

6. Changes in sleeping or eating habits

7. Frequent borrowing of money or stealing

If you wonder whether *you* are becoming dependent on a drug, ask youself the following questions. The more times you answer yes, the more likely it is that you are developing a physical or psychological dependency on the drug.

1. Do you take the drug on a regular basis? Have you been taking it for a long time?

2. Do you always take the drug in certain situations or when you're with certain people?

3. Do you find it difficult to stop using the drug? Do you feel powerless to quit?

4. Do you need to take a larger dose of the drug in order to get the same high you're used to?

5. Do you take the drug to feel "normal"?

6. Do you go to extreme lengths to get the drug? Do you put yourself in dangerous situations to get it?

7. Do you hide your drug use from others?

8. Do you think about the drug when you're not high, figuring out ways to get it?

9. If you stop taking the drug, do you feel bad until you can take it again?

10. Does the drug interfere with your ability to study, work, or socialize?

If your answers suggest dependency, talk to someone at your health clinic about taking care of the problem before it gets worse.

---

person is trying to do. Most people become drowsy with small doses, although a few become more active. However, when people take these drugs deliberately to alter their awareness or for social reasons, they can overcome most of the sedative effects and remain awake even with large doses. It is particularly easy for the user to overcome drowsiness if he or she has developed tolerance or if the environment is stimulating and exciting.

During the last twenty years, many new drugs have been marketed as "safe" and "nonaddicting" sedative-hypnotics, but most of these have turned out to have unwanted side effects and dangers, just as the barbiturates do (see the box titled "Signs of Drug Dependence").

Methaqualone (Quaalude is the trade name of a common methaqualone compound) is an example of a sedative-hypnotic that was initially considered to be safe and to have little potential for abuse. Now, it is clear that methaqualone can have significant adverse effects and is often abused.

Anxiolytics, also termed **tranquilizers**, such as diazepam (Valium) can also be classified as CNS depressants. In low doses, the anxiolytics reduce anxiety without causing extreme drowsiness but in high doses **sedation** is inevitable.

In most countries a variety of barbiturates are available. They are all similar in chemical composition and action,

---

Setting   The environment in which something is done.

"High"   The subjectively pleasing effects of a drug, usually felt quite soon after the drug is taken.

Euphoria   An exaggerated feeling of well-being.

Absorption   The passage of substances through the skin, lungs, or gastrointestinal tract into the blood.

Endorphin   A chemical produced naturally in the brain that has pain-killing effects.

Depressant   Something that decreases nervous or muscular activity.

Sedative-hypnotics   Another term for CNS depressants. These drugs cause drowsiness or sleep.

Barbiturate   A common sedative-hypnotic drug.

Anxiolytic   A drug that can reduce tension and anxiety without putting the user to sleep; a tranquilizer.

Tranquilizers   The common term for anxiolytics; CNS depressants that reduce tension and anxiety; can also refer to antipsychotic drugs.

Sedation   The induction of a calm, relaxed, often sleepy state.

but they do differ in how quickly they act and how long their action lasts. Drug users call barbiturates "downers" or "downs" and refer to specific brands by names that describe the color and design of the capsules: "reds" or "red devils" for Seconal, "yellows" or "yellow jackets" for Nembutal, "blue heavens" for Amytal, and "trees" for Tuinal (a combination of secobarbital and amobarbital). People usually take barbiturates in capsules, but injecting them is also common. Injection of any drug carries a risk of abscess—a persistent infection at the needle site or at other places in the circulatory system.

Medical Uses   Barbiturates, methaqualone, and other sedative-hypnotics are widely used for treating people with insomnia, as daytime sedatives, and for control of seizures. They are also used to modify the effects of other drugs (for example, to reduce the excessive physical activity that often accompanies the use of CNS stimulants). Some CNS depressants are used for their calming properties in combination with **anesthetic agents** before operations and other medical or dental procedures.

From Use to Abuse   People usually have their first experience with CNS depressants either by way of medical prescription or by way of friends in the drug subculture. Abuse for the medical patient may begin with repeated use for insomnia and progress to dependency through bigger and bigger doses at night coupled with a few capsules at stressful times during the day.

The abuse of Valium and Xanax, a similar but newer anxiolytic, often involves increasingly frequent doses during the day. Dependency becomes apparent when the person tries to reduce or stop the medication and feelings of anxiety ensue. The anxiety is "treated" with another dose, and the process escalates.

Most CNS depressants, including alcohol and the barbiturates, can lead to classical physical dependence, with pronounced tolerance and withdrawal symptoms. Tolerance, sometimes for up to fifteen times the usual dose, can develop during a year or two of repeated use. Tolerance to the depression of the respiratory system caused by these drugs develops more slowly than tolerance to the behavioral effects of the dose. As with heroin and alcohol, the margin between a dose that does what the user wants and a lethal overdose narrows dangerously. Withdrawal symptoms are more severe than those accompanying opiate dependence and are similar to the DTs of alcoholism. They begin as anxiety, shaking, and weakness but may turn into convulsions and possible cardiovascular collapse, which may result in death.

A recent study at the Addiction Research Foundation in Ontario, Canada, demonstrated that long-term use of Valium and other tranquilizers in the benzodiazepine family on a regular basis can lead to dependence even at ordinary prescribed doses. In the study, Valium users who were given a placebo and thus deprived of the drug experienced classic withdrawal symptoms, including headache, insomnia, sweating, feelings of anxiety, and difficulty in concentrating. The researchers concluded that physicians should be more careful about prescribing these drugs, even though they can prevent withdrawal by cutting the dose gradually and weaning the patient off the drug.

Many CNS depressant drugs show **cross-tolerance**. For example, an individual who has developed tolerance to effects of alcohol can often tolerate higher doses of barbiturates. This principle of cross-tolerance is sometimes used in treating withdrawal symptoms from sustained use of a CNS depressant drug. Withdrawal from alcohol, for instance, can be treated by substituting high doses of a less toxic cross-tolerant drug such as diazepam.

While intoxicated, people on depressants cannot function very well. They are mentally confused and are frequently obstinate, irritable, and abusive. They commonly have poor general health and may suffer from (sometimes permanent) brain damage, with impaired ability to reason and make judgments. Furthermore, the lack of coordination caused by these drugs often results in injuries and accidents.

Overdosing with CNS Depressants   Barbiturates and other sedative-hypnotics are major agents of self-destruction. Barbiturate overdose is one of the most frequent methods of suicide among American women and accounts for over 3,000 known deaths each year in the United States. Many accidental deaths result when people use barbiturates and alcohol together. Even if a single dose of either would not have been fatal, combined depressant effects of both can halt breathing. Alcohol and barbiturates are not unique in this respect; combinations of many depressants can exert more deleterious effects than a single depressant used alone. Barbiturate dependents, like alcoholics and opiate addicts, often become preoccupied with having enough of the drug and sometimes resort to criminal activities to make sure they do. Violent behavior has also been linked with barbiturate dependence and with the use of methaqualone.

Central Nervous System Stimulants   CNS **stimulants** speed up the activity of the nervous system. Under their

---

Anesthetic agents   Drugs that produce loss of sensation with or without loss of consciousness.

Cross-tolerance   The capacity of one drug to prevent withdrawal symptoms when another drug is abruptly discontinued.

Stimulant   Something that increases nervous or muscular activity.

Codependency

A codependent is a person who is in a continuing relationship with a drug-abusing person and whose actions help or enable that person to remain dependent. Codependency, also called enabling, removes or softens the effects of the drug use on the user. People often become enablers spontaneously and naturally. When someone they love becomes dependent on a drug, they want to help, and they assume that their good intentions will persuade the drug user to stop. Unfortunately, alcoholics and drug-dependent people have a system of denial that is strengthened rather than diminished by well-meaning attempts to help.

The habit of enabling hinders a drug-dependent person's recovery because the person never has to experience the consequences of his or her behavior. Frequently, the enabler is dependent too—on the pattern of interaction in the rela-

tionship. People who need to take care of people often marry people who need to be taken care of. Children in these families often develop the same pattern of behavior as one of their parents, either by becoming helpless or by becoming a caregiver. This is why treatment programs for drug dependency, such as Alcoholics Anonymous, Narcotics Anonymous, and Cocaine Anonymous, involve the whole family.

Have you ever been an enabler in a relationship? You may have if you have ever done any of the following:

- Given someone one more chance to stop abusing drugs, then another, and another . . .
- Made excuses or lied for someone to his or her friends, teachers, or employer
- Joined someone in drug use and blamed others for your behavior

- Lent money to someone to continue drug use
- Stayed up late waiting or gone out searching for someone who uses drugs
- Felt embarrassed or angry about the actions of someone who uses drugs
- Ignored the drug use because the person got defensive when you brought it up
- Not confronted a friend or relative who was obviously intoxicated or high on a drug

There are a number of books available in bookstores on codependency. A good one is *Codependent No More* by Melody Beattie (see the Recommended Readings). If you come from a codependent family or see yourself developing relationships like this, consider acting now to make changes in your patterns of interaction.

influence, heart rate accelerates, blood pressure rises, blood vessels constrict, the pupils of the eyes and the bronchial tubes dilate, and gastric and adrenal secretions increase. There is greater muscular tension and sometimes an increase in motor activity. Small doses usually make people feel more awake and alert, less fatigued and bored. The most common CNS stimulants are cocaine, amphetamine, nicotine (discussed in Chapter 9), and caffeine.

Cocaine   Usually derived from the leaves of coca shrubs that grow high in the Andes Mountains, cocaine is a potent CNS stimulant. For centuries natives of the Andes have chewed coca leaves both for pleasure and to increase their endurance. For a short time in the nineteenth century, some physicians were enthusiastic about the use of cocaine to cure alcoholism and addiction to morphine, which was used as a painkiller. As is so often the case with new drug treatments, enthusiasm waned after the adverse side effects became apparent.

Cocaine—also known as "coke" or "snow"—quickly produces an intense euphoria, which makes it a popular recreational drug. A 1988 study indicated that the number of casual users of cocaine in the United States had decreased since 1985, but the number of heavy users—those who use it daily or at least weekly—had risen sharply. Cocaine is expensive, costing about $600 an ounce for high-quality supplies, and cheaper substitutes such as methamphetamine are sometimes used. Alternatives don't produce the same pleasure, however, so they're not as desirable.

■ **Exploring Your Emotions**

Do you think there is such a thing as responsible use of illegal psychoactive drugs? Are they a legitimate recreational activity if used with restraint? If you think so, where do you draw the line between legitimate and illegitimate use?

Table 11-1 Why Crack Cocaine Poses Particular Problems

Crack Cocaine	Comparison Drugs
Rapid onset of effects.	Drugs ingested or sniffed have much slower onset.
Initial effect usually intense euphoria.	Other drugs less intense.
More "brain rewarding" than any other drug.	Preferred over all other drugs in animal self-administration studies.
Short duration of effects with abrupt termination of pleasurable effects.	Almost all other drugs have more gradual termination of their effects. "Let-down" less intense.
Often no obvious side effects.	Alcohol and other CNS depressants often cause slurring of speech, etc. Opiates often cause drowsiness.
No odor.	Marijuana and alcohol have distinctive odors.
Can be smoked.	"Regular" cocaine does not vaporize and thus is usually sniffed or injected.
No attractive chemical alternative.	Therapists can substitute other CNS depressants for alcohol, methadone for heroin, etc.

METHODS OF USE   Although cocaine can be swallowed and absorbed into the bloodstream from the stomach and intestine, it is usually sniffed, snorted, or injected intravenously since those methods of administration provide more rapid increases of cocaine concentrations in the blood and hence more intense effects. Another method of administration involves heating the cocaine with ether or other chemicals and then inhaling its vapors. In "free-basing," as this practice is called, the user risks burns from sudden combustion.

A chemically similar method of processing cocaine involves baking soda and water. This yields a ready-to-smoke form of free-base cocaine, often called crack. Crack is typically available as small beads or pellets smokable in glass pipes or sprinkled on tobacco or marijuana. The tiny but potent beads can be handled more easily than cocaine powder and marketed in smaller, less expensive doses. Thus, processing cocaine into crack has increased cocaine availability to young people and others who couldn't afford to buy more expensive preparations

(see Table 11-1). This increased availability of smaller, cheaper doses was a major factor in the surge of cocaine use in the 1980s and the growth of a crime-ridden crack subculture in American cities.

EFFECTS   The effects of cocaine are usually intense but short-lived. The euphoria lasts from five to twenty minutes and ends abruptly, to be replaced by irritability, anxiety, or slight depression. When the cocaine is absorbed via the lungs, either by smoking or inhalation, it reaches the brain in 10 seconds or so, and the effects are particularly intense. This is part of the appeal of both free-basing and smoking crack. The effects from intravenous injections occur almost as quickly—20 seconds. Since the mucous membranes in the nose briefly slow absorption, the onset of effects from sniffing or snorting takes two or three minutes. Heavy users who want to maintain the effects inject cocaine intravenously every 10 to 20 minutes.

■ **Exploring Your Emotions**

Cocaine can cause sudden death in healthy people, although such cases are very rare. If you were at a party where people were using cocaine, would you point out the risks? Would you use it yourself?

The larger the dose of cocaine and the more rapidly it is absorbed into the bloodstream, the greater the immediate—and sometimes lethal—effects. Sudden death from cocaine is most commonly the result of excessive CNS stimulation that causes convulsions and respiratory collapse, cardiac arrhythmias (irregularities in heartbeat), excessive constriction of the arteries to the heart causing ischemia (lack of oxygen to heart muscle), and possibly heart attacks or strokes. Fatalities can occur in young, athletic people who have no underlying health problems. Fortunately, these deaths are quite rare, although they generate widespread publicity when they involve professional athletes or other celebrities.

Cocaine users sometimes try to alter or control their experience by using "speedball" mixtures, which combine cocaine with a depressant, such as a barbiturate, or with an opiate. However, the rapid changes thus imposed on the CNS are sometimes fatal. Comedian John Belushi died from a combination of intravenous cocaine and heroin.

Cocaine constricts the blood vessels and it acts as a local anesthetic. It is still used for minor nose surgery where bleeding is a problem. However, in the chronic cocaine snorter, this therapeutic "benefit" can occasion-

Vasoconstriction   A constriction of the blood vessels.

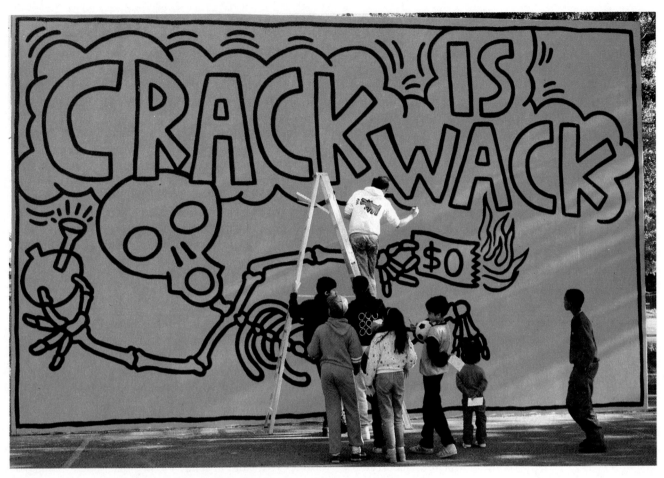

With the introduction of crack cocaine in the 1980s, the use of drugs and the incidence of associated crime rose dramatically in the United States, especially in the cities. This playground backboard, painted by the late Keith Haring, attempts to raise awareness among young people about the consequences of crack use.

ally progress to a "cost" of the drug. The repeated **vasoconstriction** produces a typical inflammation of the nasal mucosa, which can lead to persistent bleeding and ulceration of the septum between the nostrils.

Cocaine users may become paranoid or violent. The early stereotype of the crazed, homicidal "dope fiend" was the cocaine user, not the heroin addict. However, even for the chronic cocaine user, the "dope fiend" stereotype seldom applies.

DEPENDENCE   Because cocaine is metabolized so quickly and because tolerance builds up rapidly, it has to be taken frequently to produce the desired effect. Psychological craving and withdrawal reactions are probably also factors in chronic use. When steady cocaine users stop taking the drug, they may feel depressed and lethargic. The depression is temporarily relieved by taking more cocaine, so continued use is reinforced (see the box titled "Drugs in America: The Human Cost"). Some binge cocaine users go for weeks or months without using any cocaine and then take large amounts repeatedly. This pattern underscores the importance of psychological factors in chemical dependencies and refutes older conceptions of "addiction" that insisted on physiological tolerance or withdrawal symptoms.

COCAINE-AFFECTED BABIES   Since cocaine rapidly crosses the placenta, as virtually all drugs do, the fetus is vulnerable when a pregnant woman takes the drug. The babies of women who use cocaine in any form during pregnancy are more likely to have birth defects and other problems than are the babies of women without a cocaine habit. These defects include brain damage; heart defects; kidney problems; and malformed heads, arms, and fingers. The type of defect depends on when during pregnancy cocaine was taken. If cocaine is used during the first trimester of pregnancy, for example, when the limbs are forming, the likely result will be malformed arms and fingers. When cocaine is taken toward the end of pregnancy, the infant is more likely to be stillborn (born dead), premature, or born physiologically dependent on cocaine.

■ **Exploring Your Emotions**

Recently, a court ruled that a mother can lose custody of her child because it was born addicted to drugs. What do you think about this ruling? What are the mother's and the child's rights in this situation?

Cocaine-dependent infants often experience withdrawal after birth. They are typically irritable, jittery, and do not eat or sleep properly. They don't seem to be able to respond or relate to people the way normal babies do, and they're very difficult to comfort or console. These characteristics affect their social and emotional development because it's difficult for adults to interact with them. Many cocaine-affected infants show multiple developmental and medical problems as they get older. Cocaine is also easily passed on to nursing infants through breast milk.

An alarming number of babies are being born now who were exposed to cocaine before birth. A survey by the U.S. Department of Health and Human Services reported that nearly 9,000 "crack babies" were born in eight major cities in 1989. New York City reported the highest number, followed by Los Angeles, Chicago, and Miami. It was estimated that caring for those babies would cost $500 million for hospital and foster care through age 5 and preparing them for school would cost an additional $1.5 billion. The report recommended that state and local governments develop prenatal care and education programs for women at risk of cocaine addiction. Clearly, this is one of the major problems our society faces in the 1990s.

Amphetamines Amphetamines are a group of synthetic chemicals that are potent CNS stimulants. Some common amphetamines are dextroamphetamine (Dexedrine), *d-1-*amphetamine (trade name Benzedrine), and methamphetamine (trade name Methedrine). Popular names for these drugs change often and are different in different parts of the country. Some of the more common ones are "uppers" and "speed." The properties of amphetamines are also shared by another group of synthetic chemicals, which include methylphenidate (trade name Ritalin), phenmetrazine (trade name Preludin), and diethylpropion (trade names Tenuate and Apisate). These drugs are most commonly taken orally, although sometimes they are "mainlined" intravenously.

EFFECTS Small doses of amphetamines usually make people feel better, more alert and wide-awake, and less fatigued or bored. Small doses can produce some improvement in activities requiring extreme physical effort or endurance, such as certain athletic contests or military maneuvers. Amphetamines generally increase motor ac-

tivity but do not measurably alter a normal, rested person's ability to perform tasks calling for complex motor skills or high-level thinking. When amphetamines do improve performance, it's primarily by counteracting fatigue and boredom. Amphetamines in small doses also increase the heart rate and blood pressure and change sleep patterns.

Amphetamines are sometimes used to curb appetite, but after a few weeks the user develops tolerance, and higher doses are necessary. Sometimes, too, when people stop taking the drug, their appetites rebound, and they gain back the weight they lost. One over-the-counter diet drug, propanolamine, has become popular. However, all these appetite-suppressing drugs have the intrinsic limitation of not permanently changing eating behavior. Amphetamines have other medical uses, but many physicians doubt their usefulness and consider other approaches more worthwhile and not as risky.

TREATING CHILDREN'S BEHAVIOR PROBLEMS WITH AMPHETAMINES Amphetamine-like drugs, such as Ritalin, have been used to reduce the distractibility, impulsivity, and other behavior problems of children or young adults who are diagnosed as having attention deficit disorder (ADD) with hyperactivity. There is now considerable evidence that in individuals who have been accurately diagnosed as having this disorder, CNS stimulants effectively improve attention span and overall school performance while reducing aggressive and distractible behavior. However, establishing an accurate diagnosis is not easy and usually requires a comprehensive evaluation. In some instances, CNS stimulants have been used indiscriminately for a variety of learning and behavioral problems. As one would expect, the results have been mixed, with some individuals showing a worsening in behavioral and other problems. This illustrates the role of drug specificity and the importance of careful diagnosis and monitoring; drug effects useful in some people are injurious in others.

MDMA, or Ecstasy, is an amphetamine-related drug that is often mistakenly referred to as a designer drug. As suggested by its chemical name, 3,4 methylenedioxymethamphetamine, the basic pharmacological effects of MDMA are similar to those of amphetamine. With large enough doses, there can be adverse effects similar to those of amphetamine. Although proponents of MDMA claim that it has unique pharmacological properties and behavioral effects, the differences between a drug like MDMA and other chemically related drugs are often related to dosage.

FROM USE TO ABUSE Much amphetamine abuse begins as an attempt to cope with a passing situation. A student cramming for exams or an exhausted long-haul truck

Drugs in America: The Human Costs

It's old news that drugs are big business in America. Sales of illegal drugs totaled an estimated $100 billion in 1986, more than the sales of the largest American corporation and more than the total earnings of all American farms combined. About 60 percent of the illegal drugs produced in the world eventually find their way to the United States, where they are resold in small quantities for hundreds of times their purchase price.

Drugs are a way of life for many of the people, mostly minorities, who live in America's inner cities. Where violence, broken families, and hopelessness prevail, drugs provide the only escape; and where lack of opportunity dooms people to endless poverty, the drug business is the only economy. Selling drugs, especially cocaine, is seen as the ticket to quick cash, the good life, the American dream. It is also the route to disease, violence, and death.

Since the advent of the crack epidemic in the mid-1980s, drug-related health problems have multiplied. Hospitals in the inner cities are being overwhelmed by cases involving cocaine. A 1988 survey of 19 major cities by the National Institute on Drug Abuse found that record numbers of cocaine-related illnesses were treated in hospital emergency rooms. In some hospitals, typically located in large cities like New York and Los Angeles, physicians say that perhaps half of their emergency patients are drug users.

Drug overdoses and drug-related violence, particularly gunshot wounds, are common reasons for going to the emergency room; but the most frequent medical complications reported are chest pains, erratic heartbeats, and seizures,

potentially fatal conditions that are frequently induced by cocaine. Cocaine use is also related to automobile accidents and fatalities. Almost 25 percent of all people killed in traffic accidents in New York City between 1984 and 1987 tested positive for cocaine.

Two of the most devastating and fastest growing drug-related health problems are AIDS and cocaine-affected babies born to drug-using mothers. Intravenous (IV) drug users, their sexual partners, and their children represent an increasing proportion of cases of AIDS. Of the AIDS cases reported in the first six months of 1989, 23 percent were female or heterosexual male IV drug users. This represents a 5 percent increase since 1985. Cases of sexually transmissible diseases are also increasing, at least in part because people are selling sex for drugs.

Blacks and Hispanics account for a disproportionate number of AIDS cases as the disease shifts from a primarily gay male population to the urban poor. In New York City, 84 percent of women with AIDS are black or Hispanic, as are 90 percent of the children with AIDS. Among blacks and Hispanics, both men and women, between the ages of 25 and 44, AIDS is the leading cause of death.

The number of babies exposed to drugs during pregnancy multiplied three to four times between 1985 and 1990. About 11 percent of all newborns now suffer prenatal exposure to illicit drugs. Babies whose mothers use crack cocaine must be stabilized after birth and nursed through withdrawal. Their hospital stays average 42 days, as opposed to 3 days for a normal infant. In many cases, they are abandoned at birth or soon thereafter. If they aren't abandoned,

they go home to a drug environment in which they are at great risk for neglect and abuse. The full extent of the developmental problems they will experience as they grow up is still not known.

The costs of health care for drug-related conditions are staggering. The lifetime medical care costs of a person with AIDS are now estimated at between $60,000 and $200,000, and the costs of treating all people with AIDS in 1989 were estimated at $3.5 billion. By 1992 they will be about $7.5 billion. Despite reimbursements from Medicaid, Medicare, and private insurance companies, many hospitals cannot meet their costs of treating AIDS cases. Even greater financial burdens will occur as the AIDS population changes and includes more people with low incomes or no insurance. The cost of treating one infant born to a crack-addicted mother may be as high as $125,000, again borne mostly by the hospital. The costs of providing this kind of care have put some hospitals on the brink of collapse.

Clearly, there are no easy solutions to the drug problem today. "Just Say No" approaches may be effective among some groups of young people, but they are unlikely to have much influence in inner cities, where life is dominated by a drug subculture. Wider economic and social issues—poverty, joblessness, violence, crime, urban neglect and decay, and many others—have to be addressed in any successful approach to the drug problem in the United States.

Based on The nightmare drugs, *Mayo Clinic Health Letter*, November 1989; Hispanics ignore AIDS threat as death toll rises, leaders say, *San Jose Mercury News*, January 19, 1990; Sandra G. Boodman, Kids and crack, *Washington Post Health*, September 12, 1989.

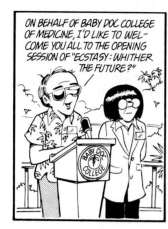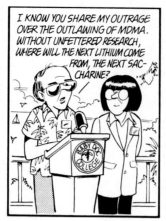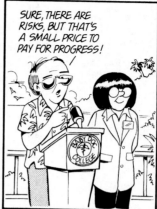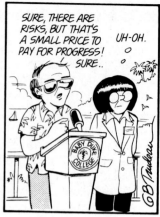

driver can go a little longer by "popping a benny," but the results can be disastrous. The likelihood of making bad judgments significantly increases. An additional danger is that the stimulating effects may wear off suddenly, and the user may precipitously feel exhausted or fall asleep ("crash").

Another problem is **state dependency**, the phenomenon whereby information learned in a certain drug-induced state is difficult to recall when the person is not in that same physiological state. Test performance may deteriorate when students use drugs to study and then take tests in their normal, nondrug state.

DEPENDENCE   Repeated use of amphetamines, even in moderate doses, often leads to tolerance and the need for larger and larger doses. The result can be severe disturbances in behavior, including paranoid **psychosis** with illusions, hostility, delusions of persecution, and unprovoked violence. It is just like a nondrug psychosis except that it ends if the person stops taking the drug.

Some users inject large doses of amphetamines into their veins. Each injection immediately produces a feeling of intense pleasure, an orgasmic "rush," followed by sensations of vigor and euphoria that last for several hours. As these feelings wear off, they are replaced by feelings of irritability and vague uneasiness. The discomfort strongly motivates the user to take another injection. The situation is somewhat similar to the injection of opiates. The result is a "run," a period of repeated injections of amphetamines. During a run, the individual often goes without sleep and without enough food or liquids. He or she is also prone to develop **paranoid behavior**.

A run ends when the user is too uncomfortable or too disorganized, or simply when the drug is all gone. The exhausted user will sleep for a day or two, then be lethargic or depressed. Injecting amphetamines instantly relieves the lethargy or depression, so the user is inclined to begin another run.

Continued high-dose amphetamine use is often associated with pronounced psychological dependence. Chronic abusers frequently spend much of their time obsessively seeking drugs. People ending a run sometimes try to combat the stress and discomfort by using heroin or other CNS depressants. At least in this respect, amphetamines can be a stepping-stone to other drugs.

■ **Exploring Your Emotions**

Have you ever misused or abused a drug, even coffee or an over-the-counter remedy? If so, what were your reasons and motivations? Was it hard to stop?

Paranoia is only one of the hazards of amphetamine use. Others include malnutrition and loss of weight, damage to blood vessels, strokes, and other changes in the heart and blood vessels. As with opiates, the injection method brings an added danger, the risk of diseases caused by unsterile conditions.

Caffeine   Caffeine is probably the most popular psychoactive drug and also one of the most ancient. It is found in coffee, tea, cocoa, soft drinks, headache remedies, and over-the-counter drugs like No-Doz. In ordinary doses caffeine produces greater alertness and a sense of well-being. It also cuts down on feelings of fatigue or boredom, and using caffeine may enable a person to keep at physically exhausting or repetitive tasks longer. Such

---

State dependency   Situation where information learned in a drug-induced state is difficult to recall when the effect of the drugs wears off.

Psychosis   A severe mental disorder in which there is a distortion of reality. Symptoms might include delusions or hallucinations.

Paranoid behavior   Behavior caused by false beliefs (delusions).

use is usually followed, however, by a sudden letdown. Caffeine does not noticeably influence a person's ability to perform complex intellectual tasks unless fatigue, boredom, alcohol, or other factors have already affected normal performance.

Caffeine mildly stimulates the heart and respiratory system, it increases muscular tremor, and it enhances gastric secretion. Higher doses may cause nervousness, irritability, headache, disturbed sleep, and gastric irritation or peptic ulcers. In women excessive caffeine consumption may aggravate the symptoms associated with premenstrual syndrome. Some people, especially children, are quite vulnerable to the adverse effects of caffeine. They become "wired"—hyperactive and exquisitely sensitive to any stimulation in their environment. In rare instances, the disturbance is so severe there is misperception of their surroundings—a toxic psychosis.

Drinks containing caffeine are rarely harmful for most individuals, but some tolerance develops and withdrawal symptoms of irritability and headaches do occur. Thus, although we don't usually think of caffeine as a dependency-producing drug, it is. Excessive caffeine consumption causes excessive anxiety in many people. People with certain psychiatric problems often feel better when they decrease or eliminate their intake of caffeine (see Table 11-2). These caffeine-related health risks are dose-related. People who are susceptible to them can usually avoid problems by simply decreasing their daily dosage. Recently, caffeine-free coffee and cola drinks have become popular; these are useful for people who are sensitive to the adverse effects of caffeine. Interestingly, caffeine is useful in treating certain kinds of headaches—especially migraines. However, caffeine withdrawal headaches are common in users who reduce their daily consumption.

Marijuana and Other Cannabis Products　Marijuana is the most widely used illicit drug in the United States (cocaine is second), although use is not as high as it was in the late 1970s (see the box titled Students' Reasons for Avoiding Drugs). The National Institute on Drug Abuse reports that nearly 62 million Americans over the age of 12—about one in three—have tried marijuana at least once. In 1985 over 50 percent of high school seniors and roughly 75 percent of young adults under 25 had tried marijuana. The marijuana available today is generally more potent than that used in the 1970s.

Marijuana is a crude preparation of various parts of the Indian hemp plant, *Cannabis sativa*, which grows in most parts of the world. THC (tetrahydrocannabinol) is the main active ingredient in marijuana. Concentrations of THC vary widely, depending on where the plant is grown and how it is cultivated, harvested, and cured. Hashish is a potent cannabis preparation derived mainly from the thick resinous materials of the flowering tops

Table 11-2 The daily dose. This chart will help you calculate your daily caffeine intake. But remember, caffeine content varies widely, depending on the product you use and how it's prepared.

Beverages	Serving Size	Caffeine (mg)
Coffee, drip	5 oz	110–150
Coffee, perk	5 oz	60–125
Coffee, instant	5 oz	40–105
Coffee, decaffeinated	5 oz	2–5
Tea, 5-minute steep	5 oz	40–100
Tea, 3-minute steep	5 oz	20–50
Hot cocoa	5 oz	2–10
Coca-Cola	12 oz	45

Foods	Serving Size	Caffeine (mg)
Milk chocolate	1 oz	1–15
Bittersweet chocolate	1 oz	5–35
Chocolate cake	1 slice	20–30

Over-the-counter Drugs	Dose	Caffeine (mg)
Anacin, Empirin, or Midol	2	64
Excedrin	2	130
NoDoz	2	200
Aqua-Ban (diuretic)	2	200
Dexatrim (weight control aid)	1	200

Source: Caffeine update: The news is mostly good. *University of California, Berkeley, Wellness Letter*, July 1988.

and upper leaves of the plant. It contains high concentrations of THC. THC can be synthesized, but it is a very expensive process. Because of the cost, pure THC is virtually never available on the illicit market. Drugs sold as THC are almost always something else, such as methamphetamine.

Marijuana is usually smoked, but can also be ingested. Although it is usually thought of as a psychedelic, the classification of marijuana is a matter of some debate. For this reason, it is treated separately here.

Short-Term Effects and Uses　As is true with most psychoactive drugs, the effects of a low dose of marijuana are strongly influenced by set and setting—what the user expects and what his or her previous experience with the drug has been. At low doses, marijuana users typically experience euphoria, heightening of subjective sensory experiences, slowing down of the time sense, and a relaxed, "laid-back" attitude. These pleasant effects are the reason why this drug is so widely used. With moderate doses, these effects become stronger, and the user can also expect to have impaired memory function, disturbed

Students' Reasons for Avoiding Drugs

Much has been made of young people's reasons for using and abusing drugs. What about their reasons for *not* using drugs or for stopping once they start? Here are the five most common reasons students give for abstaining from drug use:

1. Concern about health risks, including developing dependency

2. Peers don't approve of drug use

3. Role models (parents, older friends) don't use drugs

4. Fear of getting caught and shaming others

5. Individual doesn't view self as drug user

And here are the four most common reasons students give for discontinuing marijuana use:

1. Health reasons

2. Disliked the effects

3. Mental or emotional problems

4. Athletic training or lifestyle changes

The majority of students don't use drugs. Their reasons show a healthy respect for the risks and growing sense of self-responsibility.

Adapted from R. A. Selan, *Stanford Report,* 1990, and D. F. Duncan, *Journal of Drug Education,* 1988.

---

thought patterns, lapses of attention, and subjective feelings of depersonalization.

The effects of marijuana with higher doses are determined mostly by the drug itself rather than by set and setting. Very high doses produce feelings of depersonalization in which the mind seems to be separated from the body, as well as marked sensory distortion and changes in the body image (such as a feeling that the body is very light). People who have not had much experience with marijuana sometimes think these sensations mean that they are going crazy and become anxious or even panicky. Such reactions resemble a bad trip on LSD, but they happen much less often, are less severe, and do not last as long.

Physiologically, marijuana chiefly acts to cause increases in heart rate and dilatation of certain blood vessels in the eyes, which creates the characteristic bloodshot eyes. The user also feels less inclination for physical exertion.

Cannabis preparations were once medically prescribed for a variety of human illnesses, including insomnia, migraine, depression, and epilepsy. Now, however, none of these uses can be supported. Its medical use for sedative or euphoric effects is limited because of the perceptual and cognitive changes it brings about and also because individual reactions cannot be predicted. Somewhat more promising are current investigations into the use of THC to reduce nausea and improve appetite during cancer chemotherapy. In this situation, adverse side effects are less critical. THC and related compounds are also being studied for possible use in certain forms of glaucoma, an eye disease that causes blindness.

Long-Term Effects   Although occasional use of marijuana doesn't seem to have any lasting effect on health, the effects of long-term use are largely unknown. Widespread use has been common for only about twenty years, and some effects may take longer than that to manifest. We can predict, however, from experience with other drugs that the body systems and functions most affected in the beginning by marijuana are the ones most vulnerable to long-term injury. A small percentage of users will undoubtedly develop lung disorders, and some may show changes in brain functions. It is unlikely that all chronic cannabis users will suffer harmful effects. Individuals vary greatly in how susceptible they are to both immediate and long-term effects of drugs. When we consider the long-term effects of marijuana (and of any other drugs), we should keep in mind the time-lag factor. A period of time must pass before long-term effects of a drug can be recognized. Tobacco, for example, was long thought to be a "harmless" drug.

DEPENDENCE   Does marijuana cause dependence? Some tolerance can develop, but marijuana smoking irritates the throat and lungs. These unpleasant side effects make a steady increase in use of low-potency preparations unlikely. However, like all drugs that relieve "bad" feelings and produce "good" feelings, marijuana can become the focus of the user's life to the exclusion of other activities. The chronic marijuana user will not necessarily limit his or her drug use to cannabis. Drug uses appear to be related, and the chronic marijuana user is more likely to be a heavy user of tobacco, alcohol, and other dangerous drugs. The person who buys marijuana is in touch with the illicit drug market, and that contact may be the key to the association between marijuana use and subsequent use of cocaine and heroin.

Psychedelics   The term *psychedelics* refers to a group of drugs whose predominant pharmacological effect is to alter perception, feelings, and thoughts in the user. These drugs are also called hallucinogens, although at low doses hallucinations are not one of their major effects. They are sometimes called "psychomimetics" ("psychosis-mimicking"), but their effects are quite different from schizophrenia and other psychotic disturbances described in Chapter 3.

■ Exploring Your Emotions

Some people take drugs, especially psychedelics, to expand their consciousness or have a spiritual experience. What do you think about such drug-induced experiences? Are they meaningful? Do you think drugs can open doors in the mind?

The psychedelics include LSD (lysergic acid diethyl-amide), mescaline, psilocybin, STP (dimethoxy-methyl-amphetamine), DMT (dimethyl-tryptamine), and many others. These drugs are most commonly ingested or smoked. LSD is the most widely known of the psychedelics, and we discuss it in detail here as an example of the entire group.

LSD   LSD is one of the most powerful psychoactive drugs. A dose of 50 micrograms, an amount so small that it can hardly be perceived, will produce noticeable effects in most people. These effects include an altered sense of time, disorders of vision, an improved sense of hearing, changes in mood, and distortions in how people perceive their bodies. There is almost always dilation of the pupils, and there may also be slight dizziness, weakness, and nausea. With larger doses, users may experience a phenomenon known as **synesthesia**, feelings of **depersonalization**, and other alterations in the perceived relationship between self and external reality.

Psychedelics are particularly human drugs. As mentioned earlier, laboratory animals do not self-administer psychedelics. The reasons for this are not totally clear, but the psychedelics do not activate certain areas of the brain that are associated with stimulation and rewards.

Many psychedelics induce biological tolerance so quickly that after a few days' use their effects are reduced greatly. The user must then stop taking the drug for several days before his or her system can be receptive to it again. These drugs cause little drug-seeking behavior and no physical dependence or withdrawal symptoms.

The immediate effects of low doses of psychedelics are largely determined by set and setting. Many effects of psychedelics are hard to describe because they involve subjective and unusual dimensions of awareness—the **altered states of consciousness** for which psychedelics are famous.

Psychedelics have acquired a certain aura not associated with other drugs. Some people have taken LSD in search of a religious or mystical experience, or in the hope of exploring new worlds, or as therapy, in an attempt to solve their problems. LSD has been acclaimed not only as a "mind blower" but also as an aid to personal growth and perhaps to creativity, but only in already creative people. The issue of creativity is complex. People on LSD may make a greater number of original responses, but they are less able to synthesize them, to coordinate them into an appropriate pattern. Claims of LSD-induced increased sensitivity and powers of insight are also complex and difficult to document scientifically.

A severe panic reaction, which can be terrifying in the extreme, can occur at any dose of LSD. It is impossible to predict when a panic reaction will occur. Some LSD users report having hundreds of pleasurable and ecstatic experiences before an inexplicable "bad trip," or "bummer." If the user is already in a serene mood and feels no anger or hostility and if he or she is in secure surroundings with trusted companions, a bad trip may be less likely, but a tranquil experience is not guaranteed.

Even after the drug's chemical effects have worn off, spontaneous flashbacks and other psychological disturbances can occur. Flashbacks are perceptual distortions and bizarre thoughts that occur after the drug has been entirely eliminated from the body. Flashbacks are relatively rare phenomena, but they can be extremely distressing. They are often triggered by specific psychological cues associated with the drug-taking experience, such as certain mood states or even types of music.

Researchers in the 1970s claimed that LSD damages **chromosomes**. Evidence so far indicates that LSD in moderate doses, at least the pure LSD produced in the laboratory, does not damage chromosomes, cause detectable genetic damage, or produce birth defects.

Synesthesia   A condition in which a stimulus evokes not only the sensation appropriate to it but also another sensation of a different character. An example is when a color evokes a specific smell.

Depersonalization   A state in which a person loses the sense of his or her own reality or perceives his or her own body as unreal.

Altered states of consciousness   Profound changes in mood, thinking, and perception.

Chromosome   Microscopic bodies in the cell nucleus. The chromosomes carry the genes that convey hereditary characteristics.

What to Do Instead of Drugs

- Bored? Go for a walk or a run; stimulate your senses at a museum or a movie; challenge your mind with a new game or book; introduce yourself to someone new.
- Stressed? Practice relaxation or visualization; try to slow down and open your senses to the natural world; get some exercise.
- Shy, lonely? Talk to a counselor; enroll in a shyness clinic; learn and practice communication techniques.

- Feeling low on self-esteem? Focus on the areas in which you are competent; give yourself credit for the things you do well.
- Depressed, anxious? Talk to a friend, parent, or counselor.
- Apathetic, lethargic? Force yourself to get up and get some exercise to energize yourself; assume responsibility for someone or something outside yourself; volunteer.

- Search for meaning? Try yoga or meditation; explore spiritual experiences through religious groups, church, prayer, or reading.
- Afraid to say no? Take a course in assertiveness training; get support from others who don't want to use drugs; remind yourself that you have the right and the responsibility to make your own decisions.

Other Psychedelics Most other psychedelics have the same general effects that LSD has, but there are some variations. As in LSD use, the effects of small doses depend largely on psychological and social factors, the set, and the setting. A DMT high does not last as long as a LSD high. An STP trip, in contrast, lasts longer than an LSD trip. Ditran and related compounds cause greater intellectual impairment and confusion than other psychedelics.

Mescaline (peyote), the ceremonial drug of the Native North American Church, supposedly produces a trip different from that caused by LSD. Obtaining mescaline costs far more than making LSD, however, so most street mescaline is LSD that has been highly diluted. Psychedelic effects can be obtained from certain mushrooms (*Psilocybe mexicana* or "magic mushrooms"), certain morning glory seeds, nutmeg, jimsonweed, and other botanical products, but unpleasant side effects, such as dizziness, have limited the popularity of these products. Development and use of new psychedelics will probably continue, at least until they turn out to be less effective or to have more unpleasant side effects than older drugs. A few will probably have certain features that will make them useful for some purposes. Research on therapeutic applications of LSD practically stopped when LSD became illegal. Before then LSD was being tried with the terminally ill, with heroin addicts, in the treatment of alcoholism, and as an aid to psychotherapy. Many experts feel this research should be resumed since the therapeutic potential of hallucinogens has not been clearly determined.

Deliriants Many drugs, and other substances not usually thought of as drugs, can bring on a form of abnormal behavior called **delirium**, or **toxic psychosis**. Delirium results from a temporary impairment of brain function. Different chemicals act on the brain in different ways, but the results are generally similar. They consist of changing levels of awareness to surrounding events, decreased ability to maintain attention to a task, and variable amounts of mental confusion. The person may also experience hallucinations, especially visual ones. The belladonna alkaloids found in jimsonweed are an example of a deliriant that causes profound memory impairment.

PCP Phencyclidine, also known as "angel dust," "PCP," "hog," and "peace pill," is a widely used synthetic drug that can be considered a deliriant. PCP reduces and distorts sensory input, especially **proprioception** (awareness of the position of arms and legs, joints, and so forth), and creates a state of sensory deprivation. This drug was initially used as a human anesthetic, but was unsatisfactory because of the postoperative agitation, confusion, and delirium its use caused. However, it is still used in veterinary medicine as an animal anesthetic. Since the ingredients of PCP are readily obtainable and it can be easily made, it is often available on the illicit market and is sometimes used as a cheap adulterant for other psychoactive agents.

Following the faddish pattern of use of most psychedelics, PCP was extensively used in the mid-1960s. It declined in popularity when that generation became aware of the prevalence of adverse side effects, including convulsions, memory impairments, coma, and occasionally death. In the mid 1970s PCP again became widely used and now in the 1990s is again a major drug problem.

Inhalants   Delirium can be produced by inhaling certain chemicals such as some glues, gases in aerosols, kerosene, gasoline, butyl nitrite, and anesthetic agents such as laughing gas (nitrous oxide). Most inhaled chemicals interfere directly with brain function, but some do so indirectly by interfering with oxygen exchange in the lungs. Inhalants can be very dangerous to health; high concentrations of these substances in the blood can cause brain, liver, and kidney damage or even asphyxiation.

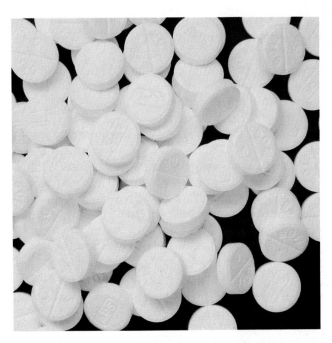

Drugs that relieve anxiety have a place in medical treatment, but they are easily abused. Valium, pictured here, can produce dependency even when taken exactly as directed.

Psychiatric Use of Drugs

Certain classes of psychoactive drugs can be useful in treating psychiatric problems, including schizophrenia, anxiety, and depression.

Antipsychotics   The antipsychotic drugs, also called **neuroleptics** or major tranquilizers, are helpful in some individuals who have schizophrenia. They include chlorpromazine (Thorazine), haloperidol (Haldol), and many others. We do not know exactly why they work the way they do, but there is no question that in psychotic individuals they reduce bizarre motor activity, decrease responsiveness to external and internal stimuli, and check hallucinations and delusions. In proper doses for the individual patient, the antipsychotic drugs accomplish these results without causing so much sedation that the individual cannot continue his or her daily activities.

Antianxiety Drugs   A different class of drugs is the anxiolytic. Benzodiazepines such as Valium and Librium are examples of this group. They can reduce anxiety, relieve muscle tension, and cut down irritability in most people without causing extreme sedation. However, they can cause drowsiness, especially when combined with other CNS depressants or when taken in tranquil, boring settings. Anxiolytic drugs are also used to treat other neurotic reactions, such as depression and phobias, as

well as many other conditions, but they are less effective in treating psychosis. They are extensively prescribed in contemporary medical practice. Physicians often prescribe them for minor problems such as transient stresses that are an inevitable part of daily life, in many cases at the request of the patient. Virtually all such unpleasant stresses are better handled by learning appropriate psychological coping techniques. In addition, anxiolytic drugs can interfere with driving and do increase the effects of alcohol. All drugs, including anxiolytics, should be avoided during pregnancy, especially during the first three months. Because many women do not realize they are pregnant until the second month, obvious difficulties can occur.

As with other psychoactive drugs, distinctions between appropriate use of anxiolytic drugs and their abuse are often difficult to make. Most medical authorities would agree that ideally these drugs should be used primarily in time-limited situations where anxiety is so high the individual's usual coping abilities are completely over-

---

Delirium   A reversible state of mental confusion sometimes marked by emotional excitement.

Toxic psychosis   A delirious state caused by brain dysfunction induced by a drug or by another agent such as fever.

Proprioception   The sensory processes that identify the position and movement of muscles, tendons, and joints.

Neuroleptics   The group of powerful drugs useful in treating schizophrenia. These drugs are also called antipsychotics.

whelmed. However, in our society these drugs are widely used where the situation is less clear-cut. Many people take anxiolytics on a frequent, often a daily, basis. The number of people who follow this pattern is far greater than the number of people who inject heroin, smoke opium, or inhale solvents.

Is this pattern of consumption drug use or drug abuse? If we agree that any drug use resulting in impairment of functioning should be considered abuse, then the anxiolytics are commonly abused. When moderate or high doses are used daily or frequently, their anxiety-reducing effects tend to accumulate, alertness decreases, and various degrees of mental and behavioral impairment result. In addition, some anxiolytics such as Valium, lead to dependence, as described earlier in the chapter. These dependencies can involve pronounced craving, marked tolerance, and withdrawal reactions including seizures.

Antidepressants   Recent research has produced many drugs for treating mood disorders. Some of these drugs, called antidepressants, are used to treat long-lasting severe **depression**. Elavil, Tofranil, and Prozac are examples of antidepressants. They are chemically different from the stimulant drugs described earlier in this chapter. Results vary, but in some individuals antidepressants cause significant restoration of positive mood, activity, and drive. As with most psychoactive drugs, it is not known precisely how they achieve these results. It is difficult for doctors to tell which individuals will benefit most from antidepressants, but studies show that these drugs work best with individuals who show "pure" severe depression with slowed body movements, reaction time, and speech pattern. The more a person's depressed behavior is combined with anxiety, hostility, or disorders in thinking, the less effective the antidepressants seem to be.

Among the newest drugs for treating severe mood disorders are the lithium salts. Lithium salts are effective in reducing **mania**. This condition is marked by exaggerated euphoria, inappropriate self-confidence, and poorly controlled overactivity. Lithium salts are also useful in treating **manic-depressive disorders**, in which the individual swings back and forth between mania and depression. As with the antidepressants, lithium salts appear to work best with people whose mood disorders are not combined with disturbances in thinking or perception. Despite the fears of many patients, lithium, antidepressants, and antipsychotic drugs do not produce dependence even when used chronically.

Drug Use in the 1990s

Drug research will undoubtedly provide new information, new treatments, and new chemical combinations in the 1990s. Refinements in the psychiatric use of drugs will probably be made, and new psychoactive drugs may present unexpected possibilities for therapy or social use. They may also present new possibilities for abuse. Making honest and unbiased information about drugs available to everyone, however, may cut down on their abuse. Lies about the dangers of drugs—"scare tactics"—can lead some people to disbelieve any reports of drug dangers, no matter how soundly based and well documented they are.

■ **Exploring Your Emotions**

Some people make a distinction between the recreational use of drugs like marijuana, cocaine, and LSD, which they think is OK, and the hard-core use of crime-associated drugs like heroin and crack, which they think is wrong. Others say that taking any drug supports the organized crime drug business and contributes to the problems of the inner city, including the rise in AIDS cases and the number of "crack babies." They point out that middle-class users often buy their drugs through the open windows of their cars on inner city streets. What do you think about this issue? Are recreational users part of the drug problem?

Although the use of some drugs, both legal and illegal, has declined dramatically since the 1970s, the use of others, such as heroin, has held steady, and the overall use of cocaine has increased. Mounting public concern has led to great debate and a wide range of opinions about what should be done. Proposals include everything from mandatory drug testing to legalization of drugs (see the box entitled "Should Drugs Be Legalized?"). In 1989 President Bush initiated a "war on drugs" focusing on law enforcement, prosecution, and treatment and edu-

---

Depression   A mild or severe emotional state characterized by dejection, low spirits, feelings of inadequacy, and inability to act.

Mania   An emotional disorder characterized by excessive enthusiasm, unstable attention, and exaggerated activity.

Manic-depressive disorders   A psychiatric disorder in which the patient's mood swings from mania to depression and back. This disturbance, which often runs in families, is also called bipolar disease.

Should Drugs Be Legalized?

In a reversal of their usual political stances, some liberals are calling for increased drug law enforcement and some conservatives are calling for controlled legalization of drugs. George Shultz, former Secretary of State under Ronald Reagan and stalwart conservative Republican believes that "we're not really going to get anywhere until we can take the criminality out of the drug business." The conservative position reflects a growing sense of pessimism over the effectiveness of the nation's drug programs, according to Shultz, as well as doubt that the present system of seizure, punishment, and treatment will ever eliminate the drug problem.

Shultz says he was influenced by the writings of Ethan A. Nadelman, assistant professor of politics and public affairs at Princeton University. Nadelman writes that drug traffickers—from the notorious foreign drug cartels to the local dealers—are the greatest beneficiaries of present anti-drug laws. He draws a tight connection between illicit drugs and crime, pointing out that crimes by drug users usually are committed to buy drugs that cost relatively more than alcohol and tobacco because they are produced illegally.

Contradicting popular wisdom, Nadelman believes that the drugs themselves are not the problem. He claims that most users of cocaine don't get into trouble with the drug itself. The nation's leaders should look at illicit drugs the same way they look at alcohol and tobacco, according to Nadelman. Some people drink and smoke to excess and require some forms of treatment, but many don't. Legalization of both tobacco and liquor have eliminated crimes associated with their sale.

Opponents of legalization respond that alcohol and tobacco are major causes of disease and death in our society and that they shouldn't be used as a model for other practices. They feel that regardless of practical issues, decriminalization would give drugs an approval that they don't now have. This factor would be particularly important in how children and teenagers regard drugs. Many opponents of legalization believe that government, as the agent of society, is responsible for helping to instill certain values and virtues in people, such as decency, dignity, self-control, duty, and responsibility. Drug-dependent people, they claim, are unlikely to make productive workers, good parents, reliable neighbors, or safe drivers—qualities considered desirable by most people.

Opponents of legalization also believe that more people would use drugs if they were legal, especially since they would be less expensive and easier to get, and that this would lead to a greater number of drug-degraded people in our society. There would still be tremendous costs associated with drugs for regulation and enforcement of controls. Opponents of legalization believe that the best ways to stop drugs are intensified prosecution and enforcement, widespread testing, community cooperation with police to reassert public control over streets and parks, and improved drug education programs in the schools.

What do you think?

Adapted from Robert G. Fichenberg. 1989. Shultz backs legalized drugs. *San Francisco Examiner.* October 31, and James Q. Wilson and John J. Dilulio, Jr. 1989. Crackdown. *The New Republic,* July 10.

cation at the local level. With drugs entering the country on a massive scale from South America, Southeast Asia, and elsewhere and distributed through tightly controlled drug-smuggling organizations and street gangs, it remains to be seen how effective these programs will be.

Drug Testing   One of the more controversial issues in American politics is drug testing in the workplace. It has been estimated that many workers, perhaps one in ten, use psychoactive drugs on the job. For some occupations, such as air traffic controllers, truck drivers, train conductors, physicians, and so on, drug use can create significant dangers, sometimes involving hundreds of people. Some people believe that the dangers are so great that all workers should be tested and that anyone found to have traces of drugs in the blood or urine should be fired or treated. Others insist that this would violate people's right to privacy and to the freedom from unreasonable search guaranteed by the Fourth Amendment. Proponents then ask whether companies who don't test for drugs should be liable for damages if their employees cause harm to others.

Some employers are already testing their employees, and the U.S. armed forces tests military personnel on a

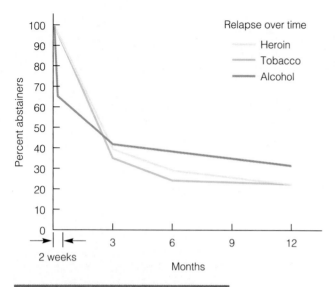

VITAL STATISTICS

Figure 11-4 Percentage of people who continue to abstain over time after giving up heroin, tobacco, and alcohol.

regular basis. However, drug testing is expensive, with costs running as high as $100 per individual test; and questions about accuracy and reliability complicate the issue. Another factor to be considered is that most jobs don't involve hazards, so employees who are on drugs aren't any more dangerous than employees who aren't on drugs. All these legal and practical issues mean that drug testing is likely to remain controversial in the 1990s.

Professional Treatment for Drug Dependence   Professional programs to help people break their drug habits are usually one of two kinds—drug substitution programs or programs based in rehabilitation centers. Neither method is consistently successful over the long term (see Figure 11-4). Nonprofessional self-help programs, such as Alcoholics Anonymous, Narcotics Anonymous, and Coke Enders, on the other hand, appear to be effective for some people.

Drug Substitution Programs   Sometimes a less debilitating drug can be substituted for one with many damaging effects, thus reducing the "costs," or risks, of the drug use. Methadone is a synthetic drug used as a substitute for heroin. When methadone is used, addicts can stop taking heroin without experiencing severe withdrawal reactions. Methadone is addictive too, but it decreases the craving for heroin and allows the individual to function normally in personal, social, and vocational activities. It also blocks the action of narcotics, so addicts don't get high even if they take heroin. Methadone maintenance treatment allows many former heroin abusers to live more useful lives.

One disadvantage of methadone is that it is metabolized fairly rapidly (although not as rapidly as heroin) and thus must be taken on a daily basis. Newer heroin substitutes, such as LAAM, are metabolized more slowly still and need to be taken only two to three times a week. Because they are relatively inexpensive to administer, drug substitute programs are a popular form of treatment.

There is a significant relapse rate from methadone and LAAM treatment programs, as is the case with all drug dependency treatment efforts. This rate is reduced when psychological and social services are provided in addition to methadone. The fact that this type of support improves recovery rates underscores the importance of psychological factors in drug dependency. A common mistake of some recovery programs is to focus on the pharmacological factors alone.

Treatment Centers   A variety of programs have been established in drug rehabilitation treatment centers. Their features can include hospitalization, detoxification, counseling, and other psychiatric services, offered over the short or the long term. There are nearly 9,000 treatment centers for drug dependency in the United States. A specific type of center is the therapeutic community, a residential program run in a completely drug- and alcohol-free atmosphere. Administered by ex-addicts, these programs use confrontation, strict discipline, and unrelenting peer pressure to attempt to resocialize the addict with a different set of values. Therapeutic communities appear to be effective for a limited segment of the addict population, mainly young, middle-class people who are highly motivated to discontinue their drug use. As mentioned earlier, self-help programs may be the best route to recovery for some types of drug abusers.

Prevention of Drug Abuse   Clearly, the best solution to drug abuse is prevention. A large part of government attempts at controlling the drug problem focus on stopping the production, importation, and distribution of illicit drugs. Creative effort also has to be put into stopping the demand for drugs. Developing persuasive antidrug educational programs offers the best hope for solving the drug problem in the future. Indirect approaches to prevention involve building young people's self-esteem, improving their academic skills, and increasing their recreational opportunities. Direct approaches involve giving information about the adverse effects of drugs and teaching tactics that help students resist peer pressure to use drugs in various situations. Developing strategies for resisting peer pressure is one of the more effective techniques.

Prevention in the 1990s will probably focus on the different motivations individuals have for using and abus-

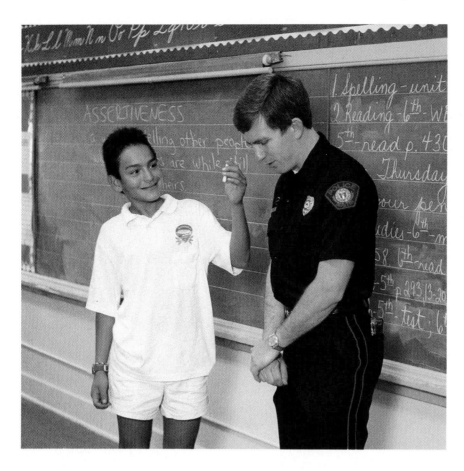

Drug education programs aimed at elementary school children seem to be most effective when they involve respected figures and when they teach specific skills for resisting drug use. This police officer is explaining the meaning and importance of assertiveness to a fifth grade class.

ing specific drugs at different ages. For example, grade school children seem receptive to programs that involve their parents or well-known adults like professional athletes. Adolescents in junior or senior high school are often more responsive to peer counselors. Many young adults tend to be influenced by efforts focusing on health education. For all ages, it is important to provide non-drug alternatives that speak to that individual's or group's specific reasons for using drugs, such as recreational facilities, counseling, greater opportunities for leisure activities, or places to socialize.

The Role of Drugs in Your Life   Where do you fit into this complex picture of drug use and abuse? Chances are good that you've had experience with over-the-counter

and prescription drugs, and you may or may not have had experience with one or more of the drugs described in this chapter. You probably know someone who has used or abused a psychoactive drug. Whatever your experience up to now, it's likely that you will encounter drugs at some point in your life. To make sure you'll have the inner resources to resist peer pressure and make your own decision, cultivate a variety of activities you enjoy doing, realize that you are entitled to have your own opinion, and don't neglect your self-esteem. Like other aspects of health behavior, making responsible decisions about drug use depends on information, knowledge, and insight into yourself. Many choices are possible; making the ones that are right for you is what counts.

Summary

- Psychoactive drugs alter a person's sensations, feelings, thoughts, or the functions of the nervous system; they help create the drug society that prevails in many countries today.

The Drug Tradition

- Naturally occurring drugs have been used throughout human history for religious, medicinal, and personal reasons; in the nineteenth century it became possible to purify and synthesize drugs, and use increased. Although drug use dropped after 1900, it surged again in the 1960s; it has been declining since the late 1970s, except for cocaine use.

Use, Abuse, and Dependence

- Reasons for using drugs include the lure of the illicit; curiosity; rebellion; peer pressure; and the desire to alter one's mood or escape boredom, anxiety, depression, or other psychological problems. These problems are magnified in the inner city, where issues of race, class, and economics are integral to the buying and selling of drugs.
- Drug misuse involves taking a drug for a purpose or in a way for which it was not intended. Drug abuse involves taking a drug to the extent that it causes physical damage to the user, impairment of the user's ability to function, or behavior harmful to others.
- Drug dependence can be physical or psychological. Physical dependence is characterized by withdrawal symptoms when the user tries to give up the drug or cut back. It often involves tolerance as well, the need for larger and larger doses to achieve the effects.
- Psychological dependence involves a craving for the mood changes that a drug provides; it is strongly affected by social factors.
- The opiates often cause dependency; CNS depressants and stimulants can also induce physical dependence.

How Drugs Affect the Body

- The effects of a drug depend on drug factors, user factors, and psychological and social factors.
- Drug factors include (1) pharmacological properties—the drug's overall effect on a person's body chemistry, behavior, and psychology, (2) dose-response function—the relationship between amount of a drug taken and the intensity of type of effect, not necessarily a direct relationship, (3) time-action function—relationship between time elapsed since a drug was taken and the intensity of its effect, (4) cumulative effects—physiological alterations over time that change the effects of the drug, and (5) method of use—ingestion, inhalation, injection, or absorption through the skin or tissue linings.
- User factors are a person's physical characteristics, such as body mass, general health, genetic factors, and other drugs being taken. Taking any drug during pregnancy can be risky or even devastating to fetal development.
- Psychological factors include *set*, the user's expectations about how he or she is going to respond to the drug, and *setting*, the physical and social environment surrounding the drug use. Setting and set are sometimes more important in determining effects than the drug itself, if low doses are involved.

Representative Psychoactive Drugs

- Opiates relieve pain, cause drowsiness, and induce euphoria; they reduce anxiety and produce lethargy, apathy, and an inability to concentrate. They include opium, morphine, heroin, methadone, and codeine.
- Central nervous system depressants slow down the overall activity of the nerves; they reduce anxiety and produce mood changes, muscular incoordination, slurring of speech, and drowsiness or sleep. They include barbiturates, tranquilizers, and alcohol. Physical dependency is possible with most CNS drugs, and withdrawal symptoms are severe. Even prescribed doses of antianxiety agents can cause dependency.
- Central nervous system stimulants speed up the activity of the nerves, causing acceleration of heart rate, rise in blood pressure, dilation of pupils and bronchial tubes, and an increase in gastric and adrenal secretions.
- The CNS stimulant cocaine produces an intense euphoria; it is usually sniffed, snorted, or injected intravenously. Crack is a less expensive, ready-to-smoke version of cocaine. Tolerance builds up quickly; psychological craving and withdrawal reactions are factors in chronic use.
- Amphetamines are CNS stimulants that make people feel more alert and less fatigued or bored; they may increase motor activity but don't necessarily improve ability to perform tasks. Amphetamines increase the heart rate and blood pressure and change sleep patterns.
- *State dependency* refers to the phenomenon in which information learned when under the influence of drugs is difficult to recall when the drug-induced state wears off.
- Amphetamine use can lead to tolerance. Paranoid psychoses, including illusions, hostility, delusions, and unprovoked violence, can result from abuse. Other dangers include damage to blood vessels, strokes, and other changes in heart and blood vessels. Psychological dependence is associated with continued high-dose use.
- Also a CNS stimulant, caffeine mildly stimulates the heart and respiratory system, increases muscular tremor, and enhances gastric secretion. Tolerance can develop and withdrawal symptoms can appear.
- Marijuana, the most widely used illicit drug in the United States, is usually smoked but can be ingested. Its classification is a matter of debate. At low doses euphoria and a relaxed attitude are common; very high doses produce feelings of depersonalization and sensory distortion. Marijuana use increases heart rate and dilation of blood vessels in the eyes. Effects of long-term use are unknown, but lung disorders and changes in brain function are possible.
- Tolerance to marijuana can develop, but the major problem is psychological dependence and contact with the illicit drug market.

- Psychedelics alter perception, feelings, and thought. LSD is the most widely known; its effects include an altered sense of time, disorders of vision, and changes in mood. Large doses may lead to synesthesia and depersonalization.
- Tolerance to psychedelics occurs, but there are no withdrawal symptoms. Immediate effects are often determined by set and setting. Panic reactions and flashbacks are among the adverse effects of LSD use.
- Deliriants cause temporary impairment of brain function—changing levels of awareness to surrounding events, decreased ability to maintain attention to a task, confusion, and perhaps hallucinations. PCP is a widely used deliriant with dangerous side effects.
- Inhalants, such as glue, kerosene, butyl nitrite, and nitrous oxide can produce delirium; their use can lead to brain, liver, and kidney damage.

Psychiatric Use of Drugs

- Antipsychotic drugs—referred to as neuroleptics or major tranquilizers—are helpful in treating schizophrenia. They reduce bizarre motor activity, decrease responsiveness to stimuli, and check hallucinations and delusions.
- Antianxiety drugs like Valium can reduce anxiety, relieve muscle tension, and cut down irritability; they also help with depression and phobias. In the past, physicians and patients probably relied excessively on them when appropriate coping techniques could have been learned instead.
- Antidepressants are used to treat long-lasting, severe depression. They can restore positive mood, activity, and drive. Lithium salts are effective in treating mania and manic-depressive disorders.

Drug Use in the 1990s

- Honest and unbiased information about drugs may help cut down on their abuse; scare tactics and exaggerations are ineffective.
- Drug testing, a controversial issue in American politics, has begun for some federal and private sector employees; it involves a basic conflict between public safety and the individual's right to privacy and freedom from unreasonable search.
- Drug substitution programs attempt to reduce the costs, or risks, of drug abuse. Methadone maintenance allows many former heroin users to lead more useful lives; the significant relapse rate is reduced when psychological and social services are also provided.
- Features of drug treatment centers include hospitalization, detoxification, counseling, and other psychiatric services. Therapeutic communities use confrontation, strict discipline, and peer pressure to resocialize addicts.
- Government attempts to control the drug problem focus on production, importation, and distribution. Persuasive antidrug educational programs are necessary; especially important is helping students develop strategies for resisting peer pressure. Providing nondrug alternatives that address an individual's or group's specific reasons for using drugs is essential.

Take Action

1. For the next week, each time you see someone taking drugs, ask yourself, "Why is this person using this drug at this time? What are the motivations?" Keep track of the incidents in your health diary. At the end of the week, look at your record and see how many times drugs were taken mainly for the drug effects and how many times they were taken more for social reasons.

2. Keep track of your own drug use for a week, noting in your health diary the name of the drug, the approximate dosage, the time of day, and what you think the reasons were for taking each dose. Don't forget to include coffee, soft drinks, and over-the-counter medications. What pharmacological categories do they fall into? Are there any patterns? Are there any signs of abuse or dependence?

3. Survey three older adults and three young students about their attitudes toward legalizing marijuana. Are there any differences? If so, what accounts for these differences?

4. Find out what facilities are available in your community to handle drug dependence. If none is available, what facilities are needed? Locate the public health agency that is responsible for your area and ask them why these needs aren't being met.

5. Contact a drug dependence treatment facility and see if you can visit it. Find out what their admission and release requirements are, what treatment approach they use, and what their rate of successful rehabilitation is. If possible, observe some of the activities. Write a brief report about your experience, including whether or not it changed your attitudes toward drugs.

Behavior Change Strategy

Changing Your Drug Habits

Many psychoactive drugs are discussed in this chapter, and a lot of them may be unfamiliar to you. For this reason, we have chosen to devote this behavior change strategy to one of the most common but least controlled drugs—caffeine. The basic elements of a behavior change strategy can be adapted to any behavior. If there is another drug you want to cut down on or stop using, you can devise your own plan based on this one and on the steps outlined in Chapter 1.

Because caffeine supports certain behaviors that are characteristic of our culture, such as sedentary, stressful, white-collar work, you may find yourself relying on coffee (or tea, chocolate, or colas) to get through a busy schedule. Such habits often begin in college. Fortunately, it's easier to break a habit before it becomes entrenched as a lifelong dependency.

Caffeine overdose can have some harmful effects on you, and knowing what they are can help motivate you to reduce your intake. You may feel increased anxiety and irritability; some people may be especially sensitive to caffeine and may find such exaggerated states hard to manage.

When you are studying for exams, the forced physical inactivity and the need to concentrate even when fatigued may lead you to overuse caffeine. But caffeine doesn't "help" unless you are already sleepy. And it does not relieve any underlying condition (you are just more tired when it wears off). So how can you change this pattern?

Diary Self-monitoring

Keep a log of how much caffeine you eat or drink. Use a standard measuring cup to measure coffee or tea; heat-resistant ones are available.

Using Table 11-2, convert the amounts you eat or drink into an estimate expressed in milligrams of caffeine. Be sure to include all forms, such as chocolate bars and pills, as well as caffeine candy, colas, cocoa or hot chocolate, chocolate cake, tea, and coffee.

Don't be surprised if your intake falls sharply from just keeping a daily diary—that's one benefit of paying attention to your habits. It's also a good conversation piece, which increases the attention you give to the behavior change strategy.

Self-assessment

At the end of the week, add up your daily totals and divide by 7 to get your daily average in milligrams. How much is too much? At more than 250 mg per day, you may well be experiencing some adverse symptoms. Are you experiencing at least five of the following? If so, you may want to cut down.

- Restlessness
- Nervousness
- Excitement
- Insomnia
- Flushed face
- Excessive sweating
- Gastrointestinal problems
- Muscle twitching
- Rambling flow of thought and speech
- Irregularities in rhythm of heartbeats
- Periods of inexhaustibility
- Excessive pacing or need to constantly move around

Set Limits

Can you restrict your caffeine intake to a daily total, and stick to this contract? If so, set a cutoff point, such as one cup of coffee. Pegging it to a specific time of day can be helpful, because then you don't

confront a decision at any other point (and possibly fail). If you find you cannot stick to your limit, you may want to cut out caffeine altogether; abstinence can be easier than moderation for some people. Remember—tea, cocoa, and so on are not caffeine-free substitutes for coffee.

Find Other Ways to Keep Your Energy Up

If you are fatigued, it makes sense to get enough sleep or to exercise more rather than drowning the problem in coffee. Different individuals need different amounts of sleep; you may also need more sleep at different times, such as during a personal crisis or an illness. Also, exercise raises your metabolic rate for hours afterward—a handy fact to exploit when you want to feel more awake and want to avoid an irritable coffee jag. And if you've been compounding your fatigue by not eating properly, try chowing down on complex carbohydrates such as whole-grain bread and potatoes instead of candy bars.

Some Tips on Cutting Out Caffeine

Here are some more ways to decrease your consumption of caffeine:

1. Keep some noncaffeine drink on hand, perhaps hot water or bouillon, to give a warm feeling to your hands and mouth.
2. Alternate between hot and very cold liquids.
3. Drink decaffeinated coffee or herbal teas.
4. Fill your coffee cup only halfway.
5. Avoid the office or school lunchroom or cafeteria and the chocolate area of the grocery store. (Often people drink coffee or tea and eat chocolate simply because it's there.)

Selected Bibliography

American Psychiatric Association. 1987. *Diagnostic and Statistical Manual of Mental Disorders: Third Edition–Revised*. Washington, D.C.: American Psychiatric Association.

Boodman, Sandra G. 1989. Up against it. *Washington Post Health,* September 5.

Cohen, Sidney. 1985. *The Substance Abuse Problems*. Vol. 2: *New Issues for the 80s*. New York: Haworth Press.

Cregler, L. L., and H. Mark. 1986. Cardiovascular dangers of cocaine abuse. *American Journal of Cardiology* 57:1185.

Duncan, D. F., and R. S. Gold. 1982. *Drugs and the Whole Person*. New York: Wiley.

Fisher, Seymour, Allen Raskin, E. H. Uhlenhuth, eds. 1987. *Cocaine: Clinical and Biobehavioral Aspects*. New York: Oxford University Press.

Ray, Oakley, and Charles Ksir. 1987. *Drugs, Society, and Human Behavior*, 4th ed. St. Louis: Mosby.

U.S. Public Health Service. 1987. *Prevention Research: Deterring Drug Abuse among Children and Adolescents*. Washington, D.C.: U.S. Department of Health and Human Services.

U.S. Public Health Service. 1988. *Progress in the Development of Cost-Effective Treatment for Drug Abusers*. Washington, D.C.: U.S. Department of Health and Human Services.

U.S. Public Health Service. 1988. *Mechanisms of Tolerance and Dependence*. Washington, D.C.: U.S. Department of Health and Human Services.

Recommended Readings

Beattie, Melody. 1987. *Co-dependent No More*. New York: Harper and Row. *A practical treatise on issues of co-dependency.*

Blum, R. H., et al. 1969. *Society and Drugs*. San Francisco: Jossey-Bass. *A well-written book that emphasizes the historical and social context of nonmedical drug use.*

Jones, R. T. 1983. Cannabis and health. *Annual Reviews of Medicine* 34:247–58. *A scholarly, balanced review of marijuana's effects on health.*

Kaplan, J. 1970. *Marijuana—The New Prohibition*. New York: World Publishing Co. *The classic book on the politics of marijuana control in the United States.*

Kaplan, J. 1983. *The Hardest Drug: Heroin and Public Policy*. Chicago: University of Chicago Press. *An excellent description of the scientific and political issues involving heroin.*

Nadelman, Ethan A. 1988. U.S. drug policy: A bad export. *Foreign Policy* 70:83–107, Spring. *Nadelman is a vocal advocate of the controlled legalization of currently illicit drugs.*

Schuckit, M. A. 1989. *Drug and Alcohol Abuse: A Clinical Guide to Diagnosis and Treatment*. 3rd ed. New York: Plenum Press. *A balanced, informative text that focuses on the clinical aspects of drug use.*

Wilson, James Q., and John Jay DiIulio, Jr. 1989. Crackdown. *The New Republic,* July 10. *This article focuses on crack and the costs of decriminalizing it.*

Contents

Making Connections

Of all your daily behaviors and habits, choosing a nutritious diet is probably the single most important action you can take to influence your health in a positive way. Some kinds of diets are linked with vitality, energy, and well-being; others are linked with a host of diseases, including cancer and heart disease. The trick is consistently making sensible choices. The scenarios presented on these pages describe situations in which people have to use information, make a decision, or choose a course of action, all related to nutrition. As you read them, imagine yourself in each situation and consider what you would do. After you've finished the chapter, read the scenarios again and see if what you've learned has changed how you would think, feel, or act in each situation.

Your grandmother has suffered from osteoporosis for many years and is now stooped over and considerably shorter than she used to be. Your mother recently started taking hormones to protect herself from bone loss. You're an average-weight, healthy, 21-year-old woman (although you do smoke). How great is your risk of developing osteoporosis? Is there anything you can do now to protect yourself?

You and your date go out to dinner one night at a popular local restaurant that has a reputation for fresh, healthy food. You order spaghetti with marinara sauce, and she decides on a salad, saying she's been eating too much junk food lately. You walk over to the salad bar with her to check it out. She starts with a plate full of lettuce and then adds marinated mushrooms, scallions, chopped green pepper, tomato, bacon bits, croutons, hard-boiled eggs, shredded cheese, avocado, and sunflower seeds, topping it off with creamy Italian dressing. When you return to your table, she says, "I'm glad I'm eating a healthy, nonfattening meal for a change. Why don't you try a salad next time? It's better for you." Is she right?

12
Nutrition Facts and Fallacies

You wanted to improve your diet, so instead of buying chocolate chip cookies at the store, you bought some all-natural granola bars. While you're eating one, you glance at the nutritional label on the side of the box and notice that it's unusually long. Looking more closely, you identify seven different sweeteners—sugar, honey, molasses, corn syrup, brown sugar, dextrose, and malt syrup—and three different kinds of hydrogenated oil. Also listed are glycerin, sorbitol, citric and malic acid, sulfiting agents, and BHA. It doesn't seem much like a health food. What does "all-natural" mean anyway?

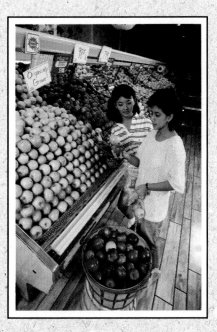

Lately you've been giving serious consideration to becoming a vegetarian for a variety of personal reasons. But when you mention it to your housemate, she advises you against it. She says it's almost impossible to get enough protein if you eliminate meat, cheese, milk, and eggs from your diet. Actually, you were just thinking of giving up meat, not all animal products. Would that still make you a vegetarian? Would you have a hard time getting enough protein?

You wander into a local health food store in search of a sandwich and find yourself in a new world. Bottles of vitamins, minerals, and dietary supplements line the shelves, along with more exotic items like nutritional yeast, lecithin, and bee pollen. You half-seriously ask a salesperson if all these things are necessary, and she responds emphatically that they are, explaining that the U.S. Recommended Daily Allowances for vitamins and minerals are far too low. "That's why we have such a high rate of disease in this country," she tells you. "Everyone has borderline deficiencies. Frankly, I'd be afraid to go one day without taking my vitamin supplements." You're taken aback by her vehemence. Looking over the shelves again, you wonder if she's right. Should you ask her what she thinks might be missing in your diet? And should you buy the products she recommends?

In your lifetime, you'll spend about six years eating foods—about 70,000 meals and 60 tons of food. You'll face an avalanche of conflicting **nutrition** advice from newspapers, magazines, books, and television programs concerning what foods you should eat. You'll hear that your nutritional habits affect your risk for the major chronic "killer" diseases, such as heart disease, cancer, stroke, and diabetes. In addition, you'll be told that a poor nutrient intake can make you more susceptible to **osteoporosis** and iron-deficiency **anemia**, while an over-zealous use of supplements can lead to toxicity from excess consumption of vitamin A, vitamin B_6, iron, copper, and other nutrients. Choosing foods that provide the nutrients you need is an important part of your daily life.

If you're confused about the ideal diet for you, this chapter can offer some help. Although the science of nutrition is relatively young, we already know what nutrients are needed for an adequate diet and what foods provide them. Understanding just these basic facts can help you eat sensibly and protect yourself against many nutrition-related problems that can ultimately affect your health. The food choices you make now, in your younger adult years, can significantly influence your health during your elderly years. A recent U.S. Surgeon General's Report states that "for most of us, the most likely [health] problems are overeating—too many kcalories for our activity levels—and an imbalance in the nutrients consumed." The report recommends diets lower in sodium (salt) and fat, especially saturated (solid) fat, with an increase in the amount of whole grains, calcium, and iron. After reading this chapter, you'll understand the reasons for the Surgeon General's recommendations.

Nutritional Requirements: Components of a Healthy Diet

Today we know that a diet adequate for human growth, development, and maintenance must contain energy to fuel the required body processes. We express the fuel potential in a diet as **kilocalories** (kcalories). One kilocalorie represents the amount of heat it takes to raise the temperature of 1 liter of water 1° C. Sometimes people use the term *calorie* (a very small energy unit), but they usually are referring to kcalories. A kcalorie contains 1,000 calories. We need about 2,000 of the larger kcalorie units per day or 2 million of the smaller calories.

Just meeting energy needs is not enough. Our bodies also require carbohydrates, proteins, fats, vitamins, minerals, and water—about 45 **essential nutrients.** The word *essential* in this context means that we must get these substances from food because, with few exceptions, our bodies cannot manufacture them. Many of the diet patterns followed throughout the world can supply these essential nutrients.

Although we can live up to 50 days without food, we can live only a few days without water. Water is the major component in both foods and the human body—you are about 60 percent water. Our needs for proteins, fats, carbohydrates, **vitamins,** and **minerals,** in terms of weight, are much less. Practically all foods contain mixtures of proteins, fats, and carbohydrates, although foods are commonly classified according to the predominant nutrient. Most plants use light from the sun to convert chemicals from the air, water, and soil into all the complex chemicals they need. Animals, including humans, must eat foods to get the nutrients needed to fuel their bodies and to maintain associated tissues and organ systems.

■ Exploring Your Emotions

Do you have emotional attachments to particular kinds of foods or meals, such as those you eat on holidays or at family gatherings? If so, do your attachments make it hard for you to evaluate those foods objectively and acknowledge that some of them may not be good for you?

Although alcohol is not an essential nutrient and has no nutritional value, it is a major energy source in the American diet; alcoholic beverages are the third leading kcalorie contributor (6 percent of total), after white bread, rolls, and crackers and cookies and cakes.

Nutrition   The science of food and how the body uses it in health and disease.

Osteoporosis   A condition, mostly affecting women, in which the bones become extremely thin and brittle.

Anemia   A deficiency in the oxygen-carrying material in the red blood cells.

Kilocalorie   Unit of fuel potential in a diet, 1 kcalorie represents the amount of heat needed to raise the temperature of 1 liter of water 1° C.

Essential nutrients   Substances your body must get from foods because (with minor exceptions) it cannot manufacture them. They include vitamins, minerals, some amino acids, glucose, linoleic acid, and water.

Vitamin   A carbon-containing substance whose lack causes a specific deficiency disease curable by that substance.

Minerals   Inorganic compounds needed in relatively small amounts for regulation, growth, and maintenance of body tissues and functions.

Amino acids   The building blocks of proteins.

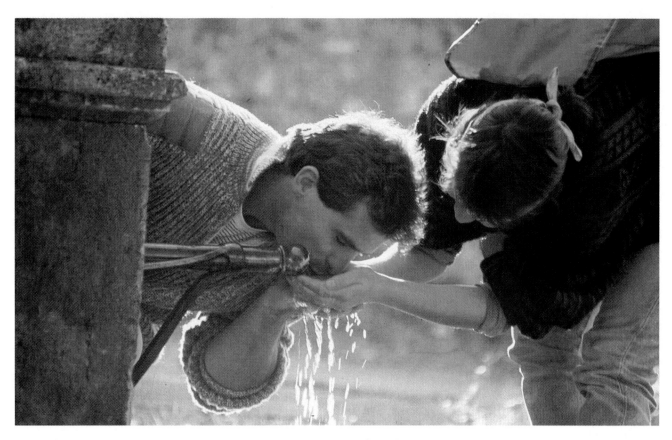

Often overlooked but absolutely crucial to life, water is an essential part of our diet.

Proteins—The Basis of Body Structure   Proteins form important parts of the body's main structural components—muscles and bones. Proteins also form important parts of blood, enzymes, some hormones, and cell membranes. The building blocks of proteins are called **amino acids.** Twenty common amino acids are found in food; nine of these are essential parts of an adult diet: histidine, isoleucine, leucine, lysine, methionine, phenylalanine, threonine, tryptophan, and valine. The other eleven amino acids can be produced by the body, given the presence of the needed building blocks supplied by foods. Protein sources are considered "complete" or of high quality if they supply all the essential amino acids in adequate amounts and "incomplete" if they do not. Meat, fish, poultry, eggs, milk, cheese, and other foods from animal sources provide complete proteins. Incomplete proteins, which come from plant sources, such as beans, peas, and nuts, are good sources of most essential amino acids, but are usually low in one or two.

Combining two vegetable proteins, such as wheat and peanuts in a peanut butter and jelly sandwich, allows each vegetable protein to make up for the amino acids missing in the other protein. The combination yields a complete protein for the meal. Actually, the focus on

amino acids and, in turn, complete protein should be on what a meal supplies, rather than on what each individual food supplies. A varied diet of plant proteins naturally provides the needed amino acids; plant proteins are also rich in many vitamins and minerals. By having plant proteins complement each other so that all essential amino acids are consumed in a meal, vegetarians can get the amino acids they need to synthesize the proteins their bodies require. Healthy vegetarian diets are discussed in detail later in this chapter.

Whenever you eat foods from animal sources you are eating protein. About two-thirds of the protein in the American diet comes from animal sources; hence, the American diet is rich in essential amino acids. Most Americans consume nearly twice the amount of protein they need per day; on the average women consume 70 grams of protein per day while needing only 45 grams, and men consume 104 grams while needing 60 grams. The amount of protein you need equals about 15 percent of the total kcalories in a diet (see Figure 12-1). Any extra protein provides no special benefit to the body. Protein consumed beyond protein needs is simply synthesized into fat for energy storage or burned for energy needs. For most of us this extra protein in the diet is not

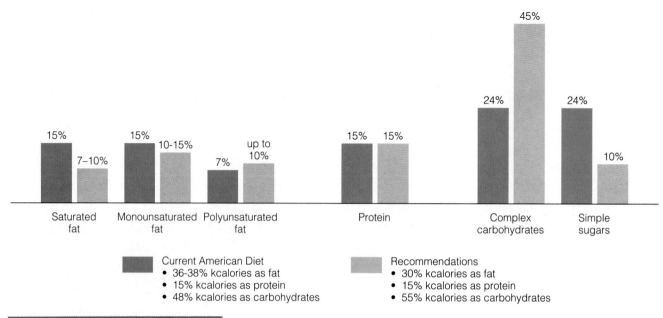

Figure 12-1 What Americans eat, compared to what they should eat—as recommended by major health authorities.

harmful: it simply reflects the standard of living and the dietary habits that we enjoy. The leading sources of protein in the American diet are (1) beef, steaks, and roasts, (2) hamburger and meatloaf, (3) white bread, rolls, and crackers, (4) whole milk, and (5) pork.

Fats—Essential in Small Amounts Fats, also known as lipids, are the most concentrated source of energy at nine kcalories per gram—compare that to carbohydrate and protein at four kcalories per gram and alcohol at seven kcalories per gram. The fats stored in your body not only represent usable energy, but also help insulate your body and support and cushion your organs. Fats in the diet help your body absorb fat-soluble vitamins from the intestine, as well as add important flavor and texture to foods. Fats are the major fuel for the body during rest and light activity; carbohydrates fuel the nervous system, brain, and red blood cells, while fats fuel most of the rest of the body's organ systems.

Certain fats are essential components of the diet. They form key regulators of body functions, such as the maintenance of blood pressure and the promotion of childbirth. About one tablespoon of vegetable oil per day in your diet supplies these essential fats. The average American diet supplies much in excess of those needs; in fact, fats make up about 38 percent of our kcalorie intake.

When we're referring to foods, we call the fats that are solid at room temperature *fats* and those that are liquid at room temperature *oils*. Both fats and oils found in food are composed of glycerol (an alcohol) plus three fatty acids. Fatty acids differ in the length of their carbon atom chains and in the number of double bonds contained between the carbon atoms. If no double bonds exist between the carbon atoms, the fatty acid is called **saturated.** Those fatty acids with one double bond are called **monounsaturated,** and those fatty acids with two or more double bonds are called **polyunsaturated.** Linoleic acid and linolenic acid, which are polyunsaturated, are the fats we referred to earlier as essential components of a diet.

Food fats are often composed of both saturated and unsaturated fatty acids; the dominant type of fatty acid determines the fat's characteristics. Oils tend to be unsaturated, while fats are mostly saturated. Olive, canola, and peanut oils contain mostly monounsaturated fatty acids. Sunflower, corn, soybean, and safflower oils con-

---

Saturated fats Fats whose molecules are filled to capacity with hydrogen.

Monounsaturated fats Fats with room for two hydrogen atoms per molecule.

Polyunsaturated fats Fats with room for four or more hydrogen atoms per molecule.

Hydrogenation A process by which liquid oils are turned into solid fats; used to extend the shelf life of certain foods.

Serum or blood cholesterol A waxy substance found in the blood and implicated in heart disease.

Fat Substitutes: Good News for Mayonnaise Lovers?

Imagine being able to reduce your fat intake by 35 percent or more—without even trying. What if you could eat ice cream, french fries, cake, and mayonnaise without worrying about saturated fats and percentages of fat calories? Two fat substitutes—Olestra (sucrose polyester) and Simplesse—have received much public and scientific attention in recent months.

Olestra

Olestra, or sucrose polyester, is made by adding fatty acids to sucrose (table sugar) molecules; with the fatty acids attached, the molecules cannot be broken down by either digestive enzymes or the bacteria that live in the intestine. As a result, Olestra cannot be absorbed and yields no kcalories. In addition, as it leaves the body, it can even pull cholesterol-containing substances in the intestine with it, thereby lowering serum cholesterol level.

Olestra should prove to be a versatile ingredient; according to the manufacturer, it can replace up to 35 percent of the fat in salad dressings and cakes. Its most exciting use might be as an ingredient for frying foods.

Why, then, haven't we seen foods that use Olestra on the supermarket shelves or in fast food restaurants? Like mineral oil, it tends to bind fat-soluble vitamins, preventing their absorption; the manufacturer proposes adding vitamin E to compensate. Also like mineral oil, it acts as a laxative. The Food and Drug Administration (FDA) doesn't allow mineral oil to be added to foods as a kcalorie-free fat; the FDA's concerns apply to Olestra as well. It's unclear when the product will be available.

Simplesse

The FDA approved the use of Simplesse in food products in February 1990. To produce Simplesse, egg and milk proteins are mixed together under heat in such a way that microscopic mist-like protein globules are produced. These globules feel like fat in the mouth. Simplesse does yield energy, but its 1.3 kcalories per gram are much less than the 9 kcalories per gram for fat. A 4-ounce serving of regular ice cream has 5 grams of fat and 250 kcalories; a frozen dessert made with Simplesse would have less than 1 gram of fat and 120 kcalories. Regular mayonnaise has 11 grams of fat per tablespoon and 99 kcalories; made with Simplesse, it would have less than 1 gram of fat and 21 kcalories.

Simplesse is most useful for replacing fat in mayonnaise, salad dressings, ice cream, and other dairy products. Cooking and frying with Simplesse alters its structure so that it no longer resembles fat. For those purposes, we'll have to wait for Olestra or some other, as-yet-undreamed-of fat substitute.

---

tain mostly polyunsaturated fatty acids. Most saturated fatty acids in the diet come from animal fat. Two plant oils—palm oil and coconut oil—that are often used in cakes and nondairy creamers are highly saturated. Hydrogenated vegetable oils are also highly saturated. The process of **hydrogenation** turns many of the double bonds in unsaturated fatty acids into single bonds and produces a more solid fat from a liquid oil. Food manufacturers use this process to extend the shelf life of fatty acids; the more double bonds a fatty acid contains, the more likely it is to break down and turn rancid. The more solid fats that result from hydrogenation make better pastry and cake products; hydrogenation also prevents oil from separating from the ground peanuts in peanut butter.

Many health experts recommend that we reduce our current fat intake from 38 percent of total kcalories to 30 percent or less of total kcalories. In addition, people who have high **blood cholesterol** levels (over 200 milligrams of cholesterol per 100 milliliters of blood serum) should specifically attempt to limit saturated fat intake. Controlling the amount of saturated fat in your diet is the most important action you can take to control your **serum cholesterol** levels. An elevated serum cholesterol level is associated with an increased risk for heart disease (see Chapter 15). Butter, shortening, and visible fats in meats are obvious sources of saturated fat in the diet, but we must also consider poultry skin, whole milk (low-fat milk and skim milk are better choices), ice cream, and many baked products. The leading sources of saturated fat in the American diet are animal flesh (hamburger, steak, roasts), whole milk, cheese, and hot dogs/lunch meats.

Remember, you need about 1 tablespoon of plant oils

How to Calculate Your Fat Intake

To calculate how much fat you consume, you first need to know the total number of kcalories and grams of fat in your diet. A paperback book listing the kcalorie and fat content of many foods is a valuable resource, since this information is not available on many food labels. Multiply the grams of fat by 9 (because there are 9 kcalories in a gram of fat). Then divide that number by the total kcalories. For example: A tablespoon of peanut butter has 8 grams of fat and 95 kcalories. So $8 \times 9 = 72$, divided by the number of kcalories (95) equals 0.76, or about 75 percent kcalories from fat.

To control the fat percentage in your diet, multiply the grams of fat in any individual food by 9. If the result is more than a third of the total kcalories, the food is relatively high in fat. You can still eat it, but make sure you limit the amount you eat—especially if it's also high in saturated fat. And make sure that you balance it with low-fat foods so that you end up with fewer than 30 percent of your total daily kcalories from fat.

---

per day; the amount of fat you eat beyond that is up to you. For many of us fat consumption deserves more careful attention because all fats provide large amounts of kcalories and saturated fats can raise serum cholesterol levels over desired standards. Today the average American obtains about 15 percent of kcalories from saturated fat. If you want to lower an elevated serum cholesterol level, your diet should obtain no more than 10 percent of its kcalories—and ideally 7 percent or less of its kcalories—from saturated fat.

■ **Exploring Your Emotions**

Are your tastes "your own," or do they derive from your childhood family customs? When you entered college, how did your eating habits change? Do you feel more comfortable with your current habits or less? Why?

Lately, the nutritional values of fish oils have been highly publicized. When the double bonds of a polyunsaturated fat start after the third carbon of the fatty acid chain, an omega-3 (ω-3) form is produced. If the double bonds start after the sixth carbon atom, then an omega-6 (ω-6) form is produced. Nutritionists recommend that Americans should try to consume fish at least once or twice a week because the omega-3 fatty acids found in fish reduce the tendency for blood to clot, decrease inflammatory responses in the body, and even lower the risk of heart disease. You'll read more about omega-3 fatty acids in Chapter 15. For now, keep in mind that the position of the double bonds in a polyunsaturated fatty acid determines that fatty acid's health benefits. Since the turn of the century, the American diet has been dominated by omega-6 fatty acids, coming primarily from corn oil and soybean oil. Now we think the pendulum should swing a little more toward omega-3 fatty acids to get a better balance of the two; hence, the recommendation to consume fish on a weekly basis.

Carbohydrates—An Ideal Source of Energy   Carbohydrates are needed in the diet primarily to supply energy for body cells that prefer this kcalorie source; such cells are found in the brain and other parts of the nervous system and in blood. During high-intensity exercise, muscles also use carbohydrate for fuel. When we don't eat enough carbohydrates to satisfy the needs of the brain and red blood cells, our bodies synthesize carbohydrates from proteins. This synthesis is expensive in terms of both **metabolism** needed (see Chapters 13 and 14) and the original cost of protein foods (compare the cost of a 1-pound loaf of whole wheat bread to that of 1 pound of lean beef). When the diet lacks sufficient carbohydrates and proteins, the body turns to its own proteins, and so severe muscle wasting occurs in a starvation diet.

Just 50–100 grams of carbohydrate a day in your diet meets your body's need for carbohydrate and in turn spares protein for more essential functions. On average, Americans consume over 200 grams of carbohydrates per day, approximately 48 percent of our total kcalories. In fact, you would have to struggle to consume a diet so low in carbohydrate that it would force the body to synthesize carbohydrate from dietary or body protein. Crash diets and very low carbohydrate diets are the only common examples.

Carbohydrates can be divided into two groups: simple and complex. Table sugar, honey, fructose, glucose, and corn syrup are simple carbohydrates and contain only one or two sugar molecules. Starches and most types of dietary fibers are complex carbohydrates; they consist of

TACTICS AND TIPS

Fourteen Ways to Reduce the Fat in Your Diet

1. Steam, boil, or bake vegetables, or stir fry them in a small amount of vegetable oil.

2. Season vegetables with herbs and spices rather than with sauces, butter, or margarine.

3. Try lemon juice on salad or use a yogurt-based salad dressing.

4. To reduce saturated fat use tub margarine instead of butter or stick margarine in baked products. When possible, use vegetable oil instead of these solid fats.

5. Try whole-grain flours to enhance flavors when making baked goods with less fat and fewer cholesterol-containing ingredients.

6. Replace whole milk with skim or low-fat milk in puddings, soups, and baked products.

7. Substitute plain low-fat yogurt, blender-whipped cottage cheese, or buttermilk in recipes that call for sour cream.

8. Choose lean cuts of meat, and trim any visible fat from meat before and after cooking.

9. Roast, bake, or broil meat, poultry, or fish so that fat drains away as the food cooks.

10. Remove skin from poultry before cooking.

11. Use a nonstick pan for cooking so added fat will be unnecessary; use a vegetable spray for frying.

12. Chill broths from meat or poultry until the fat becomes solid. Spoon off the fat before using the broth.

13. Eat a vegetarian main dish at least once a week.

14. Limit high-fat cheese intake.

---

chains of many sugar molecules. During **digestion** in the mouth and small intestine, your body breaks down starches and double sugars into the single sugar molecules of **glucose** for absorption (see Figure 12-2). Once glucose is in the bloodstream, cells take it up and use it for energy. The liver and muscles also take up glucose to provide carbohydrate storage in the form of the animal starch called **glycogen.**

Carbohydrates consumed beyond body needs are synthesized into fat and stored as such. Any type of diet where kcalorie intake exceeds kcalorie needs can lead to fat storage and weight gain. It makes little difference whether these excess kcalories come from carbohydrate, protein, fat, or alcohol.

Human digestive enzymes cannot break down the links between the sugar molecules in dietary fiber, and so the fibers pass down your intestinal tract and provide bulk for stools (feces) in the large intestine (colon). Much of this fiber can be broken down by bacteria in the large intestine; too much fiber intake can therefore lead to intestinal gas.

Carbohydrates are found in cereals, breads, fruits, vegetables, and milk; they give food its sweetness. Two slices of bread and one cup of milk supply enough carbohydrate for a day. Most health experts agree Americans should increase their intake of carbohydrates—particularly complex carbohydrates—at the expense of their intake of fats. Athletes in training can especially benefit from high-carbohydrate diets, which enhance the amount of carbohydrates stored in their muscles (as glycogen) and therefore provide more carbohydrate fuel for use during athletic events. In addition, carbohydrates consumed during athletic events can help fuel muscles and prolong the availability of the glycogen stored in muscles. A discussion of "carbohydrate loading" is included in Chapter 14.

Dietary Fiber—A Closer Look As we said, dietary fiber (also known as "bulk" or "roughage") includes plant substances that are difficult or impossible for humans to digest. All foods of plant origin contain fiber in various quantities. The expression "crude fiber" refers to an outmoded way of measuring the fiber in foods, although it still appears today on some food labels. When nutritionists make fiber recommendations for a diet, they are referring to the dietary fiber. During crude fiber analysis,

---

Metabolism The sum of the biochemical activities within your body. Substances changed by chemical reactions within your body are said to be *metabolized.*

Digestion Processes of breaking down foods in the gastrointestinal tract into compounds your body can absorb.

Glucose A simple sugar that is your body's basic fuel.

Glycogen An animal starch stored in the liver and muscles.

Figure 12-2   The digestive tract. Digestion of carbohydrates begins in the mouth, but most digestion takes place in the small intestine and stomach.

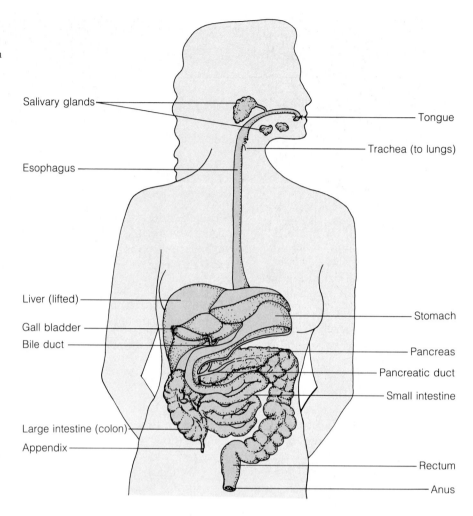

Salivary glands

Esophagus

Liver (lifted)

Gall bladder

Bile duct

Large intestine (colon)

Appendix

Tongue

Trachea (to lungs)

Stomach

Pancreas

Pancreatic duct

Small intestine

Rectum

Anus

some fiber components are destroyed and can't be measured; therefore, a crude fiber value underestimates the true fiber contribution of a food.

Fiber in the intestinal tract holds water, making feces bulkier and softer so they pass more quickly and easily through the intestines. Low-fiber diets can cause constipation and in turn lead to hemorrhoids and problems such as diverticulitis (a painful condition in which abnormal pouches in the wall of the large intestine are produced and then become inflamed). Researchers at the National Cancer Institute also feel that a low-fiber diet increases the risk for colon cancer. Under medical supervision, a very high fiber intake has a place in the treatment of diabetes and high serum cholesterol levels.

Nutritionists have recently started classifying fibers into **insoluble fibers** and **soluble fibers.** The insoluble fibers primarily take up water and therefore are most important for increasing bulk in the stool. A good source of insoluble fibers is wheat bran—the covering that surrounds each wheat grain. Some studies have linked high levels of insoluble fiber in the diet with lower incidences of colon cancer. There is even some evidence that high levels of insoluble fiber can suppress and reverse precancerous changes that can lead to colon and rectal cancer.

Soluble fiber is found primarily in oat bran and psyllium (in some laxatives). This type of fiber tends to bind cholesterol-containing compounds in the intestine and slow glucose absorption, rather than binding water. As a

Insoluble fiber   Fiber that does not dissolve in water and is not broken down by bacteria in the large intestine.

Soluble fiber   Fiber that dissolves in water or is broken down by bacteria in the large intestine.

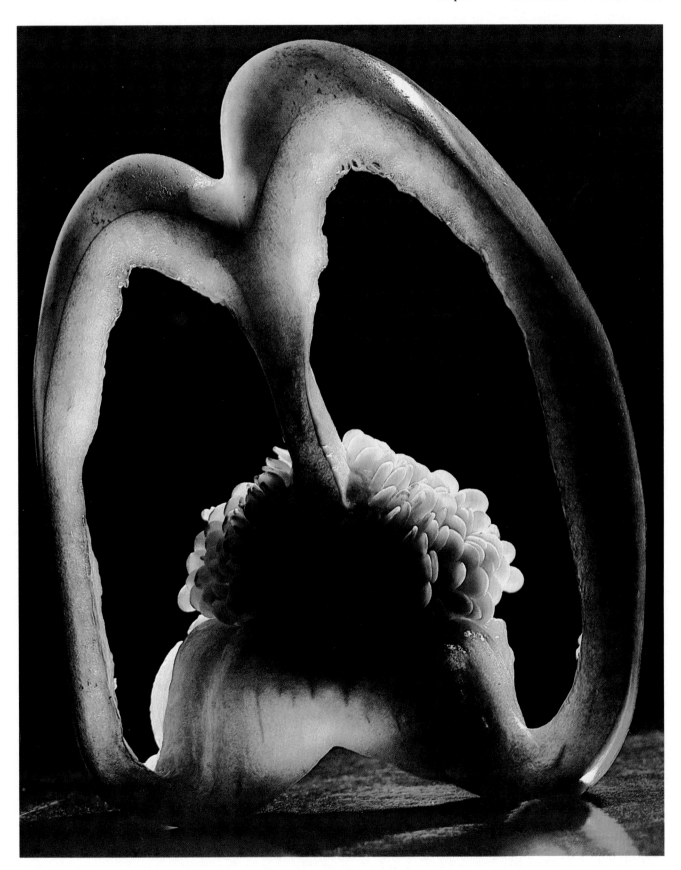

Whole foods. . . healthy, natural, and beautiful.

result, oat bran has been used to lower an elevated serum cholesterol or blood glucose level. By binding cholesterol-containing substances in the intestine, oat bran can somewhat deplete the body of cholesterol, and therefore serum cholesterol levels fall. Chapter 15 will discuss this mechanism and the latest research findings on cholesterol in more detail.

Although it's not yet clear exactly how much and what types of fiber would be ideal to consume, most authorities feel that the average American would benefit from a modest increase in daily fiber intake. We currently eat about 11–13 grams a day. A better goal would be 20–35 grams a day. Emphasizing fruits, vegetables, cereals, **legumes,** and whole grains in the diet makes this fiber goal easy to obtain. Eating a fiber-rich cereal for breakfast is one way to get a good start on this goal each day. Follow that with whole wheat bread on your sandwich for lunch and a piece of fruit. Finally, have a serving of vegetables with dinner.

Too much fiber in the diet can cause health problems, such as producing stools that are too large or binding important minerals. Thus, moderation in fiber intake, as with other nutrients, is an important dietary prescription. Stick to foods—not supplements.

Vitamins—Organic Micronutrients Vitamins are organic (carbon-containing) substances required in very small amounts to promote specific chemical reactions within living cells (see Table 12-1). Many vitamins act as catalysts—substances that initiate or speed up chemical reactions, while themselves remaining unchanged. Vitamins provide no energy to the body directly but instead are used to unleash the energy stored in carbohydrates, proteins, and fats. Nevertheless, vitamins are essential parts of a diet. A vitamin A deficiency can cause blindness, a niacin deficiency can lead to mental illness, a vitamin B_6 deficiency can cause seizures, a vitamin B_{12} deficiency can cause a severe type of amemia, and a vitamin D deficiency can cause growth retardation. A substance is considered a vitamin only if a lack of it causes a specific disease that is cured when the substance is resupplied. The best known deficiency disease is probably **scurvy,** caused by a vitamin C deficiency; it killed many sailors on long ocean voyages until people realized in the eighteenth century that eating oranges and lemons could prevent it. Even today some people develop scurvy; its presence suggests a *very* poor intake of fruits and vegetables, which are often rich sources of vitamin C.

Humans need thirteen vitamins. Four are fat-soluble (A, D, E, and K), while nine are water-soluble (C, and the eight "B-complex" vitamins: thiamin, riboflavin, niacin, vitamin B_6, folate, vitamin B_{12}, biotin, and pantothenic acid). Because patients can survive for many years without becoming ill on intravenous feeding formulated with just these substances and the other essential nutrients, it appears that no vitamins remain to be discovered. A few vitamins are also made within the body. Vitamin D is made in your skin when it is exposed to sunlight, and biotin and vitamin K are made by intestinal bacteria.

Extra vitamins can be harmful in the diet, especially when taken as supplements. Vitamin A is especially toxic during pregnancy or when high doses are taken over many months. Cases of irreversible nerve damage have recently been seen in women consuming large amounts of vitamin B_6 in an attempt to cure premenstrual syndrome. High doses of niacin are sometimes used to lower elevated serum cholesterol levels. This therapy is effective, but may cause side effects such as flushing of the skin and liver disorders. Later in this chapter we will discuss when a vitamin supplement might be advisable. For now, keep in mind that some vitamins can produce toxic results when consumed in high quantities; as always, the dose determines the poison.

Vitamin deficiency diseases are rare in the United States because vitamins are readily available from our food supply and because many foods, such as flour and breakfast cereals, are enriched with vitamins. People suffering from alcoholism run the greatest risk of vitamin deficiencies, especially from the water-soluble vitamins thiamin and folate. Vitamins (and minerals) can be lost when foods are prepared, stored, and cooked. To retain the maximum nutritional value, follow the tips listed in the box titled "Keeping the Food Value in Your Food."

Minerals—Inorganic Micronutrients Minerals are inorganic (not carbon-containing) compounds you need in relatively small amounts to help regulate body functions, aid in growth and maintenance of body tissues, and act as catalysts for the release of energy (see Table 12-2). We know of about seventeen essential minerals. The major minerals occur in the body in amounts exceeding one gram: calcium, phosphorus, magnesium, sulfur, sodium, potassium, and chloride. The essential trace minerals (which you need in minute amounts) are chromium, co-

---

Legumes   Vegetables such as peas and beans that are high in fiber and are also important sources of protein in a vegetarian diet.

Scurvy   A disease caused by lack of vitamin C in which the gums bleed and teeth are loosened.

Table 12-1 Vitamins: Their Functions and Food Sources

Vitamin	U.S. RDA[a]	Function	Food Sources
Thiamin	1.4–1.5 mg	Conversion of carbohydrates into usable forms of energy	Yeast, mushrooms, whole-grain and enriched breads and cereals, liver, pork, lean meats, poultry, eggs, fish, beans, nuts
Riboflavin	1.7 mg	Energy release; maintenance of skin, mucous membranes, and nervous structures	Dairy products, liver, whole-grain and enriched breads and cereals, lean meats, poultry
Niacin	20 mg	Conversion of carbohydrates, fats, and protein into usable forms of energy; essential for growth, synthesis of hormones	Eggs, chicken, turkey, fish, milk, grains, nuts, enriched breads and cereals, lean meats
B_6 (pyridoxine, pyridoxal, pyridoxamine)	2.0 mg	More than 60 enzyme reactions, mostly involving proteins	Milk, liver, lean meats, fish, poultry, whole grains
B_{12}	6 micrograms	Synthesis of red and white blood cells; other metabolic reactions	Liver, meat, eggs, milk
Folate	0.4 mg	Blood cell production, maintenance of nervous system	Liver, leafy vegetables, oranges, whole grains
Biotin	0.3 mg	Metabolism of fats, carbohydrates, and proteins	Cauliflower, egg yolks, nuts, cheese
Pantothenic Acid	10 mg	Metabolism of carbohydrates, fats, and proteins	Mushrooms, eggs, liver, kidneys, peanuts, whole grains, most vegetables, milk, fish
A (retinol)	5,000 International Units	Maintenance of eyes, vision, skin, linings of the nose, mouth, digestive and urinary tracts, immune function	Liver, milk, butter, cheese fortified margarine, carrots, spinach, other vegetables and fruits
C (ascorbic acid)	60 mg	Maintenance and repair of connective tissue, bones, teeth, cartilage; promotes wound healing	Peppers, broccoli, brussel sprouts, citrus fruits, tomatoes, potatoes, cabbage, other fruits and vegetables
D (cholecalciferol)	400 International Units	Aids in calcium and phosphorus metabolism; promotion of calcium absorption; development and maintenance of bones and teeth	Fortified milk, fish liver oils; sunlight on skin produces vitamin D
E (tocopherol)	30 International Units	Protection and maintenance of cellular membranes	Vegetable oils, whole grains, leafy vegetables, asparagus, peaches; smaller amounts widespread in foods
K	—	Production of prothrombin and other factors essential for blood clotting	Green leafy vegetables, other vegetables, liver; widespread in other foods

[a]General recommendations for adults and children age 4 or older (used in food labeling). More specific recommendations are made as part of recommended dietary allowances (RDA).

TACTICS AND TIPS

Keeping the Food Value in Your Food

1. Consume or process vegetables immediately after purchasing (or harvesting).

The longer vegetables are kept before they are eaten or processed, the more vitamins are lost, especially vitamin C and folate.

2. Store vegetables and fruits properly.

If you can't eat fruits and vegetables immediately after purchasing (or harvesting) but plan to do so within a few days, keep them in the refrigerator. Place them in covered containers or plastic bags to lessen moisture loss.

The best method for preservation is to freeze fruits and vegetables when possible. Blanch them first (briefly simmer them in water) to retain more flavor. Consult a cookbook for directions. This method preserves the vitamin content best because it stops the enzyme activity that destroys vitamins.

Canning fruits and vegetables preserves them, but it's a lot of work and causes a greater nutrient loss because of the high temperatures required.

3. Reduce preparation and cooking of vegetables and other foods.

The more preparation and cooking of foods that is done before eating, the greater the nutrient loss. To reduce the losses:

• Avoid soaking vegetables in water.
• When possible, cook vegetables, like potatoes, in their skins.

• Don't soak and rinse rice before cooking; you'll wash off the B-vitamins.
• Cook in as little water as possible.
• Bake, steam, or broil vegetables. Microwave cooking retains vitamins. If you stew meats, consume the broth too.
• When boiling, use tight-fitting lids to diminish evaporation of water.
• Cook vegetables in as short a time as possible. Develop a taste for a more crunchy texture.
• Cook frozen vegetables in the frozen state: don't thaw beforehand.
• Prepare lettuce salads right before eating.

---

balt, copper, fluoride, iodide, iron, manganese, molybdenum, selenium, zinc, and probably some others still under investigation.

The minerals most commonly lacking in our diets are iron and calcium—and possibly zinc. Adolescents and young adults should focus on good food choices for these nutrients. Lean meats are rich in iron and zinc, while low-fat milk is an excellent choice for calcium. Iron-deficiency anemia is a problem in this age group, and many researchers fear poor calcium intake is sowing the seeds for future osteoporosis, especially in women. See the box titled Osteoporosis: Reducing Your Risk to learn more.

Nutritional Guidelines: Planning Your Diet

A panel of scientists has made nutrient recommendations for the American diet regarding kcalories, protein, and certain vitamins and minerals. These **Recommended Dietary Allowances (RDAs)**, Estimated Safe and Adequate Daily Dietary Intakes (ESADDI), and Estimated Minimum Requirements (for sodium, potassium, and chloride) are standards for nutrient intake designed to prevent nutrient deficiencies. An ESADDI gives a range of values that will provide enough of a particular nutrient. The **Daily Food Guide** then translates these nutrient recommendations into a food group plan that, when followed, insures a balanced intake of the essential nutrients. To provide further guidance in choosing foods, **Dietary Guidelines for Americans** have been established with specific intent of preventing certain chronic "killer" diseases. Recently the Surgeon General and the National Academy of Sciences have added further clarifications to these Guidelines. Let's review each of these concepts separately.

Recommended Dietary Allowances (RDAs) The RDAs are set by the Food and Nutrition Board of the National Academy of Sciences. This group of nutrition scientists meets approximately every five years to set RDAs (see Table 12-3). Their goal is to establish recommended intakes for essential nutrients that meet the known needs of practically all healthy persons. The RDA for each vitamin and mineral is usually set by estimating the range for normal human needs, selecting the number at the high end of that range, and then adding additional

Table 12-2 Selected minerals: Their functions and food sources

Mineral	U.S. RDA[a]	Function	Food Sources
Calcium	1,000 mg[b]	Maintenance of bones and teeth; blood clotting; maintenance of cell membranes; control of nerve impulses	Milk and milk products, tofu, fortified orange juice, sardines
Phosphorus	1,000 mg	Bone growth and maintenance (teams with calcium); energy transfer in cells	Present in nearly all foods, especially milk, cheese, bakery products, and meats
Magnesium	400 mg	Transmission of nerve impulses; energy transfer; composition of many enzyme systems	Widespread in foods and water (except soft water) and especially found in wheat bran, milk products, beans, nuts, and leafy vegetables
Iron	18 mg	Component of hemoglobin (carries oxygen to tissues) and myoglobin (in muscle fibers) and enzymes	Liver, lean meats, legumes, enriched flour; absorption enhanced by presence of vitamin C
Iodine	150 micrograms	Essential part of thyroid hormones; regulation of body metabolism	Iodized salt, seafood
Zinc	15 mg	More than 70 enzyme reactions including synthesis of proteins, RNA, and DNA	Meat, eggs, liver, and seafood (especially oysters), milk, whole grains
Copper	2 mg	Iron metabolism and red blood cell formation	Liver, shellfish, nuts, dried beans

[a]General recommendations for adults and children age 4 or older (used in food labeling). More specific recommendations are made as part of recommended dietary allowances (RDA).
[b]For women, some authorities now recommend 1,000 mg daily before menopause and 1,500 mg after menopause if not following estrogen replacement therapy.

amounts to account for needed body storage and losses during food preparation. RDAs have been established for kcalories, protein, eleven vitamins, and seven minerals. ESADDIs have been established for two vitamins and five minerals. Estimated Minimum Requirements are set for three minerals.

It is important to understand two things about the RDAs. First, the aim of the RDA is to guide you in meeting your nutritional needs with food, rather than with vitamin and mineral supplements. This aim is important because only nineteen of forty or so necessary nutrients—not counting essential amino acids—have an RDA. Not enough is known about many nutrients for the Food and Nutrition Board to actually set an RDA. Second, the RDAs

are not requirements or minimums for individuals, but are recommended daily averages for groups. The RDAs were developed to guide food service personnel who feed large groups and are deliberately set higher than most people need in order to cover the range of individual variation. For a rule of thumb, the further one strays from the RDA, the greater the risk of suffering a nutritional deficiency.

Diets meeting only half the RDA are likely to be insufficient to replace daily losses of nutrients and thus over the long run can lead to a deficiency. No nutrient (even water) is absolutely needed daily. You can survive for a few days on a diet without water and about one year on a diet without vitamin A. Signs and symptoms of nutri-

Recommended Dietary Allowances (RDAs) Amounts of certain nutrients considered adequate to meet the needs of most healthy people.

Daily Food Guide Food group plan that provides practical advice to ensure balanced intake of the essential nutrients.

Dietary Guidelines for Americans Seven general principles of good nutrition intended to help prevent certain diet-related diseases.

Osteoporosis: Reducing Your Risk

Does any woman who reads a daily newspaper or monthly magazine—or who watches any television at all—*not* know about osteoporosis? Journalists and advertisers have made it almost impossible. Osteoporosis affects 20 to 25 million people in the United States, mostly women. Because their life expectancies are shorter and their rate of bone loss in adulthood is slower, men are usually not affected. Those who are tend to be alcoholics and men who age into their nineties. Osteoporosis results in loss of bone density, which leads to poor bone strength. In turn, fractures in the wrist, spine, and hip become more likely. Loss of height, back pain, and a bent spine also occur (see the illustration). Bone growth in humans stops sometime between ages 20 and 30. After age 30, and especially after menopause in women (age 50 years or so), bone loss predominates.

The slender, inactive woman who smokes is most susceptible to osteoporosis, but any man or woman who lives long enough can suffer. As men and women age into their eighties and nineties, osteoporosis becomes the rule—not the exception. Furthermore, osteoporosis not only is debilitating, but also can be fatal. Between 12 and 20 percent of all elderly people who break their hips eventually die from fracture-related complications. Spine fractures cause considerable pain and deformity and decrease physical ability. There is currently no effective therapy for severe osteoporosis.

Does Hormone Therapy Work?

Since 1985, doctors have recommended estrogen replacement therapy at menopause in order to prevent osteoporosis in women. New therapies using the hormones calcitriol (active vitamin D hormone) and calcitonin are also under study. Estrogen replacement at menopause seems to virtually stop further bone loss. We can assume, then, that estrogen replacement therapy will eliminate the risk for significant osteoporosis in women who begin it right after menopause and take it for the rest of their lives. When long-term studies are completed, we will be more certain. Estrogen replacement therapy is thought to be very safe; although breast cancer risk is slightly increased, heart disease risk is reduced. Chapters 15 and 16 explain why.

Is Calcium Therapy Another Answer?

Some women choose not to follow estrogen replacement therapy, and some women cannot take estrogen because they have estrogen-sensitive breast and uterine tumors. Will increasing calcium intake help them as much as estrogen would?

Studies from the United States and Denmark have found that taking even 2,000 mg of extra calcium (equal to 7.5 glasses of milk!) does not prevent bone loss after menopause in the spine, hip, or wrist as successfully as estrogen replacement does. Extra calcium in the diet is more effective than doing nothing at all to reduce bone loss in the total skeleton, but a high calcium intake may be no better for reducing bone loss in the spine than is just meeting the RDA. Increasing calcium intake to 1,500 milligrams per day, however, can reduce the dose of estrogen needed to prevent bone loss. In most cases it is not estrogen versus calcium but probably estrogen plus calcium that constitutes the best approach.

Are All Women at Risk?

About one-third of all women experience osteoporosis-related fractures in their lifetimes. Women who don't live beyond 75 may experience bone loss, but their bones still remain strong enough. In addition, some women have much more dense bone than other women. They probably built more bone when they were young, and so they can endure greater bone loss without experiencing more fractures. Also, some women may more easily adapt to poor calcium diets. On the other hand, a lack of regular menstruation, premature menopause, use of some medications, and prolonged bed rest are all associated with low bone-density values in women. Many factors in addition to calcium are involved in this disease.

Establishing a woman's individual risk for osteoporosis requires knowing the bone density of her spine, hip, and wrist, especially at menopause. Special bone densitometer instruments are available in medical centers for these measurements.

Osteoporosis: Reducing Your Risk (continued)

What Can You Do Now?

Although it is logical to assume that a good calcium intake in youth will promote a strong bone structure, no studies are available to support this assumption. The question is still being studied, and we hope for answers soon. Until they are available, we recommend calcium intake at or slightly above the RDA to possibly prevent—or at least minimize—later development of osteoporosis.

Regular menstruation is the overwhelming key to bone maintenance in young women, as evidenced by poor bone density in nonmenstruating female athletes.

Premenopausal women should see a physician at any sign of irregular menstruation. Although an active lifestyle, including sun exposure (to make vitamin D) and weight-bearing exercise, is important in preventing osteoporosis, exercise does not prevent the bone loss associated with irregular menstruation.

Poor calcium absorption is probably also an important link. Alcohol is toxic to bone cells, and alcoholism is probably a major undiagnosed, and so unrecognized, cause of osteoporosis. Smoking affects hormone levels in the bloodstream. Restricting alcohol intake and not smoking are necessary elements in an osteoporosis-prevention program.

At menopause, women need to discuss estrogen replacement therapy with a physician. Both men and women can keep track of bone loss by keeping track of their height, which should be measured at age 20. A decrease of more than one inch from that baseline measurement is a sign that significant bone loss is taking place. A loss in height should be the signal to see a physician and set a prevention plan in motion.

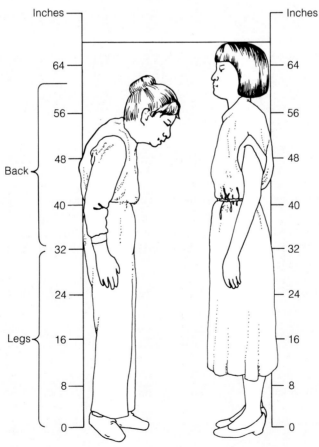

The curved spine of osteoporosis is due to multiple fractures in the vertebrae.

Table 12-3 Recommended Dietary Allowances, Revised 1989[a]

Category	Age (years) or Condition	Weight[b] (kg)	Weight[b] (lb)	Height[b] (cm)	Height[b] (in)	Protein (g)	Fat-Soluble Vitamins Vitamin A (µg RE)	Vitamin D (µg)	Vitamin E (mg α-TE)	Vitamin K (µg)
Infants	0.0–0.5	6	13	60	24	13	375	7.5	3	5
	0.5–1.0	9	20	71	28	14	375	10	4	10
Children	1–3	13	29	90	35	16	400	10	6	15
	4–6	20	44	112	44	24	500	10	7	20
	7–10	28	62	132	52	28	700	10	7	30
Males	11–14	45	99	157	62	45	1,000	10	10	45
	15–18	66	145	176	69	59	1,000	10	10	65
	19–24	72	160	177	70	58	1,000	10	10	70
	25–50	79	174	176	70	63	1,000	5	10	80
	51 +	77	170	173	68	63	1,000	5	10	80
Females	11–14	46	101	157	62	46	800	10	8	45
	15–18	55	120	163	64	44	800	10	8	55
	19–24	58	128	164	65	46	800	10	8	60
	25–50	63	138	163	64	50	800	5	8	65
	51 +	65	143	160	63	50	800	5	8	65
Pregnant						60	800	10	10	65
Lactating	1st 6 Months					65	1,300	10	12	65
	2nd 6 Months					62	1,200	10	11	65

[a] The allowances, expressed as average daily intakes over time, are intended to provide for individual variations among most normal persons as they live in the United States under usual environmental stresses. Diets should be based on a variety of common foods in order to provide other nutrients for which human requirements have been less well defined.

[b] Weights and heights of Reference Adults are actual medians for the U.S. population of the designated age. The use of these figures does not imply that the height-to-weight ratios are ideal.

tional deficiency may be subtle and develop slowly. Decreased effectiveness of the immune system, reduced organ function, and decreased ability to carry oxygen in the bloodstream may not be apparent for a long period of time. You may become ill more often and not really know why. Though your diet may be inadequate, you still may show no telltale signs; no "smoke detector" will sound the alarm. So it is best to eat a diet that meets your nutrient needs on a daily basis.

A variant of the RDA is the **U.S. Recommended Daily Allowances** (U.S. RDAs). These are usually the largest values for each age and gender category (RDAs vary according to age and gender) of the RDA values set in 1968. Percentages of the U.S. RDAs are listed on nutrition labels, such as those seen on cereal boxes.

Many countries publish their own nutrient guides, as does the World Health Organization (WHO) in conjunc-

tion with the U.N. Food and Agriculture Organization (FAO) for application worldwide. These guidelines differ somewhat from each other because some scientists disagree about requirements and because different diets can lead to different vitamin and mineral needs. U.S., Canadian, British, and WHO standards are compared in Table 12-4.

Daily Food Guide   Most of us learned the four food groups in grade school. We learned that by choosing foods from each group, we could have a healthy diet. The fundamental principles of this food guide are moderation, variety, and balance. A diet is balanced if it contains appropriate amounts of each nutrient; choosing foods from each of the food groups helps insure that. The latest version of the food group plan is called the "Hassle-free Daily Food Guide." It contains five groups:

U.S. Recommended Daily Allowances   A simplified version of the RDAs used in food products labels:

Vita-min C (mg)	Thia-min (mg)	Ribo-flavin (mg)	Niacin (mg)	Vita-min B$_6$ (mg)	Fo-late (µg)	Vita-min B$_{12}$ (µg)	Cal-cium (mg)	Phos-phorus (mg)	Mag-nesium (mg)	Iron (mg)	Zinc (mg)	Iodine (µg)	Sele-nium (µg)
30	0.3	0.4	5	0.3	25	0.3	400	300	40	6	5	40	10
35	0.4	0.5	6	0.6	35	0.5	600	500	60	10	5	50	15
40	0.7	0.8	9	1.0	50	0.7	800	800	80	10	10	70	20
45	0.9	1.1	12	1.1	75	1.0	800	800	120	10	10	90	20
45	1.0	1.2	13	1.4	100	1.4	800	800	170	10	10	120	30
50	1.3	1.5	17	1.7	150	2.0	1,200	1,200	270	12	15	150	40
60	1.5	1.8	20	2.0	200	2.0	1,200	1,200	400	12	15	150	50
60	1.5	1.7	19	2.0	200	2.0	1,200	1,200	350	10	15	150	70
60	1.5	1.7	19	2.0	200	2.0	800	800	350	10	15	150	70
60	1.2	1.4	15	2.0	200	2.0	800	800	350	10	15	150	70
50	1.1	1.3	15	1.4	150	2.0	1,200	1,200	280	15	12	150	45
60	1.1	1.3	15	1.5	180	2.0	1,200	1,200	300	15	12	150	50
60	1.1	1.3	15	1.6	180	2.0	1,200	1,200	280	15	12	150	55
60	1.1	1.3	15	1.6	180	2.0	800	800	280	15	12	150	55
60	1.0	1.2	13	1.6	180	2.0	800	800	280	10	12	150	55
70	1.5	1.6	17	2.2	400	2.2	1,200	1,200	320	30	15	175	65
95	1.6	1.8	20	2.1	280	2.6	1,200	1,200	355	15	19	200	75
90	1.6	1.7	20	2.1	260	2.6	1,200	1,200	340	15	16	200	75

Table 12-4 Dietary Standards for Adults, Determined by U.S., U.K., Canada, and World Health Organization

Classification	Kcal	Protein (grams)	Calcium (mg)	Iron (mg)	Vitamin A (RE)	Thiamin (mg)	Riboflavin (mg)	Vitamin C (mg)
United States (1980)								
Female (63 kg, 1.63 m)	2,200	50	800	15	800	1.1	1.3	60
Male (79 kg, 1.76 m)	2,900	63	800	10	1,000	1.5	1.7	60
United Kingdom								
Female	2,150–2,500	54–62	500	12	750	0.9–1.0	1.3	30
Male	2,500–3,350	63–84	500	10	750	1.0–1.3	1.6	30
Canada (1983)								
Female (55.8 kg)	2,100	41	700	14	800	0.9	1.1	45
Male (71.1 kg)	3,000	57	800	8	1,000	1.2	1.5	60
FAO/WHO (1974)								
Female	2,300	39	400–500	18	750	0.9	1.3	30
Male	3,200	46	400–500	10	750	1.2	1.8	30

Shils, M.E. and Young, U.R.: 1988, *Modern Nutrition in Health and Disease*, ed. 7, Philadelphia. Lea & Febriger.

Table 12-5 The daily food guide

This guide lets you easily turn the RDA into food choices. You can get all essential nutrients by eating a balanced variety of foods each day from the food groups listed here. Eat a variety of foods in each food group and adjust serving sizes appropriately to reach and maintain a desirable weight. Even with the addition of some plant proteins as suggested in the text, this pattern will yield only about 1,600 kcalories.

Additions of plant proteins and following the other suggestions listed should provide a diet adequate in all nutrients, except possibly iron for women who experience a heavy menstrual flow.

Group	Serving	Major Nutrients	Food and Nutritional Serving Sizes[a]
Milk and cheese (emphasize low-fat and nonfat varieties)	2 (adult) 3–4 (ages 11–24 years, pregnant, lactating) 2–3 (child)	Calcium Riboflavin Protein Potassium Zinc	1 cup milk 1⅓ oz. cheese 1 cup yogurt 2 cups cottage cheese 1 cup custard/pudding 1½ cups ice cream
Meat (poultry and beans)	2 (adult)[b] 3 (pregnant, lactating)	Protein Niacin Iron Vitamin B$_6$ Zinc Thiamin Vitamin B$_{12}$[c]	2 oz. cooked meat, poultry, fish 1 cup cooked dry beans 4 T. peanut butter 2 eggs ½–1 cup nuts
Fruits and vegetables (choose a green vegetable and fruit with vitamin C)	4	Vitamin A Vitamin C Folate Fiber	½ cup cooked fruit or vegetable ½ cup juice 1 whole fruit 1 small salad
Breads and cereals (emphasize whole grains)	4	Thiamin Iron Niacin Magnesium[d] Fiber[d] Zinc[d]	1 slice bread 1 oz. ready-to-eat cereal ½–¾ cup cooked cereal, rice, or pasta
Fats[c], sweets, and alcohol		Foods from this group should not replace any from the other groups. Amounts consumed should be determined by individual energy needs.	

[a]May be reduced for child servings
[b]Consider adding two servings of plant proteins, like beans and peanuts
[c]Only in animal food choices
[d]Whole grains especially
[e]One tablespoon of vegetable oil makes a healthful contribution to a diet

(1) a milk and cheese group; (2) a meat, poultry, fish, and beans group; (3) a fruits and vegetables group; (4) a breads and cereals group; and (5) a fats, sweets, and alcohol group (see Table 12-5). Caution is advised when choosing from the latter group, although foods within that group can supply the essential fats for your diet.

If you're worried about maintaining your ideal weight or want to lose weight while living the somewhat sedentary life of a student, the Daily Food Guide can help you create food plans that contain as few as 1,200–1,400

kcalories but meet the adolescent and young adult RDAs (age 11–24 years) for protein, thiamin, niacin, riboflavin, and other important nutrients. Unfortunately, the plans may be low in vitamin E, vitamin B$_6$, magnesium, iron, and zinc. To make up for these possible lacks, add two servings of plant proteins to two servings of meat, poultry, and fish. For fruits and vegetables, include a vitamin C source and a dark-green vegetable each day. For breads and cereals, all servings should be whole-grained. Finally, include a tablespoon of vegetable oil (if not already present in the other food products). A diet using these low-fat food choices contains only about 1,600 kcalories but meets known nutritional needs, except possibly for iron in some women who have heavy menses. For those women, foods fortified in iron, such as breakfast cereals, are indicated.

■ **Exploring Your Emotions**

How much is your diet controlled by habit and circumstances, such as what you find in the refrigerator, what you can get at the corner take-out restaurant, or what someone else cooks? If you're not really taking charge of your diet, what do you think is causing you to act that way?

If 1,600 kcalories is too many kcalories for you, first try to become more active. It's hard to design an adequate diet for young adults from foods that supply fewer than 1,600 kcalories. If you can't increase your energy output, you can include some nutrient-fortified foods, like breakfast cereals. In addition, if your diet does not include meat or other animal products, see the recommendations made in discussion of vegetarianism.

Dietary Guidelines for Americans Although the Daily Food Guide provides practical advice for avoiding nutrient deficiencies, it doesn't directly address the prevention of the diet-related chronic "killer" diseases. To do so, the U.S. Department of Agriculture and the Department of Health and Human Services have issued Dietary Guidelines for Americans, most recently in 1985. Since then, the Surgeon General, the American Heart Association (AHA), the National Cancer Institute (NCI), and the National Academy of Sciences (NAS) have added further recommendations to the basic framework of the Dietary Guidelines. What follows is a summary of the advice provided by the Dietary Guidelines with additional comments from various health-related organizations.

1. *Eat a variety of foods*—focus on the Daily Food Guide we just discussed. The NAS report suggests limiting protein intake to twice the RDA and not taking a nutrient supplement in quantities greater than the RDA in any one day. Both the NAS and the Surgeon General's Report encourage everyone, especially adolescent girls and women, to meet their RDA for calcium. Cook and store foods for maximum nutrient retention.
2. *Maintain desirable weight*—the middle ranges of the Metropolitan Life Table (see Chapter 13) can serve as a standard. Both the NAS and the Surgeon General's report emphasize balancing food intake with regular physical activity to avoid creeping overweight and eventual obesity. Excess weight increases the risk for diabetes, heart disease, cancer, and other diseases.

For those who are overweight, the recommended loss of one or two pounds a week should be accomplished by increasing physical activity and eating low-kcalorie, nutrient-rich foods—fruits, vegetables, and grains—not fat and fatty foods, sugar and sweets, and alcoholic beverages. Diets with fewer than 800 kcalories per day can be hazardous and should be followed only under medical supervision.

3. *Avoid too much fat, saturated fat, and cholesterol*—the NAS, AHA, and NCI suggest limiting fat intake to 30 percent of total kcalories. The NAS report and AHA recommend limiting saturated fat to one-third of total fat intake (10 percent of total kcalories) and dietary cholesterol to 300 milligrams per day. Again, the average American consumes 15 percent of total kcalories as saturated fat and about 400–500 milligrams of dietary cholesterol per day. Experts recommend choosing lean meat, fish, poultry, and dry beans and peas as protein sources; using nonfat or low-fat milk and milk products; limiting your intake of fats and oils high in saturated fat; trimming fat off meats; broiling, baking, or boiling instead of frying; and moderate use of fat-containing foods such as breaded or deep-fried foods.
4. *Eat foods with adequate starch and fiber*—emphasize complex, rather than simple carbohydrates. The NAS report suggests five or more servings of vegetables and fruits daily and six or more servings of breads, cereals, and legumes (beans) daily. The NCI intends this intake to yield 20–35 grams of dietary fiber per day.
5. *Avoid too much sugar*—some authorities recommend no more than 10 percent of total kcalories come from sugar. This would amount to about 40 pounds per year, as opposed to our current intake of approximately 145 pounds per year.
6. *Avoid too much sodium*—the NAS suggests limiting salt intake to 6 grams per day, which would yield 2.4 grams of sodium (salt is sodium chloride). A restriction of this magnitude would require a great change in food habits for many people, such as eliminating processed (lunch) meats, salted snack foods, most canned and prepared soups, regular cheese, and many tomato-based products. You can begin to make this change by learning to enjoy the flavors of unsalted foods, adding little or no salt during cooking or at the table, and flavoring foods with herbs, spices, or lemon juice.
7. *If you drink alcoholic beverages, do so in moderation*—both the NAS and Surgeon General's report recommend no more than two drinks daily and no alcohol use during pregnancy. Two drinks would be the equivalent of 8 ounces of wine, 24 ounces of beer, or 3 ounces of distilled spirits. Keep in mind that alcoholic beverages are high in kcalories and low in nutrients.

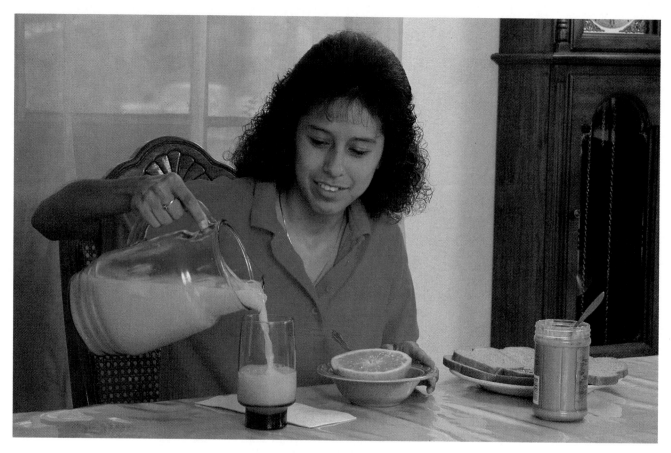

You can use the various nutrient guides to plan healthy meals and ensure that you meet all your daily nutritional needs. This young woman is off to a good start with ample supplies of vitamin C, protein, carbohydrate, and fiber.

The NCI further recommends moderation when consuming salt-cured, smoked, and nitrate-cured foods (such as bacon and sausage) because these may increase the risk of colon cancer. The NAS and Surgeon General's report adds a recommendation for obtaining an adequate fluoride intake, particularly during the growing years. This strengthens tooth structure and so reduces the incidence of dental caries. Finally, the Surgeon General's report recommends that children, adolescents, and women of childbearing age consume iron-rich foods, primarily to decrease the incidence of iron-deficiency anemia.

These guidelines do not apply equally to everyone. We vary in susceptibility to developing high serum cholesterol levels, high blood pressure (make sure you have both values checked if you haven't done this lately), obesity, cancer, and the other health problems these guidelines seek to counteract. For instance, in people who have a low energy output, high sugar intake may cause problems because they need a nutrient-dense diet—one that provides many nutrients per kcalorie. However, for people who have a very active lifestyle and practice good

dental hygiene, dietary sugar causes no apparent health problems. The same argument applies to sodium. No scientific data show that typical North American sodium intakes necessarily produce high blood pressure in persons who presently have normal blood pressure.

■ **Exploring Your Emotions**

Do you have food habits that are part of your daily routine, such as getting a soda from a particular vending machine every time you're in a certain building or snacking on M & M's when you're studying? If some of your habits are unhealthy, can you think of ways to change them?

You should consider your own health status in order to apply these guidelines appropriately. Implement appropriate changes and see if they are effective—sometimes results are disappointing even when you really follow a new diet closely. We call that a sign of nonresponse. Still, most nutrition and health researchers agree with some of the guidelines set by our major health and science institutions—the need for varying the diet;

The Compulsive Dieter's Dream Diet

So many elaborate new diets appear every year that a parody like this may give us some perspective on ourselves. This "diet" is a model of creative rationalization.

Dieting Under Stress

This diet is designed to help you cope with the stress that builds up during the day.

Breakfast
½ grapefruit
1 slice whole wheat toast, dry
8 oz. skim milk

Lunch
4 oz. lean broiled chicken breast
1 cup steamed spinach
1 cup herb tea
1 Oreo cookie

Midafternoon Snack
Rest of the Oreos in the package
2 pints Rocky Road ice cream
1 jar hot fudge sauce
Nuts, cherries, whipped cream

Dinner
2 loaves garlic bread with cheese
Large sausage, mushroom, and cheese pizza
4 cans or 1 large pitcher of beer
3 Milky Way or Snickers candy bars

Rules for this Diet

1. If you eat something and no one sees you eat it, it has no calories.

2. If you drink a diet soda with a candy bar, the calories in the candy bar are canceled out by the diet soda.

3. Food used for medicinal purposes *never* counts, such as hot chocolate, brandy, toast, or Sara Lee Cheesecake.

4. If you fatten up everyone else around you, then you look thinner.

5. Movie-related foods do not have additional calories because they are part of the entire entertainment package and not part of one's personal fuel, such as Milk Duds, buttered popcorn, Junior Mints, Red Hots, and Tootsie Rolls.

6. Cookie pieces contain no calories. The process of breaking causes calorie leakage.

7. Things licked off knives and spoons have no calories if you are in the process of preparing something. Examples: peanut butter on a knife making a sandwich and ice cream on a spoon making a sundae.

Foods that have the same color have the same number of calories. Examples are spinach and pistachio ice cream, mushrooms and white chocolate. NOTE: Chocolate is a universal color and may be substituted for any other food color.

Ethnic Choices: The Best and the Worst

Take the fat out of a traditional American dinner, and what's left may well be flavorless and dull: no gravy for the meat, no sour cream for the potato. But in a low-fat ethnic meal—say, pasta with pesto—there's still plenty of flavor.

Whether you eat at ethnic restaurants or cook ethnic food yourself, favor the low-fat choices in the "Best" column over the high-fat ones labeled "Worst."

Cuisine	Best	Worst
Italian	pasta with red clam sauce, meatless marinara, pesto, or mushroom sauce; pizza with fresh vegetable toppings	sausages and meatballs, white cheese sauces, garlic bread
Chinese	stir-fried chicken, seafood, and vegetables; soft noodles, steamed rice	fried won tons and egg rolls, egg fu yung, fried rice, "crispy" entrees, lobster sauces
Mexican	chicken, seafood, and vegetable burritos and enchiladas	refried beans; pork and cheese chimichangas
French	poached or steamed fish, chicken in wine or other light sauces, niçoise salads	pâté, quiche, duck, hollandaise-type sauces, dishes with *beurre* or *crème*
Greek	beef shish kebab, salads, couscous, tabouli, pita bread	lamb, spanakopita, deep-fried falafel
Japanese	sushi, chicken and fish teriyaki, tofu and vegetables	tempura and other deep-fried dishes
Indian	Tandoori chicken, vegetable curry, fish	fried breads, coconut milk
Thai/Indonesian	grilled beef or chicken sate, chicken salads	sauces with coconut milk
Cajun	seafood or vegetable gumbo or jambalaya, grilled fish	andouille and other sausages, fried fish

Excerpted from IN HEALTH. Copyright © 1988 Hippocrates Partners.

controlling body weight; reducing total fat and saturated fat intake for adults; eating more fruits, vegetables, and cereal grains; and moderating alcohol intake. However, many scientists do not think that general recommendations for the public can be justified for sugar, complex carbohydrates, fiber, salt, specific vitamins, and cholesterol. Rather, they believe, as we do, that these recommendations need to be individualized according to a person's current health status. Nevertheless, we all should consider some of the implications of these general dietary recommendations, such as emphasizing low-fat dairy products, lean meats and plant proteins, fruits and vegetables, and ample breads and cereals.

How many times a week do you eat at your favorite fast food restaurant? The Appendix at the end of this chapter lists kcalories, fat, protein, and carbohydrate contents as well as U.S. RDAs for many of the fast foods we grab when we neglect to plan for a nutritious meal. If you look at the last column, you'll see that very few of them have a percentage of kcalories as fat that is less than 40 percent.

Despite reported trends in the American diet away from saturated fats (whole milk and cream being replaced by low-fat and skim milk, for instance), not all the dietary news is good. In fact, whole milk and whole-milk beverages continue to be one of the five major contributors of kcalories to the U.S. diet. The other four are white bread, rolls, and crackers; doughnuts, cakes, and cookies; alcoholic beverages; and hamburgers, cheeseburgers, and meatloaf. Some of these foods have some nutritional value, but were the American diet truly moving toward the ideals we've just discussed—a decrease in alcohol, sugar, and saturated fats, along with an increase in fiber—we wouldn't expect to find these foods at the top of the list. We suggest replacing them with low-fat milk; whole-wheat bread and whole-grain cereals; lean meat, tuna, beans, and other vegetable proteins; and oranges and broccoli. What would your list look like?

The Vegetarian Alternative   Some people choose a diet with one essential difference from the diets we've already described—food of animal origin (meat, poultry, fish, eggs, milk) are eliminated or restricted. Today, several million Americans follow a vegetarian diet. Most do so

---

■ **Exploring Your Emotions**

Do you feel good after you eat a healthy meal? Are your good feelings physical or emotional or both?

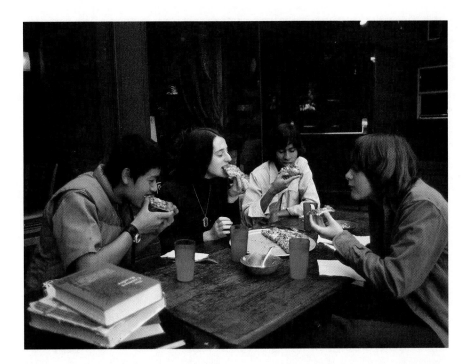

Pizza makes a convenient lunch, but it's not a good choice on a daily basis. The cheese is high in saturated fat, and the white-flour crust is filling without providing needed nutrients. These students could improve their meal by adding a salad or having fresh fruit for dessert.

because they think foods of plant origin are healthier, more natural, and take less energy to produce. Some do so for religious, ethical, or philosophical reasons. If you choose to be a vegetarian, you can be confident you can meet your nutritional needs by following a few basic rules. However, we feel vegetarian diets for children and in pregnancy deserve individual professional guidance.

There are a variety of vegetarian styles. **Vegans** eat only plant foods. **Lactovegetarians** eat plant foods and dairy products. **Lactovovegetarians** eat plant foods, dairy products, and eggs. Finally, **lactovopescovegetarians** eat plant foods, dairy products, eggs, and fish. The wider the variety of the diet eaten, the easier it is to meet nutritional needs.

Including some animal protein in a diet makes diet planning much easier. Most vegetarians consume at least dairy products, if not dairy products and eggs. A four-food-group plan has been developed for lactovegetarians; it includes six servings from a protein group that has nuts, grains, legumes, and seeds in it. Three or more servings from a vegetable group, one to four servings from the fruit group, and two or more servings from the milk and/or eggs group complete the plan.

This plan differs somewhat from the typical Daily Food Guide pattern for omnivores, but it shares some similarities. The vegetarian who follows this plan has to find protein sources in foods other than meats. You can't just

cut meat out of your diet and eat everything else. You need high-quality protein sources to replace the meat, and you can find them in the nuts, grains, legumes, and seed group. It becomes your new meat group. By following this plan, the lactovegetarian should have no problem getting an adequate diet. Consuming fruits with most meals is especially helpful, because any vitamin C present will improve iron absorption (the iron in plants is more difficult to absorb than is that in animal sources).

In contrast to those who eat dairy products, the vegan has to do much more special diet planning. Although a vegan diet is often rich in vitamin A, vitamin C, and folate, grains and legumes are especially necessary for good-quality protein. Furthermore, this diet needs good sources for riboflavin, vitamin D, vitamin B_{12}, calcium, iron, and zinc. Riboflavin can be obtained by eating green leafy vegetables, whole grains, yeast, and legumes. Vitamin D is most easily obtained by spending at least one-half hour a day out in the sun or—if that is not possible—a supplement of 400 I.U. is recommended. Vitamin B_{12} is found only in animal foods, so the vegan will have to take a vitamin supplement or consume a special yeast, soy milks, breakfast cereals, or other foods that are fortified with vitamin B_{12}. The body can store up to four years' worth of vitamin B_{12}, and so it takes a long time for vitamin B_{12} deficiency to develop. But when the deficiency does develop, it can damage nerves irreversibly.

Vegans   Vegetarians who eat no animal products at all.

Lactovegetarians   Vegetarians who include milk and cheese products in their diet.

Lactovopescovegetarians   Vegetarians who include eggs, dairy products, and fish in their diet.

Lactovovegetarians   Vegetarians who eat no meat, poultry, or fish, but do eat eggs and milk products.

The Japanese Advantage: Low Meat Consumption, High Life Expectancy

The Japanese, who seem to be besting the competition in nearly every field these days, now are outliving the rest of the world, too. With a diet heavy on soybean curd, seaweed, and raw fish, and a universal system of medical coverage, the Japanese have outstripped Sweden, the United States and other countries in life expectancy. A Japanese male born in 1987 can expect to live more than 75 years; a Japanese female born then can expect to live to be nearly 81.

Both figures represent one of the most dramatic increases in life expectancy of any nation since the end of World War II, when Japanese men could expect to live only 50 years and Japanese women 53 years. The Japanese have been living longer than Americans since the 1970s, but only in the 1980s have they surpassed the Swedes to top longevity charts. Average life expectancy for Americans is 70 years for men and 77 years for women.

Japanese postwar gains in life expectancy can be traced largely to the elimination of many deadly diseases, including dysentery and tuberculosis, and to major advances in nutrition and medical care that have given this country the lowest infant death rate in the world. Meanwhile, since 1955 the United States has slipped from sixth to eighteenth among industrialized nations. But the primary reason for Japanese longevity, according to experts, is a diet that is low in fat and total caloric intake and high in fiber from various roots, vegetables, and seaweed. As a result, the Japanese have one of the lowest levels of cholesterol and heart disease in the world. Heart disease is the leading cause of death in the United States, and the U.S. death rate from heart attacks is several times higher than in Japan.

"They have a heavy fish-based diet. We've been using that argument in this country to say why it would be better to eat more fish, better than chicken or turkey even," said Dr. William Castelli, director of the Framingham, Mass., study that has followed several thousand people for thirty-eight years to assess their risk of heart disease relative to smoking, high blood pressure, and other factors. The Japanese particularly favor fatty fish such as tuna, mackerel and sardines, which recently have been found to keep cholesterol in check.

"The U.S. has a much higher standard of living," said Shigemi Kono, head of the Institute of Population Problems in the Ministry of Health and Welfare. "But we live longer, and the reason is the Japanese diet is kind of ideal—less fat, less cholesterol," said Kono. "I used to tell my American friends, 'You eat too much meat, so your blood is sticky.'"

But Castelli and others here are worried about recent changes in the Japanese diet, particularly

To obtain calcium, the vegan can consume fortified soy milk, tofu, green leafy vegetables, and nuts. Iron is found in whole grains, dried fruits, nuts, and legumes. Zinc is found in whole grains and legumes. Of all of those nutrients, calcium is the most difficult to consume in adequate amounts. Supplements may be needed.

With respect to essential amino acids, even vegans do not have to consciously plan their diet to include complementary proteins. As long as vegans eat proteins from a wide variety of sources and include a couple of protein sources at each meal, the need for essential amino acids will be met. A good rule of thumb is that 60 percent of the protein should be from grains; 35 percent from legumes, which include black-eyed peas, peanuts, split peas, garbanzos, **tofu** (soybean curd), lentils, and many other types of beans and peas; and 5 percent from dark-green leafy vegetables.

It takes a little planning and common sense to put together a good vegetarian diet. If you are a vegetarian or are considering becoming one, devote some extra time and thought to your diet. It's especially important that you eat as wide a variety of foods as possible to ensure that all of your nutritional requirements are filled.

A Personal Plan: Making Intelligent Choices about Food

Now that you understand the basics of good nutrition and a healthy diet, you can put together a diet that works

Tofu   A custardlike food made from soybeans.

The Japanese Advantage:
Low Meat Consumption, High Life Expectancy (continued)

among the young, who often prefer Western-style ham-and-egg breakfasts or McDonald's Big Macs and french fries to the more traditional Japanese meals of rice, soy bean curd, or tofu and fish. As a result, cholesterol levels have been rising, and so has Japan's heart attack rate.

Fifteen years ago, the average Japanese man had a cholesterol level of 180 milligrams per deciliter of blood plasma; today the average is getting close to 200 mg. In the U.S., the typical American has a cholesterol level of about 215 mg., down somewhat from the past but still well over the 150 mg. level that Castelli said would all but eliminate the risk of heart attack.

The U.S. diet is healthier than the Japanese diet in at least one respect—Americans consume much less salt. But the Japanese have recently begun to make improvements. In the last few years, the government has warned

people that Japan's traditionally salty diet has resulted in one of the highest death rates from strokes— blood vessel hemorrhages in the brain. It is nearly twice the U.S. rate. The Japanese consumed about 20 to 25 grams of salt a day fifteen years ago. Today, they consume on average only about 13 grams, which is still higher than the 10 grams the average American ingests each day.

High salt consumption may also help explain one of Japan's great public health mysteries—its unusually high rate of stomach cancer. Unlike most other cancers, Japan's stomach cancer rate is well above that found in the U.S. Others

theorize that the mystery can be explained by the fact that Japanese prefer their food—much like their baths—extremely hot in temperature, and that such hot food can irritate the stomach lining. As for the hot baths, the Japanese have an almost religious devotion to them. And many firmly believe that long soaks in mineral-rich hot springs, of which there are thousands in Japan, are the real reason for Japanese longevity.

From "Japanese Outpace the World in Life Expectancy: Experts Credit Their Low-Meat Diet," by Margaret Shapiro. *Washington Post Health*, March 8, 1988. p. 11.

V I T A L S T A T I S T I C S		
Average Years a Baby Born Today Will Live		
Country	**Men**	**Women**
Japan	75.2	80.9
United States	70.1	77.6

for you. There probably is an ideal diet for you based on your particular nutrition and health status, but there is no single type of diet that provides optimal health for everyone. The Japanese diet is often promoted as a healthful alternative for Americans. At the same time, it is associated with one of the highest rates of stomach cancer in the world, which offsets its lower risk for colon or breast cancer. Overall, many cultural dietary patterns encompass the practices recommended by nutrition experts: eating a variety of foods, maintaining a desirable body weight, and maintaining a physically active lifestyle. For you, the key is to focus on the likely causes of health problems in your life and to make specific dietary changes to address those. Some tips for applying the Dietary Guidelines to practical situations are provided in a nearby box. And advice on choosing an expert to help you plan the best diet is given later in this chapter. Beyond this, there are some specific areas that may be of

concern to you, such as food additives and vitamin supplements, and we turn to those next.

Reading Food Labels to Learn More about What You Eat To make intelligent choices about food, you should learn to read and understand food labels. Under current government regulations, food labels must contain information about nutritional content if the manufacturer makes a nutritional claim about the food or if nutrients are added to the food. Some manufacturers elect to add a nutrition label even though they aren't required to. As mentioned before, this label expresses nutrient quantities as percentages of the U.S. RDA. Information about kcalories, protein, carbohydrate, fat, and sodium content, as well as the presence of various vitamins and minerals, is also provided. In addition, almost all foods must list their ingredients in descending order based on weight, so you can learn quite a lot about them from their labels.

TACTICS AND TIPS

Applying the Dietary Guidelines to Practical Situations

If you usually eat this	Instead, try this
White bread	Whole-wheat bread—not as many nutrients have been lost in refinement/processing
Sugared breakfast cereal	Low-sugar cereal; use the kcalories you save for a side dish of fruit
Cheeseburger and french fries	Hamburger (hold the mayonnaise) and baked beans (for less fat and the benefits of plant proteins)
Potato salad at the salad bar	Three-bean salad
Doughnut	Bran muffin or bagel (no cream cheese)
Soft drinks	Diet soft drinks (save the kcalories for more nutritious foods)
Boiled vegetables	Steamed vegetables (more nutrient retention)
Canned vegetables	Frozen vegetables (fewer nutrients lost in processing)
Fried meats	Broiled meats (watch the fat drain away)
Fatty meats, like ribs	Lean meats, like ground round; have chicken and fish often
Whole milk and ice cream	1 percent milk and sherbet or frozen yogurt (reduce saturated-fat intake)
Mayonnaise or sour cream salad dressing	Oil and vinegar dressings, or diet varieties (to save kcalories)
Cookies for a snack	Popcorn (air popped with minimal margarine)

You can also get other important information, such as the kind of fat they contain (lard, palm oil, coconut oil, butter, and so on), that can guide your food choices. A sample label is shown in the box titled Decoding A Nutrition Label along with an explanation of what it means.

Additives in Food: Are They Dangerous?   Additives make up less than 1 percent of our food. The most widely used are sugar, salt, and corn syrup. These three, plus citric acid, baking soda, vegetable colors, mustard, and pepper account for 98 percent by weight of all food additives used in the United States. Today, some 2,800 substances are intentionally added to foods for one or more of the following reasons: (1) to maintain or improve nutritional quality, (2) to maintain freshness; (3) to help in processing or preparation; or (4) to alter taste or appearance.

Nutrition quality is improved when vitamins and minerals are added to enrich (replace those lost in processing) or fortify (add nutrients not normally present in such quantities). Breads and cereals are enriched with B vitamins lost or destroyed during the milling and processing of grains. Common examples of fortification include the addition of vitamin D to milk, vitamin A to margarine,

vitamin C to fruit drinks, and iodide to table salt.

The purpose of many additives is to maintain freshness. A lot of foods last as long as they do on the shelf or in the refrigerator because of additives that retard spoilage, preserve natural color and flavor, and keep fats and oils from turning rancid. Nitrates and nitrites, for example, protect meats from contamination from the toxin responsible for botulism. Nitrate consumption from cured foods and natural vegetables (such as spinach and carrots) is associated with the synthesis of cancer-causing agents in the stomach. However, the cancer risk appears to be low, except for people with low stomach acid output (some elderly people, for example). Consequently government agencies have chosen not to ban nitrate or nitrite use in foods, but rather to change manufacturing practices to reduce cancer risk.

Antioxidants, such as BHA and BHT, prevent changes in color, flavor, or texture that occur when foods are exposed to air. While some studies show that BHT prevents certain forms of cancer in animals, other studies link BHT to some other forms of cancer. The FDA is reviewing use of BHT and BHA, but any risk to the diet from these agents is far less than that from food-poisoning organisms. Meanwhile, some companies have

---

Antioxidants   Agents such as vitamin E and sulfites that prevent destruction of food products by oxygen and enzymes.

Decoding a Nutrition Label

Use of word natural is unregulated and meaningless. The "low fat" claim means the label must list saturated and unsaturated fatty acids as well as cholesterol, but "low fat" itself has no legal definition.

This figure must be within 20 percent of the actual calorie count. Thus a serving of this cereal could contain anywhere from 88 to 132 calories.

To determine the percentage of fat calories, multiply the grams of fat (6) by the number of calories in a gram of fat (9). Then divide the result—54—by the total calorie count (110). The resulting percentage of fat calories, 49, is quite high for cereal, since grains alone are low in fat, and well above the 30 percent recommended as the maximum in a healthful diet.

Must be included if nutrition information is given

Optional

Ingredients are listed in descending order according to weight. Be careful: you can't tell how much of a particular ingredient is used. But often, if you add together the various forms of sweetener in a product—in this case, sugar, brown sugar, corn syrup, malt syrup and honey—sweeteners become the primary ingredient. Foods with a standard of identity do not require an ingredient list.

Soybean oil is polyunsaturated; coconut oil is saturated. The label does not have to specify which oil was used in this product.

Label is a composite of information typically printed on a cereal box.

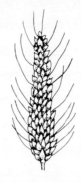

BREAKFAST CEREAL
ALL-NATURAL—LOW FAT

Serving Size	1 ounce
Calories	110
Protein	2g
Carbohydrates	23g
Total Fat	6g
Polyunsaturated fatty acid	4g
Saturated fatty acid	2g*
Cholesterol	0mg
Sodium	180mg
Potassium	55mg

*Applies if coconut oil is used

PERCENTAGE OF U.S. RECOMMENDED DAILY ALLOWANCE

Protein	4
Vitamin A	25
Vitamin C	*
Thiamine	25
Riboflavin	25
Niacin	25
Calcium	15
Iron	15
Vitamin D	10
Vitamin B6	25
Folic Acid	25
Vitamin B12	25
Phosphorus	4
Magnesium	4
Zinc	2
Copper	4

*Contains less than 2% of the U.S. R.D.A.

INGREDIENTS: Whole wheat, rolled oats, sugar, corn, brown sugar, partially hydrogenated soybean and/or coconut oil, malted barley, salt, corn syrup, coconut, whey, malt syrup, honey, artificial flavor, artificial food coloring (Yellow No. 5), BHT, MSG.

VITAMINS AND MINERALS: Vitamin A palmitate, niacinamide, iron, vitamin B6, riboflavin (vitamin BH12), thiamine mononitrate (vitamin B1), zinc oxide, folic acid, vitamin D and vitamin B12.

CARBOHYDRATE INFORMATION

Dietary Fiber	1g
Complex carbohydrates	16g
Sucrose and other sugars	6g
Total carbohydrates	23g

One ounce is two-thirds of a cup. Most people eat double that amount for breakfast. When comparing similar products be sure to compare equal serving sizes.

Sugars, fiber and complex carbohydrates are lumped together. Further information is optional. (This label offers additional details below.)

Cholesterol is associated with fat in foods of animal origin only.

The potassium listing is optional.

The label must list the first eight nutrients here. Listing the additional nutrients is optional, unless the product makes a special claim involving them.

All food additives must be listed on the label, but sometimes it is impossible to recognize them. MSG, or monosodium glutamate, a flavor enhancer which some people are allergic to, is a source of sodium. It must be listed on the label. But hydrolized vegetable protein, which contains MSG, may be designated as natural flavoring.

BHT is a preservative. It acts as an antioxidant.

With the exception of Yellow No. 5, to which some people are allergic, food colors and flavors do not have to be listed by name.

Despite the fact that this product contains corn and oats and whole wheat, it is an insignificant source of fiber. Complex carbohydrates are important in the diet; sucrose and other sugars provide calories and sweetness.

From *The New York Times*, July 12, 1989, p. B8.

TACTICS AND TIPS

To Protect Yourself from Pesticide Residues . . .

- Thoroughly rinse and scrub fruits and vegetables, with a brush, if possible. Peel them, if appropriate, even though you'll peel away some of the nutrients.
- Remove outer leaves of leafy vegetables, such as lettuce and cabbage.

- Trim fat from meat and poultry and skin (which contains most of the fat) from poultry and fish, and discard fats and oils in broths and pan drippings. Pesticide residues in feed concentrate in the animals' fat. Trim skin and fatty deposits from fish.

- Throw back the big fish—the little ones have less time to take up and concentrate pesticides and other harmful residues.

Adapted from Food and Drug Administration: *Safety first: protecting America's food supply,* p. 26, November 1988.

---

stopped using BHA and BHT and substituted other preservatives, such as vitamin C, citric acid, or vitamin E.

Sulfites protect vegetables from turning brown. Their use has been severely limited by the FDA in the last few years because some people develop allergic reactions after eating foods treated with them. These reactions include difficulty in breathing, wheezing, hives, diarrhea, vomiting, abdominal pain, and dizziness after exposure. As of January 9, 1987, the FDA requires manufacturers to declare the presence of sulfites on labels of packaged foods containing at least 10 parts per million of sulfites. Labels on wine bottles must also have a sulfite warning.

Food irradiation causes "ionizing" radiation by creating ions, or free radicals, in foods. These highly reactive free radicals can destroy cell membranes, break down DNA, and link proteins. The gamma radiation used does not make the food radioactive; however, the energy is strong enough to break chemical bonds. By altering DNA, enzymes, and a variety of proteins, irradiation can prevent the growth of microorganisms, parasites, and insects without creating much heat in the food product. The process is sometimes referred to as "cold sterilization."

Proponents of food irradiation claim that it is a safe and effective means of preservation that extends the shelf life of foods, destroys microorganisms, slows the rapid ripening of harvested produce, and reduces the need for pesticides, some of which are harmful. However, researchers have also shown that irradiation can cause unpleasant flavors, discoloration, and changes in texture. In addition, decreases in thiamin, vitamin A, and vitamin E content of foods have been detected after irradiation. Consumer acceptance of food irradiation in the United States remains very low; nevertheless, the FDA continues to condone it.

Still other additives help in food processing or preparation. They give body and texture to foods, help blend food components, improve baking qualities, control acidity or alkalinity, help retain moisture, and prevent caking or lumping. For example, emulsifiers suspend fat in water, in turn giving a uniform consistency to cakes. Thickeners create smoothness and prevent ice crystals from forming in frozen foods such as ice cream. Leavening agents, such as yeast and baking powder, make baked goods rise by releasing carbon dioxide during the cooking process.

Finally, some additives alter taste and appearance. Products to improve flavor or appearance include coloring agents, natural and synthetic flavors, and flavor enhancers such as monosodium glutamate (MSG) and sweeteners. Some artificial flavors are chemically identical to their natural counterparts, while others such as saccharin are not.

The amount of an additive that can be used in food processing must be kept to the lowest amount needed to do the job and is also limited to $\frac{1}{100}$ to $\frac{1}{1000}$ of the dose that is found safe to administer to animals. If the additive is known to cause cancer in animals, then it generally cannot be intentionally used in foods at all. Thus, although additives such as sulfites, MSG, and the yellow dye tartrazine do cause reactions in sensitive individuals, food additives pose no significant health hazard to most people because the levels used are well below any that could produce toxic effects. Check food labels if you think you are sensitive to MSG or tartrazine. Foods containing these products can always be replaced by others free of the additives.

If you consume a variety of foods in moderation, the chance of suffering negative health consequences from

---

Food irradiation   A sterilizing process used to preserve food by means of ionizing radiation.

To Protect Yourself from Food Poisoning . . .

- Thoroughly wash hands with hot soapy water before and after handling food, especially raw meat, fish, poultry, or eggs, which may contain Salmonella bacteria.
- Don't let groceries sit in a warm car; bacteria will grow in warm temperatures. Get them home to the refrigerator or freezer promptly.
- Don't buy food in containers that leak, bulge, or are severely dented. Deadly botulism food poisoning may be present.
- Make sure counters, cutting boards (use plastic ones), dishes, and other equipment are thoroughly cleaned before and after use, especially if they have come in contact with raw meat, fish, poultry, or eggs.
- Wash fresh fruits and vegetables carefully to remove dirt.
- If possible, use separate cutting boards for meat and for foods that will be eaten raw, such as fruits or vegetables.
- Cook foods thoroughly, especially beef, poultry, fish, pork, and eggs. Cooking kills most microbes.
- Store foods below 40° or above 140° F. Do not leave cooked or refrigerated foods, such as meats or salads, at room temperature for more than two hours.
- Avoid coughing or sneezing over foods, even when you are healthy, and cover any cuts on your hands.
- Use only pasteurized milk.
- Cook stuffing separately from poultry; or wash poultry thoroughly, stuff immediately before cooking, and then transfer the stuffing to a clean bowl immediately after cooking.

food additives is minimal. The same is true of environmental contaminants. The presence of mercury in swordfish may concern you, for example, but it's a health risk only if your diet is dominated by swordfish. The small amount of mercury in most swordfish isn't harmful if you're exposed to it infrequently. Some practical tips for limiting the amount of pesticides in your diet are provided in a nearby box.

The Food Supply: Is It Safe?   Although many people are concerned about additives and environmental contaminants, by far the greatest threat to the safety of the food supply comes from bacteria and other microorganisms that cause food poisoning. Millions of cases of diarrhea are caused each year in the United States by food-borne organisms. Thousands of cases of more severe food poisoning are caused by salmonella-contaminated milk, cheese, poultry, or eggs. Although food poisoning is usually not serious, some groups—such as children and the elderly—are more at risk for severe complications such as rheumatic diseases, seizures, blood poisoning, and other ailments.

It usually isn't possible to tell from taste, smell, or sight that a particular food is unsafe. Your last bout of "flu" may very well have been food poisoning. The symptoms of both are the same: diarrhea, vomiting, fever, and weakness. When food poisoning occurs, the microbe may be causing illness directly, by invading the intestinal wall (as is the case with salmonella poisoning), or indirectly, by producing a toxin that makes you sick (as is the case

with botulism). Because the soil that our food grows in contains billions of bacteria in every square inch (only some of them disease-causing), we are always exposed to the possibility of food poisoning. To decrease the risk of food poisoning when you are handling or preparing food, follow the tips listed in the nearby box.

If you think you may be having a bout of food poisoning, drink plenty of clear fluids to offset the effects of diarrhea and rest in bed to speed recovery. To prevent further contamination, wash your hands often and avoid handling food until the diarrhea disappears. A fever higher than 102° F, blood in the stool, or dehydration deserves a physician's evaluation, especially if the symptoms persist for more than two to three days. In cases of suspected botulism poisoning (primarily from improperly canned foods, especially meats and vegetables), consult a physician immediately because use of an antitoxin may help you recover sooner.

Overall, the American food supply is outstandingly safe, whether you're concerned with additives, pesticides, or bacteria. With reasonable precautions in preparing food and avoiding substances to which you seem to be sensitive, you can be confident that the food supply is not causing you harm. By far the greatest dietary risks to your health come from overconsumption of calories, fat, and sodium.

Who Should Take Vitamin or Mineral Supplements?
Another dietary concern you may have is whether or not to take vitamin or mineral supplements. To answer this

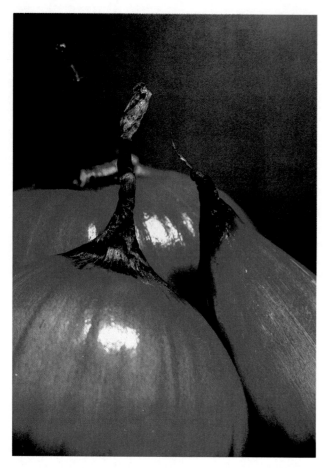

A balanced diet rich in fruits and vegetables helps you get all the fiber, vitamins, and minerals you need without resorting to supplements.

question, first look closely at your diet. Does it follow the Daily Food Guide, especially emphasizing whole grains, low-fat dairy products, leafy and dark-green vegetables, foods containing vitamin C, and a serving of vegetable oils? If so, men are probably meeting their nutrient needs; some women (those with heavy menstrual flows) may still need more iron to compensate for that lost. Secondly, do you regularly consume a fortified breakfast cereal? Most breakfast cereals have extra vitamins and minerals added, some even matching the adult U.S. RDA.

Nutrition scientists generally agree that most people can obtain needed vitamins and minerals from a healthy diet. Improve your diet where needed. After that, consider whether you need a supplement. We advise talking to a registered dietitian and your physician as well, because there is some risk to consuming even standard multivitamin and mineral supplements, not necessarily megadoses. These risks include iron toxicity in individuals genetically prone to a certain liver disease (hemochromatosis) and birth defects during the early months of pregnancy.

Recently a panel of scientists from the American Institute of Nutrition and the American Society for Clinical Nutrition suggested certain cases when vitamin and mineral supplements should be considered.

- Women with excessive bleeding during menses may need iron.
- Women who are pregnant or breastfeeding may need extra iron, folate, and calcium.
- People with very low kcalorie intakes need the range of vitamins and minerals.
- Some vegetarians may need extra calcium, iron, zinc, and vitamin B_{12}.
- Newborns, under the direction of a physician, need a single dose of vitamin K.
- People with certain illnesses or diseases, and those on certain medications, may need supplementation of specific vitamins and minerals at the direction of a physician. Examples include extra potassium when using thiazide diuretics and possibly extra vitamin D for the treatment of osteoporosis.

If you're taking supplements because of an illness or drug therapy, you need to be directed by a physician because some vitamins and minerals counteract the actions of certain medications. Vitamin B_6 can counteract the action of L-dopa (used to treat Parkinson's disease), and high intakes of vitamin E can inhibit vitamin K metabolism and in turn increase the action of anticoagulants (blood thinners) such as warfarin.

If you decide to take a vitamin and mineral supplement, the Council on Scientific Affairs of the American Medical Association recommends a supplement containing between 50–150 percent of the adult U.S. RDA for vitamins. We suggest the same guidelines for minerals. A balanced formulation in a multivitamin and mineral supplement is important because it minimizes the chances of vitamin and mineral competition and therefore an eventual vitamin and mineral imbalance. For instance, a high amount of copper in a supplement can inhibit zinc absorption, and a large amount of folate can mask the symptoms of a vitamin B_{12} deficiency, preventing early diagnosis of that potentially life-threatening disorder.

In sum, most of us can rely on a healthy diet for our nutrient needs. Few people need to resort to regular use of a nutrient supplement, and those who do should do so under professional guidance.

Getting Reliable Nutrition Advice   If you have a question about nutrition, it's probably most convenient to ask a faculty member in the nutrition department on your campus. Local registered dietitians and home economists are also helpful resources, as is your family physician.

Most large communities contain a service called "Dial a Dietitian" where you can phone a registered dietitian and receive nutrition information free of charge.

You should look for the credential "Registered Dietitian (R.D.) when seeking a nutritionist, because these individuals are specially trained to translate nutritional needs into healthful, tasty diets. The R.D. certification is earned only after bachelor's level nutrition training, extensive professional experience, and passing of a comprehensive examination. In many states, people can pass themselves off as dietitians or nutritionists without any training whatsoever; an R.D. credential guarantees that the person has a good nutrition background.

Whenever people need detailed nutrition advice, they usually also require a physician's consultation; a possible exception is moderate weight loss in an otherwise healthy individual. People who find they have high blood cholesterol levels, high blood pressure, or diabetes; feel they suffer from food allergies (sensitivities) or digestive problems; or are beginning to develop osteoporosis should have a careful evaluation by a physician. The presence of one disease is often the result of still another disease, and a physician needs to evaluate the total health of a person to make a proper diagnosis. A complete and accurate diagnosis then allows the registered dietitian to design the proper diet.

Experts on quackery suggest that you steer clear of anyone who says that everyone needs vitamin supplements. In addition, avoid anyone who suggests that most diseases are caused by faulty nutrition or who suggests that large doses of vitamins are effective against many diseases. (See Chapter 22 for a full discussion of quackery.) Individuals who suggest hair analysis as a basis for determining the body's nutritional state should be avoided because hair analysis is not reliable for this purpose. Anyone who uses a computer-scored nutrition deficiency test as the basis for prescribing vitamins should be avoided. And above all, any practitioner—licensed or not—who sells vitamins in his or her office should be thoroughly scrutinized.

Summary

- Choosing foods that provide needed nutrients is an important part of daily life. Food choices made in youth can significantly affect health in the elderly years.

Nutritional Requirements: Components of a Healthy Diet

- The fuel potential in our diet is expressed in kcalories.
- To function at its best, the human body requires about 45 essential nutrients in specific proportions. People get the nutrients needed to fuel their bodies and maintain tissues and organ systems through the foods they eat; the body cannot synthesize most of them.
- Proteins, made up of amino acids, form muscles and bones and help make up blood, enzymes, hormones, and cell membranes. Foods from animal sources provide complete proteins; plants provide imcomplete proteins, but combinations yield complete proteins. The American diet is rich in protein, which should constitute about 15 percent of the total kcalorie intake.
- Fats, a concentrated source of energy, also help insulate the body and cushion the organs; 1 tablespoon of vegetable oil per day supplies essential fats. Dietary intake should be limited to 30 percent of total kcalories. Americans need to reduce consumption of saturated fats and replace them in part with fish oils, which have health benefits.
- Carbohydrates supply energy to the brain and other parts of the nervous system as well as to red blood cells. The body needs 50–100 grams of carbohydrates a day; much more is usually consumed. During digestion, carbohydrates are broken down into glucose for energy; some is stored as glycogen.
- Dietary fiber includes plant substances difficult or impossible for humans to digest. Insoluble fibers like wheat bran hold water and increases bulk in the stool; they may prevent rectal and colon cancer. Soluble fibers like oat bran bind cholesterol-containing compounds in the intestine and slow glucose absorption; they may help lower elevated serum cholesterol and blood glucose levels.
- The thirteen vitamins needed in the diet are organic substances that promote specific chemical reactions within living cells. Deficiencies can cause serious illnesses and even death.
- The seventeen minerals needed in the diet are inorganic substances that regulate body functions, aid in growth and maintenance of body tissues, and act as catalysts for release of energy. The minerals most commonly lacking in the diet are iron, calcium, and zinc.

Nutritional Guidelines: Planning Your Diet

- Various scientific and governmental groups have established nutrition guidelines for preventing nutrient deficiencies, for providing balanced nutrient intake, and for preventing specific diseases.

- Recommended Dietary Allowances (RDAs) are recommended intakes for essential nutrients that meet the needs of healthy persons. They are a guide to foods, not to supplements, and are averages for groups.
- The Daily Food Guide contains five food groups; choosing foods from each every day helps insure appropriate amounts of necessary nutrients. The fundamental principles of the Daily Food Guide are moderation, variety, and balance.
- The Dietary Guidelines for Americans address prevention of diet-related diseases like cardiovascular disease, cancer, and diabetes. The guidelines advise: (1) eat a variety of foods, (2) maintain desirable weight, (3) avoid too much fat, (4) eat adequate starch and fiber, (5) avoid too much sugar, (6) avoid too much sodium, and (7) drink alcohol in moderation, if at all.
- Although not all nutritionists agree with all the Dietary Guidelines and some feel they should be individualized, most agree that variety, weight control, fat reduction, increased carbohydrate/fiber intake, and restricted alcohol intake are important.
- A vegetarian diet can meet human nutritional needs. Although including dairy products makes diet planning easier, a vegan can meet all needs through careful planning and a wide variety of foods.

A Personal Plan: Making Intelligent Choices about Food

- No single diet provides wellness for everyone; people should focus on the likely causes of health problems in their lives and make dietary changes to address them.
- Food labels express nutrient quantities as percentage of U.S. RDA and provide ingredients in descending order based on weight.
- Food additives maintain or improve nutritional quality, maintain freshness, help in processing, and alter taste or appearance. They make up less than 1 percent of our food; the chance of suffering negative health consequences is minimal.
- Food poisoning from food-borne organisms is a greater threat to health than are additives and environmental contaminants; many cases of "flu" are probably actually food poisoning. Specific precautions in handling and preparing food can help prevent food poisoning.
- Most people don't need vitamin and mineral supplements. Those who do include pregnant and breastfeeding women, vegetarians, and people who are ill or taking certain medications.
- Reliable nutritional advice can be obtained from registered dietitians; some people will also need consultation with a physician.

Take Action

1. In your health diary or a notebook, keep track of everything you eat and drink for three or four days. Then see how well your average daily intake meets the guidelines in the Daily Food Guide.

2. Buy an inexpensive cookbook or nutrition paperback that contains a table detailing the nutrient composition of common foods. Using the U.S. RDA table in this chapter, write down the amount of each essential nutrient required by someone in your age group (calories, protein, vitamin A, iron, and so on).

Then, using the table of nutrient composition, calculate the nutrient value of the foods you recorded for three or four days in your health diary. Compare the amounts you actually consumed with your requirements. Finally, put together a few days' worth of meals that satisfy your nutritional requirements without exceeding them by too much, being sure to use foods you really like. Try following this diet for a while. Use the book you bought when you want to evaluate other foods in your diet.

3. Read the list of ingredients on three or four canned or packaged foods that you enjoy eating. If any ingredients are unfamiliar to you, find out what they are and why they have been used.

4. Find out what kind of nutritional and dietary guidelines are used to prepare the food served in your school. Are they consistent with what you've learned in this chapter? If not, try to find out more about the guidelines that have been used and why they were chosen.

Behavior Change Strategy

Improving Your Diet

If you want to alter your diet, some of the major health behavior change strategies we have already examined can help you. Here are some suggestions for behavior management that you can use to lower your fat consumption, raise your fiber intake, or make other changes in your diet.

Establishing a Baseline

Let's say that you want to do two things to your diet: (1) cut out all candy while walking between classes or while on errands in town and (2) eat more fresh fruits and raw vegetables.

Begin by keeping track of your candy consumption. In a diary jot down the time of day and what occurred before and after you ate the candy. On a chart such as the one shown here, keep track of the number of candy eating events. Because you also want to add more fruits and vegetables to your diet, also keep notes on the kinds of foods you have been eating at meals. You can include this information on the same chart that you are already using (on the right-hand vertical axis), or you can simply keep two graphs.

Intervention

Once you have established your baseline levels, begin to make some changes in those routines that seem to precede your eating candy. For example, you might find that you have been eating candy from a vending machine that you walk by every day after class. If this is the case, try another route that allows you to avoid the machine. If you find that you usually are hungry at one particular time of day and that you rarely have lunch or a healthful snack with you, try to

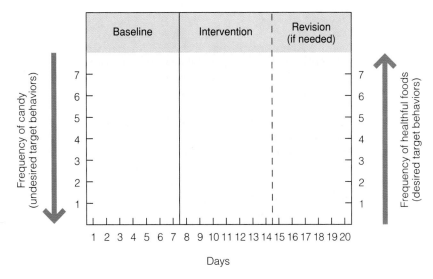

keep a healthful snack on hand so that you won't be caught off guard and be pushed toward eating candy (which always seems to be available). Putting fresh or dried fruit in a backpack or pocket every morning can help. You can use the same sort of strategy to increase the number of fruits and vegetables in your diet: specifically, you will need to shop for these food items *in advance* and prepare them *ahead of time* so that they are readily available.

Revision (If Needed)

You may discover that your initial plan works perfectly or that it works well for three weeks but then loses its effectiveness. Watch out for programs that become stale and lose their strength, and, of course, revise an ineffective program entirely once you have given it a real try. The critical data from your diary can help you to decide how to revise your program. Plotting the data on a prominently displayed chart can encourage you to continue.

Social Eating Events

Avoiding an attractive candy vending machine may be a lot easier than cutting back on late-night pizza

binges; the former involves only you while the latter involves you and your friends. It's harder to make adjustments in social eating patterns, but there are some strategies that you can try. First, tell your friends that you would prefer to try something new to eat instead of pizza, such as popcorn. Being assertive in such matters can be very helpful; you may discover some allies who share your views about the type of food you want to eat. Second, try to cut down on these group activities without eliminating them entirely. Of course, you can try to change or limit the kinds of food you eat at these times, but it's generally very difficult to refrain from joining in once you're actually in the social situation.

Systematic Changes in Other Habits

Many people take up sports activities or begin to increase their routine activity levels (walks after meals, etc.) at the same time that they try to adjust their diet. While it isn't a good idea to try to make too many significant changes at one time, you may want to experiment with other changes while you're making adjustments in your diet.

Selected Bibliography

Albin, R. L., and others. 1987. Acute sensory neuropathy from pyridoxine overdose. *Neurology* 37:17.

Block, G., and others. 1985. Nutrient sources in the American diet: Quantitative data from the NHANES II survey. *American Journal of Epidemiology,* 122:13.

Council on Scientific Affairs. 1987. Vitamin preparations as dietary supplements and as therapeutic agents. *Journal of the American Medical Association* 257:1929.

Davies, L. 1988. Practical nutrition for the elderly. *Nutrition Reviews* 46:83.

Fishman, J. A. 1988. Control of hypertension through life-style and nutrition. *Topics in Clinical Nutrition* 3:47.

Lanza, E., and others. 1987. Dietary fiber intake in the U.S. population. *American Journal of Clinical Nutrition* 46:790.

Olson, J. A., and Hodges, R. E. 1987. Recommended dietary intakes (RDI) of vitamin C in humans. *American Journal of Clinical Nutrition* 45:693.

Recker, R. R., and others. 1988. Calcium absorpability from milk products and imitation milk and calcium carbonate. *American Journal of Clinical Nutrition* 47:93.

Stegink, L. D. 1987. The aspartame story: A model for the clinical testing of a food additive. *American Journal of Clinical Nutrition* 46:204.

Wardlaw, G. M. 1988. The effect of diet and life-style on bone mass in women. *Journal of the American Dietetic Association* 88:17.

Recommended Readings

Committee on Diet and Health, National Research Council, 1989. *Diet and Health,* Washington, D.C.: National Academy Press. *A well-referenced review of nutrition and its relationship to chronic diseases, such as heart disease and cancer.*

Robertson, L., Carol Flinders, and Bronwen Godfrey, 1976. *Laurel's Kitchen.* Petaluma, CA: Nilgiri Press. *The classic on vegetarian cooking and nutrition, with solid nutritional information and innovative recipes.*

U.S. Department of Health and Human Services—Public Health Service, 1988. *The Surgeon General's Report on Nutrition and Health.* Washington, D.C.: U.S. Government Printing Office. *A comprehensive guide to the role of nutrition in disease prevention.*

Wardlaw, G. M., and Insel, P. M., 1990. *Perspectives in Nutrition.* St. Louis: Mosby. *An easy-to-understand review of major concepts in nutrition—from infancy to elderly years.*

Yetiv, J., 1986. *Popular Nutrition Practices: A Scientific Appraisal.* Toledo, Ohio: Popular Medicine Press. *A thoroughly referenced analysis of more than 100 topics of contemporary interest.*

Appendix
The Facts about Fast Food

	SERVING SIZE	CALORIES	PROTEIN	CARBOHYDRATES	FAT: TOTAL	POLYUNSATURATED FAT	MONOUNSATURATED FAT AND SATURATED FAT	CHOLESTEROL	SODIUM	POTASSIUM	PHOSPHORUS	VITAMIN A	VITAMIN C	THIAMINE	RIBOFLAVIN	NIACIN	CALCIUM	IRON	ZINC	FAT/KCAL %
	grams		grams	grams	grams	grams	grams	mg	mg	mg					% U.S. RDA					
Kentucky Fried Chicken																				
per piece:	Original Recipe																			
Center breast	115	283	27.5	8.8	15.3	1.97	3.84	92.5	672	N/A	N/A	*	*	6.13	10.15	57.5	3.61	5.37	N/A	49
Wing	55	178	12.2	6.0	11.7	1.76	2.99	64.0	372	N/A	N/A	*	*	*	4.86	18.51	4.79	6.83	N/A	59
Drumstick	57	146	13.1	4.2	8.5	1.26	2.19	67.0	275	N/A	N/A	*	*	3.06	7.09	16.19	2.12	5.87	N/A	52
per piece:	Extra Crispy Recipe																			
Center breast	120	353	26.9	14.4	20.9	2.02	5.27	93.0	842	N/A	N/A	*	*	6.4	9.18	50.4	3.49	4.8	N/A	53
Wing	57	218	11.5	7.81	15.6	1.82	4.04	63.0	437	N/A	N/A	*	*	2.28	4.36	14.25	2.14	2.88	N/A	64
Drumstick	60	173	12.7	5.9	10.9	1.27	2.75	65.0	346	N/A	N/A	*	*	3.2	8.47	14.10	*	3.37	N/A	57
"Chicken Littles" sandwich	47	169	5.7	13.8	10.1	3.44	2.0	17.6	331	N/A	N/A	*	*	10.92	6.88	10.93	2.26	9.62	N/A	54
Biscuit (1)	66	232	4.2	27.1	11.9	1.91	2.88	1.1	539	N/A	N/A	*	*	19.21	13.1	13	8.25	10.15	N/A	46
Mashed potatoes and gravy	98	71	2.42	11.86	1.61	.16	.45	<1.0	342	N/A	N/A	*	*	*	2.44	5.94	2.2	2.26	N/A	20
Regular french fries	77	244	3.2	31.1	11.9	.66	2.61	1.6	139	N/A	N/A	*	26.15	9.74	2.71	9.92	*	3.42	N/A	44
Corn-on-the-cob	143	176	5.1	31.9	3.1	1.46	.5	<1.0	<21	N/A	N/A	5.43	3.81	9.53	6.64	9.30	*	4.37	N/A	16
Cole slaw	91	119	1.5	13.25	6.57	3.36	.96	4.61	197	N/A	N/A	6.19	35.94	2.43	*	*	3.28	*	N/A	50

* Contains less than 2% of the U.S. RDA of these nutrients.
N/A — not available

	SERVING SIZE	CALORIES	PROTEIN	CARBOHYDRATES	FAT: TOTAL	POLYUNSATURATED FAT	MONOUNSATURATED FAT	SATURATED FAT	CHOLESTEROL	SODIUM	POTASSIUM	PHOSPHORUS	VITAMIN A	VITAMIN C	THIAMINE	RIBOFLAVIN	NIACIN	CALCIUM	IRON	ZINC	FAT/KCAL %
	grams		grams	grams	grams	grams	grams	grams	mg	mg	mg					% U.S. RDA					
Wendy's																					
Wendy's Big Classic	270	580	24	47	34	N/A	N/A	N/A	80	1015	580	N/A	20	25	30	25	30	15	30	N/A	53
Small hamburger	106	260	13	31	9	N/A	N/A	N/A	30	510	210	N/A	2	4	25	15	20	10	15	N/A	31
Small cheeseburger	124	320	17	31	15	N/A	N/A	N/A	50	805	210	N/A	2	4	25	80	20	10	15	N/A	42
Chicken Sandwich	219	430	26	41	19	N/A	N/A	N/A	60	705	460	N/A	10	15	30	20	70	10	80	N/A	40
Single cheeseburger with everything	245	490	26	36	28	N/A	N/A	N/A	85	1100	485	N/A	15	25	30	90	30	10	25	N/A	51
Single hamburger with everything	227	430	22	36	22	N/A	N/A	N/A	70	805	485	N/A	15	25	30	20	30	10	25	N/A	46
Bacon Swiss Burger	261	710	37	58	44	N/A	N/A	N/A	90	1390	560	N/A	15	30	40	25	40	15	30	N/A	56
Philly Swiss Burger	201	510	30	46	24	N/A	N/A	N/A	65	975	360	N/A	*	10	30	20	30	10	25	N/A	42
Chef salad	331	180	15	10	9	N/A	N/A	N/A	120	140	590	N/A	110	110	15	25	6	25	15	N/A	45
Chili	256	230	21	16	9	N/A	N/A	N/A	50	960	565	N/A	20	15	8	10	15	6	25	N/A	35
Bacon/cheese Potato	350	570	19	57	30	N/A	N/A	N/A	22	1180	1380	N/A	15	60	15	10	15	20	15	N/A	47
Chili/cheese Potato	400	510	22	63	20	N/A	N/A	N/A	22	610	1590	N/A	15	60	20	15	20	25	20	N/A	35
Crispy Chicken Nuggets	93	310	15	14	21	N/A	N/A	N/A	50	660	230	N/A	*	*	10	8	45	2	6	N/A	61
French fries	106	310	4	38	15	N/A	N/A	N/A	15	105	675	N/A	*	20	10	2	15	*	6	N/A	44
Frosty dairy dessert	243	400	8	59	14	N/A	N/A	N/A	50	220	585	N/A	10	*	8	30	*	30	6	N/A	32

* Contains less than 2% of the U.S. RDA of these nutrients.
N/A — not available

	SERVING SIZE	CALORIES	PROTEIN	CARBOHYDRATES	FAT: TOTAL	POLYUNSATURATED FAT	MONOUNSATURATED FAT	SATURATED FAT	CHOLESTEROL	SODIUM	POTASSIUM	PHOSPHORUS	VITAMIN A	VITAMIN C	THIAMINE	RIBOFLAVIN	NIACIN	CALCIUM	IRON	ZINC	FAT/KCAL %
	grams		grams	grams	grams	grams	grams	grams	mg	mg	mg					% U.S. RDA					
Jack in the Box																					
Dbl. cheeseburger	149	467	21	33	27	3.1	11.6	12.3	72	842	N/A	N/A	8	*	10	20	30	40	15	N/A	52
Jumbo Jack®	222	584	26	42	34	8	13	11	73	733	N/A	N/A	*	*	24	17	9	14	17	N/A	52
Bacon cheeseburger	230	705	35	48	39	7	15	15	85	1127	N/A	N/A	*	*	32	31	15	28	22	N/A	50
Gr. sourdough burger	223	712	32	34	50	7.9	17.8	15.9	109	1140	N/A	N/A	14	*	43	28	40	19	24	N/A	63
Swiss and bacon burger	187	678	31	34	47	7	18	20	92	1458	N/A	N/A	*	*	17	20	17	22	12	N/A	62
Chicken Fajita Pita	189	292	24	29	8	1.4	3.6	2.9	34	903	N/A	N/A	10	*	50	10	30	25	15	N/A	25
Chicken Supreme	231	575	27	34	36	7.6	13.4	14.3	62	1525	N/A	N/A	*	*	20	8	60	10	20	N/A	56
Fish Supreme	228	554	20	47	32	7.4	11.0	13.5	66	1047	N/A	N/A	30	*	10	15	25	45	15	N/A	52
Egg roll (each)	57	135	5	14	6.3	2.7	.6	2.4	10	301	N/A	N/A	3.3	2.6	5	3.3	5	1.6	5	N/A	42
Chicken strip (each)	31.25	87.25	7.25	7	3.5	.2	1.5	3.5	17	187	N/A	N/A	3.75	*	1	2	2.5	2.5	2	N/A	36
Taquito (each)	28	72	3.2	8	3.2	.5	1.12	1.12	7.4	93.4	N/A	N/A	*	*	.8	1	2.2	3.4	3.6	N/A	40
Reg. french fries	109	353	3	43	19	2.7	7.8	7.9	13	262	N/A	N/A	*	8	8	3	9	*	5	N/A	48
Onion rings	108	382	5	39	23	1.3	9.3	11.1	27	407	N/A	N/A	*	5	14	7	9	3	8	N/A	54
Chocolate shake	332	330	11	55	7	<1.0	2.1	4.3	25	270	N/A	N/A	*	*	10	35	2	35	4	N/A	19
Chef salad	332	325	30	10	18	1.3	5.2	8.4	142	900	N/A	N/A	73	46	29	27	30	44	8	N/A	50

* Contains less than 2% of the U.S. RDA of these nutrients.
N/A — not available

	SERVING SIZE	CALORIES	PROTEIN	CARBOHYDRATES	FAT: TOTAL	POLYUNSATURATED FAT	MONOUNSATURATED FAT	SATURATED FAT	CHOLESTEROL	SODIUM	POTASSIUM	PHOSPHORUS	VITAMIN A	VITAMIN C	THIAMINE	RIBOFLAVIN	NIACIN	CALCIUM	IRON	ZINC	FAT/KCAL %
	grams		grams	grams	grams	grams	grams	grams	mg	mg	mg					% U.S. RDA					
Arby's																					
Arby's regular roast beef	147	353	22.2	31.6	14.8	2.4	5.1	7.3	39	588	368	N/A	*	2	15	25	35	8	20	25	38
Beef-n-cheddar	197	455	25.7	27.7	26.8	7.1	12.1	7.6	63	955	335	N/A	8	*	25	30	40	6	20	25	53
Chicken breast sandwich	184	493	23.0	47.9	25	10.3	9.6	5.1	91	1019	330	N/A	*	8	15	30	40	8	20	10	46
Roast chicken club	234	610	31.0	40.0	33	14	11	8	80	1500	430	N/A	*	*	35	35	45	15	20	15	49
Turkey deluxe	197	375	23.8	32.5	16.6	7.8	4.7	4.1	39	1047	346	N/A	6	8	15	25	60	8	15	10	40
Ham-n-cheese	156	292	22.9	19.2	13.7	2.7	6.3	4.7	45	1350	312	N/A	5	*	10	15	30	20	15	6	42
Super roast beef	234	501	25.1	50.4	22.1	5.4	8.2	8.5	40	798	503	N/A	15	60	25	35	45	10	25	25	40
French fries	71	246	2.1	29.8	13.2	4.7	5.5	3.0	0	114	240	N/A	*	*	4	*	10	*	6	*	48
Potato cakes	85	204	1.8	19.8	12.0	4.3	5.5	2.2	0	397	289	N/A	*	35	4	*	8	*	8	*	53
Jamocha shake	326	368	9.3	59.1	10.5	1.6	6.4	2.5	35	262	525	N/A	6	4	4	45	25	25	15	10	26
Burger King																					
Hamburger		275	15	29	12	7	7	5	37	509	235	12	3	5	16	15	20	4	16	N/A	39
Cheeseburger		312	17	30	15	8	8	7	48	651	247	19	7	5	16	17	20	10	16	N/A	43
Whopper w/cheese		711	32	47	43	26	26	17	113	1164	568	36	21	19	25	29	35	21	28	N/A	54
Bacon double cheeseburger		510	33	27	31	16	16	15	104	728	363	33	8	*	20	25	31	17	21	N/A	55
Whaler fish sandwich		488	19	45	27	21	21	6	77	592	369	25	1	*	18	12	20	5	9	N/A	50
French fries		227	3	24	13	6	6	7	14	160	360	11	*	N/A	7	2	11	*	7	N/A	52
Onion rings		274	4	28	16	13	13	3	0	665	173	20	*	*	*	*	*	12	7	N/A	53
Chicken Tenders		204	20	10	10	8	8	2	47	636	200	24	2	*	5	5	35	2	7	N/A	44
Choc. shake		374	8	60	11	N/A	N/A	N/A	N/A	225	590	26	*	*	8	30	*	25	9	N/A	26
Chef salad		180	17	7	9	N/A	N/A	N/A	120	570	550	26	100	23	19	13	20	16	9	N/A	45
Garden salad		90	6	7	5	2	2	3	15	125	440	13	100	60	4	6	6	15	7	N/A	50

* Contains less than 2% of the U.S. RDA of these nutrients.

N/A — not available

	SERVING SIZE	CALORIES	PROTEIN	CARBOHYDRATES	FAT: TOTAL	POLYUNSATURATED FAT	MONOUNSATURATED FAT	SATURATED FAT	CHOLESTEROL	SODIUM	POTASSIUM	PHOSPHORUS	VITAMIN A	VITAMIN C	THIAMINE	RIBOFLAVIN	NIACIN	CALCIUM	IRON	ZINC	FAT/KCAL %
	grams		grams	grams	grams	grams	grams	grams	mg	mg	mg					% U.S. RDA					
McDonald's																					
Egg McMuffin	138	290	18.2	28.1	11.2	1.29	6.2	3.82	226	740	N/A	N/A	10	0	30	20	20	25	15	N/A	35
Cheeseburger	116	310	15	31.2	13.8	.93	7.66	5.17	53	750	N/A	N/A	8	4	20	15	20	20	15	N/A	40
Quarter Pounder w/cheese	194	520	28.5	35.1	29.2	1.51	16.5	11.18	118	1150	N/A	N/A	15	6	25	20	35	30	20	N/A	50
Big Mac	215	560	25.2	42.5	32.4	1.5	20.9	10.05	103	950	N/A	N/A	8	2	30	25	35	25	20	N/A	52
Filet-O-Fish	142	440	13.8	37.9	26.1	10.76	10.22	5.16	50	1030	N/A	N/A	2	*	20	8	15	15	10	N/A	53
McDLT	234	580	26.3	36	36.8	8.5	16.7	11.5	109	990	N/A	N/A	15	10	25	20	35	25	20	N/A	57
McChicken	190	490	19.2	39.8	28.6	11.6	11.5	5.4	426	780	N/A	N/A	2	4	60	15	45	15	15	N/A	53
Med. fries	97	320	4.4	36.3	17.1	.7	9.21	7.17	12	150	N/A	N/A	*	20	15	*	15	*	4	N/A	48
Choc. shake	304	390	11	62.6	10.6	.37	5.06	5.13	41	240	N/A	N/A	6	*	8	30	2	35	4	N/A	24
Chef salad	283	230	20.5	7.5	13.3	.91	6.52	5.91	128	490	N/A	N/A	80	20	20	20	20	25	8	N/A	52
Garden salad	213	110	7.1	6.2	6.6	.53	3.16	2.90	83	160	N/A	N/A	80	20	6	10	2	15	6	N/A	54

* Contains less than 2% of the U.S. RDA of these nutrients.
N/A — not available

Contents

Making Connections

If you're like most people, you'll probably gain weight as you get older, and that weight will be a burden on your health as the years go by. Maintaining your ideal weight will require conscious effort and informed, sensible lifestyle choices. The scenarios presented on these pages describe situations in which people have to use information, make a decision, or choose a course of action, all relating to weight management. As you read them, imagine yourself in each situation and consider what you would do. After you've finished the chapter, read the scenarios again and see if what you've learned has changed how you would think, feel, or act in each situation.

Your brother has been dating a woman who talks about her diet all the time, even though she doesn't appear to you to be overweight. She skips a lot of meals to keep her weight under control, but periodically she goes off her diet in a big way. You've even seen her eat a whole small pizza by herself at one sitting. Recently, your brother told you he thought she had some kind of eating problem but he didn't know what it was. He asked if you had any clues. Do you?

You and your roommate have both gained a little weight and have decided to watch your diets. When you go to the cafeteria, she thinks you should get the Vegetarian Fiesta Delight—pinto beans, corn tortillas, spicy rice, and salsa. You think that's too starchy. You vote for broiled pork chops with gravy and a salad, because it's high in protein and low in carbohydrates. Which would be the better choice?

13
Weight Control

One of your friends is extremely overweight—you'd guess by at least 50 pounds—but he doesn't seem to be interested in doing anything about it. He says everyone in his family has the same basic body shape and is just naturally very large, so there's no point in his trying to lose weight. And, in fact, when you see a picture of his parents and younger brother, you note that they're even heavier than he is. Is it true that his weight problem is genetic, and is there anything he can do about it?

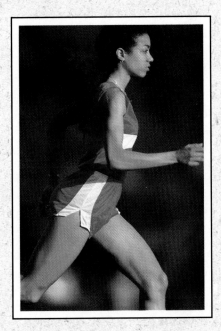

Your roommate is driving you crazy—she eats whatever she wants and never gains any weight, while you watch every bite and are just barely able to maintain the weight you want. She says her secret is walking and riding her bike everywhere she goes, but you're skeptical that it could make that much difference. She suggests you stop taking the bus for a month and see what happens. Was she just born to be skinny? Should you give her idea a try?

You're curious about a "safe and easy" weight loss program you've heard advertised on the radio. In this program, you follow an individualized plan that's drawn up for you by a health counselor, eat the prepackaged foods sold by the program, and take vitamin, mineral, and amino acid supplements. The program guarantees that you'll lose 30 pounds in six weeks. It's expensive, but it sounds too good to pass up. Should you give it a try?

There *is* a "secret" to weight control: Maintain a moderate level of total **kcalories**, minimize fat kcalories, and get lots of exercise. Unfortunately, this simple formula is not so exciting as the latest fad diet or the "scientific breakthrough" that promises slimness without effort. If only kcalories didn't count or a beautifully proportioned body could be had with only a few minutes a day of exercise, then the continuing stream of diet books, special programs, dietary supplements, and medical procedures for weight loss that assault the American public year after year might disappear. Obesity would not be the public health problem or the personal agony that it is for so many. Fad diets and promises of being able to get something for nothing are the fool's gold of weight control.

Yet more and more Americans are going on diets. At any given time, more than one-third of the American public is engaged in dieting behavior. Research shows that many girls start dieting during adolescence and that the rate of dieting reaches 60 percent or more during the college years. Males too are getting caught up in the dieting craze. Furthermore, this bad habit is taking hold at younger and younger ages; many have started dieting in high school or even grade school. Twenty-two percent of tenth-grade girls reported frequent dieting, and another 10 percent engaged in fasts. Unfortunately, such behavior can undermine the development of a truly healthy lifestyle that will naturally and easily allow someone to maintain an appropriate body weight.

Dieting can lead to difficulties in managing weight. Restricting kcalories lowers metabolism and makes the body more efficient at storing energy from food as body fat. Dieting puts the emphasis on food, instead of on the combination of balancing kcalories consumed and kcalories expended through physical activity. Restrained eaters worry excessively about weight, food, and eating. The slightest infraction of self-imposed dieting rules can result in guilt, anxiety, self-blame, and periodic abandonment of efforts to eat in a healthy way. Dieting is not a desirable component of a healthy lifestyle, nor does it make weight control easier.

Lifestyle and Weight Control

At the turn of the century, Americans consumed a diet very different from that of the 1990s, and they got lots more exercise. Our grandparents and great-grandparents ate many more complex carbohydrates, especially bread, potatoes, pasta, rice, beans, and legumes, along with fresh vegetables and whole grains. They also ate fewer simple or refined carbohydrates (sugars) and less fat. Americans today actually eat somewhat *fewer* kcalories overall (down about 3 percent), but they eat more fat (up by 31 percent) and more refined sugars (up 50 percent). In large part this change reflects the trend toward more processed foods and away from fresh, unprocessed foods and especially complex carbohydrates.

Despite the increased interest in exercise and jogging during recent years, Americans today get far less exercise than did their great-grandparents. In earlier times, people walked or rode bicycles more often than they drove. Most worked on farms or did manual labor. They were able to eat more and weigh less because they didn't have the dubious benefits of labor-saving devices. Today, not only do most occupations require less vigorous physical activity, but they also tend to give rise to stress. Alcohol and food are often the quickest and easiest means of relieving such stress. Eating refined sugar, usually in the form of candy, ice cream, cookies, and pastries, is a favorite way of coping with stress. Simple sugars together with fats make up over 50 percent of all kcalories consumed in the 1990s, compared to less than 25 percent in 1900.

People from other countries often deplore the prevalence of obesity in this country. Americans can afford to eat more meat than can people in the rest of the world, who still consume mostly complex carbohydrates. Gasoline here is cheap in comparison to its cost elsewhere, and most Americans view automobiles as a necessity. American cities are not particularly safe for walking or riding bicycles, which are still the primary means of transportation for most people in the world. The typical American lifestyle does not naturally promote healthy eating or adequate exercise. No wonder so many have such difficulty maintaining a good weight, and no wonder dieting has practically become an American institution.

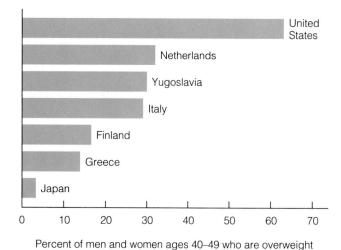

Percent of men and women ages 40–49 who are overweight

VITAL STATISTICS

Figure 13-1 Degree of overweight in people aged 40–49 in population samples of seven countries.

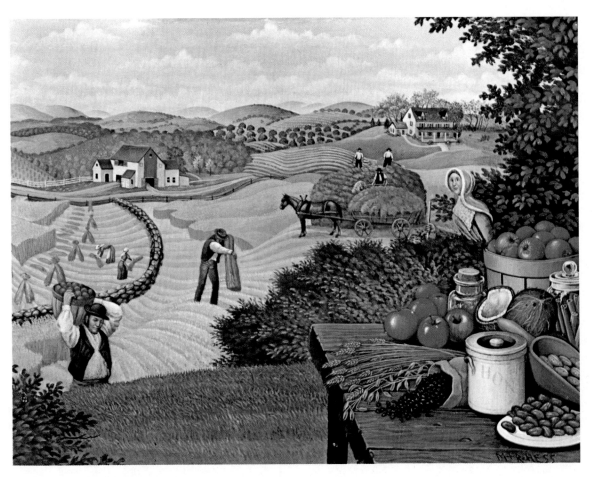

Working hard all day on the farm and eating whole foods gave our great-grandparents a health advantage we lack today. A great part of the American weight problem can be traced to sedentary habits and overrefined foods.

Even though more children and adolescents are developing weight problems than ever before, most young people arrive at early adulthood with the advantage of having a "normal" body weight (that is, neither too fat nor too lean). In fact, many young adults get away with terrible eating and exercise habits and don't develop a weight problem. Yet! As the rapid growth period of adolescence slows and the steady state of growth maintenance takes over in adulthood, however, adopting a healthy lifestyle is necessary to maintain normal weight without undue effort. As family and career obligations increase and less time and perhaps motivation are available for other things, living a healthy lifestyle becomes a greater and greater challenge. The time to develop such a lifestyle is early in adulthood, when good habits and behavior patterns have a better chance of taking a firm hold.

Adopting a Healthy Lifestyle

Four factors are crucial to the kind of lifestyle that will naturally yield a good body weight: what goes into your mouth, what you do with your body, what goes on in your head, and how you cope with life. In other words,

Kilocalorie (kcalorie)   A measure of the energy the body gets from food or uses in exercise. Technically, it is the energy used to raise 1 liter of water 1° C.

Eating Smart—Little Things Add Up

It's easier to incorporate small switches and substitutions in your eating habits than to initiate radical changes. These simple suggestions for a more healthful diet can reduce your fats and calorie intake considerably while still satisfying your appetite. To put these numbers in perspective, if you consume 2,000 calories a day, you should eat no more than about 66 grams of fat—that way fat will contribute less than 30% of your daily kcalories.

Instead of Eating	Substitute	To Save*
1 croissant	1 plain bagel	35 kcalories, 10 grams fat
1 whole egg	1 egg white	65 kcalories, 6 grams fat
1 oz. cheddar cheese	1 oz. part-skim mozzarella	35 kcalories, 4 grams fat
1 oz. cream cheese	1 oz. cottage cheese (1% fat)	74 kcalories, 9 grams fat
1 T whipping cream	1 T evaporated skim milk, whipped	32 kcalories, 5 grams fat
3.5 oz. skinless roast duck	3.5 oz. skinless roast chicken	46 kcalories, 7 grams fat
3.5 oz. beef tenderloin, choice, untrimmed, broiled	3.5 oz. beef tenderloin, select, trimmed broiled	75 kcalories, 10 grams fat
3.5 oz. lamb chop, untrimmed, broiled	3.5 oz. lean leg of lamb, trimmed, broiled	219 kcalories, 28 grams fat
3.5 oz. pork spare ribs, cooked	3.5 oz. lean pork loin, trimmed, broiled	157 kcalories, 17 grams fat
1 oz. regular bacon, cooked	1 oz. Canadian bacon, cooked	111 kcalories, 12 grams fat
1 oz. hard salami	1 oz. extra-lean roasted ham	75 kcalories, 8 grams fat
1 beef frankfurter	1 chicken frankfurter	67 kcalories, 8 grams fat
3 oz. oil-packed tuna, light	3 oz. water-packed tuna, light	60 kcalories, 6 grams fat
1 regular-size serving fast-food French fries	1 medium-size baked potato	125 kcalories, 11 grams fat
1 oz. oil-roasted peanuts	1 oz. roasted chestnuts	96 kcalories, 13 grams fat
1 oz. potato chips	1 oz. thin pretzels	40 kcalories, 9 grams fat
1 oz. corn chips	1 oz. plain air-popped popcorn	125 kcalories, 9 grams fat
1 T sour-cream dip	1 T bottled salsa	20 kcalories, 3 grams fat
1 glazed doughnut	1 slice angel-food cake	110 kcalories, 13 grams fat
3 chocolate sandwich cookies	3 fig bar cookies	4 grams fat
1 oz. unsweetened chocolate	3 T cocoa powder	73 kcalories, 13 grams fat
1 cup ice cream (premium)	1 cup sorbet	320 kcalories, 34 grams fat

*The values listed are the most significant savings; smaller differences are not shown. Weights given for meats are edible portions.
Reprinted permission of: University of California, *Berkeley Wellness Letter*, P.O. Box 10922, Des Moines, IA 50340

nutrition, physical activity, thinking and emotions, and habits and behavior patterns are the keys to successful maintenance of normal weight. These four factors are discussed in detail in this section.

Nutrition　Too often nutrition is a topic studied in a class on health, and too seldom does it become personally relevant to most people's lives. Knowing about nutrients and a balanced diet may help, but actually making healthy food choices day to day is what really counts.

What goes into your mouth directly affects health and body weight. In particular, refined sugars and too much dietary fat undermine good health in the long run, whereas eating more complex carbohydrates and keeping total kcalories at a moderate level produces a healthy body weight with little effort.

Sugar　Some people equate sugar with fatness, even though there is no evidence that fat people consume

Table 13-1 Calories, sources, and recommendations for food components

Food Component	Kilocalories per gram	Principal Sources	Recommended Intake of Total Calories

Protein
    Complete
    Incomplete
	4	Poultry, fish, meat, cheese, eggs, milk and milk products, tofu, legumes	15%

Carbohydrate
    Complex
    Simple
	4	Vegetables, dried beans, peas, whole grains, pasta, bread, cereal, starches, fruit, sugar, honey, molasses, syrups	55%

Fat
    Monounsaturated
    Polyunsaturated
    Saturated
	9	Vegetable oils, butter, margarine, salad dressings, nuts, coconut, lard, cream, cream cheese	<30% (10% for each of the three types)

more sugar than thin people. Sugar is a health problem primarily because it causes tooth decay. Still, for some who are trying to maintain a good body weight, sugar can be a problem. Sugar is a major component of many favorite foods in the American diet. Ice cream, for example, is 63 percent sugar, 27 percent fat, and only 10 percent protein. An ounce of milk chocolate is 59 percent sugar, 33 percent fat, and 8 percent protein. Under such names as corn syrup, corn sweetener, honey, molasses, fructose, sucrose, and dextrose, sugar is added to processed foods such as breads, crackers, cereals, sauces, salad dressings, fruit-flavored yogurt, soft drinks, pastries and baked goods, and bacon and cured meats.

Some people believe sugar to be addictive. In fact, carbohydrate in the diet increases the levels of **serotonin**, a neurotransmitter in the brain, and is associated with a calming, even sedative, effect. Perhaps this is why some people crave chocolate, especially when feeling stressed. An excess of sugar, however, may trigger binge eating. Eating a lot of simple sugar at once produces a quick rise in the level of sugar in the blood; insulin is then released, and the blood sugar level plunges. The result is increased appetite, and then the cycle repeats itself if more sugar is consumed. The solution is to avoid eating a lot of simple sugar or to eat it in the context of a meal.

Fat   Most experts agree that the real problem in the American diet is not a "sweet tooth" but rather overcon-sumption of dietary fats. Although no more than 30 percent of total kcalories (and preferably less) should come from fat, Americans get 36 to 38 percent of their kcalories from fat sources (see Table 13-1). Oils, margarine, butter, cream, and lard are almost pure fat. Meat and processed foods contain a great deal of "hidden" fat, while nuts, seeds, and avocados are plant sources of fat. Most fat in the American diet comes from fatty red meats, dairy products, and processed foods, including snack foods like potato and corn chips (see Table 13-2). You can substantially decrease your fat consumption by moving closer to a vegetarian (complex carbohydrate) diet: eating more fruits, vegetables, grains, and legumes and decreasing overall meat consumption. Learn to substitute leaner choices (fish or poultry without the skin) for high-fat choices such as bacon, sausage, and ribs.

The "Supermarket" Diet   A high sugar consumption, combined with a high-fat diet, spells double trouble. Laboratory rats that were fed either a high-sugar diet, a high-fat diet, or a "supermarket" diet of both high sugar and high fat all gained weight. Rats on a high-sugar diet did not gain as much weight as those on a high-fat diet; the rats eating a supermarket diet of chocolate chip cookies, peanut butter, bananas, and so forth gained 269 percent more weight than did a control group of rats who only ate ordinary rat chow. Although extending such results to humans is questionable, it's hard to resist the suspicion

---

Serotonin   A neurotransmitter in the brain that has a calming effect; carbohydrate deprivation causes serotonin depletion.

Table 13-2 Foods and Their Fat

Percentage Fat	Food
95–100	Butter, margarine, mayonnaise, salad oil, olives, Italian dressing, heavy cream
90–95	Pecans, macadamia nuts, baking chocolate
85–90	Walnuts, egg yolk, avocado, sour cream
80–85	Almonds, cream cheese, frankfurter, pork spareribs
75–80	Peanut butter, sunflower seeds, salami, bacon, half and half
70–75	Cheddar cheese, lamb chop
65–70	American cheese, mozzarella cheese, tuna fish in oil, ground chuck
60–65	Sweet chocolate, coconut, eggs, potato chips
55–60	Veal chop, milk chocolate, pie crust
50–55	Roast beef, pork chop, roast chicken with skin
45–50	Ice cream, whole milk, club steak, salmon
40–45	Granola, banana bread, buttered popcorn, french fries, chili, Ritz crackers
35–40	Lasagna, hamburger on a bun, chocolate chip cookies
30–35	Chicken (skinless dark meat), 2% milk
25–30	Pizza, ground round, sea bass
20–25	Chicken (skinless white meat), liver, turkey, chicken noodle soup, chocolate pudding
15–20	Halibut, oatmeal
10–15	Plain popcorn, pretzels, bread, fig bar, low-fat cottage cheese
5–10	Tortilla, brown rice, sherbet, haddock, honeydew melon, raisins
0–5	Skim milk, white rice, egg white, spaghetti, potatoes, most fruits and vegetables, beer, wine, most cereals, clear soups

that the composition of the diet eaten is a factor in weight gain.

Protein   Americans worry far too much about the protein content of their diet. Proteins, or more specifically, the amino acids that form proteins, are used by the body for constant building and repair of cells and for producing enzymes and hormones used in the body. Most people need not trouble about getting too little protein. Although the typical American eats an average of 100–150 grams of protein every day, an adult male needs only 60 grams of protein a day and an adult female only 45 grams. Special dietary supplements that provide extra protein are totally unnecessary for most people; and, in fact, protein not needed by the body for growth and tissue repair will be stored as body fat.

Complex Carbohydrates   People concerned about their weight often eliminate bread, pasta, and potatoes—the starches or "carbs" in the diet—in the mistaken belief that cutting these kcalories will help control weight. In fact, complex carbohydrates from these sources as well as from fresh vegetables, legumes, and other whole grains help maintain proper weight. In contrast to fat kcalories, which the body can easily convert to body fat, kcalories from complex carbohydrate actually cost the body kcalories to digest. Furthermore, eating a large amount of complex carbohydrates makes you feel full. In fact, eating a high-carbohydrate/low-fat diet can even result in weight loss without conscious restriction of kcalories and without exercise! The real problem in terms of obesity is not eating too many complex carbohydrates, but adding high-fat sauces and toppings to them. Changing the composition of your diet in favor of a higher carbohydrate-to-fat ratio may require retraining your taste buds so that you get used to bread without butter, potatoes without sour cream, and pasta with a vegetable sauce instead of a cream sauce or cheese.

Hunger and Satiety   What you put in your mouth also affects your experience of hunger and satiety. One theory says that the brain senses hunger when the blood sugar gets too low and that this sensation triggers eating. The resulting increase in blood sugar presumably produces **satiety**—feelings of fullness. However, blood sugar level varies under normal conditions, and it's not clear exactly how variations in blood sugar affect hunger. Another theory says that low levels of serotonin in the brain are associated with feelings of hunger and high levels with satiety. People who eat a diet high in fat and low in complex carbohydrates tend to have lower than normal levels of serotonin in their brains. Theoretically, eating a diet low in fat and high in complex carbohydrate should help us avoid feelings of hunger.

■ **Exploring Your Emotions**

Do you sometimes overeat? If so, what motivates you or triggers your behavior? Are you more likely to overeat in certain situations, at certain times of the day, or with particular people? Do you overeat when you're in a particular frame of mind? How do you feel afterwards?

Most people infer that they're hungry when their stomach growls or when they get the "shakes" from not eating. However, research suggests that many people are unable to recognize stomach contractions as a signal of their hunger. They might confuse anxiety or physiological arousal with feeling hungry. Telling such people to "eat only when hungry" is poor advice. It's better to say, "stop eating when full," since people are much better at knowing when they feel full than when they feel hungry. Unfortunately, many people who know they're full keep eating because the food tastes good. We all need to mentally monitor feelings of fullness and be guided by adequate portion control in order to maintain normal weight.

Eating Habits   Equally important to weight control is eating small, frequent meals—three a day or more, plus planned, appropriate snacks if desired. Some people skip breakfast and even lunch, thinking they're saving kcalories. When they do finally eat, they're often so hungry they can't stop eating for the rest of the night. Gradually their eating pattern gets shifted to later and later in the day, until finally they "can't" eat breakfast in the morning. They're still full from the night before! In addition, waiting to eat until late in the day often results in shopping for a meal on an empty stomach and feeling stressed and fatigued from a day without sufficient body fuel. Insufficient energy contributes to poor performance. Failure to do a job well then leads to feelings of stress. This stress can result in making poor food choices, overeating, and possibly drinking too much alcohol. Eating eventually takes on the appearance of being an effective means of self-soothing and distraction from problems. This cyclical pattern sets the stage for future problems with food.

A healthier approach is to develop a *structure* to guide eating. This structure involves having a more-or-less regular time for meals. (Weekends and vacations may differ from week days.) It also means establishing a set of *decision rules* that guide food choices. These rules indicate what choices are "allowed" for breakfast, lunch, and dinner, when high-fat or high-sugar choices may be indulged in, what are the preferred substitutions for the less healthy choices, and so forth. For example, the rule governing breakfast choices might be, "Choose a sugar-free, high-fiber cereal with nonfat milk most of the time. Once in a while (no more than once a week) a poached or soft-boiled egg is okay. Save pancakes and waffles for special occasions." The decision rule governing dinner entrees might be, "Choose chicken or fish most of the

time. Avoid cream sauces. Once in a while if a steak is desired, make it a small fillet or flank steak."

Decreeing some food "off limits" is generally not a good idea. Doing so sets up a struggle to be vigilant and resist the urge to eat that food, but almost everyone eventually succumbs to the forbidden food rather than feel deprived. The guiding principle should be "everything in moderation." If a particular food becomes troublesome, it could be placed off limits temporarily until control over it is regained.

Exercise and Physical Activity   It's becoming more and more apparent that exercise is an all-purpose remedy for modern ailments and a source of endless benefits. As described in Chapter 14 and other chapters, regular, aerobic exercise strengthens the heart and cardiovascular system, confers greater endurance and energy, provides a means of managing stress, and helps prevent osteoporosis. It also burns kcalories and keeps the **metabolism** geared to using food for energy instead of storing kcalories.

Well-meaning weight control experts have misled many people about the value of exercise. It's been said that exercise isn't worthwhile because "you must chop wood for 10 hours or play volleyball for 32 hours to lose just one pound of fat." This assertion neglects the metabolism boost that results from exercise—and that lasts even beyond the period of exercise. The body burns more kcalories when metabolism is more active.

Furthermore, calculating the number of kcalories burned for any given activity is more complex than it might seem. Heavy people burn more kcalories than do lighter ones, and the level of a person's physical fitness affects kcalorie burn. Because of these factors, kcalorie-expenditure tables are at best only a general guide to the relative kcalorie-burning value of any activity (see Table 13-3).

You may have heard that exercise increases risk of sudden death. Although that risk exists for people who have been sedentary or who have undiagnosed heart conditions, the risk of continuing to lead a sedentary lifestyle is still greater. Everyone needs to learn how to undertake an appropriate program of exercise, gradually increase the workout load, and never do anything in conjunction with exercise that would add stress—like use drugs. It's important to anticipate and prepare for the problems posed by cold weather, precipitation, or very hot, humid weather.

Satiety   Feelings of fullness after eating, perhaps associated with blood sugar levels or with serotonin levels in the brain.

Metabolism   Refers to the sum of all of the vital processes in which energy and nutrients from foods are made available to and utilized by the body.

Table 13-3 Kilocalories used in ten minutes of various activities

	Body Weight				Body Weight		
	125 Pounds	175 Pounds	250 Pounds		125 Pounds	175 Pounds	250 Pounds
Personal Necessities				*Light Work*			
Sleeping	10	14	20	Assembly line	20	28	40
Sitting (watching TV)	10	14	18	Auto repair	35	48	69
Sitting (talking)	15	21	30	Carpentry	32	44	64
Dressing or washing	26	37	53	Bricklaying	28	40	57
Standing	12	16	24	Farming chores	32	44	64
Locomotion				House painting	29	40	58
Walking downstairs	56	78	111	*Heavy Work*			
Walking upstairs	146	202	288	Pick and shovel work	56	78	110
Walking at 2 mph	29	40	58	Chopping wood	60	84	121
Walking at 4 mph	52	72	102	Dragging logs	158	220	315
Running at 5.5 mph	90	125	178	Drilling coal	79	111	159
Running at 7 mph	118	164	232	*Recreation*			
Running at 12 mph	164	228	326	Badminton	43	65	94
Cycling at 5.5 mph	42	58	83	Volleyball	43	65	94
Cycling at 13 mph	89	124	178	Baseball	39	54	78
Housework				Basketball	58	82	117
Making beds	32	46	65	Bowling (nonstop)	56	78	111
Washing floors	38	53	75	Canoeing (4 mph)	90	128	182
Washing windows	35	48	69	Dancing (moderate)	35	48	69
Dusting	22	31	44	Dancing (vigorous)	48	66	94
Preparing a meal	32	46	65	Football	69	96	137
Shoveling snow	65	89	130	Golfing	33	48	68
Light gardening	30	42	59	Horseback riding	56	78	112
Weeding garden	49	68	98	Ping-Pong	32	45	64
Mowing grass (power)	34	47	67	Racquetball	75	104	144
Mowing grass (manual)	38	52	74	Skiing (downhill)	80	112	160
Sedentary Occupation				Skiing (water)	60	88	130
Sitting writing	15	21	30	Skiing (cross country)	98	138	194
Light office work	25	34	50	Squash	75	104	144
Standing, light activity	20	28	40	Swimming (backstroke)	32	45	64
Typing (electric)	19	27	39	Swimming (crawl)	40	56	80
				Tennis	56	80	115

Note: Heavier people use *more* kcalories than lighter people, because more energy is needed for the extra weight. This table is for *continuous* activity (not for the minutes of resting during an activity). Energy used varies greatly with the *intensity* of doing the activity.

Source: Reprinted with permission from K. D. Brownell, 1987, *The LEARN Program of Weight Control* (Philadelphia: University of Pennsylvania), pp. 64–65.

Research strongly suggests that exercise is crucial for successful long-term maintenance of normal weight. Although weight loss can be achieved without exercise, research also shows that rate of weight loss is accelerated and lean body tissue (muscle mass) is better preserved when exercise is a component of a weight-loss effort. The key question is, What kind of exercise is best for you?

Aerobic Exercise Aerobic exercise—running, swimming, bicycling, aerobic dancing, walking briskly, and the like—has traditionally been the "gold standard" for weight control. For maintaining normal weight, research has found that mild exercise is better than strenuous, marathon exercise sessions because it can be comfortably sustained for a longer time. Walking from 45 to 60 minutes or more five days a week will contribute to a weight-loss effort. Regular brisk walking on a daily basis for a total of 30 minutes or so will help maintain normal weight for most people. Of course, more vigorous exercise can add fun and satisfaction to your life.

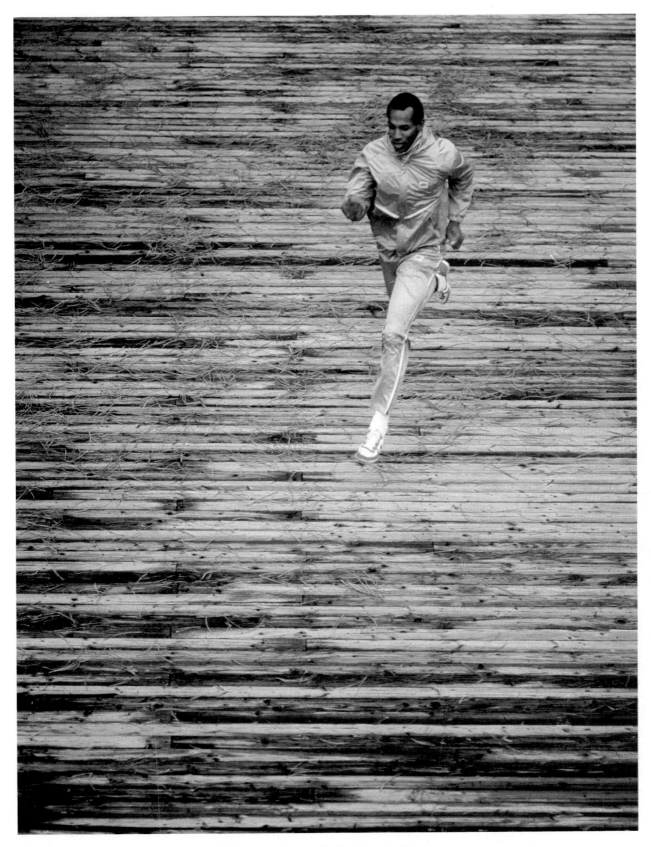

Exercise is an essential component of any effective weight control plan. Running is just
one of innumerable activities that can help you get in shape.

Resistance Weight Training Long the domain of body builder fanatics and macho-types, weight training was thought to be good for building muscle bulk but not for burning kcalories or contributing to weight loss. Only recently has it gained favor as a means of weight management. Research suggests that weight training results in improved maintenance of lean body tissue during diet-induced weight loss. Women have tended to reject weight training because of fears it will *add* body weight, particularly muscles. In fact, such fears are largely unwarranted, because females lack the necessary hormones to add muscle bulk easily. Furthermore, it takes a lot of effort and long hours in the gym to add much bulk. On the other hand, an exercise program that includes a workout with weights can not only increase muscle strength but also add muscle definition that makes the body look better. Joining a gym or having access to expensive equipment is not necessary. You can start on a good weight-resistance training program if you have a few pairs of dumbbells and know how to use them appropriately.

The Well-Rounded Exercise Program No one kind of exercise is "best." All kinds of exercise contribute in some degree to fitness, health, or well-being. As explained in Chapter 14, a well-rounded exercise program for a healthy lifestyle would include not only aerobic exercise and resistance weight training, but also exercises, sports, and activities that contribute to flexibility, strength, relaxation, and enjoyment. Living a healthy lifestyle also means taking advantage of routine opportunities to get exercise, such as taking the stairs instead of the elevator, biking instead of driving, and so forth.

Getting and staying motivated for exercise gets harder as you get older and acquire more and more obligations. The sooner you establish good habits, the better. The key to success is to make exercise an integral part of the lifestyle you enjoy now and will enjoy in the future. Chapter 14 contains many suggestions for becoming a more active, physically fit person.

Thinking and Emotions What goes on in your head is the third component of a healthy lifestyle and successful weight control. Cognition, or thinking, involves perception, memory, judgment, beliefs, attitudes, and expectations—and the way all these come together to give meaning to events. The way you think about yourself and your world influences how you feel and how you act. Likewise, how you feel (your emotions) and how you behave give rise to additional thoughts and beliefs. The relevance of cognition and emotion to human adaptation and behavior has only recently gained (some would say *regained*) a central focus in psychology. Certain kinds of thinking produce negative emotions, which in turn undermine the maintenance of a healthy lifestyle.

■ **Exploring Your Emotions**

How do you feel about your body weight, shape, and size? Do you have strong feelings about what an ideal male and female body should look like? Where do you think you've learned these ideals?

Research on people who have a weight problem indicates that low self-esteem and the negative emotions that accompany it are significant problems. However, feelings of low self-esteem are more likely the result of being overweight and having other problems in life, than the cause of the weight problem itself. This low self-esteem often results in part from mentally comparing the actual self to an internally held picture of the "ideal self." The greater the discrepancy, the larger the impact on self-esteem and the more likely the presence of negative emotions.

Often our internalized "ideal self" is the result of having adopted perfectionistic goals and beliefs about how we and others "should" be. Examples of such beliefs include, "If I don't do things perfectly, I'm a failure," "It's terrible and awful if I'm not loved by everyone," and "Something bad that happened to me in the past is going to affect me now and perhaps forever." Some psychologists argue that these *irrational beliefs* actually cause emotional disturbance. The remedy is to challenge such beliefs and replace them with more realistic ones.

The beliefs and attitudes you hold give rise to self-talk, an internal dialogue you carry on with yourself about events that happen to and around you. Positive self-talk includes leading yourself through the steps of a job and then praising yourself when it's successfully completed. Too often self-talk is "negative." It takes the form of self-deprecating remarks, self-blame, and angry and guilt-producing comments. Negative self-talk generally undermines efforts at self-control and leads to feelings of anxiety and depression.

Your beliefs and self-talk influence how you interpret what happens to you and what you expect in the future, as well as how you feel and react. A healthy lifestyle is supported by having realistic beliefs and goals and by engaging in positive self-talk and problem-solving efforts.

Coping Strategies The fourth component of a healthy lifestyle is adequate and appropriate coping strategies for dealing with the stresses and challenges of life. One strategy that some people adopt for coping is eating. (Others use drugs, alcohol, smoking, spending, gambling, and so on, to cope.) So, when boredom presents itself, eating can provide entertainment. Food may be used to alleviate loneliness or as a pickup for fatigue. Eating provides distraction from difficult problems and is a means of punishing the self or others for real or imagined transgressions.

Play Plans for Exercise and Weight Loss

Peter Wood has developed a variety of ways in which people can reduce weight and avoid unpleasant dieting. One strategy involves using so many kcalories each day in play activities—doing things that are fun and interesting. When people get into the habit of expending a few more kcalories each day, in time they can lose many pounds. Here are three plans, each designed to use up a different number of kcalories. Plan A is a minimum plan, while Plans E and J are more vigorous.

Play Plan A
(25 kcalories per day)

Choose *one* playful act *each* day from the accompanying list. These are *extra* play kcalories to *add* to your usual routine.

Walk a quarter mile (3 blocks).

Cycle a mile, slowly.

Swim for 3 minutes.

Dance (aerobic) for 5 minutes.

Clean windows for 6 minutes.

Rake leaves for 6 minutes.

Scrub floor for 6 minutes.

Feel free to try different activities on different days.

Playful Hints . . .

- Get off to a good start—don't overdo.
- Find a companion who will exercise with you.

Play Plan E
(150 kcalories per day)

Choose *one* activity every day.

Walk at moderate speed for 30 minutes.

Cycle for 25 minutes.

Swim for 15 minutes.

Dance (aerobic) for 25 minutes.

Dance (disco) for 30 minutes.

Play volleyball for 30 minutes.

Play table tennis for 30 minutes.

Clean windows to music for 30 minutes.

Scrub floors to music for 30 minutes.

Playful Hints . . .

- Think "play" whenever you have to go somewhere: Can you walk over, not ride? Is the bike handy? Why not walk to and from the restaurant? You can even jog a little on the way.
- If you don't drive, you won't have a parking problem (or a parking ticket).

Play Plan J
(500 kcalories per day)

Choose *one* activity each day:

- Walk five miles in 75 to 90 minutes.
- Run for 45 minutes.
- Cycle for 60 minutes.
- Play racquetball for 60 minutes.
- Dance (aerobic) for 60 minutes.
- Play soccer for 60 minutes.
- Roller skate for 65 minutes.
- Mow the lawn for 60 minutes.
- Saw wood for 50 minutes.

This high level of fitness should be approached slowly. It involves playing vigorously for about an hour a day, or 4 percent of our 24-hour day. The player is very fit, eats a lot, and has banished weight problems.

Playful Hints . . .

- Remember, drink more water than you feel you need when it's hot.
- To avoid injuries, do your stretching exercises and vary your plan.
- This level of play will keep you slim and fit forever.

Peter Wood, 1983, *The California Diet and Exercise Program* (Mountain View, Calif.: Anderson World Books).

People who lead healthy lifestyles have learned more effective ways to get their needs met. They have learned to communicate assertively and to manage interpersonal conflict effectively and don't shrink from problems or overreact. The person with a healthy lifestyle knows how to create and maintain relationships with others and has a solid network of friends and loved ones. Food is used appropriately—to fuel life's activities and growth and for personal satisfaction, not to manage stress.

The healthy lifestyle that naturally and easily results in a good body weight is one characterized by good nutrition, adequate exercise, positive thinking and emotions, and effective coping strategies and behavior patterns. All these factors interact in determining exactly how a person acts in certain situations. Figure 13-2 presents two simple "behavior chains" that illustrate how thinking, feeling, coping strategies, environmental cues, and behavior can work together to produce weight gain or weight loss.

Are You an Emotional Eater?

1. I tend to eat more when there's too much work to do. (True/false)

2. I sometimes find myself prowling about, looking for I know not what, then end up in the kitchen eating something. (True/false)

3. I prefer a restaurant with a relaxed atmosphere that helps me eat away the day's worries. (True/false)

4. I'm liable to eat more if I'm annoyed after a bad morning. (True/false)

5. I tend to eat more if the mood is not relaxed. (True/false)

6. When I'm troubled, eating has a soothing effect. (True/false)

7. I like to eat when I'm lonely, frustrated, or anxious. (True/false)

If you answered "true" to four or more of these statements you may regard yourself as an "emotional eater." About 13 percent of men and 27 percent of women fall into this category. They are usually overweight despite attempts to reduce by diet and tended to be chubby in childhood. They may benefit from psychologic guidance, switching from fad to practical diets, and developing more interest in work, hobbies, and sport.

From *Healthline*, November 1989, Vol. 8, No. 11.

Overcoming a Weight Problem

Not everyone arrives at young adulthood at normal weight. About 30 percent of obese adults become so before the age of 18, and 80 to 85 percent of obese teenagers become obese adults. Some young adults of normal weight have a lifestyle that inevitably leads to weight-control problems. When weight is a problem, especially for younger people, decisive action needs to be taken immediately.

■ Exploring Your Emotions

How do you feel about obese people? Do you make personal judgments about them? Do you do the same about extremely thin people?

Assessing Your Weight and Body Composition   One of the first questions a young person has to have answered is, "Am I really overweight, and if so, what should I weigh?" Answering this question isn't as easy as you might expect. Several different approaches are possible, each with its own problems.

Height-Weight Tables   The most common means of assessing **overweight** is to refer to a height-weight table. Many often contradictory height-weight tables exist, and these give ranges of "ideal," "recommended," or "desirable" weights, adjusted for sex and height and sometimes frame size. Most experts agree that these tables have inherent problems. First, the ranges of weights recommended in height-weight tables as "healthy" (that is, associated with minimum mortality) are too narrow. A much greater range of "healthy" weights exists than has generally been recognized. Although research has established that significant health risk is associated with extreme overweight or underweight, a large "gray area" lies between any of the currently recommended ranges of weight and these extremes.

Second, although weights associated with minimum mortality have been found to rise with age, most height-weight tables rarely take age into account. They lump all ages 25 through 59 together, and individuals under the age of 25 are not even considered. Yet overweight in those under 30, even when it is of a lesser degree than that considered "severe" in someone older, has been shown to be a significant health risk and to predict later obesity.

Third, although more recent tables have attempted to

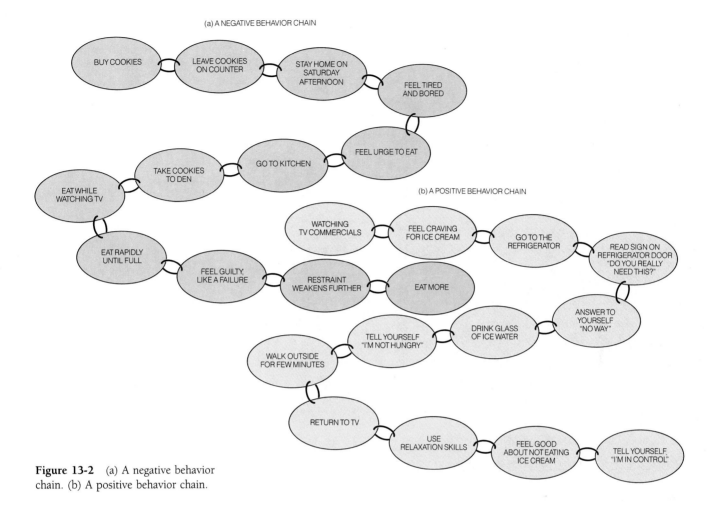

Figure 13-2 (a) A negative behavior chain. (b) A positive behavior chain.

provide a means of assessing frame size, they have done so with little success. In some recent tables, the reference values for elbow breadth as a measure of frame size were obtained by arbitrarily using the 25th and 75th percentiles within height categories and were not based on estimates of mortality. Furthermore, getting a reasonably accurate measurement of elbow breadth is quite difficult and requires special measuring apparatus.

Even if these problems were correctable, however, the present height-weight table recommendations are based on data that are unrepresentative of large sections of the population and that may indeed be inaccurate. Most tables were based on actuarial data obtained by self-report from insured individuals—mostly middle- and upper-class white males. Minorities and women are underrepresented in the data base. (Despite all these objections,

a height-weight chart is provided in Table 13-4 so you can see the standards used by one major life insurance company.)

Using height-weight tables, researchers define **obesity**—a condition of excessive body fat—as 20 percent or more above a person's upper limit for weight, adjusted for sex and height. (Some researchers use 30 percent because 20 percent gives too many false positives.) But height-weight tables reflect total body weight rather than body composition—the proportion of body fat to lean body mass. A more accurate assessment of obesity requires that body composition be assessed and body fat be measured.

However this measurement is obtained, the "normal" fraction of total body weight that is fat in male subjects aged 18 is approximately 15 to 18 percent. The corre-

---

Overweight Body weight above the recommended range according to a height/weight table, adjusted for sex, height, and possibly frame size and age. This is an arbitrary classification based on population norms.

Obesity A complex health-impairing disorder characterized by an excessive accumulation of body fat. It can be defined as (1) being 20 percent or more above the upper limit of recommended weight using height-weight tables, (2)

having over 25 percent of body weight as fat (males) and over 30 percent as fat (females), or (3) having a BMI over 28 (males) or 32 (females).

Table 13-4 Life insurance company desirable weight table

		W O M E N					M E N		
		Frame*					Frame*		
Height					Height				
Ft	In	Small	Medium	Large	Ft	In	Small	Medium	Large
4	10	102–111	109–121	118–131	5	2	128–134	131–141	138–150
4	11	103–113	111–123	120–134	5	3	130–136	133–143	140–153
5	0	104–115	113–126	122–137	5	4	132–138	135–145	142–156
5	1	106–118	115–129	125–140	5	5	134–140	137–148	144–160
5	2	108–121	118–132	128–143	5	6	136–142	139–151	146–164
5	3	111–124	121–135	131–147	5	7	138–145	142–154	149–168
5	4	114–127	124–138	134–151	5	8	140–148	145–157	152–172
5	5	117–130	127–141	137–155	5	9	142–151	148–160	155–176
5	6	120–133	130–144	140–159	5	10	144–154	151–163	158–180
5	7	123–136	133–147	143–163	5	11	146–157	154–166	161–184
5	8	126–139	136–150	146–167	6	0	149–160	157–170	164–188
5	9	129–142	139–153	149–170	6	1	152–164	160–174	168–192
5	10	132–145	142–156	152–173	6	2	155–168	164–178	172–197
5	11	135–148	145–159	155–176	6	3	158–172	167–182	176–202
6	0	138–151	148–162	158–179	6	4	162–176	171–187	181–207

Based on a weight-height mortality study conducted by the Society of Actuaries and the Association of Life Insurance Medical Directors of America, Metropolitan Life Insurance Company, revised 1983.

*Weight at ages 25 to 59 based on lowest mortality. Height includes 1-in. heel. Weight for women includes 3 lb. for indoor clothing. Weight for men includes 5 lb. for indoor clothing.

sponding figure for females is 20 to 25 percent. Individuals engaged in vigorous, regular exercise may have much lower proportions in the range of 3 to 5 percent for males and 10 to 15 percent for females. Using the body composition approach, researchers have defined obesity as a body-fat content greater than 25 percent of total body weight for males and greater than 30 percent for females. This condition is also termed **overfat.** Several methods have been devised for measuring body fat, although again, none is perfect.

Underwater Weighing One of the most accurate methods for assessing fatness is *hydrostatic weighing* or weighing under water. Since the density of fat is different from that of lean tissue these masses can be estimated by either measuring the amount of water displaced or by comparing the difference between the underwater and the dry weighings. In addition to being an intimidating method of assessment, especially for those who have a fear of water, underwater weighing is neither convenient nor a widely available procedure. And it is not without error. The outcome of the measurement can be affected by eat-

ing foods that create internal gas or engaging in activities that affect fluid retention or cause dehydration. Furthermore, the norms used for assessing the outcome were developed by testing middle-aged sedentary males. Such norms are useless when judging an athletic female.

Skinfold Measurement A more convenient substitute is the *skinfold thickness technique* (actually "fatfold"), which measures the thickness of fat under the skin. It should be performed by a highly trained technician who grasps a fold of skin at a predetermined location between the thumb and forefinger of the left hand and lifts it firmly away from the underlying muscle. Calipers that exert a pressure of 10g/mm² are then attached to the fold and allowed to come together for a specified number of seconds so that a reading can be recorded. Repeated measurements are taken from several specific areas of the body, and the results are computed using a formula to determine the percentage of body weight that is fat.

This technique has been criticized because the distribution of body fat is nonuniform and taking the measurements can be difficult. Although nearly half of total body

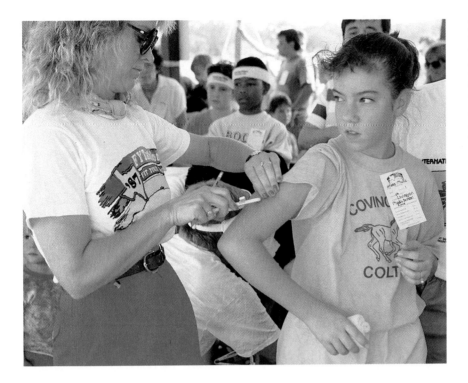

Measuring the thickness of the fat layer under the skin is one way of assessing body composition, but it has several limitations. One problem is that people are sometimes measured against inappropriate standards. This girl, for example, has more subcutaneous fat than would one of her male peers, simply because she's female.

fat is *subcutaneous* (directly under the skin), the relation between specific subcutaneous **adipose tissue** (such as that between thumb and forefinger) and fat in other subcutaneous sites and body compartments is uncertain. Error that results from pinching up muscle along with fat and skin or misapplying the calipers is a serious problem in skinfold measurement. Furthermore, the calipers can go out of adjustment, producing additional error. Most importantly, there are age, sex, and ethnic differences in skinfolds, and appropriate norms are not always used to take these differences into account.

Electrical Impedance Analysis Body fat can also be assessed by the newly popular technique of electrical impedance analysis. Electrodes are attached to the body in several areas, and a harmless electrical current is transmitted from electrode to electrode. The electrical conduction through the body favors the path of the lean tissues over the fat tissues. A computer can calculate percentage fat from these current measurements.

Like the other methods, electrical impedance analysis is subject to error. Electrical impedance equipment is calibrated with the same equations used in underwater weighing, making it subject to the same criticisms about norms. Furthermore, the margin for error with this equipment may be even greater than with skinfold or hydrostatic techniques. If the person being analyzed does anything that affects water retention or the electrolyte balance of the body—such as use diuretic medications or do vigorous exercise—additional error can be introduced. For an accurate measurement, the person being measured needs to avoid consuming alcohol for 48 hours and avoid eating for at least 3 hours before the test.

Although other techniques exist for determining the proportion of body weight attributable to fat and lean body mass, all inherently retain some amount of error or raise other questions of validity.

Body Mass Index Yet another approach to the definition of overweight and obesity has been taken by the National Center for Health Statistics. **Body mass index** (BMI) is normally defined as body weight (in kilograms) divided

---

Overfat A condition in which a person has more body fat (adipose tissue) than is considered to be healthy. The amount differs according to gender (females naturally have more body fat than males), race, and ethnicity.

Adipose tissue Connective tissue in which fat is stored.

Body mass index (BMI) A measure of relative body weight nearly independent of height and correlating highly with more direct measures of body fat. It is calculated by dividing total body weight in kilograms by the square of body height in meters.

Figure 13-3   Body Mass Index (BMI).

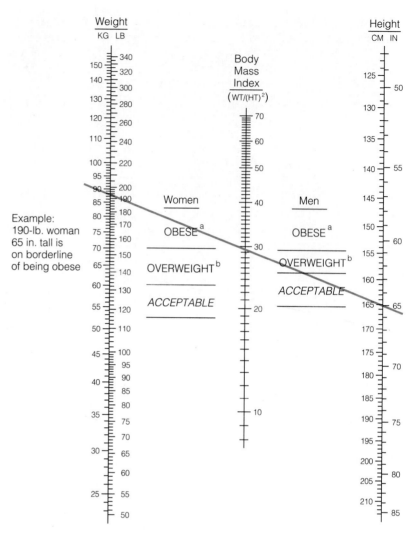

Note: To determine BMI, place a ruler or other straight edge between the body weight column on the left and the height column on the right and read the BMI from the point where it crosses the center. In the example, a 190-lb. woman, 65 inches tall (5 foot, 5 inches) would be on the borderline between overweight and obese, with a BMI of 29.5.
[a] *Obesity:* BMI above 30 kg/m^2.
[b] *Overweight:* Body mass index (BMI) of 25 to 30 kg/m^2.

by the square of the height (in meters) or BMI = kg/m^2. Although this measure cannot determine how much body weight comes from fat tissue and how much from muscle, bone, and water, BMI correlates highly with direct measures of body fat and is nearly independent of height.

The National Center for Health Statistics has defined overweight as a body mass index (BMI) greater than the 85th and 95th percentile of 20- to 29-year-old men and women respectively. This corresponds to a BMI of 28 for men and 32 for women (see Figure 13-3). (Conversely, a BMI of less than 19 points is an unhealthy underweight

condition.) You should know that these are statistical definitions and are not derived from mortality data. What is not reflected in these criteria is that overweight as defined by BMI at younger ages has a detrimental effect on life expectancy and is a serious health problem. A stricter range of BMI should be employed for those in their late teens and twenties. A BMI higher than 25 for young persons signals the need for immediate corrective action.

A Radical Answer   Unfortunately, all of this discussion begs the question, "What should you weigh?" Height-weight tables, body composition analyses, and BMI measurements can best serve as general guides or estimates for body weight. They can't account for individual genetic, racial, or ethnic differences that cause variations from "average" population weights but that may still be healthy. Perhaps it's time for a radical idea: To answer the question of what you "should" weigh, let your lifestyle be your guide. Don't focus on a particular weight as your goal. Focus on living a lifestyle that includes eating moderate amounts of healthful foods, getting plenty of exercise, thinking positively, and learning to cope with stress. Then let the pounds fall where they may. For most people, the result will be close to the recommended weight ranges discussed earlier. For some, their weight will be somewhat higher than societal norms—but right for them. By letting a healthy lifestyle determine your weight, you can avoid the dieting hysteria and fixation on body weight that grips this country.

What Contributes to a Weight Problem? As far as knowing what influences body weight we're still pretty much in the Dark Ages, but we are making progress. Today we know that physical factors, as well as psychological, cultural, and social factors, play a significant role. In particular, heredity and metabolism have been linked to a tendency toward obesity.

Genetic Factors Obesity can be produced in animals through selective breeding. That is, animals can be bred for higher or lower fat content, and the same principles may hold true for humans. A recent study comparing 540 adult Danish adoptees and their biological parents concluded that genetic influences played an important role in determining fatness in adults. The best predictor of a woman's weight was her own mother's weight. Furthermore, if both parents are overweight, 73 percent of their offspring are likely to be overweight. If only one parent is overweight, 41 percent of the offspring are likely to be overweight. If neither parent is overweight, only 9 percent tend to be overweight.

■ **Exploring Your Emotions**

Is anyone in your family overweight? If so, can you identify factors that contribute to this weight problem? How would you feel about suggesting ways the problem could be addressed?

Genes influence body type, body size, body weight, and obesity, and the occurrence of obesity in families has long been reported. Even the pattern of fat distribution on the body (that is, whether it tends to accumulate on the hips, at the waist, in the abdomen, etc.) is a function

of heredity. Women tend to accumulate fat in the hips and buttocks, whereas for men it is above the waist, especially in the abdominal ("potbelly") area. The amount or functioning of brown adipose tissue, which is the source of thermogenesis (heat production) and is a factor in some kinds of obesity, may also be determined by heredity. Heredity may also be the culprit in certain types of glandular, chromosomal, neurological, or metabolic dysfunctions that produce some kinds of obesity. Nevertheless, probably no more than 5 percent of all obesity problems are attributable to such causes.

Remember that genes are not destiny. With increased exercise and decreased food consumption, even those with a genetic tendency toward obesity can maintain a healthy body weight. (This weight may be higher than the culturally defined ideal, however.) Giving up efforts at weight control and failing to strive for your best body weight because of genetic factors is to exacerbate the problem: An unhealthy lifestyle plus a genetic tendency toward obesity can lead to a very significant weight problem and elevated health risk.

Set Point Theory A controversial explanation for why some people have such difficulty managing weight is called *set point theory*. This concept holds that every person has a "natural" or genetically determined weight or set point that his or her body works to preserve. Actually, set point is believed to be a range of weight (such as 130–150 pounds) rather than a particular number. Presumably the body sends out physiological and/or psychological signals to keep weight from going above or below the set point range. Those who accept this theory believe that the only way to change set point is through increased exercise.

Just what mechanism controls set point or where that mechanism is located in the body hasn't been clarified. Although some research suggests that gaining or losing weight beyond the set point range is difficult and that even when weight does go outside the range, it tends to return to the original level, scientific support for this theory is minimal. Some experts contend that body weight is governed not by an unidentified mechanism that controls energy intake and expenditure but rather by an interplay of both physiological and environmental factors that produces a "settling" point for weight. Dr. Kelly Brownell of the University of Pennsylvania has argued that, because of the implications for how overweight persons view their obesity, set point theory should not be promoted without proof. Until better evidence for set point theory exists, it should not be taken seriously.

Metabolism The idea that the body settles at a particular weight can better be explained by considering how metabolism influences weight. *Metabolism* is the sum of all

Some Facts about Weight Control

Diet Aids Don't Work

Over-the-counter appetite suppressants contain the decongestant phenylpropanolamine, or PPA, which disrupts hunger signals to the brain and dries out the mouth, making food taste bland and unappetizing. Side effects can include nervousness, irritability, insomnia, and high blood pressure.

If you don't mind chewing tasteless food and living with a bad disposition, such products *can* curb your appetite, but not for long. Once you're off the pills, a step that's medically advisable after three months, any weight you lost will probably sneak right back.

Diet chewing gums and candy, to be taken before meals, are more benign—but less helpful. They contain benzocaine, which numbs the mouth's nerve endings, making them less sensitive to sweet. You'll keep your taste for fat.

Diet Sodas May Not Help

Though one study did actually show that artificial-sweetener users consumed 165 fewer kcalories a day, another found that women using such sweeteners were even *more* likely to gain weight than those who didn't. Many people save 30 or so kcalories by stirring a packet of artificial sweetener into their after-dinner coffee, then use that virtue as an excuse to order chocolate mousse.

There's No Such Thing as Cellulite

The orange-peel dimpling that often occurs around women's thighs and hips is just plain, ordinary fat. Strands of tissue near the skin separate fat compartments and anchor them to deeper muscles. When these fat cells are extremely full they bulge, leaving little valleys—the "cellulite"—in between. Skip the loofah sponges, the horsehair mitts, and other touted remedies. The way to get rid of the dimples is to lose weight, preferably before age 35 or 40, when your skin is still elastic enough to shrink back.

You Can't Slim Just One Body Part

Do leg-lifts and you may burn enough calories to lose some fat, but not necessarily from around your thighs. In fact, by toning the muscles beneath a layer of fat, they could make your legs even bigger. Only good old aerobic exercise, sustained for 15 or 20 minutes, melts body fat. Rubberized sweatsuits, sauna belts, and cellophane wraps simply dehydrate you.

The one real treatment for localized fat is liposuction, a surgical process that removes fat cells from under the skin. It's expensive, risky, and sometimes painful.

You Can't Lose Weight Forever

On most diets the first few pounds come off quickly because less food means fewer carbohydrates and less salt—both of which lead to water losses. At the same time metabolism slows. Plus, as more weight comes off, you spend less energy to move. For every 25-pound drop, you need 100 fewer kcalories a day. To keep losing weight, keep upping your exercise.

Some People are Born to be Thin

It's not fair, but when it comes to metabolic rates, we're not all created equal. In general, metabolic rates are faster in infants, adolescents, and pregnant women; in men, who typically have more muscle than women; and in tall, thin people, whose larger surface area radiates more heat. Even when two people are the same sex, height, and weight, one's metabolism may burn 1,400 kcalories a day, the other person's 1,000. No one knows why.

Everybody Gets Fatter with Age

Between the ages of 20 and 50, the typical body both adds fat and loses muscle. The fat content of a man's body usually doubles, while a woman's increases by half. It happens because the metabolism slows by two percent each decade; and unless you maintain or increase your activity level, you'll inevitably get fatter. A small weight gain may not be bad. Some evidence suggests that people who *slowly* gain weight with age may not be adding to their risk of disease or premature death.

of the vital processes in which energy and nutrients from foods are made available to and utilized by the body. **Basal metabolic rate**, or BMR, is the minimum level of energy required by the body to simply stay alive while completely at rest, without considering digestion. **Resting metabolic rate**, or RMR, is the BMR plus the energy needed to digest food.

Metabolic rate differs from person to person, depending on a variety of factors. Not only do people inherit or develop a wide variation in metabolic rates, but there are also important sex differences in metabolism. The average BMR for women is between 5 and 10 percent lower than that for men, partly because women naturally have a larger percentage of body fat and smaller muscle mass than most men. There are also substantial differences in metabolism between lean and obese people. When thin people eat, they dissipate kcalories through heat loss to a greater degree than do fatter people. Compared to lean people, obese people are better at storing energy and more efficient in expending energy.

In addition to individual differences in metabolism, the body has the ability to alter the rate of metabolism and to defend a particular level of weight or energy balance. If a person begins to starve or undertakes a fast of more than a day or two, his or her metabolism will slow down. This tendency toward metabolic slowdown is even greater for the person who has a history of dieting. Restrictive dieting or caloric deprivation can cause metabolism to slow down dramatically, and this slowdown is most marked in people whose initial metabolic rate is already low—possibly the majority of obese people. Repeated dieting causes metabolic rate to fall more rapidly and rebound more slowly. Thus weight is lost more slowly and regained more rapidly with each diet—the so-called yo-yo effect.

Fat Cell Theory According to fat cell theory, the quantity of fat stored in the body is the result of the number of fat cells that a person has and their size. People with an above-average number of fat cells may have been born with them or may have developed them at certain critical times because of overfeeding. Childhood-onset obesity, or hyperplasia, is thought to be the result of developing too many fat cells. Adult-onset obesity, or hypertrophy, is the result of developing bigger, rather than more, fat cells. Some very obese people are thought to have a combination of both too many fat cells and extraordinarily large fat cells. As the theory goes, having extra fat cells

creates a biological pressure to keep these fat cells full, but the scientific evidence for this is not clear.

At one time researchers thought that the number of fat cells stabilized some time in adolescence and that additional fat cells could not be developed after that; nor could fat cells once developed be lost. We now believe that new fat cells can be developed at almost any time in life, most likely in response to prolonged overeating when existing fat cells reach the limit of their fat storage capacity. Similarly, it seems that the number of fat cells can be decreased if weight is kept off for an extended period. More research is needed to determine the actual relevance of fat cell theory to the development and maintenance of obesity in humans.

Overeating Although "common sense" tells us overeating is involved in weight gain, research has not been able to prove that all or even most obese people eat more than normal people. Of course, it is true that the obese overeat in the sense that their caloric intake is too great to keep them thin, but they don't necessarily eat abnormally large amounts of food. Indeed, many overweight people maintain their weight on relatively modest intakes. Something other than excessive kcalorie consumption must explain the situation, perhaps a metabolism that is either naturally efficient in storing kcalories or that has adapted to maintaining weight on lower intakes.

Psychological Problems At one time most health professionals believed that obesity was the result of psychological problems. Yet research has shown that overweight people are no more neurotic than are people of normal weight and do not suffer more psychiatric disturbance. No particular personality characteristics are consistently linked with obesity, although some obese people tend to be more dependent and passive than average. Although the obese may be more emotional in certain circumstances, by and large negative emotions are the result of concern about weight and failed efforts to reduce. Dieting per se can cause emotional disturbances—the most common complaints being anxiety, irritability, depression, and a preoccupation with food.

Obese Eating Style When they found few personality differences between the obese and others, psychologists attempted to identify an obese eating style. Few consistent differences were found. Both lean and fat people reported eating in the absence of hunger, eating rapidly,

---

Basal metabolic rate (BMR) The minimum level of energy required by the body to simply stay alive while completely at rest, but without having eaten.

Resting metabolic rate (RMR) BMR plus the energy needed to digest food.

TACTICS AND TIPS

Scaling Down

If you want to shed pounds while eating a balanced diet, the key is watching your portion sizes. But study after study has shown that people are very poor estimators of portion sizes, and most of us have trouble accurately describing or even remembering what we've eaten the day before. Indeed, during the first week or so of your new eating program it may be wise to keep a diary of what you eat—measured as precisely as possible. Don't forget to include estimated amounts of toppings, gravies, and garnishes. If your eating plan allows only three ounces of skinless chicken breast, do you know what a three-ounce portion looks like on the plate? It's not much bigger than a pack of playing cards or the palm of your hand.

In order to stick to an eating plan, a kitchen scale is as wise an investment as a bathroom scale. Use it when you cook, especially for such calorie-dense foods as meat, fish, or cheese. Train your eye to remember what a reasonable portion looks like so that eventually you won't have to rely on scales or calorie counters. Be sure your kitchen is equipped with measuring cups and spoons, and follow recipes to the letter.

UC Berkeley Wellness Letter, April 1988. Vol. 4, No. 7.

and having frequent snacks. Only one thing seemed to differentiate the obese—good-tasting food kept them eating longer.

Externality Theory   Although few real differences in eating style have been found, investigators thought that the obese might be more sensitive to external cues to eat. To support this externality theory, they looked for evidence that time of day, elapsed time between eating episodes, sight of food, and association of eating with particular cues might account for differences between lean and obese. In fact, environmental cues are intimately linked to eating behavior, but this was found to be true for people in every weight category. Overweight people on the average are more responsive than lean people to food cues in the environment, but many people of normal weight are too.

Lifestyle and Weight   Most weight problems are in fact lifestyle problems. Researchers have found a strong relationship between socioeconomic status (SES) and obesity as well as other eating disorders. The prevalence of obesity goes down as SES level goes up, but bulimia and anorexia (discussed later in this chapter) are more likely in children of families oriented toward high achievement. One major study found that the rate of obesity in women was 30 percent for the lower SES group, 16 percent of the middle group, and only 5 percent for the higher group. More women are obese at lower SES levels than are men, but men are somewhat more obese at the higher SES levels than are women. These differences may reflect the greater sensitivity and concern for a slim physical appearance among upper SES women. It may also reflect the greater acceptance of obesity among low-income and certain ethnic groups, as well as different subcultural values related to food choices.

In addition to poor nutrition and lack of adequate exercise, an unhealthy lifestyle is characterized by too many obligations and too few rewards. Sometimes the seeds of an unhealthy lifestyle are planted early, in the family of origin. When a family advocates setting high goals for accomplishment, being a perfectionist, putting work first, and not balancing obligations with personal rewards, it establishes the basis for a lifestyle that may support a weight problem.

Social and cultural influences further complicate the picture. Food is used to show friendship and caring; it is part of the social fabric and is involved in celebrations and social gatherings. In our society, eating well and sharing food with friends are highly valued activities. Food is a symbol of love and caring.

Resources for Getting Help   What should you do if you are overweight? Several approaches are possible.

Doing It Yourself   Research by Dr. Stanley Schachter at Columbia University indicates that people are far more successful than was previously thought at losing weight and keeping it off. Schachter found that about 64 percent of the people he studied achieved long-term success without joining a formal program or getting special help. Supporting Schachter's findings, a 1979 Public Health Service survey indicated that around 50 percent of the general public succeed with long-term weight management.

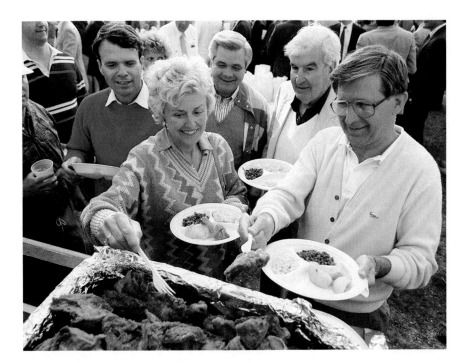

Eating is so intimately bound up with the social fabric of everyday life that people trying to change their diets often meet unexpected obstacles and difficulties. Fried chicken is obviously an integral part of this company picnic, not easily avoided even by those who are aware of its high fat content.

TACTICS AND TIPS

Getting Started on a Sensible Diet

You *can* pull off a successful diet without special guidance. The way to start is by determining how much food you really ought to be eating. To figure out your kcalorie needs, multiply the weight you'd *like to be* by one of the following numerals:

- Sedentary
  (walk sometimes but never run or swim)
  10 for a woman; 13 for a man
- Moderately active
  (exercise three times a week)
  13 for a woman; 15 for a man
- Very active
  (exercise vigorously almost every day)
  15 for a woman; 20 for a man

The number you'll get is an estimate of the kcalories you'll need to maintain your ideal weight.

Say, for instance, that you're a medium-height, moderately active woman. You want to reclaim your trim high school weight of 120 pounds. The calculation would go: 120 × 13 = 1,560 kcalories—call it 1,600.

You need to know that number so you don't cut back *too much*. An overly strict dieter may not get enough vitamins and minerals, and will be sluggish and grouchy—a sure route to failure. Experts advise cutting your daily energy intake to no less than 1,100 or 1,200 kcalories.

To lose 1 pound a week, delete 500 kcalories a day, no matter what you weigh. The easiest way to do that is to avoid as much fat as you can—in cheese, mayonnaise, potato chips, salad dressing, cooking oil, red meats, and ice cream.

(Passing up one chocolate-covered extra-rich ice cream bar will save you 450 kcalories.) Satisfy snack cravings with fresh fruit or low-fat yogurt.

If you want to try for a 2-pound-a-week loss but can't ditch 1,000 kcalories a day without going under 1,200 kcalories, try cutting back by 500 and then getting more exercise to burn off the rest. Generally, losing no more than 2 or 3 pounds a week is best because your body gets time to adjust—no sudden shocks to the system.

When you hit your target weight, you can have bigger portions—to reach your ideal 1,600 kcalories—as long as you don't cut your exercise.

Excerpted from IN HEALTH. Copyright © 1989 Hippocrates Partners.

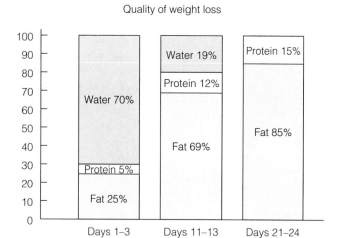

Quality of weight loss

Figure 13-4 Quality of weight loss. Most weight lost during the first three days of any weight loss program is water.

Other research by Dr. Robert Colvin of Southern Illinois University and Dr. Susan B. Olsen of the Southwest Bariatric Clinic of Phoenix investigated the characteristics that distinguished those who lost at least 20 percent of body weight and maintained this loss for two years or more. Although some (mostly women) had used diet alone to lose weight, some had used exercise alone, and others had used a combination of diet and exercise, virtually all maintained their success by making exercise a permanent part of their lifestyle. They also kept tabs on their weight and habits. In addition, they learned to develop their own diet, exercise, and maintenance plans, and they became more involved in and excited by activities other than eating—such as careers, projects, and special interests.

If you need to lose weight, focus on adopting the healthy lifestyle we've described. The "right" weight for you will naturally evolve, and you won't have to diet. However, if you must diet, do so in combination with exercise, and avoid very low kcalorie diets. (A nearby box discusses fallacies—and facts—about crash diets.) Realize that most low-kcalorie diets cause a rapid loss of body water at first. When this phase passes, weight loss declines. As a result, dieters are often misled into believing that their efforts are not working. They then give up, not realizing that smaller losses later in the diet are actually better than the initial big losses, because later loss is mostly fat loss, whereas initial loss was primarily fluid.

A study conducted to analyze quality of weight loss demonstrates how this process works. Subjects were put

on a 1,000-kcalories-per-day diet and exercised for 2½ hours a day; the program lasted 24 days. Figure 13-4 illustrates the results. During the first few days, subjects averaged 1.8 pounds weight loss per day, but 70 percent was due to fluid loss. As the program continued, weight loss due to fluid became progressively less. By the middle three days, subjects were losing an average of 0.5 pounds per day, but only 19 percent was due to fluid loss. Finally by days 21-24, weight loss due to fluid dumping had ceased, and 89 percent of the 0.4 pounds lost per day was due to fat loss.

Diet Books   Many people who try to lose weight by themselves fall prey to one or more of the dozens of diet books on the market. Although a very few of these do contain useful advice and tips for motivation, most make promises they can't fulfill. Some guidelines for evaluating and choosing a diet book can be offered:

1. Reject books that advocate an unbalanced way of eating. These include books advocating a high-carbohydrate-only diet, such as *Bloomingdale's Eat Healthy Diet*, or those advocating low-carbohydrate/high-protein diets, such as *The Complete Scarsdale Medical Diet* and *Dr. Atkin's Diet Revolution*.

2. Reject books that claim to be based on a "scientific breakthrough" or to have the "secret" to success. Examples include *The T-Factor Diet* and *The La Costa Book of Nutrition*.

3. Reject books that use gimmicks, like combining foods in special ways to achieve weight loss, rotating levels of kcalories, or purporting that a weight problem is due to food allergies, food sensitivities, or yeast infections. Examples include *The Beverly Hills Diet*, *Fit for Life*, *The Rotation Diet*, *The Two-Day Diet*, *The Diet-Type Weight-Loss Program*.

4. Accept books that advocate a balanced approach to diet plus exercise and sound nutrition advice. Some books to consider include *The I-Don't-Eat (But-I-Can't Lose) Weight Loss Program*, by Steven Jonas and Virginia Aronson, *Maximize Your Body Potential*, by Joyce D. Nash, and *The Weighting Game*, by Lawrence E. Lamb.

Dangerous Do-It-Yourself Options   Using commercially available supplements for modified fasting can be a dangerous option, especially if they are the sole source of nutrition, because there is no medical monitoring by a physician. Such approaches include powders used to make shakes that substitute for some or all of the daily food intake, as well as food bars. Many provide fewer than 800 kcalories a day. Although the products available today are much improved over the liquid-protein supplements that contributed to many dieters' deaths in the

Myths about Crash Diets

Myth "Crash" or very low kcalorie diets will lead to a permanent loss of body weight and to a swift loss of body fat in a short time ('Lose 10 pounds in 10 days!').

Fact Any rapid weight loss in the first several days of dieting is due to body water, not fat. Going "on a strict diet" is usually followed by going "off a diet," and a return of the lost weight, sometimes even more weight than before.

Myth Very restricted dieting (for example, only eating fresh fruits or milk products) can be safe and effective in losing weight rapidly.

Fact Such diets are very unsafe because the body needs a complete balance of four basic food types (beans, grains, and nuts; fruits and vegetables; milk products; and poultry, fish, eggs) to ensure sufficient intake of complex carbohydrates, proteins, and fats as well as vitamins, minerals, and electrolytes daily.

Myth Fasting is the most powerful strategy to use in taking off excessive weight rapidly.

Fact Complete fasting can be very dangerous for several reasons. First, the body can lose almost as much lean body mass (from 30 to 50 percent), such as muscle tissue, as fat tissue. This protein malnutrition can seriously disrupt liver, kidney, and lung functioning as well as the nervous system. Also, fasting can reduce the body's level of antibodies that are essential in fighting disease. Fasting also reduces the storage of glycogen (glucose) in the body's muscles. Reduced glycogen can lower physical activity levels and may encourage diabetes. Finally, fasting stimulates the liver to release more poor-quality cholesterol into the bloodstream (low-density lipoprotein, or LDL) and reduces availability of the better-quality cholesterol (high-density lipoprotein, or HDL cholesterol).

Myth Skipping meals helps lose weight.

Fact Actually, skipping meals, such as breakfast, commonly leads to overeating at the next meal, *and, more importantly*, contributes to energy and mood changes that make it more difficult to lose weight. Eating *more* often, such as minimeals four to six times a day ("grazing"), and avoiding fats and refined sugars encourage weight loss by controlling appetite and increasing energy levels so that vigorous aerobic-type physical activities can be performed.

1970s, only careful medical evaluation and monitoring can significantly reduce the risk of such an approach. Furthermore, dietary supplements teach reliance on patented products, not on sound, lifelong eating habits. And although weight loss can be rapid, muscle tends to be lost too, and weight is often regained.

Choosing a Weight Control Program If losing weight on your own does not seem feasible, you may decide to turn to a commercial weight loss program. Many such programs now include nutrition education, an emphasis on exercise, and a focus on changing behavior and lifestyle—all believed necessary for successful, long-term weight management. But programs differ widely. You should understand the differences and how they might affect your own needs and preferences, as well as your chances for success. A nearby box gives tips on evaluating programs.

After evaluating the legitimacy of a weight loss program, consider your own needs and preferences. If you have never tried a formal approach before, Weight Watchers is a good choice. The inspirational group approach works for many people, the dietary recommendations are regarded highly by the experts, and best of all, Weight Watchers is one of the least expensive programs. If large groups turn you off, however, consider The Diet Center. The Diet Center (and its clones) offers one-to-one individual counseling and frequent—usually daily—contact. Some nutrition experts quarrel with The Diet Center's dietary recommendations and the fact that it pushes its own brand of vitamin supplements (at a higher price than can be found elsewhere). Still, The Diet Center is a solution for many. Suppose you hate shopping for and preparing meals. Nutri/System takes away the need to choose and minimizes shopping and preparation by supplying you with prepackaged diet food. If you have a compulsive overeating problem, Overeaters Anonymous may be an alternative. Patterned after Alcoholic Anonymous, it teaches the twelve steps. Different programs may work for different individuals; Table 13-5 compares nine types of programs.

Table 13-5 How popular diet programs compare

	Approach	Staff
OPTIFAST	Clients eat powdered meal replacements, to which vitamins and minerals have been added. 4-phase program: modified fast, 420 calories per day for adults; realimentation, 800 calories; stabilization, according to individual needs; maintenance: calories determined during stabilization. Individual and group counseling; behavior modification taught, exercise encouraged.	R.D., M.D., psychologist at most locations; all clients must be under M.D. supervision.
DIET CENTER	4-phase program includes: reducing, 915 calories for women and 1,045 for men; maintenance, 1,500 for women and 1,700 for men. Highly restrictive food plan relies on vitamin/mineral supplements. Dairy foods forbidden during reducing phase. Starches limited unrealistically. Individual counseling; behavior modification taught, exercise encouraged.	Counselors are (nonprofessional) clients trained in Diet Center philosophy, who've lost weight under the program; health professionals at headquarters only; includes one R.D. and medical consultants.
WEIGHT WATCHERS	3-phases: Quick Start Plus, 1,000 calories for adults; reducing, 1,200 for women and 1,600 for men; maintenance, according to individual needs. Food plan has wide variety of foods. Group counseling; behavior modification taught, exercise encouraged.	Counselors are (nonprofessional) clients trained in Weight Watchers philosophy, who've lost weight under the program; health professionals at headquarters only; includes R.D.'s, psychologist, M.D., and other consultants.
TAKE OFF POUNDS SENSIBLY (TOPS)	Nonprofit, mutual support group where members meet to discuss sensible, safe weight loss and management. No standard food plan; members follow individual diets prescribed by their personal physicians. No individual counseling; local chapters are self-directed, so each one has its own approach.	Elected (nonprofessional) volunteer members direct local activities.
NUTRI/SYSTEM	Clients eat special prepackaged entrees and use "flavor sprays" as snack substitutes. Both supplied exclusively by company. 2 phases: reducing, 1,000 calories for adults; maintenance, according to individual needs. Individual and group counseling; behavior modification taught, exercise encouraged.	Locations include R.N. and psychological counselor (B.S. in psychology); professional health staff including R.D.'s at headquarters.
OVEREATERS ANONYMOUS	Nonprofit, mutual support group. Program based on 12 steps of Alcoholics Anonymous; members admit they have a weight problem, then take one-day-at-a-time steps to avoid overeating. No nutritional guidance provided; members encouraged to consult their own M.D.'s or R.D.'s.	Volunteer (nonprofessional) members direct local activities.
REGISTERED DIETITIANS IN PRIVATE PRACTICE	R.D. tailors diet regimen and calorie levels to client's individual needs. Individual and group counseling; behavior modification taught, exercise encouraged.	Registered dietitian; may work in association with other health professionals, such as M.D., psychologist, exercise physiologist.
HOSPITAL WEIGHT LOSS CLINICS	Treatment programs, and thus calorie levels, vary greatly. Individual and group counseling; behavior modification taught, exercise encouraged.	R.D. generally on staff; other health professionals, such as M.D., R.N., and psychologist, may be involved.
RESIDENTIAL FACILITIES, SPAS	Varies greatly. A serious residential facility focusing on weight loss and general good health may have highly educational programs. A more socially oriented spa may provide "pampering," i.e., steam room, massage, etc., with option of eating low-calorie foods.	Varies greatly; residential facility typically has R.D., medical director, exercise physiologist, either on staff or as consultant. Spas may not have any health professionals.

Table 13-5 How popular diet programs compare (continued)

Length	Availability	Prices	Comments
Modified fast, 12 weeks maximum; realimentation, 6 weeks; stabilization, 8 weeks; maintenance, no limit.	About 500 centers across U.S. Headquarters in Minneapolis.	Varies; typically $1,500–$2,500 for six months; includes powdered meals.	Clients must be 30% above ideal body weight. *Borderline recommended,* only for people with significant excess weight or those who need to lose weight to alleviate a medical condition.
Reducing, until goal weight is reached; stabilization, 3 weeks maximum; maintenance, one year with staff supervision.	2,100 locations in U.S. and Canada Headquarters in Rexburg, Idaho.	$35–$75 per week ($2,000–$4,000/year); does not include meals.	*Not recommended* because of highly restrictive diet.
Quick Start Plus, 4 weeks; reducing, until goal weight achieved; maintenance, 6 weeks; if successful, then become a lifetime member.	Every major U.S. city and many smaller ones (24 countries worldwide). Headquarters in Jericho, N.Y.	$25 to join, plus $7.50 per week ($390/year).	Clients must want to lose at least 10 pounds. *Generally recommended* because of sensible food plan and well-rounded approach, but beware of unrealistic expectation of fast initial weight loss.
No limit	Every U.S. state (11,580 chapters worldwide) Headquarters in Milwaukee.	$12/year plus local chapter fee (avg. 50¢/month).	Main focus on group support. *Borderline recommended* due to lack of professional guidance, lack of consistent approach for all chapters. Prospective members should evaluate each chapter individually.
Varies; until goal weight achieved.	800 locations in U.S. and Canada. Headquarters in Willow Grove, Penn.	Company declined to quote price range, but said cost varies according to how much weight each client wants to lose, among other factors. Entrees and flavor sprays cost an extra $40–$50 per week.	*Not recommended* due to total initial reliance on company-supplied packaged foods.
No limit.	7,000 chapters in more than 30 countries. Headquarters in Torrance, Calif.	No membership fee; local chapters may set small fees for meetings.	Main focus on self-discovery of reasons for overeating. 1981 study showed that 22.5% kept lost weight off after two years. *Borderline recommended* due to lack of professional guidance, lack of consistency in approach for each chapter. Each one must be evaluated individually.
Varies according to goal weight desired.	Every state; many R.D.'s have offices in hospitals.	Usually hourly rate; varies according to area of country; range, $20–$75/hour.	*Generally recommended* due to highly individualized, personalized, professional approach. To receive a list of registered dietitians in your area, write to Holly F. David, R.D., public relations director of Consulting Nutritionists in Private Practice. Address: 32 Broadway South, Westbrook, Conn. 06498.
Varies according to goal weight desired.	Most major hospitals.	Varies according to area of country; can be on per-visit or complete-program basis. May be less expensive than seeing an R.D. in private practice.	*Generally recommended* because programs are directed by health professionals, but beware that many hospitals offer commercial programs, such as Optifast. Hospital programs must be evaluated individually.
Varies from 2–3 days to 4 weeks or longer.	Scattered throughout U.S., many in SW, NE, SE regions.	Varies greatly; range, $50–$350 per day.	Residential facilities and spas provide opportunity to immerse self in program away from daily stresses and distractions. *Borderline recommended* due to inconsistency in approach among facilities and spas. Each must be evaluated individually.

Environmental Nutrition, August 1987.

Using a particular brand of diet or health products helps some people lose weight, but making sound lifestyle choices is the real key to maintaining an ideal body weight.

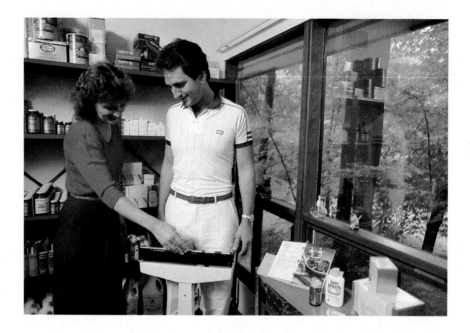

Traditionally, registered dietitians (R.D.s) have considered dietary counseling and weight management their territory. More and more dietitians are going into private practice or conducting weight control programs, sometimes through hospitals or clinics. Dietitians are especially good at teaching innovative ways of managing food, but they sometimes become unduly focused on food and forget about the other aspects of weight management.

More physicians are also getting into the weight control game. The pill-pushing and shot-giving "diet docs" of a few years ago are beginning to be edged out by physicians who genuinely want to bring appropriate medical management to their obese patients. Often the new brand of diet doctor is a member of an interdisciplinary team consisting of at least a dietitian and a mental health counselor. Most physicians working with obesity specialize in techniques appropriate only for severe obesity—drugs, surgery, or supplemented fasting.

Extraordinary Measures   **Morbid obesity** is a serious medical condition defined as being 100 pounds or more above ideal weight. It is associated with a six- to twelve-fold increase in mortality rates, as well as with a variety of medical problems and conditions, including skin rashes, joint and bone problems, hypertension, obstetrical problems, coronary artery disease, anesthesia-related

complications, endocrine dysfunctions, and so forth. The serious morbidity and mortality risk associated with morbid obesity justifies, in most cases, the use of extraordinary measures to try to correct it. One such measure is the use of a very low kcalorie diet (VLCD). These diets, which provide 300–600 kcalories per day, are designed to prevent inappropriate loss of lean body mass by providing large amounts of dietary protein (70–100 grams a day) of high biological value. They appear to be safe when limited to periods of three months or less under careful medical supervision. However, weight regain after a VLCD is widely believed to be a serious problem.

Getting Psychological Help   Although some people do seek individual psychotherapy for treatment of obesity, it is not clear whether psychotherapy alone can help. Often people choose this potential solution when they feel they have tried everything else and failed, or when the emotional disturbance from failed dieting efforts becomes unbearable. Although no empirical evidence supports the notion, some clinicians feel that some obesity is associated with early child abuse, particularly sexual abuse. Likewise, other eating disorders—**anorexia nervosa** and **bulimia**—may sometimes have their origins in early childhood experiences. No evidence exists that merely exploring the historical roots of such problems

---

Morbid obesity   A relatively rare but serious medical condition defined as being 100 pounds or more above ideal weight.

How to Evaluate Commercial Weight Loss Programs

The National Council Against Health Fraud disparages commercial weight control programs that:

1. Promise or imply dramatic, rapid weight loss (substantially more than 1 percent of total body weight per week).

2. Promote diets that are extremely low in kcalories (below 800 kcalories per day; 1,200-kcalorie diets are preferred) unless under the supervision of competent medical experts.

3. Attempt to make clients dependent upon special products rather than teaching how to make good choices from the conventional food supply. (This does not condemn the marketing of low-kcalorie convenience foods which may be chosen by consumers.)

4. Do not encourage permanent, realistic lifestyle changes including regular exercise and the behavioral aspects of eating wherein food may be used as a coping device.

(Programs should focus upon changing the causes of overweight rather than simply the effects, which is the overweight itself.)

5. Misrepresent salespeople as "counselors" supposedly qualified to give guidance in nutrition and/or general health. Even if adequately trained, such "counselors" would still be objectionable because of the obvious conflict-of-interest that exists when providers profit directly from products they recommend and sell.

6. Require large sums of money at the start or require that clients sign contracts for expensive, long-term programs. Such practices too often have been abused as salespeople focus attention upon signing up new people rather than delivering continuing, satisfactory service to consumers. Programs should be on a pay-as-you-go basis.

7. Fail to inform clients about the risks associated with weight loss in general or the specific program being promoted.

8. Promote unproven or spurious weight loss aids such as human chorionic gonadotropin hormone (HCG), starch blockers, diuretics, sauna belts, body wraps, passive exercise, ear stapling, acupuncture, electric muscle stimulating (EMS) devices, spirulina, amino acid supplements, and so forth.

9. Claim that "cellulite" exists in the body.

10. Claim that use of an appetite suppressant or a "bulking agent" enables a person to lose body fat without restricting accustomed caloric intake.

11. Claim that a weight control product contains a unique ingredient or component unless it is unavailable in other weight control products.

From *Nutrition Forum*, March 1988, Vol. 5, No. 3.

helps reduce overeating or relieve eating disorders. Together with a program specifically focused on managing obesity, bulimia, or anorexia nervosa, individual psychotherapy may be beneficial.

Eating Disorders

Problems of body weight and weight control are not limited to excessive body fat. A growing number of people, especially teenagers and young adults, experience what are called "eating disorders," problems associated with food and eating. Western society's emphasis on extreme thinness as the ideal for females places many young women in conflict about their weight. Although the typical woman under the age of 30 has become heavier by 5–6 pounds, the ideal body weight as reflected by winners of the Miss America Pageant and magazine centerfolds has declined since the 1960s. This widening gap between reality and ideal for most young women is reflected in their high rates of body dissatisfaction.

■ **Exploring Your Emotions**

Have you ever been tempted to engage in self-starvation or purging? If so, what kinds of pressures made you feel that way, and what seemed to be the benefit you would derive from it? How do you feel about the fact that most anorexics and bulimics are women?

Research has found that the majority of adolescent girls and young women in the United States and Western Europe dislike their bodies and report that they have dieted to lose weight. The proportion of young women who say that they "feel fat" and would like to lose weight generally ranges from approximately 50 to 80 percent. Yet most of these young women are within the normal weight range. By self-report, low-kcalorie diets appear to be the most popular weight loss regime among this population. A random sample of 400 college students found that 47 percent reported using such a diet since starting college. Although investigators have found that dieting increases the risk for binge eating, we still don't know what proportion of dieters who binge proceed to a level of severity that interferes with their lives. Likewise we don't know the degree to which a preoccupation with body shape, body-image dissatisfaction, and extreme dieting contribute to the development of eating disorders.

Anorexia Nervosa   A person suffering from anorexia nervosa doesn't eat enough food to maintain a reasonable body weight. (Weight that is 15 percent below normal—and lower—is now viewed as potentially unhealthy.) Anorexics maintain themselves on starvation diets and often combine eating very little with being very physically active. Onset of this disorder generally occurs during adolescence and is believed to be related to maturational problems brought on by the stresses of puberty. It is hypothesized that a "weight phobia" is central to anorexia nervosa and that anorexics avoid many of the social consequences of adolescence by reducing weight, obliterating secondary sexual characteristics, and returning to a prepubertal role. Some research suggests that genetic factors also play a role in anorexia nervosa, but the mechanism for this is unknown.

Anorexia is more prevalent among females, particularly in the middle and upper social classes. Factors that may be conducive to the development of anorexia include high and competitive achievement standards, ambivalence about feminine role definitions and sexuality, and being reinforced for dependent behavior. Anorexia affects between 1 and 3 million Americans, mostly women. It is life-threatening and ends in death between 15 and 20 percent of the time.

The diagnostic criteria for anorexia nervosa set forth by the American Psychiatric Association in their *Diagnostic and Statistical Manual of Mental Disorders, Third Edition—Revised* (DSM-III-R) include:

1. Refusal to maintain body weight over a minimal normal weight for age and height (for example, weight loss leading to maintenance of body weight 15 percent below that expected); or failure to make expected weight gain during period of growth, leading to body weight 15 percent below that expected.
2. Intense fear of gaining weight or becoming fat, even though underweight.
3. Disturbance in the way in which one's body weight, size, or shape is experienced; for example, the person claims to "feel fat" even when emaciated, believes that one area of the body is "too fat" even when obviously underweight.
4. In females, absence of at least three consecutive menstrual cycles when otherwise expected to occur (primary or secondary amenorrhea—a woman has amenorrhea if her periods occur only following hormone administration.)

Typically, the anorexic is a "restricting" person who rigidly sticks to a starvation-like diet. She also commonly uses vigorous and prolonged physical activities to reduce body weight. Anorexics tend to differ in personality from women who are of normal weight or who suffer from other problems such as bulimia nervosa. Researchers describe the anorexic as somewhat obsessive, usually introverted, emotionally reserved and socially insecure, very self-critical, self-denying and deferential to others, and overly rigid and stereotyped in her thinking. Whereas the bulimic tends to be more socially outgoing, more labile (up and down) in emotional state, and more socially deviant (for example, more likely to smoke, abuse alcohol, and other drugs), the anorexic tends to favor health foods, be obsessive about health issues, and take charge of the preparation of meals (even though she rarely eats them).

Most research on treating anorexia deals with behavioral and pharmacologic approaches, although the place of the latter in treatment is not entirely clear. Most therapists agree that there are two stages to the treatment of the anorexic patient: first, restoration of body weight to

---

Anorexia nervosa   An eating disorder characterized by a refusal to eat enough food to maintain normal, healthy body weight and/or the use of measures to produce severe weight loss. Anorexics do experience hunger and appetite but resist the impulse to eat.

Bulimia   An eating disorder characterized by alternating binging and purging by means of vomiting, laxatives or diuretics, or excessive exercise. Bulimics can be normal weight or overweight.

as near normal as possible, usually accomplished in a specialized inpatient setting; and second, longer-term therapy directed toward preventing relapse. Anorexia is a long-term illness, lasting as long as 10 years in some individuals. Treatment for anorexia (and bulimia) is most successful when it begins early, but the symptoms are often not recognized until the eating habits are well established.

Bulimia   Unlike anorexia nervosa, which has been recognized as a distinct, if relatively rare, syndrome dating back at least to the seventeenth century, bulimia is a new development. Although early reports of bulimic behavior date back to the late 1800s, detailed reports of bulimic symptoms began to appear only around 1940. The term *bulimarexia* was first used in 1979 to identify a behavior pattern similar to but different from anorexia in a large number of female students seeking treatment at Cornell University. Bulimia, which literally means "ox hunger," typically involves trying to stay on a strict low-kcalorie diet, but inevitably going on a food-eating binge or eating more than intended, and then deliberately forcing oneself to vomit or purge before the food is digested. In an article coining the term *bulimia nervosa*, Gerald Russell listed criteria for bulimics: (1) the patients suffer from powerful and intractable urges to overeat, (2) they seek to avoid the fattening effects of food by inducing vomiting or abusing purgatives or both, and (3) they have a morbid fear of becoming fat.

According to the American Psychiatric Association's *DSM-III-R* manual, the diagnostic criteria for bulimia nervosa are:

1. Recurrent episodes of binge eating (rapid consumption of a large amount of food in a discrete period of time).
2. A feeling of lack of control over eating behavior during the eating binges.
3. Regularly engaging in either self-induced vomiting, use of laxatives or diuretics, strict dieting or fasting, or vigorous exercise in order to prevent weight gain.
4. A minimum average of two binge eating episodes a week for at least three months.
5. Persistent overconcern with body shape and weight.

Bulimia has been confined almost exclusively to women, the majority of whom are in their twenties. Like anorexia, it affects women from upper socioeconomic classes the most. More and more, however, bulimia is affecting males and older women. Studies show the average age of onset for females to be approximately 18 with a range from 9 to 45. The illness usually lasts about 5 years.

The onset of bulimic symptoms often follows a period of restrictive dieting. This concern with dieting is often associated with a developing interest in the opposite sex. Traumatic events such as loss or separation from a significant person are also associated with the onset of bulimic behavior as are feelings about sexual changes or arguments with significant others. In one study, 40 percent of the respondents attributed the onset of bulimia to difficulty in handling specific emotions, especially depression, loneliness, boredom, and anger. Interpersonal conflicts were also mentioned as precipitating factors.

Research is just beginning to shed light on the personality characteristics of bulimics. They may have problems identifying and describing internal states such as hunger, satiety, and various emotions. They appear to have highly variable moods that fluctuate from persistent fatigue and depression to feelings of agitation accompanied by impulsive behaviors. Their thinking is characterized by cognitive distortions that may contribute to feelings of depression and low self-esteem. They experience self-doubt and uncertainty as well as feelings of ineffectiveness. They have high self-expectations and tend to be very harsh, critical, and punitive in their evaluations of themselves. Despite being highly sensitive to signs of rejection or disapproval from others, they generally seek interpersonal relationships.

Research on treatment has concentrated on two approaches. The first, a psychological approach, aims at interrupting the restricted eating pattern through cognitive-behavioral therapy. The goal is to interrupt the revolving cycle of dietary restriction, binge eating, and purging by reinstating normal dietary habits while challenging the distorted beliefs that accompany the disorder. The second treatment approach, a pharmacological one, uses antidepressants to relieve the depression that is assumed to underlie the disorder. The main problem with this approach is that the medication may be vomited along with food. Research on the effectiveness of these approaches to treatment is just beginning, but preliminary results point to a good prognosis with cognitive-behavioral therapy.

Eating disorders are characterized by underlying emotional and psychological problems, but in a sense they can be seen as the logical extension of the concern with weight that pervades American society. Most people don't succumb to irrational or distorted ideas about their bodies, but many do become obsessed with dieting. The challenge facing Americans today is achieving a healthy body weight without excessive dieting—by adopting and maintaining sensible eating habits, an active lifestyle, realistic and positive attitudes and emotions, and creative ways to handle stress.

Summary

- The "secret" of maintaining ideal body weight is balancing kcalories consumed, especially fat kcalories, and kcalories expended in physical activity. Although millions of Americans—especially young women—are on diets at any given time, dieting is not a component of a healthy lifestyle.

Lifestyle and Weight Control

- The overweight problem that plagues American society can be traced to the sedentary, high-stress American lifestyle and the overly refined and processed foods that make up much of the American diet.
- Poor eating and exercising habits begin to catch up with people as the rapid growth of adolescence slows down and career and family obligations take up more time. The best time to get a healthy lifestyle in place is early adulthood, when good habits and behavior patterns have a better chance of taking hold.

Adopting a Healthy Lifestyle

- The four key factors in maintaining normal weight are nutrition, physical activity, thinking and emotions, and coping strategies.
- Making healthy food choices on a day-to-day basis is one of the key components of weight control.
- Although sugar causes tooth decay and may be addictive for some people, the real problem in the American diet is too much fat. A high-fat, high-sugar diet (the "supermarket diet") produces even more weight gain than a high-fat or high-sugar diet alone.
- Protein is amply supplied in the typical American diet, making protein supplements unnecessary for most people. Excess dietary protein is stored as body fat.
- Eating more complex carbohydrates is a key component in maintaining proper body weight. The body has to expend energy to digest complex carbohydrates, and eating starchy foods makes you feel full.
- Many people have trouble recognizing signs of hunger and knowing when they're full, both of which are important factors in maintaining proper weight. Additionally, many people continue eating after they're full because the food tastes good.
- Eating small, frequent meals is another important factor in weight control. It's a good idea to have a structure to guide eating (regular meal times) and decision rules to guide food choices (allowed foods). No foods should be placed permanently off limits; moderation in everything should be the rule.
- The second factor in maintaining proper body weight is physical activity. In addition to its many other benefits, exercise burns calories and keeps the metabolism geared up to active levels.
- Exercise is important to a weight loss or maintenance program because the body responds to dieting alone with lowered metabolic rates. Although weight can be lost without exercise, the rate of loss is increased—and the body is kept in better shape—if exercise, especially aerobic exercise, is part of the plan.
- The third factor in maintaining proper body weight is thinking and emotions. Many people have an internalized "idealized self," based on perfectionistic irrational beliefs, with which they frequently compare themselves. Such comparisons can lead to low self-esteem and other emotional problems and to negative "self-talk."
- Finally, maintaining proper body weight depends on having a repertoire of appropriate techniques for coping with stress and other challenges. Productive techniques include communicating effectively, being appropriately assertive, managing interpersonal conflicts constructively, keeping up relationships, and maintaining a sensible lifestyle.

Overcoming a Weight Problem

- People who have or think they may have a weight problem need to begin by determining by how much they're overweight and how much they should weigh.
- Using height-weight tables, researchers define obesity as being 20 percent or more above a person's upper weight limit, adjusted for sex and height. Using body composition techniques, researchers define obesity as a body fat content greater than 25 percent of total body weight for males and greater than 30 percent for females.
- Techniques for analyzing body composition include hydrostatic weighing, skinfold measurement, and electrical impedance analysis. Another technique that measures body weight but that correlates highly with direct measures of body fat is the body mass index.
- Rather than concerning themselves with elaborate measurements, individuals should focus on the four factors that go into maintaining normal weight. By living a healthy, balanced life, people can avoid the unhealthy dieting hysteria that has so many Americans in its grip.
- Physical, psychological, social, and cultural factors can all play a role in weight problems.
- Genetic factors influence many physical characteristics, but people can control whether they actually become obese by modifying their behavior and adopting a healthy lifestyle.

- Set point theory suggests that the body has a certain natural weight and resists moving away from it by very much. Although this theory seems to explain a commonly observed tendency, it may be that weight is controlled by an interplay of biological and environmental factors rather than simply by a genetically determined set point.
- Rate of metabolism is an important factor in weight control. Repeated dieting can cause the metabolic rate to decrease more rapidly and rebound more slowly, making it harder to lose pounds and easier to regain them with every dieting attempt.
- Fat cell theory suggests that obese people were born with more or larger fat cells than normal-weight people or developed them during childhood. Now it is thought that the number of fat cells can be increased at any time during life by overeating and decreased by keeping weight off.
- Overeating is not the main cause of obesity, nor are psychological problems or particular personality characteristics consistently associated with overweight. Obese people do not have a distinctive eating style, such as eating rapidly or frequently.
- Most weight problems are lifestyle problems. There is a strong association between weight problems and socioeconomic status, overweight being more common among people of lower SES and eating disorders being more common among people of higher SES. Many people are successful at losing weight and keeping it off. They use a combination of diet and exercise, take control of their lifestyles, and enjoy many things in life besides eating.
- A person who diets should be sure to exercise as well and should not follow a very low calorie diet. Such diets cause a rapid loss of weight—mostly water—at first and a much slower subsequent loss of fat, which leads many people to give up.
- A wealth of popular diet books are available in bookstores, but they should be carefully evaluated because many advocate useless or dangerous steps. Also dangerous are supplements for modified fasting if used without medical monitoring.
- Commercial weight control programs vary widely. Some are helpful but others are simply money-making ventures that rely on ineffective gimmicks. Registered dietitians and nutrition-conscious physicians are taking a more active role in weight control programs for individuals.
- The health risks associated with morbid obesity justify such extraordinary measures as surgery and very low calorie diets supervised by physicians. Psychological counseling can be used to support weight control programs but by itself does not solve a weight problem.

Eating Disorders

- Our society emphasizes unrealistic thinness as the body ideal for females. Many adolescent girls report being dissatisfied with their bodies, believing themselves to be "too fat."
- Anorexia nervosa is an eating disorder characterized by self-starvation, increased physical activity, distorted body image, intense fear of gaining weight, and cessation of menstrual periods. It requires intensive treatment that focuses first on restoring body weight and then on addressing underlying psychological problems and changing eating habits.
- Bulimia is an eating disorder characterized by intense concern with body weight, recurrent episodes of uncontrolled binge eating followed by feelings of guilt and depression, and frequent purges, either by self-induced vomiting or by using laxatives or diuretics. Bulimia is usually treated with either cognitive-behavioral therapy or with drug therapy.
- Although eating disorders are extreme conditions, many Americans are obsessed with dieting. The challenge is to maintain normal body weight by balancing diet and exercise.

Take Action

1. Investigate the commercial weight control programs that operate in your community. Evaluate them in terms of the eleven criteria listed in the box in this chapter. Are any of them questionable? Are any acceptable? Look at the frozen diet dinners in your supermarket, such as Weight Watchers and Lean Cuisine. How do they compare in terms of calories, fat content, and nutritional value?

2. Interview some people who have successfully lost weight and kept it off. What were their strategies and techniques? Do you think their approach would work for others?

3. Find out what percentage of your body weight is fat by taking one of the tests described in this chapter at your campus health clinic, sports medicine clinic, or health club. If you have too high a proportion of body fat, consider taking steps to reduce it.

4. Monitor your diet for a week to see exactly how much fat and sugar you consume. If these amounts are excessive, make a list of specific steps you can take to reduce them, such as those suggested in the boxes in this chapter.

Behavior Change Strategy

A Weight Control Plan

The behavior management plan described in Chapter 1 provides an excellent framework for a weight control program. Following are some suggestions about specific ways you can adapt that general plan to controlling your weight.

Goal-setting

Choose a reasonable weight you think you would like to reach over the long term, and be willing to renegotiate it as you get further along. Set a short-term goal of losing 10 pounds. Focus on reaching that goal, and when you do, set a new short-term goal of another 10 pounds. Keep doing this until you get close to your long-term goal. Decide whether you want to renegotiate your original number. Likewise, when setting behavioral goals, break them down into small, reasonable steps—big enough to be a challenge but not so big that you can't accomplish each step. Don't try to convert to a new behavior pattern all at once. Shape yourself into a new way of behaving by designing small, manageable steps that will get you to where you want to go.

Self-monitoring

Keep a chart, diary, or record of your weight and behavior change progress. Try keeping a record of everything you eat. Write down what you plan to eat, the quantity, and the caloric content as well. Do this *before* you eat it. You'll find that just having to record something that is "not okay" to eat is likely to stop you from eating it. If you also note what seems to be triggering your urges to eat (for example, you feel bored, it's lunchtime, someone offered you something, it was there so you ate it), you'll become more aware of your weak spots and be better able to take corrective action.

Stimulus control

Figure out what makes you want to eat. Then engineer your environment so that these cues are eliminated (or avoid them if you can't get rid of them). Go through your pantry and refrigerator and throw out or give away "trouble" food—ice cream, candy, cookies, etc. Avoid driving past the doughnut shop that always beckons you to stop. Ask your friends or fellow students not to offer you snack food. Anticipate problem situations and plan ways to handle them more effectively.

Social support

Get others to help. Get someone to join your efforts to adopt a healthy lifestyle. Make an appointment with someone to exercise together. Talk to friends and family about what they can do to support your efforts. Give them lots of praise for helping.

Reward yourself appropriately

Use lots of self-praise; think good thoughts. (Definitely avoid self-criticism, even when you slip.) Plan special non-food treats for yourself—a walk, a movie, an afternoon's reprieve from studying—when you accomplish a small step or short-term goal. Don't wait for the long-term goal to reward yourself. Reward yourself often and for anything that counts toward success.

Cognitive strategies

Give yourself credit for even the smallest successes. Don't discount anything you can possibly count as progress. Tell yourself what you need to do next to stay on track. Think about your accomplishments and achievements. Give yourself lots of self-praise. Avoid demanding too much of yourself. Don't be a perfectionist; let yourself be human. Above all, don't criticize yourself!

Learn to recover from slips

When you have a slip (and you will, because you are human), learn from it. Decide what you might do to reduce the risk of its happening again. Identify the "high-risk" situations that set you up to backslide. Figure out how you can avoid such situations or change your response so that you win.

Selected Bibliography

Agras, W. S. 1987. *Eating Disorders: Management of Obesity, Bulimia, and Anorexia Nervosa*. New York: Pergamon Press.

Bray, G. A., Ed. 1989. Obesity: Basic aspects and clinical applications. *The Medical Clinics of North America*, 78(1). Philadelphia: W. B. Saunders.

Brownell, K. D., and J. P. Foreyt, Eds. 1986. *Handbook of Eating Disorders*. New York: Basic Books.

Kirkley, B. G., and J. C. Burge. 1989. Dietary restriction in young women: Issues and concern. *Annals of Behavioral Medicine*, 11(2):66–72.

Nash, J. D. 1987. Eating behavior and body weight: Physiological influences. *American Journal of Health Promotion*, 1(3):5–15.

Nash, J. D. 1987. Eating behavior and body weight: Psychological influences. *American Journal of Health Promotion*, 2(1):5–14.

Recommended Readings

Brody, J. 1985, 1987. *Jane Brody's Good Food Book.* New York: Norton. *Good nutrition information; easy to read.*

Jonas, S., and V. Aronson. 1989. *The I-Don't-Eat (But-I-Can't-Lose) Weight Loss Program.* New York: Rawson Associates. *An easy-to-read, accurate and balanced eating plan for people trying to lose weight or merely trying to begin a more healthful way of eating.*

Lamb, L. E. 1989. *The Weighting Game.* Secaucus, N.J.: Lyle Stuart. *Informational, not motivational. Provides straight talk about weight loss.*

Nash, J. D. 1986. *Maximize Your Body Potential.* Palo Alto, Calif.: Bull Publishing. *Winner of an award from the American Medical Writers Association, this book was designated "the most helpful book on lifetime weight management" by the Journal of Nutrition Education. Includes information on nutrition, exercise, cognition, and behavior change.*

Roth, G. 1984. *Breaking Free from Compulsive Eating.* New York: New American Library (Signet). *A book for bulimics and binge eaters; outlines a program for resolving the conflicts at the root of eating disorders.*

Contents

Making Connections

Exercise has nearly limitless benefits. It helps you control your weight, manage stress, boost your immune system, and protect yourself against heart disease, cancer, and perhaps even premature death. But knowing how and when to exercise can make a big difference in your benefits and enjoyment. The scenarios presented on these pages describe situations in which people have to use information, make a decision, or choose a course of action, all related to exercise and fitness. As you read them, imagine yourself in each situation and consider what you would do. After you finish the chapter, read the scenarios again and see if what you've learned has changed how you would think, feel, or act in each situation.

You just joined an aerobics class and notice that some of the students have water bottles that they keep on the side of the room. In between routines they seem to drink quite a lot of water. You thought you weren't supposed to drink while you were exercising, though you're not sure why. Most of the students don't bring water bottles. Should you bring one or not?

You and some friends are planning a cross-country ski vacation and have been looking at the trail maps from the ski resort. You all do resistance weight training at the gym and consider yourselves in excellent shape. One friend wants to tackle the longest and most arduous of the trails, but you're wondering if you should start out with something easier until your muscles get accustomed to the movements involved in cross-country skiing. Your friend says that because you're young and lift weights, you ought to be able to ski the toughest trail. Is he right? What should you plan for your trip?

14

Exercise for Health, Fitness, and Performance

Your roommate wanted to work some exercise into her crowded schedule, so she decided on swimming during the morning lap swim hours, 6 to 8 A.M. At first she loved it and swam for 45 minutes every day. But it's gotten harder for her as the mornings have gotten darker and colder. Last week it was raining every morning when she woke up, and she just couldn't face it. She's been down on herself about losing her motivation, and you'd like to help her out with some support or advice. What can you tell her about getting her fitness program back on track?

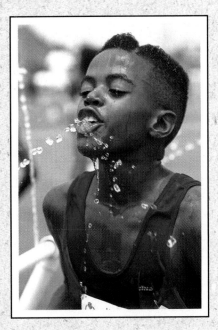

Your mother decided she wanted to get in shape, so you suggested she join a health club in her community and take their low-impact aerobics classes. She investigated one club but was intimidated by the whole scene. She said the manager wanted her to sign a three-year contract without taking it home to discuss with anyone else. She thought the instructors were more interested in looking at themselves in the mirror than in helping the students learn the exercises and dance routines. Your mother is discouraged about clubs now but doesn't know what else to do. Are all health clubs like that? What advice can you give her?

Your roommate was a star football player in high school and is going out for the freshman team. He told you he started taking steroids last summer because he's under pressure from back home to make the team. He's offered to get you some steroids to help you out with your body building program. You heard they were dangerous, but he says the health risks aren't significant in the short term. He hasn't experienced any ill effects and feels more competitive than ever. Should you give them a try?

Physical fitness is in. Millions of Americans are walking, jogging, and working out in gyms and fitness centers. They're talking about weight training, aerobic exercise, cardiorespiratory capacity, and body composition. Colleges are stressing regular exercise programs, and businesses are providing recreational and fitness facilities for their employees.

But the "fitness boom" is not without its casualties. Some people start an exercise program without enough thought and drop it a few months later because it's too time consuming, inconvenient, or boring. Some rush into sports or activities without proper training or knowledge, only to get benched with a sprained ankle or sore knee a week or two later. Many "weekend warriors" suffer overuse injuries from trying to squeeze all their activities into a 48-hour period.

Most of these difficulties arise because people don't have the basic knowledge and understanding they need to exercise properly and get the most from it. Many choose inappropriate activities or do too much too soon. When their program doesn't work out, they become frustrated and discouraged about exercise in general. At the same time, some people remain on the sidelines because they simply don't know where to begin. If you have ever been confused about the best way to get in shape and stay in shape, this chapter will help you understand the basics of exercise so you can put together a physical fitness plan that will work for you. If approached correctly, exercise and sports can contribute immeasurably to health and well-being, add fun and joy to life, and provide the foundation for a lifetime of fitness.

What Is Physical Fitness and Why Is It Important?

Physical fitness is the ability to adapt to the demands and stresses of physical effort. It has many components, some related to general health and others related more specifically to particular sports or activities. General health-related components include the following:

- Cardiorespiratory endurance
- Flexibility
- Muscular strength, power, and endurance
- Body composition (proportion of fat to lean body mass)

In addition to some or all of these, physical fitness for a particular sport or activity might include the following:

- Coordination
- Speed
- Agility
- Balance
- Skill

Although some components may overlap, each is largely independent and requires specific types of exercise. Your body has the ability to adapt to physical stress and improve its function; that is, through specific physical activities, you can increase your heart and lung capacity, develop stronger muscles, become more flexible, improve your performance in particular sports, and so on. In general, your level of physical fitness is an accurate reflection of the amount and intensity of your physical activity.

Why is physical fitness so important? Part of the answer to this question lies in your genetic inheritance. Your body is a wonderful moving machine, designed to be active. Your bones, joints, and ligaments provide a support system for movement; your muscles perform the motions of work and play; your heart and lungs nourish and cleanse all your cells as you move through your daily life. Millions of years of evolution have made your body a precision tool capable of astonishing feats of speed, strength, endurance, and skill, all in the service of survival. But your body is made to work best when it *is* active. Left unchallenged, bones lose their density, joints stiffen, muscles become weak, and body chemistry and systems begin to degenerate. To be truly well, you must be active.

Unfortunately, modern life for most Americans provides few built-in occasions for vigorous activity—people don't have to hunt, fight, or work strenuously all day for their dinner, as human beings did in the past. Technological advances have made our lives increasingly inactive and sedentary; we drive cars, ride escalators, watch television, and push papers around at school or work. Growing evidence points to lack of physical activity as a prime contributing factor to the array of perplexing degenerative diseases we now see in our society—heart disease, cancer, stroke, obesity, diabetes, and hypertension, among others. For example, a study of almost 17,000 male Harvard alumni revealed that the death rate from heart disease, respiratory disease, cancers, suicide, and all causes of death combined was significantly higher in sedentary men than in active men. Overall, sedentary people have been found to have up to 50 percent more health problems than people with active lifestyles.

■ **Exploring Your Emotions**

Do you exercise because you like it or because you think you should? Are there any forms of exercise that you do just for the love of it?

New evidence for the risks of a sedentary life comes from a major physical fitness study reported in the *Journal of the American Medical Association* that followed 13,000 men and women for eight years. Inactive men in this study were almost 3½ times more likely to die over the course of the eight years than active men, and inactive women were over 4½ times more likely to die than active women. Being sedentary was found to be as risky as having hypertension, high cholesterol, high blood-sugar levels, or obesity. An encouraging finding is that even mild exercise, such as a brisk walk for 30 to 60 minutes a day, was enough to make a substantial difference in an individual's risk of death. The conclusion is obvious: Exercise and physical activity are good for your health.

There is another basic reason to be physically fit, of course: It's fun and it feels good. Some people are active not because they're thinking about health benefits but simply because they enjoy it, whether they're skiing, swimming, hiking, playing basketball, or engaging in any of innumerable other activities. Sports provide the opportunity to be active, to develop strength and skills, to improve and excel, to challenge yourself or an opponent, to share victory and defeat with fellow team members, to compete and win. Many people who play sports feel that physical performance is an integral part of an active and exciting lifestyle.

As one of the most important—and most controllable—factors in a person's general health, exercise is mentioned in many other contexts in this book. It can help you to manage stress, to maintain your emotional well-being, to control your weight, to boost your immune system, and to protect yourself against serious diseases later in life. It does all this by improving the overall functioning of your body in ways detailed more fully in the rest of this chapter.

Why Is Exercise So Good for You?

The health benefits of exercise can be divided into five general categories—improved cardiorespiratory functioning and health, more efficient metabolism and better control of body fat, improved psychological and emotional well-being, improved muscular strength and flexibility, and improved health over the whole life span.

Improved Cardiorespiratory Functioning **Cardiorespiratory endurance** (or **aerobic**) **exercise**—which improves heart and lung functioning—is the most important kind of exercise. As aerobics expert Kenneth Cooper remarked, "You can live without big muscles or a nice figure, but you can't live without a healthy heart." This type of exercise helps your body become a more efficient machine, better equipped to cope with challenges. The

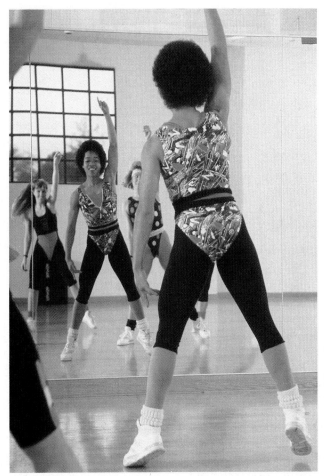

Aerobic exercise conditions the heart, improves the functioning of the entire cardiorespiratory system, and has many other health benefits as well. An effective personal fitness program should be built around an activity like running, biking, swimming, or aerobic dance.

many specific effects of aerobic exercise on the cardiorespiratory system are outlined in Table 14-1. (*Aerobic* means "requiring oxygen." In *anaerobic* exercise, such as sprinting, the body doesn't take in enough oxygen to supply the body, and the person is left breathless after the activity.)

The primary effect of endurance exercise is to improve the ability of the heart, lungs, and circulatory system to carry oxygen to the body's tissues. The heart pumps more blood per beat, resting heart rate slows down, the number of red blood cells increases, blood supply to the tissues improves, and resting blood pressure decreases. A

Physical fitness The extent to which the body can respond to the demands of physical effort.

Cardiorespiratory endurance The extent to which the heart and lungs can respond to physical exercise.

Aerobic exercise Endurance exercise; emphasizes increased use of oxygen.

Table 14-1 Effects of endurance exercise on the cardiorespiratory system

Endurance Exercise Tends to Increase	Endurance Exercise Tends to Decrease
1. Efficiency of the heart	1. Blood levels of triglycerides, total cholesterol, and low-density lipoprotein cholesterol
2. Size of blood vessels	2. Glucose intolerance
3. Blood supply to the heart	3. Obesity and body fat
4. Efficiency of distribution of blood to the tissues	4. Platelet stickiness (overadhesiveness in this type of blood cell has been implicated in the development of coronary artery disease)
5. Return of blood to the heart	5. Arterial blood pressure
6. Enzymes in the tissues that help supply energy	6. Heart rate
7. Efficiency of blood coagulation factors	7. Vulnerability to dysrhythmias of electrical conduction in the heart
8. High-density lipoprotein (HDL) cholesterol	8. Overreaction by "stress" hormones
9. Blood volume and number of red blood cells	9. Strain associated with psychic stress
10. Efficiency of the thyroid gland	
11. Growth hormone production, which increases the use of fats	
12. Tolerance to stress	

Source: Adapted from W. L. Haskell. 1984. Cardiovascular benefits and risks of exercise: the scientific evidence. In R. H. Strauss, ed., *Sports Medicine.* (Philadelphia: Saunders), p. 65.

fit cardiorespiratory system doesn't have to work as hard at rest and at low levels of exercise, because it functions more efficiently. A healthy heart can better withstand the stresses and strains of daily life and meet the occasional emergencies that make extraordinary demands on the body's cardiorespiratory resources.

Endurance exercise also has a positive effect on the balance of lipids, or fatlike substances such as cholesterol and triglycerides, that are circulating in the blood. As explained in Chapter 15, lipids are involved in the formation of plaques, or fatty deposits, on the inner lining of the coronary arteries. Cholesterol is carried in the blood by **lipoproteins,** which are classified according to size and density. Cholesterol carried by low-density lipoproteins (LDLs) tends to stick to the walls of coronary arteries, and high-density lipoproteins (HDLs) tend to pick up excess cholesterol in the bloodstream and carry it back to the liver for excretion from the body. Some researchers say that the relative amounts of HDLs and LDLs in the blood may be the most important factor involved in the development of coronary heart disease. Recent studies have shown that people with low levels of HDL have an increased risk of coronary heart disease even if their total cholesterol is low. The good news is that one excellent way to increase your HDLs and lower your LDLs is to exercise.

Endurance exercise also protects the cardiorespiratory system from the effects of stress. Many studies have shown that excessive stress and anxiety are associated with poor cardiorespiratory health. Psychological stress prompts increased secretion of **epinephrine** and **norepinephrine,** the so-called fight-or-flight hormones, which are thought to speed the development of atherosclerosis, or hardening of the arteries. Excessive hostility has also been found to be associated with an increased risk of heart disease. Exercise decreases the secretion of hormones triggered by emotional stress, and it can diffuse hostility by providing an emotional outlet for pent-up anger.

More Efficient Metabolism and Better Control of Body Fat   A second major effect of endurance exercise is to improve the efficiency of the body's metabolism, the complicated process by which the body converts chemical or food energy into mechanical or work energy. This process involves hormones, oxygen, fuels, and enzymes. A physically fit person is better able to generate useful energy, to use fats as fuel, and to regulate hormones. A more efficient metabolism may be the mechanism by which an active life protects against cancer, a recent and unexplained finding. According to one theory, the bodies of physically active people process food faster and get rid of cancer-causing agents before they can create a problem.

A related effect of endurance exercise, of course, is simply to expend calories and thus help regulate energy balance and body weight. Without exercise, it is extremely difficult to eat a nutritious diet and maintain an ideal body weight. Sedentary people may gain weight on a good diet simply because they are taking in more cal-

Table 14-2 Calorie expenditure for selected activities

To determine how many calories you burn when you engage in a particular activity, multiply the calorie multiplier given below by your body weight and then by the number of minutes you exercise.

Activity	Cal./min./lb.	× Body Weight	× Min.	= Activity Cal.
Aerobic dance (vigorous)	.062	_____	___	_____
Basketball (vigorous, full court)	.097	_____	___	_____
Bicycling (13 mph)	.071	_____	___	_____
Canoeing (flat water, 4 mph)	.045	_____	___	_____
Cross-country skiing (8 mph)	.104	_____	___	_____
Gardening (digging)	.062	_____	___	_____
Gardening (raking)	.024	_____	___	_____
Handball (skilled, singles)	.078	_____	___	_____
Horseback riding (trot)	.052	_____	___	_____
Jogging (5 mph)	.060	_____	___	_____
Rowing (vigorous)	.097	_____	___	_____
Running (8 mph)	.104	_____	___	_____
Soccer (vigorous)	.097	_____	___	_____
Swimming (55 yds/min.)	.088	_____	___	_____
Table tennis (skilled)	.045	_____	___	_____
Tennis (beginner)	.032	_____	___	_____
Walking (4.5 mph)	.048	_____	___	_____

Adapted from Ivan Kusinitz and Morton Fine. 1987. *Your Guide to Getting Fit.* (Mountain View, Calif.: Mayfield).

ories than they are using. Table 14-2 shows the number of calories burned in a variety of physical activities.

Improved Psychological and Emotional Well-Being
Most people who participate in sports or vigorous exercise have noted a number of social, psychological, and emotional benefits of being active. The joy of a well-hit cross-court backhand, the euphoria of a run through the park, or the rush of a downhill schuss through deep snow powder provides pleasure that transcends health benefits alone. Competent performance of a physical activity serves as proof that you can master skills and control your efforts, which in turn enhances your self-image. Exercise improves the appearance of your body, which also tends to make you feel better about yourself. Sports offer

an arena for harmonious interaction with other people as well as opportunities to strive and excel. Physically fit people have plenty of energy, since their bodies are functioning so efficiently, and their lives can be full and varied.

■ **Exploring Your Emotions**

Has exercising ever made you feel elated? What kind of exercise was it, and how long were you doing it when you felt that way?

Beyond these personal and interpersonal benefits, positive feelings are associated with exercise that have a phys-

---

Lipoproteins (*low-density lipoproteins, LDL; high-density lipoproteins, HDL*) Substances in blood, classified according to size, density, and chemical composition, that transport fats.

Epinephrine A hormone secreted principally by the adrenal medulla with a wide variety of functions, such as stimulating the heart, making carbohydrates available in the liver and muscles, and releasing fat from fat cells.

Norepinephrine A hormone released from the adrenal medulla and nerve endings of the autonomic nervous system. Has many of the same effects as epinephrine.

iological basis in hormones and body chemicals. Exercise decreases the secretion of stress-related hormones, as noted earlier, and it alleviates depression and anxiety by providing an emotional outlet. Additionally, researchers have recently identified a group of substances resembling morphine, called **endorphins,** that are secreted by the brain. These substances seem to have many functions: they play a role in decreasing pain, in producing euphoria, and in suppressing fatigue. Some researchers credit endorphins with the "runner's high" that some people claim to experience during exercise. More research is needed to determine exactly what the nature of endorphins is and what role they play in our sense of well-being.

Improved Muscular Strength and Flexibility   Most of the benefits already discussed are benefits of cardiorespiratory endurance exercises, but exercises designed to improve muscular strength and endurance, joint flexibility, and posture are also crucial to your physical well-being. Back pain, for example, plagues a large percentage of the population. In most cases, it can be directly traced to weak abdominal and spinal muscles with poor muscular endurance; poor flexibility in the spine, hips, and legs; and chronically poor posture.

A basic principle in human functioning is "Use it or lose it!" If muscles aren't used, they degenerate. If joints aren't moved, they become stiff. But if you do specific exercises for strength and flexibility, your functioning both in sports and in everyday life is improved. Muscular strength, for example, is an advantage whether you're hitting a baseball, unscrewing the lid of a jar, or moving your furniture into a new apartment. Stronger muscles make it easier to move the skeleton, and they're also less susceptible to injury and disability, especially in the long term. Similarly, flexible joints that are pain free and capable of normal movement are less likely to impede your activities, whether you're sprinting to class or running a marathon. Good posture helps to keep your internal organs in position and your body systems functioning properly. And an attractive, fit, healthy-looking body helps you feel good about yourself and project self-confidence and radiant well-being.

Improved Health over the Life Span   Exercising regularly may be the single most important thing you can do in your twenties to improve the quality of your life in your forties, fifties, sixties, and beyond. All the benefits described continue to accrue but gain new importance

as the resilience of youth begins to wane. Physically fit individuals are less likely to develop the diseases and disabilities now associated with middle age in our society, including heart disease, stroke, diabetes, and high blood pressure. They may be able to avoid fatigue, weight gain, memory loss, and other problems associated with aging. Their cardiorespiratory systems tend to resemble those of people ten or more years younger than themselves. With flexible spines, strong hearts and muscles, lean bodies, and a repertoire of physical skills they can call on for exercise and enjoyment, these people have the potential to maintain their physical and mental well-being throughout their entire lives.

A specific benefit of exercise for older people, especially postmenopausal women, is the protection it seems to provide against the effects of **osteoporosis,** a disease that results in loss of bone density and poor bone strength (see Chapter 12). Weight-bearing exercise, which includes almost everything except swimming, builds bone during the teens and twenties, when bones are still growing. Older people with denser bones can endure the bone loss that comes with osteoporosis better than can people whose bones are not as dense. With stronger bones, they're less likely to suffer the bone fractures that debilitate so many older people.

Designing Your Exercise and Fitness Program

The best exercise and fitness program has two primary characteristics: it promotes your health and it's fun for you to do. Exercise doesn't have to be a chore. On the contrary, it can provide some of the most pleasurable moments of your day, once you make it a habit. A little thought and planning will help you achieve these goals.

■ **Exploring Your Emotions**

Choosing a physical activity you like can make all the difference in your commitment and motivation. What forms of exercise do you like? What is it about them that you enjoy? Are there other forms with the same characteristics that you could try?

Begin by choosing an activity that makes sense for you. Are you competitive? If so, you probably won't enjoy running around a track; try racquetball, basketball, or

---

Endorphins   Substances resembling opium that are secreted by the brain. They seem to be involved in modulating pain.

Osteoporosis   A bone disease characterized by the loss of bone mineral. It is particularly prevalent in postmenopausal women.

Walk Your Way to Fitness

If you are one of those many people who dislike jogging and swimming, who never learned to ski or play tennis, and who don't want to spend money on an expensive health club, there is no need to despair of ever becoming more physically fit. Regardless of real or imagined limitations due to age, weight, or lack of athletic prowess, you can still get into great shape. You can walk your way to fitness!

Many people aren't aware of the physical conditioning value and aerobic effects of walking. They may think walking just isn't demanding enough to qualify as a worthwhile fitness activity. In reality, however, walking—if done briskly enough and long enough—can be just as good as jogging or any other endurance exercise for developing a high level of cardiorespiratory fitness. It promotes increased lung action, stimulates the circulation, lowers elevated blood pressure, and activates many large muscle groups.

Walking is also one of the best ways to lose weight, especially when combined with a moderate, low-fat diet. It burns calories, curbs the appetite, and raises the metabolic rate, perhaps for as long as four hours. Like many other forms of exercise, walking helps reduce the effects of stress. And for anyone who is extremely overweight, who is advanced in years, who has limiting physical conditions such as knee problems, or who has been sedentary for a long time, walking is the preferred way to fitness.

How much do you have to walk to experience health benefits? To achieve a cardiorespiratory effect, you have to exercise in the upper half of your target zone for 30 to 40 minutes or in the lower half for 60 minutes, at least three to five times a week (see page 385). Check your heart rate while you're walking by carefully counting your pulse at the wrist or throat. (Count for 15 seconds and multiply by 4). If necessary, stop walking long enough to do this and then resume walking. Adjust your pace as required to keep your heart rate high enough.

Some experts think that shorter, high-intensity workouts are better for cardiorespiratory benefits and that longer walks at a more moderate, comfortable pace are better for burning fat and losing weight. But anything is better than nothing. If walks of 5 to 10 minutes are all you can do at first, take several short walks during the day and gradually build up to longer walks. You can walk as seldom as three times a week or as often as every day.

Walkers who want to pick up the pace in order to raise their heart rates further or burn more calories have a few choices. They can look for hills to climb or carry some extra weight in a knapsack. They can walk on a treadmill in a fitness center, setting it for a faster pace or adjusting it to a slight incline. Or they can bend their arms at a 90-degree angle at the elbow, form a comfortable fist with their hands, and let their arms swing loosely like two pendulums in coordination with their steps as they walk. All these techniques increase the vigor of the workout.

As a form of regular exercise, walking offers many advantages over other activities and sports. It's comfortable, convenient, affordable, safe, and likely to wear well. You can fit it into your daily living pattern with a minimum of hassle and equipment, and you can take it with you wherever you go. More than most other forms of exercise, walking lends itself to sharing, socializing, and enjoying nature. And because it's so easy and pleasurable, you're likely to continue including it in your routine long after you've dropped more exotic or strenuous sports.

squash instead. Do you prefer to exercise alone? Then consider cross-country skiing, triathlon, or road running. If you don't have a favorite sport or activity, try something new. Take a physical education class, join a health club, sign up for jazz dancing. You're sure to find an activity that's both enjoyable and good for you.

Be realistic about the constraints presented by some sports, such as accessibility, expense, and time. For example, if you have to travel for hours to get to a ski area, skiing isn't a good choice for your regular exercise program. If you don't have large blocks of time available, you may have trouble squeezing in eighteen holes of golf. And if you've never played tennis, it will probably take you a fair amount of time to reach a reasonable skill level; you may be better off walking or jogging to get a good workout (see the box "Walk Your Way to Fitness"). Try to choose activities that contribute to your general health and well-being, especially your cardiorespiratory endur-

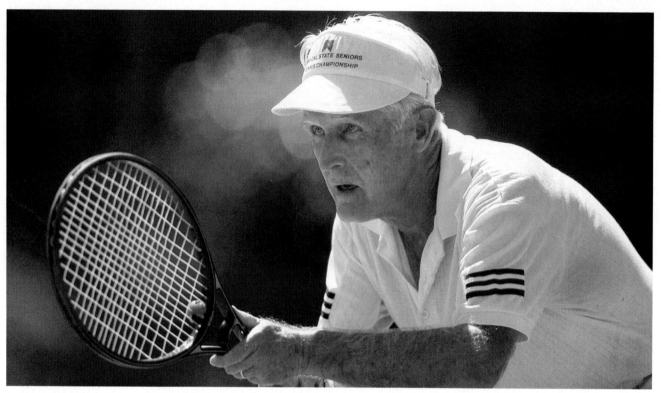

It makes sense to choose sports that will add enjoyment to your life for years to come. In this older tennis champ we can see the rewards of a lifetime of fitness and smart exercise habits.

ance (as discussed in detail in the next section). If your activities don't develop several aspects of fitness, such as flexibility, be sure to supplement them with exercises that do. Participating in a variety of activities will help you become generally fit.

If you are over 35 or have questions about your health, get a medical examination before beginning an exercise program. Diabetes, asthma, heart disease, or extreme obesity are conditions that may call for a modified program. If you have an increased risk of heart disease because of smoking, high blood pressure, or obesity, have an exercise **electrocardiogram (ECG)** before beginning a program. This checkup can help ensure that your program is a benefit to your health rather than a potential hazard.

As discussed earlier, fitness has many components—cardiorespiratory endurance, flexibility, strength, agility, and so on. Each component has value, and each requires specific exercises. Lifting weights develops muscle strength, for example, but it doesn't condition the heart and lungs. Running is excellent for increasing cardiorespiratory capacity, but it contributes little to strength and power. In addition, different sports and activities call for different skills, and to become proficient in them, you have to practice the specific movements they require, as explained in the box "Exercise for Performance."

It's virtually impossible to stay in shape for all the activities in which you might want to participate—swimming, skiing, tennis, ice skating, roller skating, dancing, hiking, golf, volleyball, basketball, and so on. What you can do instead is choose a few activities and exercises and do them regularly as part of a general conditioning program. Then if you want to add an activity or try a new sport, you'll be in good shape to begin. A general conditioning program that supports an active lifestyle and promotes good health should contain the following components: cardiorespiratory endurance exercises, flexibility exercises, muscle strengthening exercises, and training in specific skills.

Electrocardiogram (EKG or ECG) A recording of the changes in electrical activity of the heart.

Memory drum theory A theory that states that motor movements are imprinted in the motor cortex, then "replayed" by reflex when a person wishes to repeat the movement.

Motor cortex A portion of the brain responsible for movement.

Exercising for Performance

Many people, particularly young adults, enjoy sports and want to improve their skills. They swim, ski, or play basketball for the fun of it, not because the activity improves their heart or lung capacity (although it does). The skills needed in many sports and physical activities are somewhat different from those emphasized in a cardiorespiratory fitness program, and an understanding of physical performance can make workouts more effective and enjoyable. Components of fitness related to sports performance fall into two general categories—those related to strength and those related to skill.

Strength, Power, and Speed

Many sports require strength—the ability to exert force—and power—the ability to apply force rapidly. Strength is largely a function of muscle size, which is increased by subjecting the muscle to increased loads—that is, more intense exercise. Power is a function of both strength and skill.

How do muscles work during physical activity? When you want to perform a movement, your nervous system calls on specific muscle fibers (bundles of muscle cells), depending on the force required. Muscles are divided into two categories, fast-twitch and slow-twitch, according to such factors as their size and strength. In general, fast-twitch muscles are stronger and more powerful than slow-twitch fibers but fatigue more rapidly. Slow-twitch fibers have much more endurance but are considerably weaker and slower.

Your body calls on low-twitch fibers for low-intensity or repeated contractions, such as those in-volved in maintaining your body in an upright position or in performing light exercise such as walking. Fast-twitch fibers are called on for high-intensity contractions, such as heavy weight lifting or sprinting. Successful power athletes, such as sprinters, baseball players, and discus throwers, have a greater percentage of fast-twitch fibers in their active muscles; endurance athletes, such as marathon runners and cross-country skiers, tend to have more slow-twitch fibers.

When you are building strength and power for a particular sport or type of exercise, you need to train the fibers you will be using in the activity. The muscle fibers used in speed sports are trained by high-intensity exercises. Football, for example, is an explosive sport that requires high-intensity training, such as that provided by sprinting. You wouldn't get in shape for football with slow jogs. Low-intensity, prolonged exercise, on the other hand, requires more prolonged muscle contractions. To get in shape for alpine skiing, you would need to do endurance training, such as that provided by running, cross-country skiing, and cycling. Many sports call for both explosive strength and endurance and so require a full range of training, such as exercises for strengthening particular parts of the body, jogging, sprinting, and, perhaps most important, stretching to improve flexibility and prevent injury.

Skill, Coordination, Balance, and Reaction Time

Playing a sport also requires skill. You have to learn the precise movements involved in playing your chosen sport, and this learn-ing involves a complex interaction of sensory, neurological, and muscular activity. When you want to hit a tennis ball, for example, your brain must translate input from your eyes, ears, and various receptors in your muscles, joints, skin, and inner ear in order to initiate movements in your musculoskeletal system. Movement begins in a part of your brain called the motor cortex, which sends commands to nerve cells within your spinal cord that control specific muscles. Another part of your brain, the cerebellum, constantly compares the intended movement with your actual movement so that each movement sequence is coordinated.

According to a theory formulated by F. M. Henry of the University of California, Berkeley, and known as the **memory drum theory**, the **motor cortex** functions in a manner analogous to the running of a computer program. Muscle fibers are programmed to contract in an incredibly precise order that is regulated in terms of time, intensity, and duration. The skill sequence is somehow "imprinted" on the motor cortex in the same way that a magnetic imprint is made on a computer floppy disk. The purpose of practicing a skill is to imprint a precise movement sequence in the brain. Repeated practice of the correct movement, involving specific actions, coordination, balance, reaction time, and so on, will eventually result in an almost reflex performance of the skill. This is the process that produces a smooth forehand or backhand stroke in tennis, a "grooved swing" in golf or baseball, and all the skilled actions required in specific sports. The more you practice these movements, the better you will become at them.

Table 14-3 Recommended quantity and quality of exercise for healthy adults

Mode of Activity

Aerobic or endurance exercises, such as running-jogging, walking-hiking, swimming, skating, bicycling, rowing, cross-country skiing, rope skipping, and various game activities.

Frequency of Training

3 to 5 days per week

Intensity of Training

60 percent of capability range plus resting pulse rate, or 50 percent to 85 percent of maximum oxygen uptake

Duration of Training

15 to 60 minutes of continuous aerobic activity. Duration depends on the intensity of the activity.

Source: American College of Sports Medicine. 1978. *Sports Medicine Bulletin* 13:1–4.

Cardiorespiratory Endurance Exercises   Exercises that condition your heart and lungs should have a central role in your fitness program. The best exercises for developing **cardiorespiratory endurance** are those that stress a large portion of the body's muscle mass for a prolonged period of time. These include walking, jogging, running, swimming, bicycling, and aerobic dancing. Games such as racquetball, tennis, basketball, and soccer are also good if the skill level and intensity of the game are sufficient to provide a vigorous workout.

Specific recommendations have been made by the American College of Sports Medicine for the kind and amount of exercise that provide the optimal workout for your heart and lungs. They have defined three dimensions of training that should be taken into consideration: frequency, intensity, and duration of exercise. Frequency refers to the number of times per week you exercise; intensity refers to how hard you work; and duration refers to the length of your exercise session. Basic recommendations for quantity and quality of exercise are outlined in Table 14-3.

Frequency of Training   The optimal workout schedule for endurance training is three to five days per week. Beginners should start with three and work up to five days.

Training more than five days a week often leads to injury for recreational athletes. Training less than three days a week provides little health benefit, and you risk injury because your body never gets a chance to adapt fully to regular exercise training.

Intensity of Training   The most misunderstood aspect of conditioning, even among experienced athletes, is training intensity. Intensity is the crucial factor in attaining a training effect—that is, in increasing the body's cardiorespiratory capacity. A primary purpose of endurance training is to increase **maximal oxygen consumption (MOC)**. MOC represents the maximum ability of the cells to use oxygen and is considered the best measure of cardiorespiratory capacity. Intensity of training is the crucial factor in attaining a training effect—that is, in increasing the body's cardiorespiratory capacity—and in improving MOC.

■ **Exploring Your Emotions**

How much of your free time do you spend exercising and engaging in physical activities? Do you feel comfortable with that amount of time? Would you feel comfortable spending more time exercising? Less time?

However, it's not true that the harder you work, the better it is for you. Working too hard can cause injury, just as not working hard enough provides little benefit. One of the easiest ways to determine exactly how intensely you should work involves measuring your heart rate. It is not necessary or desirable to exercise at your maximum heart rate—the fastest heart rate possible before exhaustion sets in—in order to improve your cardiorespiratory capacity. Beneficial effects occur at lower heart rates with a much lower risk of injury. To find out how you can determine the intensity at which you should exercise, refer to the box "Determining Your Target Heart Rate."

After you begin your fitness program, you may improve quickly, because the body adapts readily to new exercises at first but slows after the first month or so. The more fit you become, the harder you will have to work to improve. By monitoring your heart rate, you will always know if you are working hard enough to improve,

---

Endurance exercise   Rhythmical, large-muscle exercise for a prolonged period of time. Partially dependent on the ability of the cardiovascular system to deliver oxygen to tissues. Also known as aerobic or cardiorespiratory endurance exercise.

Maximal oxygen consumption (MOC)   The body's maximum ability to transport and use oxygen.

Capability range (CR)   The capacity of the heart to increase its rate above a resting level.

Heart rate reserve   The capacity of the heart to increase its rate above a resting level. Same as capability range.

Determining Your Target Heart Rate

To determine your *target heart rate*—the rate at which you should exercise to experience cardiorespiratory benefits—first determine your resting heart rate—your heart rate after ten minutes of complete rest. Then establish your maximum heart rate by one of three methods: (1) take a treadmill test in a physician's office, hospital, or sports medicine laboratory; (2) subtract your age from 220 (3) refer to the accompanying table. The latter two methods are fairly accurate for most people, but they can be grossly inaccurate for some people. For example, a 20-year-old college student may have a maximum heart rate as low as 180 beats per minute or as high as 215 beats per minute.

The difference between your resting and maximum pulse rates is your **capability range (CR)**, or **heart rate reserve**. For example,

Maximum heart rate   200
Resting heart rate   − 70
Capability range   130 beats

The training effect occurs when the heart rate is higher than the resting heart rate by an amount that is 60 to 80 percent of the CR. For example,

Capability range   130
Minimum intensity   × .6
60% CR   78
Resting heart rate   + 70
Target heart rate   148 beats per minute

Target heart rates for people in age groups between 20 and 60 are shown in the table.

Measure your pulse either at your wrist or at one of your carotid arteries, located on either side of your Adam's apple. Begin counting immediately after you have finished exercising. The pulse rate usually drops rapidly after exercise, so you will obtain the most accurate result by counting beats for 15 seconds and then multiplying by 4. To build cardiorespiratory endurance, you must exercise at your target heart rate for a minimum of 15 to 20 minutes.

Maximum and target heart rates predicted from age			
Age	Predicted Maximum Heart Rate	Target Heart Rate 60%	80%
20–24 years	200	149	174
25–29	200	149	174
30–34	194	145	170
35–39	188	142	165
40–44	182	138	160
45–49	176	134	155
50–54	171	131	151
55–59	165	128	146
60–64	159	124	142
60+	153	121	137

Source: Derived from Metropolitan Life Insurance Company charts and Karvonen formula (target heart rate = 0.6 or 0.8 $[HR_{max} − HR_{rest}] + HR_{rest}$).

not hard enough, or too hard. For most people, a fitness program involves attaining an acceptable level of fitness and then maintaining that level. There is no need to keep working indefinitely to improve; doing so only increases the chance of injury. After you have reached the level you want, you can maintain fitness by exercising at the same intensity approximately three times per week.

Many people use a relatively new approach to exercise known as **periodization of training**, or *cycle training*. This technique involves varying the intensity of the workout from one session to the next so that you're rested on the days you exercise the hardest. For example, the intensity schedule of a week-long series of workouts might be (1) hard, (2) easy, (3) moderate, (4) easy, (5) moderate, (6) rest, and (7) rest. A hard workout might be practiced at 80 percent of the heart rate reserve, a moderate workout at 70 percent, and an easy workout at 60 percent (see the box "Determining Your Target Heart Rate.") Cycle training allows your body to adapt rapidly to intense workouts by giving it time to recover between strenuous sessions.

Duration of Training   The length of time you should spend on a workout depends on its intensity. If you are walking, swimming slowly, or playing a stop-and-start game like tennis, you should participate for 45 to 60 minutes. High-intensity exercises such as running that keep your heart rate in the target zone for at least 20 minutes can be practiced for a shorter period of time. The recreational athlete should start off with less vigorous activities and only gradually increase intensity. For most people, continuous endurance exercise should last from 15 minutes (high-intensity activities) to 60 minutes (low-intensity activities).

You can use these three dimensions of cardiorespiratory endurance training—frequency, intensity, and duration—to construct a fitness program that protects your heart and lungs and provides all the benefits described earlier in this chapter. Build your program around 15 to 20 minutes of continuous aerobic activity at your target heart rate three to five times a week. Then add exercises that develop the other components of fitness.

Flexibility Exercises   Flexibility, or stretching, exercises are perhaps the most neglected part of fitness programs, but they are extremely important. They are necessary to maintain the normal range of motion in the major joints of the body and to keep muscles from contracting and shortening. Some exercises, such as running,

actually decrease flexibility because they require only a partial range of motion. It's important to do stretching exercises at least three to five times a week to develop this component of fitness.

Stretching should be performed statically. "Bouncing" is dangerous and counterproductive. Stretch to the point of tightness in the muscle and hold the position 10 to 30 seconds (up to 60 seconds if your muscles are tight). You should feel a pleasant, mild stretch as you let the muscles relax; stretching shouldn't be painful. There are large individual differences in flexibility, so don't feel you have to compete with others during stretching workouts. Flexibility increases gradually over a period of time as you incorporate stretching exercises into your fitness program. You can set apart a special time for these exercises or do them before or after your aerobic exercise. You may develop more flexibility if you do them after exercise, because your muscles are warmer then and can be stretched farther. A sequence of appropriate stretching exercises is given in the box "Exercises for Flexibility."

Muscle Strengthening Exercises   Exercises that develop muscular strength and muscular endurance should also be included in any program designed to promote health. Your ability to maintain correct posture and to move efficiently depends in part on adequate muscle fitness. Strengthening exercises also increase muscle tone, which improves the appearance of your body. A lean, healthy-looking body is certainly one of the goals and one of the benefits of an overall fitness program.

Muscular strength and endurance can be developed in many ways, from weight training to calisthenics. (Taking **anabolic steroids** is *not* a safe or healthy way to increase muscle strength or endurance; in fact, it runs counter to all the practices that promote good health discussed in this chapter. See the box "Anabolic Steroids—Not Worth the Risk.") Common exercises such as sit-ups, push-ups, pull-ups, and wall-sitting (leaning against a wall in a seated position and supporting yourself with your leg muscles) maintain the muscular strength of most people if they practice a few exercises for the major muscle groups three to five days a week. To condition and tone your whole body, choose exercises that work the major muscles of the shoulders, chest, back, arms, abdomen, and legs.

To increase strength (rather than simply maintain it) you must do **resistive exercise**—exercises in which your muscles must exert force against a significant resistance. Resistance can be provided by weights, exercise machines, or your own body weight. Your muscles become

---

Periodization of training   A training technique that systematically varies the volume and intensity of the workouts.

Anabolic steroids   Synthetic male hormones used to increase muscle size and strength.

Resistive exercise   Exercise that forces muscles to contract against increased resistance; for example, weight training.

Exercises for Flexibility

1. Shoulder blade scratch (shoulders, arms)

Reach back with one arm as if to scratch your shoulder blade. Use your other hand to extend the stretch. Alternate arms.

2. Towel stretch (triceps, shoulders, chest)

Grasp a rolled towel at both ends and slowly bring it back over your head as far down as possible. Keep your arms straight. (The closer your hands are, the greater the stretch.)

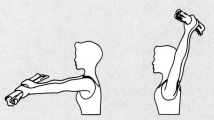

3. Alternate knee-to-chest (lower back)

Bring one knee up to your chest. Curl your head toward your knee. Keep the other leg on the floor.

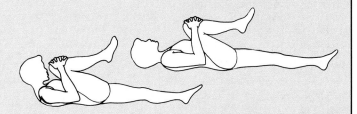

4. Double knee-to-chest (lower back)

Same as alternate knee-to-chest (3), except bring both knees up to your chest.

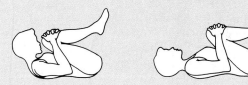

5. Sole stretch (groin)

With the soles of your feet pressed together, pull your feet toward you while pressing your knees down with your elbows.

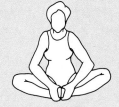

6. Seated toe touch (hamstrings)

Sit with your legs straight. Fold one leg in front and gradually reach for the toes of your other foot. Eventually you will be able to grasp your feet at the instep. Keep your head down. Alternate legs.

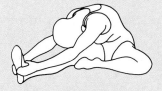

Exercises for Flexibility (Continued)

7. Seated foot-over-knee twist (hips)

Seated as depicted, turn at the hips to face the rear. Hold your ankle to keep your foot on the floor. Alternate legs.

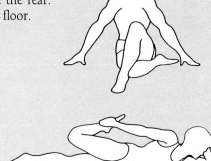

8. Prone knee flexion (quadriceps)

Lying on your side with one arm tucked behind your head, use the other arm to slowly pull one foot up toward your buttocks. Flex the leg up until you feel the stretch in your quadriceps.

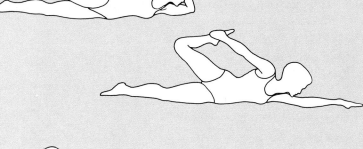

9. Wall lean (lower legs)

Lean against the wall with one leg bent and the other straight. Keep your back straight and your heels on the floor. Bend the knee of the straight leg—this changes the stretch from the calf muscle to the Achilles tendon. Alternate legs.

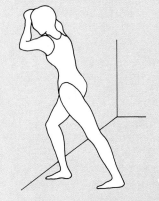
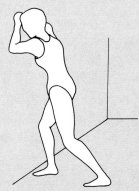

10. Stride stretch (hips, hamstring)

Assume the racer's starting position and stretch one leg backward. Keep your head down. Alternate legs.

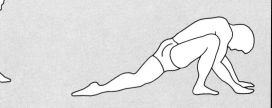

Source: I. Kusinitz and M. Fine. 1987. *Your Guide to Getting Fit* (Mountain View, Calif.: Mayfield).

stronger when you subject them to **overload**, an exercise stress that is more severe than what they are used to. By pushing your muscles to temporary fatigue and by gradually increasing the amount of resistance or the number of times they must resist, you force them to adapt to greater physical stress. If you use heavy resistance with few repetitions (one to ten), you build muscle strength and size. If you use lighter resistance and do more repetitions, you improve muscular endurance (the ability to exert force over a longer period of time). Strength training improves performance in most sports and has become a prominent part of the training program of many athletes. In general, you have to train at least twice a week for an hour to experience significant results. You also have to allow recovery time between workouts—two to four days—to train properly and avoid injury.

There are three different kinds of strengthening exercises. **Isometric exercises** involve applying force without movement, such as when you contract your abdominal muscles. This static type of exercise is valuable for toning and strengthening muscles. Isometrics can be practiced anywhere and don't require any equipment. Try holding your stomach in for ten to thirty seconds several times during the day (but don't hold your breath—that can restrict blood flow to your heart and brain). Within a few weeks, you'll notice the effect of this isometric exercise.

Isokinetic exercises involve exerting force at a constant speed against an equal force exerted by a specialized strength training machine. Proponents of this type of exercise claim that training at faster speeds produces a training effect more specific to the rapid movements used in sports. Isokinetic machines are considerably more expensive than traditional weight training equipment and so are not as widely available.

Isotonic exercises involve applying force with movement, as, for example, in weight training exercises such as the bench press. These are the most popular type of exercises for increasing muscle strength and seem to be most valuable for developing strength that can be transferred to other forms of physical activity. They include exercises using barbells, dumbbells, weight machines, and the body's own weight, as in push-ups or sit-ups.

Examples of isotonic exercises for various muscle groups include the bench press for the chest; the overhead press, the behind-the-neck press, and upright rowing for the shoulders; barbell and dumbbell curls for the arms; pull-ups and chin-ups for the upper back; sit-ups

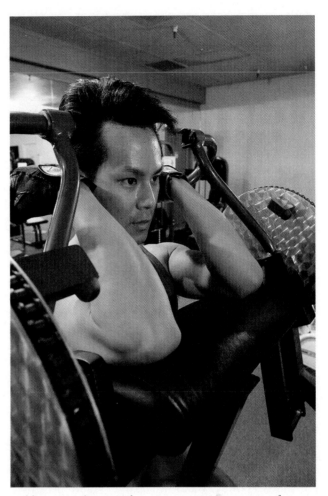

Building muscular strength is an important component of a fitness program. Weight training is just one way to increase strength, improve muscle tone, and enhance the overall appearance of the body.

and crunches for the abdominals; and squats and leg presses for the legs. Exercises are repeated until the muscles are fatigued, and muscle contraction—the lifting or pushing part of the exercise—is always accompanied by an exhalation. Level of exertion is gradually increased over a period of weeks. To learn how to do these exercises properly so they increase your muscle strength and don't cause injury, you should receive instruction from a trainer in a gym, a health club, a physical education class, or a Y or community recreation department.

Training in Specific Skills   The fourth element in your fitness program is learning the skills required in the

---

Overload   Subjecting the body to more stress than it is accustomed.

Isometric exercise   Application of force without movement. Also called *static* exercise.

Isokinetic exercise   Application of force at constant speed. A form of isotonic exercise.

Isotonic exercise   Application of force with movement.

Anabolic Steroids—Not Worth the Risk

Anabolic steroids are drugs that resemble male hormones such as testosterone and are widely used by athletes in such sports as track and field, weight lifting, and football. Athletes take them in the hope of gaining weight, strength, power, speed, endurance, and aggressiveness. Although research findings are divided, most experts feel that they are effective in improving some types of athletic performance, but only at a cost to health. A recent, alarming trend is young nonathletes taking these drugs to improve appearance and sex appeal.

Male hormones, principally testosterone, are partially responsible for the tremendous developmental changes that occur in boys during puberty and adolescence. Male hormones have both androgenic and anabolic effects. **Androgenic effects** are characterized by changes in primary and secondary sexual characteristics such as enlargement of the penis and testes; changes in the voice; hair growth on the face, armpit, and genital areas; and increased aggressiveness. The **anabolic effects** of androgens include accelerated growth of muscle, bone, and red blood cells, and enhanced neural conduction. Anabolic steroids have been manufactured to enhance the anabolic properties (tissue building) of the androgens and to minimize the androgenic (sex-linked) properties. However, no steroid has completely eliminated the androgenic effects.

Anabolic steroids can have dangerous side effects. Although they improve athletic performance, the benefits are not worth the health risks. The principal side effects of anabolic steroids can be subdivided into (1) normal physiological actions of male hormones that are inappropriate in the recipient, and (2) toxic effects caused mainly by oral forms.

The *physiological side effects* include reduced testosterone production, testicular function, and sperm cell production. Libido (sex drive) may increase or decrease. Anabolic steroids increase fluid retention. Steroid use by women and immature children may induce masculinizing hair growth on face and body, deepening of the voice, oily skin, increased sweat gland activity, acne, and baldness. In women, some of these changes are irreversible. Women may also experience clitoral enlargement and menstrual irregularity. Children initially experience accelerated maturation followed by premature closure of growth centers in the long bones.

Anabolic steroids can result in testicular atrophy and decreased sperm production. These changes may also reverse themselves after usage stops, but prolonged use may permanently disturb the delicate hormone regulatory system.

Anabolic steroids may also harm the immune system. These drugs are thought to block the action of hormones called corticosteroids involved in breakdown and repair after a heavy workout. In reaction, the body increases production of corticosteroids and their receptors. Corticosteroids suppress the immune system, which fights off diseases. Athletes often get colds or flu when going off steroids because of the increased corticosteroids.

Oral anabolic steroids, such as methandrostenolone (Dianabol), present the greatest risk of toxicity, particularly to the liver, because their structure has been altered to make them more biologically active. Such steroids concentrate in the liver much earlier and in greater quantity than the injectable varieties. Prolonged use has been linked to severe liver disorders such as blood-filled cysts, liver cancer, and bile duct obstruction.

Several factors in steroid use are linked to increased risk of coronary heart disease: high levels of cholesterol and triglycerides, high blood pressure, and low levels of high-density lipoproteins (HDLs). Many weight-trained athletes use steroids from ten to more than twenty years, risking premature death from atherosclerosis. Hypertension (high blood pressure) is also common, probably due to fluid retention.

A variety of other side effects have been reported including muscle cramps, gastrointestinal distress, headache, dizziness, sore nipples, and abnormal thyroid function. Some of these side effects even show up in people who have only taken low doses for short periods of time.

Anabolic effects   Effects of anabolic steroids that tend to build tissues such as muscle.

Androgenic effects   Effects of anabolic steroids that cause changes in secondary sexual characteristics, such as hair growth, aggressiveness, and deepening of the voice.

Synovial fluid   Fluid found within many joints that provides lubrication and nutrition to the cells of the joint surface.

sports or activities in which you choose to participate. These skills are specific and therefore unrelated to other activities. In other words, if you want to learn them, you have to practice them and not something else. Taking the time and effort to acquire competence means that instead of feeling ridiculous, becoming frustrated, and giving up in despair, you achieve a sense of mastery and add a new physical activity to your repertoire.

The first step in learning a new skill is to get help. Sports like tennis, golf, sailing, skiing, and most others require mastery of basic movements and techniques, so instruction from a qualified teacher can save you hours of frustration and increase your enjoyment of the sport. Take a class, sign up for lessons, or get private instruction.

Skill is also important in conditioning activities such as jogging, swimming, and cycling. Know your own capacity and learn to gauge the intensity of exercise that will result in improvement without injury. Some instruction on technique from a coach or fellow participant can often help you to move and train more efficiently. Even if you learned swimming, tennis, golf, soccer, or some other sport as a child, additional instruction now can help you refine your technique, get over stumbling blocks, and relearn skills that you may have learned incorrectly.

Finally, as discussed earlier, choose activities and sports that suit your personal tastes, your time constraints, and your pocketbook. Be sure to vary your program enough so you don't get bored by doing the same thing over and over.

■ Exploring Your Emotions

In our society, boys and men tend to be more active in sports and physical activities than girls and women. Why do you think that is? How do you feel about it?

Putting It All Together   Now that you know the basic components of a fitness program, you can put them all together in a program that works for you. Remember to include the following:

- Cardiorespiratory endurance exercise—do 15 to 20 minutes of aerobic exercise at your target heart rate three to five times a week
- Muscle strengthening exercise—work the major muscle groups three to five times a week
- Flexibility exercise—do stretches three to five times a week
- Skill training—incorporate some or all of your aerobic or strengthening exercise into an enjoyable sport or physical activity

A summary of the fitness benefits of a variety of activities is provided in Table 14-4 to help you plan your program.

In any program, it's important to *warm up* before you exercise and *cool down* afterwards. Warming up enhances your performance and decreases your chances of injury. Your muscles work better when their temperature is slightly above resting level. Warming up helps your body's physiology gradually progress from rest to exercise. Blood needs to be redirected to active muscles, and this takes time. Your heart needs time to adapt to the increased demands of exercise. Warm-up helps spread **synovial fluid** throughout joints, which helps protect surfaces. (This is like an automobile: warming up a car spreads oil through the engine parts before you shift into gear.)

A warm-up session should include low-intensity movements similar to those in the activity that will follow. Low-intensity movements include hitting forehands and backhands before a tennis game, skiing down an easy run before tackling a more difficult one, and running a 12-minute mile before progressing to an 8-minute one. Some experts also recommend warm-up stretching exercises for flexibility.

Cooling down after exercise is important to restore circulation to its normal resting condition. When you are at rest, a relatively small percentage of your total blood volume is directed to muscles, but during exercise as much as 85 percent of the heart's output is directed to them. During recovery from exercise, it is important to continue exercising at a low level to provide a smooth transition to the resting state. Cooling down helps maintain the return of blood to your heart.

There are as many different adequate fitness programs as there are different individuals. Consider these examples:

Maggie is a person whose life revolves around sports. She's been on volleyball teams, softball teams, and swim teams, and now she's on her college varsity soccer team. She follows a rigorous exercise regimen established by her soccer coach. Soccer practice is from 4 to 6 P.M. four days a week. It begins with warm-ups, drills, and practice in specific skills, and it ends with a scrimmage and then a jog around the soccer field. Games are every Saturday. Maggie likes team sports, but she also enjoys exercising alone, so she goes on long bicycle rides whenever she can fit them in. She can't imagine what it would be like not to be physically active every day.

Janine is a young mother of twins. Her life is so busy caring for them that she hardly has time to comb her hair, much less spend a lot of time exercising. To keep in shape, she joined a health club with a weight room, exercise classes, and child care. Every Monday, Wednesday, and Friday morning, she takes the twins to the club and attends the 7 o'clock "wake-up" low-impact aerobics class. The teacher leads the class through warm-ups, a 20-minute aerobic workout, exercises for the arms, legs, abdomen, buttocks,

Table 14-4 Fitness benefits of selected activities

Sports and activities are classified here as high (H), moderate (M), or low (L) for their ability to develop five different components of physical fitness: cardiorespiratory endurance (CRE), body composition (BC), muscular strength (MS), muscular endurance (ME), and flexibility (F). In the Skill Level column, low (L) means little or no skill is required to obtain fitness benefits from the activity; moderate (M) means average skill is required; and high (H) means much skill is required. In the Fitness Prerequisite column, low (L) means there is little or no fitness prerequisite; moderate (M) means some preconditioning is required; and high (H) means substantial fitness is required. In the last column, 1 means the activity is self-paced; 2 means pacing is by a combination of yourself and others; and 3 means it's paced by someone other than yourself.

Sports and Activities	Components					Skill Level	Fitness Prerequisite	How Paced
	CRE	BC	MS	ME	F			
Aerobic dance	H	H	M	H	H	L	L	3
Backpacking	H	H	H	H	M	L	M	1
Badminton (skilled, singles)	H	H	M	M	M	M	M	2
Ballet	M	M	M	H	H	M	L	3
Ballroom dancing	M	M	L	M	L	M	L	3
Baseball (pitcher and catcher)	M	M	M	H	M	H	M	3
Basketball	H	H	M	H	M	M	M	3
Bicycling	H	H	M	H	M	M	L	1
Bowling	L	L	L	L	L	L	L	1
Calisthenic circuit training	H	H	M	H	M	L	L	1
Canoeing and kayaking	M	M	M	H	M	M	M	1
Cross-country skiing	H	H	M	H	M	M	M	1
Fencing	M	M	M	H	H	M	L	3
Field hockey	H	H	M	H	M	M	M	3
Folk and square dancing	M	M	L	M	L	L	L	3
Football/touch	M	M	M	M	M	M	M	3
Frisbee/ultimate	H	H	M	H	M	M	M	2
Golf (riding cart)	L	L	L	L	M	L	L	1
Handball (skilled, singles)	H	H	M	H	M	M	M	3
Hiking	H	H	M	H	L	L	M	1
Hockey/ice and field	H	H	M	H	M	M	M	3
Horseback riding	M	M	M	M	L	M	M	1

Table 14-4 Fitness benefits of selected activities (continued)

Sports and Activities	Components					Skill Level	Fitness Prerequisite	How Paced
	CRE	BC	MS	ME	F			
Interval circuit training	H	H	H	H	M	L	L	1
Jogging and running	H	H	M	H	L	L	L	1
Judo	M	M	H	H	M	M	L	3
Karate	H	H	M	H	H	L	M	3
Modern dance (moving combinations)	M	M	M	H	H	L	L	3
Popular dancing	M	M	L	M	M	M	L	3
Racquetball (skilled, singles)	H	H	M	M	M	M	M	2
Rock climbing	M	M	H	H	H	H	M	1
Rope skipping	H	H	M	H	L	M	M	1
Rowing	H	H	H	H	H	L	L	1
Sailing	L	L	L	M	L	M	L	1
Skating/ice and roller	M	M	M	H	M	H	M	1
Skiing/alpine	M	M	H	H	M	H	M	1
Soccer	H	H	M	H	M	M	M	3
Squash (skilled, singles)	H	H	M	M	M	M	M	2
Surfing	M	M	M	M	M	H	M	2
Swimming	H	H	M	H	M	M	L	1
Table tennis	M	M	L	M	M	M	L	3
Tennis (skilled, singles)	H	H	M	M	M	M	M	2
Volleyball	M	M	L	M	M	M	M	3
Walking	H	H	L	M	L	L	L	1
Waterskiing	M	M	M	H	M	H	M	2
Weight training	L	M	H	H	H	L	L	1
Wrestling	H	H	H	H	H	H	H	3
Yoga	L	L	L	M	H	H	L	1

Adapted from Ivan Kusinitz and Morton Fine. 1987. *Your Guide to Getting Fit.* (Mountain View, Calif.: Mayfield).

and legs, stretches, and a relaxation exercise. Janine is exhilarated and ready for the rest of the day before 9 A.M.

Tom is an engineering student with a lot of studying to do and an active social life as well. For exercise, he plays tennis. He likes to head for the courts around 6 P.M., when most people are eating dinner. He warms up for 10 minutes practicing his forehand and backhand against a backboard, and then plays a hard, fast game with his regular partner for 45 minutes to an hour. After he walks back to his room, he does some stretching exercises while his muscles are still warm. Then he showers and gets ready for dinner. Twice a week he works out at the gym, with particular attention to keeping his arms strong and his elbows limber. On Saturday nights, he goes dancing with his girlfriend.

■ **Exploring Your Emotions**

Was exercise part of your family life when you were growing up? How much do your parents exercise? Do you think you're influenced by their attitudes and habits? How will you motivate your own children to exercise?

Each of these people has worked an adequate or more-than-adequate fitness program into a busy daily routine. How can you include exercise in your life?

Getting Started and Keeping on Track

Once you have a program that fulfills your basic fitness needs and suits your personal tastes, adhering to a few basic principles will help you improve at the fastest rate, have more fun, and minimize the risk of injury. These principles include buying appropriate equipment, eating and drinking properly, and managing your program so it becomes an integral part of your life.

Selecting Equipment   When you're sure of the activities you're going to do, buy the best equipment you can afford. Good equipment will enhance your enjoyment and decrease your risk of injury. Part of the "fitness fad" has been a wave of new equipment and clothing for every sport imaginable. Some of it is truly revolutionary: new skis allow you to go faster with better control, new tennis racquets make it easier to hit the ball over the net, and new materials make sports clothing more comfortable and fashionable. Unfortunately, some new products are either overpriced or of poor quality. A flashy but overweight tennis racquet can produce an elbow injury, and a shoe that can't absorb shock can cause leg pains.

Before you invest in a new piece of equipment, investigate it. Is it worth the money? Does it produce the results its proponents claim for it? If you're choosing exercise equipment, does it work your body actively or passively? Passive devices such as rubberized suits and massage machines provide no conditioning effect and may be dangerous. Look for equipment that provides a genuine workout, such as stationary bicycles, cross-country skiing machines, or stair-climbers. Ask the experts (coaches, physical educators, and sports instructors) for their opinion. Better yet, educate yourself. Every sport, from running to volleyball, has its own magazine. A little effort to educate yourself will be well rewarded.

Footwear is perhaps the most important piece of equipment for almost any sport. Buy shoes that fit properly and that are appropriate for the activity. Running shoes, court shoes (for tennis, racquetball, basketball,

and so on), and shoes for aerobic dance and exercise have different characteristics. Figure 14-1 shows the characteristics of an ideal running shoe.

Eating and Drinking for Exercise   Most people do not need to change their eating habits when they begin a fitness program. Many athletes and other physically active people are lured into buying aggressively advertised vitamins, minerals, and protein supplements. The truth is that in almost every case a well-balanced diet (see Chapter 12) contains all the energy and nutrients needed to sustain an exercise program.

A balanced diet is also the key to improving your body composition when you begin to exercise more. One of the promises of a fitness program is a decrease in body fat and an increase in lean, muscular body mass. As mentioned earlier, the control of body fat is determined by the balance of energy in the body. If more calories are consumed than are expended through metabolism and exercise, then fat increases. If the reverse is true, fat is lost. The best way to control body fat is to follow a diet containing adequate but not excessive calories and to participate in aerobic exercise.

The one change in diet that some long-distance runners and other athletes make is to increase the proportion of carbohydrates they consume. Diets that are higher than average in carbohydrates can benefit athletes because carbohydrates increase the amount of **glycogen** present in the body. Glycogen, a carbohydrate stored in muscles and the liver, is vitally important for sustaining physical activity over long periods of time. When levels of this substance are low, the athlete feels sluggish, weak, and tired. One of the most exciting discoveries in sports medicine in recent years has been that consuming carbohydrate drinks during exercise can improve performance and that drinking them immediately after exercise rapidly replenishes glycogen. For a more detailed discussion of

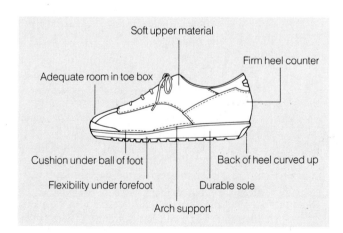

Figure 14-1   What to look for in a running shoe.

the role of carbohydrates and other substances in exercise and athletic performance, see the box "Carbohydrate Loading—Does It Work?"

One of the most important principles to follow when you're exercising is to drink enough water. Your body depends on water to sustain many chemical reactions and to maintain correct body temperature. Sweating during exercise depletes your body's water supply and can lead to dehydration if fluids aren't replaced. Serious dehydration can cause reduced blood volume, increased heart rate, raised body temperature, muscle cramps, heat stroke, and other serious problems. Drinking water before and during exercise is important to prevent dehydration and enhance athletic performance.

Thirst alone is not a good indication of how much you need to drink, because thirst is quickly depressed by drinking even small amounts of water. Most of your weight loss immediately after exercise is from loss of fluids. If you rely only on thirst, it can take 24 hours or more to replace these fluids. Ideally, you should restore your body fluids before you exercise vigorously again. As a rule of thumb, try to drink about 8 ounces of water (more in hot weather) for every 30 minutes of heavy exercise. Bring a water bottle with you when you exercise so you can replace your fluids while they're being depleted. Water—preferably cold—or diluted carbohydrate drinks such as Gatorade are the best fluid replacements. You do not need to replace electrolytes, such as sodium and potassium, during exercise because the body is very efficient at sparing them.

Managing Your Fitness Program   How can you tell when you're in shape? When do you stop improving and start maintaining? How can you stay motivated? These are important questions if your program is going to become an integral part of your life and if the principles behind it are going to serve you well in the years ahead.

Consistency: The Key to Physical Improvement   It's important to be able to recognize when you have achieved the level of fitness that is adequate for you. This level will vary, of course, depending on your goals, the intensity of your program, and your natural ability. Your body gets into shape by adapting to increasing levels of physical stress. If you don't push yourself by increasing the intensity of your workout—by adding weight, pushing your joints past their normal range of motion, running a little faster or a little longer—no change will occur in your body.

But if you subject your body to overly severe stress, it will break down and become distressed, or injured. Overdoing exercise is just as bad as not exercising hard enough. No one can become fit overnight. Your body needs time to adapt to increasingly higher levels of stress. The process of improving fitness, of training, involves a countless number of stresses and adaptations. If you feel extremely sore and tired the day after exercising, then you have worked too hard. Injury will slow you down just as much as a missed workout.

Consistency is the key to getting into shape without injury. Steady fitness improvement comes when you overload your body consistently over a long period of time. The best way to ensure consistency is by keeping a training diary in which you record the details of your workouts—how far you ran, how much weight you lifted, how many laps you swam, and so on. This record will help you evaluate your progress and plan your workout sessions intelligently.

How to Tell When You're in Shape   When are you "in shape"? It depends. One person may be out of shape running a mile in five minutes; another may be in shape running a mile in twelve minutes. As mentioned earlier, your ultimate level of fitness depends on your goals, your program, and your natural ability. The important thing is to set goals that make sense for you.

If you are interested in finding out exactly how fit you are before you begin a program, the best approach is to get an assessment from a modern sports medicine laboratory. Such laboratories can be found in university physical education departments and medical centers. Here you will receive an accurate profile of your capacity to exercise. Typically, your endurance will be measured on a treadmill or bicycle, your body fat will be estimated, and your strength and flexibility will be tested. This evaluation will reveal whether your physical condition is consistent with good health, and the personnel at the laboratory can suggest an exercise program that will be appropriate for your level of fitness.

Assessing your own fitness is more difficult because endurance, strength, coordination, agility, and other components of fitness are specific to activities or tasks. It's meaningless to count how many pull-ups or push-ups you can do when you're interested in having the muscle strength to play tennis, ski, or jog. Endurance for running doesn't translate directly into endurance for swimming or bicycling—you have to practice the activities themselves to improve in them. Nevertheless, a very

Glycogen   A complex carbohydrate, found largely in the liver and skeletal muscle, that serves as a carbohydrate storage depot.

Carbohydrate Loading—Does It Work?

Manipulation of the diet in hopes of enhancing athletic performance has a long and checkered history. As recently as twenty years ago, football players were encouraged on hot practice days to get "toughened up" for competition by consuming salt tablets liberally before and during practice and by not drinking water. It is now widely recognized that this practice can be fatal. Today's athletes still search for ways to maximize their potential, but they can take advantage of scientific evidence that some substances—notably carbohydrates—do enhance athletic performance, at least in some athletes in some situations, without posing a threat to their health.

Carbohydrate is an indispensable fuel for essentially all types of athletic performance because the energy demand in athletics exceeds what can be supplied by fat or protein. There is ample evidence that the depletion of stored carbohydrate (glycogen) in the muscles is a cause of fatigue in exercise that lasts longer than 60 to 90 minutes. Glycogen depletion may contribute to diminished performance in brief, high-intensity competition as well. A reduction in the levels of sugar (glucose) in the blood during prolonged exercise has also been associated with early fatigue. It's hardly surprising, then, that dietary carbohydrate has been manipulated before and during exercise in hopes of improving performance.

One of the better known ways to manipulate carbohydrates in the diet is carbohydrate loading, the practice of gradually reducing the duration of athletic training sessions during the week before an important competition while pro-

gressively increasing the consumption of dietary carbohydrates. The athlete consumes 20 to 40 percent of dietary calories as carbohydrate for the first three days of the carbohydrate-loading regimen and then 70 to 85 percent for the three or four days immediately preceding competition. This procedure is designed to maximize the storage of muscle glycogen before competition and to thereby extend the duration of high-level performance before the onset of fatigue. For the average athlete, carbohydrate loading has been shown in both laboratory and field situations to significantly increase endurance time. Although some persons experience gastrointestinal discomfort or a feeling of sluggishness with high-carbohydrate diets, most athletes and exercise physiologists vouch for the efficacy and reliability of carbohydrate loading.

Carbohydrate loading works by increasing the amount of glycogen stored in the muscles *before* a competitive event. Performance can also be improved by increasing the level of glucose in the blood *during* competition—by consuming carbohydrate drinks. The more concentrated a solution is, the longer it takes to empty out of the stomach into the intestine and be absorbed into the bloodstream. Carbohydrate drinks—solutions of glucose, fructose, or sucrose, for example—supply the athlete with a continuous source of energy, thus improving endurance performance. Drinks containing about 5 to 8 percent carbohydrates are ideal because they maintain cardiovascular function and body temperature regulation as well as water does. Elite endurance athletes who consume 150 to 250

milliliters of 5–8 percent carbohydrate solution every 20 minutes during exercise may experience a 30 percent improvement in endurance. Less well trained athletes can expect a more modest improvement of 5 to 7 percent in an event lasting more than 45 minutes. Most commercial "sports rehydration drinks" include carbohydrates in the appropriate concentration ranges. However, beverages containing more than 3 to 4 percent fructose or more than 10 percent glucose or sucrose tend to cause gastrointestinal distress and are not well tolerated by most athletes.

Other substances have been investigated for their effect on athletic performance, including sodium bicarbonate, caffeine, and various vitamins and minerals, but none of them has proven as safe or useful as have carbohydrates. Sodium bicarbonate, for example, is effective in neutralizing lactic acid, which accumulates in muscles during performance and leads to fatigue, but it also produces nausea and diarrhea. Caffeine provides some performance enhancement but can cause cardiac arrhythmias, nausea, and light-headedness, which can actually impair performance. And vitamins and minerals have positive effects only in people who are deficient in them, a fairly rare condition in American athletes. Manipulating dietary carbohydrates, on the other hand, appears to be a safe, effective way to enhance athletic performance.

Adapted from David R. Lamb. 1989. Dietary substances and athletic performance. *Healthline*, October.

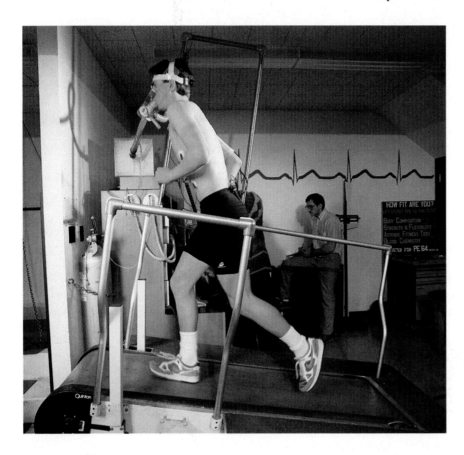

An accurate assessment of fitness involves measuring cardiorespiratory endurance, usually on a treadmill, and testing strength and flexibility. This student will also have his body composition evaluated in an underwater weighing tank.

rough estimate of your cardiorespiratory fitness can be obtained by checking your time in the 1.5 mile run or walk. Use Table 14-5 to find out in general terms whether your level of fitness is consistent with good health.

Dealing with Athletic Injuries Injuries can happen even to the most careful physically active person. Although annoying, most are neither serious nor permanent. However, an injury that isn't cared for properly can escalate into a chronic problem, sometimes serious enough to permanently curtail the activity. It's important to learn how to deal with injuries so they don't derail your fitness program.

Some injuries require medical attention. Consult a doctor for head and eye injuries, possible ligament injuries, broken bones, and internal disorders such as chest pain, fainting, and intolerance to heat. Also seek medical attention for apparently minor injuries that do not get better within a reasonable amount of time.

For minor cuts and scrapes, stop the bleeding and clean the wound. Treat soft tissue injuries (muscles and joints) immediately with ice packs. Elevate the affected part of the body above the level of the heart, and compress it with an elastic bandage to minimize swelling. Use ice for 48 hours after the injury or until all swelling

Table 14-5 Standards for the 1.5-mile run/walk (min:sec)				
	High	**Good**	**Fair**	**Poor**
Males				
20–29	9:45	12:00	13:00	15:00
30–39	10:00	12:15	13:30	16:00
40–49	10:30	12:30	14:00	16:30
50–59	11:00	13:30	15:00	18:30
60 +	11:15	14:30	16:30	19:00
Females				
20–29	11:00	13:15	14:15	16:15
30–39	11:15	13:30	14:45	17:15
40–49	11:45	13:45	15:15	17:45
50–59	12:15	14:45	16:15	19:45
60 +	12:30	15:45	17:45	20:15

Note: This test should not be attempted without at least six weeks of conditioning. Check with your doctor if you are over 35.

Evaluating the Clubs

Are you looking for a health and fitness club to help you get or stay in shape? If so, some general guidelines will help you weed out the clubs that are just in it for the profit and find one that can really meet your needs. The general advice that follows is offered by *Consumers Guide.*®

High-pressure Selling

When you enter a health club, you can expect a tour followed by a high-pressure sales pitch. Be ready for it. Instructors and managers are well schooled in making an effective representation. They want your business.

Consumers Guide® sees nothing wrong with the health club manager's making a strong case emphasizing the value of exercise. But that's it. Under no circumstances should you feel badgered, embarrassed, belittled, threatened, detained, or mocked. If you feel any excessive amount of pressure, leave or at least ask for more time. If you are told this is a once-in-a-lifetime deal or that the rates go up tomorrow, forget it. It's a high-pressure outfit interested in the dollar figure, not yours.

The Contract   Read the contract carefully. If you want more time, take it. If you feel you should read it at home or want to discuss it with anyone else, do so. If the health club won't permit you to take the contract home, steer clear of that organization. Make sure the contract commits you to no more than two years; one year is preferable. All contracts should provide for a minimum three-day cooling-off period; look for a "use of facility" clause permitting you to use the club during those three days.

Key Considerations

During the tour, explanation of facilities, and closing, you should be aware of the following:

1. Is there a discussion of your individual problems? This should take place prior to signing the contract. Is there a discussion of your physical limitations, risk factors, and the possibility of stress tests? Do they recommend that you talk to your doctor before you embark on an exercise program?

2. Is the person conducting the tour an instructor, a manager, or what? Does he or she seem to be well trained and not just well built? Ask if he or she is a physical education or physical therapy graduate with additional training in fitness. If not, does the club have an in-service training program emphasizing cardiovascular fitness? Do you sense that the person has a genuine interest in you? Is he or she able to explain how the machines operate, their value and limitations? Are the aerobics instructors safety conscious and concerned about their students? Do they teach them how to monitor their heart rates?

3. Does the spa manager or instructor emphasize cardiovascular fitness, or is the focus on muscle strength and muscle endurance? If the emphasis is on muscle strength and endurance, you can eliminate that club. The primary focus should be on cardiovascular fitness.

4. Visit the club *at a time of day when you plan to use it*. This is crucial. Every club has a peak usage time. Waiting in line to run on the treadmill, ride a bicycle, or lift weights can be a serious inconvenience. Consider time and use of facilities as important factors.

5. Before signing anything, talk to several of the people who are exercising (or who have just finished, if you don't want to interrupt their work). Ask what they think of the program, what the emphasis is, and whether personal attention is given.

6. Observe the facility. Is it clean, well ventilated, and properly maintained? Is equipment in good condition? Is there shock-absorbent flooring for aerobics workouts—a suspended wood floor, high-density matting, or carpet over cushioning? High-impact activity should never be done on tile, linoleum, or cement.

7. Find out how long the club has been in your area. The longer the better, and if under the same management, that's another plus. Approach a new club with caution—especially "pre-opening" sales. There have been cases where con artists have held pre-opening sales for clubs that never opened.

8. Find out if the club belongs to the Association of Physical Fitness Centers. This trade association for full-service health spas is dedicated to upgrading the industry. The Association has established a code of ethics that covers programs, facilities, employees, and consumers' rights. You can also check on the club with the Better Business Bureau to see if any complaints have been filed against it.

9. The spa needs you more than you need the spa. Don't forget that. A club is an extra. It can provide you with some social contacts, motivation, and a special plan to exercise—if you need these things.

Source: Adapted from Carol Krucoff. 1989. Joining the club. *Washington Post Health*, September 5, p. 20.

is gone. (Don't leave ice on one spot for more than 20 minutes at a time.) Some experts recommend taking over-the-counter medication that decreases inflammation, such as aspirin or ibuprofen, to treat soft tissue injuries.

Don't use heat on an injury at first because heat draws blood to the area and increases swelling. After the swelling has subsided, apply heat to speed up healing. Heat helps relieve pain, relax muscles, and reduce stiffness. Check with your physician about whether moist heat (hot towels, heat packs) or dry heat (heating pads) is better for your particular injury. Whirlpools are a good way to combine heat and gentle massage.

To rehabilitate your body after a minor athletic injury, follow these four steps: (1) reduce the initial inflammation using the RICE principle (rest, ice, compression, elevation), (2) restore normal joint motion, (3) restore normal strength and endurance, and (4) restore functional capacity. This fourth step involves gradually reintroducing the stress of the activity until you are capable of returning to full intensity. Before returning to full exercise participation, you should have a full range of motion in your joints, normal strength and balance among your muscles, normal coordinated patterns of movement, with no injury compensation movements, such as limping, and little or no pain.

To prevent injuries in the future, follow a few basic guidelines: (1) stay in condition; haphazard exercise programs invite injury; (2) warm up thoroughly before exercise; (3) use proper body mechanics when lifting objects or executing sports skills; (4) don't exercise when you're ill or overtrained; (5) use the proper equipment; and (6) don't return to your normal exercise program until athletic injuries have healed. Professional athletes appear to recover quickly from their injuries because they treat them promptly and correctly. You can keep your fitness program on track by doing the same.

Staying with Your Program   Once you have attained your desired level of fitness, you can maintain it by exercising on a regular basis at a consistent intensity, three to five times a week. You must work at the intensity that brought you to your desired fitness level. If you don't, your body will become less fit because less is expected of it. In general, if you exercise at the same intensity over a long period, your fitness will level out and can be maintained easily. Sometimes it's easiest to stay with a program if you spend money to take a class or join a club. Community and Y programs are affordable for nearly anyone, but health clubs can be overpriced and their services of questionable value; see the box "Evaluating the Clubs" for some hints on choosing a good one.

What if you run out of steam? Although good health is an important *reason* to exercise, it's a poor *motivator* for consistent adherence to an exercise program. If you don't enjoy your program, you won't continue it for very long. It's easy to say, "Missing this workout isn't going to matter." Unfortunately, that missed workout can stretch into several weeks or months. But if you *select a physical activity that you like and look forward to, you will be much more faithful.* A variety of specific suggestions for staying with your program are given in the behavior change strategy at the end of this chapter. It's also a good idea to have a goal, anything from fitting into the same size jeans you used to wear to successfully skiing down a new slope. Remember, you can have goals without striving to improve your fitness.

Varying your program is another way to stay interested. Consider competitive sports at the recreational level—swimming, running, racquetball, volleyball, golf, and so on. Find out how you can participate in an activity you've never done before—canoeing, hang gliding, windsurfing, backpacking. Try new activities, especially ones that you will be able to do for the rest of your life. Get maps of the recreational or wilderness areas near you and go exploring. Fill a canteen, pack a good lunch, and take along a wildflower or bird book. Every step you take will bring you closer to your ultimate goal—fitness and health that last a lifetime.

Summary

- A physical fitness plan that works requires a basic knowledge and understanding of exercise.

What Is Physical Fitness and Why Is It Important?

- The components of overall *physical fitness*, the ability to adapt to the demands and stresses of physical effort, include cardiorespiratory endurance; flexibility; muscular strength, power, and endurance; and body composition. Components of fitness for a specific activity might include coordination, speed, agility, balance, and skill.

- The body can improve its functioning; the level of physical fitness generally reflects the amount and intensity of physical activity.

- The body works best when it *is* active, but modern lifestyles are increasingly sedentary, which means higher risks for degenerative diseases and early death. By improving the overall functioning of the body, exercise can help in managing stress, maintaining emotional well-being, controlling weight, boosting the immune system, and protecting against serious diseases.

Why Is Exercise So Good for You?

- Cardiorespiratory endurance (or aerobic) exercise improves the ability of the heart, lungs, and circulatory system to carry oxygen to the body's tissues. This efficiency means that the heart doesn't have to work as hard in daily life and can meet emergency needs.
- Exercise has a positive effect on the balance of lipids in the blood; exercise increases HDLs and lowers LDLs. Exercise also decreases the secretion of hormones triggered by emotional stress and helps diffuse hostility.
- Endurance exercise improves the efficiency of the body's metabolism, helping to regulate energy balance and body weight.
- Exercise has social, psychological, and emotional benefits. Positive feelings associated with exercise have a physiological basis in hormones and body chemicals. Endorphins, secreted by the brain during exercise, help decrease pain, produce euphoria, and suppress fatigue.
- Exercises designed to improve muscular strength and endurance, joint flexibility, and posture are also essential to fitness.
- Beginning to exercise regularly can improve health over the life span. Physical fitness helps prevent heart disease, stroke, diabetes, and high blood pressure; it may help prevent fatigue, weight gain, memory loss, and other problems associated with aging. Exercise is especially helpful in preventing osteoporosis.

Designing Your Exercise and Fitness Program

- The best exercise and fitness programs promote health and are fun to do. Activities should be chosen to fit the personality; accessibility, expense, and time need to be considered as well. Activities should contribute to cardiorespiratory endurance, but also to muscle strength, flexibility, and specific skills for individual sports or activities.
- Cardiorespiratory endurance exercises stress a large portion of the body's muscle mass for a prolonged period of time.
- To be effective, endurance exercise should be undertaken three to five days a week.
- Intensity of training is crucial to increasing the body's maximal oxygen capacity; monitoring the heart rate helps ensure that a workout is done at the appropriate intensity. Periodization of training involves varying the intensity of the workout from day to day so that the most intense exercise follows a period of rest.

- The amount of time spent on a workout should be determined by its intensity. Continuous endurance exercises should last from 15 minutes (high-intensity activities) to 60 minutes (low-intensity activities).
- Flexibility, or stretching, exercises are necessary to maintain the normal range of motion in the major joints of the body and to keep the muscles from contracting and shortening.
- Exercise to develop muscular strength and endurance are necessary for correct posture, efficient movement, and muscle tone. Resistive exercises are necessary to increase muscle strength; these include isometric exercise (applying force without movement), isokinetic exercise (exerting force at a constant speed against an equal force exerted by a training machine), and isotonic exercise (applying force with movement).
- Learning the skills required for specific sports or activities helps people achieve a sense of mastery and add new physical activities to their exercise programs. Getting help from a class or instructor is usually necessary.
- Warming up exercises decrease chances of injury by helping the body gradually progress from rest to exercise as blood is redirected to active muscles. It helps spread synovial fluid through the joints.
- Cooling down after exercise involves continuing to exercise at a low level to provide a smooth transition to the resting state, where little of the total blood volume is directed to the muscles.

Getting Started and Keeping on Track

- Good equipment enhances enjoyment and decreases risk of injury. Footwear is especially important; it should fit properly and be appropriate for the activity.
- A well-balanced diet contains all the energy and nutrients needed to sustain a fitness program. Increasing the proportion of carbohydrates can benefit some athletes by increasing the amount of glycogen present in the body.
- When exercising, it's important to drink enough water, which is necessary to prevent dehydration and maintain correct body temperature.
- People in a fitness program need to recognize when they have reached an adequate level of fitness. Subjecting the body to severe stress will cause injury. Consistency leads to steady improvement.
- The ultimate level of fitness depends on the goals, the program, and natural ability. Fitness levels can be evaluated at sports medicine laboratories.
- Injuries that require medical attention include head and eye injuries, possible ligament injuries, broken bones, and internal disorders such as chest pain, fainting, and intolerance to heat.
- Rest, ice, compression, and elevation (RICE) are the

appropriate treatments for muscle and joint injuries. Heat can be used after swelling has subsided. Before the fitness program can be resumed at its former intensity, it's necessary to restore normal joint motion, strength, and endurance and to reintroduce the stress of the activity—working up to full intensity.

- A desired level of fitness can be maintained by exercising three to five times a week at a consistent intensity. Ways to stay motivated include having specific goals, enjoying the activity, and maintaining interest by varying the program.

Take Action

1. In your health diary, list the positive behaviors and attitudes that help you avoid a sedentary lifestyle and stay fit. How can you strengthen these behaviors and attitudes? Then list the negative behaviors and attitudes that block a physically active lifestyle. Which ones can you change? How can you change them?

2. Habit helps us conserve energy as we go through our daily lives,

but it also blinds us to areas we could change. Make a list of ten ways you can incorporate more physical activity into your life by changing a habit, such as walking instead of riding the bus, taking the stairs in a certain building instead of the elevator, and so on.

3. Go to your school's physical education office and ask for a comprehensive listing of all the

exercise and fitness facilities available on your campus. Visit the facilities you haven't yet seen and investigate the activities that are done there. If there are sports or activities you'd like to try, consider doing so.

4. Investigate the fitness clubs in your community. How do they compare with each other, and how do they measure up in terms of the guidelines provided in this chapter?

Behavior Change Strategy

Planning a Personal Exercise Program

Although most people recognize the importance of incorporating exercise into their lives, many find it difficult to do. No single strategy will work for everyone, but the general steps outlined here should help you create an exercise program that fits your goals, preferences, and lifestyle. A carefully designed contract and program plan can help you convert your vague wishes into a detailed plan of action. And the strategies for program compliance outlined here and in Chapter 1 can help you enjoy and stick with your program for the rest of your life.

Step 1: Set Goals

Setting specific goals to accomplish by exercising is an important first step in a successful fitness program because it establishes the direction

you want to go in. Your goals might be specifically related to health, such as lowering your blood pressure and risk for heart disease, or they might relate to other aspects of your life, such as improving your tennis game or the fit of your clothes. If you can decide why you're starting to exercise, it can help you to keep going.

Think carefully about your reasons for incorporating exercise into your life, and then fill in the goals portion of the Personal Fitness Contract.

Step 2: Select a Sport or Activity

As discussed in the chapter, the success of your fitness program depends upon the consistency of your involvement. You should select activities that encourage your commitment: the right program will

be its own incentive to continue; poor activity choices provide obstacles and can turn exercise into a chore.

When choosing activities for your fitness program, you should consider the following:

- Is this activity fun? Will it hold my interest over time?
- Will this activity help me reach the goals I have set for myself?
- Will my current fitness and skill level allow me to participate fully in this activity?
- Can I easily fit this activity into my daily schedule? Are there any special requirements (facilities, partners, equipment, etc.) that I must plan for?
- Can I afford any special costs required for equipment or facilities?

Personal Fitness Contract

I, _____, am contracting with myself to follow an exercise program to work at the following goals.

Fitness Goals

(Note as many as appropriate.)

1. _____
2. _____
3. _____
4. _____
5. _____

Program Plan

Activities	Components (Check ✓) CRE	BC	MS	ME	F	Intensity	Duration	Frequency (Check ✓) M.	Tu.	W.	Th.	F.	Sa.	Su.
1. _____														
2. _____														
3. _____														
4. _____														
5. _____														
6. _____														
7. _____														
8. _____														
9. _____														
10. _____														

I will begin my program on _____ .

I agree to maintain a record of my activity, assess my progress periodically, and, if necessary, revise my goals.

Signed _____   Date _____

Witness _____

Note: You should conduct activities for achieving CRE goals at your target heart rate.

Adapted from Ivan Kusinitz and Morton Fine (1987), *Your Guide to Getting Fit* (Mountain View, CA: Mayfield).

- (If you have special exercise needs due to a particular health problem.) Does this activity conform to my special health needs? Will it enhance my ability to cope with my specific health problem?

Refer to Table 14-4, which summarizes the fitness benefits and other characteristics of many activities. Using the guidelines listed above, select a number of sports and activities. Fill in the "Program Plan" portion of the Fitness Contract, using Table 14-4 to include the fitness components your choices will develop and the intensity, duration, and frequency standard you intend to meet for each activity. Does your program meet the criteria of a complete fitness program discussed in the chapter?

Step 3: Make A Commitment

Complete your Fitness Contract and Program Plan by signing your contract and having it witnessed and signed by someone who can help make you accountable for your progress. By completing a written contract you will make a firm commitment and will be more likely to carry through to your goals.

Step 4: Begin and Maintain Your Program

Start out slowly to allow your body time to adjust. Be realistic and patient—meeting your goals will take time. The following guidelines may help you to start and stick with your program:

- Set aside regular periods for exercise. Choose times that fit in best with your schedule and stick to them. Allow an adequate amount of time for warm-up, cool-down, and a shower.
- Take advantage of any opportunity for exercise that presents itself

(for example, walk to class, take the stairs instead of the elevator).

- Do what you can to avoid boredom. Do calisthenics to music or read while riding your stationary bicycle.
- Exercise with a group that shares your goals and general level of competence.
- Vary the program. Change your activities periodically. Alter your route or distance if biking or jogging. Change racquetball partners or find a new volleyball court.
- Establish minigoals or a point system and work rewards into your program. Until you reach your main goals, a system of self-rewards will help you stick with your program. Rewards should be things you enjoy and that are easily obtainable.

Step 5: Record and Assess Your Progress

Keeping a record that notes the daily results of your program will help remind you of your ongoing commitment to your program and give you a sense of accomplishment. Create daily and weekly program logs that you can use to track your progress. You should record the activity type, frequency, and duration. Keep your log handy and fill it in immediately after each exercise session. Post it in a visible place to both remind you of your activity schedule and offer incentive for improvement.

Here are some additional tips to help make your program a success:

- If in the first few weeks you find that your program is unrealistic, revise the goals and activity information on your contract. Expect to make many adjustments in your program along the way.
- Don't expect your progress to be even and regular. You will notice fluctuations: on some days your progress will be excellent, while on others you will barely be able to drag yourself through the scheduled activities.

- Don't rush yourself. Overzealous exercising can result in discouraging discomforts and injuries. Your program is meant to last a lifetime, so begin slowly and increase your activity level gradually.
- If you notice that you are slacking off, try to list the negative thoughts and behaviors that are causing noncompliance. Devise a strategy to decrease the frequency of negative thoughts and behaviors. Adjust your program plan and reward system to help renew your enthusiasm and commitment to your program.
- Review your goals. Visualize what it will be like to reach them, and keep these pictures in your mind as an incentive to stick to your program.

Adapted from Ivan Kusinitz and Morton Fine. 1987, *Your Guide to Getting Fit*. (Mountain View, Calif. Mayfield).

Selected Bibliography

American College of Sports Medicine. 1986. *Guidelines for Graded Exercise Testing and Exercise Prescription*. Philadelphia: Lea and Feibiger.

Brooks, G. A., and T. D. Fahey. 1987. *Fundamentals of Human Performance*. New York: Macmillan.

Dintiman, G. B., S. E. Stone, J. C. Pennington, and R. G. Davis. 1984. *Discovering Lifetime Fitness: Concepts of Exercise and Weight Control*. St. Paul, Minn.: West.

Fahey, T. D., ed. 1986. *Athletic Training: Principles and Practice*. Mountain View, Calif.: Mayfield.

Nieman, D. C. 1990. *Nutrition and Sports Medicine: An Introduction*. Palo Alto, Calif.: Bull Publishing.

Paffenbarger, R. S., R. T. Hyde, A. L. Wing, and C. H. Steinmetz. 1984. A natural history of athleticism and cardiovascular health. *Journal of the American Medical Association* 252:491–95.

Rejeski, W. J., and E. A. Kenney. 1988. *Fitness Motivation: Preventing Participant Dropout*. Champaign, Ill.: Human Kinetics.

Recommended Readings

Cooper, K. 1983. *The Aerobics Program for Total Well-being*. New York: Bantam. *A comprehensive guide to shaping up your heart and lungs.*

Fahey, T. 1989. *Basic Weight Training*. Mountain View, Calif: Mayfield. *A practical guide to developing training programs tailored to individual needs.*

Kan, E., and M. Kraines. 1987. *Keep Moving! It's Aerobic Dance*. Mountain View, Calif.: Mayfield. *Discusses the fitness principles and techniques every aerobic dancer should know.*

Kusinitz, I., and M. Fine. 1987. *Your Guide to Getting Fit*. Mountain View, Calif.: Mayfield. *A step-by-step guide to developing a personalized fitness program.*

Maglischo, E. W., and C. F. Brennan. 1984. *Swim for the Health of It*. Mountain View, Calif.: Mayfield. *Includes discussions of conditioning and stroke techniques for people who want to use swimming to improve their health and physical fitness.*

Contents

Making Connections

Cardiovascular disease is so common in our society that you or someone you know is very likely to fall victim to it, perhaps in middle age. But the habits you adopt now can make a big difference in whether you keep your healthy heart or develop one of the debilitating cardiovascular diseases. The scenarios presented on these pages describe situations in which people have to use information, make a decision, or choose a course of action, all related to cardiovascular health. As you read them, imagine yourself in each situation and consider what you would do. After you've finished the chapter, read the scenarios again and see if what you've learned has changed how you would think, feel, or act in each situation.

You've been trying to improve your diet lately, and you've noticed quite a few products in the store labeled "no cholesterol." You've been pleasantly surprised to find that some of your favorite snack foods, like potato chips and peanut butter, are cholesterol-free. Still, chips seem so greasy and peanut butter seems so oily, it's hard to believe they're that good for you. Does "no cholesterol" mean a food is a healthy choice?

You recently realized that your family has a strong pattern of cardiovascular disease. Your grandfather had a heart attack when he was 51, one of your uncles had a heart attack at 53, and another uncle had a stroke at 47. When you pointed this pattern out to your brother, he said, "So? What are we supposed to do? I'll worry about it when I'm 45." Is your brother smart not to get too worried about heart disease now? Is it true that there isn't anything he can do about it?

15
Cardiovascular Health

Your dad was told he had high blood pressure last year and was given some medication to take for it. When you went home for vacation, you discovered that he didn't think he needed the medication any more and had stopped taking it. He said he was jogging, playing tennis, and eating a sensible diet and had never felt better in his life. Your mom wants him to take the medication again, but he says the symptoms he had have gone away. Is your dad right to stop taking the medication since he feels all right now? What advice can you give him?

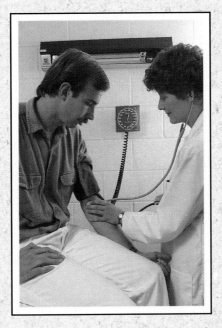

One day when you were visiting your grandmother, a strange thing happened. She was standing in the kitchen when suddenly she became so dizzy she had to sit down. When you asked her what was wrong, she was only able to mumble some sounds you couldn't understand. Then just as suddenly, she was fine again. You were greatly relieved that she recovered but concerned about what had happened. You wanted her to call her doctor, but she said it was just one of her spells and nothing to be alarmed about. Is she all right? What should she do if it happens again? What should you do?

One of your housemates worries about her health a lot and is constantly buying new health foods. You notice that lately she's been buying different breakfast cereals containing oat bran. In fact, you've been noticing many oat bran products on display at the supermarket. Your housemate says it's good for your heart but she doesn't know why. Is this another fad, or is there something to it? How can oat bran be good for your heart?

When a heart attack hits, it can strike with the sudden savage force of a sledgehammer. It can also sneak up on you at night, masquerading as indigestion with slight pain or pressure in your chest. Although no adult is completely immune, there is much you can do at an early age to reduce the risk. People who are most vulnerable to early heart attacks or strokes are smokers, those with uncontrolled high blood pressure, those with high cholesterol levels, and those who are overweight and underactive.

Cardiovascular disease (CVD) is the number one killer in the United States today, affecting approximately 66 million people—one-quarter of the population. It will continue to hold this position until most of us change our lifestyles, beginning in our teens. In fact, many Americans have been doing just that, and the results of these behavior changes can be seen in declining death rates from heart attacks and strokes. In the last twenty years heart attacks have declined 25 percent and strokes nearly 40 percent (see Figure 15-1).

Exactly what is CVD, and how does it do its damage? More important, how can you take steps now to make sure you keep your heart healthy throughout your life? This chapter provides some answers to these questions.

The Cardiovascular System

The **cardiovascular system** consists of the heart and the blood vessels (veins, arteries, and capillaries); together, they pump and circulate blood throughout the body. The blood carries dissolved materials, such as oxygen, carbon

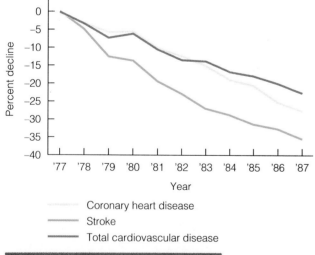

VITAL STATISTICS

Figure 15-1 Cumulative percentage decline in age-adjusted death rates for major cardiovascular diseases, United States: 1977–1987.

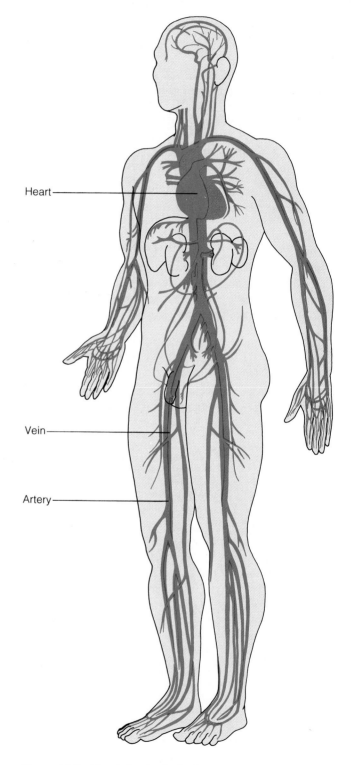

Figure 15-2 Circulation in the body.

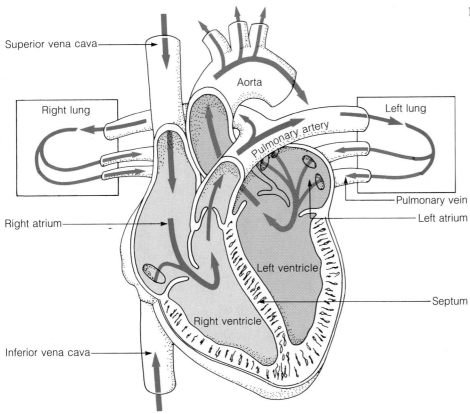

Figure 15-3 Circulation in the heart.

Superior vena cava

Aorta

Right lung

Left lung

Pulmonary artery

Pulmonary vein

Right atrium

Left atrium

Left ventricle

Septum

Right ventricle

Inferior vena cava

dioxide, nutrients, hormones, enzymes, wastes, and so on, to and from the body's cells. In human beings, the blood travels through two separate circulatory systems, each with its own pump—the right or left side of the heart. The right side of the heart pumps blood to and from the lungs; this is called the pulmonary circulation. The left side of the heart pumps blood through the rest of the body; this is called the systemic circulation (see Figure 15-2).

The heart itself is a four-chambered muscle, shaped like a cone and about the size of a fist. The wall of the heart has three layers. The interior layer, called the **endocardium**, is a membrane lining the chambers of the heart. The middle layer, the "muscle," is called the **myocardium**. The outer layer, a membrane called the **epicardium**, covers the heart. Separating the two sides of the heart is a membrane called the cardiac septum.

Each side of the heart contains two separate spaces: the **atria** (plural of atrium), or auricles, which are the thin-walled upper chambers, and the **ventricles**, the thick-walled lower chambers. Blood circulates through the heart in two distinct patterns (see Figure 15-3). Used blood returns from the body via the **vena cava**, the largest vein in the body, and enters the right atrium, from which it flows into the right ventricle. When the ventricle contracts, the blood is forced through the pulmonary artery into the lungs. Here, it picks up oxygen and discards carbon dioxide.

The cleaned and oxygenated blood then passes via the pulmonary veins into the left atrium and from there into the left ventricle. The muscular wall of the left ventricle is very powerful, and when it contracts, it forces blood out through the **aorta**, the body's largest artery, into the systemic circulation. The left ventricle contracts with

Cardiovascular disease (CVD)   Diseases of the heart and blood vessels: hardening of the arteries, high blood pressure, and heart attacks.

Cardiovascular system   The heart and blood vessels.

Endocardium   A membrane lining the cavities of the heart.

Myocardium   A muscular wall of the heart.

Epicardium   A membrane covering the heart.

Atria   The two upper chambers of the heart in which blood collects before passing to the ventricles; also called auricles.

Ventricles   The two lower chambers of the heart from which blood flows through arteries to the lungs and other parts of the body.

Vena cava   Large vein through which blood is returned to the right atrium of the heart.

Aorta   The large artery that receives blood from the left ventricle and distributes it to the body.

enough force to drive the blood to all the tissues of the body. Two blood vessels supply blood to the heart itself, directly to the myocardium. These blood vessels, branching from the aorta, are the coronary arteries. The total volume of blood varies depending on a person's size, but a man weighing about 150 pounds has about 5 quarts of blood. This total volume is circulated about once every minute.

Your heart beats every time the ventricles contract (called **systole**), pumping blood to the lungs via the pulmonary artery and to the body via the aorta. Between beats, the heart relaxes (called **diastole**), and blood flows from the atria into the ventricles. Valves prevent the blood from flowing in the wrong direction. The heart movements create vibrations that produce the familiar "lub-dub" sound of your heartbeat.

Blood vessels are classified by size and function. Veins carry blood *to* the heart, arteries carry it *away* from the heart. Arteries have thick, elastic walls that enable them to expand and relax as blood is pumped into them under pressure from the heart. Veins have thinner walls. After leaving the heart, the aorta branches into smaller arteries, which in turn branch into even smaller arteries. The smallest arteries, called **arterioles**, branch still further into **capillaries**, minute vessels only one cell thick.

The exchange of nutrients and waste products takes place between the capillaries and the tissues, so that the oxygen- and nutrient-rich blood becomes oxygen-poor, waste-carrying blood. This blood empties out of the capillaries into small veins called **venules**, then into larger veins, and finally into the large veins that return it to the heart. From there the cycle is repeated.

Who is at Risk for Cardiovascular Disease?

Not everyone is equal when it comes to cardiovascular disease. Although it is the leading cause of death in the United States, some segments of the population have a much higher risk of developing it than others.

- Men have a greater risk of heart attack and stroke than women, who seem to be protected from heart disease by estrogen until they reach menopause (see Figure 15-4). Even after menopause, when their risk increases, it never reaches that of men.

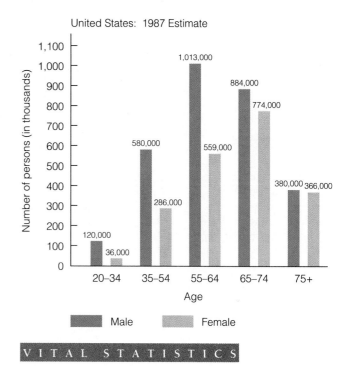

United States: 1987 Estimate

Figure 15-4   Estimated prevalence of coronary heart disease, age 20 and over, United States, 1987 estimate.

- Black Americans suffer twice the incidence of CVD that whites do. One factor in this difference is the higher incidence of high blood pressure among blacks—38 percent of black men and 39 percent of black women aged 18 to 74 have high blood pressure, compared with 33 percent of white men and 25 percent of white women. Another factor is sickle-cell anemia, which often causes strokes and which occurs almost exclusively among blacks.
- The risk of heart attack increases dramatically after age 65. About 55 percent of all heart attack victims are age 65 or older, and almost four out of five who suffer fatal heart attacks are over 65. However, the behaviors that increase the risk factors leading to heart attack or stroke often begin early in life.
- Genetic factors make some people more susceptible to CVD than others. For example, high cholesterol levels and abnormal blood clotting tendencies appear to run in families. A family history of premature heart attacks is a risk factor for CVD.

Systole   Contraction of the heart.

Diastole   Relaxation of the heart.

Arterioles   The smallest arteries that end in capillaries.

Capillaries   Very small blood vessels that distribute blood to all parts of the body.

Venules   Small veins.

Hypertension   Sustained abnormally high blood pressure.

V I T A L   S T A T I S T I C S

CVD in America: A Statistical Summary

Prevalence* 65,890,000 Americans have one or more forms of heart or blood vessel disease.

- High blood pressure— 60,990,000.
- Coronary heart disease— 5,000,000.
- Rheumatic heart disease— 2,180,000.
- Stroke—2,060,000.

Cardiovascular Disease (CVD) Deaths 976,706 in 1987.

- Other 1987 mortality: cancer 477,190; accidents 94,840.
- One-fifth of all people killed by CVD are under age 65.

Heart Attack Caused 513,700 deaths in 1987, 52.6 percent of all CVD deaths.

- Heart attack is the leading cause of death in America today.
- 5,000,000 people alive today have a history of heart attack, angina pectoris (chest pain), or both.
- More than 300,000 people a year die of heart attack before

they reach a hospital—studies indicate 50 percent of heart attack victims wait more than two hours before getting to an emergency room.
- This year as many as 1,500,000 Americans will have a heart attack, and more than 500,000 of them will die.
- Five percent of all heart attacks occur in people under age 40, and 45 percent occur in people under age 65.

Stroke Killed 149,200 people in 1987, 15.3 percent of all CVD deaths.

- Approximately 2,060,000 stroke victims are alive today.
- Approximately 500,000 people suffer strokes each year.
- Stroke is the third largest cause of death, ranking only behind heart attack and cancer.

High Blood Pressure Afflicts an estimated 60,990,000 Americans age 6 and older.

- Hypertensive disease killed

30,900 people in 1987; however, high blood pressure is a factor in many of the other CVD deaths.
- Many people who have high blood pressure don't get treatment.
- Only a minority of people with high blood pressure have it under control.
- The cause of 90 percent of the cases of high blood pressure isn't known; however, high blood pressure is easily detected and usually controllable.

Rheumatic Heart Disease Afflicts 2,180,000 Americans.

- Rheumatic fever and rheumatic heart disease killed about 6,100 Americans in 1987.
- Modern antibiotic therapy has sharply reduced mortality; in 1950, more than 22,000 Americans died of these diseases.

(Estimates based on 1987 provisional statistics for the U.S.)
*The total number of cases of a given disease existing in a population at a specific time.

- People who are overweight or obese are at higher risk for CVD because their hearts have to work harder to pump blood through their bodies. Recent evidence indicates that where fat is located on the body may affect risk. Fat around the hips isn't a problem; fat around the waist appears to increase risk.
- People with diabetes are at risk for CVD because the disease affects the levels of cholesterol in the blood. Diabetes and obesity both have a genetic component as well as a behavioral component.

In addition to these factors, other behaviors and conditions increase the risk of CVD, including **hypertension,** high blood cholesterol, cigarette smoking, a sedentary lifestyle, and certain personality traits such as hostility.

The more risk factors a person has, the higher the chances of heart attack, stroke, or other manifestation of CVD (see Figure 15-5).

Cardiovascular disease was once considered a disease of old age. This is no longer the case, since many men in their forties now die from CVD. Although the influence of heredity is strong, many of these early deaths can be traced to the lifestyle common among many Americans. In most cases, early death can be prevented only by early intervention. To protect themselves from disease and premature death, many Americans need to change their patterns of daily living, especially their smoking habits, diets, exercise programs, and reaction to stress. Later in this chapter, we discuss steps you can take now to lower your risk of developing CVD.

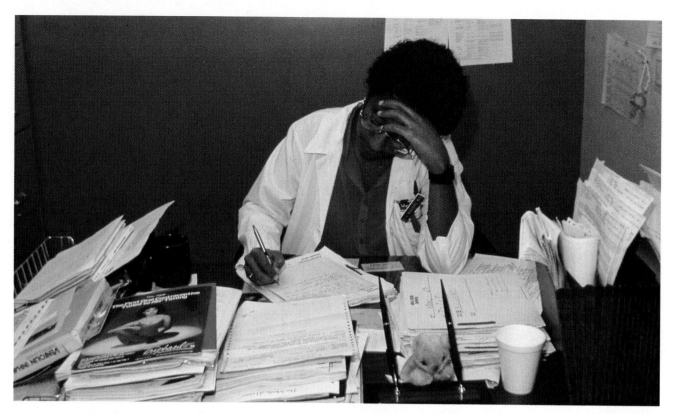

Women are less susceptible to cardiovascular disease than men. Even though this woman has to cope with the same on-the-job stresses as men in her profession, she is less likely to have a heart attack in middle age than they are.

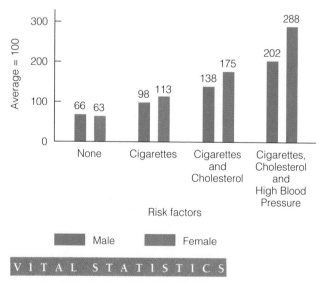

VITAL STATISTICS

Figure 15-5 Danger of heart attack by risk factors present. This chart shows how a combination of three major risk factors can increase the likelihood of heart attack. For purposes of illustration, this chart uses an abnormal blood pressure level of 150 systolic and a cholesterol level of 260 in a 55-year-old male and female.

Major Forms of Cardiovascular Disease

The chief forms of CVD are atherosclerosis, high blood pressure, stroke, congestive heart failure, congenital heart disease, and rheumatic heart disease. Except for congenital heart disease and rheumatic heart disease, the various forms are interrelated and have elements in common; we treat them separately here for the sake of clarity.

Atherosclerosis One of the most common cardiovascular diseases is **atherosclerosis**, the principal form of **arteriosclerosis**, or hardening of the arteries. Atherosclerosis is a slow, progressive process that often begins in childhood. Arteries become narrowed by deposits of fat, cholesterol, and other substances. As these deposits, called **plaques**, accumulate on the walls of the arteries, the arteries lose their elasticity and are unable to expand and contract (see Figure 15-6). The flow of blood through the narrowed arteries is restricted. **Platelets** in the blood may get stuck on a plaque and form a blood clot (**thrombus**), which further restricts the flow of

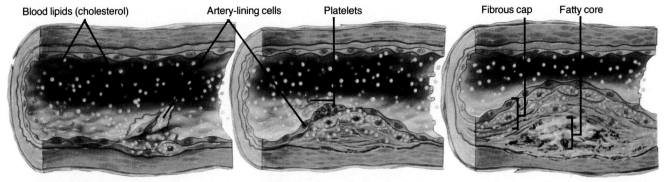

Blood lipids (cholesterol)   Artery-lining cells   Platelets   Fibrous cap   Fatty core

1   Plaque buildup begins when excess fat particles, called *lipids,* collect beneath cells lining the artery that have been damaged by smoking, high blood pressure, or other causes.

2   Platelets, one of the body's protective mechanisms, collect at the damaged area and cause a cap of cells to form, isolating the plaque within the artery wall.

3   The narrowed artery is now vulnerable to blockage by clots that can form if the cap breaks and the fatty core of the lesion combines with the clot-producing factors in the blood.

Figure 15-6   Stages of plaque development.

blood, blocking the artery and depriving the heart, brain, or other organ of the vital oxygen carried by the blood. When a coronary artery is blocked, the result is a *coronary thrombosis,* which is one type of heart attack. When a cerebral artery (leading to the brain) is blocked, the result is a *cerebral thrombosis,* a type of stroke.

What causes atherosclerosis? Although there are many possible contributing factors, three of the main factors are cigarette smoking, high levels of blood cholesterol, and hypertension (high blood pressure). Hypertension not only contributes to atherosclerosis (and vice versa) but is also a disease itself, afflicting more than 60 million people. For this reason, we discuss hypertension separately following the discussion of atherosclerosis.

Cigarette Smoking   The single most important risk factor for atherosclerosis is smoking. Cigarette smoke may be involved in the formation of plaque, and it also appears to destroy **heparin**, the body's natural anticoagulant. With less heparin, blood cells are more prone to clot, and clots tend to form on and around plaques, increasing their size. Cigarette smokers have more than twice the risk of heart attack that nonsmokers have (see Chapter 9). They also are more likely than nonsmokers to die suddenly (within an hour) if they have a heart attack.

■ **Exploring Your Emotions**

How do you feel about the idea of cutting back on fats in your diet—hamburger, french fries, chips, ice cream, pastries? Are these some of your favorite foods? If so, why do you think you like them so much?

You don't have to smoke to be affected by cigarettes: passive smoke (smoke from other people's cigarettes) in high concentrations is strongly implicated in the development of atherosclerosis, as it is in the development of lung cancer. Living or working with smokers for a long period of time may in itself be a risk factor for atherosclerosis and heart disease.

Cholesterol   Cholesterol is a fatlike substance, or lipid, that is essential to the normal functioning of your body. It is a key component of cell membranes and is used in the production of the sex hormones and bile. Most of the cholesterol circulating in your blood (blood cholesterol) is manufactured in your liver, but a portion of it comes from your diet (dietary cholesterol). Dietary cholesterol is found only in animal products, such as meat, poultry, fish, butter, and eggs. Foods that are rich in cholesterol

Atherosclerosis   The principal form of arteriosclerosis; in atherosclerosis, the inner layers of artery walls are made thick and irregular by deposits of a fatty substance. The internal channel of arteries become narrowed, and blood supply is reduced.

Arteriosclerosis   Hardening of the arteries.

Plaque   A deposit of fatty (and other) substances on the inner wall of the arteries.

Platelets   Microscopic disk-shaped cell fragments in the blood. These disintegrate on contact with foreign objects and release chemicals that are necessary for the formation of blood clots.

Thrombus   A blood clot that forms in a blood vessel and remains attached there.

Heparin   A natural substance in the body that prolongs clotting time.

or in saturated fats, including not just animal products but palm oil, coconut oil, and hydrogenated vegetable oils, can drive up the level of cholesterol in your blood.

THE ROLE OF CHOLESTEROL IN CVD Cholesterol is a major component of plaque, but its role in atherosclerosis and heart disease is not completely understood. What is known is that high blood cholesterol increases the risk of heart attack and that the higher the cholesterol, the greater the risk. Middle-aged men with a cholesterol level above 240 milligrams per deciliter of blood (mg/dl) are especially at risk. It's also known that when middle-aged men as a group reduce their cholesterol, they experience a 2 percent drop in the rate of heart attacks for every 1 percent drop in cholesterol.

In countries where the diet is high in saturated fat, such as Finland, the Netherlands, and the United States, the population tends to have high blood cholesterol levels and high heart disease rates. Where intake of saturated fat is lower, such as in Greece, Italy, Japan, and Yugoslavia, blood cholesterol levels are low and heart disease rate is low. The case of Japan is particularly striking because smoking and hypertension, the other major risk factors for heart attacks, are common there, but blood cholesterol and heart disease are both low. Japanese people who live in the United States and eat the typical high-fat American diet have higher cholesterol levels and more heart attacks.

A CLOSER LOOK AT CHOLESTEROL Until recently, guidelines about recommended levels of blood cholesterol were based on *total* cholesterol, but now scientists know that the levels of the various *components* of cholesterol are what counts. Cholesterol is transported in the blood in three different forms: very-low-density lipoproteins (VLDL), **low-density lipoproteins (LDL)**, and **high-density lipoproteins (HDL)**. LDL—the "bad" cholesterol—carries cholesterol out to the periphery of the body, sometimes in amounts that lead to deposits and buildup in the artery walls. But HDL—the "good" cholesterol—draws cholesterol out of the walls and returns it to the liver for recycling (see Figure 15-7).

If your LDL levels are too high, you are in danger; but if your HDL levels are too low, you may be in even more danger. High HDL levels predict cardiovascular health more strongly than high LDL levels predict disease. For this reason, some scientists believe it is more important to raise your HDL than to lower your LDL.

WHAT SHOULD YOUR CHOLESTEROL LEVEL BE? Cholesterol levels under 200 mg/dl are generally considered desirable. Levels between 200 and 239 are considered borderline high, and 240 and above are considered high. People in the high category are clearly at increased risk for coronary heart disease, and people in the borderline high category are at increased risk if they have other risk factors, such as overweight or smoking.

Blood cholesterol is measured with a simple blood test, but measuring it can be tricky. Natural fluctuations are normal over the course of the day, so experts recommend multiple measurements. Anyone whose first measurement is under 200 need not have another measurement for five years. But if the first measurement is over 200, a second and perhaps a third measurement should be taken and the measurements averaged. If total cholesterol measures over 200, or if a person has two or more risk factors, then LDL and HDL should also be measured.

Portable cholesterol screening units in the community, such as at a local drugstore, mall, or YWCA, can give accurate readings if they follow established guidelines for quality control of the instruments, training of the staff, education of participants, and referral in case of high readings. However, the advantage of having your cholesterol measured in your physician's office is that you can get adequate interpretation of the results and appropriate follow-up.

A NATIONAL PLAN FOR LOWERING CHOLESTEROL In response to growing concern about the disastrous rate of heart disease in our country, the federal government established the National Cholesterol Educational Program (NCEP) in 1985. This program seeks to (1) make all Americans aware of their cholesterol levels, (2) change the national diet so it contains less saturated fat and thereby reduce the average American's cholesterol levels by 10 percent, and (3) treat people with high cholesterol, at first with diet and then, if necessary, with drugs.

The program recommends that all adults have their cholesterol measured at least once every five years, beginning at age 20. It also recommends that all Americans over the age of two adopt the American Heart Association's "prudent diet." This diet limits daily fat intake to 30 percent of total calories, divided equally among saturated, monounsaturated, and polyunsaturated fats, and limits dietary cholesterol to 250 to 300 mg daily, slightly more than the amount in one egg (see Chapter 12).

The NCEP program is endorsed by the American Heart

Low-density lipoproteins (LDLs) Blood fats that result in cholesterol accumulating on artery walls, which eventually block the flow of blood to the heart and brain.

High-density lipoproteins (HDLs) Blood fats that help transport cholesterol out of the arteries and thus protect against heart diseases.

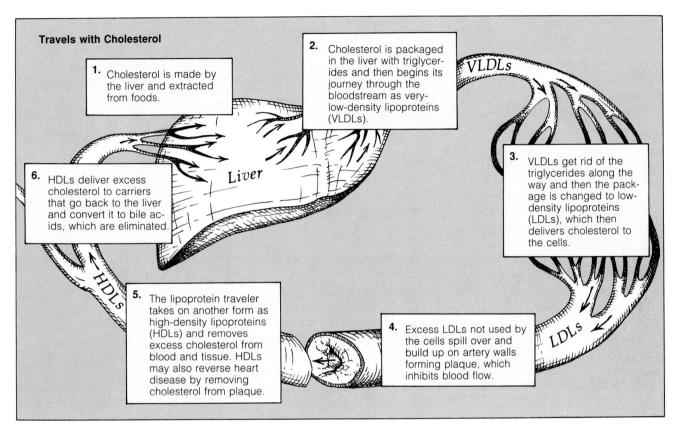

Travels with Cholesterol

1. Cholesterol is made by the liver and extracted from foods.

2. Cholesterol is packaged in the liver with triglycerides and then begins its journey through the bloodstream as very-low-density lipoproteins (VLDLs).

VLDLs

3. VLDLs get rid of the triglycerides along the way and then the package is changed to low-density lipoproteins (LDLs), which then delivers cholesterol to the cells.

6. HDLs deliver excess cholesterol to carriers that go back to the liver and convert it to bile acids, which are eliminated.

Liver

HDLs

5. The lipoprotein traveler takes on another form as high-density lipoproteins (HDLs) and removes excess cholesterol from blood and tissue. HDLs may also reverse heart disease by removing cholesterol from plaque.

4. Excess LDLs not used by the cells spill over and build up on artery walls forming plaque, which inhibits blood flow.

LDLs

Figure 15-7 Travels with cholesterol.

Association, the American Medical Association, and other groups and is being transformed into government policy and cultural change. Over 70 percent of the respondents in recent federal surveys have altered their diet to reduce the risk of heart disease, and two-thirds have taken a blood cholesterol test. Despite widespread acceptance and awareness, however, the cholesterol crusade has recently come under increased scrutiny and criticism. For a closer look at this issue, see the box "Cholesterol: Crusades and Controversies."

Hypertension High blood pressure is often called a "silent killer" because it usually has no specific symptoms or early warning signs. It's possible to have high blood pressure for years without realizing it. During those years, it may be causing damage to vital organs, particularly the heart, the brain, the kidneys, and the eyes, increasing the risk of heart attack, congestive heart failure, stroke, and kidney failure.

Blood vessels in the kidneys, for example, may rupture from constant pressure, making it difficult if not impossible for them to clear waste material from the bloodstream. In the eyes, pressure on the capillaries in the retina may cause swelling and tiny hemorrhages, eventually resulting in blindness. Having your blood pressure

taken on a regular basis is the key to avoiding the complications of hypertension. Hypertension cannot be cured, but it can be treated and controlled. An estimated 60 million Americans have high blood pressure, and only a small percentage have it under control.

Blood Pressure Defined Blood pressure is the force exerted by the blood on the walls of the blood vessels, especially the arteries. This force is created by the pumping action of the heart. Every time the heart contracts, or beats (systole), blood pressure increases. When the heart relaxes between beats (diastole), the pressure decreases. Blood pressure can fluctuate considerably, depending on different factors. For example, when you're excited or afraid or when you're exercising, the heart pumps more blood into your arteries and your blood pressure goes up.

■ **Exploring Your Emotions**

How do you feel about the fact that food companies use people's health concerns to market and sell their products? Do you often buy foods because of the health claims they make? How do you evaluate such claims?

Selling Cardiovascular Health to Americans

"No Cholesterol!" "As Always, Cholesterol Free!" "Excellent Source of Oat Bran!" "Lower in Saturated Fat!" The stream of health facts on food labels is swelling to a flood of disease-prevention claims as more and more food manufacturers imply their products can prevent heart disease and other ailments. When health experts and government panels began recommending several years ago that Americans lower their intake of saturated fats and cholesterol, the food industry responded with aggressive marketing and advertising campaigns for many of their products.

Some claims have bordered on the illegal, since the Food and Drug Administration doesn't allow food manufacturers to claim that their foods prevent or reduce the risk of certain diseases. Others simply mislead. The labels of some brands of peanut butter, for example, proclaim that the product "contains no cholesterol." This is true, since no food from vegetable sources supplies cholesterol—all peanut butter is cholesterol-free. Not so prominently stated is the fat content of peanut butter—76 percent—a far cry from the 30 percent recommended for Americans in the American Heart Association's "prudent diet." The fine print also reveals the presence of partially hydrogenated oil, a saturated fat that can raise the level of cholesterol in your blood.

Labels on other products, such as margarine, vegetable oils, and potato chips, have also sprouted heart motifs and banners stating "no cholesterol." Some labels feature a seal of approval or a quote from a study or scientific panel—"A low-fat, high-soluble-fiber diet can lower cholesterol." Others mislead by prominently displaying their percentage of fat by weight. One brand of turkey bologna, for example, proclaims itself "82 percent fat free." But that's not the same as percentage of kcalories contributed by fat, the figure that matters for your diet. A little computing reveals that 75 percent of the total kcalories in this bologna come from fat.

No product has received more attention recently than oat bran, which has been touted as a cholesterol-buster for years. A boost to oat bran promoters came in 1986 when a study conducted at Northwestern University found that oat bran, together with a low-fat diet, lowered blood cholesterol about 3 percent. When the federal government warned Americans to keep their cholesterol down, the rush was on.

Cereal manufacturers moved to reposition their products in the market and to rename and relabel them. New cereals appeared—Post Oak Flakes, Kellogg's Cracklin Oat Bran, Common Sense Oat Bran, Oat Bran Options, Nutrific Oatmeal Flakes. The Quaker Oats Company launched a highly visible TV ad campaign, and Cheerios sailed past Kellogg's Cornflakes as the top-selling breakfast cereal in the country. Sale of oat-bran cereals rose 240 percent in one year.

Aside from breakfast cereals, some 300 new items containing oat bran appeared, including oat-bran bread, pasta, pretzels, popcorn, potato chips, Belgian waffles, pilaf, cookies, snacks, and beer. When 132 shoppers were asked in a survey if they would buy oat-bran Coke or oat-bran Life Savers, 32 percent said they would. Books and cookbooks about oat bran made their way to the best-seller list.

Then in January 1990 a study appeared in the *New England Journal of Medicine* contradicting the oat-bran message. It reported that oat bran was found to have no more cholesterol-lowering qualities than do low-fiber products such as white flour. Despite the fact that the study involved only twenty subjects and that they had relatively low cholesterol to begin with, and despite the fact that the oat-bran–cholesterol link was widely supported in a number of studies conducted over many years, this single study caused a media uproar. Featured in the nightly TV news and in newspaper headlines, it caused cereal stocks to drop and consumers to clamor for answers. Forced into a defensive position, food companies mobilized to control the damage and wait out the storm.

What this story tells us is *not* that oat bran doesn't lower cholesterol. Scientific research indicates that it does. What the story tells us is that food companies are exploiting health concerns to sell their products. It tells us that a news-hungry media can blow any story up out of proportion. And it tells us that the American consumer is confused and worried about cholesterol and vulnerable to marketing tactics that promise health benefits and quick fixes. In the short term, the controversy about oat bran may have a chilling effect on a wide range of products that make health claims. In the long run, it may encourage Americans to approach so-called miracle products with more caution. Knowing the facts about health issues can help everyone interpret labels and put product claims in perspective.

Based on Oat-bran heartburn, *Newsweek*, January 29, 1990, and Forget about cholesterol? *Consumer Reports*, March 1990.

When blood pressure exceeds normal limits most of the time, a person is considered to have high blood pressure. It can result from either increased output of blood by the heart or increased resistance to blood flow in the arteries due to narrowing and hardening. When a person has high blood pressure, it indicates that the heart is working harder than normal to force the blood through the arteries and that the arteries are under greater strain. Over time, high blood pressure causes the heart to enlarge and weaken and speeds up the process of atherosclerosis.

Measuring Your Blood Pressure   Blood pressure is measured with a stethoscope and an instrument called a **sphygmomanometer**. A sphygmomanometer consists of an airbag or cuff and a column of mercury marked off in millimeters. The cuff is wrapped around the upper arm and inflated by squeezing an attached rubber bulb. The inflated cuff depresses the brachial artery in the arm, stopping the flow of blood. Air pressure supports the column of mercury. As air is slowly released from the cuff, the column of mercury falls. When the cuff is no longer tight enough to prevent the passage of blood through the artery, the examiner will hear a thudding sound with the stethoscope as blood flow resumes. The height of the mercury when the sound is first heard is the reading of the systolic blood pressure, the pressure when the ventricular heart contraction is occurring. After noting the systolic blood pressure, the examiner continues to release air until the sound can no longer be heard. The pressure at this point is diastolic blood pressure, the blood pressure when the heart is relaxed. Blood pressure is expressed as two numbers—for example 120/80. The first and larger number is the systolic blood pressure, and the second number is the diastolic blood pressure.

As with most physiological measurements, including blood pressure, the word *normal* has no single meaning. Because blood pressure readings can be quite variable, depending on anxiety, excitement, setting, and a number of other factors, it's best to compute an average based on at least three measurements on different days. Average blood pressure readings for young adults in good physical condition are 110 to 120 systolic over 70 to 80 diastolic. Newborns have an average systolic pressure of 20 to 60. Blood pressure goes up with age.

High blood pressure in adults is defined as a systolic pressure equal to or greater than 140 mm Hg and/or a diastolic pressure greater than or equal to 90 mm Hg.

What Causes Hypertension?   In about 90 percent of the cases of hypertension, the cause is unknown. High blood pressure of unknown cause is called **essential hypertension**. In the other 10 percent of the cases, the condition is a symptom of another problem, such as a defect in a kidney or another organ. In these cases, referred to as **secondary hypertension**, blood pressure usually returns to normal when the underlying problem is corrected surgically.

The enzyme **renin** seems to be associated with some cases of essential hypertension. This enzyme, produced by the kidneys, promotes the formation of **angiotensin** proteins, which cause the arteries to constrict. Some people with essential hypertension have higher than normal levels of renin in their blood, indicating that it may be causing constriction of their arteries. People with high renin levels have an increased incidence of heart attacks, strokes, and kidney failure.

Other people with essential hypertension have lower than normal levels of renin in their blood. For them, hypertension may be caused primarily by increased blood volume. This condition could result either from decreased sodium excretion by the kidneys or from increased secretion of aldosterone, a hormone produced by the adrenal glands that causes the kidneys to retain water.

Atherosclerosis is another cause of hypertension, since it narrows the arteries and restricts the blood flow. It also increases friction within arteries, elevating blood pressure. Conversely, hypertension contributes to atherosclerosis, as mentioned earlier, probably by causing injury to the artery walls and promoting further plaque growth. Recent studies have suggested that stress may sometimes be a cause of sustained high blood pressure as well. When the sympathetic nervous system is activated by stressors, either internal or external, heart rate increases, arteries constrict, and the blood exerts greater force on artery walls (see Chapter 2). Chronic stress has been implicated in heart disease.

Hypertension also has a strong genetic component, although the specific mechanisms are still unknown. Separating genetic from environmental factors has traditionally been a knotty problem in all areas of human biology. Essential hypertension most likely has many causes, including diet, obesity, alcohol abuse, physical and emotional stress, and psychological and genetic factors. Environmental factors alone probably do not produce hypertension in someone without a genetic predisposition to it.

Sphygmomanometer   An instrument for measuring blood pressure.

Essential hypertension   Persistent elevated blood pressure without known or specific cause.

Secondary hypertension   High blood pressure caused by disease such as kidney dysfunctioning or tumor.

Renin   An enzyme found in the kidney.

Angiotensin   A naturally occurring substance that constricts blood vessels.

Cholesterol: Crusades and Controversies

The national plan to educate people about cholesterol has come under fire from various quarters almost since it began. Critics point out that the studies on which the NCEP's guidelines are based involved only middle-aged men with very high levels of cholesterol. They question the necessity of lowering cholesterol for other groups, such as women, older people, and young men. Women, for example, have never been explicitly studied in a clinical trial, although such a trial was begun by the National Heart, Lung, and Blood Institute, which coordinates the NCEP, in late 1989. Women generally have a different cholesterol and heart disease profile than men, with higher levels of HDL and lower rates of heart attack, at least before menopause.

The elderly too were excluded from clinical trials up to late 1989, even though they suffer the vast majority of heart attacks. Cholesterol rises with age (for unknown reasons), and many older people have high cholesterol, but the link between cholesterol level and coronary disease weakens with age, particularly in men. Because federal agencies advise against routine cholesterol screening in the elderly, such screenings aren't paid for by Medicare.

Prominent individuals, such as Dr. Michael De Bakey, chancellor of the Baylor College of Medicine, and Dr. Thomas N. James, a past president of the American Heart Association, question the recommendation that elderly people try vigorously to lower cholesterol. Dr. James also doubts whether children and others not at high risk ought to follow the dietary recommendations for lowering cholesterol. Other countries with similar rates of CVD have declined to cast so wide a net. They consider it unreasonable to test huge numbers of seemingly healthy people, then medically supervise major dietary changes and perhaps lifetime treatment with costly drugs in order to avoid a possibly modest number of heart attacks.

There is also concern about the possible long-term side effects if patients resort to a lifetime of cholesterol-lowering drugs. Earlier drugs were so unpleasant that many patients gave them up. Newer ones, such as lovastatin, are easier to take, but they haven't been tested for long-term effects. Critics also believe the emphasis on cholesterol diverts attention from other factors, such as cigarette smoking, which is the number one risk factor for CVD. Finally, in looking at the studies, they

point out that although lowering cholesterol is associated with a lowered number of heart attacks, it isn't associated with reduced mortality and it is associated with an increase in gastrointestinal surgery, two trends that puzzle researchers.

Proponents of the cholesterol-lowering plan concede that not every aspect of their advice is based on irreproachable clinical data. Concerns about applying the guidelines to the entire population have prompted their new study. However, they argue that cholesterol reduction does no harm, that reducing saturated fats in the diet has other benefits, and that the guidelines may well prevent heart attacks in many people. They believe that early lifestyle changes are the only way to change the rate of heart disease in the United States. Many people can reduce their cholesterol levels by an average of 10 percent if they follow a diet low in saturated fat and so will never have to resort to drugs.

What is the average American to make of all this? Some things are clear. First of all, the focus on cholesterol shouldn't distract people from the importance of other factors, such as smoking and high blood pressure. Second, although not everyone needs to make dietary

---

Treating Hypertension   Treatment of hypertension often consists of **antihypertensive drugs** and changes in diet. One group of antihypertensive drugs is the **diuretics**, which increase fluid secretion by the kidneys. Use of diuretics is recommended for low-renin patients whose

hypertension is thought to be due primarily to increased blood volume. Another group of antihypertensive drugs called beta-blockers block certain sympathetic nerves that cause arteries to narrow. Vasodilators cause the muscle in the walls of the arteries to relax, permitting the

---

Antihypertensive drugs   Prescribed drugs that lower blood pressure.

Diuretics   Drugs that increase the secretion of salts and water by the kidneys.

Cholesterol: Crusades and Controversies (continued)

changes (genetic and other factors allow some people to eat just about anything they want without raising their cholesterol levels), most Americans do not benefit from a diet high in kcalories and saturated fat. Cutting down on high-fat dairy products, meat, and baked goods is probably a reasonable goal for the population as a whole.

Still remaining are questions about how low cholesterol levels should be at various ages, when and how drugs should be used, and how important HDL is in judging the risk of heart disease. One thing that is clear is that fretting endlessly about cholesterol levels in old age can detract from the enjoyment of life. No one can offer eternal life to the elderly. What people can do is avoid death in middle age by taking all the risk factors for heart disease—especially smoking, blood cholesterol, and high blood pressure—more seriously.

Based on Gina Kolata, Major study aims to learn who should lower cholesterol, *The New York Times*, September 26, 1989, p. C1, and Timothy Johnson, The cholesterol controversy. *Harvard Medical School Health Letter*, December 1989.

What We Know about Cholesterol

Key Findings from Studies

- In middle-aged men, high blood cholesterol levels increase the risk of a heart attack.
- A 50-year-old man with a cholesterol level of 180 and no other risk factors has a 10 percent chance of suffering a heart attack over ten years. With a cholesterol level of 260, the risk rises to 17 percent.
- High-risk men who reduced cholesterol 10 percent with drugs had a 20 percent reduction in heart attacks.
- Reducing cholesterol levels 20 percent slowed or reversed the formation of artery-clogging plaques.
- Diet alone can reduce cholesterol levels by an average of 10 percent.
- Cholesterol reduction has not been shown to extend life. In various clinical trials of middle-aged men, the reduction in heart attacks or cardiac deaths has been offset by deaths from other causes.

Remaining Uncertainties

- The effects of lowering cholesterol in women and the elderly have not been explicitly studied. The advice to them to lower cholesterol is by analogy from middle-aged men.
- The long-term health effects of cholesterol-lowering drugs are unknown.
- Whether there are health problems stemming from cholesterol reduction is unknown.

Source: *The New York Times*, September 26, 1989, p. C1.

---

artery to dilate (widen). ACE inhibitors, a relatively new group of drugs to treat hypertension, interfere with the body's production of angiotensin.

Mild hypertension (less than 160/90) can frequently be treated by changes in diet alone, such as restricted salt intake in salt-sensitive people, reduced kcaloric intake, or both. Although not everyone's blood pressure is affected by salt consumption, blood pressure in some people goes up as soon as they eat salt. These salt-sensitive people must restrict their salt intake to control

their blood pressure. Restricting salt intake tends to curb fluid retention, thus reducing blood volume.

Overweight people are more susceptible to elevated blood pressure because added weight places greater demands on the cardiovascular system. Adipose (fatty) tissue, such as organ and muscle tissue, requires blood to nourish it. In overweight people, the heart must pump more blood through a more extensive system of blood vessels. Potbellies in men appear to increase the risk of heart attack.

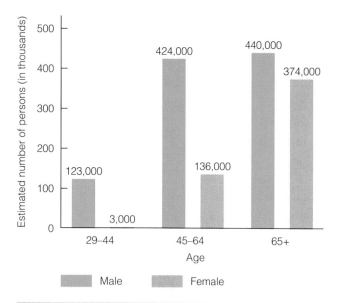

Figure 15-8 Estimated annual number of Americans, by age and sex, experiencing heart attacks.

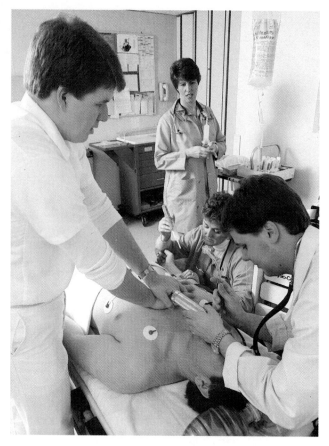

Heart attack victims who receive prompt attention from trained personnel have the best chance of survival. These emergency room technicians are administering CPR to a patient and stabilizing his vital signs.

Heart Attacks Over a million Americans have a heart attack every year (see Figure 15-8). Although a heart attack may come without warning, it is the end result of a long-term disease process. The most common form of heart disease is coronary artery disease caused by atherosclerosis. When one of the coronary arteries—the arteries that branch off the aorta and supply blood directly to the heart muscle—becomes blocked by a blood clot, a heart attack results. A heart attack caused by a clot is called a **coronary thrombosis**, a **coronary occlusion**, or a **myocardial infarction**. In myocardial infarction, part of the heart muscle (myocardium) may suffocate from lack of oxygen.

If the heart attack is not fatal—that is, if enough of the muscle is undamaged to permit life to continue—the muscle begins to repair itself. It does so through a process called **collateral circulation**, in which small blood vessels open to take over the functions of the blocked artery and to move more blood through the damaged area. As healing takes place, scar tissue replaces part of the injured muscle.

Angina Arteries narrowed by disease may still be open enough to deliver blood to the heart. At times, however—chiefly during emotional excitement, stress, or physical exertion—the heart requires more oxygen than narrowed arteries can accommodate. When the need for oxygen exceeds the supply, the heart's electrical system may be disrupted, also causing a heart attack. Chest pain, called **angina pectoris**, is a signal that the heart is not getting enough blood to supply the oxygen it needs. Angina pain

is felt as an extreme tightness in the chest and heavy pressure behind the breastbone or in the shoulder, neck, arm, hand, or back. This pain, although not actually a heart attack, is a warning that the load on the heart must be reduced. Angina may be controlled in a number of ways (with diet and drugs), but its course is unpredictable. Over a period of months or years, the narrowing often goes on to full blockage and a heart attack.

Arrhythmias Of the more than 500,000 heart attack deaths each year, about 60 percent happen within the first hour from an abnormal heartbeat called an arrhythmia, which usually results from damaged heart muscle. Sudden death can be caused by failure of the heart's electrical system, which normally sends electrical impulses through the heart at a rate of 60 to 100 times per minute. A normal heart rhythm can often be restored using a defibrillator, which gives an electrical shock to the heart. This must be done within three to four minutes unless blood flow is restored through **cardiopulmonary resuscitation (CPR)**.

TACTICS AND TIPS

What to Do in Case of a Heart Attack

When it comes to a heart attack, delay spells danger. Minutes make a difference, so it's important to know what to do.

Know the Signals of a Heart Attack

- Uncomfortable pressure, fullness, squeezing, or pain in the center of the chest lasting two minutes or more.
- Pain may spread to shoulders, neck, or arms.
- Severe pain, dizziness, fainting, sweating, nausea, or shortness of breath may also occur. Sharp, stabbing twinges of pain are usually not signals of a heart attack.

Know What Emergency Action to Take

- If you are having typical chest discomfort that lasts for two minutes or more, call the local emergency rescue service immediately.
- If you can get to a hospital faster by car, have someone drive you. Find out which hospitals have twenty-four-hour emergency cardiac care and discuss with your doctor the possible choices. Plan in advance the route that's best from where you live and work.
- Keep a list of emergency rescue service numbers next to your telephone and in a prominent place in your pocket, wallet, or purse.

Know How to Help

- If you are with someone who is having the signals of a heart attack, take action even if the person denies there is something wrong.
- *Call* the emergency rescue service, or
- *Get* to the nearest hospital emergency room that offers twenty-four-hour emergency cardiac care, and
- *Give* mouth-to-mouth breathing and chest compression (CPR) if it is necessary and if you are properly trained.

Source: American Heart Association.

Helping the Heart Attack Victim Most people who suffer a fatal heart attack do so within two hours from the time they experience the first signals (see the box "What to Do in Case of a Heart Attack"). Therefore, recognizing the signals and responding immediately by getting to the nearest hospital or clinic with twenty-four-hour emergency cardiac facilities is critical. If the person loses consciousness, emergency cardiopulmonary resuscitation (CPR) should be initiated by a qualified person. Damage to the heart muscle increases with time. If the victim gets to the emergency room quickly enough, reperfusion therapy can be performed. This technique involves injecting a clot-dissolving agent to dissolve a clot in the coronary artery. These relatively new "clot-busting" drugs, such as streptokinase, urokinase, and tissue plasminogen activator

(TPA), are being used successfully to treat not only heart attacks but also some types of stroke. The sooner these drugs are used, the more effective they are likely to be.

Detecting and Treating Heart Disease Whether a person has already had a heart attack or not, physicians have a variety of diagnostic tools to evaluate the condition of the heart and the arteries. To determine whether a person is at risk of a heart attack, physicians give a stress or exercise test, in which the patient runs on a treadmill while being monitored for heart rhythm abnormalities with an **electrocardiogram (ECG)**. Characteristic changes in the heart's electrical activity while under stress are associated with certain heart conditions, such as restricted blood flow to the heart muscle.

Coronary thrombosis A clot in a coronary artery, often causing sudden death.

Coronary occlusion Partial or total obstruction of a coronary artery, as by a clot; usually resulting in myocardial infarction.

Myocardial infarction A heart attack in which the heart muscle is damaged through lack of blood supply.

Collateral circulation The movement of blood by a system of smaller blood vessels when a main vessel is blocked.

Angina pectoris A condition in which the heart muscle does not receive enough blood, causing severe pain in the chest and often in the left arm and shoulder.

Cardiopulmonary resuscitation (CPR) A technique involving mouth-to-mouth breathing and chest compression to keep oxygen flowing to the brain.

Electrocardiogram (ECG) A test to detect abnormalities by measuring the electrical activity in the heart.

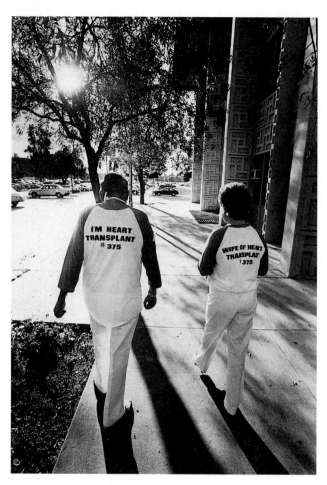

Heart transplants are performed when the heart is so damaged that no other treatment is possible. This heart transplant candidate, selected as a good prospect for successful surgery, bides his time at the medical center waiting for a heart to become available for him.

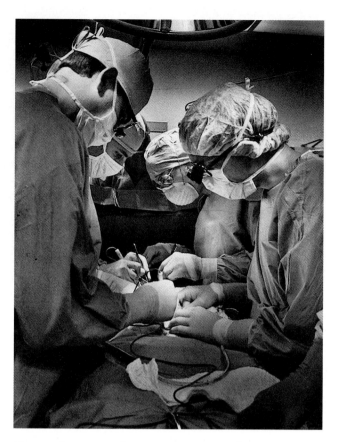

The complex process of giving someone a new heart requires hours of effort by a team of experts. The rate of success for heart transplants has improved greatly since drugs were developed to keep the body from rejecting the new organ. Still, transplants are clearly a poor substitute for a healthy heart of one's own.

Other tools allow the physician to visualize the patient's heart and arteries. One test involves threading a catheter through major arteries and into the heart and injecting dye through the catheter. An x-ray picture of the heart, called an angiogram, shows which arteries are clear and which are narrowed with plaque. Another test involves injecting a radioactive tracer into the body and measuring it as it courses through the circulatory system. This test shows whether blood is reaching the heart properly or is slowed by blocked arteries.

If tests indicate that a problem exists or if a person has already had a heart attack, a variety of treatments may be tried, ranging from changes in the diet and drug therapy to surgery designed to improve blood supply to the heart muscle. The most common type of surgery is **coronary bypass surgery**, in which a healthy blood vessel, usually a vein from one of the patient's legs, is implanted to bypass a blockage. During the surgery, a heart-lung machine maintains circulation.

Another technique was developed in the late 1970s, called **percutaneous transluminal angioplasty (PCTA)**. The technique involves threading a catheter with an inflatable balloon tip through the artery until it reaches the area of blockage. The balloon is then inflated, flattening the fatty plaque and widening the arterial opening. The procedure, which is becoming increasingly common, has several advantages over bypass surgery: it is done under a local anesthesia and does not involve surgery or the use of a heart-lung machine. It is also less expensive and requires only a day or two of hospitalization. Angioplasty is being used to treat blockages in the arteries of the legs and the **carotid artery**, the major vessel carrying blood to the brain.

A nonsurgical treatment that may lower the risk of heart attack is taking aspirin ever other day. Aspirin has an anticlotting effect; it discourages platelets in the blood from sticking to arterial plaque and forming clots. However, frequent use of aspirin can lead to ulcers or gastrointestinal bleeding, and aspirin is also implicated in certain types of stroke. Taking aspirin also has no effect on blood cholesterol levels, the formation of plaque, or any of the other risk factors for heart disease.

Whatever treatment is used, the person with heart disease is also advised to make behavior and lifestyle changes, such as changing the diet to lower blood cholesterol and quitting smoking. Otherwise, the arteries simply become clogged again, and the same problems recur a few years later.

Stroke   For brain cells to function as they should, they must have a continuous and ample supply of oxygen-rich blood. If brain cells are deprived of blood for more than a few minutes, they die. A **stroke**, also called a *cerebrovascular accident*, occurs when the blood supply to the brain is cut off. Stroke can be particularly serious because injured brain cells, unlike those of other organs, cannot regenerate themselves.

Types of Strokes   There are three major types of stroke. The most common is the *thrombotic stroke*, caused by a blood clot, or *thrombus*, that forms in one of the cerebral arteries (see Figure 15-9). This condition, called **cerebral thrombosis**, is likely to occur when the cerebral arteries become damaged by atherosclerosis. If a cerebral artery is clogged with plaque, the formation of clots is more likely. The risk of stroke is much higher among people with hypertension than among those with normal blood pressure, since high blood pressure accelerates the process of atherosclerosis.

A second type of stroke, the *embolic stroke*, occurs when a wandering blood clot, or **embolus**, is carried in the bloodstream and becomes wedged in one of the cerebral arteries. This event is called a **cerebral embolism**.

The third type of stroke, the *hemorrhagic stroke*, is the least common but most severe type of stroke. It occurs when a blood vessel in the brain bursts, spilling blood into the surrounding tissue and causing damage to it. When a **cerebral hemorrhage** occurs, cells normally nourished by the artery are deprived of blood and cannot function. People who suffer from both atherosclerosis and high blood pressure are more likely to suffer cerebral hemorrhage than are those who have only one condition or neither. About one in six strokes is caused by a brain hemorrhage rather than a blood clot.

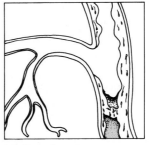

(a) Thrombus

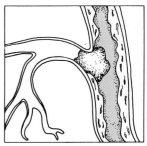

(b) Embolism

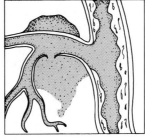

(c) Hemorrhage

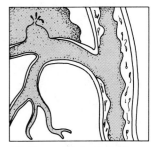

(d) Aneurysm (ruptured)

Figure 15-9   Causes of stroke. Five out of six strokes are caused by blood clots (A and B), but a hemorrhagic stroke (C and D) is more serious.

Bleeding of an artery in the brain may also be caused by a head injury or by the bursting of an **aneurysm**. An aneurysm is a blood-filled pocket that bulges out from a weak spot in an artery wall. Aneurysms in the brain may remain stable and never break. But when they do, the result is a stroke.

Effects of a Stroke   The interruption of the blood supply to any area of the brain prevents the nerve cells there from functioning, in some cases causing death. Of the 400,000 Americans who have strokes each year, approximately 150,000 die. Those who survive usually have some lasting disability. Which parts of the body are affected by the stroke depends on the area of the brain

---

Coronary bypass surgery   Surgery in which a vein is grafted from a point above to a point below an obstruction in a coronary artery, improving the blood supply to the heart.

Percutaneous transluminal angioplasty (PCTA)   A technique in which a catheter with a balloon on the tip is inserted into an artery; the balloon is then inflated at the point of obstruction in the artery, pressing the plaque against the artery wall to improve blood supply.

Carotid artery   The major blood vessel carrying blood to the brain.

Stroke   An impeded blood supply to some part of the brain resulting in the destruction of brain cells (also called *cerebrovascular accident*).

Cerebral thrombosis   A clot in a vessel that supplies blood to the brain.

Embolus   A blood clot that breaks off from its place of origin in a blood vessel and travels through the bloodstream.

Cerebral embolism   Blockage of a blood vessel in the brain, caused by blood clots or other material carried in the blood from other parts of the body.

Cerebral hemorrhage   Bleeding in or near the brain.

Aneurysm   A sac formed by a distension or dilation of the artery wall.

affected. Nerve cells control sensation and most of our bodily movements, so a stroke may cause paralysis, walking disability, speech impairment, or memory loss. The severity of the stroke and its long-term effects depend on which brain cells have been injured, how widespread the damage is, how effectively the body can restore the blood supply, and how rapidly other areas of the brain can take over.

Detecting and Treating Strokes   Strokes can be treated, but effective treatment requires prompt recognition of symptoms and correct diagnosis of the type of stroke that has occurred. Warning signs of a stroke include the following:

- Sudden numbness or weakness of the face, arm, and leg on one side of the body
- Loss of speech or difficulty speaking or understanding speech
- Dimming or loss of vision, especially in only one eye
- Unexplained dizziness, particularly if other symptoms are present

Some stroke victims have a **transient ischemic attack (TIA)**, or mini-stroke, days, weeks, or months before they have a full-blown stroke. They produce temporary strokelike symptoms, such as weakness or numbness in an arm or leg, speech difficulty, or dizziness, but these symptoms are brief and don't seem to cause permanent damage. TIAs should be taken as warning signs of a stroke and reported to a physician.

Until recently, there was very little that could be done to treat strokes, but now they are treated with the same urgency as heart attacks. A person who has had or is having a stroke should be rushed to the hospital for diagnosis and treatment. Tests may include an electrocardiogram (which measures the electrical activity of the heart), an **electroencephalogram** (which measures nerve cell activity in the brain), and a **computerized tomography (CT)** scan (a painless technique that can assess brain damage). The CT scan uses a computer to construct a picture of the brain from x-rays beamed through the head.

If the tests reveal that the stroke is caused by a blood clot, the person can be treated with the same kind of clot-dissolving drugs that are being used to treat coronary artery blockages. If the clot is dissolved quickly enough, damage to the brain is minimized and symptoms may disappear. The longer the brain goes without oxygen from a blood clot, the greater the risk of permanent brain damage.

If tests reveal that the stroke is caused by a cerebral hemorrhage, drugs may be prescribed to lower the blood pressure, which is usually high. Careful diagnosis is crucial, since administering clot-dissolving drugs to a person suffering a hemorrhagic stroke would cause more bleeding and potentially more brain damage.

If detection and treatment of stroke come too late, rehabilitation is the only treatment. Although damaged or destroyed brain tissue cannot regenerate, the brain can find new pathways, and some functions can be taken over by other parts of the brain. Some spontaneous recovery starts immediately after a stroke and continues for a few months.

Rehabilitation consists of various types of therapy: physical therapy, which helps strengthen muscles and improve balance and coordination; speech and language therapy, which helps those whose speech has been damaged; and occupational therapy, which helps improve hand-eye coordination and everyday living skills. Progress varies from person to person and can be unpredictable. Some people recover completely in a matter of days or weeks, but most stroke victims who survive struggle with disabilities of one kind or another for the rest of their lives.

Congestive Heart Failure   A number of conditions, including high blood pressure, heart attack, atherosclerosis, rheumatic fever, and birth defects, can cut down on the heart's pumping efficiency. When the heart cannot maintain its regular pumping rate and force, fluids begin to back up and collect in the lungs and other parts of the body. When this extra, collected fluid seeps through capillary walls, edema (swelling) results. Fluid accumulating in the lungs causes swelling there, and this condition is called **pulmonary edema**. Pulmonary edema, in turn, causes shortness of breath. The entire process is **congestive heart failure**.

Congestive heart failure can be controlled. Treatment includes reducing the workload on the heart, modifying salt intake, and using drugs that help the body eliminate excess fluid. Drugs used to treat congestive heart failure include digitalis, which increases the pumping action of the heart; diuretics, which help the body eliminate excess salt and water; and vasodilators, which expand the blood vessels, decrease the pressure, and allow blood to flow more easily, which in turn makes the heart's work easier.

Heart Disease in Children   Although most cardiovascular disease occurs in adults—and usually in middle-aged or older adults at that—it can occur in children, usually as congenital heart disease or as a result of rheumatic fever.

Congenital Heart Disease   Out of every 125 children born in the United States, one has a defect or malformation of the heart or major blood vessels. These conditions are referred to collectively as **congenital heart disease**.

The most common congenital defects are holes in the wall that divides the lower chambers of the heart. Holes

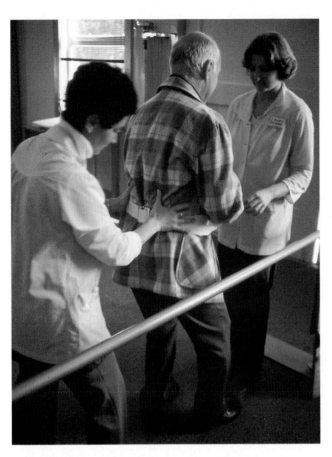

Rehabilitation after a stroke can be a long and arduous process. Complete recovery eludes many stroke victims.

may also occur in the wall between the upper chambers. With these defects the heart produces a distinctive sound, making diagnosis relatively simple. One such defect is **coarctation of the aorta**, which is a narrowing, or constriction, of the aorta. Heart failure may result unless the constricted area is repaired by surgery.

Most of the common congenital defects can now be accurately diagnosed. Important in saving lives is the early recognition that the newborn infant who shows blue appearance, respiratory difficulty, or failure to thrive may be suffering from congenital heart disease.

Rheumatic Heart Disease   Ninety percent of heart trouble in children can be attributed to **rheumatic fever**, a disease process that begins with strep throat (caused by the streptococcus bacterium) and continues one to five weeks later with damage to the heart muscle and heart valves and inflammation of the sac around the heart. The most common symptoms of strep throat are the sudden onset of a sore throat, painful swallowing, fever, swollen glands, headache, nausea, and vomiting. Strep infections can be diagnosed by rapid laboratory detection tests. The symptoms of rheumatic fever are generally vague, making diagnosis difficult. Among the symptoms observed in children are loss of weight or failure to gain weight; a low but persistent fever; poor appetite; repeated nosebleeds without apparent cause; jerky body movements; pain in the arms, legs, or abdomen; fatigue; and weakness. Rheumatic fever can usually be prevented by treating strep throat, when it occurs, with antibiotics.

Cardiovascular Disease, Personality, and Lifestyle

Historian Arnold Toynbee comments, "At the earliest moment at which we catch our first glimpse of man on Earth, we find him not only on the move but already moving at an accelerated pace. The crescendo of acceleration is continuing today. In our generation it is perhaps the most difficult and dangerous of all current problems of the human race." And nutritionist Jean Mayer says, "We are again in the age of the great pandemics. Our plague is cardiovascular." We are social animals. We respond to the world with our hearts, our arteries, and our internal juices. Even while we lie in bed, a random thought can make our heart race and our blood pressure rise. No wonder many of us will eventually become disabled or die from cardiovascular disease, at a national cost estimated in the billions of dollars (see Figure 15-10).

The most widely publicized research linking cardiovascular disease with lifestyle comes from cardiologists Meyer Friedman and Ray Rosenman, who wrote *Type A Behavior and Your Heart* (1974). They studied men in the aircraft industry and concluded that men who have early heart attacks have much in common. They tend to be people with few hobbies; they find routine jobs at home

---

Transient ischemic attack (TIA)   A small stroke; usually a temporary interruption of blood supply to the brain causing numbness or difficulty with speech.

Electroencephalogram (EEG)   A test that measures nerve cell activity in the brain.

Computerized tomography (CT) scan   A test using computerized x-ray images to create a cross-sectional depiction of tissue density.

Pulmonary edema   Accumulation of water in the lungs.

Congestive heart failure   A condition resulting from the heart's inability to pump out all the blood that returns to it. Blood backs up in the veins leading to the heart, causing an accumulation of fluid in various parts of the body.

Congenital heart disease   Disease present at birth due to malformation of the heart or its major blood vessels.

Coarctation of the aorta   A congenital defect in which the aorta is narrowed or constricted.

Rheumatic fever   A disease, mainly of children, characterized by fever, inflammation, and pain in the joints; often damages the heart muscle.

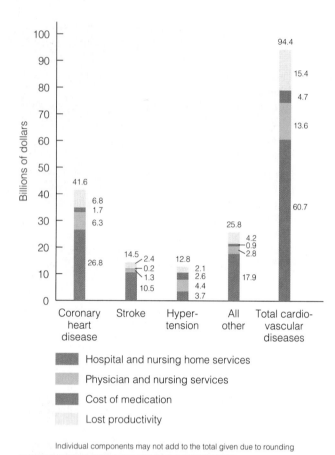

Hospital and nursing home services

Physician and nursing services

Cost of medication

Lost productivity

Individual components may not add to the total given due to rounding

VITAL STATISTICS

Figure 15-10 Estimated cost of major cardiovascular diseases by type of expenditure, United States, 1990 estimate. (Individual components may not add to the total given due to rounding.)

bothersome because they feel the time could be spent more profitably. They walk rapidly, eat quickly, and attempt to do several things at one time. They are impatient, often anticipating what others will say, frequently interrupting before questions or replies are fully completed. These Type A's seem to aspire to some vague, ill-defined achievements in their social environments. Further research into the Type A personality has indicated that "hostility and cynicism" are the more important features of the coronary-prone person (see the box "Getting to the Heart of Type A's").

■ **Exploring Your Emotions**

Research suggests that hostile or cynical people have a greater risk of developing cardiovascular disease than do more trusting people. Would you characterize yourself as a hostile or cynical person? If not, do you know anyone you would characterize that way? What do you think causes a person to have this type of personality?

What can you do now, while you're young, to improve your chances of avoiding CVD in middle age? Here are a number of important steps you can take:

• Have your blood pressure measured regularly, at least yearly if you are under 30 years old, even if it is on the low side of normal. Follow your physician's advice on how to lower it if it's high.
• Have your blood cholesterol measured if you've never had it done. Talk to your physician about interpreting the results.
• If you smoke, quit. If you live or work with people who smoke, encourage them to quit—for their sake and yours. *Remember, smoking, high blood pressure, and high cholesterol are the three most important risk factors for cardiovascular disease that you can do something about.*
• Bring your diet into line with the recommendations of the American Heart Association. Reduce the amount of saturated fat in your diet and increase monounsaturated fat (such as olive and peanut oils) and polyunsaturated fat (such as corn, safflower, and sesame oils). Eat more fiber-rich vegetables, fruits, and starches. See the box "Lowering the Risk of Heart Disease—Without Drugs" and the Behavior Change Strategy at the end of the chapter for some specific dietary suggestions.
• Keep your weight under control.
• Exercise regularly. Aerobic exercise has been shown to raise levels of HDL, the "good" cholesterol. It may also strengthen your heart and improve your circulation. It helps you control your weight, too.

■ **Exploring Your Emotions**

Have you taken any steps to lower your chances of developing cardiovascular disease later in life, such as cutting back on fat or having your blood cholesterol measured? If you haven't, why haven't you? When do you think you will?

• Develop effective ways to handle stress and anger. Refer to Chapter 2 for suggestions about how to manage stress and avoid its negative consequences.
• Monitor any medical problems you have, such as diabetes, and keep them under control.
• Know your risk factors, both personal and familial.

In a sense, some of us choose our diseases when we choose the way we live. On the other hand, sometimes it's difficult to see that other choices are possible. Our competitive society, with its emphasis on status and material wealth, fosters certain values and behaviors. It's hard to resist the influences that lead to a competitive, stressful—sometimes joyless—lifestyle. If we can see that other choices are possible, or if we can learn to mediate the negative effects of the "fast track," we can perhaps make cardiovascular disease less inevitable in our lives.

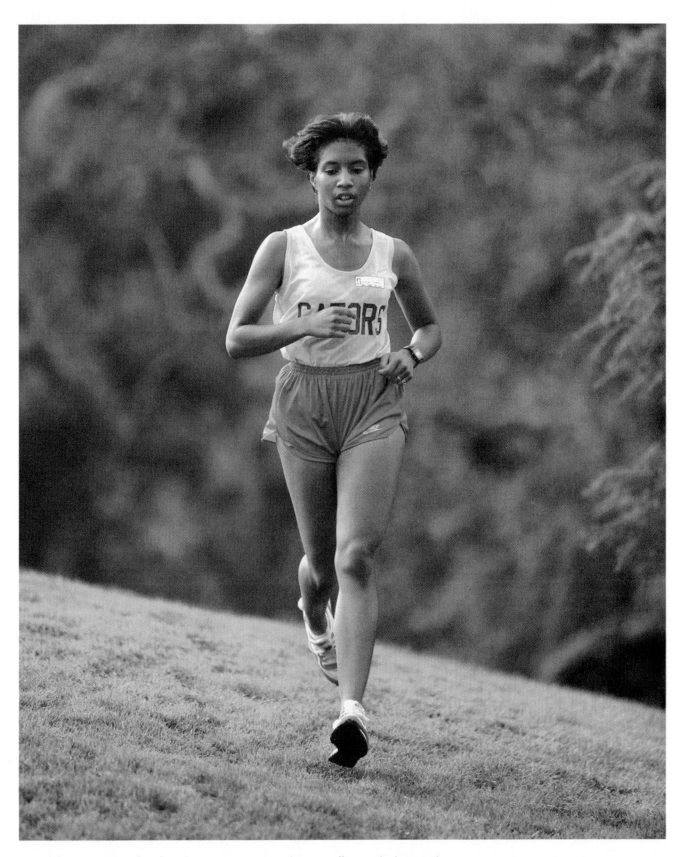

One of the primary benefits of aerobic exercise is its conditioning effect on the heart and lungs. A lifetime of sensible exercise habits offers protection against cardiovascular disease later in life.

Getting to the Heart of Type A's

What takes a toll on your heart is not hurrying or workaholism but hostility, argues Redford Williams, M.D., director of the Behavioral Medicine Research Center at Duke University and author of *The Trusting Heart: Great News About Type A Behavior.*

We all know Type A people, who tend to rush around, hate lines, and get easily irritated. They have long been thought to run a greater risk of heart disease. How solid is that link?

At the end of the 1970s, Type A behavior was widely accepted as a risk factor for heart disease. But a number of studies done in the early 1980s failed to support the link. So researchers started looking more closely at various components of Type A behavior, particularly hostility and its relationship to disease. It is now pretty clear that only the hostility and anger associated with Type A behavior actually contribute to heart disease. The other Type A traits, such as rushing around, workaholism and competitiveness, don't. Of course, being in a hurry often triggers anger. But it's the quickness to anger, the persistent hostile outlook and the cynical mistrust of other people rather than impatience per se that appear harmful. Preliminary studies indicate that the increased risk for heart disease associated with being chronically hostile is similar to that created by having high cholesterol or high blood pressure.

What makes hostility and anger so hazardous?

They can increase your blood pressure, for one. Studies show that the blood pressure of people prone to hostile Type A behavior rises much more when they encounter the irritations of daily life. Hostility also stresses the body physiologically, causing the release of adrenaline and other chemicals that put the nervous system on alert. People who don't exhibit Type A behavior tend to calm down much faster than their high-strung counterparts, taking the stress off their bodies and hearts. Type A personalities seem to lack the physiological ability to stem the stress response.

Are hostile people born that way, or do they learn that behavior?

Studies of twins suggest that 30 to 50 percent of the behavior pattern is rooted in the genes. But the way children are reared has a lot to do with whether that pattern will dominate in later life. Children who don't get unconditional parental love and care and lots of physical contact are more likely to be mistrusting, easy-to-anger adults, for example.

Everybody gets mad. What type of anger is typical of Type A people? And what form of cynicism?

I am not talking about justified anger when someone does something to legitimately warrant your temporary wrath. There's no evidence that feeling that way is bad for your health. I am talking about people who have hostility just beneath the surface all the time, who are ready to blow for the most minor reasons.

As for cynicism and mistrust, again sometimes they are justified. But persistent feelings of cynicism and chronic mistrust of others, with a hostile component, are associated with the behavior pattern leading to health problems.

What Type A warning signs should you watch for?

People in an express checkout line who count the items being bought by the person in front of them have a mistrusting Type A nature, especially if they get mad and impatient when that person is over the limit. People who seethe when the elevator doesn't come even if they are not in a rush also exhibit hazardous Type A behavior. Impatience and quick anger with children are another telling sign. Type A's seem to have negative tapes playing constantly in their heads that blame other people for life's minor irritations.

Can Type A's change their ways?

Yes. Research a few years ago showed clearly that men who had suffered a heart attack and who then underwent a behavior-modification program could become less hurried and less hostile. The men who went through that program had fewer second heart attacks and lower death rates than those who did not. But you needn't wait for a heart attack to change your behavior. The first thing to do may sound simplistic, but it requires real effort: Control your thoughts. If cynical, mistrusting thoughts cause you a lot of stress, you need to stop having them. Realize how futile those thoughts are and how angry and hostile they make you feel. You may also want to keep a hostility log, writing down every time you have those thoughts. Trusting other people to make some decisions for you can help you overcome feelings that others are out to get you. Finally, though it sounds trite, try to enjoy life more. You only have a relatively short stay in this world, so why go around being angry all the time? Focus on what is important in your life.

Source: Conversation with Steven Findlay, *U.S. News & World Report*, May 15, 1989, p. 68.

Lowering the Risk of Heart Disease—Without Drugs

After your recent checkup your internist calls to tell you that your cholesterol reading is 290—substantially higher than desirable—and that if you can't get it below 240 within the next few months, she'd recommend drug therapy. Does that mean you'll need pills for the rest of your life to keep your cholesterol level down and decrease your risk of heart disease? Probably not.

Some believe that 85 to 95 percent of persons with initial cholesterol levels in the 275–300 range can decrease them to below 240, and that many will even be able to reach the more desirable level of 200 or less, *without drug therapy*. It might not be a cinch, but the benefits will be worth the effort: not only reduction of heart disease risk, but also, for those suffering from overweight, diabetes, or high blood pressure, improved control of those conditions.

Dietary Therapy

The first and often the only step needed to lower cholesterol is to revamp the diet. In fact, even if drugs become necessary, dietary therapy should be maintained. A cholesterol-lowering diet actually requires that you make only two basic adjustments: eat less saturated fat and dietary cholesterol and eat more carbohydrates (see the accompanying table).

From now on, be a discriminating food shopper. Search for items that are low in fat (many labels will specify the amount of fat per serving). Reasonable dietary goals would be less than 85 grams of fat for an average-size man eating 2,500 kcalories and 60 grams for a woman eating 1,800 kcalories. On this "prudent diet," there's no need to feel deprived or discouraged. If you have a family, and everyone adopts this "prudent diet," it will be easier to stick to and you'll all benefit.

Many people wonder if exercise is also a good way to lower cholesterol levels, and the surprising answer is no. If the diet doesn't change, exercise isn't going to make much difference. But that doesn't mean that starting an exercise program is useless; on the contrary, it's highly recommended. Regular aerobic exercise will increase the blood level of HDL (high-density lipoprotein, the "good" cholesterol); and, because it is usually adopted as part of a lifestyle change (smoking cessation, better diet, weight loss), it will help keep heart disease at bay.

Fish and Fish Oils

Many mothers used to insist that their kids take a tablespoon of cod-liver oil every day. Although many of these mothers had little nutritional knowledge, current research appears to support their belief about fish and even about cod-liver oil. What they didn't know—and neither did anyone else—was that it's extremely healthful for another reason.

The health benefits of seafood first garnered medical attention in 1978, when two Danish scientists, Hans Bang and Jorn Dyerberg, observed that cardiovascular disease was rare among Eskimos. They hypothesized that the reason was that Eskimos consume large amounts of seafood, which contain a special kind of fat commonly called omega-3 fatty acids.

Since 1978, scientific evidence has increasingly supported the notion that omega-3s are healthy for the heart. Studies have shown that fish and fish-oil supplements inhibit platelet stickiness. Platelets are small cells that float in the bloodstream and help blood to clot. That's fine when a person is cut. Unfortunately, these platelets can also help form clots in the coronary arteries and result in a heart attack. Fish oils have been shown to interfere with the platelets' tendency to stick to plaque, thereby decreasing the risk of heart attacks. One study, for instance, found that heart disease mortality among men who reported eating one ounce of fish a day was *half* that of men who never ate fish. Researchers concluded that eating as few as two fish dishes per week may protect against CVD. Another study demonstrated that cod-liver oil supplements may actually slow the development of atherosclerosis despite a high cholesterol level.

Omega-3s may also decrease blood pressure and blood viscosity and increase HDL. Moreover, they can almost always significantly lower the concentration of certain fats (triglycerides) in the blood and reduce blood cholesterol as well. In fact, one study demonstrated decreases far more dramatic on a fish and fish-oil diet than on a low-fat, low-cholesterol diet. It must be noted, however, that the patients consumed a whopping amount of omega-3s daily—the equivalent of about one-and-a-half pounds of salmon per day, or forty to sixty of the commonly available fish-oil capsules per day. Taking this amount of omega-3s would not only be impractical, but might even have side effects, such as bleeding tendencies, weight gain (fat, even if derived from fish is fattening), vitamin E deficiency, and vitamin A and D toxicity if large amounts of cod-liver oil are used.

(continued)

Labels on fish-oil supplements suggest that healthy persons take three to six capsules (1–2 grams of omega-3s) per day. That amount is probably safe, but its health value is speculative since no long-term studies of fish-oil consumption have been done. So most researchers recommend eating more seafood rather than taking supplements, especially since the beneficial effects of fish may be due not only to the oil but to other substances in fish as well. Ideally, two or three fish dishes per week should replace meat or other foods high in saturated fats. Especially good sources of omega-3s are salmon, mackerel, sardines, tuna, and herring. The fish should be broiled, baked, or poached; frying adds fat and calories. Finally, shellfish, which have traditionally been off-limits to cholesterol-restricted persons, have a minimal effect on serum cholesterol. So lobster, crab, shrimp, clams, oysters, and scallops can be enjoyed with a clear conscience.

Oat Bran and Other Fiber

Oat bran has recently replaced calcium as the latest cure-all, and food manufacturers have been rushing to supply "oat bran everything" to the health-hungry public. Is it all just advertising hype, or is there some validity to the claims made for oat bran?

Although many claims have been overblown, scientific studies show that a high-fiber diet can indeed lower cholesterol levels, enhance control of diabetes, improve bowel habits, and possibly induce weight loss. But many foods besides oat bran contain soluble fiber, the type that helps lower cholesterol levels and is

Recommended dietary changes to lower blood cholesterol levels	
Decrease Intake	Increase Intake
Whole milk	Nonfat and low-fat milk
Hard cheeses, cream cheese	Cottage cheese, low-fat yogurt
Beef, pork, sausage, bacon	Fish, skinless chicken, turkey
Butter, high-fat mayonnaise	Margarine, mustard
Ice cream	Sherbet, frozen yogurt
Palm and coconut oils	Olive and vegetable oils
Many luncheon meats	Turkey, chicken meats
Many prepared baked goods	Fruits, vegetables
Egg yolks (egg whites are OK)	Beans, cereals, pasta, bread

found in beans, cereals, fruits, and vegetables. Insoluble fiber, present in large amounts in wheat bran and in lesser amounts in celery and many other vegetables, has no effect on cholesterol levels, but does exert the other benefits we've mentioned.

Decreases in cholesterol levels effected by soluble fiber have ranged from very small (around 5 percent) to quite substantial (up to 25–30 percent). The degree of change depends on the initial cholesterol levels, other dietary changes, the amount and type of fiber supplement, and the compliance of the patient in eating the altered diet and the fiber supplement.

Psyllium

A fiber found in the husks of psyllium seeds, psyllium is the active ingredient in Metamucil and other stool softeners (e.g., Fiber-all). A recent study, supported by other findings, showed that persons taking a teaspoon of this supplement (stirred into 8 ounces of water) three times daily for eight weeks lowered their cholesterol

levels by 15 percent—from 247 to 211. Eight of the fourteen subjects complained of mild gastrointestinal side effects (primarily cramping during the first two weeks), but no serious adverse reactions occurred. Psyllium has a long history of safe use for various ailments such as irritable bowel syndrome and constipation. It is well tolerated and relatively cheap, and thus seems well suited to long-term treatment of high cholesterol levels, if dietary therapy does not work.

To sum up: the vast majority of patients burdened with high cholesterol can probably avoid drug therapy and conquer the problem with diet alone. The delicious low-fat cuisines of many peoples around the world (whose fat intake is usually less than that recommended in this country) demonstrate that a low-cholesterol diet is hardly a punishment. When your cholesterol level has plummeted fifty points or so on a hearty, tasty diet, you'll be motivated to eschew greasy food and keep new eating habits that are kind to your heart.

Source: Jack Yetiv, M.D. 1989. Lowering the risk of heart disease—without drugs, Health-line, May.

Summary

- Although cardiovascular disease is still the number one killer in the United States, changes in the American lifestyle have led to declining death rates from heart attacks and strokes.

The Cardiovascular System

- The cardiovascular system, which consists of the heart and blood vessels, pumps and circulates blood throughout the body; the pulmonary and systemic circulation systems are controlled by the right and left sides of the heart.
- The four-chambered heart is about the size of a fist; the atria are the thin-walled upper chambers, and the ventricles are the thick-walled lower chambers.
- The heart beats when the ventricles contract (systole), pumping blood to the lungs via the pulmonary artery and to the body via the aorta and the entire arterial system. When the heart relaxes between beats (diastole), blood flows from the atria into the ventricles.
- The exchange of nutrients and waste products takes place between the capillaries and the tissues. The total volume of the body's blood is circulated about once a minute.

Who Is at Risk for Cardiovascular Disease (CVD)?

- Men have a greater risk of heart attack and stroke than do women; black Americans have twice the rate of CVD as whites, probably because of sickle-cell anemia as well as the high incidence of high blood pressure.
- Although behaviors that increase the risk of CVD begin early in life, the risk of heart attack increases dramatically after age 65. Genetic factors like high blood cholesterol levels and abnormal clotting tendencies also increase susceptibility to CVD.
- Also at risk are people who are overweight or obese and people who have diabetes.
- Hypertension, high blood cholesterol, cigarette smoking, sedentary lifestyle, and personality traits like hostility—all usually behavioral components of one's lifestyle—increase the risk of CVD.

Major Forms of Cardiovascular Disease

- Atherosclerosis is the process whereby arteries become narrowed by deposits of fat, cholesterol, and other substances. As plaques accumulate, arteries lose elasticity and the ability to expand and contract. Platelets may get stuck on a plaque and form a blood clot, which can block the artery and deprive organs of blood.
- Smoking may be involved in the formation of plaque and appears also to destroy the body's natural anticoagulant abilities; passive smoking is also a risk factor.

- The higher one's blood cholesterol level and intake of saturated fats, the higher the risk of CVD. High LDL levels and low HDL levels indicate CVD risk.
- The federal government established the National Cholesterol Educational Program to make Americans aware of their cholesterol levels, change the national diet to contain less saturated fat, and treat people with high cholesterol.
- High blood pressure often has no symptoms but may be causing damage to vital organs; it cannot be cured, but it can be treated and controlled.
- Blood pressure is the force exerted on the blood vessels when the heart pumps. Blood pressure increases with the systole and decreases with the diastole. Hypertension occurs when blood pressure exceeds normal limits most of the time. Increased output of blood or increased resistance in the arteries both raise blood pressure.
- Blood pressure is recorded as systolic pressure (pressure when ventricles contract) over diastolic pressure (pressure when the heart is relaxed). High blood pressure is defined as systolic pressure of 140 mm Hg or higher and diastolic pressure of 90 mm Hg or higher.
- In essential hypertension, the cause is unknown; with secondary hypertension, the condition is caused by another problem. The enzyme renin seems to be associated with essential hypertension; high levels may cause artery constriction, and low levels may lead to increased blood volume.
- Atherosclerosis causes hypertension by narrowing arteries and restricting blood flow; conversely, hypertension contributes to atherosclerosis, perhaps by injuring the artery walls and promoting plaque growth. Stress can also be a cause of high blood pressure.
- How genetics contributes to hypertension is not yet clear, but environmental factors alone probably don't produce hypertension if a genetic predisposition isn't present.
- Antihypertensive drugs include diuretics, which increase fluid secretion by the kidneys; beta-blockers, which inhibit artery constriction; vasodilators, which allow the arteries to dilate; and ACE inhibitors, which interfere with the body's production of angiotensin.
- Mild hypertension can sometimes be treated by (1) restricting salt intake to curb fluid retention and reduce blood volume and (2) losing weight so that the heart need not pump more blood through a more extensive system of blood vessels.
- Heart attacks are the end result of a long-term disease process. A coronary thrombosis occurs when one of the coronary arteries becomes blocked by a blood clot.

- After a heart attack, the muscle begins to repair itself through collateral circulation, where small blood vessels open to move more blood through the damaged area.
- Angina pectoris is the chest pain that occurs when—because of narrowed arteries—the heart doesn't get enough blood to supply the oxygen it needs.
- Arrhythmia is an abnormal heartbeat (usually resulting from damaged heart muscle); if the heart's electrical system fails, sudden death can occur.
- It's important to recognize the signals of a heart attack and immediately get the victim to an emergency cardiac facility. Reperfusion therapy—the injection of a clot-dissolving agent—can dissolve a clot in the coronary artery.
- Heart disease can be diagnosed through use of stress or exercise tests, electrocardiograms, catheters, angiograms, and radioactive tracers.
- The most common surgical treatment for heart disease is coronary bypass surgery. Percutaneous transluminal angioplasty uses a catheter with an inflatable balloon to widen the arterial opening. Taking aspirin can inhibit platelets in the blood from sticking to arterial plaque and forming clots.
- Any medical or surgical treatment must be accompanied by behavior and lifestyle changes, including quitting smoking and changing the diet to lower blood cholesterol.
- A stroke occurs when the blood supply to the brain is cut off; injured brain cells cannot regenerate themselves.
- A thrombotic stroke occurs when a clot forms in one of the cerebral arteries, usually because of atherosclerosis. An embolic stroke occurs when a blood clot is carried in the bloodstream and becomes wedged in a cerebral artery.
- A hemorrhagic stroke occurs when a blood vessel in the brain bursts and spills blood into surrounding tissue. Head injuries and burst aneurysms also cause bleeding in the brain.

- Strokes usually lead to some lasting disability, such as paralysis, walking disability, speech impairment, or memory loss. Effective treatment depends on prompt recognition of symptoms and correct diagnosis of the type of stroke.
- Transient ischemic attacks, which produce temporary stroke symptoms, are warning signs of a stroke and should be reported to a physician. Diagnostic tests include electrocardiograms, electroencephalograms, and CT scans.
- Strokes caused by a blood clot can be treated with clot-dissolving drugs; antihypertensive drugs are prescribed for cerebral hemorrhages. Rehabilitation helps the brain find new pathways; some brain functions are taken over by other parts of the brain.
- Congestive heart failure occurs when the heart's pumping efficiency is reduced and fluids build and collect in the lungs or other part of the body. The extra fluids cause swelling or edema; pulmonary edema causes shortness of breath.
- Treatment for congestive heart failure includes reducing the workload on the heart (through digitalis and vasodilators), modifying salt intake, and using diuretics to eliminate excess fluid from the lungs.
- Defects or malformations of the heart or major blood vessels at birth constitute congenital heart disease. These include holes in the wall that divides the chambers of the heart and a constricted aorta. Early recognition of congenital heart disease is essential.

Cardiovascular Disease, Personality, and Lifestyle

- Hostility and cynicism are the characteristics of the Type A personality most associated with CVD.
- To avoid CVD, it's important to have blood pressure checked regularly; have blood cholesterol measured; quit smoking; alter diet to reduce saturated fat and eat fiber-rich vegetables, fruits, and starches; keep weight under control; exercise regularly; learn to handle stress and anger; monitor medical problems; and know personal and familial risk factors.

Take Action

1. Blood pressure varies considerably at different times and under different conditions. Go to a local drugstore or community center and have your blood pressure taken on three or four different occasions. Average the measurements to get an accurate idea of your blood pressure. Refer to Appendix 1 in Chapter 21 for information on home blood pressure monitoring.

2. The CPR courses given by the Red Cross and other groups provide invaluable training that may help you save a life some day. Anyone can take these courses and become qualified to administer CPR. Investigate CPR courses in your community and sign up to take one.

3. Do some research into your family medical history. Is there cardiovascular disease in your family, as indicated by premature deaths from heart attack, stroke, or congestive heart failure? Such a history is a risk factor for you. Keep that in mind as you consider whether you need to make lifestyle changes to avoid CVD.

Behavior Change Strategy

Reducing the Saturated Fat in Your Diet

Although the amount of dietary cholesterol you consume (in foods like eggs and organ meats) affects your blood cholesterol level, the amount of saturated fat you consume affects it even more. The American Heart Association recommends that no more than 10 percent of the kcalories in your diet come from saturated fat. To see how your diet measures up, monitor yourself for a week, keeping track of everything you eat. Keep your record in your health diary, writing the foods you eat (including meals and snacks) on the left side of the page and leaving room on the right for information about each food.

If you don't already have one, buy an inexpensive book with nutritional tables that show the calorie and fat content of a variety of foods. Look for one that breaks down fat content into saturated, monounsaturated, and polyun-saturated fats. Remember, the biggest sources of saturated fats are animal products, such as red meat, cheese, milk, cream, yogurt, and butter; the "tropical oils," such as palm and coconut oil; and heavily hydrogen-ated vegetable oils. For fast foods, use the appendix to Chapter 12 of this book.

Each day, after you have noted the foods you ate, enter the kcalories and the grams of saturated fat, and then compute the percentage of saturated fat using the formula explained in Chapter 12. (Multiply grams of fat by 9 and divide the total by the total kcalories. The result is the percentage of fat.) At the end of each day, average all the percentages, and at the end of the week, average the daily percentages. Is it about 10 percent, or is it more?

You can also monitor and compute the percentages of monounsaturated and polyunsaturated fats in your diet. Foods high in polyunsaturated fat include corn oil, cottonseed oil, safflower oil, soybean oil, mayonnaise made with any of these oils, margarine, sunflower seeds, and walnuts. Foods high in monounsaturated fat include olive oil, peanut oil, sesame oil, margarine, almonds, cashews, hazelnuts, peanuts, pecans, pistachio nuts, and avocados. Try to keep each of these groups at about 10 percent of your total kcalories too.

If your diet includes more than your fair share of saturated fat, you can take steps to reduce it. Begin by looking at the tips in the box

"Lowering the Risk of Heart Disease—Without Drugs." Start to become more aware of what type of food you order in restaurants, buy at the supermarket, and prepare for meals. Do you usually go for hamburgers, hot dogs, steaks, and chops? Choose lean meat, chicken, or fish instead, and broil or bake it instead of frying it. Do you have salami and cheese on rye for lunch? Try turkey for a change. Is ice cream your downfall? Sliced fruit in season with low-fat yogurt and honey is a delicious alternative.

If there is a lot of saturated fat in your diet, you may have to change some of your habits for a while—you may have to avoid fast food restaurants or forego pizza at night with your friends. Put your best effort into finding attractive, satisfying, and enjoyable activities as substitutes, such as trying out restaurants that serve low-fat dishes. If you can recruit some friends to join you in your campaign, it will be easier to stick with it. Remember, cardiovascular disease often starts when people are in their teens or early twenties. By cutting down on saturated fat now, you'll be doing yourself a favor that will give you benefits your whole life.

Selected Bibliography

American Heart Association. 1990. *Heart and Stroke Facts.*
Belsey, R., and D. Baer. 1990. Cardiac risk classification based on lipid screening. *Journal of the American Medical Association* 263: 1250–52.
Raloff, J. 1989. Do you know your HDL? *Science News,* Sept.
Wilson, P. 1989. Impact of national guidelines for cholesterol risk factor screening. *Journal of the American Medical Association* 262: 41–44.

Recommended Readings

Fletcher, A. 1990. Eat Fish, Live Better, New York: Harper and Row. *The author reviews the findings related to fish and heart disease. It includes an extensive glossary describing common and uncommon varieties of fish.*
Healthline, July 1990. Entire issue is devoted to preventing heart disease.

830 Menlo Avenue, Suite 100, Menlo Park, Ca. 94025.
Williams, R. 1989. The Trusting Heart, New York: Times Books. *Dr. Williams, an expert in Behavioral Medicine discusses the biological correlates of anger and hostility that can lead to heart disease.*

Contents

Making Connections

Although cancer is not the leading cause of death among Americans—cardiovascular disease has that distinction—it is a particularly dreaded disease that many people fear above all others. Cancer-causing agents and risks seem to abound in our society, but there are steps you can take to protect yourself, starting now. The scenarios presented on these pages describe situations in which people have to use information, make a decision, or choose a course of action, all related to cancer. As you read them, imagine yourself in each situation and consider what you would do. After you've finished the chapter, read the scenarios again and see if what you've learned has changed how you would think, feel, or act in each situation.

You keep seeing ads for a new tanning center downtown that encourages you to "enjoy the healthy glow of summer year round" and promises a "safe tan without burning." You're planning to go on vacation and wouldn't mind being tan before you get there. On the other hand, you've heard that sunlight isn't that good for your skin. What do they do at the tanning center to make the tan "safe?" Can you trust what they say?

Lately it seems that everywhere you go—the supermarket, the gas station, the liquor store, your favorite restaurants—you notice signs warning that certain chemicals and other substances are "known to cause cancer." You know your state recently passed a law that these signs had to be posted where carcinogens were present, but you're shocked at how often you see them. Are there really that many carcinogens around? How dangerous are they? What can you do to avoid them?

16
Cancer: A Closer Look

The last time you visited your grandparents, you noticed that your grandfather sprinkled some dry flakes on top of his breakfast cereal in the morning. He said that it was wheat bran and that he added it to his diet because his dad had died of colon cancer. "It wouldn't be a bad idea for you to have some, too," he tells you. "After all, you inherited some genes from him the same as I did." Is your grandfather saying a tendency to get cancer of the colon is inherited? What does wheat bran have to do with it? Should you take his advice?

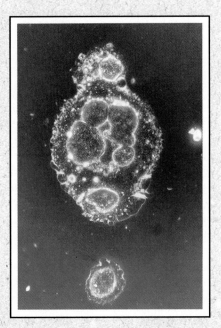

Your grandmother had severe osteoporosis and your mother has been talking to her physician about taking estrogen to protect herself against the disease, now that she no longer menstruates. Her physician says that hormone replacement therapy is believed to be safe and that the amounts of estrogen involved are very low. Nevertheless, he advised your mother to stop smoking to lower her chances of developing cancer in her reproductive system. Your mother doesn't know what smoking has to do with her uterus. Is her physician giving her good advice?

A friend of yours tells you that her recent Pap test was abnormal. She's supposed to have minor surgery to remove some cells or, she says, they could turn into cancer. Her gynecologist told her that in the future she can protect herself against cancer of the cervix to some extent by making sure her sexual partner uses a condom. You're shocked. Is the gynecologist suggesting that cervical cancer is a sexually transmissible disease? How can condoms protect you against cancer?

The word *cancer* comes to us from the Greek word for crab, *karkinos*. We are all familiar with cancer as a tumor—a malignant and invasive growth that tends to recur after removal and to reappear at distant sites. The ancient Greek physicians who first studied cancer noticed that in some cases a malignant tumor, with its hard mass and claw-like extensions, resembled a crab. In the modern world, cancer has retained its reputation as an alien invader and is the most feared of all noninfectious diseases. It may not be the most common cause of death, but it is correctly seen as a progressive fatal condition that often cannot be successfully treated.

What Is Cancer?

Cancer is an abnormal and uncontrollable growth of cells or tissue that leads to death if untreated. Most cancers take the form of tumors, although not all tumors are cancers. A tumor is simply a mass of new tissue that serves no physiological purpose. It can be benign, like a wart, or malignant, like most lung cancers; the terms **malignant tumor** and **malignant neoplasm** are synonymous with *cancer*. **Benign tumors** are made up of cells similar to the surrounding normal cells and are enclosed in a membrane that prevents them from penetrating other tissues. They are dangerous only if their physical presence interferes with bodily functions. A benign brain tumor, for example, can cause death if it blocks the blood supply to the brain. A malignant tumor, or cancer, is capable of invading surrounding structures, including blood vessels, the lymph system, and nerves. It can also spread, or *metastasize,* to distant sites via the blood and lymphatic circulation and so produce invasive tumors in almost any part of the body. A few cancers like leukemia, or cancer of the blood, don't produce a mass and so aren't properly called tumors. But since the leukemic cells do have the fundamental property of rapid and inappropriate growth, they are still malignant and therefore cancers.

■ **Exploring Your Emotions**

In the past, there was often a stigma attached to cancer, and many people tried to hush up cases of cancer or cancer deaths. What is your reaction when you hear someone has cancer? Is it different from your reaction when you hear that someone has had a heart attack?

Metastasis occurs because cancer cells do not stick to each other as strongly as normal cells and so may not remain at the site of the original or *primary tumor.* They break away easily and can pass through the lining of small blood vessels to invade nearby tissue. They can also drift to distant parts of the body, where they establish new colonies of cancer cells. This traveling process is called metastasizing, and the new tumors are called *secondary tumors,* or *metastases.*

Traveling cancer cells can follow two courses. They can produce secondary tumors in the lymph nodes and be carried through the lymph system to form secondary sites elsewhere, or they can invade blood vessels and circulate through the vessels to colonize other organs. This ability of cancer cells to metastasize makes early cancer detection critical. To control the cancer and prevent death, every cancerous cell must be removed. Once cancer cells enter either the lymph or the blood system, it is extremely difficult to stop their spread to other organs of the body.

Every case of cancer begins as a change in a cell that allows it to grow and divide when it should not. Normally (in adults), cells divide and grow at a rate sufficient to replace dying cells. When you cut your finger, for example, the cells around the wound divide more rapidly to heal the wound. When the wound is healed, the rate of cell growth and division returns to normal. In contrast, a malignant cell divides without regard for normal control mechanisms and gradually produces a mass of abnormal cells—a tumor.

As the tumor increases in size it will eventually be noticed, because it will produce a sign or symptom that is determined by its location in the body. In the breast, for example, a tumor may be detected as a lump and diagnosed as cancer by x-ray or biopsy (surgical removal and examination of a sample of tissue). In less accessible locations, like the lungs or bowel, tumors may be noticed only after considerable growth has taken place and then be detected by an indirect symptom—for instance as a persistent cough or unexplained bleeding or pain. In the case of leukemia there is no lump, but the changes in the blood will eventually be noticed as increasing fatigue, infection, or abnormal bleeding.

Types of Cancer   The behavior of tumors arising in different body organs is characteristic of the tissue of origin. (Figure 16–1 shows the major cancer sites and the incidence of each type.) Since each cancer begins as a single (altered) cell with a specific function in the body, the cancer will retain some of the properties of the normal cell for a time. So, for instance, a cancer of the thyroid gland may produce too much thyroid hormone and cause hyperthyroidism as well as cancer. Usually a cancer loses its resemblance to normal tissue as it continues to divide, and it becomes a group of rogue cells with increasingly unpredictable behavior.

Malignant tumors are classified according to the types of cells that give rise to them. The most common cancers

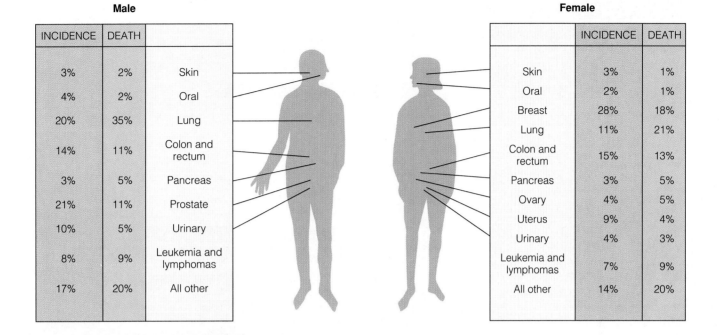

Male		
INCIDENCE	DEATH	
3%	2%	Skin
4%	2%	Oral
20%	35%	Lung
14%	11%	Colon and rectum
3%	5%	Pancreas
21%	11%	Prostate
10%	5%	Urinary
8%	9%	Leukemia and lymphomas
17%	20%	All other

Female		
	INCIDENCE	DEATH
Skin	3%	1%
Oral	2%	1%
Breast	28%	18%
Lung	11%	21%
Colon and rectum	15%	13%
Pancreas	3%	5%
Ovary	4%	5%
Uterus	9%	4%
Urinary	4%	3%
Leukemia and lymphomas	7%	9%
All other	14%	20%

VITAL STATISTICS

Figure 16-1   Cancer incidence by site and sex, and cancer deaths by site and sex. Percentages shown are estimates for 1989, excluding nonmelanoma skin cancer. The "incidence" column indicates what percentage of all cancers occurred in each site; the "death" column indicates what percentage of all cancer deaths were attributed to each type.

are carcinomas, sarcomas, lymphomas, and leukemia (the suffix *-oma* means "tumor"). **Carcinomas,** the most common form of cancer, arise from the **epithelial layers** (outside layers) of cells which are usually the most actively growing cells in the adult body. Important epithelial layers include the skin, the epithelium of glandular organs (breast, uterus, prostate), and cells lining the respiratory tract (lungs, bronchial tubes), gastrointestinal tract (mouth, stomach, colon, rectum), and urinary tract. Carcinomas metastasize primarily via the lymph vessels. In breast cancer, counting the number of nearby lymph nodes that contain cancer cells is one of the principal methods of predicting the outcome of the disease; as the number of involved lymph nodes goes up, the prognosis becomes increasingly bleak.

Sarcomas occur less often than carcinomas. They arise from connective and fibrous tissue like muscle, bone, cartilage, and the membranes covering muscles and fat. Sarcomas have the reputation of metastasizing primarily by way of the blood vessels. **Lymphomas** are cancers of the lymph nodes, part of the body's infection-fighting system. They are closely related to leukemias and, like them, result from changes in the white blood cells.

Leukemia is cancer of the blood-forming cells, which reside chiefly in the bone marrow. Rapid growth of these cells displaces the red blood cell precursors from the marrow and can lead to anemia. Since the malignant cells no longer fight infection, the immune system also loses its ability to defend against bacteria, viruses, and other infectious organisms.

There is a great deal of variation in how easily different cancers can be detected and how well they respond to treatment. For instance, basal cell skin cancer (one type of skin cancer) is easily detected, grows slowly, and is

---

Malignant tumor   A tumor that is cancerous and capable of spreading.

Malignant neoplasm   A cancerous growth. A new growth of abnormal cells.

Benign tumor   A tumor that is not malignant or cancerous.

Metastasis   The spread of cancer cells from one part of the body to another.

Carcinomas   Cancer that originates in epithelial tissue (skin, glands, and lining of internal organs).

Epithelial layer   A layer of tissue that covers a surface or lines a tube or cavity of the body, enclosing and protecting other parts of the body.

Sarcomas   Cancers arising from bone, cartilage, or striated muscle.

Lymphomas   Tumors originating from lymphatic tissue (neck, groin, armpit).

Leukemia   Malignant disease of the blood-forming system.

Figure 16-2   Five-year cancer survival rates for selected sites.

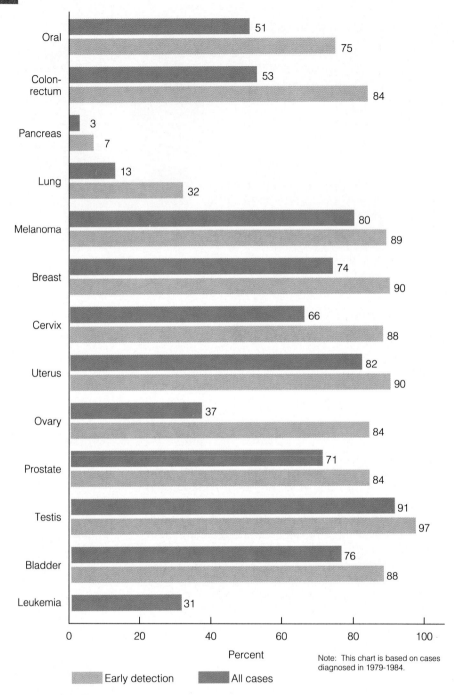

Note: This chart is based on cases diagnosed in 1979-1984.

Early detection   All cases

very accessible. Although there are almost 500,000 cases per year in the United States, virtually all are cured. On the other hand, cancer of the pancreas, fortunately far less frequent, is difficult to detect and only rarely approachable surgically. Fewer than 4 percent of patients live more than three years after diagnosis. In general, the ability of the **oncologist** to predict the progress of a specific type of tumor is still limited and empirical; since every tumor arises from a unique set of changes in a small population of cells, no general theory has emerged that would allow exact prediction of the behavior of the tumor or the course of the disease.

Incidence of Cancer   In 1989, more than 1,000,000 people in the United States were diagnosed as having cancer (if we leave out the 500,000 cases of easily cured skin cancer). Cancer is second only to heart disease as a cause of death in the United States and is the leading

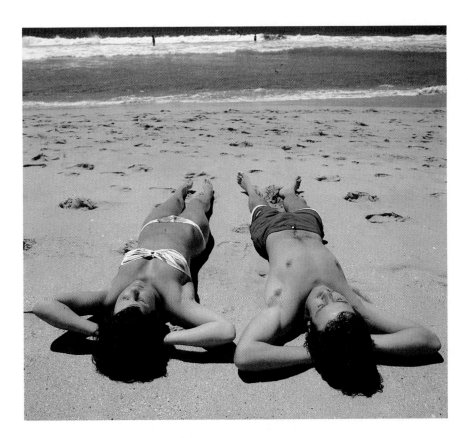

Cumulative exposure to sunlight, beginning in childhood, increases the risk of skin cancer later in life. Blistering sunburns are particularly dangerous, but tanning also poses a hazard. Sunscreens help protect the skin from the sun's radiation.

cause of death in certain age groups—for instance among women aged 30 to 54 and among children aged 3 to 14. Although one person in three will develop cancer in his or her lifetime, 49 percent of those will "survive" their cancer; that is, the five-year survival rate is 49 percent. The five-year survival rate customarily given for cancer is corrected for the noncancer deaths that occur in cancer patients over the next five years. This rate is defined as the ratio of the survival rate for the cancer group to the survival rate for an age- and sex-matched control group. In almost all cases, survival for five years is equivalent to a cure, but in very rare instances, tumors may recur even after five years. The surviving fraction has steadily increased, year by year, since the 1930s, when only about twenty percent survived. Still, about 502,000 deaths from cancer occurred in 1989—1,375 people per day, or about one every 63 seconds (see Figure 16–2).

Is the incidence of cancer increasing or decreasing? This question must be answered carefully, because the American population is rapidly aging and cancer strikes more frequently with advancing age. As the nation improves its cardiovascular health through healthier eating and more exercise, people live longer, and so are increasingly likely to die of cancer rather than of heart attack or stroke. But when cancer death rates are adjusted for the effects of an older population, death rates from the major cancer types seem to be leveling off or decreasing. The only major exception to this trend is lung cancer. Since it takes many years of smoking for the premalignant cells of the lung to become cancerous, the diagnosis of lung cancer today has increased in parallel with the increased rate of smoking of twenty years ago.

Although cancer strikes more frequently with advancing age, your behavior while you are in your twenties will help determine your cancer risk well into the future. The damage to a cell's DNA that leads to cancer may occur twenty to thirty years before the cancer is detected. For an individual, then, the most important questions are (1) which cancers are avoidable, and (2) what precautions can be taken to prevent cancer-producing changes in DNA? In this chapter we will put strongest emphasis on the risk factors for specific cancers, where they are known, and on the lifestyle changes that can prevent the "cancer fuse" from being lit.

Oncologist   A specialist in the study of tumors.

Common Cancers

A discussion of all types of cancer would be beyond the scope of this book, but in this section we look at some of the most common cancers and their causes, prevention, and treatment.

Lung Cancer Lung cancer, the most common cancer in the United States, is very difficult to detect at an early stage. (Table 16–1 lists the leading cancer sites in Americans.) Symptoms don't usually appear until the disease has advanced to the invasive stage. Signals such as a persistent cough, chest pain, or recurring bronchitis may be the first indication of the tumor's presence. A diagnosis can usually be made by studying the cells in sputum or by chest x-ray. Since almost all lung cancers arise from the cells that line the bronchi, tumors can sometimes be visualized by fiber-optic bronchoscopy, a test in which a flexible lighted tube is inserted into the windpipe and the surfaces of the lung passages are directly inspected. Smoking is not the only cause of lung cancer, but it is by far the most important. Most of the other causes, including exposure to asbestos particles or radon gas, are greatly intensified by simultaneous smoking. The best protection against lung cancer, then, is not to smoke.

■ **Exploring Your Emotions**

Does knowing that smoking is responsible for 80 to 90 percent of all lung cancers affect how you feel about smokers? About tobacco companies?

Lung cancer is not only the most common cancer, but is also one of the most deadly. Since it is usually detected after it has begun to spread and since malignant lung cells are resistant to almost all forms of chemotherapy, it isn't surprising that only 13 percent of lung cancer patients are alive five years after diagnosis. The rate of survival has improved only slightly during the past ten years. Lung cancer is most often treated by surgery; and when all the tumor cells can be removed, there are occasional cures. Otherwise, the tumor continues to grow, somehow outwitting the usual cell-killing agents.

There is a small ray of hope. About 25 percent of lung cancers are a type called oat cell or small cell lung cancer. There have been encouraging recent developments in treating oat cell cancers; they can now be treated fairly successfully without surgery, using modern chemotherapy combined with radiation. A large percentage of

cases respond with **remission** and in some cases the remission lasts for years.

Colon and Rectal Cancer The second most common cancer in the U.S. is colon and rectal cancer (also called colorectal cancer). This cancer is clearly linked both to diet and to genetic susceptibility (which is discussed in the next section). In countries where diets are low in fat and high in fiber, the incidence of this cancer may be only 10 or 20 percent of that in the United States. Probably one-third of the population is uniquely susceptible to colon cancer because of heredity, but we don't yet know enough to be able to accurately identify those at greatest risk. Even for those most susceptible, however, attention to diet, particularly to insoluble fiber such as that found in wheat bran, can minimize the risks of colon cancer. High-fiber diets can slow or even reverse precancerous changes in colon cells, just as cessation of smoking can reverse precancerous changes in the lung.

Colon cancer rarely occurs before the age of 40. Most colon cancers arise from preexisting polyps, or small growths on the wall of the colon, which may gradually drift toward malignancy over a period of years. The tendency to form polyps appears to be determined by genes, and so you should be particularly vigilant if colon cancer has occurred among your close relatives. Polyps may bleed as they progress; if the bleeding is detected in time, the polyp may be directly visualized by a fiber-optic device and sampled or even removed without the need for major surgery. The standard warning signs of colon cancer are bleeding from the rectum or change in bowel habits, but improvements in early detection require more aggressive measures than simply waiting for danger signs. A rectal examination can detect some rectal tumors, and a stool occult blood test, done during a routine physical exam, can detect small amounts of blood in stool long before obvious bleeding would be noticed.

Colon and rectal cancer is more curable than lung cancer, particularly if it is caught before it spreads beyond the bowel to other parts of the body. The five-year survival rate is 55 percent overall—about 85 percent if the tumor is localized and about 40 percent if it has spread. With increasing recognition of the genetic basis for these cancers, with improvements in diet, with more sophisticated stool tests, and with increasing education, there is reason to hope that the overall survival rate can be brought close to 85 percent.

Breast Cancer Breast cancer is the second most common cancer in women, and about one in ten women in

---

Remission Condition in which there are no symptoms or other evidence of disease.

VITAL STATISTICS

Table 16-1 Leading cancer sites, 1989[a]

Site	Estimated New Cases 1989	Estimated Deaths 1989	Warning Signals	Comment
Lung	155,000	142,000	Persistent cough or lingering respiratory ailment.	The leading cause of cancer death among men and women.
Colon and rectum	151,000	61,000	Change in bowel habits; bleeding	Considered a highly curable disease when digital and proctoscopic examinations are included in routine checkups.
Breast	143,000	43,000	Lump or thickening in the breast.	Until recently, the leading cause of cancer death in women; now surpassed by lung cancer.
Prostate	103,000	28,500	Urinary difficulty.	Occurs mainly in men over 60; the disease can be detected by palpation and urinalysis at annual checkup.
Kidney and bladder	70,200	20,000	Urinary difficulty; bleeding—in which case consult physician at once.	Protective measures for workers in high-risk industries are helping to eliminate one of the important causes of these cancers.
Stomach	20,000	14,000	Unexplained indigestion continuing for more than a week.	A 40 percent decline in mortality in 25 years, for reasons unknown.
Uterus (including cervix)	47,000[b]	10,000	Unusual bleeding or discharge.	Uterine cancer mortality has declined 65 percent during the last 40 years with wider application of the Pap test. Postmenopausal women with abnormal bleeding should be checked.
Oral (including pharynx)	31,000	9,000	Sore that does not heal; difficulty in swallowing	Many more lives should be saved because the mouth is easily accessible to visual examination by physicians and dentists.
Skin	27,000[c]	8,200	Sore that does not heal; change in wart or mole.	Skin cancer is readily detected by observation and diagnosed by simple biopsy.
Leukemia	27,300	18,000	Leukemia is a cancer of blood-forming tissues and is characterized by the abnormal production of immature white blood cells. Acute leukemia strikes mainly children and is treated by drugs that have extended life from a few months to as much as 10 years. Chronic leukemia strikes usually after age 25 and progresses less rapidly.	
Other blood and lymph tissues	52,000	27,400	These cancers arise in the lymph system and include Hodgkin's disease and lymphosarcoma. Some patients with lymphatic cancers can lead normal lives for many years. Five-year survival rate for Hodgkin's disease increased from 25 percent to 54 percent in 20 years.	

[a]All figures rounded to nearest 100.
[b]Totals do not include cases in which the carcinoma is confined to the epithelium (over 45,000 new cases).
[c]Totals do not include nonmelanoma skin cancers (500,000 new cases annually).

Source: Incidence estimates are based on rates of cancer in the United States from American Cancer Society. 1989. *ACS: Cancer Facts and Figures—1989* (New York: American Cancer Society).

Table 16-2 Factors that influence breast cancer risk	
Increase in Risk	**Decrease in Risk**
Family history of breast cancer	Short number of menstrual years; early menopause
High-fat, high-calorie diet; obesity	
Early onset of first menstruation; late menopause	Early pregnancy
	Many children
Late age for first pregnancy	Breastfeeding of infants
No children, unmarried	Bilateral removal of ovaries early in fertile life
Live births with no nursing	
Failure of ovulation	Low socioeconomic status
Prolonged high-dose estrogen treatment	Rural residence
Chest irradiation	
Adapted from Jay Roth. 1985. *All About Cancer* (Philadelphia: Stickley), p. 189.	

the United States will develop breast cancer during her lifetime. The great majority of tumors occur in women over 50; but since these tumors are curable when caught early, attention to screening methods is advisable even for younger women. The five-year survival from time of diagnosis for all stages of breast tumors, is 75 percent; for small localized tumors, the survival rate can approach 90 percent. These statistics have changed little in the past twenty years, but the incidence of breast cancer is increasing slowly, perhaps due to the increasing fat content of the American diet and increasing obesity.

Risk Factors for Breast Cancer   Breast cancer has been called a "disease of civilization," because incidence is high in industrialized Western countries and remains low in less developed non-Western countries (as is the case for lung cancer and coronary heart disease too). Although there is a genetic component in breast cancer, other major risk factors are dietary and hormonal (see Table 16–2). This connection has led some researchers to point to a link with the Western standard of living, especially the high-calorie, high-fat diet made possible by industrialized food production.

These dietary and hormonal risk factors include obesity (formerly the privilege of the wealthy), early first menstruation (thought to be related to the robustness of well-fed children), late menopause (also thought to be related to dietary improvements over the last century), late first motherhood (a choice of many women today), and not breastfeeding (an option when cow's milk and formula are available). The key to these factors may be the female sex hormone estrogen, which circulates in the body between puberty and menopause and becomes low during breastfeeding. Fat cells can produce estrogen too, so the

hormone may be involved in the link between obesity and breast cancer.

The role of estrogen as a cancer promoter has been debated for years (see the discussion of cancer promoters later in this chapter). Beginning in the 1950s it was prescribed to counter the symptoms of menopause, a treatment called estrogen replacement therapy (ERT). In the 1970s and 1980s estrogen was further shown to help prevent osteoporosis and to provide protection against cardiovascular disease by lowering total cholesterol levels and increasing the proportion of high-density lipoproteins, the "good" cholesterol.

But higher rates of cancer of the **endometrium** (the lining of the uterus) among women on ERT led to further studies, which confirmed that this cancer was linked to estrogen. Subsequent research suggested that estrogen in combination with one of the progestins (other female hormones) would counter this effect, and ERT was replaced by combined therapy, called hormone replacement therapy (HRT), which many postmenopausal women now receive.

Although estrogen is linked to endometrial cancer, it is not definitively known whether it is also linked to breast cancer. Some studies show estrogen apparently preventing some breast cancer, some show it apparently causing some, and some show it apparently having no effect. The evidence about the role of progestins in causing or preventing breast cancer is also contradictory, although the addition of progestins does seem to offset the beneficial cardiovascular effects of estrogen alone. Since findings have not been conclusive, experts recommend that women consult with their physicians on an individual basis about whether hormone replacement is an appropriate treatment for them. Critical to the decision are

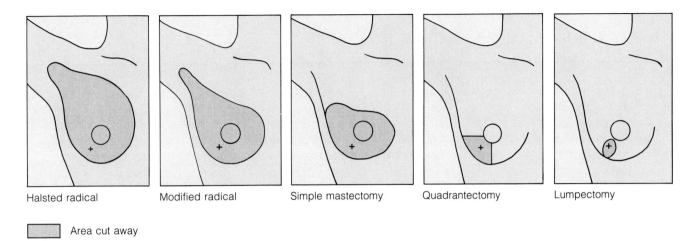

Halsted radical   Modified radical   Simple mastectomy   Quadrantectomy   Lumpectomy

▢ Area cut away
+   Primary Tumor

Figure 16-3   Types of breast surgery.

the woman's other risk factors, such as whether she smokes, whether she has previously had cancer, how old she is at menopause, and whether she has a family history of severe osteoporosis.

Although genetic factors and some hormonal factors (such as never giving birth) cannot be changed, important dietary factors in breast cancer are within the control of the individual. Maintaining a normal weight and decreasing both fat and calories in the diet can minimize the chances of breast cancer, even in someone at risk due to heredity.

Detecting and Treating Breast Cancer   The American Cancer Society recommends a three-part personal program for early detection of breast cancer. Monthly breast self-examination is recommended for all women over 20 (see the box "Breast Self-Examination"), and a clinical breast exam performed by a physician should be part of a regular health checkup. These two steps, consistently observed, will detect the majority of tumors at an early stage.

There are some tumors, however, that may already have metastasized by the time the lump becomes detectable through physical examination. Finding these tumors before they have spread requires examination with a sensitive low-dose x-ray technique called mammography. Women are advised to have a baseline **mammogram** between the ages of 35 and 40 for comparison with future mammograms. Between the ages of 40 and 50, they are advised to consult with their physicians about whether or how often to have mammograms. After age 50, mammograms are recommended annually.

If a lump is detected, either by physical examination or mammogram, it will be biopsied (removed and examined in the laboratory) to see if it is cancerous, either by needle in the physician's office or surgically. Nine times out of ten, the lump is found to be a cyst or other harmless growth, and no further treatment is needed. If the lump is found to contain cancer cells, a variety of surgeries may be called for, ranging from a lumpectomy (removal of the lump alone) to a mastectomy (removal of the breast) (see Figure 16–3). To determine if the cancer has spread, lymph nodes from the underarm are biopsied. If it has, growth of cancer cells can often be slowed by some type of additional therapy, such as hormonal therapy or chemotherapy.

Individual survival chances in cases of breast cancer vary greatly. For example, a postmenopausal woman whose tumor is discovered early—before it can even be felt—and who has no family history of breast cancer and no evidence of spread, has quite a good outlook. A person in this situation has perhaps better than a 90 percent chance of surviving five years.

Uterine, Cervical, and Ovarian Cancer   Cancers of the female reproductive system—uterine, cervical, and ovarian cancer—arise in related organs and can best be discussed as a group. The cervix is the neck of the uterus, the narrow end that opens into the vagina, and the uterus is in contact with the ovaries, which are deep in the abdomen. There are more cases of uterine cancer, but ovarian cancer and cervical cancer are more deadly. Most early detection, however, is directed at cervical cancer, for reasons we will discuss later.

Endometrium   Tissue lining the uterus.   **Mammogram**   An x-ray of the breasts.

Breast Self-Examination

Early detection of breast cancer is possible through monthly self-examination. (a) Sit in front of a mirror, raise your arms, and check for unusual dimples in the skin or depression of the nipples. This check should also be done with your arms lowered. Then lie down and place a flat pillow or a folded towel under the shoulder of the same side as the breast to be examined. (b) Keep the left arm at the side while you examine your left breast. Check the outer side of the breast, moving your hand up into the armpit. (c) Using the flat part of your fingers, inspect the lower part of the breast and then (d) the upper part. Next (e–h) raise the left arm and repeat the procedure, beginning at the breast bone. Repeat with the right breast. If you detect a lump or unusual mass, you should contact a physician immediately. (If you find a similar lump or mass in the same place in the other breast, it probably is normal tissue.) Breasts should be examined one week after the end of every menstrual period.

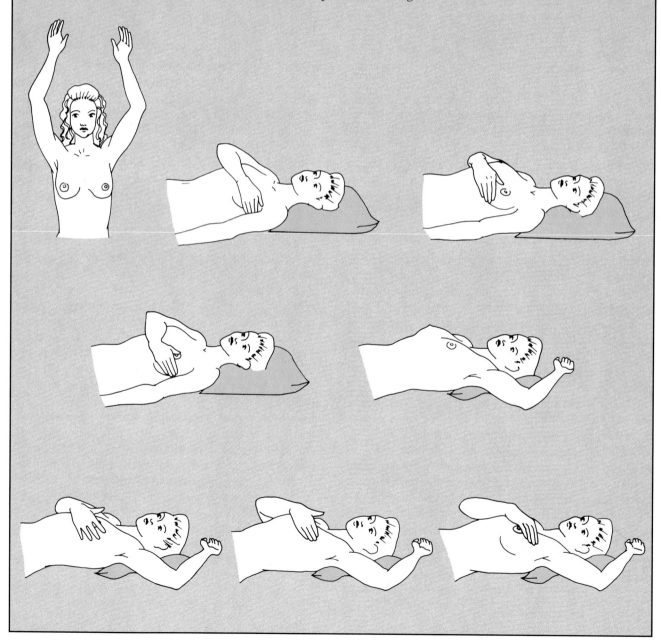

Cancer of the body of the uterus, also called endometrial cancer, is a disease of mature women, and diagnosis is usually made between the ages of 55 and 69. The risk factors are a history of infertility, obesity, and prolonged estrogen therapy. Fortunately, this cancer is often detectable during a standard pelvic exam, and it is highly curable by surgery; 88 percent of patients are alive at five years after diagnosis, with no evidence of disease.

Invasive cervical cancer, on the other hand, attacks younger women and eventually kills about half of those who are diagnosed with it. But, in a sense, cervical cancer is one of the great success stories of cancer control during the last few decades. As the use of the **Pap smear** has become almost universal in the United States during the past forty years, the death rate of cervical cancer has dropped by over 70 percent. The early noninvasive form of cervical cancer can now be identified by the presence of abnormal cells in Pap smears, with little expense or inconvenience to the patient. The abnormal cells can then be removed before they reach the dangerous invasive stage. The risk factors for cervical cancer are quite different from those for uterine cancer, and some recent insights into this disease are discussed in the box "Cervical Cancer and Papillomavirus: Evidence for a Link."

Even though ovarian cancer is rare compared to uterine cancer, it causes more deaths than any other cancer of the female reproductive system. It cannot be detected by Pap smear or any other simple screening method and is often noticed only late in its development, when surgery and other therapies are unlikely to be successful. The incidence of ovarian cancer increases with age, as does the incidence of most cancers, reaching its peak at ages 65 through 84. To make a dent in mortality from ovarian cancer will require either a sensitive new screening test or a much more effective chemotherapy. Recently, medical scientists have suggested that use of a blood test, together with ultrasound imaging of the ovaries, might be able to detect early ovarian cancer if applied to women in the high-risk group. However, this approach is fairly speculative at the moment. New forms of chemotherapy that might be effective in ovarian cancer are discussed later in the chapter.

Prostate Cancer The prostate gland is situated at the base of the bladder in men. It produces seminal fluid and when enlarged can block the flow of urine. Prostate cancer is the most common cancer in men and the cause of more deaths in men than any but lung or colon cancer. There are 103,000 new cases in the United States each year. Prostate cancer is chiefly a disease of aging, and 80 percent of cases are diagnosed in men over the age of

65. Diet and lifestyle probably influence the rates of this cancer, but compared to the other cancers we have discussed, the risk factors are somewhat obscure.

The best method for controlling prostate cancer is through early detection, and the methods of screening are becoming increasingly sophisticated. Most cases are first detected by rectal examination during a routine physical. The doctor can directly palpate the prostate gland through the rectum and determine whether it is enlarged and whether lumps are present. Although a rectal exam is unpleasant, it is quick, inexpensive, and the only practical way to detect the early stages of both prostate and rectal cancers.

Ultrasound is used increasingly as a follow-up, to detect lumps too small to be palpated and to determine their size, shape, and properties. A needle biopsy of suspicious lumps can be painlessly performed, and a pathologist can determine whether the biopsied cells are malignant or benign by examining them under a microscope. If the cells are malignant, the prostate is surgically removed, and additional treatment in the form of radiation, hormones, or anti-cancer drugs may be applied. Of course, early detection leads to a better outcome. Survival rates for all stages have improved steadily since 1940, and in the last 20 years they have increased from 48 percent to 71 percent.

Oral Cancer Oral cancer—cancers of the lip, tongue, mouth and throat—can be traced principally to cigarette and cigar smoking, excess alcohol consumption, and, increasingly, use of smokeless or chewing tobacco. These risk factors can work together to boost the likelihood of oral cancer in an individual. Sigmund Freud, a lifelong cigar smoker, was a prominent sufferer of oral cancer, as is Fidel Castro, never without a cigar in his hand. Oral cancers do have the virtue of being fairly easy to detect, though they are often hard to cure. The five-year survival rates vary from 32 percent for throat cancer to 91 percent for lip cancer, and the principal methods of treatment are, once again, surgery and radiation therapy.

Skin Cancer Skin cancer is the most common cancer of all when cases of the highly curable forms are included in the count. (Usually, these forms are not included, precisely because they are so curable.) Treatments are usually simple, successful if the cancer is caught early, and nearly painless. Although death from skin cancers is uncommon, considerable scarring can occur if they are not found and treated early while they are still small and relatively easy to remove.

Pap smear A scraping of cells from the cervix for examination under a microscope to detect cancer.

Cervical Cancer and Papillomavirus: Evidence for a Link

Unlike most cancers, which have their peak incidence after the age of 60, cancer of the cervix often occurs in younger women in their thirties or even in their twenties. Since early cancer can be devastating to family life, and since there is an excellent system of diagnosis and treatment for very early cervical cancer, this danger can and should be avoided.

Screening for the changes in cervical cells that precede cancer is done chiefly by means of the Papanicolaou test, commonly known as the Pap test. In this procedure, cells from the uterine cervix are spread on a slide, stained for easier viewing, and examined under a microscope to see whether they are normal in size and shape. If cells are abnormal, additional Pap tests are done at intervals; sometimes the cells spontaneously return to their normal size and shape, but in about one-third of cervical dysplasias, the changes progress toward malignancy. If this happens, the abnormal cells must be removed, either by excising them surgically, by treating them with ultracold, or by destroying them with localized laser treatment. Usually the patch of abnormal cells is small and can be completely removed by minor surgery.

Without timely surgery, the malignant patch of cells goes on to invade the wall of the cervix and spreads to adjacent lymph nodes and to the uterus. At this stage cytotoxic (cell-killing) chemotherapy may be used to kill the fast-growing cancer cells, but chances for a complete cure are much lower. Even when a cure can be achieved, it often means surgical removal of the uterus and therefore sterility.

How does cervical cancer get started, and what can be done to prevent it? A great deal of clinical and epidemiological data suggests that the critical event may be infection of the cervical cells by one of the human papillomaviruses (here abbreviated as HPV). This is the same group of viruses that cause common warts as well as venereal, or genital, warts. Of the sixty or so viruses in this family only a few are associated with cervical cancer, and these are distinct from those that cause either common warts or genital warts. It is worth keeping in mind that individuals with genital warts are also likely to be infected with the cancer-associated members of the family. The initial infection probably begins when the virus is introduced into the cervix by an infected sexual partner. In fact, cervical cancer is strongly associated with early sexual activity and multiple partners; women who do not have sexual relations—nuns, for instance—are not at risk for cervical cancer. Although few studies have been done, it seems likely that regular use of condoms reduces the risk of transmitting papillomavirus infection. The precautions taken to guard against AIDS may decrease the incidence of cervical cancer as well.

Although papillomavirus DNA is almost always found in cervical cancer cells, only a very small fraction of HPV-infected women ever get cervical cancer. There must be added factors, or cofactors, working in parallel with the HPV infection to produce a cancer. All the data are not yet in, but at this point it seems that the most important cofactors are (1) smoking and (2) infection with another common sexually transmitted virus, the genital type of herpesvirus. Both smoking and herpesvirus can cause cancerous changes in cells in the laboratory, and they can speed and intensify the cancerous changes begun by the papillomaviruses. In fact, it has recently been shown that nicotine and other mutagenic chemicals, carried from the lungs by the circulation of blood, can be identified in the cervical secretions of women who smoke.

There is another important system controlling the potential damage done by viral infections, and that is the immune system. It is very likely that normal cellular immunity plays the most important role in controlling the initial HPV infection and in preventing progression from a symptomless infection to cervical dysplasia, and then on to malignancy. Chemicals that suppress elements of the immune system, as substances in tobacco appear to do, are associated with an increase in dysplasia and cancer. Stress, poor nutrition, and frequent infections are additional factors that can inhibit normal immune function; these all appear to be secondary risk factors in cancer of the cervix.

So, from the point of view of prevention, it would be best to avoid the behaviors and infections that are associated with this cancer and to use condoms. Knowledge of the risk factors should provide strong motivation for you to have a Pap test at recommended intervals, to be sure that you don't have a potentially dangerous dysplasia, and to take action, with your physician's advice, if you do.

No one knows the exact mechanisms that lead to the formation and growth of skin cancers, but abnormal cellular changes in the most superficial layers of the skin known as the epidermis are consistently found. The role of sunlight in producing these changes, which can be temporary or permanent, has been well documented. Both severe, acute sun reactions (sunburns) and chronic, low-level sun reactions (suntans) can lead to skin cancer later. People with fair skin have lower natural protection against skin damage from the sun and have a higher risk of developing certain skin cancers. Chronic exposure to certain chemicals can also increase the risk of developing skin cancers, and there is a genetic component as well.

The incidence of skin cancer, especially malignant melanoma, has increased dramatically worldwide in the last four decades. The trend could worsen, according to some experts, if the ozone layer continues to be depleted. This thin layer of the atmosphere, which protects people from the ultraviolet radiation present in natural sunlight, is being damaged by the release of chlorofluorocarbon compounds from industrial processes on earth, particularly those involved in refrigeration and air conditioning. Protection of the ozone layer is an important environmental issue that needs to be addressed more comprehensively in the 1990s if skin cancer rates are to decline.

Types of Skin Cancer   There are three main types of skin cancer, named for the kind of skin cell from which they develop:

- **Basal cell carcinoma** is the most common skin cancer and is usually found in chronically sun-exposed areas such as the face, neck, arms, and hands. It usually appears as a small, shiny, pink, fleshy bump that grows slowly and persists beyond the time (several weeks) that usual skin inflammations and pimples take to resolve. Basal cell carcinoma is usually not painful, although occasionally it will bleed, crust, or form an open sore on the skin.
- **Squamous cell carcinoma** is the second most common type of skin cancer and is seen most often on ears, face, lips, and mouth, although it can occur anywhere. It may appear as a persistent, sharply outlined, red, scaly, platelike patch, as an open sore, or as a hard, rough bump.
- **Melanoma**, the third most common type of skin cancer, is the most dangerous, because it spreads so rapidly. It can occur anywhere on the body, but the most common sites are the back, chest, abdomen, and lower

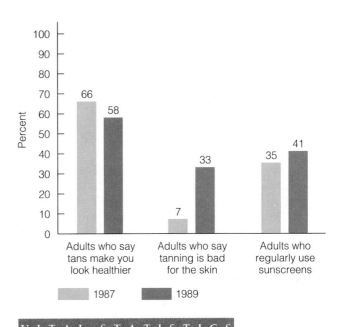

VITAL STATISTICS

Figure 16-4   Sunshine risk: some people are listening.

legs. A melanoma usually appears at the site of a preexisting mole. The mole may begin to enlarge, become mottled or varied in color (colors can include blue, pink, and white), or develop an irregular surface or irregular borders. Tissue invaded by melanoma may also itch, burn, or bleed easily.

Preventing and Detecting Skin Cancer   One of the major steps you can take to protect yourself against all forms of skin cancer is to avoid lifelong overexposure to sunlight. Blistering, peeling sunburns from unprotected sun exposure are particularly dangerous, but suntans also increase your risk of developing skin cancer later in life (see Figure 16–4). Tanning salons cannot offer safe tanning because tanning in any form increases the risk of skin cancer. People of every age, including babies and children, need to be protected from the sun with **sunscreens** and protective clothing. For a closer look at sunlight and skin cancer, see the box "Protecting Your Skin from the Sun."

The only sure way to avoid a serious outcome from skin cancers is to make sure they are recognized and diagnosed early. In most successfully treated cases, patients themselves bring their melanoma or other skin cancer to their physician's attention. Make it a habit to ex-

Basal cell carcinoma   Cancer of the deepest layers of the skin.

Squamous cell carcinoma   Cancer of the surface layers of the skin.

Melanoma   A malignant tumor of the skin that arises from pigmented cells, usually a mole.

Sunscreen   Substance used to protect the skin from ultraviolet rays; usually applied as an ointment or a cream.

Protecting Your Skin from the Sun

Experts are becoming more and more convinced that there is no such thing as a "safe tan," and more and more people are getting the message that the sun causes skin cancer and premature aging of the skin. But that doesn't mean you shouldn't lead an active outdoor life. Proper clothing and use of sunscreens can protect your skin against most sun-induced damage.

In many situations—bicycling, painting the house, playing volleyball at the beach—you can protect your forearms, chest, and back with loose, long-sleeved shirts made of closely woven cotton fabric. Beware of thin white shirts and wet clothing that clings to the body, since they are minimally protective. Hats with brims help deflect sun from ears, forehead, and upper cheeks, and hair can protect the neck and ears.

When you can't cover your skin, use a sunscreen—a lotion or cream that filters out the sun's ultraviolet (UV) rays. These products are rated according to how long you can stay out in the sun before you burn, compared to using no sunscreen. A product with a sun protection factor (SPF) of 8, for example, would allow you to remain in the sun without burning eight times longer, on average, than if you didn't apply sunscreen. Thus, if you're fair-skinned and would normally burn in ten minutes, a screen with SPF 8 would allow you eighty minutes before burning.

Sunblocks are opaque creams or pastes containing zinc oxide or titanium dioxide that prevent any light at all from reaching the skin. These *physical* sunscreens, which can protect sensitive areas such as the nose and lips but are messy to use, don't have any SPF ratings. *Chemical* sunscreens allow some UV rays to pass through to the skin, even those with SPFs of 15. Some high-SPF chemical screens now contain a physical block, such as zinc oxide. When used as directed, a screen rated 15 is usually adequate. But people tend to apply only about half the amount of sunscreen that the FDA uses to determine SPF, making a 15 only as effective as an 8. If you're fair-skinned and will be outside all day, either use a high-protection screen (SPF 30 or more) or plan to apply sunscreen frequently.

Researchers once thought that ultraviolet B (UVB) rays, which are mainly responsible for sunburn and skin cancer, were the only dangerous component of sunlight and that the longer-wavelength ultraviolet A (UVA) rays helped you tan without harming the skin. Tanning salons, which use high-intensity light sources emitting predominantly UVA radiation, based their claims to "safe tanning" on this notion of safe UV radiation. But now it appears that UVA radiation is harmful too. It penetrates into the skin more deeply, causing premature aging, and it sensitizes the skin so that sunlight is more likely to cause skin cancer. Thus, tanning salons do not offer a safe way to tan, for this reason and others (UVA rays can damage unprotected eyes and can cause adverse reactions if you're taking certain drugs, such as antibiotics, tranquilizers, antihistamines, birth control pills, or oral diabetes medication.

Most sunscreens on the market today protect mainly against UVB, and the SPF number pertains only to UVB. Usually, sunscreens offer protection through such ingredients as padimate O, a derivative of para-aminobenzoic acid (PABA). The fullest protection against UVA is offered by a group of chemical compounds known

---

amine your skin regularly. Most of the spots, freckles, moles, and blemishes on your body are normal; you were born with some of them, and others appear and disappear throughout your life. As you age, you may develop "liver" spots, patches of darkened skin that look like freckles— these are harmless. But if you notice an unusual growth, discoloration, or sore that does not heal, see your physician or a dermatologist immediately. The following characteristics may signal that a lesion is a melanoma.

A asymmetry
B border irregularity
C color change
D diameter greater than 6 mm

Additionally, if someone in your family has had numerous skin cancers or melanoma, you may want to consult a dermatologist for a complete skin examination and discussion of your particular risk.

Protecting Your Skin from the Sun (continued)

as dibenzoylmethanes. Photoplex is a sunscreen that contains one of these chemicals, and more should be coming on the market soon. Of the more common ingredients in sunscreens, benzophenones (such as oxybenzone) offer some protection against UVA rays.

Sunscreens wear and wash off from perspiration and swimming, so they should be reapplied frequently during peak sun hours. A sunscreen labeled "water-resistant" protects you after you have spent forty minutes in the water; a "waterproof" sunscreen protects you after eighty minutes in the water. If you're not wearing a sunscreen, you're not protected from the sun when you're swimming, because UV rays penetrate at least 3 feet in water.

Here are some guidelines to follow when selecting and using a sunscreen:

1. Choose a screen with SPF 15. If you're fair-skinned and will be outdoors for long hours, use one with an even higher SPF. Look for the seal of approval from the Skin Cancer Foundation, which tests sunscreens with SPF 15 or higher for safety and effectiveness in blocking UVB. About eighty

brands now carry the seal. However, new products may not yet have applied for this seal.

2. For greatest protection against both UVA and UVB rays, use Photoplex. Otherwise, look for a "broad spectrum" sunscreen (such as Presun 15, Supershade 15, Sundown 15, or Total Eclipse 15), which contains two or more ultraviolet-absorbing ingredients. Many ingredient combinations work in concert to block a broader range of light waves and also wash off less easily.

3. Apply the screen at least thirty to forty-five minutes before exposure to the sun. Studies show that this allows it to penetrate the skin for optimal effectiveness.

4. Apply it frequently and generously. A single application won't remain potent. If you swim or tend to sweat a lot, look for a waterproof or water-resistant screen.

5. Take into account the time of day and your location. UV rays are strongest between 10 A.M. and 3 P.M., so adjust your sunscreen strength and reapplication schedule accordingly. Intensity of rays also increases the closer you are to the equator and the higher the altitude.

Snow and sand reflect sun rays, making them more intense, and up to 70 percent of UV radiation can penetrate clouds. If you're fair-skinned, you may need to wear protective clothing, a hat, and a physical sunscreen on your nose and lips.

6. Don't assume that because your skin isn't red, it isn't getting burned. A sunburn is most evident six to twenty-four hours after sunning.

7. If you're taking medication, ask your doctor or pharmacist about possible reactions to sunlight and interactions with sunscreens.

Remember, your risk of skin cancer rises with your cumulative, unprotected exposure to sunlight over the course of your whole life, but with adequate protection, you can enjoy the outdoors and still have healthy skin now and in later years.

Based on Sunscreens: The full spectrum, *University of California, Berkeley, Wellness Letter*, July 1989; Myth: Tanning booths give you a safer tan, *University of California, Berkeley, Wellness Letter*, February 1989; and Judy Koperski, Preventing skin cancer, *Healthline*, March 1986.

If you do have an unusual skin lesion, the physician will sometimes be able to determine whether it is benign, precancerous, or cancerous by a physical examination. In other cases, a biopsy is necessary for a definite diagnosis. If the lesion is cancerous, it is usually removed surgically, a procedure that can almost always be performed in the physician's office using local anesthesia. Occasionally, other forms of treatment may be used. Even for melanoma, the outlook after removal in the early

states is good, with a five-year survival rate of 95 percent and a ten-year rate of 90 percent. If the tumor is removed later, after it has begun to invade the surrounding tissues or other areas of the body, the survival rate drops sharply. But since prevention requires a minimum of time and attention, it pays to be alert.

Other Cancers Some other cancers are worth special mention. Testicular cancer is relatively rare, accounting

---

Testicle Self-Examination

To detect testicular cancer, the American Cancer Society recommends the following self-examination.

1. Perform the examination after a warm bath or shower, when the scrotal skin is most relaxed. (*Scrotal* refers to the scrotum, the pouch in which the testicles normally lie.)

2. Cup each testicle in the palm of one hand and examine it by feeling with the fingers of your other hand. The normal testicle is smooth, egg-shaped, and somewhat firm to the touch.

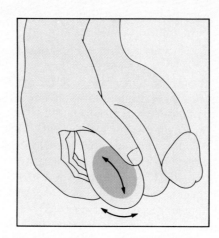

3. At the rear of each testicle is a tube called the *epididymis*, which carries sperm away from the testicle. This is a normal part of your body; its presence does not indicate cancer.

4. If there is any change in shape or texture of the testicles—or any lumps, especially hard ones—consult a physician immediately.

Repeat this examination every six or eight weeks. It is important that you know what your own testicles feel like normally so that you will recognize any changes.

---

for only 1 percent of cancer in men, but it is the most common cancer in men 29 to 35 years of age. Self-examination can permit early detection of testicular cancer (see the box "Testicle Self-examination"). Males with undescended testicles are at high risk for testicular cancer, and for this reason the condition should be corrected in early childhood.

There were 47,000 cases of bladder cancer in the United States in 1989. Bladder cancer is about three times as common in men as in women, and smoking is responsible for about half the cases in men. Other risk factors include urban living and exposure to certain industrial chemicals, such as the benzene in gasoline and petroleum products. The first symptoms are likely to be blood in the urine and/or increased frequency of urination. These symptoms should motivate a quick trip to your physician for a thorough exam, since the survival rate for early-stage bladder cancer is 88 percent.

Pancreatic cancer is the fifth leading cancer killer; it is both hard to detect and usually deadly, and the principal known risk factor is, again, smoking. Beyond that, little is known about the disease or how to prevent it. Until medical science advances, there is relatively little to do in terms of lifestyle adjustment or early detection.

Kaposi's sarcoma is a rare form of cancer that was seldom seen, and then only in older people, before the AIDS epidemic. A consequence of the immune system's inability to function properly, this cancer is characterized by purple or brownish lesions that resemble bruises but are painless and do not heal. Kaposi's sarcoma is discussed further in Chapter 17.

What Causes Cancer?

Although scientists don't know everything about what causes cancer, they have identified both genetic and environmental factors. In many cases, these work together.

Take Good Care of Your DNA Mutational damage to a cell's **DNA**, particularly to the DNA of growth-control genes, can lead to rapid and uncontrolled growth of cells (see the box "Oncogenes and Cancer"). Agents that produce mutational damage, known as mutagens, include radiation, viral infection, and chemical substances in the air we breathe and the food we eat. We also know that many mutational steps are required before a normal cell takes on all the properties of a cancer cell. Scientists will argue for the next few years over which mutations cause cancer and how many are required. But it is increasingly clear that minimizing mutational damage to our DNA will protect us from many cancers. Unfortunately, a great many substances produce cancer-causing mutations, and we can't escape them all. By identifying the important **carcinogens** and understanding how they produce their effects, we can do ourselves and our DNA a favor.

Cancer Initiators and Cancer Promoters Agents that cause mutational changes in the DNA of **proto-oncogenes** are known as "initiators" of cancer. Other chemical agents, incapable of producing mutations directly, may still act as "promoters" of cancer. Promoters accelerate the growth of cells temporarily, without damaging or permanently altering DNA. In speeding up cell growth, promoters increase the odds that any damage done to DNA will be permanently preserved; they do so by causing the cell to replicate its DNA before damage can be repaired. For this and other complex reasons, growing cells are more likely to undergo mutational change than are non-growing cells.

For example, estrogen, a natural hormone, stimulates growth of the cells of both uterus and breast; estrogen is not a mutagen, but large amounts of estrogen given over a prolonged period can lead to an increased incidence of cancer in both these organs, as described earlier. This is not to say that estrogen is a "bad" hormone, but, like any growth-promoting substance, it must be used sparingly. The estrogen supplements given to postmenopausal women to prevent osteoporosis are given in such low doses that the risk of cancer from them is thought to be negligible. There are many other examples of the cancer-promoter phenomenon, and in general we can say that any abnormal stimulus to cell growth is likely to increase the risk of cancer.

Hereditary Cancer Risks   Certain types of cancer have a genetic basis; in other words, an individual may inherit an increased risk for a particular type of cancer from one or both parents. The molecular basis for this inheritance is not completely clear, but it seems to have something to do with a special class of proto-oncogenes called "suppressor genes." These genes normally act as a brake on cell growth. Suppressor genes are normally inherited as a pair, with one gene copy on each **chromosome** of a chromosome pair. Some individuals are born with one of these suppressor genes already damaged; loss of the second suppressor gene through a later mutation will then "release the brake" and lead directly to more rapid cellular growth and division. As discussed earlier, this is a precondition for development of cancer.

■ **Exploring Your Emotions**

Has anyone in your family had cancer or died of cancer? If so, how was it handled? What were you told about it? How do you think it has affected you?

Perhaps the most dramatic example of the effects of inheriting an altered suppressor gene is seen in those individuals who have inherited an increased risk of colon cancer. It appears that about one-third of the population has an increased tendency to form colon polyps, which

can progress to cancer; most of these people seem to have an alteration in one copy of a specific pair of suppressor genes. Eventually, as our understanding increases, we should be able to identify these individuals, perhaps by laboratory tests for presence of the altered DNA. Their risk of cancer can then be reduced by both paying careful attention to diet and increased monitoring.

Carcinogens and Anticarcinogens   As noted earlier, agents that cause cancer are called *carcinogens*, whether they act as initiators or promoters. Some occur naturally in the environment, like the ultraviolet rays from the sun or the radioactive radon gas that seeps out of the earth and into the basements of houses in some areas. Others are manufactured or synthetic substances that show up occasionally in the general environment but more often in the work environment of specific industries.

Another important source of carcinogens is the food we eat. The complexity of substances in our diet, both cancer-promoting and cancer-preventing, is truly staggering. Scientific understanding of dietary effects on cancer is still evolving and difficult to summarize. Some of the carcinogens are discussed in the following pages, and some general dietary guidelines are provided in Table 16–3 and the box "A Dietary Defense against Cancer."

■ **Exploring Your Emotions**

Do you fear cancer? Does it seem mysterious to you? Do you believe you can do anything to avoid it?

A few dietary compounds, like **beta-carotene**, a precursor of vitamin A, look so promising in cancer prevention that the National Cancer Institute (NCI) has set up long-term clinical trials to determine their efficacy. Beta-carotene, carotenoids, and vitamin A itself seem to prevent cancer at the level of cancer promotion; that is, they slow the growth of epithelial cells. Other elements of the diet prevent cancer at the level of cancer initiation. Both vitamin C and vitamin E are antioxidants and can intercept and reduce many of the chemical agents capable of causing mutagenic damage to DNA. Because it takes so long for most cancers to develop, it may be ten or twenty years before the outcome of the NCI trials can tell us whether we should all add these supplements to our diet; in the meanwhile, be sure to include the RDAs of these vitamins in your diet (see Chapter 12).

DNA   Deoxyribonucleic acid, a chemical substance that carries genetic information.

Carcinogens   Any substances that cause cancer.

Proto-oncogene   A gene involved in controlling the growth of a cell.

Chromosomes   Material in the nucleus of a cell that transmits genetic information. Abnormal chromosomes are common in cancer cells.

Beta-carotene   A vitamin-A precursor found in plants.

Oncogenes and Cancer

Cancer research has produced some exciting and promising insights in the last few years, particularly into the behavior of **oncogenes**, genes that appear to be related to the uncontrolled cell growth characteristic of cancer. The development of a cancer doesn't occur in a single step but requires several sequential changes. For example, cancers of the colon, cervix, and breast are often preceded by a **preneoplastic** state, with an extensive area of cells showing more rapid and disordered growth than normal. Usually only one malignant tumor arises out of these millions of abnormal, but not yet malignant, cells. In the last fifteen years we have begun to understand that the "behaviors" that distinguish a tumor cell from a normal cell can be traced to a group of genes whose role is to control the growth of a cell. In their normal state these genes are known as proto-oncogenes, and they specify a set of proteins that are involved in the many mechanisms of cell growth control. It seems reasonable that damage or mutation to these critical genes

could easily result in a cell that divides when it should not and that travels and flourishes in places that would be forbidden to a normal cell. Not every gene can become an oncogene—only those that have a fairly direct role to play in cell growth.

The first oncogene, named *src* for sarcoma, was discovered by two California scientists, Michael Bishop and Harold Varmus, in the mid-1970s. They shared the 1989 Nobel Prize in medicine for their discovery. The src gene was discovered in a virus that causes cancer in chickens. The gene was found to be responsible for allowing the virus to transform an infected normal cell in the chicken into a tumor. To their great surprise, Bishop and Varmus found that noninfected chicken cells had a gene very similar to the src gene in the virus. Further work showed that the similar gene in the chicken was itself a proto-oncogene, implicated in control of cell growth. Changes in this gene could convert it into an active oncogene and start a cell down the road toward malignancy. Just

as Dr. Jekyll becomes a brutish Mr. Hyde under the influence of certain chemicals, so can a mutational change in the DNA of a mild-mannered proto-oncogene produce an oncogene and start a normal cell down the path of "lawless" growth. It appears that proto-oncogenes may be the final common pathway that mediates the carcinogenic action of chemicals, radiation, and other environmental carcinogens.

Since the discovery of src, over forty additional oncogenes have been found, and more remain to be discovered. As the action of each oncogene is sorted out, we gain new insights into the normal control mechanisms of the cell. One of the first lessons we have learned is that there are many levels of control on a cell's ability to grow and migrate and that a single oncogene rarely if ever acts alone to produce a cancer. In a true cancer there is always more than one oncogene at work. However, a single oncogene can give a cell a growth advantage over its normal neighbors. As that cell grows and replicates its DNA, it

---

Ingested Chemicals   Since World War II, new methods of marketing and distributing foods have greatly increased the length of time it takes food to travel from its source to the consumer. To prevent it from becoming spoiled or stale during this process, the food industry adds preservatives and numerous other additives, including stabilizers, binders, and emulsifiers (see Chapter 12). Some of these compounds are antioxidants and may actually decrease any cancer-producing properties the food might

have. Other compounds, like nitrates and nitrites, are potentially more sinister.

The food-processing industry adds both sodium nitrate and sodium nitrite to foods such as beer and ale, ham, bacon, hot dogs, bologna, and other luncheon meats. The nitrates inhibit the growth of bacteria, which could otherwise cause food poisoning, and they preserve the pink color of the meat, which has no bearing on taste but looks more appetizing to many people. While nitrates are

---

Oncogene   A gene involved in the transformation of a normal cell into a cancer cell.

Preneoplastic   Characterized by abnormal growth but not yet in a state of malignancy.

Nitrosamines   Chemical substances that can cause cancer.

Monoclonal antibodies   Antibodies harvested from cloned lymphocytes.

Oncogenes and Cancer (continued)

has an increased chance to accumulate other activated oncogenes and increase its malignant potential. In a premalignant population of cells, like those that line the bronchi of a long-term smoker, the great majority of cells will never accumulate the critical set of oncogenes that would allow them to become malignant. However, a tumor will arise from a rare cell or two that do complete all the steps. All current evidence indicates that new oncogenes are activated as premalignant cells move down the path to malignancy, and that at some critical point the accumulation of altered genes pushes one or a few cells over the line into true malignancy.

The time that elapses from the first activated oncogene to diagnosis of the resulting cancer may be ten, twenty, or even forty years. During these long intervals the body can sometimes recover from changes that might lead to cancer, either by DNA repair or by immune mechanisms. For instance, the cell will attempt to repair damage to its DNA and can often do so before the DNA is replicated. In cells

that are dividing fairly rapidly due to chronic irritation from smoke, chemicals, infection, or other causes, damage to DNA is much more likely to go unrepaired and so produce a mutation that will be passed to all the daughter cells. Also, by means that are not completely understood, the immune system can recognize some types of neoplastic cells and destroy them before they can produce a detectable tumor. The practical consequences of these recovery mechanisms is very important. As one example, in the lungs of smokers are millions of preneoplastic cells accumulating new oncogenes. If the individual stops smoking, the DNA repair and immune mechanisms have more time to work; if no cancer has occurred within three to five years after smoking is stopped, the ex-smoker has greatly improved his or her chances of surviving to a normal age without developing lung cancer.

Study of the activation of specific oncogenes may eventually suggest methods to block activation of critical oncogenes and so block

malignancy indefinitely. One suggestion has been to tailor the diet to include antioxidants and fiber and to decrease fat. The National Cancer Institute is conducting several long-term human studies to test these ideas, but since the development of tumors may take ten to twenty years, the answers will not come quickly.

This same focus on oncogenes will also lead eventually to much more effective diagnosis and therapy of established tumors. For instance, a great deal of effort is being put into development of **monoclonal antibodies** that can specifically target the protein product of certain oncogenes. When cell toxins are attached to the antibodies, they should be able to target and kill tumor cells. In the laboratory, targeted killing of tumor cells is dramatic, but this success has yet to be translated into clinical usefulness. Nevertheless, normally cautious scientists feel that an oncogene-based blueprint exists for understanding and preventing or curing most cancers and that the goal may be met in only a few decades.

not themselves carcinogenic, they may combine with amines in the body, particularly in the stomach, and be converted to **nitrosamines**, which are highly potent carcinogens. The actual impact of nitrosamines derived from the diet is under active study, but as of now, these compounds do have definite potential to cause stomach and other cancers.

Dietary Factors and Alcohol   A "fatty diet" (a diet high in saturated fats, such as those found in red meats) appears to contribute to both colorectal cancer and breast cancer. Scotland, for instance, has the highest incidence of colorectal cancer in the world, and Scots consume more fatty meat than any of their European neighbors. In Japan, by contrast, fish is the staple dietary protein, not fatty meat, and colorectal cancer is uncommon. Japanese who have

emigrated to the United States, where fatty meats are a major part of the diet, are as susceptible to colorectal cancer as other Americans.

Recent studies have shed some light on the mechanism by which dietary fats promote colorectal cancer. It appears that intestinal bacteria metabolize dietary fat to produce a class of compounds that are highly mutagenic. The presence of these compounds in the gut is correlated with increased formation of precancerous polyps. The levels of these carcinogenic fat derivatives can be lowered by increasing dietary fiber, vitamin C and vitamin E.

Some populations, particularly vegetarians, have little colorectal cancer. The vegetarian diet is typically high in insoluble fiber, and this link, plus laboratory evidence, suggests that colorectal cancer may be related to lack of fiber in the diet. While fiber does not supply nutrition,

Table 16-3 Selected foods that may have a role in cancer

Substance	Major Dietary Sources	Suspected Role in Cancer	Comment
Possible Protectors			
Beta-carotene (transformed into vitamin A by the body)	Yellow, orange, and green leafy vegetables and fruit, such as carrots, cantaloupe, broccoli, yams, spinach	Deficiency may increase risk of lung, stomach, cervical, bladder, and other cancers.	This antioxidant is thought to be more anticarcinogenic than dietary vitamin A. Extra carotene is stored in most tissue for future use. Not toxic.
Vitamin A	Liver, butter, milk, cheese, egg yolk, fish oil	Deficiency may cause abnormal cell growth, possibly leading to cancerous tumors.	Much of its protectiveness is due to beta-carotene (above). Avoid vitamin A supplements—megadoses can be toxic.
Vitamin C	Citrus fruits, tomatoes, broccoli, strawberries, potatoes, peppers, kale (C is destroyed by improper storage or long cooking)	Deficiency of this antioxidant may increase risk of cancer of stomach and esophagus. Presence may block conversion of nitrites and nitrates to cancer-causing agents.	Adult RDA is 60 milligrams, supplied by 4 ounces of fresh orange juice. Unused C is excreted. Megadoses (over 1 gram daily) can cause diarrhea and may result in kidney stones.
Vitamin E	Nuts, vegetable oils, liver, margarine, whole grains, wheat germ, dried beans	An antioxidant. Shown to protect lab animals against some cancers.	Adult RDA is supplied by one tablespoon of margarine.
Selenium	Seafood, liver, meats, grains, egg yolks, tomatoes	An antioxidant. Shown to protect lab animals against some cancers.	No RDA. Plentiful in most diets. Supplements can be extremely dangerous.
Fiber	Found only in plant foods, such as fruits, vegetables, whole grains	Promotes healthy bowel function. May lower risk of colon and rectal cancer.	Choose whole-grain breads and cereals. Eat fruit and vegetables with skins when possible.
Cruciferous vegetables	Vegetables of the cabbage family, e.g., broccoli, kale, brussels sprouts, cauliflower	Contain antioxidants that may block production of potential cancer-causing agents in lab animals.	Eat at least 2–3 servings each week. Excellent sources of fiber, minerals, and vitamins.
Possible Villains			
Fats	Meats, poultry skin, whole milk and milk products, vegetable oils	Excess consumption of fats may contribute to cancers of the digestive and reproductive systems and to obesity, another risk factor for cancer.	Choose low-fat dairy products and lean meats; trim all visible fat and discard poultry skin; don't fry meats. Eat fish. Avoid high-fat processed foods.
Alcohol	Beer, wine, liquor	Heavy drinking, especially combined with smoking, contributes to cancers of the mouth, throat, liver, and bladder. May also be a factor in breast cancer.	Drink only in moderation, if at all: no more than two drinks a day.
Nitrites	Used to preserve cured meats, such as bacon, hot dogs, sausages, ham	Promotes cancers of stomach and esophagus in lab animals.	Avoid eating cured meats habitually. Use low-temperature cooking methods; for example, microwaved bacon is lower in carcinogens, especially if you drain the fat.
Aflatoxins	Poisons formed in moldy peanuts, peanut butter, seeds, corn, and other crops	If eaten in large amounts, can cause liver cancer, a rare disease in this country.	Discard moldy, shriveled, discolored peanuts. Refrigerate freshly ground peanut butter; discard entire jar if moldy.
Browned foods	Meats grilled, barbecued, or fried at high temperatures	These cooking methods create cancer-causing agents. Most dangerous when cooking fatty meat over a heat source.	As often as possible, choose other cooking methods—steam, bake, roast, or microwave. Scrape off charred material.

Source: *University of California, Berkeley, Wellness Letter*, October 1987.

TACTICS AND TIPS

A Dietary Defense against Cancer

Based on hundreds of studies, the National Cancer Institute estimates that about one-third of all cancers are in some way linked to what we eat. This means that you can affect your risk of developing cancer by changing your diet in certain ways. The following dietary modifications are recommended as a way to reduce your chances of getting cancer:

1. Eat more high-fiber foods such as fruits and vegetables and whole-grain cereals.

2. Include dark-green and deep-yellow fruits and vegetables rich in vitamins A and C.

3. Include cabbage, broccoli, brussels sprouts, kohlrabi, and cauliflower.

4. Be moderate in consumption of salt-cured, smoked, and nitrite-cured foods.

5. Cut down on total fat intake from animal sources and on other fats and oils.

6. Avoid obesity.

7. Be moderate in consumption of alcoholic beverages.

Source: American Cancer Society

it has many other useful properties. It provides bulk, which dilutes any carcinogens that may be present. It also reduces transit time of waste through the intestine, so that carcinogens have less time to act on the epithelial cells. Fiber also binds bile acids and other lipids that act to promote development of colorectal cancer. However, we still don't know whether fiber and vitamin supplements can overcome the carcinogenic effect of a high-fat diet.

Breast cancer is also much more common in countries with a high level of dietary fat; Japan, with its traditional low-fat diet, has one of the world's lowest rates of breast cancer. However, in the presence of the many additional dietary and environmental differences between these countries, it has been difficult to establish a direct causal link between dietary fat intake and breast cancer. Nonetheless, it is likely that a major reduction in dietary fat content, begun early in life, could substantially lower breast cancer incidence in the United States.

The link between alcohol intake and breast cancer is more certain; a moderate alcohol intake is associated with a 50 percent increase in the rate of breast cancer. However, the most striking carcinogenic effect of alcohol is seen in oral cancers. As we mentioned earlier, alcohol and smoking interact as risk factors for oral cancer; heavy drinkers and smokers have a risk up to fifteen times greater than the people who don't drink or smoke.

Environmental and Industrial Pollution Pollutants in urban air have long been suspected of contributing to the incidence of lung cancer. Fossil fuel combustion products, such as complex hydrocarbons, have been of special concern. This subject has been difficult to study, due to the overwhelmingly greater influence of smoking on lung cancer rates. As mentioned earlier, at least 80 percent of lung cancers are caused by smoking, which first became popular in urban areas. Nonetheless, the available evidence suggests that atmospheric pollution plays a limited but measurable role in causing lung cancer.

The possibility that carcinogenic compounds are present in ground water is also under investigation. The process of chlorination, for instance, can modify organic compounds commonly present in water, and these chlorinated compounds are found to be carcinogenic in rats. One large controlled study showed a modest excess risk of bladder cancer among people who had used chlorinated surface water for long periods of time. Of course, this small excess risk must be balanced against the great benefits of chlorination in preventing bacterial and parasitic contamination of drinking water.

Although it is essential to keep a close watch on pollutants in our air and water, the best available data indicates that less than 2 percent of cancer deaths are caused by such general environmental pollution. This estimate is based on still limited data, and it could be modified by further research. On the other hand, exposure to dangerous materials in specific industries is a much greater problem. Occupational exposures to specific carcinogens may account for as many as 5 percent of cancer deaths. Table 16–4 lists some of the more important industrial and environmental carcinogens.

Workers in the rubber, plastics, paint and dye, cable, and petrochemical industries have historically been at greater risk of cancer than the rest of the population. Shipyard workers, for instance, who were exposed to high levels of asbestos during construction of ships in World War II, have experienced a high incidence of particular types of lung cancer. With increasing regulatory control of many identified carcinogens, we can anticipate that these industrial sources of cancer risk will continue to diminish, at least in the United States. By contrast, in eastern Europe, where environmental concerns were for

Agents	Where Found	Cancers They May Cause
Arsenic	Mining and smelting industries	Skin, liver, lung
Asbestos	Brake linings, construction sites, insulation, powerhouses	Lung, pleura, peritoneum
Benzene	Solvents, insecticides, gasoline	Bone marrow
Benzidine (outlawed in Great Britain and U.S.S.R., still used widely in U.S.)	Manufacturing rubber, dyestuffs	Bladder
Coal combustion products	Steel mills, petrochemical industry, asphalt, coal tar	Lung, bladder, scrotum
Nickel compounds	Metal industry, alloys	Lung, nasal sinuses
Radiation	Ultraviolet rays from the sun, medical treatments	Bone marrow, skin, thyroid
Synthetic estrogens	Drugs	Vagina, cervix, uterus
Tobacco	Cigarettes, cigars, pipes	Lung, bladder, mouth, esophagus, pharynx, larynx
Vinyl chloride	Plastics industry	Liver, brain

Table 16-4 Occupational and environmental carcinogens: ten suspects

a long time sacrificed to industrial productivity, cancer rates due to industrial pollution continue to climb.

Radiation   All sources of radiation are potentially carcinogenic—including medical x-rays, radioactive substances (radioisotopes), and the ultraviolet rays of the sun. The most striking historical example of this has been the increased rates of cancer, especially leukemia, seen in the survivors of the atomic bombing of Hiroshima and Nagasaki. Surviving children were particularly susceptible to even low doses of radiation, and excess new cancers are still occurring forty-five years later. A recent review of excess deaths from this bombing has caused authorities to once more raise the estimates of cancer and leukemia risk from exposure to radiation. The large number of excess leukemias seen in Hiroshima survivors is a warning to us that any unnecessary exposure of children or fetuses to ionizing radiation should be strictly avoided. Most physicians and dentists are quite aware of the risk of radiation, and heroic efforts have been made to reduce the amount of radiation needed for mammograms, dental x-rays, and other necessary medical x-rays.

Another source of environmental radiation is radon gas. Radon is a decomposition product of radium, which is found in small quantities in some rocks and soils. Since radon is inhaled with the air we breathe, it comes into intimate contact with the cells of the lung, where its radiation can produce mutations. Radon and smoking together create a risk of lung cancer that is more than additive, as studies of miners in both the United States and China have recently shown. Fortunately, in most of our homes and classrooms, radon is rapidly dissipated into the atmosphere, where it presents no threat. But in enclosed spaces, such as mines, some basements, and airtight houses built of brick or stone, it can rise to dangerous levels (see Chapter 24).

■ **Exploring Your Emotions**

How often do you have medical and dental x-rays? Are you confident that your health-care professionals are up-to-date on cancer risk from radiation? Do you feel comfortable asking them about it?

Sunlight is a very important source of radiation, but since its rays only penetrate a millimeter or so into the skin, it could be considered a "surface" carcinogen. Most cases of skin cancers are the relatively benign and highly curable basal cell cancers, but a substantial minority are the potentially deadly malignant melanomas (about 27,000 per year). As discussed earlier, all types of skin cancer are increased by early and excessive exposure to the sun, and severe sunburn early in childhood appears to carry with it excessive risk of melanoma later in life.

Detecting, Diagnosing, and Treating Cancer

Early cancer detection often depends on our willingness to be aware of changes in our own body or to make sure we keep up with recommended diagnostic tests. Although treatment success varies with individual cancers, cure rates have increased—sometimes dramatically—in this century.

Detecting Cancer   Unlike those of some other diseases, early signs of cancer are usually not apparent to anyone but the victim. Even pain is not a reliable guide to early detection, since the initial stages of cancer may be painless. Self-monitoring is the first line of defense, and the American Cancer Society recommends that you pay close attention to the following signs, which you can remember with the acronym "CAUTION":

- **C**hange in bowel or bladder habits
- **A** sore that does not heal
- **U**nusual bleeding or discharge
- **T**hickening or lump in the breasts or elsewhere
- **I**ndigestion or difficulty in swallowing
- **O**bvious change in a wart or mole
- **N**agging cough or hoarseness

Although none of these signs is a sure indication of cancer, the appearance of any one should send you to see your physician. By being aware yourself of the risk factors in your own life, including the cancer history of your immediate family and your own past history, you can often bring a problem to the attention of a physician long before it would have been detected at a routine physical.

The American Cancer Society is probably the best authority on which tests for cancer detection should be made routine. Their recommendations are summarized in Table 16-5. These routine tests are intended for people who have no signs of cancer. Self-examination of breast or testicles is probably the most useful self-screening procedure. Men and women over 40 should have a yearly rectal examination by a physician and a stool blood test every year after age 50.

Smokers can benefit from an annual sputum cytology examination. Precancerous changes in the cells that line the lung can be spotted in smears of the cells from sputum. If the cells are sufficiently abnormal, a follow-up examination by fiber-optic bronchoscopy may allow early detection of small tumors.

Trends in Diagnosis and Therapy   Detection of a cancer is only the beginning, of course; and the methods for determining the exact type, stage, and location of the tumor, and for treating it, continue to improve. Knowledge of the exact location and size of a tumor, for instance, leads to much more precise and effective surgery or radiation therapy. This is especially true in cases where the tumor may be hard to reach, as in the brain. High-technology diagnostic imaging by **magnetic resonance imaging** (MRI) is one example of such technology. It uses a huge electromagnet to detect tumors by sensing the vibrations of different atoms in the body. **Computerized tomography** (CT scanning) uses x-rays to examine the brain and other parts of the body. The process allows construction of cross sections, which show a tumor's shape and location more accurately than is possible with the conventional x-ray technique. For patients undergoing radiation therapy, CT scanning may enable the therapist to pinpoint the tumor more precisely and so provide more accurate radiation dosage while sparing normal tissue. Ultrasound has also been used increasingly in the past few years to visualize tumors. Prostate ultrasound, a rectal probe using ultrasonic waves to produce an image of the prostate, is currently being investigated for its ability to increase the early detection of small, hidden tumors that would be missed by a digital rectal exam.

Treatment methods for cancers are currently based almost exclusively on surgery (removing the tumor), chemotherapy, and radiation therapy. In the last two techniques, cells that can't be surgically removed are killed either by interfering chemically with their growth or by killing them directly with concentrated ionizing radiation. Newer, more experimental methods of treatment are also showing promise. Immunotherapy, for instance, uses the body's own immune system to control cancer; interferon, interleukin-2, and several other biological-response modifiers that stimulate the immune system are under study. They have already been shown to be more effective than conventional therapy in treating certain leukemias, kidney cancer, and melanoma. Several laboratories are also working on vaccines for melanoma,

---

Magnetic resonance imaging (MRI)   A method of visualizing body structures in cross-section without radiation by detecting the vibration of atoms in a magnetic field; used to detect tumors.

Computerized tomography (CT) scan   A test using computerized x-ray images to create a cross-sectional depiction of tissue density.

Table 16-5 Summary of tests recommended by the American Cancer Society for the early detection of cancer in asymptomatic people

Site of Cancer	Test or Procedure	Population		
		Sex	Age	Frequency
Colon or rectum	Sigmoidoscopy	M & F	Over 50	Every 3–5 years after 2 negative exams 1 year apart
	Stool guaiac test	M & F	Over 50	Every year
	Digital rectal examination	M & F	Over 40	Every year
Uterus or cervix	Pap test	F	20–65; under 20, if sexually active	At least every 3 years after 2 negative exams 1 year apart
	Pelvic examination	F	20–40	Every 3 years
			Over 40	Every year
	Endometrial tissue sample	F	At menopause; women at high risk[a]	At menopause
Breast	Breast self-examination	F	Over 20	Every month
	Breast physical examination	F	20–40	Every 3 years
			Over 40	Every year
	Mammography	F	Between 35–40	Baseline
			Under 50	Consult personal physician
			Over 50	Every year
Lung	Chest x-ray		Not recommended	
	Sputum cytology		Recommended for people at risk	
Other[b]	Health counseling and cancer checkup	M & F	Over 20	Every 3 years
		M & F	Over 40	Every year

[a]History of infertility, obesity, failure of ovulation, abnormal uterine bleeding, or estrogen therapy.
[b]To include examination for cancers of the thyroid, testicles, prostate, ovaries, lymph nodes, oral region, and skin.

which have been quite effective in animal models. Other molecules recently made available through genetic engineering include factors that stimulate the growth of both red and white blood cells (erythropoietin and colony-stimulating factors, respectively). These substances allow chemotherapy patients, whose blood-forming cells have been severely reduced, to replace these vital cells much faster than formerly.

All of these newer techniques offer the hope of reducing mortality from the common cancers and extending the lives of those who do have cancer. However, we should keep in mind that there is as yet no technique on the horizon that promises an all-encompassing cancer cure. As is the case with so many other diseases, prevention is still by far the most potent protection against cancer.

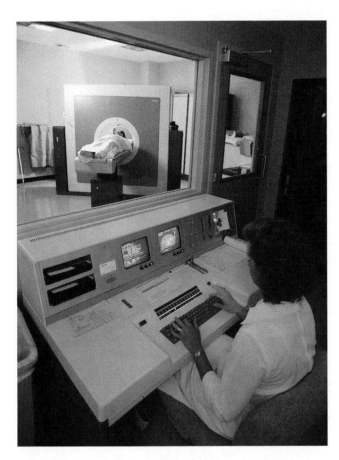

Computerized tomography—also known as CT or CAT scanning—is a diagnostic technique that provides a computer-assisted image of a relatively inaccessible part of the body, such as the brain.

Preventing Cancer

Because your behaviors and behavior changes can radically lower your cancer risks, you can take a very practical approach to cancer prevention. Primary prevention involves measures you can take to avoid cancer-causing agents in the environment, such as those in the following list. Secondary prevention involves having cancers that do develop discovered as quickly as possible by following the cancer test recommendations of the American Cancer Society, particularly for breast, colorectal, testicle, and cervical cancers (see Table 16–5). Both levels of prevention are important to your long-term health. Among the primary prevention measures recommended by the American Cancer Society are the following:

- Stop smoking and avoid breathing the smoke from other people's cigarettes. Smoking is responsible for 80

to 90 percent of all lung cancers and for about 30 percent of all cancer deaths. People who smoke two or more packs of cigarettes a day have lung cancer mortality rates fifteen to twenty-five times greater than those of nonsmokers. The carcinogenic chemicals in smoke are transported throughout the body in the bloodstream, making smoking a cocarcinogen for many forms of cancer other than lung cancer.

- Protect your skin from the sun. Almost all cases of nonmelanoma skin cancer are considered to be sun-related, and sun exposure is a major factor in the development of melanoma as well. Wear protective clothing when you're out in the sun and use a sunscreen with an SPF rating of 15 or higher. Don't go to tanning salons; they do not provide "safe tans."

- Drink alcohol only in moderation, if at all. Oral cancer and cancers of the larynx, throat, esophagus, and liver occur more frequently among heavy drinkers of alcohol. Risk is even higher among heavy drinkers who smoke.

- Avoid smokeless tobacco. Chewing tobacco and snuff, both highly habit-forming because of their nicotine content, are associated with cancer of the mouth, larynx, throat, and esophagus.

- Avoid excessive exposure to radiation. Most medical x-rays are adjusted to deliver the lowest dose possible without sacrificing image quality. Radiation from radon, on the other hand, may pose a threat. The American Cancer Society believes there is a problem with exposure to radon in some homes. Remedial steps should be taken in these cases.

- Avoid occupational exposure to carcinogens. A number of industrial agents are associated with cancer, including nickel, chromate, asbestos, vinyl chloride, and others. Risks increase greatly when combined with smoking.

- Watch your weight and exercise regularly. The risk for colon, breast, and uterine cancers increase for obese people. A high-fat diet may be a factor in the development of certain cancers, although the link between obesity and cancer hasn't been fully explained. Maintaining normal weight through a healthy diet and regular exercise lowers the risk.

- Control your diet. Based on hundreds of studies, the National Cancer Institute estimates that about one-third of all cancers are in some way linked to what we eat. Choose a low-fat, high-fiber diet containing cruciferous vegetables and foods rich in vitamins A and C; avoid salt-cured, smoked, and nitrate-cured foods. See the specific suggestions in the box and table on dietary factors in cancer.

Although other factors are important, lifestyle is a strong predictor of cancer risk. Mormons and Seventh-

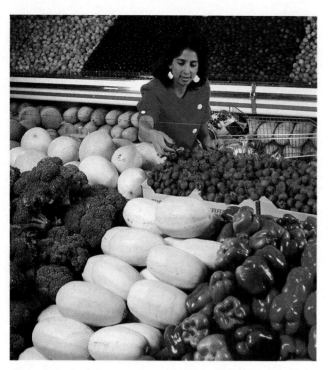

The American Cancer Society recommends a high-fiber diet containing cruciferous vegetables and rich in vitamins A and C. Broccoli, strawberries, and red and green peppers are all excellent choices.

Day Adventists, for example, are much less likely to develop cancer than the general population. Church doctrine of both groups forbids tobacco and alcohol use. Members also maintain a strong support network, which may influence both the incidence and the outcome of disease. A recent study determined that middle-aged Mormon men in the lay priesthood of that faith have reduced their risk of cancer to less than half that of the general population. Important factors in this risk reduction appear to be avoidance of tobacco and alcohol, regular exercise, and proper sleep. By making similar changes in lifestyle, other groups have every reason to expect to achieve the 50 percent cancer mortality reduction seen among Mormons and set as a goal for the nation by the National Cancer Institute for the year 2000.

■ **Exploring Your Emotions**

Although many people are aware that certain behaviors help prevent cancer—such as using sunscreen and modifying their diets—a large percentage of them don't act on their knowledge. Do you follow through with behavior changes when you learn that certain things you do increase your risk of cancer? If so, how do you make the changes? If not, why do you think you don't?

Summary

- Cancer, a dreaded disease, often cannot be successfully treated.

What Is Cancer?

- A malignant tumor can invade surrounding structures and spread—metastasize—to distant sites via the blood and lymphatic system, producing additional tumors throughout the body.
- The ability of cancer cells to metastasize makes early detection critical. To prevent death, every cancerous cell must be removed.
- Normal cells in adults grow and divide at a rate sufficient to replace dying cells; a malignant cell divides without regard for normal growth. As tumors grow, they produce signs or symptoms that are determined by their location in the body.
- Carcinomas, the most common cancers, begin in the epithelial or outer layers of cells, which are the most actively growing cells in the adult body. Carcinomas metastasize primarily via the lymph vessels.

- Sarcomas, which metastasize primarily via blood vessels, arise from connective and fibrous tissue. Lymphomas, cancers of the lymph nodes, result from changes in the white blood cells.
- Leukemia is cancer of blood-forming cells in the bone marrow.
- One person in three will develop cancer, and the five-year survival rate for those who do is 49 percent. The five-year survival rate is the ratio of the survival rate for a cancer group to the survival rate for an age- and sex-matched control group.
- Actions can be taken in young adulthood to prevent DNA damage and, hence, later cancers.

Common Cancers

- Symptoms of lung cancer usually don't occur until the tumor has reached the invasive stage. Diagnostic tests include examination of sputum cells, chest x-ray, and fiber-optic bronchoscopy. Smoking, the primary cause of lung cancer, also intensifies the effects of other causes like radon gas or asbestos.

- Because lung cancer is usually detected only after metastasis has begun and because malignant lung cells usually resist chemotherapy, the five-year survival rate for this cancer is only 13 percent. Oat cell lung cancers can now be treated fairly successfully with chemotherapy and radiation.
- Colorectal cancer is clearly linked to both diet and heredity. Although it's difficult to identify those at highest risk because of heredity, high-fiber diets can prevent and even reverse precancerous changes in colon cells.
- Early detection of colon cancer requires rectal examinations and stool occult blood tests. The five-year survival rate for colorectal cancer is as high as 85 percent if the tumor is found while it's still localized.
- Breast cancer affects about one in ten women in the U.S.; most tumors are curable when caught early, so screening is important for everyone. The five-year survival rate for all stages of breast tumors is 75 percent.
- Although there is a genetic component to breast cancer, diet and hormones are also risk factors. Specific risk factors include obesity, early first menstruation, late menopause, late first motherhood, and not breastfeeding. Estrogen may be a link in these factors—even in the connection between obesity and breast cancer.
- Early detection of breast cancer depends on monthly self-examination; a clinical breast exam every one to three years, depending on age; and regular mammograms after age 40. Malignancies are treated by surgery and—if the cancer has spread—chemotherapy or hormonal therapy.
- Endometrial cancer, usually diagnosed between ages 55 and 69, is highly curable; risk factors include infertility, obesity, and prolonged estrogen therapy.
- Because use of Pap smears has become nearly universal, the death rate from cervical cancer has dropped by 70 percent in forty years. Abnormal cells can be detected and removed before they reach the invasive stage.
- Ovarian cancer is dangerous because it can't be detected by a Pap smear or simple screening method.
- Prostate cancer is chiefly a disease of aging; diet and lifestyle probably are factors in its occurrence. Early detection is possible through a rectal examination, sometimes followed by ultrasound. Surgery is performed to remove malignancies; chemotherapy and radiation may also be used.
- Oral cancer is caused primarily by cigarette and cigar smoking, excess alcohol consumption, and use of smokeless tobacco. Oral cancers are easy to detect, but often hard to treat.
- Most skin cancers can be cured, especially if caught early. Abnormal cellular changes in the epidermis, often a result of exposure to the sun, cause skin cancers, as does chronic exposure to certain chemicals.

- Skin cancers occur as basal cell carcinoma, squamous cell carcinoma, and melanoma.
- Skin cancer prevention means avoiding overexposure to the sun. Early diagnosis leads to more successful treatment. Characteristics of skin cancer are asymmetry, border irregularity, color change, and a diameter greater than 6 mm.
- Malignant skin lesions are surgically removed, usually in a physician's office. Even with melanoma, survival rates are high if the cancer is caught in its early stages.
- Testicular cancer can be detected early through self-examination. Bladder cancer, often associated with smoking, has a high survival rate if detected at an early stage. Pancreatic cancer is hard to detect and usually fatal. Kaposi's sarcoma has become more common as a result of the AIDS epidemic.

What Causes Cancer?

- Mutational damage to a cell's DNA can lead to rapid and uncontrolled growth of cells; mutagens include radiation, viral infection, and chemical substances in food and air. Cancer prevention requires identifying carcinogens and avoiding them as much as possible.
- Cancer initiators cause mutations in the DNA of proto-oncogenes; cancer promoters accelerate the growth of cells temporarily, without damaging or permanently altering DNA. If cell growth is speeded up, the cell replicates damaged DNA before it can be repaired.
- The genetic basis of some cancers appears to be related to suppressor genes, which normally limit cell growth; people can inherit altered suppressor genes.
- Some carcinogens occur naturally in the environment; others are manufactured substances. Carcinogens also occur in food.
- Foods can contain cancer-preventing compounds as well as carcinogens. Some compounds in food, like beta-carotene, appear to have cancer-preventing properties; they slow the growth of epithelial cells. Substances like vitamins C and E, both antioxidants, intercept agents that cause DNA damage.
- While additives and preservatives are added to food to preserve freshness, dangerous chemicals can also make their way into the food supply.
- High-fat diets appear to contribute to colorectal and breast cancer; high-fiber diets, on the other hand, seem to help prevent colon cancer.
- High alcohol intake puts people at risk for oral cancer. Alcohol and tobacco interact as carcinogens.
- Carcinogenic chemicals that are inhaled over a long period of time can cause changes in lung tissue cells.
- All sources of radiation are potentially carcinogenic. Radon in combination with smoking is especially dangerous.

Detection, Diagnosis, and Treatment

- Self-monitoring is essential to early cancer detection; the appearance of any early signs necessitates a visit to a physician. (The signs can be remembered by using the acronym CAUTION.) Individuals should know their own risk factors, including family and personal medical history.
- The most important cancer screening tests include self-examination of breasts and testicles, yearly rectal exams (after age 40), and yearly stool blood tests (after age 50). Smokers should have yearly sputum cytology tests.
- Methods for determining the exact type, stage, and location of a tumor and for treating it continue to improve. Magnetic resonance imaging and computerized tomography allow more precise visualization of tumors than do standard x-rays. Ultrasound is also being used more frequently in cancer detection.
- Treatment methods consist of surgery, chemotherapy, and radiation therapy. Immunotherapy, vaccines, and genetic engineering also hold promise as effective treatments.

Preventing Cancer

- Primary prevention involves avoiding cancer-causing agents in the environment. Secondary prevention involves early detection of cancers that do occur.
- Primary prevention includes (1) not smoking and avoiding smoke, (2) protecting skin from the sun, (3) drinking alcohol in moderation, if at all, (4) avoiding smokeless tobacco, (5) avoiding excessive exposure to radiation, (6) avoiding occupational exposure to carcinogens, (7) watching one's weight and exercising, and (8) controlling one's diet.
- Lifestyle is a strong predictor of cancer risk. Studies have shown that an altered lifestyle can reduce cancer risk as much as 50 percent.

Take Action

1. In your health diary, list the positive behaviors that help you avoid cancer. How can you strengthen these behaviors? Also list the behaviors that tend to increase your risk of cancer. What can you do to change these behaviors?

2. Interview your parents or grandparents about your family medical history. Are there any cases of cancer in your family, and has anyone died of cancer? In your health diary, make a list of your inherited risks for various types of cancer, such as lung, breast, or colon cancer. Also list risks from your own personal history, such as early onset of menstruation or a previous cancer. Compile a list of genetic, hormonal, dietary, and other behavioral factors (from number 1, above) that influence your overall risk of developing cancer. Take action to change any that you can.

3. Go to a drugstore and look at the variety of sunscreens available there. Read the labels to see what ingredients they use, and compare them to those mentioned in the box "Protecting Your Skin from the Sun." Then evaluate your own risks. You have a higher than average risk of developing skin cancer, including melanoma, if you spend a lot of time in the sun unprotected, live in a sunny climate, or have fair skin, blond or red hair, a high incidence of moles, and/or a tendency to burn rather than tan. Select a sunscreen that will give you optimal protection from the sun, and use it regularly.

Behavior Change Strategy

Phasing in a Healthier Diet

Is it hard to break bad eating habits? Of course, and it doesn't happen in a day. But two nutritional scientists at the Oregon Health Sciences University in Portland have devised a plan for improving eating habits in three phases. Although Dr. William Connor and Sonja Conner designed their diet (described in their book *The New American Diet*) to reduce the risk of heart disease, their plan and many of their specific suggestions work as an anticancer diet as well. The guiding principle is to avoid doing anything radical, but instead to increase gradually your consumption of fruits, vegetables, and grains while you reduce your intake of fat, cholesterol, and known and suspected carcinogens.

Begin by monitoring your diet for one or two weeks, noting in your health diary both the health-protecting and the cancer-promoting foods you eat. Remember, protective foods include the following:

- Cruciferous vegetables (members of the cabbage family)—cabbage, broccoli, cauliflower, brussels sprouts
- Yellow and orange fruits for vitamin A—apricots, cantaloupe, cherries, peaches, nectarines, mangos, watermelon, persimmons, papayas
- Yellow and orange vegetables for vitamin A—carrots, yams, sweet potatoes, winter squash, pumpkin
- Dark-green leafy vegetables for vitamin A—broccoli, spinach, Swiss chard, kale, collard greens, sorrel
- Citrus and other fruits and vegetables for vitamin C—oranges, grapefruits, lemons, tomatoes, strawberries, red peppers, broccoli
- Nuts and vegetable oils for vitamin E
- Whole grains and dried beans for fiber—brown rice, kasha, bulgur, whole-grain breads, garbanzo beans, lentils, pinto beans

And cancer-promoting foods include the following:

- Cured meats containing nitrites or nitrates—bacon, hot dogs, ham, pastrami, bologna, sausage, liverwurst
- Meats that are grilled, barbecued, or charred at high temperatures
- Alcohol
- Foods that provide excessive calories and animal fat—red meat, poultry skin, whole milk and whole-milk products.

After you have recorded your diet, analyze it to see how often you consume the foods listed. Do you have cruciferous vegetables two to three times a week? Are carrots, peaches, or apricots part of your diet? Do you eat bacon only occasionally? Do you limit your intake of alcohol? Once you have some idea of how much your diet protects you against cancer and how much it puts you at risk, try implementing the following three-phase diet-change plan:

Phase I: Substitutions

Avoid egg yolks, butter, lard, organ meats, bacon and other cured meats, and any burnt meat. Start using vegetable oils for all purposes rather than animal fats. Switch to low-fat milk products and other low-fat foods. Discard chicken skin and meat fat. Reduce consumption of beer and wine. Keep using favorite recipes, but decrease salt and fat content.

Phase II: New Recipes

Reduce the amount of red meat and cheese you eat; replace with chicken and fish. Cut down on fats, including vegetable fats. Begin to replace meats and fats with grains, beans, fruits, and vegetables, especially those high in vitamins A and C and members of the cabbage family. Choose low-fat dishes when eating out. Replace recipes that cannot be altered.

Phase III: A New Way of Eating

Eat meats and cheeses as side dishes, in small amounts, rather than as main courses. Increase consumption of beans and grains as protein and fiber sources. Save rich foods such as chocolate and bakery goods for special treats only, no more than once a month. Make a habit of trying new grains and beans, fruits, and vegetables (select some from the lists given above, or see what the supermarkets and ethnic stores in your community offer). Keep developing a new repertory of recipes.

A diet like this can provide benefits to your cardiovascular system, help you lose weight gradually and permanently, and give you some insurance against cancer later in life. Try making these changes over the course of a few months to improve your overall health and your chances for a cancer-free future.

Based on Phasing in a healthier diet, *The University of California, Berkeley, Wellness Letter,* October 1987.

Selected Bibliography

Baltrusch, H. J., and M. Waltz. 1985. Cancer from a behavioral and social epidemiologic perspective. *Social Science & Medicine* 20:789–94.

DeVita, V. T., Jr., S. Hellman, and S. A. Rosenberg. 1989. *Cancer: Principles and Practice of Oncology.* 3d ed. Philadelphia: Lippincott.

Food and Drug Administration. 1987. *Mammography Benefits.* FDA Drug Bulletin.

Recommended Readings

American Cancer Society. 1989. *Cancer Facts and Figures.* New York: American Cancer Society. *Available in every library, this is a condensed and authoritative summary of the current cancer statistics, renewed each year. If you're interested in exploring further any of the topics in this chapter, this is a good place to start.*

Cairns, J. 1978. *Cancer: Science and Society.* San Francisco: Freeman. *A slightly dated but beautifully written and nontechnical treatment of the cancer problem.*

National Cancer Institute Fact Book. 1989. Bethesda, Md.: Office of Cancer Communications. *A source book of detailed and up-to-date information on the cancer problem.*

Moore, M., and E. Potts. 1987. *Choices: Realistic Alternatives in Cancer Treatment.* New York: Avon. *An exploration of the current choices in cancer therapy, from the patient's perspective.*

Contents

Making Connections

Although everyone knows about the AIDS epidemic, many people think that diseases like syphilis and gonorrhea are a thing of the past. But in fact, cases of all the sexually transmissible diseases are increasing, and it's more important than ever to know how to protect yourself from these infections. The scenarios presented on these pages describe situations in which people have to use information, make a decision, or choose a course of action, all related to sexually transmissible diseases. As you read them, imagine yourself in each situation and consider what you would do. After you've finished the chapter, read the scenarios again and see if what you've learned has changed how you would think, feel, or act in each situation.

Your brother and his wife have been trying to have a baby for three years, without success. It seems that your sister-in-law had pelvic inflammatory disease while she was in college and her oviducts were permanently damaged. How did she get this disease, and how can it be avoided?

A friend of yours just found out that his former girlfriend is being treated for gonorrhea. She told him she didn't know where she got it or how long she'd had it, but her doctor advised her to inform her former sexual partners and tell them they should be examined also. Your friend feels fine and has no symptoms of any kind, so he's pretty sure he's not infected. He's inclined not to bother seeing a doctor. Is he making a mistake?

17

Sexually Transmissible Diseases

You recently heard that someone you work with at the bookstore tested positive for the AIDS virus. You normally socialize with him and other co-workers before work and during coffee breaks. One of the other employees thinks he shouldn't be using the same coffee pot, kitchen facilities, or bathroom as the rest of you. You figure he's got enough to deal with without being hassled at work too. On the other hand, you're not sure if you could catch the virus from him or if there are measures you should be taking to protect yourself. What should you do?

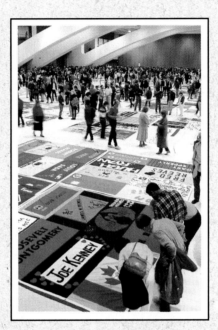

You've been dating someone whom you know has been involved in sexual relationships before. As you get closer to an intimate sexual relationship with him, you find yourself wondering about his previous experience. You'd really like to ask him if he's ever been exposed to any sexually transmissible diseases and if he's sure he doesn't have any now. Is it acceptable to bring up this subject? How? What if your questions offend him or make him angry?

You recently noticed a sore on your genitals, but it didn't hurt and you really didn't want to go to the doctor, so you didn't do anything about it. Finally, to your relief, it went away. Now your sexual partner has a very similar sore, and even though you're sure it will go away, your partner is inclined to see a physician about it. Does it make sense to have an examination when the sore is likely to heal on its own anyway? Should you go too?

No single health issue has commanded as much public attention in recent years as **acquired immunodeficiency syndrome**, or **AIDS**. This fatal, incurable disease currently ranks fifteenth as a cause of death among Americans, and the AIDS epidemic is considered the number one health priority in the United States. Former Surgeon General C. Everett Koop made AIDS a household word with his public education campaign and his "straight talk" about condoms. His efforts set a precedent that deserves to be repeated for all the **sexually transmissible diseases (STDs)**—gonorrhea, syphilis, herpes, and several others—because their incidence is also climbing among Americans.

STDs are a particularly insidious group of diseases. People can become infected and pass the infection on to a sexual partner without ever feeling sick or even knowing they have a disease. Not until years later does the cost of careless sex practices become apparent. Then an infected person may find that undiagnosed gonorrhea or chlamydia has left scarred oviducts resulting in infertility or an ectopic pregnancy; or that hepatitis B has led to cancer; or that genital herpes or syphilis has caused a birth defect in a child; or, in the case of AIDS, that the immune system has been fatally weakened and can no longer provide protection from disease.

Why is the incidence of STDs rising? Several factors have been suggested as contributing to this serious public health situation. One is the sheer number of sexually active people. The "baby boom" generation came of age and passed through their most active sexual years in the 1960s, 1970s, and 1980s. Many people became sexually active at a younger age than earlier generations had, and they tended to have more partners. Other changes occurred as well. American society began to show greater acceptance of premarital sex, the media promoted more open attitudes toward sexuality, and contraceptive information and services became more generally available. Oral contraceptives (which don't provide protection against STDs) grew in popularity and largely replaced condoms (which do provide protection). Finally, there was an increase in alcohol and drug abuse, which has a powerful influence on sexual behavior.

Despite educational efforts, the STDs remain epidemic (see Table 17–1). Their seriousness is compounded and magnified by other concerns, such as the extent of undetected infections, especially among younger people; reduced government funding and resources for STD-related programs; increasingly limited access to affordable health care for many people; and a growing population of peo-

VITAL STATISTICS

Table 17-1 STD prevalence: new cases of selected STDs every year in the United States

Disease	Number of Persons
Genital chlamydia	3,000,000
Gonorrhea	2,000,000
Genital herpes	500,000
Genital warts (females)	500,000
Syphilis	100,000
AIDS	1988: 32,196
	1989: 35,238

Note: Figures for AIDS are reported new cases (regardless of means of transmission); other figures are estimates.

Sources: *Mayo Clinic Health Letter*, October 1987, and Charles Green, AIDS epidemic could peak in mid-1990s, researcher says, *San Jose Mercury News*, February 17, 1990.

ple who exchange sex for drugs, especially crack cocaine, without regard for whether or not they're spreading disease. It has probably never been so important that people have a clear understanding of what the STDs are, how they are transmitted, and, most important, how they can be prevented. The crucial message is that they *can* be prevented. This chapter is designed to reinforce responsible attitudes toward prevention, diagnosis, and treatment of STDs and to provide information about healthy, safe sexual behavior.

The Major STDs

What are the most severe and dangerous STDs? In general, six different diseases pose major health threats: AIDS, syphilis, gonorrhea, chlamydia, herpes simplex, and human papilloma virus (HPV), which causes genital warts. These diseases are considered "major" because they are serious in themselves, cause serious complications if left untreated, and/or pose risks to a fetus or newborn. Additionally, pelvic inflammatory disease (PID) is a common complication of gonorrhea and chlamydia and merits discussion as a separate disease.

AIDS   Since its first appearance in the United States in 1980, when it was regarded as an intriguing medical

---

AIDS, acquired immunodeficiency syndrome
A fatal, incurable, sexually transmissible viral disease.

Sexually transmissible diseases (STDs)   Diseases that can be transmitted by sexual contact; some can also be transmitted by other means.

AIDS Milestones

The AIDS epidemic hit a milestone in July 1989, when the number of diagnosed cases in the United States reached 100,000. Since that time (when this graph was compiled), many more have died, including photographer Robert Mapplethorpe, choreographer Alvin Ailey, tax crusader Paul Gann, actress Amanda Blake, and teenage spokesperson Ryan White.

DRAMATIC RISE IN AIDS CASES

1. July 1981: Outbreak of skin cancer linked to "gay pneumonia" epidemic. 30 cases total.

2. April 1982: Cases among intravenous drug users are reported.

3. July 1982: Rare disease detected among hemophiliacs. The epidemic is finally named—acquired immune deficiency syndrome.

4. December 1982: First AIDS case linked to blood transfusion is detected.

5. February 1983: French researchers isolate virus that causes AIDS. Their work is largely ignored.

6. August 1983: Reagan administration officials say AIDS is "No. 1 health priority."

7. April 1984: National Cancer Institute researchers announce they have discovered virus that causes AIDS. Turns out to be the same as French virus.

8. October 1984: San Francisco public health officials close gay bathhouses.

9. March 1985: Blood banks begin testing donations for human immunodeficiency virus.

10. July 1985: The AIDS diagnosis of movie star Rock Hudson is disclosed, setting off an avalanche of media attention to the disease.

11. September 1986: Surgeon General C. Everett Koop releases his controversial report on the AIDS epidemic.

12. February 1987: Pianist Liberace dies of AIDS. Controversy rages about mandatory AIDS testing.

13. May 1987: President Reagan appoints AIDS commission and delivers his first and only speech on the AIDS epidemic.

14. January 1988: AIDS cases reach 50,000.

15. June 1988: President Reagan's AIDS commission turns in report calling for expedited research and prevention programs, a federal ban on AIDS discrimination.

16. December, 1988: Former ABC television anchor Max Robinson dies of AIDS.

17. June 1989: Underground tests on promising AIDS drug "Compound Q" are revealed.

18. July 1989: Number of AIDS cases surpasses 100,000.

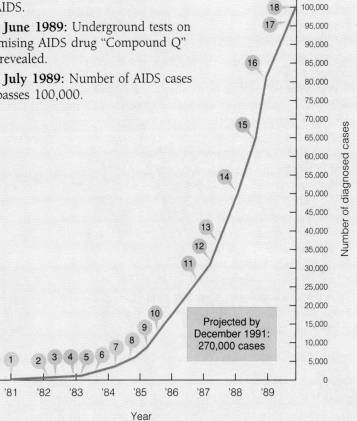

Projected by December 1991: 270,000 cases

mystery, AIDS has quickly moved to the forefront of public and medical attention as an all-too-familiar disease of progressive immune failure and premature death. Because of its long incubation period (the time when the virus is multiplying but the person doesn't experience any symptoms), people who were diagnosed with the disease in the early 1980s had actually been infected many years earlier. By the time there was widespread awareness of the disease, it was already too late for many individuals.

By January 1988, 50,000 cases of AIDS had been reported. This number doubled by July 1989, only 18 months later, and half of these 100,000 individuals had died. The number of cases continues to increase exponentially. By 1992, almost 500,000 Americans will have died or progressed to later stages of the disease. Between 1 and 1.5 million Americans are believed to be infected with the virus, but not yet ill enough to realize it. According to the World Health Organization, there will be 15 million people in the world infected with the AIDS virus by the year 2000.

This bad news is offset somewhat by an encouraging slowdown in the growth of AIDS in the United States in 1989, largely as a result of changes in sexual behavior among gay men. The number of new AIDS cases in the United States rose by 9 percent in 1989, the smallest increase ever reported. This trend has led some experts to predict that the epidemic will peak in the middle 1990s. Nevertheless, AIDS cases are expected to continue increasing each year and to increase disproportionately among drug users and minorities.

People with AIDS have been identified all over the United States and in 100 other countries around the world. The largest group of patients in the United States (61 percent) is made up of homosexual and bisexual males (see Figure 17–1). The second largest group consists of **intravenous** drug abusers. Smaller percentages are found among other groups: people who received blood or blood products between 1977 and 1985 donated by people infected with the virus; the sexual partners of infected individuals; children born to infected mothers; and a few individuals with no apparent risk factors. Of all AIDS cases, approximately 90 percent are male and 10 percent are female. Despite earlier fears that the virus would quickly spread to non-drug-abusing heterosexuals, there has been relatively little spillover into other populations.

■ **Exploring Your Emotions**

How would you feel about having daily (but nonintimate) contact with someone with AIDS? Considering what is now known about transmission of AIDS, are your feelings justified?

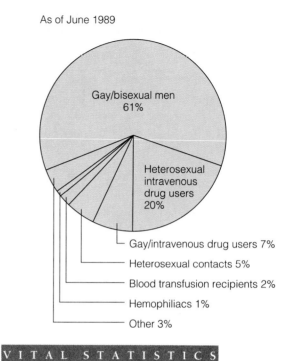

As of June 1989

VITAL STATISTICS

Figure 17-1   Transmission routes of AIDS.

What Is AIDS?   AIDS is a fatal condition that affects the immune system, the body's natural defense against disease, making an otherwise healthy person susceptible to a variety of infections, certain forms of cancer, and various neurological disorders. Caused by a virus named the **human immunodeficiency virus (HIV)**, the disease today is coming to be more widely known as HIV infection.

Under normal conditions, when a virus or other disease-causing microorganism enters the body, it is targeted and destroyed by the body's immune system. But HIV attacks the immune system itself, invading and taking over the cells that initiate and control the body's entire system of defense. Once these cells have been sidetracked from their duties, the immune system can no longer respond adequately to infection. HIV uses the genetic machinery of the immune cells to produce the protein it needs for survival. As it replicates, it produces more viruses and further cripples the immune system. In a healthy person, there are normally about twice as many **helper T-cells** (the immune cells that marshal the body's defenses) as **suppressor T-cells** (the immune cells that halt the formation of **antibodies** when the invading organism has been destroyed). In a person with HIV infection, this ratio is often reversed. (See Chapter 20 for a more detailed explanation of the process by which HIV disarms the immune system.)

How Is the Virus Transmitted?   HIV lives only within cells and body fluids, not outside the body. It cannot live in

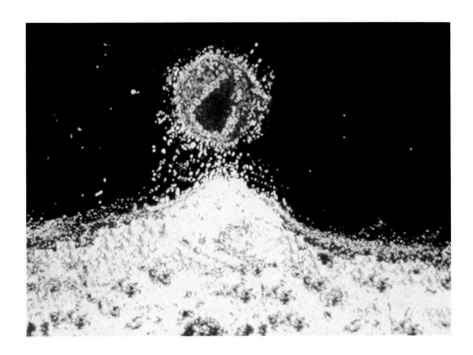

The AIDS virus attacks the body's immune system, using immune cells to reproduce itself and destroying them in the process. This micrograph shows an HIV virus as it bursts out of an infected lymphocyte (white blood cell), ready to attack another cell.

the air, in swimming pools, on toilet seats, in food, or on objects such as knives, forks, or glasses. The primary body fluids that carry the virus are blood and blood products (such as **plasma**), semen, and vaginal secretions. HIV is transmitted through the exchange of these fluids—that is, when infected blood, semen, or vaginal secretions are passed from an infected person to an uninfected person and enter the uninfected person's bloodstream. HIV has not been found in saliva, urine, or tears.

In homosexual and bisexual men, and to a lesser degree in heterosexual men and women, transmission occurs through sexual activity. The virus passes through vaginal and rectal membranes, especially if they are torn during sexual activity, and gains entry to the bloodstream. In intravenous drug users, transmission occurs through the sharing of contaminated needles or syringes with traces of blood on or in them: the virus passes directly into the bloodstream of the user.

Hemophiliacs who develop AIDS were probably infected by contaminated blood, as were other infected individuals who received blood transfusions prior to 1985. The blood supply in all licensed blood banks and plasma centers in the United States is now screened for HIV antibodies to prevent the virus from being transmitted via this route. Nevertheless, the Centers for Disease Control (CDC) has predicted that by 1992, 20,000 cases of transfusion-related AIDS will be diagnosed as a result of contamination that occurred before 1985. Children with AIDS were most likely infected through contact with their mothers' blood prenatally or during birth (see Figure 17–2). Most are the children of HIV-infected mothers, mainly women who are drug abusers or the sexual partners of drug abusers. Estimates of the number of HIV-infected babies who will be born by 1991 range from 10,000 to 20,000.

AIDS has not spread by ordinary contact to physicians, nurses, family members, or volunteers caring for people with the disease. This fact serves to dispel the fear that the disease might be transmitted through casual contact, a common concern in the earlier years of the epidemic.

Intravenous Within or into a vein; as the injection of drugs or medication directly into the vein.

HIV antibody blood test A test currently being used to determine if an individual has been infected by the human immunodeficiency (HIV) virus.

Helper T-cells (lymphocytes) Blood elements that interact directly with foreign elements to fight off infection; important in the immune system's functioning.

Suppressor T-cells (lymphocytes) Involved in the inhibiting of helper T-cells and other blood elements for proper balance in the immune system.

Antibody A globular protein produced in the blood in response to a foreign substance with which it combines.

Plasma The clear, colorless component of blood containing dissolved salts and proteins; blood minus the blood cells.

Hemophiliacs People who have a hereditary blood disease in which their blood fails to clot and abnormal bleeding occurs, which requires transfusions of blood with a specific factor to aid coagulation.

As of August 1987

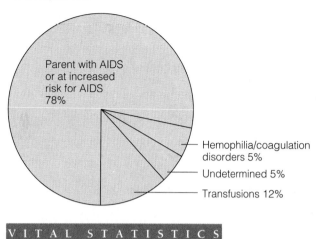

Parent with AIDS
or at increased
risk for AIDS
78%

Hemophilia/coagulation
disorders 5%

Undetermined 5%

Transfusions 12%

VITAL STATISTICS

Figure 17-2   Transmission routes of AIDS in children.

A person is not in danger of getting AIDS by being in the same classroom, dining room, or even household with someone who has the disease or is HIV-positive. Before this was generally known, many people with AIDS, including children, were the targets of ostracism, hysteria, and outright violence. Today, it is an acknowledged responsibility of all to treat people with AIDS with respect and compassion, whether they are infants, children, or adults, and whether they were infected at birth or through sexual activity, drug abuse, or a contaminated blood transfusion.

Symptoms   Signs and symptoms suggesting AIDS include unexplained, persistent swollen glands, drenching night sweats, fever, chills, significant weight loss of more than 10 pounds in less than two months (unrelated to illness, dieting, or increased physical activity), and immobilizing fatigue. Obviously, some of these symptoms can also occur with minor colds or flu.

Because the immune system is weakened, people with AIDS are highly susceptible to infections, both common and uncommon. The infection most often seen in people with AIDS is *Pneumocystis carinii* **(PCP)**, a protozoal infection that produces pneumonia. Its symptoms are shortness of breath, a persistent dry cough, sharp chest

pains, and, in severe cases, difficulty in breathing. PCP is the largest single cause of death in AIDS patients.

■ **Exploring Your Emotions**

Would you volunteer in a program designed to provide emotional support or assistance with daily living to people with AIDS? Why or why not?

The second most common problem seen in people with AIDS is **Kaposi's sarcoma**, a rare form of cancer. This disease produces purple or brownish lesions that resemble bruises but that are painless and do not heal. They may occur anywhere on the skin or inside the mouth, nose, or rectum. New studies show that HIV may exist in the brain, causing progressive neurological disease. Unexplained **dementia** (mental deterioration) and **meningitis** have also been diagnosed in people with AIDS.

Diagnosis   Early diagnosis of HIV infection is important to minimize the impact of the disease, medically, psychologically, and socially. Up until a few years ago, there were no known ways to combat the disease. Now, drugs exist that can be used to slow the progress of the virus and to fight specific infections, especially if they are discovered early.

The surest diagnosis of HIV infection is the detection of the virus itself in human tissues through laboratory tissue culture procedures, but the techniques for this method are costly and not available everywhere. For public health purposes (and for the purpose of screening blood donations), the **HIV antibody test** is used. This test determines whether a person has antibodies to HIV circulating in the bloodstream, a sign that the virus is present in the body. If an individual repeatedly tests positive on the HIV antibody test and the diagnosis is confirmed in follow-up tests, the person is considered both infected and infectious. (For a discussion of the issues involved in testing, see the box "Who Needs an AIDS Test?") There is a very strong correlation between the presence of HIV antibodies and presence of the symptoms of AIDS. Most people who test positive and have symptoms meet the CDC criteria for a diagnosis of AIDS.

Pneumocystis carinii   An organism that causes a particular type of pneumonia present in people who develop AIDS.

Kaposi's sarcoma   A form of cancer characterized by purple or brownish lesions that are generally painless and occur anywhere on the skin; usually appears in people who develop AIDS.

Dementia   Deterioration of the mental state or reduction of intellectual functioning due to organic brain disease.

Meningitis   An inflammation of the membranes of the spinal cord or brain.

Human immunodeficiency virus (HIV)   The AIDS virus. A virus that attacks white blood cells (T-helper lymphocytes) in human blood.

Who Needs an AIDS Test?

This troubling question involves us both as individuals and as a society. Dread of AIDS is universal, and many Americans (with or without good reason) now wonder whether they or others in their families or among their friends have been infected with the AIDS virus. How can they find out? Should everybody be tested? Only those in high-risk groups? Only those who wish to be tested? Some insurance companies already require a test for all applicants for life and health insurance, and some states screen marriage license applicants. Is that the way to stop the epidemic?

The test itself is fairly simple. A blood sample is drawn from the arm and analyzed in a laboratory. If the first stage of the testing proves positive, it is followed by a confirmatory test. The accuracy of the combined tests is high. In a high-risk population, virtually all people who test positive will truly be infected. In a low-risk population, however, the false positives will outnumber the true positives. Thus for every infected person correctly identified in a low-risk population, an estimated 10 non-carriers will test positive. Such testing of low-risk groups creates more problems than it solves. False negatives may occur, too. Indeed, it has been recently discovered that in rare instances carriers of the virus may not start to produce antibodies for years.

Testing Positive: Many Risks, a Few Benefits

People in high-risk groups would seem to have the most to gain from being tested. If the test is positive, early diagnosis allows the individual to consult with a physician about being treated with AZT or other drugs, including experimental ones. The physician can also offer advice and perhaps provide preventive treatment for some opportunistic diseases. People who are at high risk and are contemplating parenthood should certainly be tested. The chances of an infected mother transmitting the AIDS virus to a fetus or a newborn run from one in three to one in two; and infected babies almost always develop the disease and die. Besides, pregnancy may accelerate the disease in an infected but still healthy woman. No one infected with HIV should become pregnant or father a child; thus a test can be crucial.

Even when testing is appropriate, there are drawbacks. If the test is positive, the emotional price will be high. There is no known cure for the infection, nor any proven measure to prevent the infection from ultimately developing into the disease. So far, full-blown AIDS has proved invariably fatal. No one knows what percentage of people who carry the virus will actually develop the disease, but many experts believe that almost all will. Those who test positive will need extensive counseling; some have become chronically depressed or even suicidal. At best, their futures are compromised and their lives altered. People who undergo testing therefore need to have access to adequate counseling.

There are also social and financial risks in getting a positive result in an HIV antibody test. According to a report in the *Journal of the American Medical Association,* confidentiality is essential, yet not always easy to ensure. One young man tested positive in a small Midwestern town, only to learn that his doctor had notified the local health department, which did not keep the information confidential. The man was then fired from his job and evicted from his home, and the loss of his job meant loss of health insurance.

So are there benefits of being tested, besides the chance to seek early treatment in the event of a positive result? If you have engaged in high-risk behavior, there are two good reasons to be tested. First, if you know you are infected you can avoid passing the virus to others. This means either abstention from sex or limiting sexual activity to safer practices. Second, you can inform your sexual partner or partners and encourage them to protect others.

Of course, anyone not in a long-term and strictly monogamous relationship should practice safer sex and encourage sexual partners to do the same. You don't have to have an AIDS test to alter your behavior, nor does taking the test necessarily change a person's attitudes and actions. There are people who take the test and test positive but refuse to change their practices, even though this is morally (and perhaps legally) unjustifiable.

A Negative Test Result Can Be Risky, Too

If the test result is negative, every-

(continued)

Who Needs an AIDS Test? (continued)

one involved will be relieved, but there are pitfalls here, too. Individuals who do not wait at least twelve weeks after their last possible exposure to the virus may test negative but develop antibodies later. So to be absolutely certain, some people who test negative feel obliged to repeat the test. A negative test can be damaging, too, if it leads to a sense of invulnerability: "I've taken risks and didn't get it, so this proves I'll be okay." Whether the test result is negative or positive, the practical result has to be the same: safer sexual practices.

Getting the Test

If you decide in favor of testing, try to ensure confidentiality, and make certain that counseling will be available. If you live in New York City, Washington, D.C., or San Francisco, you can be tested at a clinic where anonymity is the rule: you will be required to fabricate a name or use a number. If you live in Alabama, Arizona, Colorado, Idaho, Minnesota, Missouri, South Carolina, or Wyoming, you have to give your right name and show identification. In Wisconsin and Kentucky positive tests are usually reported to the health

department. In Idaho and Colorado contact tracing is mandatory. That is, you will be asked for the names of your past sexual partners, who will then be notified if your test is positive.

To find out where to be tested and to discuss other issues, you can start by calling your physician, your local or state health department, or the national AIDS hotline (800-342-AIDS, or 800-344-SIDA for Spanish speakers). You can also call the American Social Health Association hotline (800-342-7514). This organization offers only general advice, but can give you the number of your state's AIDS coordinator. In New York City, San Francisco, and other big cities, you can locate so-called alternative test sites (which provide free or low-cost testing) through your local health department. Don't bill your insurance company for the test, whatever the result. Insurance companies "bank" such information, and you may, in effect, be blacklisted for future life or health insurance. If you are at low risk and test positive, have the test repeated at another lab.

Mandatory mass screenings are opposed by most health authorities as wasteful and impractical, although some would support rou-

tine testing (with refusal rights) for certain high-risk groups. Potential problems include coercion, invasion of privacy, violation of human rights, and lack of confidentiality. So far, the only effective form of general mandatory HIV screening being practiced is not for individuals but for donated blood, tissue, organs, and semen.

How Testing Can Help

Despite its drawbacks, HIV testing is a useful tool. People who want the test should be able to get it, provided that

- They understand the risks.
- They remember that the knowledge gained is wasted unless it leads to responsible behavior.
- Confidentiality (or anonymity) is the rule.
- Intensive counseling is available.

Indeed the greatest benefit of testing, for the individual as well as society, appears to be the education that accompanies it and the subsequent change in behavior. Ironically, or perhaps fortunately, the education can be provided without any testing program at all.

Adapted from University of California, *Berkeley, Wellness Letter,* August 1988.

Reporting All cases of AIDS, as defined by the CDC, must be reported to public health authorities. This measure is meant to help public health officials track the disease and keep their records of its progress up-to-date. Reporting requirements vary from state to state; although all states require that cases of AIDS be reported, most do not require that incidences of positive HIV tests alone be reported.

The issue of confidentiality is an important one. Despite public education campaigns, people who have AIDS

or who have tested HIV-positive are often stigmatized and subjected to discrimination. For this reason, physicians, hospitals, and public health departments must keep all information about testing, diagnosis, and treatment of AIDS completely confidential. If people believe they are risking their jobs, friends, or social acceptability by being tested, they are unlikely to come forward. At the same time, it is essential that sufficient information be disclosed through reporting to protect individuals and society at large. People have a right to know the incidence of the disease in their community or city, for example, and the CDC has to keep accurate records of the epidemic.

Treatment   Early hopes for a cure faded as the complexity and virulence of AIDS became apparent. But in recent years, a number of effective anti-AIDS drugs have been developed that can slow the advance of the virus. People infected with HIV may now live ten years before becoming sick with AIDS. Researchers expect that before too long, AIDS may be a manageable chronic disease that people will be able to control with medication, similarly to the way people control heart disease, diabetes, or cancer.

Probably the best known drug for AIDS is **Azidothymidine**, or **AZT**, which can both delay the onset of the disease in HIV-positive, symptom-free people and slow AIDS devastation in people who have the full-blown disease. AZT inhibits the replication of HIV and prolongs the person's life. However, it has significant toxic side effects, including anemia severe enough to require transfusions. And at $8,000 for a year's supply, AZT is also prohibitively expensive for many people. Political and consumer pressure has been put on the manufacturer to reduce the price, and the cost is expected to come down.

The only drug that can prevent an AIDS-related infection is aerosolized **pentamidine**, which is being used to prevent *Pneumocystis carinii* pneumonia. As mentioned earlier, this rare form of pneumonia is the major cause of death in people with AIDS. Aerosolized pentamidine was recently licensed by the FDA for use against this disease. Another drug, Compound Q, has been shown to kill HIV-infected cells selectively in the test tube without harming healthy cells. Unofficial human trials are now being conducted, and the manufacturer is under pressure to shortcut established procedures and release the drug more quickly. However, the medical community urges caution, partly because toxicity studies have not been completed.

Hopes for a vaccine against AIDS were bolstered in late 1989 when researchers at Tulane University successfully inoculated eight monkeys against a simian version of the AIDS virus. Because of formidable obstacles to developing a human AIDS vaccine, however, such a vaccine probably won't be a possibility until the year 2000 or later.

With treatments still limited, most efforts right now are being directed to offering care for people with AIDS. Volunteer agencies and groups have rallied to this cause

and become the core of local and national efforts. Many of them provide counseling, long-term emotional support, and assistance with the increasing difficulties of daily life for those with the disease. A highly visible and moving effort has been the "Names Project," a quilt put together from panels made by individuals in memory of their loved ones. When displayed in cities across the United States, the quilt brings together thousands upon thousands of otherwise diverse people whose lives have been touched and torn apart by the devastation of AIDS.

Prevention   Although AIDS is currently fatal and incurable, it *is* a preventable disease. You can protect yourself by avoiding behaviors that may bring you into contact with the HIV virus. In heterosexual relationships, the amount of risk is largely determined by whether one's partner is from one of the three high-risk groups—bisexual men, intravenous drug users, or prostitutes. In homosexual relationships, risk depends on one's partner and on the chosen sexual behaviors. The more times intercourse occurs with an at-risk partner, the higher the risk of contracting the virus. Behaviors with the highest risk are the following:

- Casual sex with multiple partners who might carry the AIDS virus
- Anal intercourse, with or without a condom, with someone who might carry the AIDS virus
- Vaginal or oral sex without a condom with someone who might carry the virus
- Sharing drug needles and syringes

Although AIDS is most often transmitted through sexual contact, people cannot rely on their sexual partners to protect them from the disease: protection is the *individual's* responsibility. Similarly, if a person is infected with HIV or thinks infection may be possible, it is important that the person inform all sexual partners and curtail sexual activity to prevent the spread of the disease. A list of practices that can help people protect themselves is given in the box "Preventing AIDS Infection."

The cornerstone of all efforts to prevent the continued spread of AIDS is education—in schools, homes, communities, and the media. Educational efforts mounted thus far have met with partial success. The public education campaign dating from the mid-1980s was fairly effective in the gay community, where many men responded to new information by changing their sex habits and behaviors.

Azidothymidine (AZT)   A drug used in the treatment of AIDS that inhibits reproduction of the AIDS virus.

Pentamidine   A drug used to treat *Pneumocystis carinii* pneumonia; in aerosolized form, it can prevent the disease.

TACTICS AND TIPS

Preventing AIDS Infection

The following measures will lower the risk of contracting AIDS and help prevent its spread. Individuals should remember too that it's OK to say no to sex and drugs. For those who don't have a long-term monogamous relationship, abstinence is the only truly safe option.

People who are sexually active should

• Limit their sexual partners, preferably to one person who

also prefers a monogamous relationship.
• Use latex condoms during sexual relations.
• Avoid sexual contact that could cause cuts or tears in the skin or tissue.
• Practice "safer sex" activities that allow intimate skin-to-skin contact without exposure to body fluids.

People who use IV drugs should

• Not share intravenous needles,

syringes, or anything that might have blood on it.
• Decontaminate needles and syringes with household bleach and water. (Boiling needles and syringes does not guarantee that the AIDS virus will be destroyed.)

People who are at risk for HIV infection should

• Not donate blood, sperm, or body organs.

But other segments of the population have been harder to reach, notably drug addicts and their sexual partners and children. In this group, the number of new cases is increasing rapidly. In the years ahead, the number of people with AIDS is expected to increase among all at-risk populations, including gay men, but the proportions will slowly change. An ever-growing population of addicts, most of whom will be poor, inner-city blacks and Hispanics, will account for an increasing proportion of the total number of cases. Already, AIDS is devastating some of these groups. In New York City, for example, the city with the highest incidence of AIDS in the country, 84 percent of women with AIDS are black or Hispanic, as are 90 percent of children with AIDS. AIDS is currently the leading cause of death among blacks and Hispanics of both sexes between the ages of 25 and 44. Reaching these populations is one of the greatest AIDS-related challenges our society faces in the 1990s.

■ **Exploring Your Emotions**

What do you think the government's role should be in AIDS care and prevention? Do you think the government should spend more on prevention programs geared toward expanded drug treatment programs or increased financial aid to cities bearing the medical costs of caring for AIDS patients?

Educational efforts are now being directed not just at adults in the community but at children and teenagers

in schools. The former surgeon general's report emphasized that education about AIDS should start in early elementary school and at home. Of course, the social and psychological implications of the disease make it necessary to tailor education programs very carefully to fit the intended audience. Programs for children and teenagers should be designed to minimize misinformation and unnecessary anxiety and to maximize awareness of the seriousness of the disease. Both of these groups should know which high-risk behaviors must be avoided in order to prevent infection. With intensified research into treatments and possibly a cure or vaccine for AIDS, we can hope that in the future our efforts will be directed less toward containing this epidemic and more toward eliminating it.

Syphilis Compared to AIDS, the other major STDs don't seem as serious, and in fact attention has been diverted from them in the last ten years as the AIDS epidemic has grown. Unlike AIDS, the other STDs either can be treated or are not fatal, or both. However, as mentioned at the beginning of this chapter, all STDs need to be taken seriously as health threats that, if left untreated, can lead to infertility, cancer, birth defects, disability, and/or death.

The most serious of these STDs is **syphilis**, a disease that affected millions until drugs developed in the twentieth century finally provided relief—first, before World War I, arsenic compounds, and then, in the 1940s, penicillin. Dreaded throughout history but not well under-

Syphilis A sexually transmissible disease caused by a spiral-shaped, corkscrew bacteria called a spirochete.

Reflections on AIDS

by Robert C. Gallo,
National Cancer Institute

We've learned in the past ten years that some of our most strongly held beliefs of just a decade ago were dead wrong. If you turn the clock back . . . ten years, to 1979, there was a widespread notion that epidemic diseases were things of the past, at least in the so-called developed nations. Vaccines and antibiotics had apparently tamed the microbial world. . . . Another view held then was that a worldwide outbreak of infectious disease was impossible unless the microbe was casually transmitted. A virus that needed the intimate contact of sexual intercourse or the exchange of blood, it was thought, or a virus that was transmitted congenitally from mother to child, would simply travel too slowly to become a widespread threat. . . .

Look at those statements today. With an estimated 500,000 AIDS cases in the world—more than [100,000] in this country alone—it's obvious that infectious diseases have not gone away. That's lesson number one. Before AIDS we hadn't had a worldwide epidemic since the end of World War I, when influenza killed more than 20 million people. But the lull didn't mean that we were so clever, that we'd vanquished infectious disease. Throughout history epidemic diseases have appeared and disappeared, and there have been many periods, some lasting hundreds of years, when no major outbreaks were known to have occurred.

Second, we've learned that viruses spread by close contact certainly can become global, if you allow for two conditions that people didn't allow for earlier. The first is that the virus remains infectious not for days but for years; obviously a virus that is passed on only by acts of intimacy and exchanges of blood can't travel far if people are infectious for just a short time. The second condition is that the virus is capable of lying low for long periods without producing obvious symptoms; if people can unsuspectingly carry and transmit a virus for ten years, the infection can spread far and wide.

If you now take a virus like that and introduce it to an increasingly mobile society, then the possibilities of global spread are greatly increased. I suspect that until the 1950s the AIDS virus was probably isolated in small pockets of Central Africa. But when people started moving from rural communities to large cities, they brought the virus with them. And by the 1960s, technological advances like the passenger jet began to bring people around the world into closer contact. By then, also, the medical use of blood had become global. Blood products for hemophiliacs, for example, were being sent from the United States to Japan. As a result, a virus that might once have remained relatively rare and isolated became common and global. . . .

It's been said that HIV is the most intensely studied virus in the history of medicine. Never has so much been learned about a disease in so short a time as was learned about AIDS between 1982 and 1984. The disease was defined epidemiologically, clinically, and pathologically. The cause of AIDS was found. By 1984 a virus was definitely identified by both . . . the Pasteur Institute in Paris and by our laboratory here. A test that came out of our work was developed that same year to screen the blood supply. . . . And the first inhibitor of the virus, the drug AZT, was tested.

Much of this work was possible only because of the recent advances in immunology and molecular biology. If the AIDS epidemic had occurred, say, in the 1960s, we might still have been looking for the cause ten years later. Even if we had known the cause, we'd have been in the infancy of understanding how the virus works: how it infects a cell, reproduces, and causes a disease. Certainly we wouldn't have had a blood test so soon. And if a test to detect the virus hadn't been developed in 1984, where would the virus be now? The blood supply was already contaminated. There would have been nothing to stop the virus from establishing itself in the general population. It can take the virus ten years to announce its presence in a given person. People infected by blood transfusions, not knowing they were carrying the virus, would have spread it to their sexual partners, mothers would have spread it to their children, and those people in turn could have been blood donors themselves.

Since those early discoveries, advances have come at a slower, though steady, pace. Within the past year we've made progress on

---

Reflections on AIDS (continued)

Kaposi's sarcoma, a common tumor in homosexual men with AIDS. [In late 1989] it was shown that if a person infected with HIV is also infected with human leukemia virus, the development of AIDS is strikingly enhanced. . . . To my knowledge, this is the first clear evidence of a cofactor in AIDS. . . . We're also looking at a new herpes virus, HHV-6, as a potential cofactor in AIDS. The virus is nearly ubiquitous: at least 60 percent of Americans are infected the first year or two of life, and 80 percent of adults have antibodies indicating chronic infection. . . .[T]he herpes virus may well accelerate [the course of AIDS].

The greatest part of my time now is spent on vaccines. And this work is progressing slowly, for a number of reasons. The first is that this virus is extremely complicated, much more so than, say, the poliovirus. . . . Vaccine design is yet another problem. The majority of vaccines today use whole, killed viruses to stimulate antibodies to the real thing. But we probably will never be able to use whole, killed viruses for an AIDS vaccine because you'd have to be damn well sure you'd killed every last virus, and you probably never will. . . . Finally, the virus mutates, which makes it an especially elusive target.

What lies ahead? [Behavior modification and education are] a necessity, but [they're] insufficient. . . . Too many drug addicts are already infected in this country; the epidemic in central Africa is too far along. I think an AIDS vaccine will be possible but not immediately. I believe in . . . drugs specifically designed to disrupt the virus's life cycle. AZT, for example, inhibits an enzyme crucial for viral replication. It works, though it's not the answer, and better things are coming.

I'm cautiously hopeful about CD4, which prevents the virus from binding to and entering cells. I'm hopeful about developing drugs that block enzymes needed for the final shaping of new virus proteins. Further down the road will be other drugs that inhibit virus enzymes and maybe, in time, their genes. HIV [and other new viruses] . . . pose enormous challenges—not only scientific and medical challenges, but social, political, and moral ones. Will we meet them? I certainly think so. And I hope we won't have to wait another ten years to find out.

Excerpted from Robert C. Gallo, My life stalking AIDS, *Discover*, October 1989.

---

stood, syphilis was known by a variety of names, including the "evil pox," the "great pox" (as distinguished from smallpox), and the "great imposter" (because its symptoms resemble those of so many other ailments).

Death and disability from syphilis declined dramatically after penicillin treatment was introduced, but in recent years there has been an upsurge in the number of cases, especially among teenagers, homosexuals, and minority populations. There are 100,000 new cases every year, including congenital cases (infants infected by their mothers), which increased fourfold in the years 1985 through 1987. Additionally, new statistical data show that people with herpes often have syphilis too, and many people with AIDS have had syphilis in the past. At the moment, no significant information directly links syphilis with the other STDs, except what is suggested about sexual behavior.

What Is Syphilis?   Syphilis is caused by a spirochete called ***Treponema pallidum,*** a thin, corkscrew-shaped bacterium that moves by rotating on its long axis. It requires warmth and moisture to survive and dies very quickly outside the human body. The disease is usually acquired through sexual contact, although unborn children can contract it through the placenta from an infected mother. The organism passes through any break or opening in the skin or mucous membranes and can be transmitted by kissing, vaginal or anal intercourse, or oral-genital contact.

Syphilis is characterized by sores or lesions known as **chancres** (pronounced "shang-kers") containing large numbers of bacteria; they make the disease highly contagious when they are present. Left untreated, an individual can remain contagious for as long as 18 months.

Treponema pallidum   The spiral-shaped organism that causes syphilis.

Chancre   The sore produced by syphilis in its earliest stage.

Paresis   Central nervous system damage, sometimes a result of syphilis, involving paralysis and mental degeneration.

Chlamydia trachomatis   A sexually transmissible organism that produces a wide variety of sometimes acute infections; now reaching epidemic scale in the United States.

In later stages, when the lesions have disappeared and the person is no longer contagious, the disease can cause devastating damage to almost any system of the body.

Symptoms   Syphilis progresses through three stages as the organism becomes established in the body.

FIRST STAGE: PRIMARY SYPHILIS   Within ten to ninety days (usually about three weeks) of contact with an infected partner, a single chancre about the size of a dime appears at the site where the organism entered the body, most commonly the genital area. Chancres can also appear in the mouth or armpit or on the tongue, lips, breasts, or fingers. These hardened sores are painless unless they become infected and may not even be noticed, especially if they are inside the vagina, rectum, or urethra. They generally heal within a few weeks.

SECOND STAGE: SECONDARY SYPHILIS   Approximately six weeks after a chancre first appears, an untreated person begins to show signs and symptoms of secondary disease. By now, the bacteria have had time to multiply sufficiently to produce fever, malaise, sore throat, headache, hoarseness, a depressed appetite, swollen lymph glands, and loss of hair. The second stage may also be characterized by a rash that appears anywhere on the body but most typically on the palms of the hands and the soles of the feet. The rash may also affect the mucous membranes of the lips, cheeks, tongue, tonsils, throat, and vocal chords, where grayish-white patches of mucus surrounded by dull red borders appear. These sores break down and ooze a clear fluid that contains large numbers of bacteria, making this stage highly contagious.

With or without antibiotic treatment, skin lesions of secondary syphilis usually heal in two to ten weeks. There may be relapses in which lesions recur if the person is untreated or if the treatment was inadequate. Most relapses occur toward the end of the first year following infection. Relapses are rare after two years and are believed not to occur after four years. They are generally uncommon after adequate penicillin treatment.

THIRD STAGE: LATENT SYPHILIS   By definition, people without symptoms but with evidence of having had syphilis in the past have latent syphilis. Some experts divide this stage into two periods, early latency and late latency, on the basis of the time when untreated people are likely to have relapses. The U.S. Public Health Department defines early latency as one year from the onset of infection; others consider early latency to extend beyond this time.

In this stage of the disease, the organism invades the internal organs and the central nervous system. The principal manifestation of central nervous system damage is a condition called **paresis**, which involves partial or complete paralysis and chronic, progressive mental degeneration leading to death. Symptoms may include facial tremors, slurred speech, impaired vision, headaches, epileptic convulsions, exaggerated reflexes, defective memory, delusions, depression, and dementia (insanity).

In infected pregnant women, the syphilis organism can be transmitted across the placenta after the tenth week of gestation. If the mother is not treated before the eighteenth week, the probable result is stillbirth or congenital deformity. The infected child may be crippled, blind, or deaf or have facial abnormalities such as cleft lip and palate. These children do not pass the disease on to the next generation because they are usually not infectious by the time they reach puberty.

Diagnosis and Treatment   To diagnose primary syphilis, clinicians take a specimen from the surface of the chancre and examine it under the microscope. A special microscopic examination, called the dark field, permits direct visualization of the *Treponema* organism if it is present. Diagnosis of secondary syphilis is made from blood tests and clinical observation of the symptoms. Two or three tests are used, including the Venereal Disease Research Laboratory (VDRL) test and the Fluorescent Treponema Antibody (FTA) reaction test.

Penicillin remains the drug of choice for the treatment of syphilis in all stages. Recommended treatment schedules have been prepared by the Centers for Disease Control (CDC) according to the stage of the disease. For those allergic to penicillin, tetracycline and erythromycin can be effective substitutes. Sexual partners have to be treated as well. Follow-up tests should be performed four weeks after the completion of treatment and every three months thereafter for one year to ensure that the bacterium has been eradicated. Partners should also be involved in follow-up testing.

A person who has had syphilis should not have sexual contact with others until at least one month after treatment is completed. Because of the seriousness of the disease, it is absolutely vital that the entire course of prescribed medication be completed and not discontinued when the symptoms have disappeared. The fact that there is an effective treatment for syphilis should not lead to a casual attitude about the disease. As with all STDs, it makes much more sense to avoid it altogether with responsible, intelligent sexual behavior.

Chlamydia   Gonorrhea and chlamydia have similar symptoms and are often mistaken for each other, but chlamydia is now the more common disease. In fact, **Chlamydia trachomatis** currently causes the most prevalent bacterial infection in the United States, with 3 to 4 million new cases reported every year. Chlamydia is the most common STD among heterosexual whites and is on the rise among other groups. Between 10 and 20 percent of sexually active adolescent girls have chlamydia, an in-

Myths about STDs

Myth If you have syphilis or gonorrhea, you will know it.

Fact Some infected people show no signs of having syphilis or gonorrhea until many years later.

Myth STDs in the genitals cannot be transmitted to the mouth and the reverse.

Fact Transmission of STD infections from mouth to genitals and the reverse does occur.

Myth AIDS can be spread through casual contact.

Fact AIDS is transmitted only through clearly identifiable sexual activities and by blood-to-blood contact. There is no evidence that saliva, sweat, or tears transmits the AIDS virus.

Myth You cannot have more than one STD at a time.

Fact More than half of the women who visited one STD clinic had two or more STDs.

Myth There is a high risk of acquiring AIDS from a blood transfusion.

Fact The nation's blood supply is now screened for AIDS and is considered safe.

Myth Birth control pills protect you from STDs.

Fact Birth control pills may increase a woman's chance of contracting various STDs when exposed.

Myth Once you have been cured of an STD, you cannot get it again.

Fact You can get an STD infection any time you come into contact with it whether you have had it or not.

Myth AIDS cannot be prevented.

Fact You can prevent AIDS the same way you prevent other STDs—do not allow semen, blood, urine, feces, or vaginal secretions to enter your body. Use condoms for all types of sexual intercourse. Avoid all forms of blood-to-blood contact, including the sharing of hypodermic needles, razors, and toothbrushes.

Myth Syphilis, gonorrhea, AIDS, and herpes can be contracted by contact with a toilet seat.

Fact The germs of these diseases cannot live in the open air.

cidence that is two to three times greater than that among women over 20. Teenage boys also have higher rates than do adult men. The rise in the incidence of chlamydia may be a matter not only of more actual cases but of increased awareness and improved diagnostic techniques.

Although men, women, and children are all susceptible to chlamydia, women bear the greatest burden because of the possible complications and consequences of the disease. In men, chlamydia is the leading cause of urinary tract infection and is also responsible for approximately 50 percent of the 500,000 cases of **epididymitis** (inflammation of the testicles) seen annually in the United States. *In most women, chlamydial infection produces no early symptoms,* a factor that contributes to the devastation it can cause. If left undetected for two months or more, it can lead to severe symptoms and cause extensive damage, such as inflammation of the cervix and oviducts (Fallopian tubes), a condition known as pelvic inflammatory disease (PID). PID is a leading cause of infertility; some women become infertile after a single bout of the disease. (PID is discussed in greater detail later in this chapter.)

Infants too can be infected with chlamydia. They can acquire the infection through contact with the organism in the birth canal during delivery if they are born to infected mothers. In newborns, chlamydia can cause eye infections, pneumonia, and (less often) ear infections. In fact, chlamydia is the most common cause of eye infections and pneumonia in infants under 6 months of age, accounting for 30 to 40 percent of such cases. Over 150,000 babies are born each year to infected mothers and are at high risk for contracting chlamydia infections.

Symptoms In men, chlamydia symptoms include painful urination and a slight watery discharge from the penis. In women, symptoms include a discharge from the cervix, painful urination, and painful inflammation of the oviducts, which is symptomatic of PID at this point. Most women, gay men with rectal infections, and up to 30 percent of heterosexual men infected with chlamydia have few or no symptoms, increasing the likelihood that they will inadvertently spread the infection to their partners.

Diagnosis   Doctors often diagnose chlamydia only after they have excluded the presence of gonorrhea during the examination. A definitive diagnosis is made after the organism is grown in tissue culture, which may take a week, or through a microscopic antibody test, which takes about half an hour. Researchers are working to perfect an even more efficient in-office test that doctors can use as part of a regular checkup. Because of the seriousness of an undetected infection, some physicians may add a laboratory test for chlamydia to a routine Pap test. If they get suspicious results, they follow up with more specific tests. Screening pregnant women and treating those with chlamydia is a highly effective way to prevent infection of babies during birth.

Treatment   Once chlamydia has been diagnosed, the infected person and his or her sexual partner or partners are given antibiotics, either tetracycline, doxycycline, or erythromycin. *Penicillin is not effective against chlamydia.* As with all antibiotics, it is essential that the entire course of medication be completed by all infected individuals, regardless of whether the symptoms have disappeared. Otherwise, reinfection and complications are likely. It is also important to refrain from sexual intercourse until the treatment is completed.

Chlamydia is an expensive disease. In the United States, costs associated with the infection run to more than $1 billion a year, mostly for the treatment of PID and the care of infants hospitalized with chlamydial pneumonia. And on an individual level, the physical and emotional costs—damaged reproductive organs, sterility, or an infected infant—can be even more devastating.

Gonorrhea   Although **gonorrhea** was once second in prevalence only to syphilis, its incidence has now been surpassed by that of chlamydia, with which it shares several characteristics. Still, gonorrhea, also known as "drip" or "the clap," poses a major health threat to sexually active men and women as well as to children born to infected mothers. In the United States, between 1 and 2 million new cases of gonorrhea are reported every year.

Like chlamydia, untreated gonorrhea can cause PID in women and epididymitis in men, leading to sterility. It can also cause **dermatitis** (inflammation of the skin) and a type of arthritis. An infant passing through the birth canal of an infected mother may contract **gonococcal conjunctivitis,** an infection in the eyes that can cause

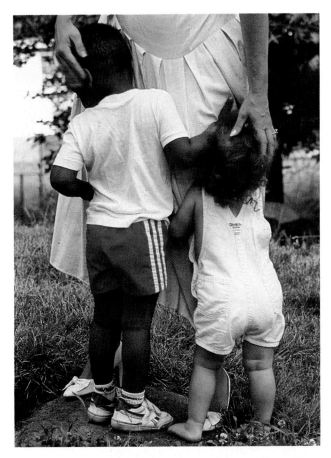

The ever-widening net cast by STDs ensnares children as well as adults. These two children with AIDS, being cared for by a foster mother, are part of a growing population of children infected with HIV in the womb.

blindness if left untreated. In some states, all newborn babies are routinely treated with antimicrobial eye drops to prevent infection from an infected mother (who may not have any symptoms).

Like syphilis and chlamydia, gonorrhea is a bacterial disease. It is caused by the bacterium *Neisseria gonorrhoeae,* which grows well in mucous membranes, including the moist linings of the mouth, throat, vagina, cervix, urethra, and anal canal. It cannot live long outside the warm, moist environment of the human body and dies within moments of exposure to light and air. Consequently, gonorrhea cannot be contracted from toilet seats, towels, or other objects.

Epididymitis   An inflammation of the small body of ducts that rests on the testes.

Gonorrhea   A sexually transmissible disease caused by a type of bacteria that usually affects mucous membranes.

Dermatitis   An inflammation of the skin evidenced by itching, redness, and various skin lesions.

Gonococcal conjunctivitis   An inflammation of the mucous membrane lining of the eyelids, caused by the gonococcus bacterium.

Symptoms In men, the incubation period for gonorrhea is brief, generally about five days. The first symptoms are a form of urethritis (inflammation of the urethra) that causes discomfort on urination and a thick, yellowish-white or yellowish-green discharge from the penis. The lips of the urethral opening may become inflamed and swollen. In some men, the lymph glands in the groin become enlarged and swollen. A small percentage of men—10 to 30 percent—will have very minor symptoms or none at all.

In women, gonorrhea is often asymptomatic. *Approximately 80 percent of women with gonorrhea have no symptoms whatsoever* and therefore don't know when they are infected. Additionally, some women with symptoms mistake the discharge from a gonorrhea infection for a normal pre-ovulation mucus discharge. When symptoms do appear in women, they are similar to those in men, including an irritating discharge and discomfort on urination. When the infection has been established for a longer period of time, generally two months or more, symptoms may include lower abdominal cramping or pain, fever, and vaginal bleeding, indicating that the woman may have PID. Any woman with discomfort and an unusual discharge should see a physician immediately to be tested for gonorrhea.

Gonorrhea bacteria can also infect the throat or rectum in individuals with the disease who engage in oral or anal sex. The symptoms of gonorrhea in the throat may be a sore throat or pus on the tonsils, and those of gonorrhea in the rectum may be pus in the feces or rectal irritation, pain, and itching. As with other infections, gonorrhea is often accompanied by a fever and swollen glands.

Diagnosis The test for gonorrhea consists of a smear test or a culture of the discharge. In men, a positive smear is generally sufficient to make the diagnosis. Asymptomatic people who suspect they might have the infection can have cultures taken. Women who suspect they may have the infection should seek examination and testing seven to ten days after they were exposed to the disease.

Accurate diagnosis of gonorrhea is especially important because of the appearance of new strains of the gonococcal organism, including antibiotic-resistant strains. **Penicillinase-producing *Neisseria gonorrhoeae* (PPNG)** was first isolated in 1976, with most cases being linked to travel in Southeast Asia, including the Philippines, Thailand, Korea, Taiwan, and Singapore. Penicillin is not an effective treatment against this form of the bacterium. Other biological changes in the organism itself produced additional resistant strains. The exact strain causing a gonorrheal infection must be accurately identified before proper treatment can be given.

Treatment When gonorrhea is diagnosed early, treatment is relatively easy. Broad-spectrum antibiotics used in combination are the preferred drugs for treating acute, uncomplicated gonorrhea and PPNG. For those allergic to penicillin, tetracycline is effective. *Using drugs prescribed for friends or sexual partners or left over from other illnesses is not an effective way to treat gonorrhea or any other STD.* As mentioned earlier, the entire course of medication must be taken, and if two people share a prescription, neither will be cured. Antibiotics may even prove harmful if taken without medical supervision. New antibiotics have been developed recently that ensure effective treatment at proper dosage levels for the specific type of gonorrheal infection.

■ **Exploring Your Emotions**

How would you feel if your sexual partner told you he or she exposed you to an STD? How would you feel if you contracted an STD?

After completion of the required course of medication, follow-up testing should be done to ensure that all traces of the infection have been eradicated. Sexual activity should not be resumed until the results of follow-up testing have been obtained. As mentioned earlier, if gonorrhea is untreated and allowed to become chronic, it can spread internally and lead to infertility as a consequence of PID.

Pelvic Inflammatory Disease A major complication in 10 to 15 percent of women who have been infected with either gonorrhea or chlamydia, or both, is **pelvic inflammatory disease (PID).** An infection of the oviducts that may extend to the ovaries, PID is often serious enough to require hospitalization and sometimes surgery. Even if the disease is treated successfully, the woman has a continuing susceptibility to recurrent infection, ectopic (tubal) pregnancy, sterility, and chronic menstrual problems. PID is responsible for a majority of the economic costs, physical damage, and personal tragedy associated with both chlamydial and gonococcal infection. It is the leading cause of infertility in young women, often un-

---

Penicillinase-producing *Neisseria gonorrhoeae* (PPNG) A strain of bacterial gonococci that produces an enzyme that inactivates or neutralizes the effects of penicillin and is therefore resistant to penicillin treatment.

Pelvic inflammatory disease (PID) An infection that progresses from the vagina and cervix to infect the pelvic cavity and Fallopian tubes.

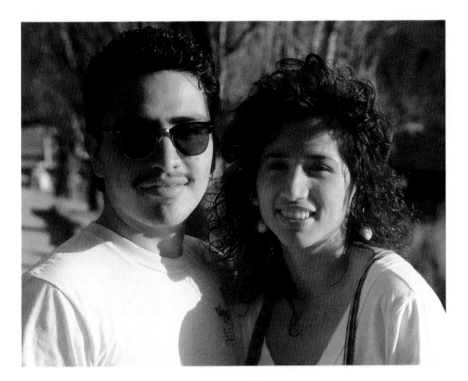

By taking a responsible attitude toward STDs, people show respect and concern for themselves and their partners. This couple's plans for the future could be seriously disrupted if one of them contracted an STD like gonorrhea or chlamydia. Either of these diseases, if untreated, could result in pelvic inflammatory disease, the leading cause of sterility in young women.

detected until later when the desire to have a child leads to further testing.

Both infectious agents, either singly or together, may be transmitted sexually by an infected partner. During or just after menstruation, these organisms appear to rise into the uterine cavity, where they may cause inflammation, or they may pass directly into the oviducts without affecting the uterus. The organisms then invade the cells. This inflammatory process spreads easily into the pelvic cavity, causing further infection and in some cases pelvic abscess.

Symptoms   Following infection with either organism, most women remain asymptomatic for some time, usually until the next menstrual cycle. Once the organisms reach the oviducts, the rate of the development of symptoms varies from one to seven days. Women with rapid onset of symptoms most often have chills, fever, loss of appetite, nausea, and/or vomiting. Most complain of abdominal pain on both sides, although the pain may be greater on one side than the other. The pain may be caused by sudden movements like sneezing or coughing. Some women may also have abnormal vaginal bleeding, prolonged menstruation, or abnormal vaginal discharge.

Diagnosis   Diagnosis of PID is usually made on the basis of symptoms. Other diagnostic techniques are based on the specific organism that is suspected of causing the disease. Laparoscopy, a surgical procedure that allows the physician to see into the oviducts, may be used to isolate the suspected organism and grow it in a culture medium. Cultures from the rectum or cervix may also be taken to assist in identifying the specific organism. Treatment is more effective when the causative organism is identified, but since gonorrhea and chlamydia are often both present, a broader-spectrum approach to treatment is usually initiated. It is also very helpful in diagnosing the disease and choosing a treatment to examine and test the woman's sexual partner(s).

Treatment   Beginning treatment of PID as quickly as possible is important in order to avoid severe damage to the reproductive organs. Antibiotics are usually started immediately; in severe cases, the woman may be hospitalized and antibiotics given intravenously. If there is no response to immediate treatment, the drugs may be changed. Thus, it is vitally important that the woman maintain contact with her health-care providers, who will carefully monitor progress. Commonly used drugs include penicillin and tetracycline. Repeat cultures are done to ensure that the bacteria have been eradicated.

When a woman has PID, it's especially important that her sexual partners be treated for infection. As many as 60 percent of the male contacts of women with PID are asymptomatic, and many men believe that unless they have symptoms, they are not infected.

Complications of PID are serious and irreversible. Scarring of the oviducts, often as a result of abscesses, can result in adhesions, chronic pelvic pain, and ectopic pregnancies; when a young woman is sterile, PID may very well be the cause.

Herpes Herpes is considered a serious STD in part because of its extremely high incidence—more than 500,000 new cases each year and over 20 million total cases in the United States—and in part because of its serious impact on newborns. Additionally, it is basically an incurable disease. Despite research and efforts to develop treatments, vaccines, and specific preventive approaches, the "arsenal" to combat this relatively common viral infection remains quite small.

After an initial herpes infection is over, new outbreaks can be triggered by a variety of factors. Each time the infection recurs, the person is contagious again, making it a difficult disease to deal with and to prevent from spreading to others. Adding to the complexity of the infection and to the confusion about its transmissibility is the fact that there are five different viruses in the herpes family that infect human beings, all with different manifestations:

- **Herpes simplex, type I**, which causes cold sores and fever blisters around the lips, mouth, and facial area
- **Herpes simplex, type II**, also known as genital herpes, which is usually seen in the genital area
- **Cytomegalovirus (CMV)**, which is asymptomic (produces no obvious symptoms) in adults but can be dangerous to fetuses in utero
- **Varicella zoster**, which causes chicken pox and shingles
- **Epstein-Barr virus**, which is implicated as the cause of infectious mononucleosis (the "kissing disease") and may play a part in "chronic fatigue syndrome"

Of the five, herpes simplex I and II and cytomegalovirus are considered sexually transmissible. Although varicella zoster and Epstein-Barr virus occasionally seem to be transmitted through sexual contact, they appear to play no significant role in STD incidence.

Symptoms Typically, herpes infections (both types I and II) appear two to twenty days after initial exposure. Symptoms can include one or more blisterlike sores on or around the mouth, the face, or the genitals. The sores are painful, fluid-filled lesions and may be accompanied by swollen glands, general muscle aches and pains, fever, a mild burning sensation during urination in men, and a vaginal discharge in women. Some women may have internal lesions on the vagina or the cervix. Because the cervix has no nerve endings, an infected woman may be completely unaware that lesions are present.

Although a direct relationship between the herpesvirus and cancer is yet to be established, women with genital herpes are five times more likely to develop cancer of the cervix. It is recommended that women who have had genital herpes inform their physicians and be sure to have a Pap test every six months. Despite the fact that herpes type I is usually found in lesions around the mouth and face and type II most often in the genital region, there have been increasing numbers of people with type I in the genital area and type II in oral and facial lesions. This reversal probably occurs when the virus is transmitted through oral-genital sex. Both types are highly contagious and do not change types because of their location.

Herpes infections are particularly dangerous to newborns because of their immature immune systems and their somewhat restricted ability to fight off a virulent virus like herpes simplex I or II. Newborns should not have direct contact with adults with cold sores, and pregnant women with herpes have to be monitored near the time of delivery to ensure that the newborn isn't exposed to the virus. If the woman's infection becomes active, the baby will usually be delivered by cesarean section to protect it from contact with lesions in the birth canal or genital area. There is no effective treatment for babies who contract the herpesvirus, which can cause severe brain damage and sometimes death in newborns.

One of the most frustrating aspects of a herpes infection is its ability to recur. After the first infection, which can last as long as three to four weeks, the virus lies dormant in the area of initial infection. (It does not travel from one location to another; rather, it tends to recur at the site of the original lesion.) Dormancy lasts for different lengths of time in different individuals. An active infection may be triggered by exposure to sun, temperature extremes, high levels of stress, acute illness, lowered

---

Herpes A type of virus, or the disease produced by the virus, such as cold sores; considered sexually transmissible.

Herpes simplex, type I A virus that causes lesions and other symptoms around the lips, mouth, and facial area.

Herpes simplex, type II A virus that causes lesions and other symptoms in the genital area.

Cytomegalovirus (CMV) A virus in the herpes family, often present in salivary glands and commonly asymptomatic. CMV infections appear as a complication in people with AIDS.

Varicella zoster The virus that causes chicken pox in children, shingles in adults.

Epstein-Barr virus A member of the herpesvirus family associated with infectious mononucleosis.

Acyclovir A drug used in the treatment of recurrent herpes infection.

Genital warts A sexually transmissible disease caused by a virus and characterized by the appearance of growths on the genital area of men and women.

Human papilloma virus The organism that causes genital warts.

TACTICS AND TIPS

Condoms Revisited

Condoms are important as a method of contraception and even more important as a method of protecting yourself from STDs. Do you remember these guidelines about using condoms from Chapter 6?

- Buy latex
- Buy fresh
- Buy lubrication (water-based only, containing nonoxynol-9)
- Buy a good design
- Wear it right

To refresh your memory about how to reduce condom failure rate by following these guidelines, refer back to the discussion of condoms and the box "Condoms—Growing in Popularity" in Chapter 6.

---

resistance from poor general health, or some other factor. Because herpes is chronic, it has a long-lasting effect on sexuality. A person with an active infection is contagious and has an obligation to prevent the spread of the disease to others. Such individuals can become aware of the factors that may trigger new outbreaks and avoid them as much as possible. Maintaining good general health is an important insurance policy against repeated bouts of infection.

Diagnosis   Of the herpes cases seen by medical practitioners, 90 percent are diagnosed on the basis of the presence of lesions, medical history, and other characteristics such as muscle aches and pains, fever, and swollen lymph glands. If doubt exists that the infection is caused by the herpesvirus, a more definitive test is available at some clinics and laboratory facilities. A sample smear is obtained from the lesion and grown in live tissue culture to determine the type of virus. This test is relatively expensive and is only done when necessary, such as when a pregnant woman is evaluating delivery options to protect her newborn.

Treatment   At present, there is no cure for herpes. Research has yet to solve the puzzle of how to intercept and destroy a virus that can lie dormant in the body without also damaging healthy surrounding tissues and organs. As scientists learn more about the characteristics of viruses in general, cures will be developed and effective preventative approaches identified for viruses that daunt us today. For the time being, treatment of herpes is directed at relieving pain, itching, and burning, avoiding secondary infection of lesions, and preventing the infection from spreading to other parts of the body. Bathing with soap and water or other drying agents, such as Epsom salts or Burrow's solution, is helpful in preventing secondary infection and speeds drying of the lesions. Avoiding certain "trigger" foods, such as chocolate,

nuts, and seeds, helps some people prevent recurrent infections.

For the past ten years, the drug **acyclovir** has been used to treat genital herpes, with varying degrees of effectiveness for different individuals. The long-term effects of acyclovir have yet to be evaluated, and the issue of viral resistance to the drug is being explored. Additional nonspecific treatments include zinc compounds, a variety of ointments, and ultrasound. None of these has stood the test of time or clinical trials, so individuals need to work closely with their personal physician to develop the best treatment for their case.

Genital Warts   In the last few years, **genital warts**, or condyloma, have attained new status in the field of STDs. Now among the most common of the STDs, condyloma presents a new challenge to the medical community because of its known relationship to cervical cancer. The precancerous condition known as cervical dysplasia often occurs among women with untreated genital warts. (See the discussion of this topic in Chapter 16.) Identification of the causative agent of condyloma has revealed a family of viruses known as **human papillomavirus (HPV)**, of which there may be as many as sixty-five different strains. Of these, twelve have been implicated in cervical cancer, and five of these are commonly isolated from genital warts. A genital wart infection is very contagious through contact with the lesions.

■ **Exploring Your Emotions**

Do you feel comfortable about having a frank discussion with a new sexual partner about your sexual histories? Under what circumstances do you feel such a discussion would be appropriate or inappropriate?

As more becomes known about these viruses, physicians are finding more of their patients have the disease; although reliable statistics are not as yet available, the CDC estimates the incidence of condyloma to be comparable to that of herpes.

Genital warts were apparently very common in the ancient world but they were thought to be caused by syphilis. In 1949, scientists isolated a virus—the same virus that caused skin warts—as the cause of what were then called venereal warts. Not until twenty years later was the specific genital wart virus isolated and given the name papillomavirus. Further research has extended the knowledge about this entire family of viruses, each member of which has its own identifying characteristics.

Most genital warts are seen in young adults, both men and women. Early diagnosis and effective treatment are often impeded by a long incubation period, a lack of awareness of symptoms in women, and a complex approach to treatment, which may not always work.

Symptoms   Genital warts look like the warts that might develop on any other part of the body. They're dry, painless growths, rough in texture and gray or pink in color. They can be flat or raised, and they vary in size. Untreated warts can grow together to form a cauliflowerlike mass. In males, they appear on the penis, more commonly in circumcised men. They often involve the urethra, appearing first at the opening and then spreading as a complication. The growth may cause irritation and bleeding, leading to painful urination and a urethral discharge. Warts may also appear around the anus or within the rectum.

In women, warts may appear on the labia, vulva, and may spread to the perineum, the area between the vagina and the rectum. Despite the spread, warts are rarely seen on the thighs or trunk of the body. They may also, however, appear on the cervix, unknown to the woman if undetected at the time of a physical examination or checkup. If the warts are small and flat, they can be difficult for the physician to see.

The incubation period for condyloma has been estimated at four to six weeks from the time of contact, and it can be as long as two to three months before any symptoms are identified. These factors contribute to the difficulty of diagnosis and often a missed diagnosis.

People can also be infected with the virus and be capable of transmitting it to their sex partners without having any symptoms at all. This is one reason why it's essential that people who do have symptoms inform their sex partners that they may be infected.

Diagnosis   To treat genital warts effectively, the physician has to differentiate the lesions from those of other diseases, particularly those of secondary syphilis. Sometimes both diseases are present, and each requires a different treatment. Sexual partners have to be treated as well; this means they have to be examined, since there is no diagnostic test that reveals whether a person is carrying the HPV.

The virus lives within the lesion itself and does not travel throughout the body. Therefore, HPV is diagnosed by the physical appearance of the lesion and the presence of the virus in it. Treatment also focuses on individual lesions rather than on a systemic approach. It isn't yet clear whether the HPV has the ability to lie dormant as the herpesvirus does.

Treatment   Currently, no one treatment for genital warts is superior to another, although new developments are more promising. Treatment decisions, again, should be made jointly with a personal physician. The traditional and long-standing treatment for genital warts is application of **podophyllin**, a toxic agent, directly to the lesion. The drug can burn surrounding tissue, so careful application is necessary. Repeat applications are often required.

Other treatment options include removal of the lesion by electrocautery, cryosurgery (freezing), surgery, and, recently, laser therapy. In 1989 the FDA approved a new drug, alpha interferon, to treat genital warts. The drug is administered in a series of injections directly into the lesion. Although the long-term effects of the treatment are still being studied, it appears to bring about a complete cure and to marshall the body's defenses against further infection as well.

Even when treated, however, genital warts can recur, probably because the treatment has eradicated the wart but not the viral infection. Follow-up care is especially important with this condition, as are avoidance of sexual contact until healing is complete, and continuing open communication with sexual partners. Because of the relationship of HPV to increased risk of cervical cancer, women who have had genital warts should have Pap tests every six months.

Other STDs

Although they are far less serious than the diseases already described, a few other diseases are transmitted sexually and are therefore included in this discussion. More annoying than threatening, these STDs still require responsible sexual behavior to prevent their spreading to others. They include trichomoniasis, a protozoal infection; *Candida albicans,* a fungal (yeast) infection; pubic lice, a parasitic infection; and scabies, also a parasitic infection.

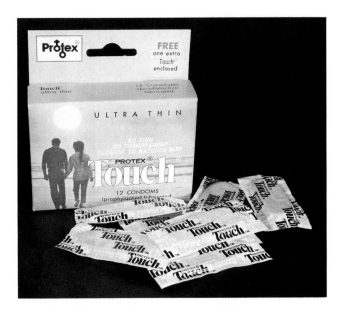

The use of condoms fell as more advanced methods of contraception, such as birth control pills and IUDs, became available. But condoms are once again gaining in popularity because of the protection they afford against STDs, especially when lubricated with the spermicide nonoxynol-9 or used in combination with spermicidal foam.

Trichomoniasis, commonly called "trich," is one of the most common protozoal infections in North America. The one-celled organism that causes trich, ***Trichomonas vaginalis***, thrives in warm, moist conditions, making women particularly susceptible to these infections in the vagina. This organism can remain alive on external objects for as long as 60 to 90 minutes, in urine for three hours, and in seminal fluid for six hours. Thus it is possible, given precise conditions, to contract trich by nonsexual means. However, it is unusual; the most likely means of transmission is sexual contact with an infected partner.

Women who become symptomatic with trich develop a greenish, foul-smelling vaginal discharge within four days of the time of contact with the organism. The discharge also causes severe itching and irritates the vagina and vulva, causing redness and pain. Although most males do not have any symptoms, some may experience slight itching, clear discharge, and sometimes painful urination. The organism has been known to survive under the foreskin of the penis without causing any symptoms.

Diagnosis of trich is simple; a microscopic examination of the discharge reveals the organism and thus determines the choice of treatment. If the organism is identified, the drug of choice is metronidazole (Flagyl). Sexual partners should be treated as well to prevent the "Ping-Pong" effect that occurs when partners pass infection back and forth to each other. It is important to complete a course of medication to avoid reinfection and to prevent the spread of the disease.

Candida albicans is an extremely common organism normally found in the vaginal tract. The problem occurs when there is an increased production of the fungus, resulting in discomfort and itching (often referred to as a "yeast infection"); symptoms can then be transmitted to a male partner. A Ping-Pong effect is common, since males do not generally experience symptoms but are capable of giving the infection back to their sexual partner. Candidiasis has also become one of the more common opportunistic infections in people with AIDS, and control of fungal infections is an integral part of their ongoing treatment.

Various factors may contribute to the increased production of fungus in the vaginal tract, and often a runaway yeast infection is a symptom of a more extensive problem. These include diabetes, metabolic changes due to pregnancy, use of oral contraceptives (in some women), antibiotic therapy, and general lowering of body resistance to infection.

Intense vaginal and vulval itching and a thick, cottage cheese-like discharge are common symptoms of candidiasis. In gay men, this infection may manifest itself in the mouth (thrush) and show as whitish patches on the mucous membrane of the insides of the cheeks and back of the throat, making eating very difficult. The two manifestations require very different approaches to treatment.

Vaginal suppositories of the antibiotic mycostatin have proven very effective in women, but other methods of treatment are dependent on a complete medical evaluation of the individual. As with any infection, following medical advice and completing the course of medication are as vital as refraining from sexual intercourse until the infection is cleared up.

Pubic lice, most commonly known as "crabs," merits mention as a pest but not necessarily as a disease or an illness. They are included here because they are so highly contagious, both sexually and nonsexually. Called pubic lice because they are attached to the pubic hairs of the

---

Podophyllin An acid used in the treatment of warts.

Trichomonas vaginalis The one-celled organism (protozoa) that causes a vaginal infection in women; may be carried by male sexual partners.

Candida albicans The organism that causes the candida (or yeast) infection.

Pubic lice Parasites that infest the hair of the pubic region.

body, these parasites have three claws in front and four pairs of small legs in back. They are often difficult to see but are the color and size of small freckles until they have fed, and then they become dark brown in color. Like mosquitoes, lice feed on human blood. Although usually found in pubic hair, they have been known to attach themselves to hair on the head, eyelashes, underarms, and even mustaches and beards. (Head lice belong to a different species than pubic lice.) Separated from their human hosts, lice are able to survive about twenty-four hours.

Easily passed from person to person, lice can also be transmitted via infested bedding, towels, clothing, sleeping bags, and even toilet seats. Intense itching is the usual symptom, and with careful examination, both the parasite and its eggs, or nits, can be seen.

Treatment is generally very easy, although the infestation can be persistent and warrant repeated applications of over-the-counter medications. These preparations are in lotion or shampoo form and include a fine comb for removing any remaining lice or nits from body hair. Washing clothing and linen carefully is also essential for preventing reinfestation. If the infestation persists, a stronger medication is available by prescription from a physician.

Scabies is another fairly common infestation. A burrowing parasite, the scabies mite deposits eggs beneath the skin in the creases of the body. These hatch in a few days, and the new mites congregate around hair follicles. Any burrowing parasite produces intense itching, especially at night. The usual sites of infestation are between the fingers, on wrists, in armpits, underneath the breasts, along the inner surfaces of the thighs, penis, scrotum, and occasionally the female genitals.

■ **Exploring Your Emotions**

How do you feel about seeking examination or treatment for an STD? Do you feel differently than you would about other symptoms?

Scabies is easily spread from person to person, not only through sexual contact but also through any direct or close contact. Scabies has been known to infest entire households and all members, including the children. Diagnosis is made by actual identification of the mite, the eggs, or the larvae in scrapings taken from the burrows in the skin of the human host. Standard treatment is prolonged hot baths with vigorous scrubbing of infected areas and the application of benzyl benzoate emul-

sion or Kwell lotion, available by prescription only. Kwell is a toxic agent and should be handled carefully and according to directions. It is especially toxic to young children and requires supervision. Itching and inflammation may occur as a result of secondary infection and should be checked by a physician.

What Can You Do?

You can take responsibility for your health and contribute to a general reduction in the incidence of STDs in three major areas: education, prevention, and diagnosis and treatment.

Education   Since the AIDS epidemic began, public and private agencies have gotten serious about educating the public and increasing their awareness of all the STDs. This campaign may already be paying off in changing attitudes and sexual behaviors, at least among certain segments of the populations. Recent surveys indicate that condom use is increasing, and the number of new AIDS cases among the gay population has been smaller in recent years than was originally feared. On the other hand, surveys also reveal that there are often lapses in safe sex practices, times when individuals revert back to unprotected sex. Such lapses are dangerous because they can mean exposure to a serious or fatal disease. Also discouraging, as mentioned earlier, is the fact that the number of AIDS cases among harder-to-reach groups, such as intravenous drug abusers and their sexual partners and children, is still increasing.

In addition to public awareness campaigns, there are other opportunities for education about STDs in our society. Colleges offer courses in human sexuality, family life, and women's health, all of which contribute to a broader understanding of sexual behavior. Free pamphlets and other literature are available from public health departments, health clinics, physicians' offices, student health centers, and Planned Parenthood, and easy-to-understand books are available in libraries and bookstores. A national STD hot line has been set up to provide free, confidential information and referral services to callers anywhere in the country.

Information about STDs is widely disseminated, but learning about STDs is still up to the individual. You must assume responsibility for learning about the causes and nature of STDs and their potential effects on you, the children you may have, and others with whom you have relationships. Once you know about STDs—their

---

Scabies   A contagious skin disease caused by a type of mite.

The STD Hot Line

The Centers for Disease Control and the American School Health Association sponsor an STD national hot line to provide confidential information and referrals about sexually transmissible diseases. Trained volunteers staff the lines between 8 A.M. and 11 P.M. (Pacific time), Monday through Friday. If you have a question or want to know where to go for diagnosis or treatment, call 1-800-227-8922. For information about AIDS only, call 1-800-342-AIDS.

---

symptoms, how they're transmitted, how they can be prevented—you are in a position to educate others. Providing information to your friends and partners, whether in casual conversation or in more serious decision-making discussions, is an important way that you can make a difference in your own and others' health.

Diagnosis and Treatment   What specifically can you do to prevent STDs? If you are sexually active, be alert for any sign or symptom of disease, such as a rash, a discharge, sores, or unusual pain (see the box "Genital Self-examination Guide"), and don't hesitate to have a professional examination if you notice such a symptom. Be alert for these signs or symptoms in your sexual partner too, and don't hesitate to question him or her if you notice something unusual.

Testing for STDs is done through private physicians, public health clinics, community health agencies, and some student health services. If you are diagnosed as having an STD, you should begin treatment as quickly as possible. Inform your partner(s) to prevent further spread of the infection and to protect him or her from the complications that can occur when treatment is delayed. Avoid any sexual activity until your treatment is complete and testing indicates that you are cured. If your sexual partner tells you that he or she has contracted an STD, you need to be tested immediately, even if you don't have any symptoms. Sometimes uninfected partners are treated to ensure that an STD won't spread or recur.

Telling a sexual partner that you have exposed him or her to an STD isn't easy. You may be afraid your partner will be angry or resentful, or you may worry that your partner will think less of you or reject you. At the same time, you may be feeling afraid, ashamed, embarrassed, or angry yourself. Feelings like these can block communication and lead to lies ("I caught it from a toilet seat"), half-truths ("No one knows how I got it, but you have to be treated too"), or rationalizations ("He'll find out sooner or later if he's got it, even if I don't tell him").

Despite the awkwardness and difficulty, it's crucial that you inform your partners quickly, openly, and honestly about any disease to which they may have been exposed.

As stressed throughout this chapter, undetected and untreated STDs can lead to serious medical complications and even death. In asymptomatic cases, the only way infected people can find out they have a disease is by being told they need to be tested. Uninformed sexual partners can go on to spread the disease to others, contributing to anguish for others as well as spiraling public health problems. The responsibility of informing partners is an ethical task too important to shirk.

With the exception of AIDS treatment, available treat-

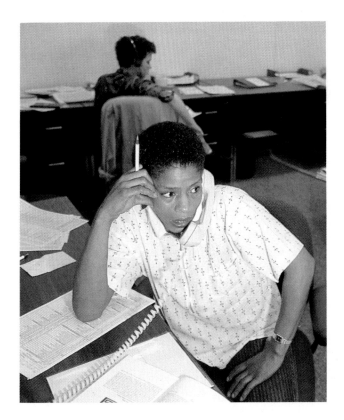

Accurate, confidential answers to personal questions are available from local and national STD hotlines. Separate AIDS hotlines, such as the one shown here, provide referrals, information, and updates on the success of the latest AIDS treatments.

Genital Self-Examination Guide

A campaign to increase public awareness of sexually transmitted disease was undertaken in 1989 by Burroughs Wellcome Company, a North Carolina-based pharmaceutical company, in conjunction with several professional organizations, including the American Academy of Family Physicians and the American College Health Association. Burroughs Wellcome, the manufacturer of AIDS drug AZT, modeled its genital self-examination (GSE) campaign after the American Cancer Society's breast self-examination campaign.

Although the GSE Guide warns readers that only a physician can make a proper diagnosis of an STD, it explains how individuals can examine themselves to determine if they have any of the signs or symptoms that might indicate an infection. To receive a copy of the guide in English or Spanish, call 1-800-234-1124. The instructions that follow are excerpted from the guide. (If you're unsure of any of the terminology, refer to Chapter 4.)

GSE for Women

Once undressed, start by examining the area that your pubic hair covers from the mons down to the area between your legs. You may want to use a mirror and position it so that you can see your entire genital area. Even with a mirror, you may find it difficult to see the

area from your urinary opening down. Do the best you can without putting yourself in an uncomfortable position.

Start by spreading your pubic hair apart with your fingers. Carefully look for any bumps, sores, or blisters on the skin. Sometimes the bumps or blisters may be red, at other times they may be light-colored. They may even look like pimples. Bumps and blisters sometimes develop into open sores. If you see anything that resembles a sore, blister, or bump, see your physician.

In addition, look for warts. Genital warts may look like warts you may have seen on other parts of your body. They may first appear as very small bumpy spots. Left untreated, they could develop a fleshy, cauliflowerlike appearance. Some warts are hard to detect with the naked eye. If you feel any bumpy growth, no matter how slight, have it checked by a physician.

Once you've examined the area covered by pubic hair (the mons and the outer lips), spread your outer vaginal lips apart and take a close look at the hood of your clitoris. Then gently pull the hood up to reveal your clitoris. Once again, look for any bumps, blisters, sores, or warts.

Next look at both sides of your inner lips for the same signs. Then move on to examine the area

around your urinary opening and your vaginal opening. This is as far as we recommend that you look. Some signs of STDs may appear up in your vagina, near your cervix, and out of view. Therefore, if you feel you may have come in contact with someone who has a sexually transmitted disease, see your physician even if you discover no signs or symptoms during your genital self-examination.

In addition to examining your entire genital area for redness, sores, blisters, bumps, or warts, be alert to other symptoms that are often associated with STDs. Some STDs may cause a vaginal discharge. Because most women have a vaginal discharge from time to time, try to be more aware of what your "normal" discharge looks like. Discharge caused by a sexually transmitted disease will appear more unusual—it may be thicker, possibly yellow. It may also have an odor. Other symptoms or signs to be aware of include a painful or burning sensation when urinating, pain in your pelvic area, bleeding between menstrual periods, or an itchy rash around the vagina.

If you notice any of the signs or symptoms described—no matter how slight—see your physician. You may or may not have a sexually transmitted disease. The only way to know for sure is to see your physician for a diagnosis. Please be aware that the symptoms of

ments are safe, effective, and generally inexpensive. If you are being treated, follow instructions carefully and complete all the medication as prescribed. Don't stop taking the medication just because you feel better or your symptoms have disappeared. Above all, don't give any of your medication to your partner or to anyone else. Doing so

will only make your treatment incomplete and reinfection more likely. Being cured of an STD doesn't mean that you will not get it again; exposure to STDs doesn't convey lasting immunity, nor does it prevent you from getting any other STD. This is all the more reason to be informed, to inform your partners, and to practice safer sex.

Genital Self-Examination Guide (continued)

STDS are sometimes so mild that you might not notice them, or the symptoms might seem to disappear; however, you are still infected and could spread disease to others. Symptoms of STDs may not appear for weeks, or even months after the sexual encounter. So if you're sexually active, be sure to see your physician and get an examination on a regular basis. Between physician check-ups, use the GSE periodically to check yourself for early warning signs. If you suspect anything, don't wait. See your physician.

GSE for Men

Once undressed, hold your penis in your hand. Start by examining the head of the penis from the urinary opening down to where it extends out a little just above the shaft. If you are not circumcised, pull down the foreskin to examine the head. Look over the entire head of the penis in a clockwise motion. Carefully look for any bumps, sores, or blisters on the skin. Sometimes the bumps or blisters may be red; at other times they may be light-colored. They may even look like pimples. Bumps and blisters sometimes develop into open sores. If you see anything that resembles a sore, blister, or bump, see your physician.

In addition, look for warts. Genital warts may look like warts you may have seen on other parts of your body. They may first appear as very small, bumpy spots. Left untreated, they could develop a fleshy, cauliflowerlike appearance. Some warts are hard to detect with the naked eye. If you feel any bumpy growth, no matter how slight, have it checked by a physician.

Once you've examined the head of the penis, move down the shaft and look for the same signs or symptoms. Then go on to the base. At the base, try to separate your pubic hair with your fingers so you can get a good look at the skin underneath. After careful examination here, move on to the underside of the penis. This area is often difficult to see, and sometimes gets overlooked. It is very important that you check this part of your body. You may want to use a mirror to be sure that you've seen the entire underside. The mirror may also be helpful as you move on to the scrotum. Handling each testicle gently, examine the scrotum for the same signs or symptoms. Also, be alert to any lump, swelling, or soreness in the testicle.

Once you've examined your entire genital area for redness, sores, bumps, and warts, be aware of these other symptoms often associated with sexually transmitted diseases. STDs may cause burning or pain when you urinate. Some STDs cause a drip or discharge from the penis. This drip may vary in both color and consistency. The drip could be thick and yellow, or it could be watery or very slight.

If you notice any of the signs or symptoms described—no matter how slight—see your physician. In addition, if you feel you may have come in contact with someone who has a sexually transmitted disease, consult your doctor even if you discover no signs or symptoms during your genital self-examination. You may or may not have a sexually transmitted disease. The only way to know for sure is to see your physician for a diagnosis.

Please be aware that the symptoms of some STDs are sometimes so mild you might not notice them, or the symptoms might seem to disappear; however, you are still infected and could spread disease to others. Symptoms of STDs may not appear for weeks, even months after the sexual encounter. So if you're sexually active, be sure to see your physician and get an examination on a regular basis. Between physician check-ups, use the GSE periodically to check yourself for early warning signs. If you suspect anything, don't wait. See your physician.

Source: *Genital Self-examination Guide,* Burroughs Wellcome Co., Research Triangle Park, North Carolina 27709.

Prevention   All STDs are preventable. The key is to think about prevention when you are about to have sex. Most people don't want to think or talk about STDs, for many reasons. Some people feel it detracts from the appeal and excitement of sex. Others take questions about sexual health from a potential partner as a personal insult. But actually, thinking and talking about STDs are expressions of caring for yourself, your partner, and all the people who make up your various communities, as well as your future children. Taking STDs seriously is practical, courageous, and loving; it means giving yourself the respect you deserve.

Everyone can reduce the risk of infection by practicing responsible sexual behaviors, but this requires some planning. The most effective preventive approach, obviously, is abstinence—not having sex. The next most effective approach is having sex with one mutually faithful uninfected partner. If you are sexually active with more than one partner, using a condom, especially one lubricated with the spermicide nonoxynol-9, reduces your risk of contracting a disease. Using spermicidal foam is also highly recommended. Unless the condom breaks or is used improperly, it provides an effective barrier against chlamydia, gonorrhea, syphilis, herpes, genital warts, and the AIDS virus. A disease can be transmitted if there is contact with an infected area that isn't protected by the condom, however, such as the scrotum, the perineum, or the anal area.

Approaches to STD prevention that are not safe include urinating or douching after intercourse, engaging in oral sex, or practicing genital play without full penetration. Birth control pills and sterilization protect you against conception and unwanted pregnancy but not against STDs. Further preventative measures include knowing the signs and symptoms of STDs, seeking treatment of any infections that do occur, and communicating openly with health-care professionals and sexual partners.

The decision to have a sexual relationship carries with it certain uncertainties and risks, both physical and emotional. It also carries the responsibility of safeguarding one's own health and that of others. You and your partner need mutual respect and honesty to make good decisions together. Caring about yourself and your partner means asking questions and being aware of signs and symptoms. It may be a bit awkward, but the temporary embarrassment of asking intimate questions is a small price to pay to avoid contracting or spreading disease. If your partner thinks less of you for being concerned, you may want to reconsider the relationship in terms of your personal values. Concern about STDs is part of a sexual relationship, not an intrusion into it, just as sexuality is part of life, not separate from it.

Summary

- Taking charge of your health includes having responsible attitudes toward prevention, diagnosis, and treatment of STDs.

The Major STDs

- The six major STDs are serious in themselves, cause serious complications if untreated, and/or pose risks to a fetus or newborn.
- Because AIDS has a long incubation period, between 1 and 1.5 million Americans are believed to be infected with the virus without knowing it.
- Most AIDS patients are homosexual and bisexual males and intravenous drug users. Also at risk are people who received blood and blood products between 1977 and 1985, sexual partners of infected individuals, and children born to infected mothers.
- AIDS, which is caused by human immunodeficiency virus (HIV), affects the immune system, taking over the cells that control the body's system of defense. The virus uses the immune system cells to nourish and replenish itself.
- The HIV virus lives only within the cells it invades; it is carried in blood and blood products, semen, and vaginal secretions. HIV is transmitted through the exchange of these fluids—in sexual activity, sharing of contaminated needles, and blood transfusions. AIDS is not spread by casual contact.

- Because AIDS weakens the immune system, people with the disease are susceptible to infections—especially *Pneumocystis carinii*. AIDS patients also typically develop Kaposi's sarcoma, dementia, and meningitis.
- Most AIDS diagnoses depend upon detecting antibodies to HIV circulating in the bloodstream.
- All cases of AIDS must be reported to public health authorities; those who have the disease or test HIV-positive have the right to confidentiality, but sufficient information needs to be available to protect individuals and society.
- By inhibiting the replication of HIV, AZT can delay the onset of the disease in symptom-free people and slow down the full-blown disease. Aerosolized pentamidine can prevent pneumocystis pneumonia.
- A vaccine for AIDS will probably not be available for at least another ten years.
- An individual can take responsibility for preventing AIDS by avoiding behaviors that lead to contact with the HIV virus.
- Education, an important part of AIDS prevention, has been successful in the gay community, but less so among drug addicts and their sexual partners. Educational programs for children and teenagers should emphasize avoiding high-risk behaviors.
- The number of cases of syphilis has been rising in recent years. Syphilis is usually contracted through sexual contact or through the placenta in an infected mother.

- Syphilis has three stages. The first stage, primary syphilis, is characterized by a chancre that appears where the organism enters the body. In the second stage, secondary syphilis, an untreated person develops fever, malaise, sore throat, swollen glands, and a rash, among other symptoms. During the third stage, latent syphilis, the organism invades internal organs and the central nervous system; partial or complete paralysis as well as mental degeneration are possible.
- The syphilis organism can cross the placenta after the tenth week of gestation.
- Primary syphilis is diagnosed from a chancre specimen; secondary syphilis is diagnosed through blood tests and clinical observation. Penicillin is usually used to treat all stages of syphilis. Sexual partners must also be treated, and follow-up testing is essential.
- Chlamydia is increasing in incidence. In men, chlamydia causes urinary tract infection and epididymitis; in women, chlamydia produces no early symptoms, which allows extensive damage to take place as a result of pelvic inflammatory disease.
- Infants born to infected mothers can acquire the infection through contact with the organism in the birth canal; the result can be eye infections, ear infections, and pneumonia.
- People infected with chlamydia are often symptom-free, which increases the likelihood that they will spread the infection.
- Diagnosis is usually made through a tissue culture test or a microscopic antibody test. Tetracycline, doxycycline, or erythromycin are used in treatment; penicillin is not effective.
- Untreated gonorrhea can cause PID in women and epididymitis in men, leading to sterility. Newborns can contract gonococcal conjunctivitis by passing through the birth canal of an infected mother.
- The incubation period for gonorrhea is usually about five days. The first symptoms in men include urethritis and a discharge from the penis. Many infected women have no symptoms at all, but after the infection has been established for two months or more, symptoms of PID may emerge.
- Diagnosis of gonorrhea is made by a smear test or culture of the discharge. New strains have emerged against which penicillin is ineffective. Proper treatment requires identifying the strain causing the infection. Follow-up testing is essential.
- Pelvic inflammatory disease, a complication of gonorrhea or chlamydia, is an infection of the oviducts that may extend to the ovaries. PID is the leading cause of infertility in young women.
- Once a woman is infected with gonorrhea and/or chlamydia, the organisms enter the uterus during or after menstruation and then enter the oviducts. When the organisms invade the cells of the oviducts, inflammation occurs and spreads throughout the pelvic cavity.
- Symptoms of PID include chills, fever, loss of appetite, nausea, vomiting, abdominal pain, and abnormal vaginal bleeding. Diagnosis is usually made on the basis of symptoms.
- Treatment of PID should be initiated as soon as possible to avoid damage to the reproductive organs; antibiotics are given, sometimes intravenously. Without treatment, or when treatment is too late, complications include scarred oviducts, which can lead to ectopic pregnancies and infertility.
- Herpes occurs frequently in the United States, has serious impact on newborns, and is basically incurable.
- Symptoms of a herpes infection include blisterlike sores on or around the mouth, face, or genitals.
- Herpes infections are dangerous to newborns because they cannot easily fight off such a virus. If a mother has an active herpes infection, the baby should be delivered by cesarean section.
- After an initial infection, the herpesvirus lies dormant in the area of the infection. Recurrences can be triggered by environmental, health, and personal factors. Because herpes is chronic, it has a long-lasting effect on sexual activity.
- Diagnosis of herpes is usually made on the basis of lesions, medical history, and the presence of other symptoms. The drug acyclovir offers relief to some patients.
- Genital warts, caused by the human papillomavirus, are associated with cervical cancer and so warrant special attention. An infection is contagious through contact with the lesions.
- Early diagnosis and effective treatment of genital warts are often impeded by a long incubation period, women's lack of awareness of symptoms, and a complex approach to treatment.
- Genital warts are dry, painless growths that appear on the penis in males and on the labia, vulva, and perineum in women. Diagnosis is made on the basis of lesions; treatment usually consists of applying podophyllin directly to lesions.
- With all STDs, it's essential to avoid sexual contact until healing is complete, to have continuing open communication with sexual partners, to take all medication completely and not share it with partners, and to obtain follow-up care.

Other STDs

- Other sexually transmissible diseases, even if more annoying than threatening, demand responsible sexual behavior to prevent their spreading to others.
- Trichomoniasis, a common protozoal infection, is usually contracted sexually, though the organism that

causes it can live on external objects for up to ninety minutes.

- Trich is diagnosed through a microscopic examination of the discharge; treatment consists of the drug metronidazole. Sexual partners also need treatment.
- *Candida albicans,* a fungus that normally lives in the vaginal tract, causes discomfort and itching (a so-called yeast infection) when increased production of the organism occurs as a result of diabetes, metabolic changes due to pregnancy, use of oral contraceptives, antibiotic therapy, or immune system problems. Men rarely have symptoms. The antibiotic mycostatin is usually used in women, and other treatment options are available.
- Pubic lice are parasites that attach to the pubic hair and feed on human blood. They can be transmitted sexually, but also through infested bedding, towels, clothing, and even toilet seats. Treatment consists of over-the-counter medications in lotion or shampoo form.
- The scabies mite is a burrowing parasite that deposits eggs beneath the skin surface. Scabies can be contracted through any close contact. Diagnosis is made through identification of the organism; treatment consists of hot baths and applications of prescription lotions.

What Can You Do?

- The AIDS epidemic has led to increased awareness about all STDs and has led public and private agencies to begin education campaigns. Although positive responses have occurred (an increase in condom use), some segments of the population continue to be hard to reach.
- Preventing STDs on an individual basis means being alert to symptoms in oneself and one's partners, seeing a physician if symptoms occur, getting treatment, informing partners, and avoiding sexual activity until treatment is complete.
- Telling a partner can be awkward and difficult but is crucial to preventing the spread of STDs.
- All STDs are preventable; the key is practicing responsible sexual behaviors—which requires planning. Those who are sexually active are safest with one mutually faithful uninfected partner. Using a condom, especially one lubricated with nonoxynol-9, helps protect against STDs; spermicidal foam also helps.

Take Action

1. In your health diary, list the positive behaviors that help you avoid exposure to sexually transmissible diseases. Consider what additions you can make to this list or how you can strengthen your existing behaviors. Then list the behaviors that may block your positive behaviors or put you at risk of contracting an STD. Consider which ones you can change and how you can begin doing so.

2. Go to a drugstore and examine the over-the-counter contraceptives. Which ones contain nonoxynol-9? Which ones provide protection against STDs? If you are sexually active, make sure you use the best protection available.

3. More and more communities have treatment and support programs for people with AIDS. Look in the yellow pages or contact local health agencies to find out what services are available where you live. If any of these agencies use volunteers, consider donating some of your time to help.

Selected Bibliography

Cates, W., Jr., and K. K. Holmes. 1986. Sexually transmitted diseases. In *Public Health and Preventive Medicine,* 12th edition. Atlanta: U.S. Public Health Service.

Centers for Disease Control. 1986. *Acquired Immune Deficiency Syndrome (AIDS) Weekly Surveillance Report.* United States cases reported to Centers for Disease Control, August 4.

Division of Sexually Transmitted Diseases. 1985. *Chlamydia Trachomatis Infections: Policy Guidelines for Prevention and Control.* Atlanta: Centers for Disease Control, May.

Green, Charles. 1990. AIDS epidemic could peak in mid-1990s, researcher says. *San Jose Mercury News,* February 17.

Holmes, King K., Per Anders Mardh, P. Fredrick Sparling, and Paul J. Wiener. 1984. *Sexually Transmitted Diseases.* New York: McGraw-Hill.

Report of the Presidential Commission on the Human Immunodeficiency Virus Epidemic. Submitted to the President of the United States, June 24, 1989.

Sacks, Stephen L. 1985. Oral acyclovir—make up your own mind. *The Helper,* Summer.

Shilts, Randy. 1989. Big gains, troubling realities. *San Francisco Chronicle,* December 25.

Recommended Readings

Hamilton, Richard. 1980. *The Herpes Book.* New York: St. Martin's. *This general volume is tailored to laypeople who want to learn more about what can be done to deal with the symptoms of herpes and how to communicate with potential or ongoing sexual partners.*

Hein, Karen, and Theresa Foy Digeronimo. 1989. *AIDS: Trading Fears for Facts.* Consumers Reports Books. *Targeted at teens, this is a most readable, concise, and to-the-point book with excellent coverage, guide to vocabulary, and resources.*

Irvington Publishers. 1988. *Contraceptive Technology, 1988–1989.* New York: Irvington. *Updated every two years, this informational handbook provides a scientific overview of reproductive health, including STDs.*

Shilts, Randy. 1987. *And the Band Played On: Politics, People, and the AIDS Epidemic.* New York: St. Martin's. *A highly readable account of the AIDS epidemic and the political response it has evoked, written by a concerned and committed reporter.*

Contents

Making Connections

One consequence of the AIDS epidemic has been to make many people more aware of the incredible job constantly being performed by the human immune system—and of the equally incredible devastation that occurs when the system falters. Clearly, it's better to keep your immune system working well than to try to heal it after it's damaged. The scenarios presented on these pages describe situations in which people have to use information, make a decision, or choose a course of action, all related to immunity and infection. As you read them, imagine yourself in each situation and consider what you would do. After you've finished the chapter, read the scenarios again and see if what you've learned has changed how you would think, feel, or act in each situation.

You've had a cold for five days and have foregone your daily run to give your body a chance to get well. One of the people you normally run with says you're making a mistake. "Exercise is always good for you," your friend claims. "It'll help you recover more quickly." You're feeling kind of weak, and your throat is still irritated. Should you get out there and run, or should you wait till you feel better?

You've come down with a sore throat, slight fever, and runny nose, and you ache all over. You figure it's a cold or the flu, and you go to bed with a box of tissues and a good book. But your roommate thinks you ought to go to the student health center to get a prescription for an antibiotic. "Why be sick for a week when you can be well in two days?" your roommate says. You're not sure an antibiotic would help. Is your roommate giving you good advice?

18
Immunity and Infection

You return from a hike in the woods one Saturday to discover a tick attached to your ankle. It appears to be bloated and full of blood. One of your friends says you should grab it and turn it counterclockwise to release it from your skin; another says you should burn it with a cigarette to make it drop off. A third thinks you should go to the emergency room to have it removed and to get some antibiotics in case you've been infected with a disease. You've never had a tick bite before. Are they dangerous? Do you need an antibiotic? What should you do?

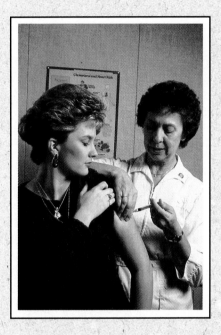

One of your classmates stayed home with a cold most of last week. This week she's back, but she's still coughing a lot and occasionally sneezing too. You think it's pretty inconsiderate of her to come to class and expose other people to her cold. Finally you say, "Why don't you take care of yourself at home until you feel better? I'll lend you my notes if it will help." She responds, "Oh, I feel all right now. All that's left of my cold is this annoying cough. But I'm not contagious or anything." Is she right, or is she probably still contagious?

You're playing Frisbee with some friends in a park when you step on something sharp. It turns out to be a nail, which has pierced the sole of your shoe and punctured your foot. It doesn't bleed when you pull it out, so you decide to continue playing. But one of your friends asks when you last had a tetanus shot, and since you're not sure, he suggests you go to the health center for a booster shot. Should you act on your friend's suggestion?

Most of the time we go about our daily lives thinking of the world as a place inhabited by beings more or less like ourselves. We seldom think of the countless, unseen microscopic organisms that live around, on, and in us. Many of them would like nothing better than to consume the very tissues and organs they call home. Only constant vigilance on the part of our immune system keeps these microorganisms at bay and our bodies intact and healthy.

Even without these "invaders," our bodies have a tendency to develop problems and diseases. The natural aging process of the human body is a prime example of the second law of thermodynamics—all things, living and otherwise, have a tendency to disintegrate or fall apart. The immune system works to keep the body from being overwhelmed not just by invaders from the outside (**infection**) but also by changes on the inside, such as cancer.

■ **Exploring Your Emotions**

Do you get a lot of colds and infections, or do you manage to stay well most of the time? Does either of your parents have a similar tendency? If so, do you think you inherited some of the characteristics of your immune system from him or her?

Most people don't pay much attention to any of these internal skirmishes unless they become sick and find themselves deprived of their usual feelings of well-being. But many people today are more knowledgeable about the complexities of immunity because they've read or heard about AIDS, which directly attacks the immune system. This chapter provides information that will help you understand immunity, infection, and how you can keep yourself well in a world of hungry microorganisms.

The Body's Defense System

Our bodies have very effective ways of protecting themselves against invasion by foreign organisms, especially **pathogens**, microorganisms that cause disease. The body's first line of defense is a formidable array of physical and chemical barriers. When these barriers are breached, the body's immune system comes into play. Together, these defenses provide an effective response to nearly all the challenges and invasions our bodies will ever experience.

Physical and Chemical Barriers   The skin, the body's largest organ, prevents many microorganisms and particles from entering the body. Although many bacterial and fungal organisms live on the surface of the skin, very few can penetrate it except through a cut or break. Wherever there is an opening in the body, or an area without skin, other barriers exist. The mouth, the main entry to the gastrointestinal system, is lined with mucous membranes, which contain cells designed to prevent the passage of unwanted organisms and particles. These surfaces are rich in antibodies (discussed in detail later in the chapter) and in **enzymes** that break down and destroy many microorganisms.

The respiratory tract is lined not only with mucous membranes but also with cells having hairlike protrusions called **cilia.** The cilia sweep foreign matter up and out of the respiratory tract. Particles that are not caught by this mechanism may be expelled from the system by a cough. If the ciliated cells are damaged or destroyed, as they are by smoking tobacco, a cough is the body's only way of ridding the airways of foreign particles. This is one reason why smokers generally have a chronic daily cough—they're compensating for damaged airways.

Routes of Infection   Despite these defenses, invaders do manage to enter the body. Disease is transmitted in one of three ways: (1) by penetration of the skin (for example, through an insect bite or cut) or by direct contact (for example, when mucous membranes come into contact with a herpes or syphilis lesion), (2) by inhalation of particles, or (3) by ingestion of contaminated food or water. Bacteria and viruses that enter the skin can cause a local infection of the tissue, or they may penetrate into the bloodstream or **lymph system** to cause more extensive **systemic infection.** Organisms that are transmitted via respiratory secretions (such as the tuberculosis and pertussis bacteria and the influenza virus) may cause upper respiratory infections or pneumonia, or they may enter the bloodstream and cause systemic infection. The great majority of respiratory infectious agents, however, such as the viruses that cause "colds," are transmitted not by coughs and sneezes but by direct contact, from hand to hand and then to mouth or nose.

Food- and water-borne organisms enter the mouth and travel to the location that will best support their reproduction. They may attack the cells of the small intestine or the colon, causing diarrhea and other symptoms, or they may enter the bloodstream via the digestive system and travel to other parts of the body. Certain bacteria, on the other hand, are present in massive quantities in the gut. (Did you know that a large portion of your daily stool is made of bacteria?) These "normal" bacteria are necessary for digestion and only cause disease when the integrity of the bowel is compromised, as when an appendix ruptures. Other "unfriendly" bacteria, such as those that cause food poisoning or botulism, disrupt the normal harmony by invading the cells that line the bowel or by producing **toxins** that cause damage.

■ **Exploring Your Emotions**

Your immune system is constantly working to keep you well. Does knowing how arduous and complex this job is motivate you to take good (or better) care of yourself? Why or why not?

Agents that cause STDs usually enter the body through the mucous membranes lining the urethra (in the male) or the cervix (in the female). HIV, the virus that causes AIDS, survives poorly by itself and requires cells present in body secretions or blood to be transmitted. This is why the virus is transmitted relatively easily in semen, cervical secretions, and blood but has never been shown to be transmitted in tears or urine, two secretions that don't contain cells.

The Immune System   Once the body has been invaded by a foreign organism, an elaborate system of responses is activated. The immune system operates through a remarkable information network involving billions of cellular defenders who rush to protect the body when a threat arises. We discuss here two of the body's responses: the inflammatory response and the immune response. But before we cover these specific defenses, let's turn to a brief description of the defenders themselves and the mechanisms by which they work.

The Immunological Defenders and How They Work   The immune response is carried out by three different groups of white blood cells, all of which are continuously being produced in the bone marrow. One group consists of the **macrophages,** or "big eaters," a type of **phagocytic** ("cell eating") **cell.** The other two groups are **lymphocytes,** white blood cells that travel in both the bloodstream and the lymph system. At various places in the lymph system there are lymph nodes (or glands), where macrophages

congregate and filter bacteria and other substances from the lymph. When these nodes are actively involved in fighting an invasion of microorganisms, they fill with cells; physicians use the location of swollen lymph nodes as a clue to the location and cause of an infection.

The two kinds of lymphocytes are known as **T-cells** and **B-cells.** T-cells are further differentiated into **helper T-cells, killer T-cells,** and **suppressor T-cells.** B-cells are lymphocytes that produce **antibodies.** The first time T-cells and B-cells encounter a specific invader, some of them are reserved as **memory T- and B-cells,** enabling the body to mount a rapid response should the same invader appear again in the future. These cells and cell products—macrophages, T-cells (helper T-cells, killer T-cells, and suppressor T-cells), B-cells and antibodies, and memory cells—are the principal players in the body's immune response.

The immune system is built on a remarkable feature possessed by these defenders—the ability to distinguish foreign cells from the body's own cells. Since the lymphocytes are capable of great destruction, it's essential that they not attack the body itself. When they do, they cause **autoimmune diseases,** such as lupus and rheumatoid arthritis.

How do the lymphocytes know when they've encountered an enemy? All the cells of an individual's body display markers on their surfaces—tiny molecular shapes—that identify them as "self" to lymphocytes who encounter them. Lymphocytes also recognize the markers displayed on the surfaces of invading microorganisms and know they've encountered "not self." Shapes that are recognized by lymphocytes as foreign and that trigger the immune response are known as **antigens.**

Lymphocytes recognize all these markers through their own sets of complementary surface markers, which work with antigens like a lock and key. When an antigen appears in the body, a lymphocyte with a complementary pattern locks onto it, triggering a series of events designed

Infection   Disease caused by a pathogen.

Pathogens   Organisms that cause disease.

Enzymes   Chemicals necessary for energy production and protein synthesis in normal animal cells.

Cilia   Microscopic hairlike structures that sweep mucus and foreign substances up out of the bronchial tubes.

Lymph system   The body system that traps pathogens and produces lymphocytes.

Systemic infection   An infection of large portions of the body.

Toxins   Poisons.

Macrophages   Large phagocytic cells that devour foreign particles.

Phagocytic cell   White blood cells that specialize in eating undesirable matter.

Lymphocytes   White blood cells continuously made in lymphoid tissue as well as in bone marrow.

T-cell   One kind of lymphocyte; arises in bone marrow, and some progeny move into thymus (giving its name).

B-cells   Lymphocytes that produce antibodies.

Helper T-cells   Lymphocytes that stimulate other lymphocytes to increase.

Killer T-cells   Lymphocytes that kill cells of the body that have been invaded by foreign organisms; also can kill cells that have turned cancerous.

Suppressor T-cells   Lymphocytes that discourage the growth of other lymphocytes.

Antibodies   Specialized proteins, produced by white blood cells, that can recognize and neutralize specific microbes.

Memory T- and B-cells   Lymphocytes that are generated during an initial infection and circulate in the body for years, "remembering" the specific antigens that caused the infection and quickly destroying them if they appear again.

Autoimmune disease   Disease in which an individual's immune system attacks the individual's own body or body parts.

Antigen   A molecule that marks an invading particle; can be recognized and neutralized by an antibody.

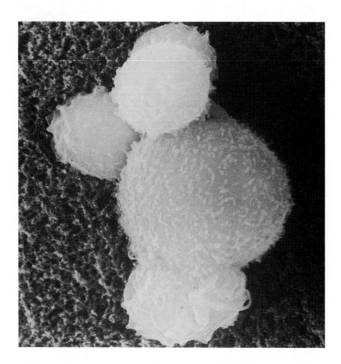

Killer T cells can recognize the antigens of both foreign cells and mutated body cells. In this electron micrograph magnified 2300 times, four killer T-cells are in the process of attacking a cancer cell.

creased heat, swelling, and redness in the affected area. White blood cells, including phagocytes, are drawn to the area and attack the invaders, in many cases destroying them. At the site of infection there may be pus, a collection of dead white blood cells and debris resulting from the encounter.

The Immune Response Another bodily response to invasion is the immune response. For convenience, we can think of this response as having four critical phases: (1) recognition of the invading pathogen; (2) amplification of defenses; (3) attack; (4) slowdown. In each of these phases, crucial actions occur that are designed to destroy the invader and restore the body to health.

1. In the first phase, macrophages are drawn to the site of the injury and consume the foreign cells; they then provide information about the enemy by displaying its antigen on their surfaces. Helper T-cells, the "commanders-in-chief" of the immune response, read this information and rush to respond.
2. Now the second phase of the immune response gets underway. Multiplying rapidly, helper T-cells trigger the production of killer T-cells and B-cells in the spleen and lymph nodes.
3. With its forces constantly amplifying, the immune system launches its attack, the third phase of its response. Killer T-cells strike at foreign cells and cells of the body that have been invaded and infected. (They destroy body cells that have mutated and become cancerous in the same way.) Puncturing the cell membrane, they sacrifice body cells in order to destroy the foreign organism within. This type of action is known as a *cell-mediated immune response,* because the attack is carried out by cells. Killer T-cells also trigger an amplified inflammatory response and recruit more macrophages to help clean up the site.

    B-cells work in a different way. Stimulated to multiply by helper T-cells, they produce large quantities of antibody molecules, which are released in the bloodstream and tissues. Antibodies are Y-shaped protein molecules that bind to antigen-bearing targets and mark them for destruction by macrophages. This type of response is known as an *antibody-mediated immune response.* Antibodies work against bacteria and

to destroy the army of invaders. The truly astonishing thing is that the body doesn't synthesize the appropriate lymphocyte lock after it comes in contact with the antigen key. Rather, lymphocytes already exist in the body with complementary markers for millions, if not billions, of possible antigens. When any of these antigens enters the body, a matching lymphocyte appears to bind with it.

The Inflammatory Response When the body has been injured or infected, one of the body's responses is the inflammatory response. Special cells in the area of invasion or injury release **histamine** and other substances that cause blood vessels to dilate and fluid to flow out of capillaries into the injured tissue. This produces in-

---

Histamine The toxin released by mast cells when the allergic antibody touches an allergen.

Opportunistic disease Illnesses caused when organisms take the opportunity presented by a primary (initial) infection to multiply and cause a secondary (additional) infection. For example, *Candida albicans* frequently infects people weakened by the AIDS virus.

Immunity Mechanisms that defend the body against infection; or the status of those mechanisms in general; or specific immunity or defenses against specific pathogens.

Adaptive or **acquired immunity** The body's ability to mobilize the cellular "memory" of an attack by a pathogen to throw off subsequent attacks. This ability can be acquired through vaccination as well as the normal immune response.

Incubation Period when a bacteria or virus is actively multiplying inside the body's cells; usually a period without symptoms of illness.

HIV: The Immune System under Siege from AIDS

The virus that causes AIDS, known as human immunodeficiency virus (HIV), destroys the immune system, short-circuiting its responses before they can be mobilized. Normally, viruses that have entered the blood or lymph system are engulfed by helper T-cells, which then trigger the immune response. But when HIV encounters and is engulfed by a helper T-cell, it takes over part of the cell's reproductive system and uses it to produce more viruses. Eventually, the helper T-cell is killed, and the immune system begins to wane. Individuals infected with HIV become susceptible to many secondary infections that people with healthy, intact immune systems have no problem overcoming. It is these **opportunistic diseases** that cause the most serious illness and death in people with AIDS.

Unfortunately, this unique ability of HIV to infect the immune system itself makes it unlikely that an effective vaccine will be developed in the near future (see Chapter 17). Because the immune response is short-circuited, the virus may be able to avoid any immune response induced by injecting the body with a vaccine. There is even concern that a vaccine would cause harm by destroying the helper T-cells that have been infected with HIV, leading to an earlier and greater impairment of the immune system. Much research is still needed before scientists can learn how to rid the body of this deadly virus.

against viruses and other substances when they are in the body but outside cells. They don't work against infected body cells or viruses that are replicating inside cells.

4. Now that the invading microorganism has been destroyed or incapacitated, the body has to call off the attack. The last phase of the immune response is the slowdown of activity. A third type of T-cell, the suppressor T-cell, regulates the levels of lymphocytes in the body and controls their activities. When the danger is over, suppressor T-cells halt the immune response and restore the body's natural balance. The box entitled "HIV: The Immune under Siege from AIDS" explains how this system is disrupted by HIV.

Immunity   In many infections, survival confers **immunity**; that is, the person will never get the same illness again. This is because some of the lymphocytes created during the amplification phase of the response are reserved as memory T- and B-cells. They continue to circulate in the blood and lymph system for years or even for the rest of the person's life. If the same antigen enters the body a subsequent time, the memory T- and B-cells recognize and destroy it before it can cause illness. This subsequent response takes only a day or two, whereas the original response lasted several days, during which time the individual suffered the symptoms of illness. The ability of memory lymphocytes to remember previous infections is known as **adaptive** or **acquired immunity.**

Symptoms and Contagion   The immune system is operating at the cellular level within your body all the time, maintaining its vigilance when you're well and fighting invaders when you're sick. How does it all feel to you, the host and playing field for these activities? How do your symptoms relate to the course of the infection and the immune response?

■ **Exploring Your Emotions**

How do you feel when you get sick? Do you feel "weak"? Guilty? Responsible? Abused? Angry? Are you impatient to get back on your feet, or do you want to prolong the time you can legitimately be excused from your normal obligations?

During **incubation**—when a virus is multiplying inside the cells or when bacteria are actively multiplying before the immune system has gathered momentum—you may not have any symptoms of the illness, but you may be contagious. During the second and third phases of the immune response, you may still be unaware of the infection, or you may "feel a cold coming on."

Many of the symptoms of an illness are actually due to the immune response of the body rather than to the actions or products of the invading organism. For example, fever is thought to be caused by the release and activation of certain substances in macrophages and other cells during the immune response. The substances travel in the bloodstream to the brain, where they cause the body's thermostat to be "reset" to a higher level.

Similarly, you get a runny nose when your lymphocytes destroy infected mucosal cells, leading to increased mucus production. You get a sore throat when your lymphocytes destroy infected throat cells. The general malaise and fatigue of the "flu" are probably caused by in-

CELL WARS

About one trillion strong, our white blood cells constitute a highly specialized army of defenders, the most important of which are depicted here in a typical battle against a formidable enemy.

VIRUS
Needing help to spring to life, a virus is little more than a package of genetic information that must commandeer the machinery of a host cell to permit its own replication.

MACROPHAGE
Housekeeper and frontline defender, this cell engulfs and digests debris that washes into the bloodstream. Encountering a foreign organism, it summons helper T cells to the scene.

HELPER T CELL
As a commander in chief of the immune system, it identifies the enemy and rushes to the spleen and lymph nodes, where it stimulates the production of other cells to fight the infection.

KILLER T CELL
Recruited and activated by helper T cells, it specializes in killing cells of the body that have been invaded by foreign organisms, as well as cells that have turned cancerous.

B CELL
Biologic arms factory, it resides in the spleen or the lymph nodes, where it is induced to replicate by helper T cells and then to produce potent chemical weapons called antibodies.

ANTIBODY
Engineered to target a specific invader, this Y-shaped protein molecule is rushed to the infection site, where it either neutralizes the enemy or tags it for attack by other cells or chemicals.

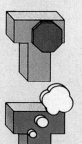

SUPPRESSOR T CELL
A third type of T cell, it is able to slow down or stop the activities of B cells and other T cells, playing a vital role in calling off the attack after an infection has been conquered.

MEMORY CELL
Generated during an initial infection, this defense cell may circulate in the blood or lymph for years, enabling the body to respond more quickly to subsequent infections.

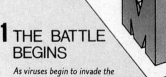

1 THE BATTLE BEGINS

As viruses begin to invade the body, a few are consumed by macrophages, which seize their antigens and display them on their own surfaces. Among millions of helper T cells circulating in the bloodstream, a select few are programmed to "read" that antigen. Binding to the macrophage, the T cell becomes activated..

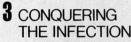

2 THE FORCES MULTIPLY

Once activated, helper T cells begin to multiply. They then stimulate the multiplication of those few killer T cells and B c[...] that are sensitive to the invad[...] viruses. As the number of B c[...] increases, helper T cells signa[...] them to start producing antibodies.

3 CONQUERING THE INFECTION

Meanwhile, some of the viruses have entered cells of the body — the only place they are able to replicate. Killer T cells will sacrifice these cells by chemically puncturing their membranes, letting the contents spill out, thus disrupting the viral replication cycle. Antibodies then neutralize the viruses by binding directly to their surfaces, preventing them from attacking other cells. Additionally, they precipitate chemical reactions that actually destroy infected cells.

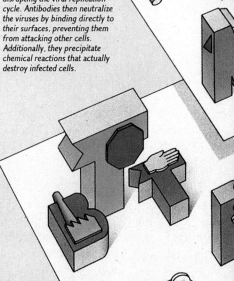

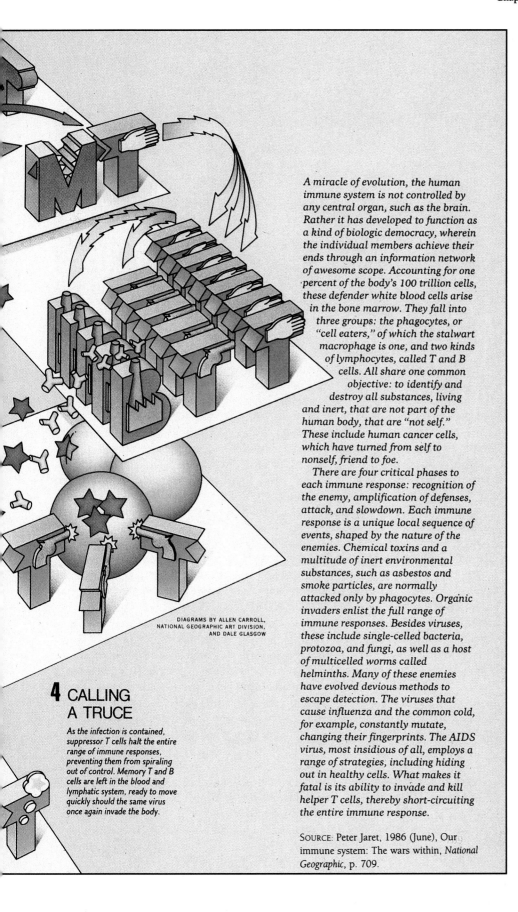

DIAGRAMS BY ALLEN CARROLL,
NATIONAL GEOGRAPHIC ART DIVISION,
AND DALE GLASGOW

4 CALLING A TRUCE

As the infection is contained, suppressor T cells halt the entire range of immune responses, preventing them from spiraling out of control. Memory T and B cells are left in the blood and lymphatic system, ready to move quickly should the same virus once again invade the body.

A miracle of evolution, the human immune system is not controlled by any central organ, such as the brain. Rather it has developed to function as a kind of biologic democracy, wherein the individual members achieve their ends through an information network of awesome scope. Accounting for one percent of the body's 100 trillion cells, these defender white blood cells arise in the bone marrow. They fall into three groups: the phagocytes, or "cell eaters," of which the stalwart macrophage is one, and two kinds of lymphocytes, called T and B cells. All share one common objective: to identify and destroy all substances, living and inert, that are not part of the human body, that are "not self." These include human cancer cells, which have turned from self to nonself, friend to foe.

There are four critical phases to each immune response: recognition of the enemy, amplification of defenses, attack, and slowdown. Each immune response is a unique local sequence of events, shaped by the nature of the enemies. Chemical toxins and a multitude of inert environmental substances, such as asbestos and smoke particles, are normally attacked only by phagocytes. Organic invaders enlist the full range of immune responses. Besides viruses, these include single-celled bacteria, protozoa, and fungi, as well as a host of multicelled worms called helminths. Many of these enemies have evolved devious methods to escape detection. The viruses that cause influenza and the common cold, for example, constantly mutate, changing their fingerprints. The AIDS virus, most insidious of all, employs a range of strategies, including hiding out in healthy cells. What makes it fatal is its ability to invade and kill helper T cells, thereby short-circuiting the entire immune response.

SOURCE: Peter Jaret, 1986 (June), Our immune system: The wars within, *National Geographic*, p. 709.

Before polio vaccines were developed by Jonas Salk and Albert Sabin in the 1950s, many people, especially children, were paralyzed or killed by this viral infection. This boy is being given oral polio vaccine as part of an inoculation program for school children.

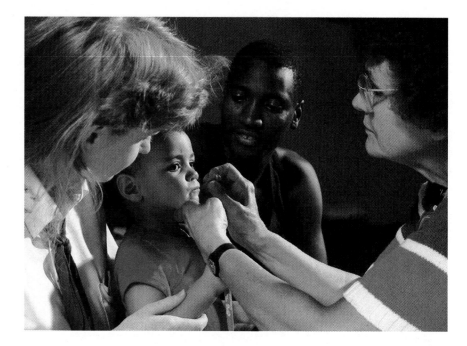

terferons, chemicals that are part of the T-cell response. And rashes can occur when the infecting organisms have spread throughout the system and break out on the skin.

You are contagious when there are active organisms replicating in your body and they can gain access to another person. This may be before a vigorous immune response has occurred, so at times you may be contagious before experiencing any symptoms. This means that you can transmit an illness to another person without knowing you're infected or catch an illness from someone who doesn't appear to be sick. On the other hand, your symptoms may continue after the invading organisms have been mostly destroyed, when you are no longer infectious.

Immunization   The ability of the immune system to remember previously encountered organisms and retain its strength against them is the basis for immunization. When a person is immunized against a disease, the immune system is "primed" with an antigen that's similar to the disease-causing organism but not as dangerous. The body responds by producing antibodies to the organism, which prevent serious infection when and if the person is exposed to the disease itself. The preparations used to manipulate the immune system this way are known as **vaccines**.

Vaccines were first used by English physician Edward Jenner late in the eighteenth century. He had noticed that people who milked cows occasionally showed an infection similar to the dreaded smallpox. These victims of cowpox—a relatively mild disease—never contracted the lethal smallpox. He rubbed scrapings from infected cow udders into the skin abrasions of people who had not had smallpox to see if this procedure would protect them.

It did: none of these people—the first to be vaccinated—contracted smallpox.

Smallpox and cowpox are caused by closely related viruses. Cowpox virus doesn't cause severe illness, but it does stimulate the lymphocytes to produce antibodies against smallpox. Without knowing the specifics of how the immune system works, Jenner had grasped the essence of the body's immune response. In the middle of the nineteenth century, French chemist Louis Pasteur developed similar procedures against other diseases, such as rabies.

Today, vaccines are made in several ways. In some cases, organisms are cultured in the laboratory in a way that weakens (attenuates) them. These "live, attenuated" organisms are used in vaccines against such diseases as measles, mumps, and rubella (German measles). In other cases, when it's not possible to breed attenuated organisms, vaccines are made from pathogens that have been killed in the laboratory but that still retain their ability to stimulate the production of antibodies. Vaccines composed of "killed" viruses are used against influenza viruses, among others. A third type of vaccine has been developed to protect against tetanus. This disease is caused by a bacterium that thrives in deep puncture wounds and produces a deadly toxin. The vaccine is made from a "toxoid" that resembles the toxin—that is, lymphocytes recognize it as being the same—but that doesn't produce the same effects. Tetanus shots are normally needed every ten years, but in the case of a deep wound, a tetanus shot may be needed if five years have elapsed since the last shot. Immunizations available in the United States are listed in Table 18-1.

Vaccines confer what is known as *active immunity*—that is, the vaccinated person produces his or her own

Table 18-1 Immunizations available in the United States

Type of Immunization	Who Should Be Immunized	Effectiveness of Immunization and Frequency of Booster Doses
Cholera	Foreign travelers	Only partial immunity; renew every 6 months for duration of exposure
Diphtheria	Children; all adults in good health with no previous immunization; travelers	Highly effective; renew every 10 years
German measles (rubella)	Mainly for children	Highly effective; need for boosters not established
Influenza	All adults of any age, especially those with chronic disease of the heart, respiratory tract, or endocrine system	Renew every year (because viral strains change easily)
Measles	Mainly for children	Highly effective; usually produces lifelong immunity; some states now require booster for school entry
Mumps	Most helpful to children and young adults who have not had mumps	Believed to confer lifetime immunity
Plague	Anyone exposed; travelers to Asia, Africa, and Tibet	Incomplete protection; boosters necessary every 3 to 6 months
Polio	Children; all adults, particularly travelers, those exposed to children, and those in health and sanitation industries	Long-lasting immunity; no booster necessary unless exposure anticipated
Rabies	Only those bitten by rabid animal	A vaccination each day for 14 to 21 days beginning soon after the bite
Rocky Mountain spotted fever	—	Not very effective
Tetanus (lockjaw)	Everyone	Very effective, renew every 10 years or when treated for a contaminated wound if more than 5 years have elapsed since last booster
Tuberculosis	High-risk people; nurses and children in contact with active tubercular cases	Variably effective
Typhoid fever	Anyone exposed; travelers	About 80 percent effective
Typhus	Anyone exposed	Renew every year (if exposed)
Whooping cough (pertussis)	Essential for children by age 3 to 4 months	Highly effective
Yellow fever	Anyone exposed; travelers	Highly effective; provides immunity for at least 17 years

antibodies to the microorganism. Another type of injection confers *passive immunity*. In this case, a person exposed to a disease is injected with the antibodies themselves, produced by other human beings or animals who have recovered from the disease. Injections of **gamma globulin**—a product made from the blood plasma of many individuals, containing all the antibodies they have

ever made—are sometimes given to people exposed to a disease against which they haven't been immunized. Such injections create a rapid but temporary immunity and are useful against certain bacterial infections, such as diphtheria, tetanus, and botulism, and against certain viruses, such as hepatitis. Gamma globulin is also sometimes used to treat antibody deficiency syndromes.

Vaccines   A preparation of killed or weakened pathogens injected or taken orally, thereby arousing the body's natural adaptive immune system to produce specific antibodies.

Gamma globulin   Serum containing specific antibodies, injected to provide temporary immunity to specific antigens.

Allergy—The Body's Defense System Gone Haywire

You probably know someone with **allergies**, or perhaps you have an allergy yourself. Allergic reactions are a response of the immune system, but in this case the response is inappropriate, annoying, and sometimes even life-threatening. Allergic reactions occur when the body recognizes a relatively harmless substance, such as dust, pollen, or animal hair, as a dangerous antigen and mounts an immune response to it. B-cells multiply, antibodies are produced, and quantities of histamine and other substances are released from cells near the location of the invasion. The resulting inflammatory response produces such symptoms as runny nose, red, itchy eyes, sneezing, congestion, hives, and asthma. The full course of the allergic reaction, as well as the latest research into this still-mysterious overreaction of the immune system, is described in the box "Stalking the Sneezemakers."

The Troublemakers—Pathogens and Disease

Now that we've discussed the beautiful and intricate system that protects us from disease, let's consider some pathogens, those disease-producing organisms that live within us and around us. When they succeed in gaining entry to body tissue, they can cause illness and sometimes death to the unfortunate host. They include bacteria, viruses, fungi, protozoa, and parasitic worms.

■ Exploring Your Emotions

Do you feel confident that you can avoid major infections, or do you feel somewhat helpless in the face of them? How do your feelings differ about your ability to avoid such infections as colds, the flu, tuberculosis, gonorrhea, and AIDS?

Bacteria   Among the microorganisms that exist everywhere in our environment are one-celled organisms called **bacteria.** Essential for life as we know it, bacteria break down dead organic matter, allowing it to be restructured for use by other organisms so that life can go on. They also perform a similar task in our intestines, helping digest food for better absorption by the body. If we view the entire digestive tract as a long hollow tube beginning in the mouth and moving down the esophagus, stomach, small and large intestine to the anus, we see that even though bacteria reside inside the intestine, they are not really a part of the body. Underneath the skin, within the bloodstream, tissues and organs, the body is devoid of bacteria, or "sterile". Bacteria found in these areas are almost always pathogenic, or disease-producing. It is here that the immune system keeps up its constant surveillance, seeking out and destroying any invaders.

Bacteria can cause infection almost anywhere in or on the body. They can cause meningitis, an infection of the spinal fluid and tissue surrounding the brain; conjunctivitis, infection of the layer of cells surrounding the eyes; pharyngitis or "sore throat"; bronchitis, infection of the airways (bronchi); pneumonia, infection of the lung itself; gastroenteritis or enterocolitis, infections of the gastrointestinal tract; cellulitis, infection of the soft tissues; osteomyelitis, infection of the bones; and so on, for each tissue and organ.

Because of their tiny size, bacteria cannot be seen with the naked eye. It was only in the seventeenth century that Anton van Leeuwenhoek invented the microscope and provided the means of understanding what had been suspected since biblical times; namely that many diseases are transmitted by "invisible creatures." Van Leeuwenhoek also described the major forms of bacteria, which he called "animalcules."

Today we know them as bacilli (rods), cocci (spheres), and spirochetes (spirals).

In the 1880s, a Danish microbiologist, Christian Gram, devised a special stain to help identify some of these organisms. Today, this same stain is still used to visualize and classify bacteria and thus to help diagnose disease. Organisms that stain dark blue are called "gram-positive"; those that stain red are "gram-negative".

Gram-positive Bacteria   In the laboratory, specimens from diseased patients are cultured; that is, they are placed on special media to aid the growth of bacteria. It is the job of the microbiologist to discover which particular bacterium is responsible for the underlying illness. This detective work often starts with the gram stain. For example, the bacterium that often inflames the tonsils and throat is the **streptococcus,** a gram-positive (stains blue) coccus (sphere) that often grows in chains. Another gram-positive coccus is **staphylococcus,** which appears

---

Allergies   Diseases caused by the body's own exaggerated response to foreign chemicals and proteins.

Bacteria   Organisms about 100–1,000 times larger than viruses, about 100 species of which can cause disease in humans.

Streptococci   Bacteria that cause infections such as strep throat, which can lead to serious cardiac damage.

Antihistamines   Drugs that interfere with histamine and its effects.

Mast cells   Body cells that release histamine.

Staphylococci   Bacteria, found on the skin, that can cause infection if allowed to multiply in food and then ingested.

Stalking the Sneezemakers

If you are a hay fever sufferer, you may well feel that pollinating plants conspire against you personally. Or you may confer "culprit" status on dust, tobacco smoke, animal dander, lobster Newburg . . . any of a host of potential allergy triggers, or allergens. Yet most allergens are harmless substances; the problem is a person's inappropriate *response* to them.

A key part of that response is the release of a chemical called *histamine*. Histamine can set off all the familiar symptoms of an allergy attack, ranging from the sniffling, tearing, and sneezing of hay fever to the itchy redness of hives or the wheezing and gasping of asthma.

Researchers have known about histamine's role in allergies since the turn of the century; **antihistamines**—drugs that counter its effects—have been the cornerstone of allergy tretament for some time. But a detailed understanding of what histamine actually does has only developed since the 1960s. In the last decade researchers have uncovered other crucial substances that conspire with histamine to trigger the allergic response.

Antigen Meets Antibody

No one knows precisely why some people get allergies and others don't. Since allergies tend to run in families, heredity must play some role. But genes cannot be the whole story. To some degree, allergies may involve luck. As the immune system develops in the womb and during infancy, the genes in immune system cells undergo a random shuffling. As a result, no two people have precisely identical immune systems, and some may be more likely to spawn allergies than others.

Allergies arise when the immune system—so efficient at identifying and destroying disease-causing organisms like foreign bacteria and viruses—gets all worked up over basically benign invaders (a pollen particle, for example). This oversensitivity involves an excess of one or more antibodies, which are proteins designed to latch onto unwelcome organisms and substances, marking them for destruction.

The antibodies that trigger allergic responses all belong to the broad class known as *immunoglobin E,* or IgE. IgE antibodies tend to take up residence on the surface of **mast cells**, which congregate in the soft tissue surrounding blood vessels in the lungs, sinuses, skin, and other areas. Among other things, mast cells contain reservoirs of histamine, which they stand ready to release on the proper signal.

If a person's mast cells are well stocked with IgE antibodies against a particular allergen, and if that allergen comes along and binds to them, the histamine floodgates open and the trouble begins.

Wide-ranging Effects

Histamine's main effect is to render nearby blood vessels more porous, allowing fluid and cells from the blood to flood the local tissue. Histamine also stimulates mucus production and, primarily in the lung, it can cause smooth muscle (the kind that functions without our awareness) to contract.

The precise symptoms that result depend on what part of the body is affected. In the nose, histamine causes flushing, congestion, and sneezing, mostly as a result of the influx of fluid from blood to tissue and the consequent blockage of airways. In the eyes, it can produce tearing, itching, and inflammation around the eyelids (conjunctivitis). In the skin, it can cause redness, swelling, and itching; and in the lungs, it can make breathing difficult by causing the muscles surrounding air passages to contract.

The most serious kind of allergic reaction, called *systemic anaphylaxis,* involves a widespread release of histamine throughout the body. Systemic anaphylaxis can cause a life-threatening loss of blood pressure known as *anaphylactic shock.* Although rare, this condition is most often brought on by bee stings or penicillin reactions in very sensitive individuals.

Allergic responses aren't the only way to cause the release of histamine. In some people, cold weather or heavy exercise can stimulate histamine release and bring on an asthma attack. In others, contact with ice can cause a skin rash.

The nervous system and emotions may also influence histamine release, by means not yet fully understood. One recent study even suggested that histamine release can be learned. In that study, guinea pigs were presented with a certain odor whenever they were exposed to a substance they were allergic to. Later, when presented with the odor but not the allergen, they still developed symptoms and had increased histamine in the blood.

(continued)

Stalking the Sneezemakers (continued)

Covert Co-conspirators

Although histamine clearly plays a major role in generating allergic symptoms, new research shows that it shares the stage with other, rarer cell products, such as *leukotrienes, prostaglandins,* and *platelet-activating factor (PAF).*

Unlike histamine, which is stored in mast cells awaiting release, these substances are manufactured on the spot, as they are needed. Like histamine, however, they contribute greatly to the inflammation of surrounding tissue, and molecule for molecule, they are considerably more potent.

Histamine and these other allergy mediators complement each other's actions in complex ways that researchers are only beginning to understand. In particular, it is hoped that further study of their interplay may lead to improved strategies for countering the "late-phase response" that affects many people with asthma or hay fever. In those individuals, an allergy or asthma attack often is followed several hours later by a milder repeat attack, which occurs even without further exposure to the offending allergen. It may be that the initial burst of mast cell products sets off a molecular chain reaction, which eventually comes full cycle and retriggers the release of histamine.

Pharmaceutical researchers are currently eyeing the possibility of drugs to block the action of the new-found mediators, the way antihistamines block histamine. So far, leukotriene blockers are showing the most promise. It seems to make sense that the more mediators we can block, the more allergy relief is in store.

And, just as the advent of antihistamines paved the way for new insights into histamine itself, leukotriene blockers and the like should help researchers refine their knowledge about which of these mediators does what, and when.

Adapted from Martha V. White and Ralph Bonheim. 1987. Allergy research: Stalking the sneezemakers. R_x *Being Well*, March-April, pp. 38–42.

---

in small clusters under the microscope. Its name means "cluster of grapes." These bacteria reside on the skin even in healthy individuals, but can cause many diseases, including boils and other skin infections. A species of these bacteria, *Staphylococcus aureus,* is responsible for toxic shock syndrome. The bacteria produce a deadly toxin that causes shock (potentially life-threatening low blood pressure), high fever, a peeling skin rash, and inflammation of several organ systems. The disease was first diagnosed in women using highly absorbent tampons, which appear to deplete the vaginal environment of magnesium. It has more recently been found in women not using tampons and in men as well.

Gram-negative Bacteria   Gram-negative organisms are more commonly bacilli (rod-shaped). They inhabit the intestines of all of us but generally are not present in the mouths or on the skin of healthy people. These organisms most often cause disease when there is a breakdown in the normal immune system or when the gut integrity is breached. They can also cause urinary tract infections.

Spirochete Infections   Spirochetes, the spiral-shaped organisms, are very difficult to grow in culture. As a result, researchers have had difficulties in understanding their life cycle as well as in diagnosing infections caused by these pathogens. Syphilis is caused by the spirochete *Treponema pallidum* (see Chapter 17). A different spirochete, *Borrelia burgdorferi,* causes the illness known as Lyme disease. Here, the spirochetes are transmitted by ticks, which usually feed on deer, mice, or rabbits but sometimes bite humans. Lyme disease, like syphilis, manifests in three distinct stages. In the first stage an expanding red rash develops from the area of the tick bite, usually about two weeks after the bite occurs. (A rash that occurs within three days is probably just a reaction to the bite itself.) Some people develop flu-like symptoms as well. The second stage occurs weeks to months later in about 10 to 20 percent of untreated patients. Symptoms involve the nervous or cardiovascular systems and can include impaired motor coordination, partial facial paralysis, and heart rhythm abnormalities. These symptoms usually disappear within a few weeks. The third stage, which occurs in about half of untreated people, can occur years after the tick bite and usually consists of chronic or recurring arthritis (an inflammation of the joints), almost always affecting the knees. Lyme disease can also cause fetal damage or death at any stage of pregnancy. See the box "Lyme Disease Alert: How Can You Be Safe?" for some guidelines on avoiding this disease.

Lyme Disease Alert: How Can You Be Safe?

In recent years, every summer has brought an increasing number of reported cases of Lyme disease. First identified as a form of arthritis in 1975 in the woodlands around Lyme, Connecticut, this disease occurs mainly in three regions: (1) wooded coastal areas of New York, New Jersey, and New England; (2) Wisconsin and Minnesota; and (3) wooded coastal areas of northern California and Oregon. Although sporadic cases have been reported in forty-three states, about 90 percent of all cases have occurred in eight states in these three areas.

Fortunately, this tick-borne disease is treatable with antibiotics and curble during its initial states, but early treatment is crucial. It's up to the individual to know how to reduce the risk of contracting Lyme disease and how to watch for signs of trouble. Here's what you need to know.

1. Lyme disease is caused by a spirochete that is transmitted primarily via certain species of deer tick. Adult ticks are about one-tenth of an in inch long, and immature ticks, called nymphs, are about the size of a pinhead. Nymphs are the chief threat to humans because they often go unnoticed until they become engorged with blood, at which point they may already have transferred the infection. Of course, not all ticks are deer ticks, not all deer ticks are infected, and not all infected deer ticks transfer the bacteria during a bite. Time is crucial: the longer the tick is attached to your skin, the greater your risk. Researchers estimate that the probability of infection is low during the first couple of hours. (A full feeding lasts 48 hours.)

2. The ticks tend to thrive in the summer months (May through August) in wooded areas and particularly in areas where suburban lawns meet woodlands. They wait on low vegetation and transfer themselves to whatever brushes by; they don't fly or jump. Dogs and cats can carry the ticks to your home and property.

3. You may not know that you've been bitten by a tick (fewer than half of all people with Lyme disease were aware they had been bitten), and you may not recognize the early symptoms of Lyme disease. If you have been in an area where Lyme disease is a problem and you notice any symptoms—a rash or a flu-like illness within the next two to three weeks—call your physician. (See the text for a full description of symptoms.)

4. If you discover a tick attached to your skin, remove it immediately. Don't try to detach it with your bare fingers; bacteria from a crushed tick may be able to penetrate even unbroken skin. Instead, use a pair of fine-tipped tweezers. In fact, if you spend much time hiking or gardening in overgrown areas, a pair of "tick tweezers" (available at many sporting goods stores) should be part of your first aid kit.

To remove a tick, grip it as close to your skin as possible and gently pull it straight away from you until it releases its hold. Don't twist it as you pull, and don't squeeze its bloated body—that may actually inject bacteria into your skin. Then thoroughly wash your hands and the bite area: apply antiseptic (such as rubbing alcohol). If you must touch the tick, cover your fingers with tissue; then wash your hands thoroughly. Save the tick in a small container or plastic bag in case identification becomes an issue. Contact your physician to see what you should do next. You may be told to wait to see if you develop symptoms, or, if you live where Lyme disease is prevalent, you may be put on antibiotics right away. There is no vaccine for the disease, and one occurrence does not protect you against new infections.

5. Whether you're hiking in the woods or playing in your yard in an area where Lyme disease has been reported, take these precautions to protect yourself from ticks:

- Cover your body as much as possible. Wear long pants and a long-sleeved shirt with buttoned cuffs. Don't go barefoot. Tuck your shirt into your pants and your pants into your socks, shoes, or boots. Wear light-colored, tightly woven fabrics: it's easier to spot ticks on white or tan slacks than on dark ones, and the ticks may not be able to grab onto the tight weave of slippery materials such as nylon. A hat may help too, since ticks like to settle on the scalp.

- In overgrown countryside, try to stay near the center of trails.

- Check yourself occasionally for ticks, especially when

(continued)

Lyme Disease Alert: How Can You Be Safe? (continued)

you're in underbrush or forests. Later do a thorough check of your entire body. Have someone look at your back and head if possible, or use two mirrors. Shower and shampoo after your outing; this may help remove ticks that haven't yet begun to feed. Check your clothes too; wash them immediately to remove any ticks that may be hidden in creases. Inspect any gear you were carrying.

- Check pets after they've been outdoors. Remove ticks from them as you would from yourself.
- Inspect children daily for ticks, especially during the summer.
- Use an insect repellent containing deet (short for N,N-diethyltoluamide) on your pants, shoes, and socks. Deet repels ticks and is relatively safe, but it can cause allergic reactions, especially in chil-

dren, and should be used sparingly.

If you take these precautions and know what to watch for, you can still enjoy the woods and countryside without taking a chance of getting Lyme disease.

Adapted from Lyme disease alert, *University of California, Berkeley, Wellness Letter*, June 1989.

As mentioned earlier, spirochetes are difficult to grow in culture; therefore, diagnosis in these diseases usually depends on the measurement of specific antibodies to the organisms in the patient's blood. This can be confusing, because once we develop antibodies we often retain them for life, regardless of whether the organism is causing disease.

Other Bacteria and Bacteria-like Organisms   A multitude of organisms aren't easily categorized by gram stain. **Tuberculosis** (TB) is caused by a bacterium that requires a special stain called "acid fast." Early in this century TB was a major killer, but it is now a treatable disease. Unfortunately, we are now seeing a resurgence, rather than a disappearance, of this disease, due to two factors: susceptibility of people with AIDS and an increased number of immigrants from countries where TB is a more common problem. The infection is transmitted via the respiratory route and almost always manifests as a pneumonia, an infection of the lungs.

Mycoplasma is an organism like other bacteria, but with an incomplete cell wall. It will not grow on the usual laboratory culture media, so special techniques are required to culture it. It is the most common cause of pneumonia in young adults and may also cause ear infections and sore throats. **Rickettsiae** are the agents of Rocky Mountain spotted fever and typhus and are transmitted by ticks, fleas, and lice.

The body's immune system can fight off many, if not

most bacterial infections. However, while the body musters its defenses, some bacteria can cause a great deal of damage. In fact, some of the body's defense mechanisms also cause damage: inflammation, caused by the gathering of white blood cells, may lead to scarring and permanent damage of tissues. In helping the body deal with these infections, science and medicine have made what is possibly their greatest contribution to humankind: antibiotics.

Antibiotics   Antibiotics are both naturally occurring and synthetic substances having the ability to kill bacteria. Most of the natural antibiotics are produced by molds. **Penicillin**, for example, was discovered by Alexander Fleming in 1929 when he noticed that bacteria growing on a culture were inhibited by a mold left in the laboratory overnight. Since that time thousands of naturally occurring substances have been screened for antibiotic activity, and many have been marketed for use in treating infected patients. Other antibiotics have been created completely in the test tube.

However they originated, most antibiotics work in a similar fashion: they interrupt the production of new bacteria by damaging some part of their reproductive cycle or by causing faulty parts of new bacteria to be made. Penicillins (plural because there are now a great many similar compounds used for this purpose) inhibit the formation of the cell wall when bacteria divide to form new cells. Other antibiotics inhibit the production of certain

---

Tuberculosis   A bacterial disease almost always infecting the lungs.

Mycoplasma   One of the smallest bacteria; has an incomplete cell wall.

Rickettsiae   Organisms that can reproduce only inside living cells; transmitted by ticks, fleas, and lice.

Penicillin   An antibiotic substance produced by the fungus penicillium.

Plasmid   A small segment of DNA carrying a few genes.

Antibiotic Overuse

Almost everyone has taken antibiotics at one time or another for strep throat, respiratory infections, or the like. However, evidence shows that these drugs are being misused and overused, and some serious medical problems may be in the making. The problems center on the possibility of creating antibiotic-resistant bacteria.

When bacteria are repeatedly exposed to small doses of antibiotics, they develop a resistance to the drug in order to survive when the drug is present. Not all the bacteria can do this, and many are readily killed by the drug. The bacteria that are not killed are the ones most resistant to the drug's effect, and they are the only ones left to reproduce. Soon, a whole colony of drug-resistant bacteria exists, able to cause illness.

To make matters worse, antibiotic-resistant bacteria that normally reside harmlessly in the digestive system can probably give up the drug-resistance portion of their genetic material, called a **plasmid,** to a more dangerous pathogenic strain of bacteria. That is, if a normal inhabitant of the gastrointestinal tract were to become resistant to antibiotics and then came in contact with, say, pneumonia bacteria, theoretically the plasmids that confer drug resistance could jump into the pneumonia bacterium. In this way, a strain of pneumonia might develop that would not respond to antibiotic therapy. It is a scientific fact that bacteria develop resistance to antibiotics upon repeated exposure; also a fact: they share resistance plasmids with other bacteria. The only missing link in the theory at present is the actual epidemic

of drug-resistant diseases. Some people think that we are on the brink of disaster.

Misuse of the drugs may stem from a lack of understanding of what antibiotics can and can't do. For example, most virus-caused diseases, such as the common cold, do not respond to antibiotics. Repeatedly taking antibiotics for a cold is a waste of money and could set the stage for a much more serious problem.

Some people use illegally obtained antibiotics or leftover prescriptions to try to treat their own diseases without the aid of a physician. Not only do they take a shot in the dark at their own cure, but also they risk breeding and passing on bacterial superstrains to others because of improper doses and procedures that promote resistance. We now have among us antibiotic-resistant gonorrhea, as well as influenza bacteria, salmonella strains that cause digestive illnesses, and strep throat bacteria that no longer respond to the standard antibiotics.

Antibiotic misuse is responsible, though less directly, for other instances of these superinfections. Many people don't realize that agriculture routinely mixes antibiotics into daily animal feeds. It was discovered that not only do small daily doses of the drugs prevent infections when animals are crowded together, but that the drugs also promote extra growth in meat animals. There is strong evidence that animals may serve as breeding grounds for superinfection bacteria that can be served to the family at the dinner table, along with the hamburgers.

Not everyone agrees that the use of antibiotics in animal feed con-

stitutes overuse. An example is the American Council on Science and Health (ACSH), an independent group that claims to evaluate consumer issues impartially. The ACSH points to the absence of epidemics caused by antibiotic-resistant bacteria as proof that such epidemics are not developing. We would be seeing pockets of such infection in the population already if such an epidemic were brewing, according to the ACSH, and until we do, the threat is only hypothetical. If antibiotics were prohibited from use in animal feed, more expensive farming methods would be necessary, fewer animals could be raised each year, and the consumer would foot the bill for the added expenses at the grocery checkout counter. The consumers must choose, the ACSH says, between paying higher meat prices and paying affordable prices but also taking a *hypothetical* risk of superbug infection.

At the opposite extreme stands the Center for Science in the Public Interest (CSPI), a consumer group that often takes an anti-industry view. They say that the consumers are bearing a great risk for the convenience of meat farmers. They point out that infections in animals can be prevented by good agriculture—that is, by less animal crowding and less stress for the animal population. Indeed, independent studies confirm that antibiotics make the biggest differences in the weight gains of animals that are under stress from overcrowding. The CSPI believes that these animals are suffering from infections caused by the stresses of their living conditions and that the antibiotics

(continued)

Antibiotic Overuse (continued)

probably enhance growth because they wipe out the organisms of disease.

The CSPI concludes that the antibiotics should be discontinued and animals should be given healthy environments to live in. If higher meat prices are the result, then so be it.

Medical organizations, so far, tend to favor the latter argument, not out of concern for the quality of life of the animals, but because evidence of antibiotic-resistant infection is beginning to surface. Recently, there was an outbreak of disease caused by just such an infection of superstrain food bacteria. Eighteen people became ill,

and one person died because the infection that was causing the illness could not be controlled. The drug-resistant strain of *Salmonella newport* was traced to a cattle herd in which animals were also falling ill with untreatable infections from the same bacteria. The antibiotics normally used to treat the salmonella infections were useless in these cases. Investigation revealed that the same drugs had been added to the animals' feed every day, and scientists concluded that the drug-resistant bacteria had developed in the animals' intestines and had been passed to people through

normal grocery store meat products.

For the moment, science seems to be ahead of the game. New, stronger antibiotics, jokingly called "gorillacillins," have been developed that can deal with some resistant strains. Whether these, too, will lose their punch after years of overuse remains to be seen. For now, it's up to the FDA and the meat industry, as well as individual consumers, to acknowledge the danger and to curb overuse of antibiotics.

Source: Frances S. Sizer. 1986. Antibiotic overuse. *Healthline*, January-February.

necessary proteins by the bacteria, and still others interfere directly with the reading of genetic material (DNA) during the process of bacterial reproduction.

When antibiotics inhibit a specific bacteria's growth, these bacteria are said to be "sensitive." Unfortunately, many bacteria become "resistant" to antibiotics through a process of mutation and selection of the strongest bacteria. So, in treating each particular bacterial infection, a physician must keep in mind just what particular bacterium might be causing the disease; otherwise the antibiotic might not help fight the infection at all. Generally, antibiotics are useful only against bacteria; against viruses (which we discuss next), they are worthless.

Viruses   Visible only with an electron microscope, **viruses,** the smallest of the pathogens, are on the borderline between living and nonliving matter. The pure virus particle appears to have no metabolism of its own. Viruses lack all the enzymes essential to energy production and protein synthesis in normal animal cells, and they cannot grow or reproduce by themselves. They must lead a **parasitic** existence inside a cell, borrowing what they need for growth and reproduction from the cells they invade. Once a virus is inside the host cell, it sheds its protein covering and its genetic material takes control of the cell and tricks it into manufacturing more viruses like

itself. (See Figure 18-1.) The normal functioning of the host cell is thereby disrupted.

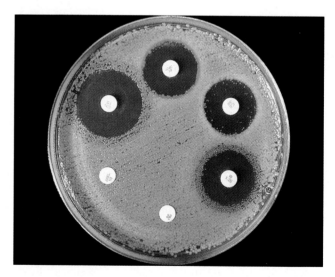

One of the dangers of antibiotic overuse is the development of bacteria resistant to drugs. Cultures of *E coli* (a bacterium normally present in the human intestine) in this laboratory dish are sensitive to four different types of antibiotics, as indicated by the wide circles where no bacteria are growing, but they are resistant to two other types, which have no effect on their growth.

Viruses   The smallest pathogenic organisms; cannot grow or reproduce by themselves.

Parasitic   Invading and surviving in the living tissue of other organisms.

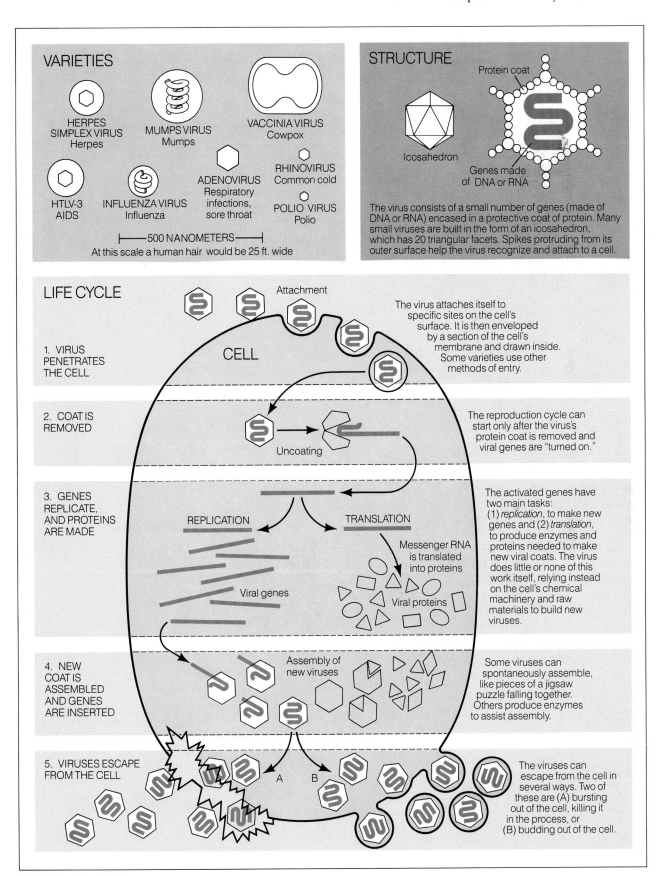

VARIETIES

HERPES
SIMPLEX VIRUS
Herpes

MUMPS VIRUS
Mumps

VACCINIA VIRUS
Cowpox

HTLV-3
AIDS

INFLUENZA VIRUS
Influenza

ADENOVIRUS
Respiratory
infections,
sore throat

RHINOVIRUS
Common cold

POLIO VIRUS
Polio

⊢——500 NANOMETERS——⊣
At this scale a human hair would be 25 ft. wide

STRUCTURE

Protein coat

Icosahedron

Genes made
of DNA or RNA

The virus consists of a small number of genes (made of
DNA or RNA) encased in a protective coat of protein. Many
small viruses are built in the form of an icosahedron,
which has 20 triangular facets. Spikes protruding from its
outer surface help the virus recognize and attach to a cell.

LIFE CYCLE

Attachment

CELL

1. VIRUS
PENETRATES
THE CELL

The virus attaches itself to
specific sites on the cell's
surface. It is then enveloped
by a section of the cell's
membrane and drawn inside.
Some varieties use other
methods of entry.

2. COAT IS
REMOVED

Uncoating

The reproduction cycle can
start only after the virus's
protein coat is removed and
viral genes are "turned on."

3. GENES
REPLICATE,
AND PROTEINS
ARE MADE

REPLICATION

TRANSLATION

Messenger RNA
is translated
into proteins

Viral genes

Viral proteins

The activated genes have
two main tasks:
(1) *replication*, to make new
genes and (2) *translation*,
to produce enzymes and
proteins needed to make
new viral coats. The virus
does little or none of this
work itself, relying instead
on the cell's chemical
machinery and raw
materials to build new
viruses.

4. NEW
COAT IS
ASSEMBLED
AND GENES
ARE INSERTED

Assembly of
new viruses

Some viruses can
spontaneously assemble,
like pieces of a jigsaw
puzzle falling together.
Others produce enzymes
to assist assembly.

5. VIRUSES ESCAPE
FROM THE CELL

A   B

The viruses can
escape from the cell in
several ways. Two of
these are (A) bursting
out of the cell, killing it
in the process, or
(B) budding out of the cell.

Figure 18-1   Viruses: varieties, structure, and life cycle.

Uncommon Facts about the Common Cold

What Causes Colds?

People often assume that "colds" (upper respiratory syndromes) are caused by exposure to the cold. Even early in this century many diseases were thought to be caused by getting chilled. Only in the 1930s did scientists discover that colds are actually caused by viruses, tiny particles that we still can't decide are "alive" or not. They are so small that more than a million could fit in one bacterium, yet they contain the basic element of life (DNA) or similar molecules known as RNA. Viruses are incomplete—they require another organism in which to reproduce. A virus tricks a cell into ingesting it and then takes over the cell's reproductive machinery, making new viruses instead of cellular proteins. At some point the cell dies, releasing the new virus particles to infect other cells. Destruction of cells lining the respiratory tract or throat for instance, can cause sore throat, cough, and runny nose.

Other symptoms are actually caused by the body's immune reaction to the virus. The body recognizes the viruses as foreign, and tries to destroy them. Special cells produce substances known as *interferons* and *leukotrienes*, which help mobilize the body's defenses. The problem is that these same substances cause fever, aches and pains, and fatigue.

Which Viruses Cause Colds?

It's no wonder colds are so common—over 200 viruses cause them. Immunity to a virus is very specific; that is, overcoming infection by one virus gives you protection against only that one, so vaccine production is difficult. This is also the reason why adults average two to five colds per year, and kids average eight to twelve per year. Colds account for 30 million days out of school, and about the same number of days off work *per year* in the United States.

Although there are so many specific cold-causing viruses, most fit into a few well-described groups.

Rhinoviruses (*rhino* means "nose" in Greek) account for up to half of all colds. These viruses like temperatures slightly cooler than the body core; hence the tendency to infect the nose. They belong to a larger group of viruses called *picornaviruses* (*pico* = small, *rna* = RNA genetic material). They are actually structurally similar to the viruses that cause polio.

There are over 100 different known rhinoviruses and probably many undiscovered varieties. Luckily, you can only get each rhinovirus once, after which you are immune. Colds from these viruses are most common in September and early October, possibly because this is when kids crowd together, back at school.

Another group is the *coronaviruses*. There are only four known varieties in this group, but they can reinfect you, because overcoming them does not give lifelong immunity. Symptoms of coronavirus colds are similar to those caused by rhinoviruses—runny nose, sneezing, often with little or no fever. Rhinovirus colds last a bit longer just over a week on average, with coronavirus colds lasting just under a week. The best way to tell the difference is that coronaviruses come more often in the winter, from December through March or April.

Adenoviruses (from the adenoids or tonsils) cause probably 5 to 10 percent of colds. These come later in the year than rhino- and coronavirus colds, usually early spring and summer. In addition to causing a dry, sore throat, fever, and runny nose, these viruses can cause an epidemic form of conjunctivitis, or "pinkeye."

A number of other viruses and even bacteria can cause syndromes similar to the common cold, but less often than those just mentioned. When a doctor says you have a "viral syndrome," you may have wondered why he or she doesn't seem to care *which* virus. The reason is that often, even despite expensive testing, the exact virus causing the disease is not identified. Even if it were, there would be no exact therapy for it. Antibiotics work in very specific ways, against portions of bacterial cell parts or reproduction. This way they do less harm to the human host than to the invading bacteria. However in general, antibiotics do not work against viruses. (We'll discuss therapeutic approaches to viruses after discussing how they are transmitted.)

Basically, colds are "caught" only from other infected people; they do not originate from getting wet or physically chilled, despite popular opinion. But people do get more colds during the frosty and wet times of year. This could be due to close contact indoors with others during these times—a great situation for a virus looking to spread. It may also be that changes in humidity or another factor during the cold days allows viruses to survive longer outside the body, accounting for increased transmission.

How Are Colds "Caught"?

Understanding transmission is very useful in preventing disease. Rhinoviruses are most easily transmitted by close personal hand-to-hand contact. Secretions from the mouth and nose of the infected person are unwittingly carried by hand to another person's hands, which then carry the virus to the nose of the next victim. Part of the human condition seems to be frequent touching of the nose and mouth. The most efficient way of interrupting this mode of transmission is frequent hand washing.

Viruses can also be transmitted in the small aerosolized particles produced by a cough or sneeze, but this requires very close contact and is not nearly as important as hand-to-hand (hand-to-nose) spread.

How to Treat a Cold

Throughout the ages, people have looked for and invented ways of treating the common cold. As early as 400 B.C., Hippocrates advocated bleeding as a cure. Much progress had been made 500 years later, when Pliny the Younger announced the best treatment as "kissing the hairy muzzle of a mouse." Even today, we can still say that there is no sure-fire cure for the common cold—not that a multitude of medicines and potions haven't been tried and touted as proven.

Consider vitamin C: Despite claims to the contrary, no one has been able, using controlled scientific testing, to show an appreciable benefit from this popular vitamin.

Interferon, genetically engineered and made to be just like the interferon your own body makes to combat colds, was given to volunteers by nasal spray. It was found, in high doses, to decrease the spread of a cold in a group of people, and also to reduce symptoms. But the dose required to show an effect caused intolerable

Is it a virus, bacteria, or allergy?	Virus	Bacteria	Allergy
Runny nose	Often	Rare	Often
Aching muscles	Usual	Rare	No
Headache	Often	Rare	No
Dizziness	Often	Rare	Rare
Fever	Often	Often	No
Cough	Often	Sometimes	Rare
Dry cough	Often	Rare	Sometimes
Raising sputum	Rare	Often	Rare
Hoarseness	Often	Rare	Sometimes
Recurs at a particular season	No	No	Often
Only a single complaint (sore throat, earache, sinus pain, or cough)	Unusual	Usual	Unusual
Do antibiotics help?	No	Yes	No
Can your physician help?	Seldom	Yes	Sometimes

side effects in the volunteers, while a well-tolerated dose was ineffective.

Numerous other drugs have been shown to be partially helpful for prevention, including one derived from an old Chinese herb. However, few of us want to take an expensive, potentially toxic drug all winter to prevent the week or two of misery we might be in for. In the meantime, research will continue the search.

Even aspirin has come under attack—some fear it may prolong the time a person sheds the virus in his or her secretions. Aspirin also is associated with an increased risk for Reye's syndrome in children. For this reason acetaminophen (such as Tylenol), rather than aspirin, should be given to children to lower a fever and reduce aches and pains. Recently, however, a preliminary study showed that ibuprofen, an aspirin-

type compound, in combination with a decongestant, actually decreased the time of viral shedding and reduced the duration of the symptoms.

Everyone has his or her own special cold remedy, but none has been proven better than chicken soup. The steam soothes a sore throat and loosens secretions, and the liquid and salt keep the patient hydrated. And loving care is probably as safe and effective as any other remedy.

So when you have a cold, it's generally OK to stay home and take "just what the doctor ordered"—rest, plenty of fluids, acetaminophen (or aspirin or ibuprofen), saltwater gargle for the sore throat, the decongestant, and chicken soup.

Source: Roger Baxter. 1988. Uncommon facts about the common cold. *Healthline*, October.

Different viruses affect different kinds of cells, and the seriousness of the disease they cause depends greatly on which kind of cell is affected. The viruses that cause colds, for example, attack upper respiratory tract cells, which are constantly cast off and replaced. The disease is therefore mild. Poliovirus, in contrast, attacks nerve cells that cannot be replaced and the consequences, such as paralysis, are severe.

More than 150 viruses are known to cause disease in humans, and illnesses caused by viruses are the most common forms of **contagious disease.** They include most of the minor ailments that cause short-lived illness and are rarely precisely diagnosed. Among these are the common cold, a variety of brief and undiagnosed respiratory infections, **influenza,** gastrointestinal upsets that cause diarrhea and can last for only twenty-four hours, and assorted aches and pains. More serious are the diseases that occur mainly in childhood and frequently cause a severe rash, such as measles, chicken pox, and mumps. Smallpox, which used to be the most severe of these diseases, has now been eliminated, thanks to a worldwide vaccination program carried out by the World Health Organization (WHO) in the 1960s and 1970s.

■ Exploring Your Emotions

How do you feel when you hear that someone has AIDS? Herpes? Chicken pox? Bronchitis? If you feel differently about these cases, what is the basis for the difference?

The herpesviruses are a large and important group of viruses. They are remarkable in that, once infected, the host is never again free of the virus (see Chapter 17). The virus lies latent within certain cells and ventures forth from time to time to produce symptoms. Normally the immune system keeps these viruses in check. However,

when the immune system is depressed—for instance, by drugs used to aid organ transplantation or by immune deficiency disease, such as AIDS—the herpesviruses may cause life threatening disease.

Infectious mononucleosis (mono) is caused by a herpesvirus called **Epstein-Barr virus.** This disease is spread by close contact and usually affects children and young adults. The virus attacks white blood cells, and its symptoms may even look like leukemia. About three weeks after contact, the infected person has a severe sore throat with painful swelling of lymph nodes in the neck, lethargy, and a fever. Antibiotics have no effect on the disease process, which is usually self-limited. Some infected people may be troubled by fatigue for weeks, even several months. The virus has been blamed for a syndrome known as "chronic fatigue," in which people can be extremely tired with muscle aches and low-grade fever for as long as several years. Recent reports in the medical literature, however, lend support to the theory that almost all patients inflicted with this disease have an emotional disorder (usually depression) as the probable cause of their fatigue.

More severe infections caused by viruses are AIDS; **poliomyelitis** (polio), a disease of the nervous system; and **hepatitis,** a liver inflammation. There are two major kinds of hepatitis. Hepatitis B, or serum hepatitis, is transmitted by blood transfusions, direct sexual contact, or hypodermic injection and is common among drug addicts. Hepatitis A is transmitted through fecal matter and spread through infected food or drink. Hepatitis A causes a less severe disease and is particularly prevalent in areas with poor hygienic conditions. It can also be spread readily wherever water is contaminated with sewage; for instance, in swimming areas close to sewage outlets. The disease is usually mild, although it is generally weakening and requires a long period of bed rest. Hepatitis B is generally more serious and may lead to extensive liver damage, a chronic carrier state, and even liver can-

---

Contagious disease   Disease that can be transmitted from one carrier to another.

Influenza   The flu—a usually mild viral disease, highly infective and adaptable; the form changes so easily that every year new strains arise, making treatment difficult.

Epstein-Barr virus   A member of the herpesvirus family associated with infectious mononucleosis.

Poliomyelitis   A disease of the nervous system, sometimes crippling; vaccines now prevent most polio.

Hepatitis   A severe liver inflammation: Type A, a less serious disease, can be transmitted through fecal matter; Type B through infected intravenous needles; Type "non-A, non-B" is less well understood.

Fungi   Molds, mushrooms, and yeasts—primitive plants.

Candidiasis   A sexually transmissible disease caused by the fungus *Candida albicans,* producing vaginitis and infant thrush (mouth sores); an opportunistic infection often accompanying AIDS.

Thrush   A yeast infection of the mouth.

Cryptococcosis   Severe systemic fungal disease.

Coccidioidomycosis   Valley fever; life-threatening systemic fungal disease.

Protozoa   Microscopic single-celled animals, often producing recurrent, cyclical attacks of disease.

Malaria   Severe, recurrent, mosquito-borne protozoal disease.

African sleeping sickness   Severe, recurrent, insect-borne protozoal disease marked by lassitude.

Amoebic dysentery   Protozoal infection of the intestines.

cer. Fortunately, all blood products are now screened for this virus and discarded if the virus is present. A third type of hepatitis, "non-A, non-B," is caused by a number of viruses that as yet have not been well characterized. Recently, a test for one of these, hepatitis C, has become available.

Certain viruses can also cause cell proliferation. The human disease resulting from this property is warts, which generally is very mild but can become extremely severe if the resistance of the infected person breaks down. There are many members of the human wart virus family, and some of them appear to be responsible for cervical cancer in women (see Chapter 16). Another virus, called HTLV-1 and distantly related to the AIDS virus, causes a rare leukemia in adults (T-cell leukemia). As our knowledge of the molecular biology of cancer increases, other tumors may turn out to be caused by viruses, but the majority of human cancers are caused by other factors.

Although most viruses cannot be treated medically, there are a few "antiviral" agents. Influenza A, for example, can be treated with a drug that actually helps cure the patient. Herpes can be treated with acyclovir, an antiviral agent that helps alleviate symptoms and decrease the length of each recurrence. However, it cannot eradicate the latent virus, so it must be taken at each recurrence. If taken daily, it can prevent recurrences as well. AIDS can be treated with AZT, which inhibits the virus and slows its progress. It affords no cure, but people tend to feel better and live longer if they take it.

■ **Exploring Your Emotions**

How do you feel about growing up in a time when sexual activity and other behaviors can lead to serious health consequences? How do you think it was different in 1970? In 1900? In 1800?

Most other viral diseases cannot be treated and must simply run their course. Over-the-counter cold remedies and pain relievers treat symptoms, not their viral cause. Acetaminophen, for example, relieves aches and pains very slightly and can bring down a fever. Decongestants relieve nasal stuffiness, but they tend to make a sore throat worse because they work by shrinking blood vessels, which in turn dries out mucosal surfaces. Antihistamines don't do much for viral upper respiratory infections; they're really helpful only if the symptoms are due to allergies. If you want to take an OTC medication for your cold or flu, it's probably better to avoid the "shotgun" approach—taking all medications at once. Take acetaminophen for a fever, decongestants for congestion, or an antihistamine for an allergy.

Fungi, Protozoa, and Parasitic Worms   The organisms referred to as **fungi** are primitive plants that may be multicellular (like molds) or unicellular (like yeasts). Mushrooms and the molds that form on bread and cheese are all examples of fungi. Only about fifty fungi out of many thousands of species cause disease in humans, and these diseases usually are restricted to the skin, mucous membranes, and lungs. Curing fungal diseases is extremely difficult. To defend themselves against treatments, some fungi form spores, which are an especially resistant dormant stage of the organism.

■ **Exploring Your Emotions**

Were you sick very much as a child? Do you remember if it was unpleasant to be sick or if there were pleasant parts to it, such as getting extra attention or staying home from school?

The most common fungal malady is **candidiasis**, a yeast infection of the vagina that can also occur in other areas of the body, especially in the mouth in infants (**thrush**). Candidiasis, which begins as a relatively mild disease that causes itching, should be treated by a physician. When untreated and persistent, the disease can become severe and inflame the mucous membranes on which it normally exists.

Another common group of fungal diseases affects the skin, including athlete's foot, jock itch, and ringworm, a disease of the scalp. These three mild diseases, although difficult to treat, rarely give rise to major problems.

Fungi can also cause systemic disease, infecting large portions of the body. Such disease is severe, life-threatening, and extremely difficult to treat. Among the systemic forms of fungal disease are **cryptococcosis** and **coccidioidomycosis**. The latter disease is also known as "valley fever" because it is most frequently seen in the San Joaquin Valley of California. Fungal infections can be especially virulent in people without a completely functioning immune system.

Another group of pathogens are the **protozoa**, microscopic single-celled animals, which are associated with such tropical diseases as **malaria, African sleeping sickness,** and **amoebic dysentery.** Many protozoa-based diseases are recurrent. The pathogen remains in the body, alternating between activity and inactivity. Hundreds of millions of Asians, Africans, and South Americans suffer from protozoal infections. The most common protozoal disease in the United States is trichomoniasis, a relatively mild vaginal infection (see Chapter 17). Another protozoal disease, which can be contracted by drinking water even in pristine wild areas, is giardiasis, characterized by diarrhea, nausea, and abdominal cramps.

Finally, the parasitic worms are the largest organisms that can enter the body to cause infection. The tapeworm, for example, can grow to a length of several feet. Worms, including such intestinal parasites as the tapeworm, hookworm, and pinworm cause a great variety of relatively mild infections. Smaller worms known as **flukes** infect such organs as the liver and lungs and, in large numbers, can be deadly. Generally speaking, worm infections originate from contaminated food or drink and can be controlled by careful attention to hygiene.

Other Immune Disorders: Cancer and Autoimmune Diseases

We've spoken at length about how the human immune system protects the body in the event of invasion by foreign microorganisms. Sometimes the body comes under attack by its own cells, most notably in cancer. In this disease cells cease to cooperate normally with the rest of the body and multiply uncontrollably. The exact causes of all cancers are mostly unknown. However, scientists are aware of several mechanisms whereby cancer cells can arise.

One of these mechanisms, simply put, is alteration of the genetic structure of a cell by a carcinogen, a substance or energy from outside the body that can predispose cells to becoming cancerous, or malignant (see Chapter 16). The immune system can often detect cells that have recently become malignant and then destroy them just as they would a foreign microorganism. But if the immune system breaks down, as it may when people get older, when they have certain immune disorders (including AIDS), or when they are receiving chemotherapy for other diseases, the cancer cells may multiply out of control before the immune system recognizes the danger. By the time the immune system gears up to destroy the cancerous cells, it may be too late.

Another immune disorder occurs when the body confuses its own cells with foreign organisms. As described earlier, the immune system must be able to recognize many thousands of antigens as foreign and then be able to recognize the same antigens again and again. Our own tissue cells also are antigenic; that is, they would be recognized by another person's immune system as foreign. A delicate balance must be maintained to ensure that one's immune system recognizes only truly foreign antigens as enemies; erroneous recognition of one's own cells as foreign produces havoc.

This is exactly what happens in what are known as "autoimmune" disorders. In this type of malady, the immune system seems to be a bit too sensitive and begins to misapprehend itself as "not-self". Rheumatoid arthritis is one such disease; the immune system attacks the joints, sometimes causing crippling arthritis. Systemic lupus erythematosus is another autoimmune disease, in which blood vessels, or the lining of the heart, lungs, or brain become inflamed when the body attacks itself.

These diseases and a number of similar disorders are treated with medicines called **anti-inflammatory medications,** which counteract some of the immune effects. In large doses, over a period of time, anti-inflammatory drugs like aspirin, ibuprofen, and certain prescription medications can slow the autoimmune process. Steroids such as prednisone have a more powerful effect on the immune system and cause the immune response to diminish to the point where the patient can actually have an immune deficiency and become susceptible to a number of serious diseases.

Giving Yourself a Fighting Chance: What You Can Do to Support Your Immune System

Pathogens pose a formidable threat to human health and lives, but many steps can be taken to prevent them from getting a foothold. Public health measures and environmental controls protect people from many diseases that are carried in water or food or by insects. A clean water supply and adequate sewage treatment help control typhoid fever and cholera, for example; and mosquito eradication programs control malaria and encephalitis. Proper food preparation prevents illness caused by food-borne pathogens. These include the parasitic roundworm *Trichina spiralis,* which causes trichinosis and is found in some uncooked meat; the salmonella bacterium, which causes food poisoning and is often found in chicken; and the deadly toxin botulinum, which causes botulism and is produced by certain bacteria in improperly canned food (usually foods canned at home). (See Chapter 12 for guidelines on preparing food safely.)

Beyond this, is there anything you can do to increase the potency of your immune response to various pathogens? In general, no. The human immune system has evolved over millions of years and is so complex, so remarkable in its ability to respond to nearly any challenge from without, that it rarely needs your conscious help. With adequate nutrition, rest, and moderation in lifestyle, most people would live a normal life span without

---

Flukes   Parasitic worms that can infest lungs and liver; can cause death.

Anti-inflammatory medications   Drugs like aspirin, ibuprofen, and corticosteroids that are often used to treat autoimmune diseases.

To Keep Yourself Well . . .

- Eat a balanced diet and maintain moderate weight. These are the best ways in which to "nourish" the immune system. No particular vitamin or mineral, including vitamin C, has been shown conclusively to prevent or treat the common cold, or any other infectious disease, for that matter (see the box entitled, "Uncommon Facts about the Common Cold.")
- Get enough sleep—six to eight hours per night. Sleep is extremely important in helping the body replenish itself. Adequate sleep allows the proper production of all immune-related cells

and products. Insufficient sleep predisposes you to a great number of illnesses and more severe infections.
- Exercise (but not while you're sick). Moderate aerobic exercise is an excellent way to reduce stress and strengthen the body, thereby preventing infection. However, exercise while you are sick—such as with a virus causing an upper respiratory infection—actually decreases your immunity and can prolong the infection, probably by facilitating the replication of the viruses. The exact mechanism of this process is unknown.

- Wash your hands. Since most viral illnesses are transmitted by hand-to-hand contact, proper hand washing with soap and hot water can often prevent transmission of disease.
- Avoid contact with people who are infectious with diseases transmitted via the respiratory route, such as influenza, chicken pox, and tuberculosis.
- Practice "safer sex" (see Chapter 17) and avoid illicit intravenous drugs to protect yourself against such diseases as hepatitis B and AIDS.

suffering dire consequences of infection. Of course, once infection has begun, some diseases can be fought with the aid of antibiotics and antiviral agents. But these medications are not helpful in *preventing* infection, except in circumstances where normal immunity is breached, such as in surgery.

Scientists have discovered, however, that even the strongest immune system (as measured by the number of helper T-cells) waxes and wanes throughout a person's life. You are most susceptible to disease at the extremes of life, namely when first born, before you have developed active immunity against most pathogens, and in old age, when the immune system, like the rest of the body, starts to deteriorate. Now, you can't avoid being young or old, but you can make sure you get appropriate vaccinations, those given to aid the immune system in case of invasion by specific pathogens. Infants should receive all required immunizations, such as diphtheria, pertussis, tetanus, measles, mumps, rubella, and polio (see Table 20–1). Adults over 65 years of age or persons with chronic respiratory diseases should receive both the pneumococcal vaccine (only once) and the influenza vaccine (every year).

One factor that is known to influence the immune response and that can also be affected by lifestyle and

■ **Exploring Your Emotions**

Have you ever noticed an association between high levels of stress in your life and a tendency to get sick? Do you feel that the two are linked?

attitudes is that nebulous entity called stress. Research has shown that the actual number of helper T-cells rises and falls inversely with stress; that is, the higher the stress, the lower the T-cell count. The term *stress* encompasses a great number of variables ranging from emotional stressors, such as anger, anxiety, depression, and grief, to physical stressors, such as poor nutrition, sleep deprivation, overexertion, and addictions, to name a few. Obviously, there's no magic potion you can take to relieve stress, since it is an integral and necessary part of life. But developing effective ways of coping with stress is essential to your overall good health (see Chapter 2).

In addition to managing the stress in your life and getting all your immunizations, you can help your body defend itself against disease by following the tips in the box entitled "To Keep Yourself Well . . . " As is the case with all your body systems, your immune system works best when you support it with a healthy lifestyle.

Summary

- The immune system works to keep the body from being overwhelmed not just by outside organisms but also by internal changes such as cancer.

The Body's Defense System

- The body's defense system against outside organisms consists of physical and chemical barriers, backed up by the immune system.
- The skin prevents microorganisms from entering the body. Cells in the mucous membranes of the mouth prevent the passage of unwanted organisms by means of antibodies and enzymes. Cilia sweep foreign matter up and out of the respiratory tract.
- Foreign organisms still manage to enter the body by penetration of the skin, inhalation, or ingestion.
- The immune response is carried out by white blood cells that are continuously produced in the bone marrow. Macrophages are cell-eating white cells that congregate in the lymph nodes and filter bacteria. Lymphocytes travel in the bloodstream and lymph system.
- B-cells are lymphocytes that produce antibodies. T-cell lymphocytes are divided into helper T-cells, killer T-cells, and suppressor T-cells. The first time T-cells and B-cells encounter an invading organism, some are reserved as memory T- and B-cells in preparation for future invasions by the same organism.
- Lymphocytes recognize tiny molecular shapes on the body's own cells as "self" and shapes on the cells of invading organisms as "not self." The latter are known as antigens. When a foreign organism appears in the body, the appropriate lymphocyte locks onto it and sets off the immune response.
- The inflammatory response occurs when cells in the area of invasion or injury release histamines and other substances that cause blood vessels to dilate and fluid to flow out of capillaries.
- The immune response has four stages: recognition of the invading pathogen; rapid replication of killer T-cells and B-cells; attack by killer T-cells; and B-cells; suppression of the immune response by suppressor T-cells.
- In many infections, survival confers immunity. Memory T- and B-cells recognize and destroy an antigen that enters the body a subsequent time.
- During a period of incubation, people rarely feel ill, though they may be contagious. Contagion exists when active organisms are replicating in the body and can gain access to another person.
- Immunization is based on the body's ability to remember previously encountered organisms and retain its strength against them. Vaccines are preparations made of antigens similar to a disease-causing organism but not so dangerous.
- Vaccines confer active immunity; injections of antibodies themselves produced by other people or animals confer passive immunity.
- Allergic reactions occur when the immune system responds to harmless substances as if they were dangerous antigens.

The Troublemakers—Pathogens and Disease

- Bacteria are one-celled organisms that break down dead organic matter; in the human digestive tract, they help digest food. Anywhere else in the body they are pathogenic. They occur as bacilli, cocci, and spirochetes.
- Gram-positive bacterial organisms like streptococcus and staphylococcus reside on the skin even in healthy individuals, but they can cause infections when they enter the body.
- Gram-negative bacteria inhabit the intestines of healthy people but cause disease when the normal immune system breaks down or when gut integrity is breached.
- Spirochetes are difficult to culture and so are not as well understood as other bacteria. Both syphilis and Lyme disease are caused by spirochetes. Lyme disease results from a tick bite and has three distinct stages; untreated, it results in chronic or recurring arthritis.
- Tuberculosis is caused by a bacterium identified by an acid fast stain.
- The mycoplasma organism has an incomplete cell wall; it causes many cases of pneumonia, ear infections, and sore throats in young adults. Carried by ticks, fleas, and mice, rickettsiae are organisms that cause Rocky Mountain spotted fever and typhus.
- Although the immune system can fight off many bacterial infections, damage can be caused by both the bacteria and the body's immune defenses. Antibiotics are both naturally occurring and synthetic substances that can kill bacteria. Most natural antibiotics, like penicillin, are produced by molds.
- Most antibiotics work by interrupting production of new bacteria—by damaging the reproductive cycle or causing faulty parts of new bacteria to be made. Bacteria can become resistant to antibiotics through mutation and selection of the strongest bacteria. Antibiotics do not work against viruses.
- Viruses, the smallest pathogens, appear to have no metabolism of their own and cannot grow or reproduce by themselves; they live a parasitic existence in the cells they invade.

- The seriousness of diseases caused by viruses depends on which kind of cell is infected. If the cells can be replaced, the disease is mild.
- Some viruses, like herpesvirus, never leave the host they infect but rather lie latent and re-emerge from time to time. They can be life-threatening in cases of immune deficiency disease.
- Viruses cause AIDS, polio, and hepatitis. Some viruses cause cell proliferation; both warts and T-cell leukemia are caused by viruses.
- Researchers have developed a few antiviral agents, such as acyclovir for herpes and AZT for AIDS.
- About fifty species of fungi can cause diseases in humans, usually restricted to the skin, mucous membranes, and lungs. The sexually transmissible yeast infection candidiasis is caused by a fungus.
- Protozoa cause several tropical diseases as well as giardiasis and trichomoniasis.

- Parasitic worm infections generally originate in contaminated food or drink.
- The immune system often detects malignant cells and destroys them as if they were pathogens. If the immune system breaks down as a result of age, immune disorders like AIDS, or chemotherapy, cancer cells can multiply before the immune system recognizes danger.
- Autoimmune diseases occur when the body identifies its own cells as foreign. Anti-inflammatory drugs and steroids can be used as treatment.

Giving Yourself a Fighting Chance

- Public health measures protect people from pathogens carried by water, food, and insects.
- The immune system needs little help other than adequate nutrition and rest, a moderate lifestyle, and protection from excessive stress. Appropriate vaccinations help protect against disease during infancy and old age.

Take Action

1. In your health diary, list the positive behaviors that help you avoid or resist infection. Consider how you can strengthen those behaviors. Then list the behaviors that tend to block your positive behaviors and put you at risk for contracting infection. Consider which of these you can change.

2. Find out from your parents or your health records which immunizations you have had, including when you last had a tetanus shot. Are your immunizations up-to-date? If they aren't, or if you're not sure, check with the health center about what they recommend.

3. Monitor yourself the next time you feel a cold coming on, keeping a record like the one shown in Chapter 1 for eating behavior. Note the symptoms, how they felt, the time and date of their occurrence, what you were doing, how you were feeling emotionally, and what you did in response to the symptoms. Keep the record until the cold is gone, noting how long it takes to run its course. Is there an association between your emotional state and how you experienced the symptoms? Between your emotional state and the length of the cold? Does taking medication (decongestant, cough syrup, etc.) make a difference in the symptoms or the duration of the cold?

4. Go to your local pharmacy and examine the cold and cough remedies. Exactly which symptoms does each one claim to alleviate, and with what active ingredient? If possible, ask the pharmacist which ones he or she recommends for various symptoms.

Selected Bibliography

Cronenberger, J. H., and J. C. Jennette. 1988. *Immunology: Basic Concepts, Diseases, and Laboratory Methods.* E. Norwalk, Conn.: Appleton and Lange.

Jawetz, E., J. L. Melnick, and E. A. Adeberg. 1987. *Review of Medical Microbiology.* E. Norwalk, Conn.: Appleton and Lange.

Mandell, G., B. Douglas, and L. Churchill. 1990. *Principles and Practices of Infectious Diseases.* New York: Churchill.

Stites, D. P., J. D. Stobo, and J. V. Wells. 1987. *Basic and Clinical Immunology,* 6th ed. E. Norwalk, Conn.: Appleton and Lange.

Recommended Readings

DeKruif, Paul. 1966. *The Microbe Hunters.* New York: Harcourt Brace. *An entertaining classic about medical discoveries; pertinent and fun to read.*

Dowling, H. F. 1977. *Fighting Infection: Conquests of the Twentieth Century.* Cambridge: Harvard University Press. *Tales of medical drama and breakthroughs, including diseases such as tuberculosis, diphtheria, and measles.*

Roueché, Burton. 1980. *The Medical Detectives.* New York: New York Times Books. *A compilation of articles from* The New Yorker *that provide insight into the medical mind. A second volume has also been published.*

Contents

Making Connections

You are aging all the time, right from the moment of birth, but the aging process gains momentum in the second half of life. Then the lifestyle behaviors that you adopted earlier begin to pay off, for better or for worse, and you start to experience directly the consequences of your choices—good health and vigor or poor health and debilitation. The scenarios presented on these pages describe situations in which people have to use information, make a decision, or choose a course of action, all related to the process and problems of aging. As you read them, imagine yourself in each situation and consider what you would do. After you've finished the chapter, read the scenarios again and see if what you've learned has changed how you would think, feel, or act in each situation.

Your mother and her sister are only two years apart, but your mother looks about ten years younger than her sister. Your aunt, an avid golfer, has deep wrinkles in her face and her skin is leathery and dry. Are her wrinkles the result of too much exposure to the sun? Are there other habits or behaviors that could account for her appearance and that you would want to avoid?

Your brother's wife has been upset lately because her parents are trying to decide whether to put her elderly grandfather in a nursing home. He's recovering from a hip injury and needs help getting around, but his mental faculties are fine and he feels he can care for himself. Your sister-in-law's parents are afraid he'll fall again and be unable to get help. The decision is traumatic for everyone involved. Is there someplace they can turn for information, counseling, and assessment? What advice can you give them?

19
Aging

You were looking at some family photos with your grandmother and came on a snapshot of her taken when she was just about your age. As you peer at it, you recognize her dark eyes, her smile, and the contours of her face. Even the way she holds her head hasn't changed. "It looks like me, doesn't it," she says, "minus all the wrinkles and gray hair. I remember clearly how I felt when that picture was taken. Inside, I'm still the same person." You hadn't thought about it very much, but when she says that you realize you think old people are qualitatively different from young people. Something happens when you become elderly, doesn't it? Isn't there a big change of some kind that transforms you into an old person?

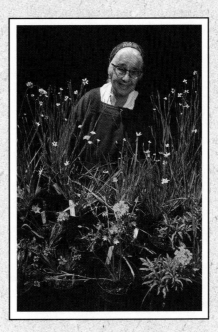

When you were home the last time, you were shocked to see a neighbor whom you had known your whole life wandering down the street in his pajamas. As you watched through the window, another neighbor ran out of her house and led him back home. When you asked your parents about it, they said he had become "demented" in his old age. "You remember how forgetful he used to be, don't you?" your father asks. What has happened to your neighbor? Is this what forgetfulness leads to in all old people? Is there anything you can or should do to avoid it yourself?

You and your housemate like your music loud and blaring, and when one of you wants to study, the other one often listens to headphones. Lately you notice your housemate doesn't seem to respond when the phone rings in another room. Could he possibly be damaging his hearing by listening to loud music, or is he just distracted? Is it OK to keep listening to the headphones?

Most people would like to live for a long time and never be old. When we see that old age grips us, we're stunned. "What has happened?" writes Aragon of ancient Greece. "It is life that has happened; and I am old." We have regarded old age as something alien, a foreign species: can I have become a different being while I still remain myself? Yes. And no. Life is a river. It changes; you change. You can't step into the same river twice, or even once. Yet there is always continuity.

Aging does not begin on the sixty-fifth birthday, and there is no precise age at which a person becomes "old." Rather, aging is the normal process of change throughout life, beginning at birth. Some people are "old" at 25; others are still young at 75. Although youth is not entirely a state of mind, your attitude toward life and attention to your health significantly determine the satisfaction you will derive from life, especially when new physical, mental, and situational challenges occur in its last quarter. What you decide, what you do, and how you interact with people today are creating the person you will be at 65 and 85. If you take charge of your health during youth, you can exert great control over the physical and mental aspects of aging, and you can better handle your response to events that might be out of your control. With foresight and energy you can shape a creative, graceful, even triumphant old age.

Generating Vitality as You Age

Circumstances, bodies, and mental facilities change. Some changes occur gradually, over a lifetime. **Biological aging**, for example, includes all the normal, progressive, irreversible changes to one's body that begin at birth and continue till death. Changes of circumstance often occur more abruptly: relocating, changing homes, losing a spouse and friends, retiring, having a lower income, switching roles and social status. Not all of these changes happen to everybody; and when they occur varies, partly depending on how people have prepared for their later days. Some never have to leave their homes and can continue friendships in the same town; some appear to be in good health until the day they die. Others have tremendous adjustments to make in entirely new surroundings with fewer financial resources, new acquaintances, increasing inability to get around, and possible loneliness and loss of self-esteem.

■ **Exploring Your Emotions**

How do you envision your old age? How will it resemble the old age of elderly people you know now, and how will it differ? What external events could affect your control of your lifestyle when you're older?

As with any other art, successful aging requires preparation. Taking stock of your mental and physical health habits right now in your teens or twenties may lead you to change strategies and practices so that you will have the best possible body and spirit sixty to seventy years down the road. By your mid-forties, you'll know your own lifestyle and how much money you need to support it. You'll want to assess your financial status and perhaps begin setting aside savings to supplement a pension and Social Security. Later, maybe in your mid-fifties you'll need to decide on health plans and retirement housing. Right now, you can pursue and cultivate hobbies you love, generate enthusiasm for activities with others and for things you love to do alone. You're already shaping many changes that will affect you during aging. They depend on what you do to and for yourself in your youth, as well as in your middle and old age. You happen to yourself!

What Happens as You Age?   Many of the characteristics we have assumed result from *chronological aging* are not due to aging at all. They are due rather to neglect and abuse of our bodies and minds. These affronts lay the foundation for later mental problems and chronic conditions like arthritis, heart disease, diabetes, hearing loss, and high blood pressure. We sacrifice our optimal health by smoking, eating a poor diet and overeating, abusing alcohol and drugs, bombarding our ears with excessive noise, and exposing our bodies to too much ultraviolet radiation from sun rays. We also jeopardize our bodies through inactivity, encouraging our muscles and even our bones to wither and deteriorate. And we endure much abuse from the toxic chemicals in our environment.

But even with the best behavior in the best environment, aging does occur. It results from biochemical processes that we don't yet fully understand. Look at Figure 19-1 to see how physiological functions decline over time and at the box "Aging and Changing: Your Body Through Time" for a summary of the bodily changes that accompany aging.

Biological aging   Changes in body parts that result from the passage of time.

Fluid intelligence   Spontaneous decision-making ability.

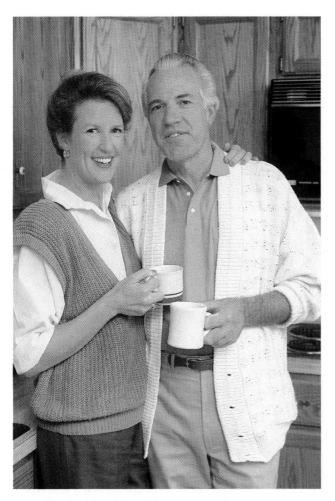

Middle age is a time of reassessment and readjustment in preparation for the second half of life. Many people in their forties and fifties who have cultivated healthy lifestyles will continue to lead vigorous lives well into old age.

Life-Enhancing Measures: Age Proofing   What you do now will influence who you are in your fifties, sixties, seventies, and eighties. Flabby muscles, "middle-age spread," loss of teeth, wrinkles, poor eyesight, stiff joints, forgetfulness, mental attitude, some chronic disease—these you can control. You can prevent, delay, lessen, even reverse the effects of some deterioration through good health habits. A few simple things you can do every day will make a vast difference to your looks, your health, your energy and vitality. The following suggestions have been mentioned throughout this text, but are profoundly related to health in later life and so are highlighted here.

Develop Physical Fitness   Exercise enhances both mental and physical health. Enough cannot be said for the positive effects of appropriate exercise throughout your life,

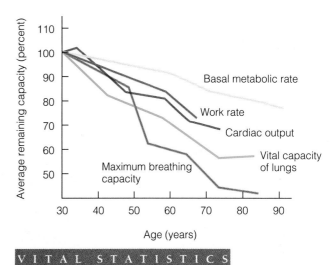

VITAL STATISTICS

Figure 19-1   Decline of basic physiological capacities with age.

particularly when weighed against the physical and mental deterioration of the elderly who have not kept their minds and bodies fit, who have not used, challenged, and stretched mind and body. The stimulus that exercise provides seems to protect against the loss of some **fluid intelligence,** our spontaneous decision-making ability. Fluid intelligence depends on rapidity of responsiveness, memory, and alertness. Contrary to former notions that this capability necessarily declines with age, studies reveal that older people who are highly fit score better on tests of intelligence than do their less fit counterparts. (In some cases, however, disease leads to the loss of mental functioning known as senility. See the box "Is 'Senility' Inevitable?") Older men who continue with racquet sports and running show faster response times than do their sedentary, age-matched control-group opposites. Exercise also appears to have some power against depression, apathy, and boredom.

Exercise is the closest thing we have to a magic anti-aging pill and the fountain of youth: it slows the aging process and lessens chances of disease. Many of the functional losses that occur between the ages of 30 and 70 are actually due to lack of exercise, not to aging itself. You need to find activities that you enjoy and can do on a regular basis. Read Chapter 14 for ideas, and build physical activity into your daily routine.

You will reap the benefits of the active and vigorous lifestyle as you age with:

- Increased resiliency and suppleness of arteries
- Better protection against heart attack and much increased chance of survival should one occur
- Sustained capacity of lungs and respiratory reserves
- Weight control through less accumulation of fat
- Maintenance of physical flexibility, balance, agility, reaction time

Aging and Changing: Your Body Through Time

Skin   Tissues throughout your body lose elasticity as you get older, so your skin doesn't snap back as well when stretched. When oil glands quit working—about ten years later for men than for women—the skin becomes drier.

Eyesight   By your mid forties you will probably become far-sighted, unable to focus clearly on nearby objects, because the ocular lens no longer expands and contracts so readily. You will lose visual acuity, the ability to distinguish fine detail. Seeing in the dark becomes more difficult, and depth perception weakens.

Hearing   The ability to hear high-pitched tones declines for most people as they age, enough so that hearing loss is now the fourth most common chronic physical disability in the United States. Even by age 35, you may not hear as well as you did at 25. These losses may be due to abuse rather than to aging, however. Extremely loud noise, such as from stereo earphones or loud machines, may contribute to hearing loss. In less industrialized and quieter societies, hearing is almost as keen in old age as it is in youth.

Taste and Smell   Sensations of taste and smell diminish with age. About two-thirds of the taste buds in the mouth die by age 70, and a large proportion of sensory receptors in the nose as well.

Hair   By age 50 half of Americans are partially gray, and hair loss in men becomes apparent. Twelve percent of men are balding by age 25, and 65 percent of men by age 65. Thickest at age 20, individual hair shafts shrink after that; by age 70, your hair will probably be as fine as when you were a baby.

Bones and Muscles   From the early twenties more minerals appear to be drawn out of the bones than are restored. As bones lose calcium, they tend to become porous, weak, prone to fractures, and slower to heal. At its extreme, the condition deteriorates to osteoporosis, a bone ailment occurring mainly in women that ends in multiple fractures of the vertebrae and pelvis. Diet and exercise may help prevent bone loss, as discussed in Chapter 12. Even without disease, height decreases with age because back muscles weaken and the discs between the bones in the spine deteriorate.

Muscles become weaker, too, although you can retard your loss of muscle strength and mass through regular hard physical work and play. As you age, more protein is being broken down and less is being synthesized, so muscle fibers atrophy and lose their ability to contract; some are lost; fat and collagen accumulate. Aging muscles are less flexible and more susceptible to strains, pulls, and cramps. After the mid forties, strength usually declines: a man may lose 10 to 20 percent of his maximum strength by 60, and a woman even more.

Your teeth, with proper care, can last a lifetime. Not aging, but disuse, abuse, and chronic degenerative disease cause teeth problems. Teeth and all their support systems respond well to the stress and stimulation of chewing hard and crunchy foods. Periodontal disease begins in early life. You can prevent it with proper dental care, as described in Chapter 21.

Heart   Your resting heartbeat stays about the same throughout

---

- Greatly preserved muscle strength
- Protection against ligament injuries, dislocation strains in the knees, spine, shoulders
- Protection against bone fractures caused by bone brittleness, demineralization, and porousness (osteoporosis)
- Increased effectiveness of the immune system
- Maintenance of mental agility and flexibility, response time, memory, hand-eye coordination

Eat Wisely   Health at every age is helped by a varied diet with perhaps special attention to lower calorie intake.

- Eat meals low in fat and high in complex carbohydrates. Concentrate on fresh fruits and vegetables; high-fiber, whole-grain cereals and breads; potatoes; brown rice; pasta.
- Eat dark-meat fish (salmon, tuna, mackerel, swordfish, rainbow trout) and poultry (no skin) instead of eggs and fatty meats.
- Use no-fat or low-fat dairy products. Substitute olive oil for other oils and fats. Say no to all but the occasional fatty, rich dessert.
- Control caloric intake so that it does not exceed your needs in maintaining an ideal weight.

Aging and Changing: Your Body Through Time (continued)

life, but the heart pumps less blood with each beat as you get older. This effect is most pronounced during exercise because your pulse can no longer rise as high as it once did. The dramatic problems of the cardiovascular system associated with aging—heart attack and stroke—are actually caused by atherosclerosis and high blood pressure, which can be largely controlled by eating right and exercising daily.

Lungs Good news: your respiratory system resists change, and your respiratory tract grows stronger with age. After a lifetime of exposure to viruses, people build up immunity and catch fewer and less severe colds by middle age. Your vital capacity—the amount of air you can expel from your lungs—should not decline if you keep fit and healthy and don't smoke. Regular and vigorous exercise can increase vital capacity in young people and reverse losses in older ones. Swimming is most effective for this.

Digestive System and Kidneys With age, your stomach will secrete less acid and smaller amounts of the enzymes that aid digestion. Digesting a meal takes longer and

may be more difficult, but your small intestines won't lose power to absorb nutrients. Kidneys deteriorate, eventually filtering wastes more slowly as they lose some filters.

Immune System With age your defense system may become less efficient, but the decline varies greatly among people. Only the progressive atrophy of the thymus gland seems invariably linked to advancing age.

Both good diet and exercise benefit the immune system. People who are in good physical shape rid themselves of respiratory infections much faster than those who are not.

Brain and Nervous System Only half as much blood travels to the brain of a 50-year-old as to that of a 10-year-old, with most of the reduction occurring before age 30. By age 85, the brain has lost 10–20 percent of its weight, mainly through nerve cell atrophy. These **neuron** losses are selective: some sites show no loss, while in the **cerebral cortex**, the site of higher mental activities, loss is significant.

Your mental ability will not necessarily decline with the loss of neurons, partly because the brain

continues to sprout new **dendrites**, communication lines to other neurons. They may be one way the brain compensates for neuron loss.

Our sleep patterns change with age. According to one expert, an 80-year-old's typical pattern is 18 minutes to fall asleep, 80 percent of the night spent asleep, six hours of total sleep time, and one hour of REM sleep.

Sexual Organs As time passes, a woman's menstrual periods tend to shorten and occur less frequently. Women in their thirties and forties, particularly those with children, tend to have fewer menstrual cramps.

A woman's sexual responsiveness peaks in her late thirties and remains on that plateau into her sixties (for example, women always retain the potential for multiple orgasm); men, however, peak in the late teens and decline from there.

The size of a woman's genitals tends to decrease over the years. As a man ages, his scrotum hangs lower, the angle of his erections begins to decline in his thirties, his sperm production declines, and the force of his ejaculations is less powerful.

• Lower your intake of salt, and increase your intake of calcium and possibly iron.

Maintain Normal Weight People can control their weight, although it takes time and can be stressful; it's especially not easy for people who have been overweight most of their lives. A sensible program of using more calories through exercise and perhaps cutting calorie intake or a

combination of both will work for most people who want to lose weight, but there is no magic formula. Obesity is not physically healthy, and it leads to premature aging.

Control Drinking Alcohol impairs both liver and kidney function, and heavy drinkers suffer brain damage as well. Alcohol taken in excess directly destroys lives, both the drinker's and others'.

Neuron A nerve cell.

Cerebral cortex The outer layer of the brain, which controls the behavior and mental activity of humans.

Dendrites A branched part of a nerve cell that transmits impulses toward the cell body.

Is "Senility" Inevitable?

Both laypeople and physicians use the term *senility* loosely. Older people are often called "senile" when they forget something or seem to be confused. But small memory lapses in old age do not necessarily show intellectual deterioration. Slight confusion and occasional forgetfulness throughout life may only mean a temporary overload of facts in the brain. Or perhaps the person who exhibits such behaviors is merely tired and not functioning as well as usual. However, people also use the term *senile* to describe significant brain deterioration in elderly individuals.

Slowly losing one's mind was once considered an inevitable part of growing old. It was once thought that if people simply lived long enough, they became senile. However, we know that most elderly people in good health remain mentally alert. Well-designed studies suggest that although "response time" may slow down, many people become smarter as they become older and more experienced.

The current *medical* term for deterioration of intellectual capacity is *dementia*—which means "deprived of mind." Its earliest symptoms may appear as a slight disturbance in someone's ability to grasp the situations he or she is in—as illustrated in the movie *On Golden Pond* when the character portrayed by Henry Fonda lost his way in the long-familiar woods near his home. As dementia progresses, memory failure becomes apparent and the affected individual may forget conversations,

events of the day, or the purpose of errands. Grooming usually decreases, confusion increases, and emotional outbursts may occur. The symptoms of dementia have many possible causes, some of which are treatable, so it is vital that we not dismiss such symptoms as "just old age." Anyone exhibiting these symptoms should be given a thorough medical examination. Even if a person suffers from incurable dementia, appropriate treatment may greatly improve the quality of his or her life.

The two main incurable forms of dementia are Alzheimer's disease and multi-infarct dementia (formerly called "cerebral arteriosclerosis" which means "hardening of the arteries of the brain"). Alzheimer's disease involves progressive, diffuse atrophy of brain tissue. Multi-infarct dementia is caused by a series of minor strokes that result in death of brain tissue in different parts of the brain. However, many *reversible* conditions have similar symptoms—such as a minor head injury, high fever, poor nutrition, or reaction to a drug. Emotional problems, particularly severe depression, can also be confused with dementia. Thus a thorough mental and neurological evaluation should be obtained for anyone showing possible signs of deteriorating brain function. The National Institute on Aging estimated that 10 to 20 percent of dementias in the elderly are reversible.

People with irreversible brain disorders can often be helped.

Carefully prescribed drugs can lessen agitation, anxiety, and depression and can improve sleeping patterns. Proper nutrition in the form of a well-balanced diet is desirable. The person should be encouraged to maintain daily routines, physical activities, and social contacts, and should not be overprotected or discouraged from trying new things. Supplying information on the time of day, place of residence, and what is going on in the immediate environment and in world events can stimulate the individuals to use those skills and information that remain.

Memory aids can also help people in their day-to-day living. Joseph D. Alter, M.D., Professor of Community Medicine at Wright State University School of Medicine, suggests posting a large calendar, lists of daily activities, written notes about simple safety measures, and labeling and directions for commonly used items. To help keep track of medications, he suggests making a chart or using a styrofoam egg carton with each day's pills arranged in a compartment in the order they are to be taken.

Maintaining constructive activity may help to slow down further deterioration of the brain. Of course, as deterioration progresses, increased supervision and even institutionalization may become necessary.

Source: Stephen Barrett, M.D. 1987. *Healthline,* May.

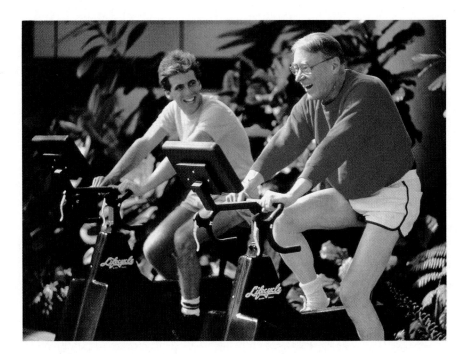

Regular exercise in youth and middle age is an important key to graceful aging. These popular exercise bicycles can be programmed to provide exactly the right workout for individuals of any age.

Don't Smoke The average pack-a-day smoker can expect to live about 12 years less than a person who doesn't smoke. Worse, smokers suffer more illnesses that last longer, and they are subject to respiratory disabilities that limit their total vigor for many years before their death. Even young cigarette smokers suffer respiratory impairment, some within a year of starting to smoke. Premature balding and skin wrinkling have been linked to cigarette smoking. Smokers at age 50 have the wrinkles of a person of 60. See Chapter 9 for more details, but remember that smoking is not part of the long or good life.

Schedule Physical Examinations to Detect Treatable Diseases Some diseases that escape notice during early stages can nevertheless take a terrible toll in premature disability and death. When detected, many can be successfully controlled by medication and some lifestyle changes. Look at the medical tests for healthy people listed in Chapter 21. Guidelines are provided for how frequently you should have them throughout your life time.

Hypertension—high blood pressure—can cause wear and tear on the **vascular system** and finally accelerate its breakdown. A simple check of blood pressure takes only a few minutes and can be done by a nurse, physi-

cians's assistant, or nurse's aide. Blood pressure higher than 140/90 is abnormal for anyone, and even small increases in blood pressure reduce life expectancy considerably.

Diabetes can escape detection for years. It accelerates the breakdown of body organs and systems, especially the circulatory system, and increases the risk of hypertension, heart attack, and strokes. When diabetes is diagnosed through blood glucose or urinalysis tests and treated early, however, chances of living a full life span improve greatly.

Much can be done to both prevent and detect cancer. Besides not smoking, appropriate diet and staying out of the sun protect you from various cancers. Self-examinations (such as breast and testicle self-examination) and examinations by a physician of sites especially susceptible to cancer could save more lives than any other means available today. Men and women over age 50 should have a yearly rectal examination by a physician. Women should have a Pap smear to detect cervical cancer at least once every three years.

You also need a test for **glaucoma** (a treatable disease of the eye that can end in blindness) at least every three years after age 40.

Hypertension Abnormally high blood pressure.

Vascular System The heart and blood vessels.

Diabetes A chronic disease characterized by too much sugar in the blood and urine.

Glaucoma Disease in which fluid inside the eye is under abnormally high pressure; can lead to blindness.

Recognize and Reduce Stress   When you are subjected to stress, your blood pressure rises, your heart rate quickens, and your body chemistry changes. These stress-induced changes increase wear and tear on your body. Cut down on the stresses in your life, perhaps by riding a bicycle instead of driving a car or by avoiding noisy, frenetic environments. Practice moderation in what you do. Prevent hearing loss by avoiding excessively loud noises. Don't wear yourself out too fast through lack of sleep, abuse or misuse of drugs, or workaholism. Practice relaxation, using the techniques described in Chapter 2. If you contract a disease, consider it your body's attempt to interrupt your life pattern and permit you to reevaluate your lifestyle, perhaps to slow down.

■ **Exploring Your Emotions**

How do you think you would react if you had to care for an elderly parent or grandparent? Could you be patient or would you lose your temper frequently? What experiences make you answer the way you do?

Ironically, the health behaviors you practice now weigh more heavily in determining how long you will live than will your behaviors in your older age. Retiring from your life's occupation with a physically healthy body will allow far more options for enjoying yourself than will retiring with frail health or disabilities. Poor health that could have been prevented drains finances, emotions, energy, and contributes to poor mental health. By attending to yourself now, you're buying some insurance for the future.

Confronting Social, Emotional, and Mental Changes

Just as you can prepare now to limit physical changes, you can also begin preparing yourself mentally, socially, and financially for a cluster of events that occurs during the fifties, sixties, and seventies and whose repercussions must be grappled with and resolved. These developmental tasks of aging are determined by biological, social, and perhaps economic changes and likewise require significant lifestyle adjustments. Although aging poses unique demands on each person, the changes cut across ethnic and socioeconomic variables. If you have aging parents, grandparents, and friends, the following information may help you understand their behavior better and spur you on to begin cultivating these appropriate and useful behaviors now.

1. Decreased energy and changes in health require the aging to *develop priorities for how to use energy*. Energy level is psychologically related to life satisfaction. A boring, tedious, uneventful, or overscheduled, "dutiful" life tailored to meet someone else's expectations is exhausting.

   Physical disabilities and chronic diseases drain and deplete energy. The poor spend more time incapacitated than do those who can afford medical care. Also, much exhaustion attributed to aging actually is caused by depression and may be directly related to poor health, poverty, poor adjustment to losses, or a lack of preparation for aging. One common disability—hearing loss—particularly affects personality: depression can result from the sense of isolation that deafness brings.

   Rather than curtailing activities to conserve energy—a strategy that can actually perpetuate the feelings of malaise and depression—the aging need to learn how to stimulate themselves and to generate energy. That usually entails saying no to the unenjoyable things and yes to enjoyable ones. It also requires close attention to needs for rest and to sleep schedules: each is unique and changes as people age. These practices are valuable exercises now as well as later.

   Carl Sandburg had it right when he wrote: "Time is the coin of your life. It is the only coin you have. Be careful lest someone else spend it for you."

2. Retirement may mean a severely restricted budget, possibly financial disaster. You need to *take stock of finances* and plan for the future while you are in your forties and fifties. Estimate what you need to meet your standard of living, calculate your projected income, and perhaps begin a savings program.

   Some creative, energetic older people may live happily on very little money, but doing so is difficult in our society. Many pleasures, such as travel, require extra money. Our culture teaches us how to buy pleasure, but not how to generate it ourselves. But there are alternatives. Many Europeans have been found to enjoy leisure time more, to need less money for their pleasure, and to take more vacations. They appear to enjoy simpler things: often they use a vacation for a walking tour, camping out at night. That's in sharp contrast to the American way of seeing how many miles can be driven in an air-conditioned car between luxury motels.

3. You need to *learn to enjoy yourself when you are alone*, another practice that is invaluable throughout life. In our culture we are not encouraged to spend time alone. Taking pleasure in being alone is considered antisocial. Many people find pleasurable ways to spend time alone—reading, writing, walking, playing

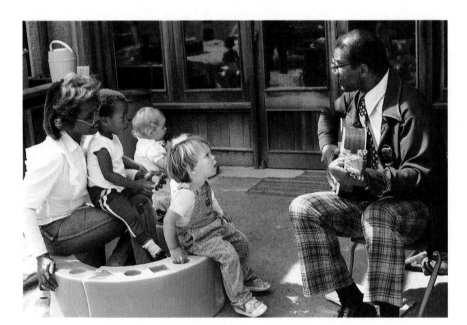

One of the challenges of aging is finding satisfying activities that provide meaningful connections with others. This retired man fills an important niche entertaining children at a day-care center.

or listening to music, gardening, quilting, photographing, keeping up with the news. Loneliness is sometimes a complaint of people who lack a sense of self and identity. A problem for many older people is that they have never established a personal identity independent from their social roles. Find out who you are by discovering the things you love to do.

4. Retirement; loss of social roles; changes in status; loss of friends, spouse, or peers; and problems of identity are linked problems. Retirement means a new social definition and a new economic situation. Although it confers the advantages of leisure time and freedom from deadlines, competition, and stress, many people do not know how to enjoy their free time. Without work and "productivity," some fall prey to loneliness, boredom, and depression.

People need to *seek new sources of nurturance and stimulation* when their usual resources disappear. People who age best tend to be involved in various activities and with other people; they are usually curious and flexible, and those who live in families fare better mentally than those who live alone. As you get older, you may want to enroll in adult education courses, read and converse more, travel, and do volunteer work. You may have to reorder your values so that on-the-job productivity and power are not the keys to your identity. Get involved as soon as possible; long before retirement, many people discover exactly how productive (to themselves and others) time can be when it's spent in a literacy program or as a "Big Brother" or "Big Sister."

5. *Resolve grief and mourning.* We all suffer losses: friends, peers, physical appearance, and health. Grief is the work of getting through the pain of loss, and it can be one of the most lonely, intense, and intimate events in a person's life.

The griever must work through shock, disbelief, denial, anger, and numbness. Usually within a year of a loved one's death, some resolution occurs: decreasing sadness, resumption of ordinary life, ability to recall the past with pleasure as well as pain. Unfortunately, most people endure grief alone in our society. Others can help by encouraging the mourner to express the grief and responding sympathetically.

Eventually we must relinquish grief. This is not a new experience: we have often said farewells to discarded self-images, broken dreams, friends who move away, parents who die. We all let go of illusions: we are not as brilliant, talented, famous, all-loving, or sensitive as we had dreamed. We lose people and possessions throughout life, not just in old age.

Death is a total loss—the loss of the self. Adapting positively to the reality of your own death is a major task of aging. Older people need to discuss their feelings about dying and death, but rarely have an opportunity to do so because the subject is still taboo and many people are uncomfortable talking about death. The acceptance of death enriches your sense of life.

6. Aging changes and slows down sexuality. Depending on the importance of sexual activity in your life, you will need to *adjust to sensory and sexual losses.* This

adjustment can be difficult. Some people, grieving for the loss of this significant aspect of themselves, go through stages of mourning, especially depression.

Loss of interest in sex and impotency are often socially, rather than biologically, induced. Some people remain sexually active into their eighties. And when sexual problems do occur, counseling usually can help. Sexuality researchers William Masters and Virginia Johnson report that they are able to restore potency in about two-thirds of their elderly male patients. Older couples can learn to accept the idea that love play and pleasure can be enjoyed in themselves and do not always have to end in orgasm. Different expectations can mean continued enjoyment of sex.

7. A major task of aging is to *adopt a flexible attitude toward whatever life brings you.* Only the right mental attitude can stave off the negative effects of some circumstances. The attitude of youth is based on striving—for more knowledge, strength, capability, and understanding of one's self. Its principal force is growth. But for older people, self-enjoyment and acceptance are more useful attitudes than self-aggrandizement and aspiration.

Aging and Life Expectancy

Human **life expectancy** is the average length of time we can expect to live. It is calculated by averaging the ages of death of a group of people over a certain period of time. Women born in the United States today have longer life expectancies than do their male counterparts. The reasons for this difference are not known, but estrogen production during a woman's fertile years appears to protect her from heart disease. Her risks increase after menopause. Increased male mortality can also be traced to smoking (lung cancer, heart and respiratory disease), more accidents, and more alcoholism. Where these factors are not operative, as among the Amish, men live as long as women even now.

Life expectancy from birth in the United States has increased dramatically in this century, as described in Chapter 1. This does not mean that every American now lives longer than in 1900; rather, far fewer people die young now, because childhood and infectious diseases are much better controlled and diet and sanitation are much improved since 1900. In 1900 only 30 percent of the population lived to be 70 years old. In 1990 closer

to 65 percent live to be 70. (For an even broader view of life expectancy through the ages see Figure 19-2.)

The young generally benefit far more from modern medical and public health measures than do the elderly. Today, a person of 20 can expect to live about twelve years longer than could a person of 20 in 1900. Recently, however, the U.S. Census Bureau reported a dramatic 3 percent decrease in death rates from the three preceding years: the life expectancy of women has been raised to 78 years and that of men to 71 years. These all-time American highs reflect new medical successes as well as health payoffs from early identification and treatment of high blood pressure, more prudent diets, and reduced cigarette smoking among middle-aged adults.

Another significant aspect of life expectancy is that as you age and survive the hazards to your life in younger years, you gain statistical life expectancy. For example, life expectancy for males born in 1990 is 71 years; but for men who were 30 in 1990, the expected remaining number of years of life is 42.5, a total of 72.5 years (30 + 42.5). For a female born in 1990, life expectancy is 78 years; but for women who were 40 in 1990, the expected remaining number of years of life is 40, or a total of 80 years. Statistically, you never run out of life expectancy. Even at age 85, men and women still have an expectation of 5.3 and 6.8 more years, respectively.

So how long can we humans expect to live in the best of circumstances? It now seems possible that biologically our maximum potential **life span** is from 100 to 120 years. Failure to achieve that span in good health results to some degree from destructive environmental and behavioral factors—factors over which we can exert considerable control. Long life doesn't necessarily mean a longer period of disability, either. People often live longer because they have been well longer. A healthy, productive old age is very often an extension of a healthy, productive middle age. However, behavior changes cannot extend the maximum human life span, which is built into our genes. Only if science could unravel the biological mystery of aging and control the aging process would this be the case.

Theories of Aging   Throughout history people have searched for and invented a great variety of "magic" preparations, devices, and practices for preserving youth. None has ever worked. More recently, science has entered the arena and directed research toward aging. Researchers would like to break through the riddles of hormones and the cell to enable people to live longer and maintain much of their youthful vigor.

Life expectancy   The average length of life of members of a species.

Life span   Theoretically projected length of life based on maximum potential of the human body in the best environment.

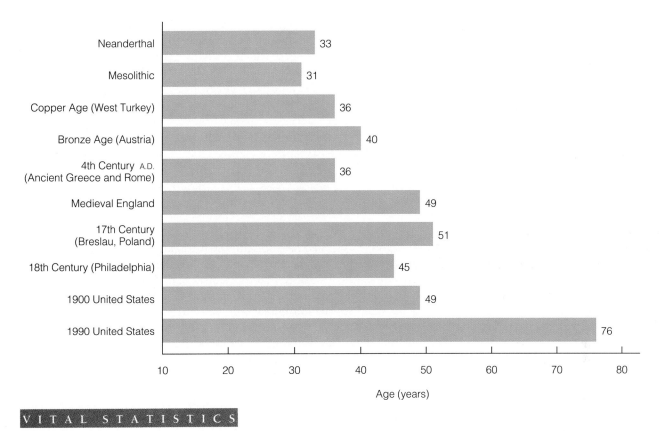

VITAL STATISTICS

Figure 19-2 Estimated changes in life expectancy through history.

Some scientists believe aging is genetically programmed: a necessary process by which the older members of a species make way for the younger members. Like a spaceship designed to fly past Mars but with no built-in instructions beyond that point, a human may be programmed to get to 85 or 90 years and to keep on going; but, after some point, its various systems begin to break down and will continue until the breakdown is total.

What causes the breakdown, the decline in energy, the body's inability to function and maintain itself? (See Figure 19-1.) No existing theory of aging accommodates all the facts, and it may be that aging is caused by a variety of different processes and affected by a variety of factors, both environmental and biological. A prime environmental factor is nutrition; evidence from animal studies indicates that it may be possible to manipulate an animal's fixed life span to some degree through diet. Biological factors may operate at both the cellular level and the system level. In other words, some aging processes may be built into individual cells; others seem to involve whole systems, such as the nervous system, the endocrine system, and the immune system.

One theory of aging based on biological factors involves the genetic makeup of the cell. The theory suggests that a cell contains "aging" genes that specify the exact number of times the cell can duplicate itself. The limiting number varies from species to species. This is why the maximum life span for fruit flies is about 100 days, for dogs about 25 to 30 years, for humans about 110 to 120 years, and for giant tortoises about 180 years. Another theory suggests that the cell's DNA somehow becomes defective after a certain point and synthesizes defective protein. The defect disables normal cell functioning, causing the cell to deteriorate.

A theory of aging involving the immune system suggests that the body begins to err in synthesizing protein and produces proteins that the immune system cannot recognize. The immune system then attacks them as it would any foreign substance, destroying cells and impairing body functions. Alternatively, the immune system itself may weaken in old age, producing fewer antibodies to fight disease. Researchers are testing drugs that would reinforce faltering immune systems.

Some of the immobility of old age results from changes in metabolic functioning. Connective tissue all over the body, such as collagen and elastic fibers, becomes stiffer and chemically immobilized with age. This is because by-products of metabolism, called cross-links, form between parallel collagen fibers, making it impossible for the two fibers to slip past each other or stretch.

Brain chemistry and hormones have also been implicated in aging. Levels of certain **neurotransmitters**—chemicals that transmit nerve impulses—are reduced in old age, preventing the brain from coordinating the functions of various glands and tissues. Experiments aimed at maintaining levels of certain neurotransmitters are being conducted to help slow down pathological aging. Sometimes sex hormones are used to prevent aging. Testosterone has been found to increase vigor and muscle tone in men who were treated with it, but it also produces side effects that make its use uncommon. Estrogen is commonly used to treat problems associated with menopause, including osteoporosis.

Should We Tamper with the Aging Process?   Significantly extended life spans would bring great social changes. While such extension appears to be inevitable, the effects of slowing the aging process will vary depending on which diseases are eliminated. If, for example, diseases of the blood vessels now associated with aging were wiped out, people might expect to live 11 years longer on the average. With the most usual causes of death eliminated, however, more people would then die of other causes, and more would survive only to face long exposure to environmental hazards and accumulated stress. Some would suffer even greater disability and dependence during the added years.

Scientific advances in lengthening lives must be matched with better control and understanding of environment and lifestyles. Researchers are aware of the problems, and they do not aim to prolong a living death. In general, they work toward adding productive and fulfilling years.

Life in an Aging America

As life expectancies increase, a larger proportion of the population will be in their later years; this change will necessitate new government policies and changes in our general attitudes toward the aged.

America's Aging Minority   People over 65 are a large minority in the American population—over 30 million people, 12 percent of the total population in the 1990s (For a statistical look at the elderly in America, see Figure 19-3). As birth rates drop, the percentage is increasing dramatically. Many older people are happy, healthy, and self-sufficient. Changes that come with age, including

negative ones, normally occur so gradually that most people adapt, some even gracefully. Only 5 percent of people over age 65 in the United States are being cared for in institutions, and generally the rest continue to live meaningful and independent lives.

■ **Exploring Your Emotions**

How do you feel about getting old? Does it scare or worry you? If so, what do you think causes you to feel that way? Can you look more closely at your feelings of fear or discomfort to see if they are realistic?

Today the status of the aging is improving more than ever before. People now in their forties and fifties will probably benefit from new knowledge about the aging process. And the enormous increase in the over-55 population is markedly affecting our stereotypes of what it means to grow old. The misfortunes associated with aging—frailty, forgetfulness, poor health, isolation—occur to fewer people in their sixties and seventies and are shifting instead to burden the very old, those over 85.

The "younger" elderly who are in good physical and mental health are gaining status in our society; politicians are listening to them; advertisers have targeted them as a good market. The elderly are, in general, better off than they have ever been in the past. They have more money than they did twenty years ago. About three-quarters of these people own their homes. Their living expenses are lower after retirement because they no longer support children and have fewer work-related expenses; they consume and buy less food. They are more likely to continue practicing their expertise for years after retirement and to be paid in cash. Thousands of retired consultants, teachers, technicians, and craftspeople work until their mid- and late seventies. They receive greater amounts of assistance, such as Medicare, pay proportionately lower taxes, and have greater net worth from lifetime savings.

As the aging population increases proportionately, however, a greater number of older people are ill and dependent and experience major social and economic problems. Tens of thousands of older Americans live in poverty, particularly minorities and women living alone. These other elderly—poverty-stricken, isolated, lonely—are just as ignored as they ever were. Their numbers are increasing: of all people above the age of 65, over 12 percent live below the "official" poverty line. About a fifth of the poor elderly live in central city poverty areas. Single black women fare worst: about 64 percent are poor.

Neurotransmitter   A substance that transmits nerve impulses.

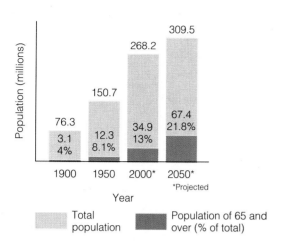

(a) Growth of the population: 65 and over

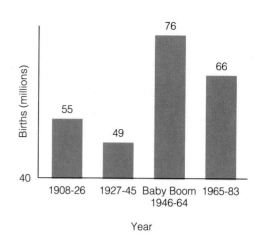

(b) Births: 1908–1983, in 19-year increments

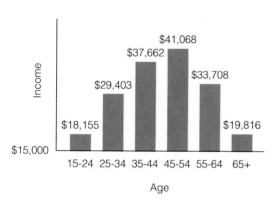

(c) Household income: Average household income by age of the household head

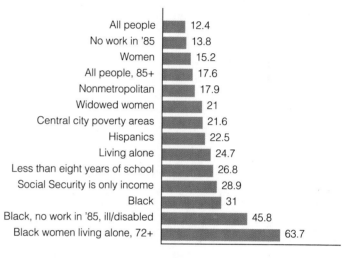

(d) Poverty and age: Percentage of elderly, 65 and over, below poverty level in 1986

VITAL STATISTICS

Figure 19-3   A statistical look at the elderly in America.

Whatever the American dream may have been, for many older citizens it has faded. Forced or persuaded into retirement, they find their income reduced to the point where they can barely subsist. They are likely to feel worthless and to be perceived in our "youthful" culture as a drag on society. Urban life and the nuclear family intensify the effects of these negative attitudes toward older people. In cultures that have *extended families,* older people stay active in society and help care for and teach the children. In today's United States, they often face isolation, or life in institutions or geriatric ghettos—bleak downtown hotels or posh retirement cities.

Even for those who don't live alone, illness can make

old age little more than a miserable, prolonged wait for death. Many disabled elderly people are dependent on others for daily care, a situation that has led to an increasing number of cases of abuse (see the box "Abuse of the Elderly"). Others are cared for in nursing homes. Whatever their circumstances, elderly people have the same needs as people at any other stage of life, including the need to feel that their lives have meaning. More and more, these needs are coming to be seen as basic human rights.

Government Aid and Policies   The government assists the elderly through several programs such as food

Abuse of the Elderly

The family: it can be a welcome refuge in difficult times. But for some people, it's a prison of neglect and abuse.

Experts are finding a "new" problem in the much-analyzed American family. It's one that most people do not like to acknowledge—but silence only makes it worse. The problem is mistreatment of the elderly. They are the fastest-growing and, in many ways, most vulnerable segment of our population.

There has been an increase of about 100,000 cases reported each year since 1981. Physical harm is evident in about half of all instances, but doctors and social workers sometimes do not recognize the problem. This makes it especially important for all of us to know the warning signs.

Scope of the Problem

This problem has been identified so recently that experts do not yet agree on basic definitions. But it now is apparent that neglect and abuse cover a wide spectrum.

The American Medical Association (AMA) estimates that 10 percent of individuals past the age of 65 may suffer some form of abuse. Within this group, about 1.1 million people can face moderate to severe abuse.

Several formal studies have now been completed, which suggest the dimensions of elder abuse in our society:

- Most victims are 75 years of age or older.
- The elderly are three times more likely to be abused if they live with someone. Men are more apt to share quarters with another person (since it is less common for wives to die first and, when this does happen, men tend to remarry). Although males more frequently are victims, females suffer greater physical harm.
- Abuse may begin with harsh words and spread to slapping, pushing, and hitting with an object. Sexual molestation also may take place.
- Three-quarters of victims are dependent upon others for daily care (bathing, dressing, eating, etc.). The caregiver may fail to address important needs of an older person (such as appropriate clothing for the season), even though resources are available. Psychological harm or misuse of the elderly person's money and possessions also can occur.
- The abuse often continues over a period of years and even decades.
- Mistreatment of the elderly is found among all ethnic and economic groups.
- Roughly half of all abusers are children or younger relatives of the victim. The victim's spouse is the abuser in about 40 percent of cases.

Case Study Profiles

Experts have several theories to explain abuse of the elderly. Many cases involve multiple causes:

- *The dependent victim.* Seventy-five percent of abuse victims must rely upon others for help with daily needs. They are vulnerable if caregivers become hostile. Conversely, some elderly persons suffer from self-neglect and do not properly care for themselves or alert others to their needs.
- *The stressed caregiver.* Helping an older person is demanding in terms of energy, time and finance. If the caregiver approaches this

---

stamps, housing subsidies, Social Security, Medicaid, and Medicare (see Table 19-1). Social Security, the life insurance and old-age pension plan, has saved many from destitution, although it is intended not as a sole source of income but as a supplement to other income. Social Security funds are currently being used to cover other government financial deficits, so the future solvency of the program is uncertain. The Medicaid program finances acute and long-term care services for the poor, including the elderly poor. Almost 40 percent of Medicaid expenditures goes for the care of 3.5 million elderly people.

The Medicare program, designed to finance acute care services for the elderly and disabled, pays about 45 percent of the medical costs of the elderly. But serious gaps in Medicare coverage require the elderly to pay for some health care expenses out of their own pockets. Chronic diseases, for example, which affect more than half of those over 75 years of age, aren't covered by Medicare. Over a million elderly people live in nursing homes, and in the year 2000, when there will be more than 2 million people over the age of 85, the nursing home business will boom. But Medicare pays less than 2 percent of nurs-

Abuse of the Elderly (continued)

task with personal problems (such as unemployment or strained relationships), abuse may become an outlet for pent-up frustration.

In about 60 percent of cases, the elderly person is a cause of stress. He or she may have long-standing conflicts with the care-giver. On top of this can come the problems of dependent old age: incontinence, falls, inappropriate language or behavior.

- *The violent family.* Many times, abuse is a learned behavior. It can operate in a cycle over several generations. Parents who abuse a child may see the youth grow up to mistreat his or her own children and then turn upon the elderly grandparents, who were abusive years earlier.

- *The "pathologic" abuser.* In rare instances, the caregiver may be unable to perform necessary duties. Mental handicaps, a history of random violence, misuse of alcohol or other drugs—such diverse conditions can lead to abuse. Some studies indicate that victims of elder abuse have been "dumped" by other relatives upon the member of the family who is least able to provide quality care.

No Single Solution Is Available

Protection is becoming an important legal issue. Mistreatment of older people is nearly as common as child abuse. But the AMA found states spend $22 per child for protective services and only $2.90 for senior citizens.

Laws have varying impact. Some states permit officials to investigate suspected cases without prior consent of the family or elderly person. Courts may require separate residences for victims and convicted abusers. But other states simply ask for voluntary reporting.

Complication: some elderly persons refuse help. They may be confused or intimidated, but they reject assistance from "outsiders." And while authorities may intervene in cases of child abuse, they are restricted from helping a competent adult who exercises the right of privacy.

Don't Be Silent

Home care for the elderly remains a highly desirable option. Often it's less expensive than institutional care, and most older people prefer familiar surroundings.

But for home care to be successful, all parties must try to understand new relationships and work together. The older person, accustomed to self-sufficiency, is now dependent. Adult children must accept new responsibility—often while still rearing children of their own. Under such pressure, an amicable relationship can be stretched. A less supportive one may collapse.

Learn the danger signs and address them early. Many communities have special services for helping the elderly. You can develop a network of doctors, social workers, and financial advisors.

If you are aware of an abusive situation, do not remain silent. You may need to contact the police. Or you may request a home call from the county health department. A visiting nurse can make a nonthreatening assessment and contact authorities if something is amiss.

It is tragic irony that victims of elder abuse often remain silent because they feel ashamed or frightened. Victims are not at fault. They deserve humane care. But they must speak out to be heard.

Source: *Mayo Clinic Health Letter*, January 1988, pp. 3–4.

---

ing home costs, and private insurers pay less than 1 percent, creating a tremendous financial burden for elderly nursing home residents and their families. (See the box entitled "Selecting a Nursing Home.")

A crucial question in aid for the elderly is, Who will pay for it? The government picks up a substantial share of the health expenses of the elderly, primarily through Medicaid and Medicare. Personal health care expenditures are about 11 percent of the U.S. gross national product, and about one-third of these expenditures go to care for the elderly. The average government expenditure for personal health services for those over age 65 is three to four times greater than that for people under age 65.

Resistance to increased health care costs on the part of the elderly themselves was illustrated in the fate of the catastrophic health insurance law that Congress passed in 1988 and repealed in 1989. Designed to protect the elderly from financial ruin due to medical expenses, this law put a cap on how much individual Medicare recipients would have to pay in one year for hospital and physician bills caused by a major illness. But unlike other Medicare programs, which are paid for by taxes from the

Many elderly people worry about what will happen to them if they have a catastrophic illness requiring expensive medical attention, hospitalization, or long-term care. Despite the efforts of activists like this woman, the United States still lacks a national health care policy.

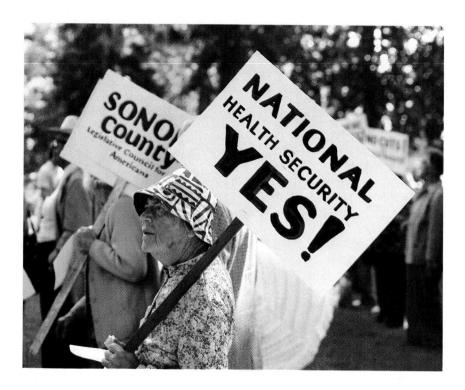

Table 19-1 Legislated benefits for the aging
1965—Medicare and Medicaid enacted.
1965—Older Americans Act establishes the Administration on Aging.
1967—Age discrimination in employment made illegal.
1972—Supplemental Security Program guarantees all older Americans a minimum income.
1972—Social Security indexed to inflation.
1973—Federal Council on Aging established.
1978—Age of mandatory retirement for most workers pushed back to 70.
1981-82—Efforts to cut Social Security and Medicare benefits defeated.
1983—Social Security reform pulls the system back from the brink of bankruptcy.
1986—Mandatory retirement at any age eliminated for almost all workers.
1988—Catastrophic health insurance under Medicare passed.
1989—Catastrophic health insurance repealed.

general population, this insurance was to be financed entirely by its elderly beneficiaries, especially those in the middle and upper income ranges. The program raised an angry outcry from senior citizens, who said it provided too few benefits at too high a cost. Congress beat a hasty retreat, repealing the law by a vote of 360–66 after having passed it a year earlier by a vote of 328–72.

Many health planners believe that instead of adding stop-gap measures to Medicare and Medicaid, the government should address the issue of health insurance for the elderly in the context of an overall national health care policy. Many difficult and complex issues need attention, including the lack of health insurance for more than 30 million Americans, the rising cost of nursing home care, the declining condition of the hospital system, and the high rate of infant mortality. Since resources are ultimately limited, difficult decisions have to be made and priorities have to be established.

In the meantime, health policy planners hope that rising medical costs for the elderly will dwindle dramatically through education and prevention. Health professionals, including **gerontologists** (or **geriatricians**), are beginning to practice preventive medicine, just as pediatricians do. They advise the aging on how to avoid and, if necessary, how to manage disabilities. They aim to instill an

---

Gerontologist (Geriatrician) A medical doctor who studies aging and specializes in the problems of the elderly.

Selecting a Nursing Home

Afraid of entering a nursing home yourself? Grieving over a decision to place a spouse or family member in one? There is cause to feel more cheerful about such decisions these days. Considerable evidence suggests that the typical nursing home has improved in quality over the past several decades. In fact, the rapid increase in the number of nursing home beds has been traced to the improved image of this institution.

The chances of an aged person living in a nursing home at some point in a lifetime are currently estimated to be at least one in four. The risk of institutionalization is greater for women than for men because women tend to live longer and to reach an age where chronic disabilities are more common. Women are also more likely to be widowed and thus to lack a spouse—and a spouse is most often the person who takes care of a disabled elderly person living at home. Moving a family member into a nursing home can be very difficult for both the client and the family. It is wise to plan ahead for this possibility, for the best nursing homes usually have long waiting lists. A little forethought and planning help to ease this transition. Before making any decisions, two questions need to be addressed. First, is the placement really necessary? And second, how should one go about selecting a home?

Alternative Community Services

Many people who currently reside in a nursing home could actually be better cared for in the community if alternative services are available. Whether or not the nursing home is the right solution for you depends on two conditions: the availability of alternative community services (such as adult day health care, home health care, personal care, or congregate housing), and on the ability of the prospective client and caregivers to cope with the burdens imposed by illness. One way to determine the need for placement is by making a thorough assessment of the individual's and caregiver's resources. This type of assessment is becoming more available at hospital outpatient clinics or through other services for the elderly. One study has shown that evaluation by a team of physicians, psychiatrists, geriatric nurse practitioners, social workers, and rehabilitation therapists resulted in 80 percent of the clients being returned home after the evaluation. A good assessment service usually provides a case manager who can monitor the client's needs and the family's resources as they fluctuate over time. This person is a nurse or social worker who directly counsels and advises the client and his or her family. The case manager can serve as a liaison and can lead families to the appropriate health and social services on an ongoing basis to meet these changing needs.

How to Select a Home

If placement in a nursing home is clearly in the best interests of the client and his or her family, they need to select a home best suited to their needs. Evaluating the quality of care these homes provide can be complicated. Does the home and its administrator have a current state license? If the client needs financial assistance and is eligible for government or other forms of assistance, select a home certified to participate in such programs. If the client needs a special diet or a specific treatment, be sure that the home can provide them. The location of the home also should be acceptable to the client, close to a general hospital, convenient for the client's personal physician, and not too distant for frequent visiting by family and friends. Once these criteria narrow the choices down to a few homes, both the client and his or her family need to visit each of them in person.

The actual quality of patient care is more difficult to assess, but your observations can be a useful guide. Start by checking the beds to make sure only those patients who *should* be in bed are actually there. Are patients unattended or unnecessarily restrained? Such problems may be indicative of poorly trained or too few staff.

Then check the overall standard of cleanliness, the quality of the amenities and furnishings, and the freedom from unpleasant odors. Check the rooms to see if many personal possessions have been brought from home. Encouraging the use of everyday objects brought from home fosters a more homelike setting and may ease adjustment to the new environment.

To evaluate the social environment, look for friendly interactions among residents, involvement in meaningful activities, and a supportive and friendly staff. The staff should know the residents' names.

Selecting a Nursing Home (continued)

From talking to staff members, one can see if they have positive attitudes toward the residents and toward their own work. Friends and relatives of other residents in the home, as well as other residents themselves, can give you some indication of the quality of care.

Financial worries may override other considerations. Understanding Medicare and Medicaid policies is a first step in finding out about any third-party payments to ease the financial strain. Become familiar with what services and supplies are covered in the basic daily rate, as well as what optional services are charged separately. Nursing homes are very expensive, and many residents exhaust all private sources of funds after admission. Those who are forced to seek Medicaid funds at some point after they have gained admission, how-ever, do have the legal right to remain at the facility. According to federal law, it is illegal to discharge a patient for lack of funds.

Certain publications can serve as further guides in selecting a nursing home:

- Health Care Financing Administration, *How to Select a Nursing Home* (HCFA-30043 booklet), December 1980. The helpful checklist can be used to system-atically compare different nursing homes.
- California Health Facilities Commission, *Choosing a Long-term Care Facility in California*, pam-phlet (1984). It gives suggestions on how to use detailed cost and operational information about the 1,200 nursing homes in the state to compare selected features of these facilities. This informa-tion covers five areas: nursing services, nonnursing expenses, employee turnover, citations issued for noncompliance with regulatory standards, and the level of profitability. It is in-tended to help consumers make a more informed decision about which nursing home to select.

Many other states' departments of health services have similar reports. And your local Area Agency on Aging or your local Health Systems Agency may be able to give you information about the nursing homes and alternative community-based services in your area.

Source: Leslie A. Grant and Colleen L. Johnson. 1986. A family guide for selecting a nursing home. *Healthline*, November.

---

ethic of bodily and mental maintenance that would pre-vent chronic disease and allow the elderly to live long, healthy, vigorous lives.

Changing the Public's Idea of Aging   Aging people may be one of our least used resources. How can we employ the knowledge and productivity of our growing numbers of older citizens, particularly those we are now losing through mandatory early retirement?

■ **Exploring Your Emotions**

How do you feel about old people? How do you think they feel about you? Are you comfortable talking with them? Are there ways you can open up or improve communication with them?

First we must change our thinking about what aging means. We must learn to judge productivity rather than age. Capacity to function should replace age as a criterion for usefulness. Instead of singling out 65 as a magic num-ber, we could consider ages 50 to 75 as the third quarter of life. Changes occur around 50 that signal a new era: children are usually grown and gone; a person has reached the maximum level of advancement in employ-ment and highest real earnings. It is often a time of some restlessness, time for "repotting" the plant that has out-grown its container. The upper end of the quarter is determined by the fact that most people today are vig-orous, in good health, mentally alert, and capable of mak-ing a productive contribution until they are at least 75 years old. That age estimate may be a bit high for some, but not for most. About 20 percent of the population—50 million people—falls within the third quarter. But 25 years from now, about 85 million will be in their third quarter.

Other formulas have been suggested for drawing the boundary line between middle and old age. Rather than counting from birth, we could count back a fixed number of years from the expected age at death. Using a current life table, we could calculate the age at which the average number of remaining years of life is 15. That would place old age around 67 today and 72 in the year 2030. An-

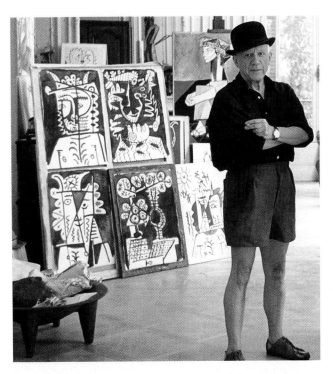

Some extraordinary individuals defy all preconceived ideas about old age. Picasso, in his seventies when this picture was taken, lived an intensely vigorous and creative life right up until his death at the age of 92.

other way to decide who is old would be to limit the group to the most elderly 10 percent of the population, which would fix the age at 75 in 2030.

Whatever way we define old age, the costs of losing what these people can contribute to our national pro-ductivity and quality of life are too high. Through their early retirement we forfeit substantial income-tax and Social Security tax revenues on their earnings. Those who retire at 62 start using their Social Security benefits earlier than otherwise.

A far better arrangement would be to make available full- and part-time volunteer and paid employment. We would benefit by providing retraining programs for both occupational and leisure time activities. We need more community-sponsored classes in remunerative activities such as real estate selling and management, horticulture, and library work, and in recreational and self-improvement activities such as music, writing, and health maintenance. Volunteer opportunities, such as preparing recordings for the blind, helping with activities for the retarded, and performing necessary tasks in hospitals, could be expanded. At the same time we could possibly change both public and private pension programs to make partial retirement possible. In such cases we could allow people to borrow against their Social Security benefits to finance their retraining or enrollment in wholly new educational programs.

There can be benefits to aging, but they don't come automatically. They require planning and wise choices earlier in life. One octogenarian, Russell Lee, founder of a medical clinic in California, perceived the advantages of aging as growth: "The limitations imposed by time are compensated by the improved taste, sharper discretion, sounder mental and esthetic judgment, increased sensitivity and compassion, clearer focus—which all contribute to a more certain direction in living. . . . The later years can be the best of life for which the earlier ones were preparation."

Summary

- People who take charge of their health in youth have greater control over the physical and mental aspects of aging.

Generating Vitality as You Age

- Biological aging takes place over a lifetime, but some of the other changes associated with aging are more abrupt. The more people prepare for aging, the more likely they are to be satisfied with their middle and old ages.
- Many characteristics traditionally considered to be consequences of aging are due rather to neglect and abuse of body and mind. Nevertheless, aging is inevitable, a result of biochemical processes.

- Exercise throughout life enhances physical and mental health; it may prevent deterioration of fluid intelligence with age. Benefits of exercise also include more supple arteries, protection against heart attack, improved lung function, weight control, physical flexibility, muscle strength, protection against injury and fractures, and increased effectiveness of the immune system.
- A varied, balanced diet with attention to lower caloric intake promotes health at every age. Low-fat, high-carbohydrate diets with an emphasis on fish and poultry, nonfat dairy products, olive oil, less salt, and more calcium are recommended. Obesity leads to premature aging.
- Alcohol impairs liver and kidney function; tobacco use

not only shortens life but also may cause severe health impairment for many years.

- Regular physical examinations help detect conditions that can shorten life and make old age less healthy; these include hypertension, diabetes, cancer, and glaucoma.

- Stress increases wear and tear on the body; getting enough sleep, avoiding drugs, and practicing relaxation help reduce stress.

Confronting Social, Emotional, and Mental Changes

- Certain developmental tasks of aging require significant lifestyle adjustments. These include (1) developing priorities for using energy and especially for generating it, (2) taking stock of finances and saving for retirement years, (3) learning to enjoy being alone and establishing an identity separate from social roles, (4) seeking new sources of nurturance and stimulation to make free time more enjoyable, (5) resolving grief and mourning and adjusting to the reality of one's own death, (6) adjusting to sensory and sexual losses, and (7) adopting a flexible attitude toward whatever life brings.

Aging and Life Expectancy

- Life expectancy, which has risen dramatically in the 1900s, is generally greater among women. Life expectancy increases with age.

- The maximum potential human life span seems to be 100 to 120 years; environmental and behavioral factors prevent most people from achieving it.

- One theory of aging deals with genetic programming; the body may be programmed to reach a certain age and keep going, but the various systems begin to break down at some point. Some aging processes may be cellular; others seem to involve entire systems.

- Cells may contain "aging" genes or may begin synthesizing defective proteins after a certain point. The immune system may attack proteins it doesn't recognize, or it may itself become weaker in old age.

- Connective tissue in the body becomes stiffer with age and leads to some of the inflexibility of old age.

- Neurotransmitters and hormones seem to be involved in the aging process.

Life in an Aging America

- People over 65 form a large minority in the United States, and their status is improving.

- Those of the aged who are ill and dependent—often those who were already poor—experience major social and economic problems; their attitudes toward themselves and society's attitudes toward them tend to be negative. Their dependency on others sometimes leads to abuse.

- Government aid to the elderly includes food stamps, housing subsidies, Social Security, Medicaid, and Medicare. Medicare does not cover all medical expenses, especially those related to chronic diseases and nursing homes. The question of paying for medical care for the elderly has received much attention, but difficult decisions still need to be made.

- Preventive medicine is as important for the elderly as for the rest of the population and may help reduce medical costs.

- The aged represent an underused resource; society needs to learn to consider productivity and capacity to function rather than age. Most people today can make valuable contributions until age 75. Society would benefit by providing retraining programs and more volunteer and paid employment. Changes in pension and Social Security programs could help make partial retirement possible.

Take Action

1. Imagine that you are very old and are looking back on your life. What do you think it will be important to you to have done with your life—had a successful career, been a good parent, found happiness, traveled, achieved self-knowledge? Make a list in your Health Diary of your life goals and priorities. Then list the kinds of things you will most regret—missed opportunities, rash decisions, choices not made. How can you begin now to work toward your goals and avoid the things you will regret? Choose one goal and take an action this week that moves you toward it.

2. Interview your parents or grandparents to find out how they want to spend their old age. Do they want to live at home, in a retirement community, with a relative? Do they plan to live on a pension, retirement account, Social Security? Have they made any concrete plans, or have they not yet confronted those decisions? Write up your interview and list any steps they have taken to plan for old age.

3. Investigate and if possible visit the different facilities in your com-

munity for the elderly—nursing homes, hospitals, senior citizen centers, recreational programs. What do you like about them and what do you dislike? Do you have suggestions for improvement?

4. Survey five college students and five older people to find out when they think people should retire. Ask them their reasons. Write up your survey and share the results with the people you included.

5. What are the most pronounced differences and similarities between a 70-year-old and a 20-year-old? List them in your Health Diary and then ask an elderly person you know if he or she agrees. Write down their list of differences and similarities and compare it to your own.

Selected Bibliography

Aging: It ain't necessarily so. *University of California, Berkeley, Wellness Letter,* June 1989.

Cole, Thomas R., and Sally A. Gadow, eds. 1986. *What Does It Mean to Grow Old? Reflections from the Humanities.* Durham: Duke University Press.

Dickinson, Peter A. 1984. *The Complete Retirement Planning Book: Your Guide to Happiness, Health, and Financial Security.* New York: Dutton.

Dychtwald, Ken, and Joe Flower. 1989. *Age Wave.* Los Angeles: Jeremy P. Tarcher.

Green, Charles. 1989. Congress votes to repeal catastrophic coverage. *San Jose Mercury News,* November 22, p. 4A.

Pifer, Alan, and Lydia Bronte. 1986. *Our Aging Society.* New York: Norton.

Rosenfeld, Albert. 1985. *Prolongevity II.* New York: Knopf.

Walford, Roy L. 1983. *Maximum Life Span.* New York: Norton.

Recommended Readings

Frome, Allen. 1984. *60 + : Planning It, Living It, Loving It.* New York: Farrar, Straus and Giroux. *Advice on senior life: practicing for retirement; better sex after 60; impact of inflation; art of living alone; making friends after 69.*

Hallowell, Christopher. 1985. *Growing Old, Staying Young.* New York: Morrow. *A highly readable and sympathetic account of most aspects of aging, with a particular look at Alzheimer's disease.*

Ogle, Jane. 1984. *Ageproofing.* New York: New American Library. *Detailed and excellent description of physiological changes throughout life. Includes nutrition and fitness guides for aging gracefully.*

Shelley, Florence D. 1988. *When Your Parents Grow Old,* 2nd ed. New York: Harper and Row. *For people caring for a parent, this is a comprehensive reference to finding help in the community, housing, home care, nursing home care, money matters, doctors, hospitals, HMOs, agencies, and organizations that can help.*

Contents

Making Connections

No one gets out of this world alive, but many of us act as if we will. Learning to accept and deal with death is a difficult but important part of life, a process that requires information, insight, and commitment just as simpler life tasks do. The scenarios presented on these pages describe situations in which people have to use information, make a decision, or choose a course of action, all related to dying and death. As you read them, imagine yourself in each situation and consider what you would do. After you've finished the chapter, read the scenarios again and see if what you've learned has changed how you would think, feel, or act in each situation.

An older neighbor has asked you to be a witness to a document he calls a "living will." He says it tells a hospital not to take any extraordinary measures to keep him alive if he's ever critically injured or ill and has no hope of recovery. "You know," he says, "it tells them to go ahead and pull the plug." You're hesitant about witnessing the document. Is it really ethical to make or carry out such a request? Isn't it illegal, too? What should you do?

Your parents recently discovered that your grandmother is terminally ill and has only six months to live. Your mother wants to bring her to your home to spend her last days with your family. Your father is against the idea, feeling it would be too difficult, too disruptive of family life, and too traumatic for your mother and your younger brother and sister, who are still living at home. Your mother doesn't want her to die in a hospital, and your father doesn't want her to die in your home. As far as you know, are there any other alternatives? What information or advice can you offer?

20
Dying and Death

Your older brother recently lost his wife to cancer after knowing she was ill for only two months. At first your brother didn't seem to be having any emotional reaction to her death at all. Surrounded by friends and relatives, he immersed himself in taking care of necessary legal and business arrangements. Now that he's wrapping that up, he's showing some emotion but not the emotion you expected. Instead of being depressed he seems to feel enraged—at the world, at himself, even at his late wife. He calls you in the middle of the night and says things that seem unrealistic to you, such as that she wouldn't have died if she really loved him. Other times he berates himself for letting her get sick or blames himself for her death. Is your brother all right? How should you respond, and what can you do to help?

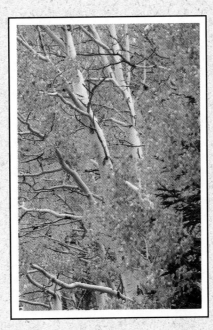

A friend of yours recently went home to attend the funeral of a teacher who had been important to her in high school. She felt the funeral was a moving and satisfying way to say good-bye to him, but she was shocked to hear later how much it had cost his widow. The woman had had to spend part of one of her husband's life insurance policies to cover the expense. Now your friend is concerned about how much it will cost her parents, who aren't wealthy by any means, when their parents die. Is it necessary to spend a fortune on a funeral? Are there alternatives? What advice can you give your friend?

Your parents are in their sixties, and your sister says she wants to talk to them sometime soon about planning for death. She wants to know how they want their bodies disposed of, whether they want to die in a hospital or at home, whether they want heroic measures taken to keep them alive, and what kinds of funerals they want. You feel extremely uncomfortable about discussing these topics with your parents, and you think they would be offended if you brought them up. Your sister reminds you that both your grandfathers died of heart attacks before they were sixty. She thinks it's important to talk to your parents now, while they're still healthy, but she won't if you strongly disagree. Are you right to want to protect your parents from this discussion, or is your sister right to bring it up? What should you do?

A man hiking a high mountain trail suddenly lost his footing and found himself hurtling toward certain death. As he plummeted past a small bush growing out of the sheer rock wall, he caught a berry in his hand and ate it. It was the most delicious berry he had ever eaten. We are each that man: each of us is hurtling toward certain death and how we deal with it has a lot to do with how freely and rewardingly we live our lives.

If you suddenly discovered you had a terminal illness, how would you spend your last year or months? How would you and your family feel about keeping you alive on **life-support systems?** What kind of final ceremony would your family have? What would they do with your possessions? Have you ever talked about these things with your family?

What Is Death?

Death, like life, is change. Matter and energy are never destroyed, but merely change from one form to another. When the body is no longer able to resist unhealthy changes in itself, is mechanically broken beyond repair, or is poisoned by the environment, it ceases to function and dies.

Defining Death   Because we now have machines that can sustain some body functions while the body itself appears to be otherwise lifeless, defining death requires that we account for various physical responses.

Traditionally, physical death has been defined as occurring when the heart stops beating and the person stops breathing. However, the brain continues to function for a short time—less than 10 minutes—after the heart stops beating. Scientists now agree that the brain, not the heart, is the key to human life. Four characteristics describe brain death, according to a Harvard Medical School committee: unreceptivity and unresponsivity, no movements or breathing without mechanical help, no reflexes, and a flat electroencephalogram for ten minutes.

Brain death is most reliably shown by a flat tracing on an **electroencephalogram.** Once the brain stops functioning, the person is medically and, in some states, legally dead. Most states either have already adopted or are considering legislation that redefines death in this way. There are a few exceptions, however. Overdoses of some

depressant drugs can produce a flat electroencephalogram trace, but people who have shown no brain life after such overdoses have recovered. And some patients whose hearts have stopped have recovered when their hearts have been directly massaged or otherwise manipulated.

Cellular death takes longer: it is a gradual process that follows the shutdown of the heart, brain, and respiration and encompasses the breakdown of metabolic processes in the cells so that organs no longer function.

Social death is defined as irreversible loss of the capacity for conscious social interaction. This perspective emphasizes the unique human capabilities—the ability to interact with one's environment and with other human beings—and narrows the definition of death so that it specifies what is essentially significant about human life.

Because the definition of death touches upon many aspects of social life, legally defining death affects criminal prosecution, inheritance, taxation, treatment of the corpse, even mourning. Legal decisions concerning organ transplantation are difficult: organs—particularly hearts—must come from other humans and cannot themselves be damaged. Thus, to provide a viable heart for transplantation requires nearly split-second timing for removing a heart from someone who has just died, as well as an extremely precise definition of death that will guarantee the heart is not taken out too early.

Why Is There Death?   No answer to the question of why death exists can satisfy us. We might think: there is death because there is life; nothing dies that hasn't lived. But that's not much comfort. Neither are we comforted by knowing that matter and energy are never destroyed but are simply changed. We want the light of consciousness; we want to know that we will be able to recognize ourselves. To know we'd be alive in some other form without the same ego wouldn't satisfy most of us.

But death does allow variety: death permits the renewal and evolution of the human species. The normal life span is long enough to ensure that we reproduce ourselves and that our species continues. It is short enough to allow new genetic combinations to be tested. This fact means that we, as a species, can adapt better to changing conditions in the environment. Seen from the viewpoint of species survival and improvement, the arrangement makes sense. But from a personal point of view, death—especially needless, accidental, or sudden death or the

---

Life-support system   Machinery and artificial body parts used to keep alive patients who would otherwise die.

Electroencephalogram   Record of fluctuating electrical potentials of the brain (brain waves) as recorded from electrodes on the scalp.

Cellular death   Total breakdown of metabolic processes occurring at the cell level.

Social death   Irreversible loss of the capacity to interact socially, usually because of unconsciousness.

death of children or adults in the prime of life—remains an emotionally unresolvable puzzle.

How Do We Feel about Death? Death is absolute loss. The thought of losing a best friend, parent, mate, or child often devastates us with outrage and pain. The thought of losing our own consciousness of this world goes against everything we have ever known. We prefer not to think about it—not so much because we don't know what will happen after death but because we must relinquish everything and everyone here. We are thrust involuntarily and unwillingly into having to puzzle out an understanding of what happens to us when we die. We can choose not to consider or accept some controversial issues, such as the likelihood of an afterlife, but not death itself.

Consequently, theories abound concerning what happens when we die. Most religions build their philosophies on the issue of death and its consequences. Some promise a better life after death if adherents behave according to the rules of their group and their god(s). Other religions teach that everyone is growing toward godhood in this life, and that we are born again and again until we reach that perfection. Some philosophers say that we cannot possibly know what happens after death and that we can only judge whether life is or is not worth living according to the rewards we find or make in this life.

■ **Exploring Your Emotions**

Think back to your first encounter with dying and death in your childhood. Who or what died—a pet, a relative, a neighbor? What were your feelings at the time, and what are your feelings as you recall the incident now? What were you told about death when you were a child? Did anyone help you with your feelings about it?

Regardless of the explanations we accept, death is painful, both to the dying person and to the ones left behind. The dying person grieves for both the loss of self and people and things left behind. While young children understand death as an interruption and an absence, their lack of a time perspective means they don't fathom death as final separation. From about ages 5 to 9 children's view of death matures considerably. Now they understand that death is final, but only for others, not for themselves. They think they will escape somehow. From about age 10 upward children begin to adjust to the inevitable: they come to see death as universal, inescapable, and irreversible. In later life, worries about deaths of loved ones may recur, particularly for those who have been married for nearly a lifetime and fear being left alone.

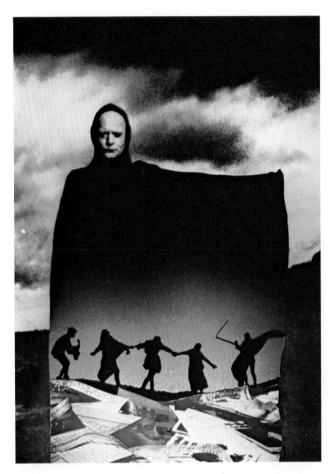

From the dawn of consciousness, people have been trying to understand and come to terms with their mortality. The Grim Reaper is only one of the many forms in which the human imagination has cast death.

Some People Appear to Welcome Death Although some people never accept death, those who have suffered great depression or a painful terminal disease often find the idea of death a relief and a release. Most of us can understand that attitude, particularly for those who are old and have lived a full life. But others—more than 30,000 annually in the United States—feel that death, even if repulsive, is preferable to living and end their lives before nature takes its course.

Forty percent of people who commit suicide are over 60, and the rate among 15- to 24-year-olds has increased over the last twenty years: 20 percent of all males and 14 percent of all females who kill themselves are in this age group. Despair is the most common motive for suicide. In one study a high level of hopelessness was the strongest sign that a person who has attempted suicide will try it again.

Adolescents don't necessarily commit suicide for the same reasons as adults. Because they lack the means, experience, and long-term patterns of grappling with and working through tough problems, they may overreact to and surrender readily to frustrations: failure on a final exam may be interpreted to mean failure in life; a disappointing relationship can be translated to mean permanent loneliness. Many young people—college students and adolescents who live away from home—are out on their own for the first time, away from home and the support group they may have grown up with, confronted by new academic or financial pressures and social adjustments.

Anxiety about schoolwork and exams is an important cause of suicide among college students. Some investigators believe that many young people have an emotionally lifeless relationship with their parents and defend themselves from it by overemphasizing the importance of their schoolwork. Suicidal high school students are more likely to be defiant and delinquent, reckless drivers, or drug and alcohol abusers. They have a high rate of antisocial behavior and have often been exposed to suicidal thoughts and suicide attempts by friends and family members. They are often at odds with their parents and may have been victims of child abuse and neglect. The disturbing rise in adolescent suicide over the last thirty years has not been well explained. Increasing family and social disorganization and rising teenage unemployment appear to contribute to it.

There is no accurate way to predict suicide, and our understanding of its meanings and motives remains limited despite much research into it. Some myths about suicide are listed in a box in Chapter 3. Suicidal adolescents, like suicidal adults, are likely to be deeply depressed, but the signs may be hard to recognize because their sadness and hopelessness are often masked by boredom, apathy, hyperactivity, or physical complaints.

When someone commits suicide, it's frightening to almost everyone involved, even to those who were barely acquaintances; it's very difficult to explain and justify. If someone you know commits suicide, it means someone you may have loved dearly has chosen to relinquish you and chosen to relinquish this life. You may feel betrayed or perhaps guilty, as though you have failed and should have done more to help. It may cause you anguish that the person who committed suicide must have suffered great pain in making such a decision alone and angry that the decision was made without shouting for help. You may also be angry that your friend or loved one didn't care enough about you to have hung on longer. Some people who commit suicide may be using death as a weapon in our death-denying culture: a suicide reminds us that we too will die, that we have the ability—and some of us, perhaps, even the desire—to kill ourselves. We don't want suicide to be an option for people we love. We want them to stick with life, fight their problems, and prevail over them.

The relatives and friends of a person who commits suicide may feel guilt and shame, which prevent normal mourning. They may avoid talking to anyone because they fear social stigma. But in fact, talking and expressing their feelings will help them recover.

Most societies have considered suicide an attack. Until 1961 it was a felony in England, and it is still a crime in the United States. One hundred fifty years ago a person committing suicide in England had to forfeit property to the state; the family lost both property and good name. Someone who committed suicide was considered to have broken a contract with society, because suicide disintegrates the fabric and structure of society; those who kill themselves have judged society, recognized its limitations, and rejected its values, usually expressing a hope of some better life. As a result, Western society has treated suicide as the act of people so deluded or in such deep despair that they couldn't think clearly. Western law has found all sorts of reasons for justifiably killing others, but no reason for killing oneself.

Some religious groups and theologians consider it an attack on God, saying that a suicidal person tries to usurp God's role by taking power over something that God has created. For Thomas Aquinas, a medieval Christian theologian, suicide is the most fatal of sins because it cannot be repented of and, consequently, the person forfeits any future life in heaven.

■ **Exploring Your Emotions**

Many people, especially young people, deny that death will ever happen to them. Do you think that you do this? Try to imagine your own death for a moment. Is it difficult to do? How does it make you feel?

Suicidal behavior in any friend, spouse, or child is frightening and hard to acknowledge. But it does not always signal a hopeless situation: therapeutic counseling can enable some suicidal people to continue leading productive lives and to put suicidal thoughts behind. For a discussion of treatment and assistance for suicidal people, see Chapter 3.

Some Americans Try to Deny Death For several generations in the United States we have tried to deny that death occurs. Some people still can't bring themselves to say "die," so they describe their relatives as having "passed away," or gone "to glory" or "to the great beyond." Families keep children away from those elderly people who are ill, often by putting them in hospitals or nursing homes. A grandparent's death is rarely a home event; we make sure it takes place in a hospital where children aren't likely to be around. They usually don't see what happens when a person dies, and they often are not told the details—or the details are hedged—because the subject is considered distasteful and is difficult for the parents to deal with. Many Americans, both adult and children, have never seen someone die. Death happens to someone else—not to you or me.

Besides "protecting" children from the actual, physical fact of the dead body, we present false ideas of it. Death, the real thing, its finality, its aftermath of grief, is largely taboo. But fake death is a game played all over television and movie screens, and it is always reversible. Children playing war, cops and robbers, or cowboys and Indians, mimic the actors, suddenly gasping and sprawling on the ground, "dead." In a minute, they get up and play the same scene over again. If we're not ignoring the fact of death altogether, we're falsifying it.

Planning for Death

Once we acknowledge the inevitability of death, we can plan for it and ease what might later be hard decisions for both our survivors and ourselves. Just as each stage of human development and growth demands that certain tasks be performed, preparing for death requires completing unfinished business, dealing with medical care needs, allocating our time and energy resources, and helping others plan what will happen after our deaths.

Some decisions can be made right now while you are young. People who find themselves facing a protracted and perhaps painful terminal illness may be too drained physically and emotionally to make decisions that could have been made ahead of time. Some decisions—about wills and ceremonies, for instance—can and should be made as early as your college years, so that an unexpected death is not made even more difficult for survivors. While other decisions perhaps cannot be made until a final illness, all of us can discuss with our closest family members the issues involved in dying and death.

Making a Will Fewer than one-fourth of all Americans get around to drawing up a will. Unfortunately, even in the case of those who feel their estate is very modest, dying without a will usually causes difficulties for the survivors. If there is any substance to the estate, the complications can be tremendous.

A will is a document you draw up that declares how you want your estate—everything you own—distributed when you die (see Figure 20-1). Until you die it can be changed, replaced, destroyed. When you die, it is a binding legal instrument that governs the redistribution of your property. Only property jointly owned—such as automobiles, bank accounts, stocks, real estate, life insurance proceeds, and death benefits—bypasses the law of **intestate** succession. So besides considering a will, you may want to transfer titles of property or add names for joint ownership to avoid having your estate pass through **probate**.

■ **Exploring Your Emotions**

If you were about to die, to whom would you leave your various belongings? Why? If you could give away your nonmaterial assets—your sense of humor, your honesty, and so on—to whom would you leave them? What impact would you like to make on the world in your lifetime?

If you die without a will—intestate—your property will be distributed in any case. An administrator appointed by the court supervises the distribution and is awarded a commission taken directly out of your estate. Usually the administrator is the closest inheriting next of kin and must post a **surety bond**, which is costly (in some states $10 per $1000 of the estate assets, renewable annually until the estate is settled). There will also be commissions (as high as 10 percent of the estate's worth) for the attorney suggested by the administrator and for an appraiser.

If you die intestate, the welfare of your children and that of your spouse will be considered as separate and not necessarily compatible with each other. A fairly rigid and predetermined formula, based on marriage and blood relationships, determines who inherits what. Anyone who is close to you in spirit only—perhaps living with you or taking care of you—if not related by blood or marriage, will get nothing. Although the distribution may be just the way you would have done it, chances are that it will not be.

You should make out a will upon reaching the **age of majority**. You can have an attorney draw it up for you for a fee, or you can get some do-it-yourself books—usually written by attorneys—that will show you how. Every will includes some standard elements. Your will should contain specific language canceling any previous will. Give your full name and where you live. Name your personal representative (the person you choose to take

---

Intestate Having made no legal will.

Probate Legal process that establishes the validity of a will.

Surety bond Guarantee—usually an amount of money—put up by a person who assumes responsibilities and debts of another, to insure against loss or damage.

Age of majority Age at which one is legally responsible for oneself.

Figure 20-1 A sample will.

Last Will and Testament

I, _____, of the city of _____, and state of _____, being of sound mind, memory, and understanding, declare this to be my last will and testament, as follows:

1. _Debts and Funeral Expenses_. I direct that all debts enforceable against my estate, and funeral expenses, be paid as soon as possible.

2. _Executor and Trustee_. I nominate and appoint _____ _____ as executor and trustee of my estate. My executor and trustee shall have the full power at his discretion to do all the things necessary for the liquidation of my estate.

3. _Spouse_. I give and bequeath to my _____ [husband or wife] all my interest in real estate and 50% of all money that I have in banks, savings and loans, certificates of deposit, and similar institutions.

4. _Children_. I give and bequeath the following items to my children. To my son, _____, I give _____.

To my daughter, _____, I give _____. To my _____, _____, I give _____.

5. _Charity_. I give and bequeath the following items to charitable organizations. To _____, I give _____. To _____ I give _____.

6. _Remainder of Estate_. I direct that the remainder of my estate be sold and that the proceeds be divided as follows: _____

7. _Death of Beneficiaries_. In the event that any of the beneficiaries named in this will die before me, or at approximately the same time as me, I direct that their children shall take their share, equally. In the event that any of the beneficiaries die before me without leaving children, I direct that the remaining named beneficiaries shall take their share, equally.

8. _Revocation of Other Wills_. I hereby revoke all prior wills, codicils, and testamentary dispositions made by me.

IN WITNESS TO THIS WILL I HAVE SET MY HAND TO THIS WILL THIS _____ DAY OF _____, 19_____.

_____

This will, consisting of _____ pages, each bearing the signature of _____ was signed on this date, and declared by _____ to be the last will and testament.

The will was signed in the presence of the following three witnesses

WITNESS   WITNESS

_____   _____

SIGNATURE   SIGNATURE

_____   _____

ADDRESS   ADDRESS

charge of your financial affairs and distribute property after your death), and lay out general directions for him or her to follow and specific instructions on how you want your property disposed of. You may specify general policy guidelines for the executor, perhaps regarding your children and regarding any ongoing business or property investments. Finally, designate who is to receive what's left.

Deciding What to Do with the Body Dying people will probably want to decide how their bodies should be disposed of: whether embalmed or not, buried, cremated, given to medicine for research, or prepared for donating organs. They can indicate whether they want a funeral or a memorial service, a wake or a party, and then plan the agenda. Some people prefer no services.

■ **Exploring Your Emotions**

How do you feel about what happens to your body after you die? Do you plan to donate organs or give your body to medicine for research? How do you feel about an autopsy? Do you have strong feelings about it? Can you determine the basis for your preferences and feelings?

Whatever your preference, wishes regarding burial, cremation, ceremony, and other issues should be expressed to the family—as well as "officially" expressed through a preplanned arrangement with a funeral home or memorial society. These decisions are easiest when considered early in life while you are still in good health.

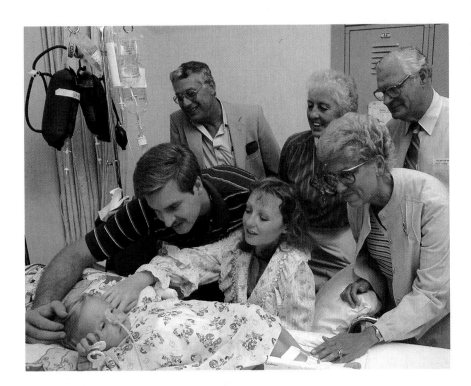

Organ transplants give hope to those who would otherwise have died. This little boy recovering from kidney transplant surgery has a chance to live a normal life thanks to a willing donor.

Donating Organs   A human body is a valuable resource. Many of its parts can be used to revitalize the living. Eye corneas can be transplanted to give sight to the blind. Kidneys can give years of vigorous life to people whose own have stopped working. Human skin is the best dressing for burn wounds. Bones can be used for grafting. Pituitary glands are desperately needed to enable some children to grow normally. In some parts of the world undiseased blood from dead bodies is used for transfusions. Jaws are needed for dental training. Although some people may find the thought of donating organs unsettling, the procedures aren't very different from those used in routine autopsies and normal preparation for burial.

The simplest and most widely used plan for donating body parts is through the **Uniform Donor card,** available from the National Kidney Foundation (see Figure 20-2). The Uniform Anatomical Gift Act, or its equivalent, has been adopted in all states and permits you to bequeath your body for immediate use after death. Several steps are involved and you need to register in these programs before the death occurs, so look into this possibility early and read the fine print about costs and requirements. In some states, permission to "harvest" usable tissues after death is communicated by a card signed and attached to the driver's license.

Burial   Traditionally in this country, people have been buried after death. However, recent exposés of the funeral industry have documented the industry's inflated costs and hard sell of unnecessary options. In response, **memorial societies** have sprung up: they are nonprofit groups of consumers who help members prearrange simple, economical burials. Because they are nonprofit they provide straight information about legal requirements, costs, and arrangements. About 175 memorial societies now operate in the United States and Canada. Membership usually runs $10 to $20 and anyone can join. You can join these societies at any time, preferably before the need is urgent so that you can decide options while you are not grieving.

Because of adverse publicity and the rise of memorial societies, the funeral industry has attempted to modify its sales approach to people in grief.

Cremation   Burning a body to its bones—**cremation**—is a clean, simple, economical way of returning earth to earth. The entire job of picking up the body, cremating, and preparing the death certificate may cost about $300. As the population increases and land prices rise, more people may prefer cremation.

Uniform Donor Card   A consent form authorizing use of the signer's body parts upon his or her death.

Memorial societies   Nonprofit groups of consumers that guide members toward simple, economical burials or cremations.

Cremation   Burning a body to its bones at very high temperatures.

UNIFORM DONOR CARD

OF_____
                Print or type name of donor
In the hope that I may help others, I hereby make this anatomical gift,
if medically acceptable, to take effect upon my death. The words and
marks below indicate my desires.

I give: (a) _____ any needed organs or parts
          (b) _____ only the following organs or parts

_____
                Specify the organ(s) or part(s)
for the purposes of transplantation, therapy, medical research
or education;
          (c) _____ my body for anatomical study if needed.

Limitations or
special wishes, if any :_____

Signed by the donor and the following two witnesses in the presence of
each other:

_____   _____
    Signature of Donor   Date of Birth of Donor

_____   _____
    Date Signed   City & State

_____   _____
    Witness   Witness

This is a legal document under the Uniform Anatomical Gift Act or similar laws.

For further information consult your physician or

KF   **National Kidney Foundation**
         116 East 27th Street, New York, N.Y. 10016

Figure 20-2   A sample organ donor card.

Planning a Ceremony   The bereaved can benefit from participating in a ceremony. A typical American Christian funeral ceremony involves **embalming** the corpse; friends viewing the body in the funeral home before the funeral service; friends and fellow church members supplying the bereaved with flowers and food; a religious ceremony; and a processional to the graveside and a final ceremony there. Other religions have different traditions, as do other ethnic groups and other countries.

New ceremonies are evolving. Some people dispose of the body immediately, so that neither embalming nor viewing the body occurs. A celebration can grow in whatever way is appropriate for all involved. Choose a place that's meaningful—indoors or out in nature. Allow the participants to decide whether they wish to speak about their feelings for the person or to be silent. Do they want a minister? a leader? Do they want to share food or dancing or song? a prayer circle?

The dying can also choose a cemetery plot and gravestone or, if cremated, indicate whether they want their ashes kept somewhere or scattered in a garden or at sea. In choosing a cemetery plot, be sure to compare advice from several sources and to consider such things as distance from the homes of relatives, costs, religious denomination, how well the graves are maintained, and the reputation of the cemetery. The gravestone can be a separate consideration.

Arranging to Pay for the Funeral   Arranging how to pay for the funeral is a significant decision because it can be quite costly. Social Security insurance allows several hundred dollars toward it. The Veterans Administration also allots approximately $400 to honorably discharged veterans for funeral and cemetery costs. Other ethnic groups, fraternal societies, and unions sometimes provide lump sum benefits to pay funeral costs. You may want to earmark a special bank account for funeral expenses so that relatives will not be strapped by paying them. Or the money can come out of the estate's assets upon the death, if the estate is large enough to cover them. Other methods of payment include prepayment plans.

Choosing Where to Die   Will you spend your last days at home tended by relatives and friends, or would dying in the hospital improve the quality of life? Although the decision about where we die is not always ours, we can and should consider all alternatives. If death is not sudden and we do have a choice, the more we know about options, the more likely we and our families are to make the most appropriate choice.

At Home   Dying at home demands considerable time and energy from relatives and may require money for hired nurses. Not so long ago almost everyone died at home, but now a very small percentage of Americans do. Dying in the hospital may be more appropriate if small children

---

Embalming   Treating a dead body to retard decomposition.

Hospice   Community-oriented, long-term treatment facility for chronic and dying patients; provides social and psychological support as well as medical care.

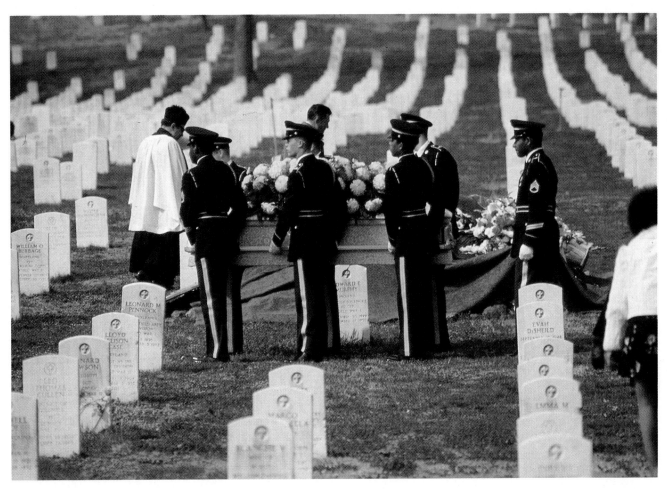

Funeral customs exist in virtually every society and mark the final rite of passage in an individual's life. Like most funerals, this military ceremony in Arlington National Cemetery includes honoring the deceased person, providing a framework for the transition from life to death, and disposing of the body.

in the home need care, if the patient needs intravenous feedings, if the patient cannot afford private nurses, or if a person plans to donate organs for transplant.

Many good books can educate caregivers about every facet of tending a patient (see, for example, *A Guide to Dying at Home* by Deborah Duda, listed at the end of the chapter). They teach about injections and other practical home care techniques; they list needed medical supplies; they discuss how to deal with morale, how to handle visitors, and other practical issues. They discuss financial considerations in hiring nurses and aides. And they are a mine of resources for help: they give information about financial aid from city, county, and state services; Social Security and survivor benefits; Medicaid; Veterans Administration aid; legal aid services; state board of health;

medical examiner, and county coroner; medical supplies through rentals; specific disease-oriented groups such as the American Cancer Society; and medical supply companies and hospital pharmacies.

Health Care at a Hospice   The **hospice** is an alternative to both home care—when relatives need some relief—and hospital care for the dying. The special needs of dying people are usually not well served by regular hospitals because the primary objectives of hospitals are short-term intense medical treatment, not long-term maintenance care. The professional staff is geared toward short-term treatment, and the social mix of patients does not lend itself to the special problems of the dying. Hospital costs are very high.

To better serve the needs of dying patients, their families and their friends, the hospice philosophy was successfully developed some years ago in England. Hospices are becoming more common in the United States (see the box "Hospices—Comfort and Care for the Dying"). They are usually administered by a team of medical, social work, mental health, legal, and spiritual practitioners who provide support, comfort, and resources for the dying. The hospice philosophy discourages inappropriate treatment and expensive life-extending medical services. Since volunteers are used widely, costs are greatly reduced. In the past they have ministered mainly to cancer patients and the terminally ill, but programs vary among the hospices.

Deciding Whether to Prolong Life   Thousands of people are alive today who would quickly die if nature took its course. Anyone who uses a heart pacemaker or an artificial kidney benefits from advanced life-support technology. Even severely disabled people, such as those who cannot use any limbs, are helped to continue living. These medical practices have miraculously and appropriately extended the lives of thousands of people.

■ **Exploring Your Emotions**

How do you think you would feel if someone you loved were terminally ill and in pain and asked to be allowed to die? What would you do? How do you think you would feel if a friend told you he or she wanted to die because of depression and an inability to cope with life's problems? What would you do?

In spite of some apparent successes, however, people are seriously objecting to the medical tradition of keeping people alive by all means and at any expense. Should a patient who cannot possibly recover, one who is not capable of knowing a meaningful life, and who may even have requested not to be kept alive for a long time in a coma, be kept alive? Some families are emotionally and financially ruined while a loved one—or any dependent—is maintained in a seemingly endless coma or in a vegetative state.

Is Euthanasia Moral?   Several issues arise in considering the feasibility of **euthanasia**, also called mercy killing. Is it moral? Some people believe that life itself is sacred, that under no circumstances should we kill or shorten any life. Some of these same people might not fight in a

war, support the death penalty, or allow abortions. They make up their own minds where to draw the line against killing or follow the suggestions of their church. They frequently also support punishment for anyone who helps someone die.

Others believe that quality, rather than quantity, of life is the issue and that under some conditions it is an act of compassion to help a person die. The most radical acceptance of euthanasia in the world is found in the Netherlands. There, a physician who meets strict criteria can give a lethal injection to a dying person who has requested death, and the physician will not be punished. A landmark case in the evolution of Dutch euthanasia occurred in 1981 when the criminal court in Rotterdam set standards for noncriminal aid in dying and laid out these rules:

1. There must be physical or mental suffering that the sufferer finds unbearable.
2. The suffering and the desire to die must be lasting, not temporary.
3. The decision to die must be the voluntary decision of an informed patient.
4. The person must have a correct and clear understanding of his or her condition and of other possibilities (treatments), must be capable of weighing these options, and must have done so.
5. There is no other reasonable (acceptable to the patient) solution to improve the situation.
6. The time and manner of death will not cause avoidable misery to others; that is, if possible, the next of kin should be informed beforehand.
7. The decision to give aid in dying should not be a one-person decision. Consulting another professional (medical doctor, social worker, psychologist, according to the circumstances of the case) is obligatory.
8. A medical doctor must be involved in the decision to prescribe the correct drugs.
9. The decision process and the actual aid must be done with the utmost care.

Will Euthanasia Be Legalized?   Another issue concerning euthanasia is its legality. In most countries, helping someone die is against the law and punishable by prison, perhaps even death. The charge can be murder or manslaughter. Although some people know they are doing the right thing in helping a loved one die, they also know that they can be prosecuted and punished. The most compassionate of crimes must also be the most secret of crimes. Few cases of euthanasia are reported; and because

---

Euthanasia   The act of helping a person die quickly, easily, and painlessly.

Hospices: Comfort and Care for the Dying

Hospice programs aim to meet a wide range of physical, social, psychological, and spiritual needs of people who require sustained medical attention. While they are known to be effective in treatment of the terminally ill, they are also open to other chronically ill patients as well. About 40 percent of cases use the hospice program to give respite to relatives; 20 percent of admissions are social isolates with no one able or willing to care for them. At the same time, 60 percent of admissions need help with better control of their pain. So hospice patients represent a mix of social and clinical needs.

Hospice programs vary from one facility to another. Some are entirely home-care oriented, while others are exclusively institutional, with no home-care services. Some have very limited bereavement follow-up service, while others offer extensive bereavement service. Many have services available on a 24-hours-a-day, seven-days-a-week basis, while some operate fewer hours.

The following list represents the ideal program toward which hospice administrators strive.

1. Service availability to home care patients and inpatients on a 24-hours-a-day, seven-days-a-week, on-call basis with emphasis on availability of medical and nursing skills

2. Home-care service in collaboration with inpatient facilities

3. Knowledge and expertise in the control of symptoms (physical, psychological, social, and spiritual)

4. The provision of care by an interdisciplinary team

5. Physician-directed services

6. Central administration and coordination of services

7. Use of volunteers as an integral part of the health-care team

8. Involvement of the patient in decision making and of family members in care giving

9. Acceptance to the program based on health needs, not on ability to pay

10. Treatment of the patient and family together

11. A bereavement follow-up service

The hospice movement underwent significant change in 1982, when services became eligible for Medicare reimbursement. This change has allowed hospices to expand their programs and has led to more standardized care.

Medicare, of course, does have rules. Guidelines cover the time a patient spends in a hospital or nursing home. Other regulations govern the total cost of services. Hospices must apply for Medicare accreditation. At present, about one-third are part of the Medicare system. Physicians in the United States are increasingly supportive of the hospice concept, but they remain less involved than their European colleagues. Experts call for more research into the benefits and limitations of hospice service. Hospices are not "high-tech," but they are "high-touch" (labor-intensive). Personnel costs must be managed carefully. Staff training and salary are important issues.

In general, people who are terminally ill are more likely to die at home if they receive hospice care than if they have traditional care in institutions. Many patients and their families appreciate having the end of life in this more natural environment. Still, this calls for a major commitment from the family. In the last weeks of a patient's life, the family may provide up to sixteen hours of care each day, with only three or four hours of respite from hospice staff who help with caregiver activities.

Many families deem this effort worthwhile. They appreciate sharing their grief with others who care and yet bring a sense of perspective to the situation. As one physician wrote to a medical journal in praise of the hospice concept:

> When your patient dies peacefully at home, you know you have not "lost the case." You have achieved the aim of medicine at the end of life. When a family member says, "You made it easier," you know you have not treated just a disease, but a family.

There are many types of hospice care throughout the United States. To find what services are available in your region, contact: National Hospice Organization, Suite 307, 1901 North Fort Myer Drive, Arlington, VA 22209, Telephone (703) 243-5900.

Based on Hospices: Comfort and Care for the Dying, *Mayo Clinic Health Letter*, March 1988.

dying patients are often heavily dosed with drugs, it is not always possible to tell exactly the cause of death.

Some people who cannot justify active administration of lethal drugs to help a person die accept the practice of **passive euthanasia**: withdrawing or not initiating life-support systems such as respirators and intravenous feedings when the dying person no longer has chances of recovery. An ethics panel of the American Medical Association has concluded that artificial feeding and the infusion of water can be stopped in cases of irreversible coma. One state's Supreme Court has ruled that mentally competent, informed patients have the right to refuse any medical treatment, including life support provided by mechanical or artificial means. Some people hail that decision as a victory for individual liberties; others call it legal suicide. What do you think?

Since 1975 American courts have by and large been affirming the right of individuals or their agents to control their deaths. Between 1976 and 1990 forty-one states enacted Natural Death Acts, which allow anyone to sign a **living will**—a document stating that if the person is suffering from a terminal illness that is certified by one (or two) physicians, the person's life should not be sustained by medication, artificial means, or heroic measures. Living wills also protect physicians from liability for acting in accordance with such wishes. Even in states that don't have Natural Death Acts, a living will can be influential. The box "Controlling Your Death" includes a sample living will.

Asking for Help   Sometimes so many things need to be decided that the dying person will ask for help. It is possible to delegate authority to another responsible, trusted person. This person is granted **power of attorney**—the legal authority to act in another person's name. It can be general or for a specific project only, and it can set a time limit (see the sample form in Figure 20-3). A dying person who wishes to give someone power of attorney for health care will want to acquaint that person with survivor benefits (Social Security, pension benefits, life insurance) and should gather together all official documents, such as the following:

- Last will and testament
- Birth and adoption certificates
- Marriage and divorce papers
- Citizenship papers
- Military service papers
- Social security numbers
- Organization memberships and benefits
- Life and accident insurance policies
- Bank accounts, stocks, bonds, savings bonds
- Safe deposit box
- Real estate papers

If a health care power of attorney has not been signed, one of the following persons, in this order, will usually be authorized to make life-and-death decisions: a court-appointed guardian, if one already exists; the spouse; an adult child; a parent; an adult brother or sister; or the nearest living relative. Any decision one of these people makes is expected to be based on the patient's wishes, if known, or made in the patient's best interests, as far as the person believes.

Previewing Tasks for the Family after the Death   To prevent legal complications, the family needs a death certificate signed by a physician, medical examiner, or **county coroner.** If a person dies unexpectedly (even though of natural causes) or from a rare or highly researched disease, the doctors may request an **autopsy.** This means that the body will be opened, the organs of interest examined, and perhaps certain parts removed for study. In cases of a natural death, family permission is required to perform an autopsy. If cause of death is unnatural, questionable, unexplained, accidental, or bizarre, the coroner will require an autopsy.

■ **Exploring Your Emotions**

How prepared do you feel to deal with the deaths of your grandparents or parents? Are there any steps you can take to make things easier for them or yourself?

Otherwise, if the person has signed a Uniform Donor's Card, find it and call the closest medical school. They will generally pick up the body, or you may have to pay

---

Passive euthanasia   The act of withdrawing life-support systems when a dying person no longer has a chance to recover.

Living will   A document stating that in case of a terminal disease or a state where recovery is impossible, a person's life should not be sustained by medication, artificial means, or heroic measures.

Power of attorney   A legal document that confers authority to do things in another person's name.

County coroner   A public official authorized to investigate unexpected deaths and deaths in unusual circumstances.

Autopsy   Examination of a body after death, usually to determine the cause of death.

Controlling Your Death: The Living Will

More and more Americans are taking legal precautions in the hope of dying with dignity. They are having their lawyers draw up living wills—signed, dated, and witnessed documents that allow them to state in advance their wishes regarding the use of life-sustaining procedures. "If you're incompetent or unconscious at the end of your life, someone will make the choice," says Fenella Rouse, executive director of the Society for the Right to Die. "If you don't want to make that decision, fine. But this is one of the ways of retaining control."

Two groups, the Society for the Right to Die and Concern for Dying, both located in New York City, have distributed millions of living-will forms over the past twenty years. Other organizations, such as the National Academy of Elder Law Attorneys in Tucson, Arizona, provide information on how to locate lawyers who specialize in drawing up such legal tools. In addition, many right-to-die advocates recommend the use of health-care proxies, or power of attorney documents, to authorize another person to make medical decisions on one's behalf in the event of an incapacitating accident or illness.

Living wills usually serve two purposes: they describe what sort of physical condition is intended to trigger the document's provisions, and they list the types of treatment the person wishes to avoid. Experts recommend making the language as specific as possible, although there are no absolute guarantees that instructions will be carried out as intended.

The main shortcoming of the living will is that it does not take effect unless a patient is terminally ill. Definitions of terminal illness vary from state to state, ranging from "imminent" death to death within a number of months. Thus, people with debilitating strokes or Alzheimer's disease or those in permanent comas are unlikely to be protected by most living-will statutes, a crucial point misunderstood by many people.

Still, living wills and health-care proxies are the best means available to enforce one's wishes. For those who choose this route, experts make the following suggestions:

- Obtain the proper forms or the help of an attorney.
- Discuss your living will and proxy with your doctor. Make sure that copies are included in your medical records.
- Be certain your living will reflects your precise wishes. Be aware of the limitations your state imposes.
- Inform your family and friends that you have signed these documents. Give copies to those most likely to be contacted in case of an emergency.
- Update the documents once a year.

Copies of the living will shown here can be obtained by writing to the Euthanasia Educational Council, 250 W. 57th St., New York, NY 10019.

Adapted from To my family. Andrea Sachs. 1990. *Time*, March 19.

**TO MY FAMILY, MY PHYSICIAN, MY LAWYER, MY CLERGYMAN
TO ANY MEDICAL FACILITY IN WHOSE CARE I HAPPEN TO BE
TO ANY INDIVIDUAL WHO MAY BECOME RESPONSIBLE FOR MY HEALTH,
WELFARE OR AFFAIRS**

Death is as much a reality as birth, growth, maturity and old age—it is the one certainty of life. If the time comes when I, _____ can no longer take part in decisions for my own future, let this statement stand as an expression of my wishes, while I am still of sound mind.

If the situation should arise in which there is no reasonable expectation of my recovery from physical or mental disability, I request that I be allowed to die and not be kept alive by artificial means or "heroic measures". I do not fear death itself as much as the indignities of deterioration, dependence and hopeless pain. I, therefore, ask that medication be mercifully administered to me to alleviate suffering even though this may hasten the moment of death.

This request is made after careful consideration. I hope you who care for me will feel morally bound to follow its mandate. I recognize that this appears to place a heavy responsibility upon you, but it is with the intention of relieving you of such responsibility and of placing it upon myself in accordance with my strong convictions, that this statement is made.

Signed _____

Date _____

Witness _____

Witness _____

Copies of this request have been given to _____

_____

_____

_____

Figure 20-3 A sample power of attorney for health care form.

POWER OF ATTORNEY FOR HEALTH CARE

I, *(your name)*, hereby appoint: *name, address and phone numbers)* as my attorney-in-fact to make health care decisions for me if I become unable to make my own health care decisions. This gives my attorney-in-fact the power to grant, refuse or withdraw consent on my behalf for any health care service, treatment or procedure. My attorney-in-fact also has the authority to talk to health care personnel, get information and sign forms necessary to carry out these decisions.

With this document, I intent to create a power of attorney for health care, which shall take effect if I become incapable of making my own health care decisions and shall continue during that incapacity.

My attorney-in-fact shall make health care decisions as I direct below or as I make known to my attorney-in-fact in some other way.

(a) Statement of directives concerning life-prolonging care, treatment, services and procedures:

(b) Special provisions and limitations:

By my signature I indicate that I understand the purpose and effect of this document. I sign my name to this form on *(date),* at *(address).*

_____

_____

Your signature

WITNESSES

I declare that the person who signed or acknowledged this document is personally known to me, that the person signed or acknowledged this durable power of attorney for health care in my presence, and that the person appears to be of sound mind and under no duress, fraud or undue influence. I am not the person appointed as the attorney-in-fact by this document, nor am I the health care provider of the principal or an employee of the health care provider of the principal.

(Date, and print names, signatures and addresses of two witnesses)

At least one of the witnesses listed above shall also sign the following declaration: I further declare that I am not related to the principal by blood, marriage or adoption, and, to the best of my knowledge, I am not entitled to any part of the estate of the principal under a currently existing will or by operation of law.

_____

_____

(Signatures)

transportation costs. Tell them what you want done with the body after the school is finished with it.

Advising friends and relatives of the death and burial plans should be done promptly to allow them time to plan to be there. A list of phone numbers and addresses should be ready beforehand. You might find volunteer friends who could help with the calls.

From Ernest Morgan's *A Manual of Death Education and Simple Burial* comes this checklist of things to be done after the death. It may take you and friends weeks or months to finish.

- Take care of yourself first.
- List immediate family, close friends, employer, business colleagues. Notify each by phone.
- If flowers are to be omitted, decide on appropriate memorial or charity to which gifts may be made.
- Write obituary. Include age, place of birth, cause of death, occupation, college degrees, memberships held, military service, outstanding work, lists of survivors in immediate family. Give time and place of memorial services. Deliver in person or by phone to newspapers.
- Notify insurance companies, including automobile insurance, for immediate cancellation and refund of premium.
- Arrange for family members or close friends to rotate answering door and phone. Keep a record of the calls.
- Arrange appropriate child care.
- Coordinate the supplying of food for the next several days.
- Consider special household needs, such as cleaning, that friends might help with.
- Arrange hospitality for visiting relatives and friends.
- Select pallbearers and notify. Choose sturdy people who can carry a heavy load.
- Notify lawyer and personal representative.
- Plan for disposition of flowers after funeral (perhaps send to a rest home).
- List people to be notified by letter or printed notice.
- Prepare message for printed notice, if needed.
- List people to receive acknowledgments of flowers, calls, and so forth. Send appropriate written or printed notes.
- Check carefully all life and casualty insurance policies and death benefits, including Social Security, fraternal, military, credit and trade unions. Check also on income for survivors from these sources.
- Check promptly on debts, mortgages, and installment payments. Some may carry life insurance clauses that cancel the debt. If payments must be delayed, consult creditors to ask for more time.
- If the deceased lived alone, notify utilities and landlord. Tell post office where to send mail. Take precautions against thieves.

Coming to Terms with Death

Most people have definite ideas about when and how they want to die. Usually we don't get to choose either the time or the means. But if you have a terminal illness that lasts a while, you will have to cope with specific issues in facing the "end game." Doing so may be the most difficult experience you ever have. You may have to adjust to becoming dependent; your activities may be reduced drastically; you may be very depressed. But there is no question that the dying benefit from having others around them—to listen, to share, to care. Most people can adapt and learn and grow if they have enough time and help, but it is a gradual process.

It shouldn't be surprising that one of the best ways to learn to cope with the reality of your own death is to participate in the deaths of your loved ones, even from childhood. With the pain of experiencing each death, you work through some fears and resolve some of your questions about the unknown.

Coping with Dying   How can you come to terms with the prospect of your own death? Responses vary greatly. In his book *Dying,* John Hinton observed that about half of dying people openly acknowledge their death and accept it. About a quarter of them speak with undisguised anguish about their death, and a quarter deny it entirely and do not speak about it at all.

■ **Exploring Your Emotions**

If you were told you had a short time to live, what would you do—withdraw, try to tie up loose ends, try to satisfy unfulfilled desires or have new experiences, try to take care of others, make no changes? Why do you think you would react this way?

After observing and interviewing hundreds of dying people, Dr. Elisabeth Kübler-Ross identified and generalized several common—though not inevitable—psychological stages people experience in coming to terms with their own deaths; she published these in her book *On Death and Dying.* Not everyone experiences every stage of emotions, nor in the same order, nor for the same duration, and some reactions may be experienced simultaneously. Working through these intense feelings enables us to accept the loss of death.

- *Stage one: denial and isolation.* Stage one is a temporary state of shock in which people deny the fact of death and isolate themselves from further confrontation with

A terminal illness allows people time to confront death directly and attempt to come to terms with it—for some, the most significant and deeply felt experience of their lives. This woman nears death from cancer in a hospice.

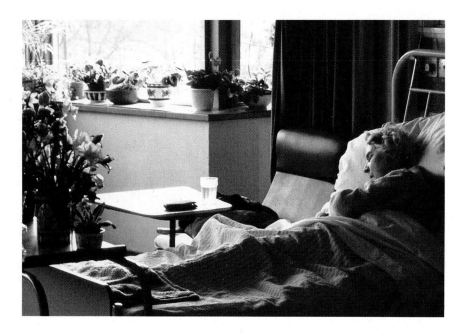

it. They say "Not me" and "You're wrong" and insist "It can't be." Denial is a useful stage because it acts as a buffer against shocks and gives the person time to collect her- or himself and mobilize other defenses.

- *Stage two: anger.* When people can no longer deny the truth, anger often follows. They ask "Why me?" and tend to lash out at family, physicians, and the hospital, blaming them for the situation. Anger at this stage is also a normal response to disability and losing control over one's life and situation.
- *Stage three: bargaining.* As a means of marshalling remaining hope, people may work to discover a way out: a common tack is to make promises to God in exchange for a prolonged life. Grasping at any straw of hope— any new treatment—makes one especially vulnerable to quackery and to charlatans.
- *Stage four: depression.* At this stage people accept their fate and often become depressed about problems they are leaving behind and unfinished work. Depression is also a kind of grief that they experience to prepare themselves for the final separation from this world. While this stage is often emotionally painful, it is an appropriate step in the process and is eased considerably when people are allowed to express sorrow in an atmosphere of nonjudgmental support and care.
- *Stage five: acceptance.* Finally, people may reach a point at which they are no longer angry, nor hoping for a miracle, nor depressed. They just accept that nothing is certain until it happens and are willing to live as much as is possible in the remaining time, to wait, and to watch. They appear both to suspend judgment about their future and to appreciate the present. They ac-

knowledge that they are powerless over the future and appear somewhat content to make the best of it. They may choose not to talk with visitors, even family, in preparation for departing. It is part of the letting go.

Other observers have mapped quite different response patterns to the dying process. One suggests that a sequence to the way people will live their final days cannot be predicted: their predicament tosses them from one emotion to the next. Another suggests that people die in a fashion that most accords with their basic personality and that the disease affects the way one dies. Dr. Edwin Schneidman observes a continual seesaw effect, dictated somewhat by personality: "a waxing and waning of anguish, terror, acquiescence and surrender, rage, and envy, disinterest and ennui, pretense, taunting and daring and even yearning for death—all these in the context of bewilderment and pain."

Seemingly contradictory theories merely underline the variety of human situations and responses, and they point out what others have observed about death: that it is a mountain with many paths to the top, and that each observer will see only those paths and that part of the mountain that experience and perspective allow him or her to see. The point is not to expect that a dying person will or should behave predictably, but rather that each person's needs should be discovered so that we can help ease the last days most effectively.

Supporting a Dying Person Modern medicine can now predict earlier and more accurately whether illnesses are terminal. Increasing numbers of people know in advance that they or others will die in weeks or months. More than ever before, people have a chance to help others experience dying gracefully and with dignity. Establishing and maintaining physical and emotional closeness with the dying person is an important part of the process. Allowing them to speak and act honestly and openly about the experience that is foremost on their mind is crucial, even though talking about death may be painful for you and others who will need to spend time with the dying person.

No rule governs who should inform a person that they are dying. Sometimes the doctor does it, sometimes a family member or a friend. Sometimes the dying figure it out and ask if their suspicions are true. Then our task is to support and help them take care of unfinished business and to deal with the array of emotions that will confront them.

A dying person's needs are not so different from anyone else's, but they are more urgent. Dying people need to know that they are valued, that they are not alone, that they are not being judged, and that those around them care and are trying to understand and to learn about this final hard place just as they are. Most need to know the truth about their physical condition. Dying people often need someone to listen to them while they talk their way through the experience and the stages of emotions—including denial—mentioned already. Friends are as important to dying people as they are to the living. As with any friendship, there are opportunities for growth on both sides.

Besides friends and family the dying person should have access to other sources of support. These might be the family physician, psychological counselors, and religious counsel. Not all therapists are equally effective and helpful, and it might take time to find the right one. Many organizations are oriented toward self-help and work with the dying and their families. Just a few groups you might want to contact are listed here. They can advise you further.

International Federation on Aging
1909 K Street NW
Washington, D.C. 20049

Forum for Death Education and Counseling
P. O. Box 1226
Arlington, VA 22210

Center for Death Education and Research
University of Minnesota
1167 Social Sciences Building
Minneapolis, MN 55445

Institute of Gerontology
520 E. Liberty Street
University of Michigan
Ann Arbor, MI 48109

The National Self-help Groups Clearinghouse is located at the

Graduate School and University Center
City University of New York
33 W. Forty Second Street
New York, New York 10036
School of Public Health and Social Welfare
U.C.L.A.
Los Angeles, CA 90024

In addition, chapters of the Self-help Group Clearinghouse can be found in many cities.

To be effective with the dying, a counselor must be compassionate, have some professional training in the principles of caring for the dying, be comfortable with the idea of death, and have a nonjudgmental philosophy. As a benevolent outsider the counselor can run interference for patients and serve as a liaison between them, their families, and physicians. A therapist can help patients accept death by working through specific fears (such as that the family may not be able to cope without them), by finding purpose in their past and a pattern to their existence, and by resolving negative feelings they may have held toward themselves and others.

Some hospitals and health organizations run group programs for the dying. They are usually chaired by a professional counselor and are designed to help patients voice their worries. Discussion is usually voluntary, and mutual support is encouraged, along with honest, open discussion. You can contact these groups by inquiring of social workers, doctors, medical services at a hospital, and other patients, and by checking local bulletin boards and newspapers.

Terminally ill people often testify that they have had the most significant experiences of their lives after they found out they were soon to die. Aware of their limited time, they are sometimes enabled to delight in and find greater meaning from the experiences of life. They become more aware of what they will lose and are able to appreciate small events that might have seemed insignificant before. Some people find deep meaning in ordering their business affairs and finally saying to loved ones important things they may have been too inhibited to say before.

Grieving   If you can allow yourself to feel and express anguish when someone close to you dies, you will be better able to accept the loss and free yourself to continue with your life. Grieving is a means to healing.

If your loved one dies after a long illness, you will probably have mixed feelings of relief that it's over and pain as you try to return to focusing on your own life. You may feel anger over unresolved issues in the relationship. And you may have feelings similar to those the

TACTICS AND TIPS

Coping with Grief

- Realize and recognize the loss.
- Take time for nature's slow, sure, stuttering process of healing.
- Give yourself massive doses of restful relaxation and routine busy-ness.
- Know that powerful, overwhelming feelings will lessen with time.
- Be vulnerable, share your pain, and be humble enough to accept support.

- Surround yourself with life: plants, animals, and friends.
- Use mementos to help your mourning, not to live in the dead past.
- Avoid rebound relationships, big decisions, and anything addictive.
- Keep a diary and record successes, memories, and struggles.
- Prepare for change, new interests, new friends, solitude, creativity, growth.

- Recognize that forgiveness (of ourselves and others) is a vital part of the healing process.
- Know that holidays and anniversaries can bring up the painful feelings you thought you had successfully worked through.
- Realize that any new death-related crisis will bring up feelings about past losses.

Source: The Centre for Living with Dying

---

dying person had: denial, isolation, guilt, anger, bargaining, depression, and acceptance. You will have so many different feelings—perhaps conflicting ones—and such intense feelings that you will need to find some resolution through talking and crying, maybe yelling. Don't try to hold back feelings and be strong and brave; no one should expect you to. However, you need not pretend to grieve if you don't have strong feelings of grief. Only be sensitive to the pain around you.

Although there is no universal pattern of stages to grief, some behaviors repeat themselves in mourning. First, you will probably feel some shock and numbness in the few days after death and through the funeral. One valuable aspect of a funeral is that activities occupy thoughts and time.

When the immediate bustle of activities following the death ends, a letdown and some silence may follow. Friends may not be as accessible as they had been while they were seeing you through the crisis. You begin to face the fact of the loss, that you really are alone, and then you may experience throbbing emotional pain.

The second stage can last a long time. During this period you may feel disorientation, despair, bewilderment, and unreasonable worry. Fears and anxiety about your own death may overwhelm you. A feeling of malaise and "why bother to go on?" takes over, and you may feel drained of energy so that you can barely make yourself do anything. Your thoughts of the dead person may seem obsessive. The depression often manifests itself as a series of physical symptoms such as insomnia, impotence, midnight sweats, anxiety attacks, and lack of appetite and physical inertia; you may become more accident-prone.

Throughout this grieving you need to express your feelings to friends or counselors so that the emotions do not overwhelm and paralyze you and make you feel hopeless. Friends, ministers, your physician, or a counselor can help or steer you to help. Usually these feelings and symptoms disappear within months, certainly within a year. If they continue longer, it may indicate that the natural self-healing process of grief has given way to a more serious depressive illness that demands medical attention.

■ Exploring Your Emotions

What do you believe happens after death—heaven or hell, eternal sleep, nothingness, return to life in another form, union with a higher consciousness, something mysterious and unknowable? Where did you get your concept or belief? What do you wish would happen after death?

Eventually, you notice that the pain eases for periods of time. Terrible lamenting turns more and more into quiet sadness. Sleep patterns, appetite, and energy, gradually return, and you can face the demands of the outside world. Most people do come to terms with bereavement pain and somehow accommodate the grief: they do not forget, but they regain the capacity to remember peacefully.

Beyond Death   Most religions spell out beliefs concerning death and provide comfort for those who believe them. They usually are based on the hope that people

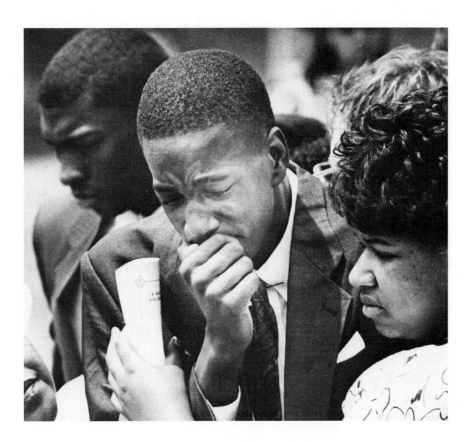

Weeping for his dead brother, this man experiences the anguish of losing a loved one who was in the prime of life. Grieving is a long and painful process, one that may continue for many months but that eventually yields to some sense of acceptance and to healing.

transcend death. Judeo-Christian traditions are held most widely in the United States. The fundamental belief about death is that the body is a temporary house, a cocoon, for the soul. The body dies, but the soul is immortal and lives forever.

Other religions hold to the idea of reincarnation, a rebirthing of the spirit in a different body. This idea negates some aspects of death and encourages people to do good so that they can return in a better body and situation. It is related to another belief based on the idea of a common cosmic consciousness shared by all people. For these believers it is an illusion to think of each person as a separate self with an individual ego. When a person dies, his or her consciousness lives on. The further we live from nature, the more difficult it is for us to be aware of this continuity and to accept our part in it.

Death in Life All who live, die. No one can control the process, so the best we can do is to live fully. This of course does not mean clutching at life in a frantic effort to squeeze out the last ounce of pleasure or meaning or accomplishment. It does mean being aware, open, sensitive, and able to experience the pain and joy of existence. Unfortunately, many people turn themselves off from life when they are quite young, perhaps because of some pain or fear they have endured. They live only in a technical sense, controlling every emotion so that they do not risk getting too close to anyone or letting anyone know they are vulnerable. Compare the fixed faces and bodies of a crowd of adults on their way to work with the faces and bodies of 2- and 3-year-olds, revealing intense, spontaneous and unrepressed delight, anger, fear, surprise. The real tragedy in life is to die without ever having lived.

Facing Death as a Way to Renew Life A confrontation with death makes us aware of the preciousness of life. European writers expressed this theme over and over again after World War II. Many of them had been condemned to death and forced to await execution. Without exception these people found that the confrontation with death liberated them from many former fears. Why? Once death is upon us, we somehow begin to see how trivial other fears are. Facing the fear of death allows us to place these other fears in perspective and to reorder our priorities. We can dare to feel compassion and affection and to express it to others without great fear of rejection. We might be able to risk a job by speaking up to an oppressive boss or to risk relationships by being truer to ourselves, less self-effacing, bolder. Knowing that life is short on this earth can help us value ourselves and others more and enable us to cut through the red tape of our fears and society's rites and forms when they interfere with more humane values.

Summary

- How people deal with death affects how they live their lives.

What Is Death?

- Brain death, today considered to be the medical definition of death, is characterized by unreceptivity and unresponsivity, no movements or breathing without mechanical help, no reflexes, and a flat electroencephalogram for ten minutes. Definitions of legal death vary from state to state.
- Cellular death (the breakdown of metabolic processes in the brain) and social death (loss of the capacity for continuous social interaction) also provide definitions of death.
- A precise definition of death is crucial when organs are going to be transplanted.
- Although death makes sense in terms of species survival and improvement, it remains an emotionally unresolvable puzzle for most people.
- Most people prefer not to think about death, but they are forced into trying to puzzle it out. Children begin to accept death as inevitable, even for themselves, from about age 10; people in later years have recurring worries about being left alone.
- Despair is the most common motive for suicide, which is high among those over 60 and increasing among those 15 to 24. Adolescents who commit suicide often have not learned long-term problem-solving skills.
- Those who are left behind by suicide often feel betrayed and guilty. Suicide is a crime in the United States; many religious groups consider it an attack on God.
- Americans seem to try to deny that death occurs by hiding it from children and by distorting its reality in television and the movies.

Planning for Death

- Preparing for death is one task in the process of human growth. Some decisions can and should be made in youth; others must wait for a final illness.
- A will is a binding legal instrument that governs the redistribution of a person's property upon death. Estates of those who die without a will pass through probate, and distribution of the property may not take place as they would have wished.
- People can and should decide in advance how they want their bodies disposed of after death.
- All states have made provisions that allow people to donate their bodies or individual organs for immediate use after death.

- In the United States bodies are usually buried after death; inflated funeral industry costs have caused people to turn to memorial societies for lower-cost burials. Cremation is another low-cost alternative.
- Funeral ceremonies often help comfort the bereaved.
- Various organizations and agencies provide funds to help pay for funerals.
- Most people would like to choose where they die and should consider all options.
- Dying at home demands much time and energy from relatives, who often need to learn home-care techniques. Hospices are alternatives to hospital and home care. Although programs vary, they depend largely on volunteers to keep costs down; their philosophy discourages inappropriate life-extending services.
- Modern technology can extend life, but many people question the use of life-extending measures in all cases. Euthanasia has both adherents and opponents. The Netherlands has the most radical acceptance of giving noncriminal aid in dying, but euthanasia is against the law in most countries.
- Passive euthanasia (withdrawing or not starting life-support systems) receives more support; individuals generally have the legal right to refuse treatment, including life support. A living will is a vehicle for expressing one's wishes about life-sustaining measures.
- A dying person can get help in making decisions by granting power of attorney to another person.
- A death certificate is necessary to prevent legal complications; in certain cases an autopsy is needed to determine the cause of death.
- The tasks to be accomplished by family and friends after someone's death often take weeks or months.

Coming to Terms with Dying

- Facing death is probably the most difficult experience anyone ever has. The dying have to adapt to many things, but they can benefit from the help of others.
- Responses to one's own imminent death vary greatly; researchers have identified stages of response, though not all stages always occur, and the order may vary: (1) denial and isolation, (2) anger, (3) bargaining, (4) depression, and (5) acceptance. Perhaps people die in accordance with their basic personality and with the disease that kills them. Those who want to help should consider the dying person's individual needs.
- Allowing a dying person to speak and act honestly and openly about the experience is crucial. Dying people need friends and family around them; they can also benefit from professional counseling.

- Grieving is a way to heal the pain of loss. Relief and anger are also associated with grief. Conflicting feelings are normal. Stages of grief include a short period of numbness and an extended period of pain and despair, depression, and obsessive thoughts. Expressing feelings during the period of grief is especially important; grief usually begins to resolve itself within a year.

- Religious beliefs about death can provide comfort to the dying and mourning.
- Turning oneself off to the joys of life is itself a form of death. Facing death often enables people to find greater meaning and joy in life.

Take Action

1. The Motor Vehicle Departments of some states are now sending organ donor forms to people with their auto registration materials. Individuals who wish to can fill them out and keep them with their drivers' licenses. In the event of a fatal automobile accident, the person's organs can be used to help others. If you have not received such materials, write to the National Kidney Foundation (116 E. 27th St., New York, NY 10016) requesting a Uniform Donor Card. When you receive it, consider the advantages and disadvantages of the donor plan. If you decide to be a donor, fill out the card and keep it with your driver's license.

2. Investigate the services available in your community to care for the dying, such as hospitals, hospices, and counseling centers. If possible, visit one or more of them. Write an evaluation of their services, including your personal reactions.

3. Investigate the services available in your community to counsel or comfort the bereaved. Write an evaluation of these services.

4. If possible, talk to your parents (or grandparents) about their wishes for their final days. Ask them if they have made out wills, living wills, or health-care power of attorney forms. If they do not wish to discuss these matters, let them know that you are open to such a discussion in the future.

Selected Bibliography

Carroll, David. 1985. *Living with Dying: A Loving Guide for Family and Close Friends.* New York: McGraw-Hill.

Cohn, Victor. 1989. D.C. Expands the Right to Refuse Treatment. *Washington Post Health,* August 22, p. 11.

Ezell, G., D. J. Anspaugh, J. Oaks. 1987. *Dying and Death: From a Health and Sociological Perspective.* Scottsdale, Ariz.: Gorsuch Scarisbrick.

Hemphill, Charles F., Jr. 1980. *Wills and Trusts: A Legal and Financial Handbook for Everyone.* Englewood Cliffs, N.J.: Prentice-Hall.

Kalish, R. A. 1985. *Death, Grief, and Caring Relationships,* 2nd ed. Monterey, Calif.: Brooks/Cole.

Kastenbaum, R. J. 1986. *Death, Society, and the Human Experience,* 3rd ed. Columbus, Ohio: Charles E. Merrill.

Krementz, Jill. 1981. *How It Feels When a Parent Dies.* New York: Knopf.

Morgan, Ernest. 1980. *A Manual of Death Education and Simple Burial,* 9th ed. Burnsville, N.C.: Celo Press.

Smith, W. 1985. *Dying in the Human Life Cycle: Psychological, Biomedical, and Social Perspectives.* New York: Holt, Rinehart, Winston.

Tatelbaum, Judy. 1982. *The Courage to Grieve: Creative Living, Recovery and Growth through Grief.* New York: Harper and Row.

Wilcox, Sandra Galdieri, and Marilyn Sutton. 1985. *Understanding Death and Dying: An Interdisciplinary Approach.* Palo Alto, Calif.: Mayfield.

Recommended Readings

DeSpelder, Lynne Ann, and Albert Lee Strickland. 1987. *The Last Dance: Encountering Death and Dying,* 2nd ed. Palo Alto, Calif.: Mayfield. *Wide selection of readings arranged by topics: death in children's lives; survivors; medical ethics; the law and death; and eleven others.*

Duda, Deborah. 1982. *A Guide to Dying at Home.* Santa Fe, N.M.: John Muir. *A practical and positive manual for caring for and tending the terminally ill and planning for death. It provides mental, emotional and spiritual support. Lists hospices and memorial societies in the United States and Canada.*

Fruehling, James A. 1982. *Sourcebook on Death and Dying.* Chicago: Marquis Professional Publications. *Provides names and addresses of organizations that supply information and help for the dying. Some information is geared to particular diseases.*

Humphry, Derek, and Ann Wickett. 1986. *The Right to Die: Understanding Euthanasia.* New York: Harper and Row. *A dispassionate attempt to explain euthanasia against the historical, cultural, and legal backgrounds. It reports court cases, the legal and religious status of euthanasia in different states and countries.*

Schneidman, Edwin S., ed. 1984. *Death: Current Perspectives,* 3rd ed. Palo Alto, Calif.: Mayfield. *Thoughtfully selected essays concerning wide variety of issues: the legal and ethical aspects of death, quality of life during dying, fresh views about suicide, personal statements of grief.*

Contents

Making Connections

J ust as people have been changing personal habits and behaviors to maintain and improve their health, they have also been taking greater responsibility for self-care when they get sick. The trend in recent years has definitely been away from total dependence on physicians' care and toward greater individual involvement in managing illnesses and injuries. This shift means people have to acquire the information and skills required for self-care. The scenarios presented on these pages describe situations in which people have to use information, make a decision, or choose a course of action, all related to self-care. As you read them, imagine yourself in each situation and consider what you would do. After you finish the chapter, read the scenarios again to see if what you've learned has changed how you would think, feel, or act in each situation.

When you were playing volleyball yesterday, you landed awkwardly on your right foot and twisted your ankle. It seemed to be OK at the time and you continued playing. But when you woke up this morning, your ankle was swollen, and it hurt a lot when you put your weight on it. You're not sure what to do. Should you wait for it to get better by itself? Elevate it and apply an ice pack? Soak it in Epsom salts? Go to the clinic to see a physician?

21
Medical Self-Care: Skills for the Health-Care Consumer

You developed an itchy skin rash over the weekend, and after a brief exam this morning your physician wrote you a prescription. She was in a hurry and rather vague about what you have, so you were curious to get the medication. But now that you've picked it up and are looking at the label, you see that it says the medication "relieves pruritus" and is "indicated for urticaria." When the pharmacist sees you reading the label, he says, "Didn't your doctor tell you how to use this? Remember, it's for topical use only." What do you have anyway? More important, how can you get better information from your physician the next time you have a complaint?

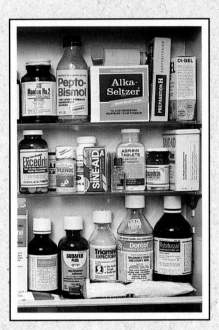

You've had a lot of sore throats in the past year, and your family physician wants you to have your tonsils removed. You've heard that tonsillectomies are unnecessary, but you don't feel comfortable questioning the medical opinions of a physician who has known you your whole life. Should you seek a second opinion? Submit to his recommendation? What are your rights and responsibilities in this situation?

You took a home pregnancy test three weeks ago and were relieved to find that you weren't pregnant. But since you still haven't gotten your period, you called the clinic to see if they might know what was wrong. The nurse said that your test result might have been a false negative and you should come in for an examination. Does that mean you might be pregnant after all?

When you think of the health-care system, do you envision physicians, nurses, clinics, hospitals, and medical laboratories? This is an accurate picture as far as it goes, but don't forget your own role in the health-care system—as a self-care provider. Even with today's dazzling medical technology, highly effective medications, and wide variety of skilled practitioners, the individual plays a crucial role in the health-care system. In fact, the professional medical-care system depends on the functioning of nonprofessional care. If people were to stop practicing self-care and seek professional care for even a small percentage of the complaints they usually manage themselves—colds, backaches, stomachaches, headaches, fatigue, and so on—the professional health-care system would be overwhelmed. Studies show that the average person has about four new medical symptoms each *month* yet consults a physician only four times a *year*. At least 80 percent of medical symptoms are self-diagnosed and self-treated.

■ **Exploring Your Emotions**

How do you feel about taking responsibility for your health? Do you feel confident about self-care? Are there ways you can increase your confidence?

Until recently, this critical role of people as the *primary* providers of health care for themselves and their families went largely unnoticed. With attention focused on the "delivery" of professional services, many individuals remained unaware of how important a part they played in their own health care. Today, people are becoming more confident of their own ability to solve personal health problems. With increased knowledge of when and how to self-treat and when to seek professional care, they can become even more competent in self-care.

The key element in this transition is the recognition that people can *manage* their own health care. Managers don't do everything themselves; they use others—consultants, advisers, experts—to help them get the job done. Once they have all the information they need, they make decisions and take responsibility for follow-through. People who manage their own health gather information—whether from physicians, friends, courses, books, magazines, or self-help groups—solicit opinions and advice, and then make their own decisions. They recognize that everyday choices about diet, exercise, and other habits are critical determinants of health. They participate in every phase of their health care and accept personal responsibility for it. They realize that the choices are theirs.

How can you develop this self-care attitude and take a more active role in your health care? The first step is to learn the skills you need to identify and manage medical problems. The second step is to learn how to make the health-care system work effectively for you. This chapter provides information that will help you become competent in both these areas.

Managing Medical Problems

Effectively managing medical problems involves developing several skills. First, you need to learn how to be a good observer of your own body and assess your symptoms. Second, you need to be able to decide when to seek professional advice and when you can safely deal with the problem on your own. Third, you need to know how to safely and effectively self-treat common medical problems.

Self-assessment   Self-care begins with careful observation of your own body. We are constantly observing our bodies, scanning for unusual sensations, aches, or pains. Symptoms are signals from our bodies. They alert us that something may be wrong.

Symptoms are often an expression of the body's attempt to heal itself. For example, the pain and swelling that occur after an ankle injury immobilize the injured joint to allow healing to take place. A fever may be an attempt to make the body less hospitable to infectious agents. A cough can help clear the airways and protect the lungs. Understanding what a symptom means and what is going on in your body helps reduce anxiety about symptoms and allows you to practice safe self-care that supports your body's own healing mechanisms.

Carefully observing symptoms also helps you identify those signals that suggest you need professional assistance to help your body heal. You should begin by noting when the symptom began, how often and when it occurs, what makes it worse, what makes it better, and if you have any associated symptoms. You can also monitor your body's "vital signs" such as temperature and pulse rate (see Appendix I, "Home Medical Tests"). These signs may give important clues as to how your body is managing an illness.

Not too long ago, the thermometer was the only tool available to evaluate medical problems at home. Now a new generation of medical self-tests are available: screening tests for colon cancer, home blood pressure machines, home blood glucose tests for diabetics, pregnancy tests, self-tests for urinary tract infections, and over a dozen other do-it-yourself kits and devices. All these tools are designed to help you make a more informed decision about when to seek medical help and when to self-treat.

Self-Care Credo

1. Health care is not only everyone's right but also everyone's responsibility.

2. *Informed self-care* should be the main goal of any health program or activity.

3. Ordinary people provided with clear, simple information can prevent and treat most common health problems in their own homes—earlier, cheaper, and often better than can doctors.

4. Medical knowledge should not be the guarded secret of a select few but should be freely shared by everyone.

5. People with little formal education can be trusted as much as those with a lot. And they are just as smart.

6. Basic health care should not be delivered, but encouraged.

From David Werner. 1977. *Where There Is No Doctor* (Palo Alto, Calif. The Hesperian Foundation).

Home medical tests offer several advantages: cost savings, convenience, privacy, an increased sense of control, and sometimes more comprehensive information. Blood pressure measurements taken at home can give a more complete picture of what your blood pressure is like throughout the day, not just during visits to the physician. Many people suffer from "white-coat hypertension"—their blood pressure may go up during the stress of a visit to the physician. Home blood pressure checks can also help hypertensives under medical supervision try nondrug treatments such as diet, exercise, or relaxation. One study even suggests that home blood pressure monitoring *itself* may lower blood pressure. Why? One theory is that checking your own blood pressure may be a form of biofeedback—as you become aware of pressure changes you can voluntarily control them. It may be that over time you experience less anxiety while checking your pressure. Or you may begin, unconsciously, to change your diet and other factors that affect blood pressure.

For diabetics, home blood glucose monitoring can be a more efficient, less expensive way to check blood glucose levels, because it allows frequent, rapid measurements without interrupting normal daily activities to go to a laboratory. Before home blood glucose monitoring was available, diabetics had to rely on urine tests, which may lag behind blood levels and therefore give misleading information about very low blood glucose levels (**hypoglycemia**) or very high levels (**hyperglycemia**). With home monitoring, diabetics can work in partnership with their physicians to keep their blood sugar levels under better control by adjusting their insulin doses, diet, and exercise. Sometimes tighter control can reduce the need for frequent visits to the laboratory or hospitalization to manage unstable diabetes.

Privacy is also an important factor in the growth of home medical tests. A self-test for pregnancy lets a woman find out for herself whether she is pregnant. Another new test allows people to check stool specimens at home for small amounts of blood. This test for "hidden" blood is recommended annually for people over age 50 as a screening test for colon cancer. If blood is found, then further tests are necessary to determine whether the bleeding is from a colon cancer or some other source.

Although home medical tests have many benefits, they are not foolproof. Just like laboratory tests, some may show abnormal results even though you are quite healthy (a **false positive** result), while others may fail to detect abnormalities (a **false negative**). Careful reading of the instructions with the test kits, including when *not* to test, as well as coaching from your physician, will minimize these problems. If you do find an abnormal test result, repeat the test. If it is still abnormal, if you are at all doubtful about the test results, or if your symptoms persist even if the tests are normal, consult your physician.

Careful self-observation and selective use of self-tests

Hypoglycemia   Abnormally low levels of glucose (sugar) in the blood. Usually occurs when a diabetic takes too much insulin.

Hyperglycemia   Abnormally high levels of glucose (a sugar) in the blood. Usually found in diabetes.

False negative   An inaccurate test result that indicates that a person is normal when he or she is actually diseased.

False positive   An inaccurate test result that indicates an abnormality in a person who is actually healthy.

Home pregnancy test kits are just one type of self-test that can be obtained without a prescription in a pharmacy. Using a home pregnancy kit, a woman can determine if she is pregnant within a week of having missed her period.

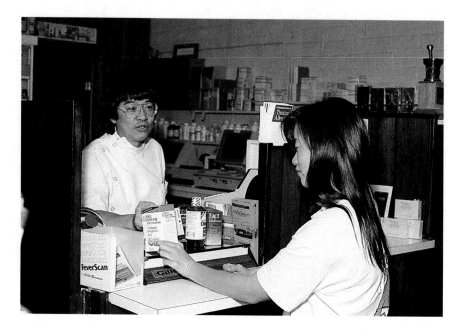

may help provide you with the type of information you need to make informed self-care decisions and participate more actively in your care.

Decision Making: Knowing When to Go to the Doctor

To self-treat or not self-treat, that is the question. When confronted with a symptom, a person must ask a series of questions: "What's going on in my body?" "Is this dangerous?" "Have I or anyone else I know had something like this before?" Some of the answers you can make to these questions are conscious and rational; others are more unconscious, emotional responses.

People often make two kinds of mistakes in deciding what to do when faced with symptoms. They may rush to their physician too often or too quickly for minor complaints they could easily and effectively manage on their own. Or they may ignore symptoms and self-treat when they should be seeking professional assistance.

For example, suppose you develop diarrhea and some mild abdominal cramping. If you immediately rush off to a clinic, you are likely to waste your time and the physician's. However, if you knew what key signs to look for (such as blood in the stool, high fever, and dehydration) and how to practice effective self-care for the symptoms (clear liquid diet, and so on), you would be in a position to make a more informed choice.

At the other extreme, people too often ignore symptoms that *should* trigger a visit to the doctor. For example, any breast lump should be medically evaluated. Although 80–90 percent of breast lumps turn out to be noncancerous, early treatment of the few that are cancerous can save lives. Informed self-care involves knowing how to

evaluate symptoms so that you don't go to a physician either too early *or* too late.

Your decision to seek professional assistance for a symptom is generally guided by your previous history of medical problems and the nature of the symptom you are experiencing. In general, you should check with a physician for symptoms that are

1. *Severe.* If the symptom is very severe or intense, medical assistance is advised. Examples include severe pains, major injuries, and other emergencies.
2. *Unusual.* If the symptom is very peculiar and unfamiliar, it is wise to check it out with your physician. Examples include unexplained lumps, changes in a skin blemish or mole, problems with vision, difficulty swallowing, numbness, weakness, unexplained weight loss, and blood in sputum, urine, or bowel movement.
3. *Persistent.* If the symptom lasts longer than expected, seek medical advice. Examples include fever for more than five days, a cough lasting longer than two weeks, a sore that doesn't heal within a month, and hoarseness lasting longer than three weeks.
4. *Recurrent.* If a symptom tends to return again and again, medical evaluation is advised. Examples include recurrent headaches, stomach pains, and backache.

Sometimes a single symptom is not a cause for concern; but when the symptom is accompanied by other symptoms, the combination may suggest a more serious problem. For example, a fever with a stiff neck suggests meningitis. A cough with green sputum and a high fever might mean pneumonia. (Guidelines for children are different from those given above; for symptoms in children, consult with a pediatrician.)

If you evaluate your symptoms and think that you need professional assistance, then you must decide how urgent the problem is. If it is a true emergency, then you should go (or be taken) to the nearest emergency room. Emergencies would include

- Major trauma or injury such as head injury, suspected broken bone, deep wound, severe burn, eye injury, or animal bite
- Uncontrollable bleeding or internal bleeding, as indicated by blood in the sputum, vomit, or a bowel movement
- Intolerable and uncontrollable pain
- Severe chest pain
- Severe shortness of breath
- Persistent abdominal pain, especially if associated with nausea and vomiting
- Poisoning or drug overdose
- Loss of consciousness or seizure
- Stupor, drowsiness, or disorientation that cannot be explained
- Severe or worsening reaction to an insect bite or sting, or to a medication, especially if breathing is difficult

Unfortunately, most visits to an emergency room (ER) are not emergencies. One study by the Indiana Hospital Association reviewed 13,523 emergency room visits. Over 50 percent were judged not to be true emergencies. In fact, even 25 percent of those patients arriving by ambulance were *not* emergencies.

There are many reasons not to go to a hospital emergency room if it is not a true emergency. Emergency rooms do not operate on a first-come, first-served basis. Patients are **triaged**, a screening process in which those patients with the most urgent needs are treated first. So if your problem is not a true emergency, you may have to wait hours while more critically ill patients are seen before you. Your past medical records are usually not available in the emergency room, and it is harder to get appropriate follow-up care. Also, many insurance policies do not cover nonemergency visits to emergency rooms, so if you go to an ER with a sore throat, cough, rash, or other mild symptom, you could end up paying the bill. And emergency room medical bills are much higher than office or urgent care center visits.

If your problem is not an emergency, but still requires medical attention, consider a call to your physician's office. Often you can be given medical advice over the phone without the inconvenience of a visit. If you do require a visit, it can often be arranged at the most convenient and appropriate time and place. Nearly 16 percent of all outpatient medical advice and 30 percent of pediatrics advice is now dispensed by telephone.

To help you make wise medical decisions, a "Self-care Guide for Common Medical Problems" is provided in Appendix II. This guide includes some specific guidelines on when to call the doctor for certain medical problems and on when and how to self-treat. To know who to call see Chapter 22 where the different types of health care professionals are discussed.

Self-treatment When confronted with a new symptom, many people try to find some pill or potion that will relieve or cure it. However, other self-treatment options are available. In most cases, your body can itself relieve your symptoms and heal the disorder. The prescriptions filled by your body's internal pharmacy are frequently the safest and most effective treatment. So patience and careful self-observation are often the best choices in self-treatment. Nondrug treatments are also sometimes highly effective. For example, massage, ice packs, and neck exercises may be, at times, more helpful than drugs in relieving headaches and other aches and pains. For a variety of disorders either caused or aggravated by stress, relaxation and stress management strategies may be the treatment of choice (see Chapter 2). So before reaching for medications, consider *all* your options for self-treatment.

Self-medication Self-treatment with nonprescription medications is an important and valuable part of our health care system. Within every two-week period, nearly 70 percent of people self-medicate with one or more drugs. If even a small percentage of people stopped using such **over-the-counter (OTC)** drugs and began making appointments with physicians for their colds, sore throats, backaches, and headaches, the physicians could not possibly handle the load. Many OTC drugs are highly effective in relieving symptoms and sometimes in curing illnesses. Physicians themselves may recommend OTC products when they can be helpful. About 60 percent of all medications are sold over the counter. (See the box, "The Market for Over-the-Counter Drugs.")

Triage A screening and sorting out of people who are sick or injured so that the most seriously ill can be treated first or so that the patient is directed to the most appropriate type of medical practitioner.

OTC (over-the-counter) Medications and products that can be purchased by the consumer without a prescription.

The Market for Over-the-Counter Drugs

American pharmacies are filled with nonprescription medications, somewhere between 100,000 and 300,000 separate products. These products mix some 700 active ingredients aimed at about 1,500 different uses, from treatment of colds to headaches to itchy skin. Because prescription drugs tend to be more expensive, the total prescription market is two and a half times the size of the OTC market, but many more types of products—and many more doses of drugs—are sold OTC.

Statistics from Kline and Co., Inc.

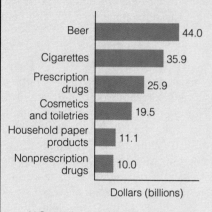

	Dollars (billions)
Beer	44.0
Cigarettes	35.9
Prescription drugs	25.9
Cosmetics and toiletries	19.5
Household paper products	11.1
Nonprescription drugs	10.0

U.S. retail expenditures: selected consumer products in billions of dollars, 1988

Type of product	1988 sales of all nonprescription drugs	1988 market share of generic, or private-label nonprescription drugs
Vitamins and minerals	$3,381	27%
Pain relievers	1,948	3%
Cough and cold medications	1,559	2%
Ointments, creams and lotions	1,370	5%
Antacids, nausea and diarrhea treatments	1,276	3%
Other products	521	17%
Tampons, pads and douches	313	1%
Allergy, asthma and sinus medication	306	2%
Total	**$10,674**	

*Note: Sales in millions of dollars

The Food and Drug Administration (FDA) has undertaken a massive review of the safety, effectiveness, and labeling of OTC products. As a result, many ineffective or unsafe OTC medications have been taken off the market. However, several other medications that formerly required a doctor's prescription are now available without prescription. So you can now walk into any pharmacy and purchase without prescription such drugs as hydrocortisone cream and antifungal agents. But with this increased consumer choice comes increased responsibility to use these medications wisely.

You need to be aware of the barrage of drug advertising aimed at you. The implicit message of such advertising is that every symptom, every ache and pain, every problem, can be solved by a product. Many of the OTC products *are* effective; but many simply waste your money and divert your attention from better ways of coping. Many ingredients in OTC's—perhaps 70 percent—have not been proven to be effective, a fact the FDA does not dispute.

It is important to remember that any drug whether bought in the supermarket or prescribed by a physician, may have side effects. However, following some simple guidelines will improve your chances of safely and effectively self-medicating:

1. Always read drug labels and follow directions carefully. A surprising number of people do not read medication labels before taking the contents. The label must by law include the names and quantities of the active ingredients, precautions, and adequate directions for safe use. Carefully reading the label and reviewing the individual ingredients may help prevent you from taking medications that have caused problems for you in the past. If you don't understand the information on the label, ask a pharmacist or doctor before using it (see Figure 21-1).

2. Do not exceed the recommended dosage or length of treatment unless you discuss this change with your doctor.

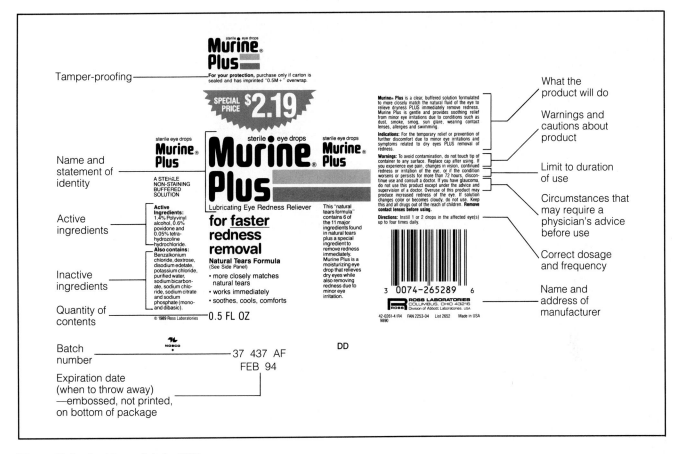

Figure 21-1   Looking at Labels: OTCs.

3. Use caution if you are taking other medications. OTC and prescription drugs can interact, either canceling or enhancing the effects of the medications. If you have questions about drug interactions, ask your doctor or pharmacist before you mix medicines (see the box titled "The Danger of Drug Interaction").

4. Try to select medications with one active ingredient rather than combination ("all-in-one") products. A product with multiple ingredients is likely to include drugs for symptoms you don't even have, so why risk the side effects of medications you don't need? Using single-ingredient products also allows you to adjust the dosage of each medication separately for optimal symptom relief with minimal side effects.

5. When choosing medications, learn the ingredient names and try to buy generic products. **Generic drugs** contain the same active ingredient as the brand-name product but generally at a much lower cost.

6. Never take or give a drug from an unlabeled container or in the dark when you can't read what the label says.

7. If you are pregnant, nursing, or have a chronic disease such as kidney disease, consult your doctor before self-medicating.

8. Many medications have an expiration date of about two to three years. Dispose of all expired medications.

9. Store your medications in a safe place away from the reach of children. Poisoning with medications is a common and preventable problem. The usual bathroom medicine chest is usually not a particularly secure or dry place to store medications. Consider a

Generic drug   Non-brand-name drug that is not registered or protected by a trademark.

The Dangers of Drug Interaction

Who needs to be concerned about drug interactions? You do, if you answer yes to some of the following questions.

- Do you have more than one physician, or do you patronize more than one pharmacy for prescription and over-the-counter (OTC) drugs?
- Do you currently take several different medicines a day?
- Do you drink coffee or alcoholic beverages?
- Do you smoke?
- Do you use sedatives or oral contraceptives?
- Do you take vitamins, antacids, pain relievers, laxatives, or other OTC medicines?
- Do you take medicine for a chronic disorder such as diabetes, high blood pressure, allergies, epilepsy, or asthma?

Literally hundreds of different drug interactions have been reported. They vary in severity and clinical importance. Such things as vitamin deficiencies, treatment failures, and even sudden death may result from a drug interaction, although many are harmless.

Drugs interact not only with other drugs, but also with foods, environmental agents, and diagnostic laboratory tests. Some interactions warrant cautionary statements on package labels, but others get little or no notice.

The next time you have an OTC cold remedy in your hand, for example, read the label. If it contains a decongestant drug and an antihistamine, the label will warn you not to take the remedy if you are taking a monoamine oxidase inhibitor and to avoid taking alcohol and the remedy at the same time.

Monoamine oxidase inhibitors (such as Nardil, Marplan and Parnate) are prescription drugs used for the treatment of mental depression. If you take one of these drugs with a decongestant drug (such as phenylpropanolamine, phenylephrine, or pseudoephedrine), the interaction between the two may precipitously elevate blood pressure, causing severe headaches and increasing risk of a heart attack or stroke. The same danger occurs when monoamine oxidase inhibitors interact with certain foods, such as aged cheddar cheese, yogurt, chicken liver, and chianti wine.

The warning about alcohol is there to prevent another kind of interaction. Antihistamines cause sedation. So does alcohol. Together, the sedative effects of both drugs are additive and likely to make you drowsy. This interaction is potentially dangerous for people who drive motor vehicles or operate machinery.

A similar, but much more dangerous interaction occurs between alcohol and other sedative drugs such as Valium, Librium, Xanax, phenobarbital, and Nembutal. The sedation caused by the combined effects of alcohol and any of these drugs may be enough to make you stop breathing as you sleep.

Other less common drug interactions may not be mentioned on the labels of OTC remedies. Aspirin, for example, may enhance the "blood-thinning" action of anticoagulant drugs (such as Coumadin and Dicoumarol) and cause bleeding. Vitamin B-6 (pyridoxine) may interfere with the action of levodopa (Dopar, Larodopa), which is used to treat Parkinsonism. Remedies for diarrhea (such as Kaopectate and Pepto-Bismol) may prevent the absorption of many drugs.

Interactions between food and drugs are common. Most often, food delays or prevents drug absorption simply by getting in the way, but specific interactions also occur. Environmental agents such as insecticides and tobacco smoke can also influence the action of certain drugs by altering the rate at which the body eliminates them.

Interactions between drugs and diagnostic laboratory tests can delay proper treatment or lead to an improper diagnosis and unnecessary treatment, hospitalization, or, perhaps, surgery. Literally scores of such tests can be affected by drugs. Always tell your physician or nurse about the medicines you take whenever a diagnostic test is conducted.

L. R. Willis, *Healthline.*

---

lockable tool chest or fishing box that can be stored out of reach of children.

10. Use special caution with aspirin. Because of recent information indicating an association with a rare but serious problem known as Reye's syndrome, aspirin should not be used for children or adolescents who may have the flu or chicken pox.

The Home Pharmacy   If you were to survey home medicine chests, what would you find? On average, there

---

Your Home Self-Care Kit

Medications:

- **Anesthetic throat lozenges, spray, or gargle**
  Sore throat

- **Antacids (aluminum hydroxide/magnesium hydroxide)**
  Indigestion and heartburn

- **Antibacterial ointment cream**
  Minor skin wounds

- **Antifungal creams/powders**
  Fungal infections (e.g., athlete's foot, ringworm)

- **Antihistamines**
  Allergies

- **Antimotion sickness medication**
  Motion sickness

- **Aspirin/acetaminophen/ibuprofen**
  Fever, headache, minor pain

- **Burow's solution**
  Minor skin irritations/rashes

- **Decongestant tablets, nose sprays, drops**
  Nasal congestion

- **Ear wax dissolver**
  Ear wax

- **Expectorant/cough suppressant (dextromethorphan)**
  Coughs

- **Eye drops and artificial tears**
  Minor eye irritations

- **Hemorrhoid preparations**
  Hemorrhoids

- **Hydrocortisone cream (0.5%)**
  Minor skin irritations/rashes

- **Hydrogen peroxide**
  Wound cleansing

- **Kaolin/pectin or attapulgite preparations**
  Diarrhea

- **Milk of magnesia or bulk laxative**
  Constipation

- **Sodium bicarbonate (baking soda)**
  Wounds, rashes, insect bites

- **Sunscreen agents**
  Prevention of sunburn

- **Syrup of ipecac**
  Poison ingestion

Supplies and Tools

- **Adhesive tape**
  Minor injuries

- **Adhesive bandages**
  Minor wounds

- **Elastic bandages**
  Strains and sprains

- **Eye cup**
  Washing out foreign bodies

- **Heating pad/hot water bottle**
  Minor pains and strains

- **Ice pack**
  Minor injuries and pain

- **Needle-nosed tweezers**
  Splinters

- **Thermometer**
  Fever

---

would be twenty-two medications, including seventeen OTC products. You would probably find an oversupply of expired medications, leftover prescription drugs, and useless medications. At the same time, certain essential medications and equipment would be absent. Most people wait until a crisis arises. They then search frantically through a poorly stocked medicine chest and often have to make an inconvenient midnight dash to a pharmacy, if they can find one open.

There are only a few essential supplies; the rest varies depending upon the particular health problems you or your family are likely to face (see the box, "Your Home Self-care Kit"). Since many of the medications deteriorate, buy small quantities of infrequently used medications and replace them about every three years.

Getting the Most Out of Your Medical Care

Self-care involves more than self-diagnosis and self-treatment. It includes knowing when to seek professional care and how to get the most out of your medical care. The key to making the health care system work for you lies in good communication with your physician and with the other members of the health-care team. Unfortunately, many people are intimidated by their doctors and afraid to communicate freely. Medical jargon can be very confusing. One study revealed that 20–30 percent of college-educated people had significant misunderstandings about the meaning of such common medical terms as *hypertension, virus, herpes, tumor, Pap smear, strep throat,* and *uterus.* Yet patients tend not to ask their physicians what such medical jargon means, because they fear appearing stupid (see the box "Understanding Medispeak"). Others are afraid to ask why a test or treatment is needed for fear of appearing to challenge the authority of the physician. Patients often conceal personal concerns about sexuality, drug abuse, emotional problems, and cancer. All these fears and others block open communication with the physician.

Physicians share the responsibility for poor communication. They may feel they are too busy or important to take the time to talk with patients. They may ignore questions, use incomprehensible medical jargon, and respond in an unsupportive way to patients' attempts to assert themselves.

■ Exploring Your Emotions

Does your physician keep you waiting for a long time in the waiting room and then in the examination room? If so, how does it make you feel? Are you able to convey your feelings?

The physician-patient relationship is undergoing an important transformation. The image of the physician as a God-like, all-knowing authority and the patient as a passive supplicant is slowly fading. What is emerging is more of a physician-patient *partnership,* in which the physician acts more like a consultant and the patient participates more actively. The necessary ingredients in a successful physician-patient partnership are a sympathetic, caring physician and a prepared, assertive patient. As physician Marvin Belsky commented, "It is not enough for the doctor to stop playing God. You've got to get off your knees."

You should try to remember that physicians are human, they have off days, they make mistakes like everyone else. You don't have to "love" your doctor as a best friend, but you should expect someone who is attentive, caring, able to listen, and able to clearly explain things to you. You also have to do your part. You need to be assertive in a firm but not aggressive manner. You need to express your feelings and concerns, ask questions, and, if necessary, be persistent. If your physician is unable to communicate clearly with you in spite of your best efforts, then you probably need to change physicians. Remember, the physician works for you.

Here are several tips that can help ensure good communication before, during, and after your visit to the doctor:

Preparing for the Visit

- Before visiting your physician, make a written list of questions or concerns that you have. Also include notes about your symptoms (when they started, how long they last, what makes them worse or better, and so on). This list prepares you to clearly state your major concerns as well as concisely answer the questions your physician is likely to ask. Have you ever thought to yourself after you walked out of the office, "Why didn't I ask about . . ."? Making a list beforehand helps ensure that your concerns get addressed.
- Bring a list of all medications (prescription and nonprescription) you are taking, or bring all these medications with you to the office so that your physician can review them. Also, if you have previous medical records or test results that might be relevant to your problems, bring them along.

During the Visit

- Take notes during the visit, or consider bringing along someone else to act as a second listener. Another set of eyes and ears may help you later recall some of the details of the visit or instructions.
- Try to be as open as you can in sharing your thoughts, feelings, and fears. Remember, your physician is not a mind reader. If you are worried, try to explain why: "I am worried that what I have is contagious, my father had similar symptoms before he died," and so on.
- Don't be afraid to ask what you may consider a "stupid" question. These questions can often indicate an important concern or misunderstanding.
- If you don't understand or remember something the physician said, admit that you need to go over it again. For example, "I'm pretty sure you told me some of this before, but I don't recall what the answer was."
- Give your physician feedback. If you don't like the way you have been treated by the physician or someone else on the health-care team, let your physician know. If you have been unable to follow the physician's advice or had problems with a treatment, tell your physician so adjustments can be made. Also, most physicians very much appreciate compliments and positive feedback, but patients are often hesitant to praise their doctors. So, if you are very pleased, let your physician know.
- When appropriate, ask your physician to write down instructions or recommend reading material for more information on a particular subject.

■ Exploring Your Emotions

People often feel overawed or intimidated by their physicians and are unable to question their opinions. Do you tend to accept everything your physician says? Do you assume he or she is always right? Do you feel comfortable saying that you would like to seek a second opinion? If not, what can you do to increase your feelings of partnership with your physician?

Understanding Medispeak

Did you ever wonder why your physician says "edema" instead of "swelling" and "hemorrhage" instead of "bleed"? Whether you call it medispeak or medicalese, the overuse of medical terminology and medical jargon can result in confusion, misinterpretation, and apprehension rather than compliance and trust. In some cases, unnecessary jargon may be used to ward off questions and challenges from listeners. In other cases, the physician may simply not be aware of what you do and don't understand.

Whatever the situation, you can avoid communication problems by becoming fluent in some basic medical terminology yourself. Begin by testing yourself on the following commonly used terms. Cover the column on the right to see how many terms you know.

1.	Adipose	Fatty
2.	Ambulatory	Able to walk
3.	Analgesic	Painkiller
4.	Antipyretic	Fever reducer
5.	Atrophy	Shrinkage or wasting of muscle or tissue
6.	Benign	Noncancerous
7.	Congenital	Condition present at birth
8.	Contraindicated	To be avoided
9.	Dermatitis	Irritation of the skin
10.	Diaphoresis	Perspiration
11.	Etiology	Pertaining to the causes of disease
12.	Febrile	Feverish
13.	Hemorrhage	Bleeding
14.	Idiopathic	Of unknown cause
15.	Lesion	Any sore or wound
16.	Malignant	Cancerous
17.	Negative test result	The patient doesn't have a disorder
18.	Parenteral	Medicine given by injection
19.	Prognosis	Expected outcome of a disease
20.	Pruritus	Itching
21.	Psychogenic	Having an emotional origin
22.	Q.I.D.	Take four times a day
23.	Sepsis	Infection
24.	Sequela	Aftereffect of a disease
25.	Subclinical	Having no symptoms
26.	Subcutaneous	Beneath the skin
27.	Syndrome	A specific collection of symptoms
28.	Systemic	Affecting the whole body
29.	Topical	On the surface
30.	Urticaria	Hives, usually from an allergic reaction

How did you do? If you knew 24 to 30 of the terms, you probably understand your physicians' explanations and instructions most of the time. If you knew 12 to 23, you're on your way to medical fluency. If you knew fewer than 12 of the terms, you may want to invest in a medical dictionary for laypeople. Ask for an explanation of terms you don't know and repeat instructions back to your physician to make sure you've understood them properly. Knowing the language is one of the keys to self-confidence when it comes to dealing with professional health-care providers.

Good communication is a crucial factor in a satisfactory physician-patient relationship. This mother is learning about asthma, a condition that individuals can often manage successfully with medication and an inhaler.

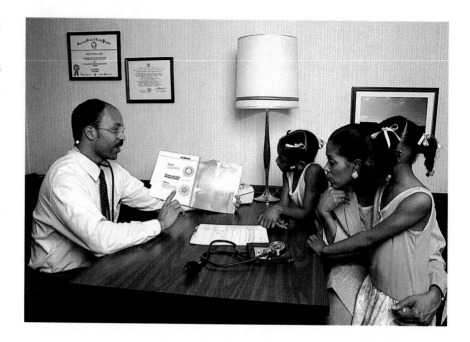

After the Visit

- At the end of the appointment, briefly repeat back—in your own words—what you understood the physician to say about the nature of the problem and what you are supposed to do. This repetition helps check your understanding, to ensure the best care.
- Make sure you understand what the next steps are. Should you return for a visit and, if so, when and why? Should you phone for test results? Are there any danger signs you should watch for and report back to your physician?

In addition to developing effective communication skills, understanding something about how a diagnosis is made, what treatment options are available, and what questions you should ask will help equip you to take a more active role in your own health care.

The Diagnostic Process Solving a medical problem is sometimes like solving a mystery. The problem is presented, clues are discovered, evidence is sought, possibilities are tracked down, and finally (we hope) a correct diagnosis is made.

There are three main sources of clues and information on which to base a diagnosis. The first is the medical history, which is the patient's own description of what has happened. The second is the physical examination of the patient. The third is the results from various diagnostic tests and procedures. All this information is then evaluated to reach a diagnosis that names and explains the problem and guides treatment.

The Medical History: Telling It Like It Is The most important part of medical diagnosis is the medical history. This is the description that you give the physician of your problem, concerns, and background. In well over 70 percent of cases, a careful history alone can lead to a correct diagnosis. Your ability to describe your illness clearly, concisely, and accurately is an essential first step in the diagnostic process. Understanding how the physician elicits your medical history can help you tell the story. Most physicians use a standard five-part procedure to elicit the medical history. Depending on the nature of the problem, you may be asked about some or all of these areas.

- *The chief complaint* To elicit the chief complaint, the physician may ask something like "What brings you here today?" Give the reason for your visit; and, if you have more than one concern, list them all briefly and concisely. Don't disguise any concerns (such as worries about cancer or sexual problems) or wait until the end of the visit to bring them up.
- *The present illness* The physician will ask a series of questions to clarify the nature, character, and time course of your major symptom. Among them are "When did it begin?" "How long does it last?" "What brings it on or makes it worse?" Be concise but as specific as possible.
- *The past medical history* You will be asked about your health in general and your medical history, including previous illnesses, hospitalizations, operations, immunizations, allergies, and medications. This information

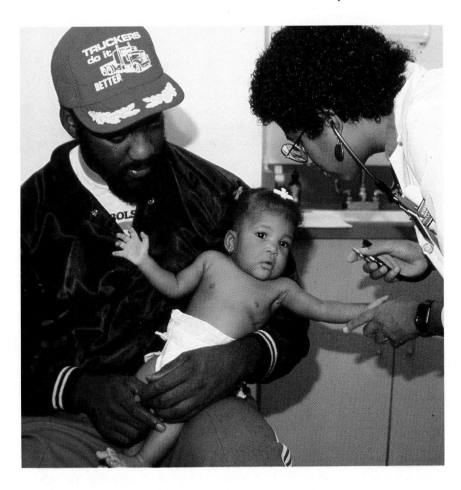

Physical examinations are particularly important for infants and are scheduled at regular intervals during the first few years of life. In addition to inoculating the child against many diseases, the physician has the opportunity to spot any problems that may be developing, and the parents have the chance to discuss their concerns.

can provide clues to what is or is not causing your current symptoms. Report all medications you're taking and be specific about allergies to medications.

- *Review of systems* The physician reviews symptoms you are experiencing in all your different body organs and physiological systems—including the gastrointestinal, urinary, nervous, cardiovascular, and respiratory systems. Although the questions asked may not seem to be related to your chief complaint, your responses may reveal information vital to managing your present illness or detecting unrecognized problems.
- *Social history* The physician may ask questions about your job, living conditions, travel experiences, family, life stresses, and health habits such as smoking and alcohol use. Clues that aid in a diagnosis might include exposure to toxic materials at work, a recent trip to a foreign country, and a family history of diseases.

Giving an accurate and concise medical history is critical to good medical care. You are the expert about how

you feel and how you experience symptoms. Through the medical history, you can share your expertise with the physician.

The Anatomy of a Physical Examination   The physician then proceeds to examine you. Depending upon your chief complaint this examination may be a complete, head-to-toes exam or may be directed to certain areas or physiological systems.

Traditionally, the physical examination consists of inspection (looking), **palpation** (feeling), and **auscultation** (listening). The physician might examine:

- *Vital signs* Pulse rate, breathing rate, temperature, and blood pressure may be measured.
- *Head, ears, eyes, nose, and throat* The physician may look at the ear canal and ear drum with a lighted instrument (**otoscope**) for signs of infection or blockage. Your hearing may be tested by whispering, a ticking

---

Palpation   The act of feeling some organ or part of the body in order to make a diagnosis.

Auscultation   The act of listening to sounds made by the body in order to make a diagnosis.

Otoscope   A lighted instrument used to view inside the ear.

watch, a tuning fork, or an electronic device. The physician may inspect the external parts of the eye; redness may indicate an infection, paleness may suggest anemia. The pupil of the eye normally constricts when light shines in. The blood vessels, retina, and optic nerve at the back of the eye can be seen with a special lighted instrument called an **ophthalmoscope.** The physician may check the mucous membranes of your nose; tapping over the sinus cavities that elicits tenderness may suggest infection. He or she may check your tongue, gums, mouth, and throat for abnormalities.

- *Neck* The physician may feel your neck for the presence of swollen lymph nodes during an infection or for irregularities in the thyroid gland, which lies just below the Adam's apple. A stethoscope can detect abnormal sounds called **murmurs** in the arteries of the neck, which may signal atherosclerotic blockage and risk of stroke.

- *Chest* The physician may tap on your chest with his or her fingers to detect possible fluid accumulation or pneumonia. You will be asked to take deep breaths in and out through your mouth as your physician listens with a stethoscope. The stethoscope can also be used to detect irregularities in heart rhythm or abnormal clicks and murmurs as the heart valves open and close. Women's breasts are checked for lumps as a possible sign of breast cancer.

- *Abdomen* The physician will use his or her fingers to probe your belly, checking your liver in the upper right side, your spleen in the upper left, your stomach in the upper middle, and intestines throughout. Any tenderness or masses will be noted. Your physician may also listen with a stethoscope to the sounds your intestines make.

- *Rectum* The physician may insert a gloved finger into your rectum to check for abnormal growths. In men, the prostate gland can be checked through the rectum for lumps, enlargement, or tenderness.

- *Genitals* In men, the penis and testicles will be checked for sores, tenderness, or growths. The physician may press a finger against the scrotal sac and lower abdomen to feel for a weakness in the abdominal wall. A bulge in the abdominal contents when you cough is a sign of a hernia. In women, a pelvic examination includes inspection, palpation, and a Pap smear, which is a test that checks for cancer in cells gently scraped off the cervix.

- *Extremities* The physician may check your legs and feet for swelling, redness, or tenderness of the joints sug-

gesting arthritis. Painless but swollen ankles and feet may be a sign of heart, liver, or kidney disease. The pulses in your feet and wrists may be checked for adequate flood flow through the arteries. Your calves may be squeezed to check for blood clots in the veins.

- *Skin* Your skin will be checked for sores, moles, lumps, and rashes. Paleness may suggest anemia; a yellow color (jaundice) may suggest a liver abnormality such as hepatitis.

- *Neurological signs* Depending on your symptoms, the physician might check your nervous system. This check might include testing your muscle strength, balance, coordination, reflexes, and sensation. For example, tapping the tendon below your kneecap normally elicits a reflex contraction of a thigh muscle. This knee-reflex action brings many parts of the nervous system into play, and a malfunction can indicate problems in the nervous system and/or quadraceps muscle in the thigh.

If you notice any pain or unusual sensations during the examination, let your physician know. Your response may provide important information. Also, if you are curious about what is being done during the exam or why, ask your physician. (But not when the physician has the stethoscope in his or her ears!)

Medical Testing   In addition to the medical history and physical examination, diagnostic testing now provides a wealth of new information to help solve medical problems. Gone are the days when medical tests meant only a microscope and a drop of blood or urine. High-tech and high-cost medical testing is now a burgeoning industry, accounting for nearly a third of our national health bill. No body fluid, orifice, or cavity is beyond the reach of a medical probe: blood and urine tests, x-rays, biopsies, taps, scans, electronic monitors, and a bewildering array of **endoscopies** (bronchoscopy, arthroscopy, sigmoidoscopy, and so on), the scoping procedures that peer into nearly every part of the body.

More than 10 billion medical tests are done in the United States each year—over forty tests per person—at a staggering cost of $140 billion, or $600 for each of us. Patients can no longer afford to take a passive role in this important phase of their medical care.

Careful scientific studies reveal that at least 25 percent of all medical tests are unnecessary. For example, one study showed that over half of the blood tests routinely ordered when a patient is admitted to the hospital for

---

Ophthalmoscope   A lighted instrument used to view the interior of the eye.

Murmur   An abnormal sound heard over a blood vessel or the heart due to some blockage of blood flow.

Endoscopy   A medical procedure in which a viewing instrument is inserted into body cavities or openings. The specific procedures are named for the area viewed: inside joints (ar-

throscopy), inside airways (bronchoscopy), inside the abdominal cavity (laparoscopy), and inside the lower portion of the digestive tract, called the *sigmoid colon* (sigmoidoscopy).

surgery were virtually useless, contributing little to patient care, but a lot to patient bills.

Of course, there are good reasons for ordering a medical test: to help your doctor diagnose symptoms accurately, monitor the progress of a known disease, or screen for a hidden one (see the box "Medical Tests for Healthy People"). Unfortunately, numerous tests are performed for other reasons. Many doctors order tests to protect themselves from malpractice. Many physicians can earn more by ordering tests and doing diagnostic procedures than by taking the same amount of time to question, examine, counsel, or think about a patient's problem.

Many patients feel that more tests means better care. People often say, "My doctor is so thorough, he did nearly every test available." Although tests can provide a measure of reassurance, a diagnosis can be made 80–90 percent of the time with only a thorough history and physical exam. Also, the tests ordered may be the wrong ones.

Consider Anne Garber, a 23-year-old woman complaining of a mild burning discomfort in her upper abdomen for about two weeks. Her doctor asked her several brief questions, examined her abdomen, and ordered "a few tests": a urinalysis, a twelve-test blood panel, a complete blood count, and an upper GI series (x-rays that outline the esophagus and stomach).

All these studies added extra costs to her bill but did little to change her suspected diagnosis of esophagitis—an inflamed esophagus caused by stomach acid backup. Nor did the tests affect her treatment—antacids. The most likely diagnosis and treatment could have been determined from her history without a lot of testing. In this respect, Anne Garber was overtested. But she was also undertested. In the previous five years, she hadn't had a Pap smear and pelvic exam, both cancer-screening tests generally recommended for women her age.

When you visit a doctor, you can help assure that medical tests are not "just what the doctor ordered" but what you really *need*. Ask the following questions, particularly when your physician recommends any expensive, uncomfortable, or potentially risky test:

- *"Why do I need the test?"* Start by asking how the test will help diagnose your problem or change your treatment. A satisfactory answer might be "I'm recommending a barium enema because you've been passing blood in your stool. A previous test shows the blood isn't due to hemorrhoids, so we need to find the source of the bleeding. It may be quite harmless, but it could be a serious problem such as a bowel cancer that needs prompt treatment."

    Ask about alternatives. For example, if you have already had the proposed test, can those earlier results be used? To this end, it is wise to keep a record of all your medical tests—when and where they were done and the results.

    Then ask your physician about the risk of waiting and not testing. Monitoring the symptoms under a doctor's supervision for a specific period of time may provide the necessary diagnostic clue, or the symptoms may simply resolve on their own.

- *"What are the risks?"* No test entirely lacks risks. Begin by weighing potential benefits against risks. To start with, the test itself may be wrong. An inaccurate result can lead to a wrong diagnosis or delayed or inappropriate treatment. A false positive may label you as "sick," provoking needless anxiety and sometimes job or insurance difficulties.

    Any time your body is penetrated by a needle, tube, or viewing instrument, you risk infection, bleeding, or damage to vital structures. Physical risks vary depending on the nature of the test, your age, past medical history, general state of health and ability to cooperate, and the skill and experience of your physician.

- *"How do I prepare for the test?"* For some tests, preparation is very important. Be sure to remind your physician about any allergies, especially to medications, anesthetics, or x-ray contrast materials. Mention medications you may be taking, bleeding problems, or whether you might be pregnant. Ask whether you should do anything special before the test, such as fasting or discontinuing medications.

- *"What will the test be like?"* Knowing how the test is done and how it will feel can decrease your anxiety and discomfort before and during a test. When you ask if a certain test will hurt, doctors often say, "Not at all" or "It only lasts a few minutes." Many physicians simply don't know how the procedure feels. Others downplay the discomfort to avoid alarming you or discouraging you from undergoing a needed test. Health professionals tend to significantly underestimate the physical and mental impact of tests on patients. Patients, however, tend to overestimate the discomfort before a test. Discomfort may vary considerably with the skill, sensitivity, and gentleness of the professional doing the test.

    During and after the test, it is important to let the doctor or assistants know what you are feeling. If you're uncomfortable, something can usually be done. Your sensations may provide the first clue to averting a developing complication.

- *"What do the results mean?"* No test is 100 percent accurate. When faced with an abnormal result, the natural tendency is to assume that you are sick. However, as noted earlier, it may be a false positive.

    A false positive can be caused by a statistical fluke in the way normal values are set. For example, the "normal," or reference, values for many blood and urine tests are often established by testing young, white, healthy volunteers—often lab technicians or

Medical Tests for Healthy People

Each year patients faithfully flock to their physicians for their annual physical exam and testing. They are questioned, tapped, probed, bled, and x-rayed—all in the name of health. But is all this testing really necessary? If you are generally healthy without symptoms, should you undergo medical testing, and, if so, which tests should you have? In order to answer such questions you need to understand the uses and limits of medical tests.

At first glance, it may seem like a great idea to undergo batteries of screening tests on a periodic basis. Then diseases can be detected even before symptoms develop, and you can be treated at an earlier, more curable stage in the disease. On this basis physicians and patients alike tend to assume that if a few tests are good, more must be better. Unfortunately, very few screening tests have been shown to be of benefit. To carefully select only those screening tests that might be useful to you, consider asking the following questions:

1. "Is the test designed to diagnose an important health problem?"

It doesn't make much sense to screen for a trivial health problem. You should be more interested in tests that detect conditions significantly influencing the quality and quantity of your life. So a screening test for pitch appreciation is unlikely to be of much benefit (unless you are a musician), while one for cancer or heart disease is more promising.

2. "Am I at significant risk for the disease or condition detected by the test?"

Many diseases occur primarily in certain groups. For example, colon cancer tends to occur in people over the age of 45 or 50, so in younger people there is little reason to screen for the disease unless special risk factors (such as family history of polyps or colon cancer) make the disease more likely. If you are not at increased risk due to your age, sex, ethnic group, or medical history, then the proposed test is unlikely to benefit you.

3. "Can the proposed screening test detect the disease or condition before symptoms alert me that something is wrong?"

Most diseases signal their presence with characteristic symptoms that, when evaluated, can lead to a diagnosis. For some diseases, however, waiting for symptoms to develop can mean that the disease will spread and perhaps become incurable. For example, early diagnosis of cervical cancer is very desirable, because a Pap smear can detect the cancer before symptoms appear, when it is most easily cured. But you don't really need a screening test for appendicitis, since the condition is usually announced promptly by abdominal pain.

4. "Do early diagnosis and treatment favorably alter the progress of the disease?"

It makes little sense to screen for a disease for which there is no effective treatment. However, even if an effective treatment is available and acceptable, it must be shown to be more effective when applied in the stage before symptoms develop. For example, if an *incurable* lung cancer is discovered six months before symptoms would have signaled its presence, the person doesn't actually survive any longer as a result of early diagnosis and treatment. The test merely informs the person of the cancer six months earlier. Fortunately, for a few diseases such as high blood pressure, breast cancer, and colon cancer, early diagnosis and treatment do make a difference.

5. "Is the proposed screening test reasonably accurate, acceptable, and inexpensive?"

One of the greatest stumbling blocks to effective screening programs is test inaccuracy, with many resulting false negatives and false positives. Unfortunately, no test is 100 percent accurate, so we must choose the best available.

The proposed test must also be acceptably comfortable and safe. For example, examining the colon with a long, flexible viewing instrument (colonoscope) may be the most effective way to detect early colon cancer. But it is unlikely that this procedure will be acceptable as a routine screening test for healthy people because of the discomfort, risk, and expense.

Expense is another consideration. Since medical resources are limited, it is generally agreed that screening tests should be shown to offer significant savings in terms of prolonged life or decreased

Medical Tests for Healthy People (continued)

suffering to justify the effort. Otherwise, health resources would be better spent elsewhere.

In summary, for a screening test to be worthwhile, it must reliably detect a significant disease before symptoms develop, the treatment must be more effective when begun before symptoms arise, and the detection and treatment must be accomplished at an acceptable risk and cost. Very few tests currently meet these requirements.

Despite disagreements and limitations, some rough guidelines can be offered to help you select which medical tests to have and approximately how often they should be performed. These guidelines represent the minimum tests recommended for people *without symptoms*. If you have symptoms or are at increased risk for certain conditions, due to your medical or family history, additional tests may be advised. Use these guidelines as a starting point, and discuss your particular needs with your physician.

And remember, if you have a normal test result, still keep on the alert for signs or symptoms that may suggest disease. While carefully selected screening tests can help you protect your health, remember that the most important factors that determine your health do not show up on medical tests at all. In truth, choosing not to smoke, drinking alcohol moderately or not at all, wearing seat belts, exercising regularly, eating wisely, managing stress effectively, and so on, will do more to protect and promote your health than all the tests in the world.

Recommended medical tests for healthy people

Test and Condition	Frequency
History and physical exam for various disorders and risks	**Age 18–39, every 5–10 years; age 40–49, every 3–5 years; age 50 and up, every 2–3 years**
Blood pressure measurement for hypertension	**Every 2–3 years**
Vision test for vision problems	Every 2–3 years if corrective lenses worn
Tuberculin skin test (PPD) for tuberculosis	**Every 5 years until age 35; every 1–2 years if high risk**
Blood glucose for diabetes	Age 18–39, every 10 years; age 40 and up, every 5–10 years
Cholesterol for heart disease risk	**Every 5–10 years**
Hearing test for hearing impairment	Age 60 and up, every 5 years
Test for hidden blood in the stool for bowel cancer	Age 50 and up, every year
Sigmoidoscopy for bowel cancer	Age 50 and up, every 5 years
For men add: Testicular self-exam for testicular cancer	Monthly until age 40
For women add: Pap amear for cervical cancer	**Age 18–49, every 3 years after 2 normal yearly exams; age 50 and up, every 3 years**
Breast self-exam for breast cancer	Monthly
Breast exam by doctor for breast cancer	Age 18–39, every 2–3 years; **age 40 and up, every 1–2 years**
Mammography for breast cancer	Once between the ages of 30 and 39; **every 1–2 years thereafter**
Rubella antibody titer for immunity to German Measles	**Once**
Hematocrit and anemia	Age 18–49, every 3–5 years

Boldface entries are the key recommendations for which there is the strongest evidence.

Source: Adapted from David S. Sobel and Tom Ferguson, 1985, *The People's Book of Medical Tests* (New York: Summit Books).

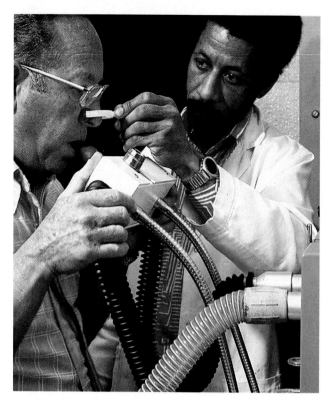

Physicians get information they need from medical tests, but patients have the right to know what the test is for, why they need it, what it will involve, and what the results will indicate. This man is undergoing a test to measure his respiratory efficiency.

medical students. The normal range is then constructed to include *only* 95 percent of those healthy people. Thus 5 percent of healthy patients will have abnormal or borderline values on any given lab test. Statistically, if you have twelve separate tests done, you run a 55 percent chance of having at least one "abnormal" result, *even though you are healthy*. If you differ significantly from the reference group, the normal range may not be appropriate for you. Conversely, normal results may be false negatives and thus do not necessarily indicate health.

Medical tests often give the impression of objectivity and precision. Yet some tests, such as x-rays, electrocardiograms, and scoping procedures, require subjective interpretation. A study of chest x-ray interpretation, for example, found that more than 70 percent of the reports contained disagreements among experienced radiologists; in 25 percent of the reports, the physicians missed important findings. Therefore, getting an experienced second opinion on diagnosis may be important, particularly when ominous symptoms are present or when risky therapies or procedures are prescribed on the basis of an abnormal test. Sometimes repeating the test can "cure" the disease.

Above all, remember that medical tests are only part of the diagnostic puzzle. Such clues must always be viewed in the context of other information about you: medical history, family, age, habits, medications, symptoms, and physical examination. Good physicians treat patients—not test results.

Medical and Surgical Treatments   Once a diagnosis is made, the treatment options can be considered. The treatments offered for diseases should reflect the wide variety of physical, chemical, and psychosocial factors that cause or aggravate the disease condition. Although some diseases can be cured or ameliorated by medical or surgical treatment, other diseases require no treatment at all or may be aggravated by attempts at therapy. Therefore, whenever a treatment is recommended, whether medications or an operation, it is important that you understand the reasons for treatments, options, risks, and expected benefits. Asking the following key questions may help ensure that you are getting the best possible care for yourself.

- *"What are my choices in treatments?"* Many conditions can be treated in a variety of ways, and your physician should be able to explain the alternative choices to you. In some cases, management with medications is a viable alternative to surgery. In other cases, lifestyle changes including exercise, diet, and stress management should be considered alongside medications or surgery before making a choice. When any treatment is recommended, also ask what the consequences are likely to be if you postpone treatment.
- *"What are the risks, costs, and expected benefits of each treatment option?"* To make an informed choice about any treatment, you need to know what each of the options would cost you. This cost includes how likely possible complications such as drug reactions, bleeding, infection, injury, or death might be. To understand a proposed treatment, you should also ask about costs, both personal (such as time loss from work) and financial (whether your insurance will pay for part or all of the proposed treatments). You also need to understand how likely it is that the proposed treatment will benefit you in terms of prolonging your life, relieving your symptoms, or improving your ability to function. No one can tell you which choice is right for you. However, to make an informed choice you need information about the treatment options. Informed *choice,* not merely informed *consent,* is an essential ingredient in quality medical care.

Prescription Medications   Thousands of lives are saved each year by antibiotics, heart medications, insulin, and scores of other drugs. Pain medications and anesthetics

Dental Self-Care

Dental diseases can be prevented through proper self-care and regular visits to the dentist. Follow these tips for healthy teeth and gums.

Brushing

Toothbrushing removes plaque and food particles from the outer, inner, and biting surfaces of your teeth. Choose a soft brush with end-rounded or polished bristles. The size and shape of the brush should allow you to reach every tooth.

A number of different toothbrushing methods are acceptable; the following is one effective way of removing plaque:

1. Place the head of your toothbrush beside your teeth, with the bristle tips at a 45-degree angle against the gumline.

2. Move the brush back and forth in short (half-a-tooth-size) strokes several times, using a gentle "scrubbing" motion.

3. Brush the outer surfaces of each tooth, upper and lower, keeping the bristles angled against the gumline.

4. Use the same method on the inside surfaces of all the teeth, still using short back-and-forth strokes.

5. Scrub the chewing surfaces of the teeth.

6. To clean the inside surfaces of the front teeth, tilt the brush vertically and make several gentle-up-and-down strokes with the "toe" (the front part) of the brush.

7. Brushing your tongue will help freshen your breath and clean your mouth by removing bacteria.

Flossing

Flossing removes plaque and food particles from between the teeth and under the gumline, areas where your toothbrush can't reach.

When flossing, follow the instructions given to you by your dentist or dental hygienist. Here are some helpful suggestions:

1. Break off about 18 inches of floss, and wind most of it around one of your middle fingers.

2. Wind the remaining floss around the same finger of the opposite hand. This finger will "take up" the floss as you use it.

3. Hold the floss tightly between your thumbs and forefingers, with about an inch of floss between them. There should be no slack. Using a gentle sawing motion, guide the floss between your teeth. Never "snap" the floss into the gums.

4. When the floss reaches the gumline, curve it into a C-shape against one tooth. Gently slide it into the space between the gum and the tooth until you feel resistance.

5. Hold the floss tightly against the tooth. Gently scrape the side of the tooth, moving the floss away from the gum.

6. Repeat this method on the rest of your teeth. Don't forget the back side of your last tooth.

Perform the self-exam for dental plaque described in Appendix 1 of this chapter periodically to see if any plaque is left on your teeth after brushing and flossing.

Source: American Dental Association.

---

make the unbearable bearable. Arthritis medications help preserve function for thousands of people. But we pay a price for having such powerful tools. Of all admissions to hospitals, nearly 5 percent are due primarily to drug reactions, and 20 percent of these patients are likely to have a second drug reaction during their hospital stay.

Part of the problem lies with physicians who overprescribe or misprescribe drugs. Mishaps also occur because patients do not receive adequate information about medications and often don't understand how to take them or fail to follow instructions given to them. Consumers must ask the following questions about their medications.

- *"Do I really need this medication?"* Many physicians often prescribe medications not because they are really necessary, but because they think that patients want and expect drugs. Ask about nondrug alternatives. Sometimes the best medication of all is no medication. Remember to mention any drugs you're taking or conditions you have that could complicate the use of medications.
- *"What is the name of the medication, and what is it supposed to do?"* Your physician should tell you why the medication is being prescribed, how the prescription might be expected to help you, and how soon you can expect results. For example, antibiotics for a strep

throat infection are given primarily to prevent later complications (rheumatic fever and heart disease) rather than to stop the sore throat pain. An anesthetic solution to gargle is intended to ease sore throat pain.

- *"How and when do I take the medication, and for how long?"* Understanding how much of the medication to take and how often and how long to take it is often critical to the safe, effective use of medications. For example, if you are taking an **antibiotic** for a bacterial infection, you may feel better within a few days but you should still take the medication as prescribed for a week or two to prevent a recurrence. Or if you stop taking **steroid** medications used to treat poison oak or poison ivy when the rash subsides rather than taking the full course of treatment, the rash can erupt again.
- *"What foods, drinks, other medications, or activities should I avoid while taking this medication?"* The presence of food in the stomach may help protect the stomach from some medications, but it can render other drugs ineffective. Other drugs you may be taking, even over-the-counter drugs and alcohol, can either amplify or inhibit the effects of the prescribed medication. The more medications you are taking, the greater the chance of an undesirable drug interaction.
- *What are the side effects, and what do I do if they occur?"* All medications have side effects. Some may be tolerable, minor annoyances while others may be life-threatening allergic reactions. You need to know what symptoms to look out for and what action to take should they develop. It is your responsibility to ask about precautions and possible side effects.
- *"Can you prescribe an alternative or generic medication that is less expensive?"* When a drug company develops a new drug in the United States, it is granted exclusive rights to produce that drug for seventeen years. After this seventeen-year period has expired, other companies may market chemical equivalents of that drug (sometimes formulated with different fillers, in different strengths, and so on). These generic medications are generally considered as safe and effective as the original brand name drug but often cost half as much (see Table 21-1). In some cases generic drugs may not be absorbed as predictably as brand-name drugs, so the physician may prefer a particular brand for certain patients—infants, children, and the elderly—or certain diseases.
- *"Is there any written information about the medication?"* Even if your physician takes the time to carefully answer all your questions about medications, you will probably find it difficult to remember all this infor-

mation. Fortunately, there are now many sources of information, from package inserts to pamphlets and books where you can read more about the medications you are taking (see Appendix III, "Resources for Self-care").

Remember, never share your prescription medication with anyone else, and never take someone else's. Store your drugs in a cool, dry place, out of direct light, and never use an old prescription for a new ailment.

Surgery   Americans are the most operated-on people in the world. Each year over 20 million operations are performed. About 20 percent of these operations are in response to an emergency such as a severe injury while 80 percent are **elective** surgeries, meaning the patient can generally choose when and where to have the operation if at all. The number of operations performed varies widely from country to country, city to city, and even surgeon to surgeon. The most important factor predicting rates of surgery in a given community is the number of surgeons, not the amount of disease. The more surgeons, the more surgery. All this suggests that you would do well to ask some questions when surgery is recommended for you or a family member to help ensure the operation is really necessary.

- *"Why do I need surgery at this time?"* Your physician should be able to explain to you the reason for the surgery, alternatives to surgery, and what is likely to happen if you don't have the operation. You should also ask about how the surgery is likely to benefit you.

  With most surgery, getting a *second opinion* is advised, and many health insurance plans now require a second opinion before all or certain elective operations. Studies show that when second opinions are required on elective surgical procedures, in 27 percent of cases the second surgeon does not agree that the recommended operation is necessary. A second opinion should be an independent opinion, not the opinion of your physician's partner or associate. Getting a second opinion is not the same as changing physicians. The second physician should not be sought as another possible surgeon, for example. Instead, he or she is only to give a disinterested opinion, in the sense that there will be no personal financial gain in recommending surgery. Consulting a nonsurgeon may also be helpful in exploring alternatives to surgery. For more information about how to get a second opinion, you can call the Second Surgical Opinion Hot Line, sponsored

---

Antibiotic   A substance derived from a mold or bacteria that inhibits the growth of other microorganisms.

Steroid   A drug of hormone origin. Certain of these medications can decrease inflammation.

Elective surgery   A nonemergency operation that the patient can choose to schedule.

Table 21-1 The most commonly used generic prescription drugs and their possible side effects

Generic Name	Brand Name	Purpose of Drug	Possible Side Effects
Amoxicillin trihydrate	Amoxil, Larotid, Polymox, Trimox, Wymox	Penicillin antibiotic commonly used to treat infections including gonorrhea	Blotchy skin rash; can provoke more severe allergic reaction in some people
Penicillin V	Penicillin-VK, Ledercillin-LK	Broad-spectrum antibiotic commonly prescribed for respiratory infections	Prolonged use may increase risk of yeast infections
Ampicillin	Amcill, Polycillin	Penicillin antibiotic used to treat common infections and meningitis	Rash and possibility of severe allergic reaction in some people
Prednisone	Deltasone, Liquid Pred	Synthetic corticosteroid used to treat inflammatory bowel disease, rheumatoid arthritis, severe asthma	Indigestion, acne
Tetracycline	Panmycin, Robitet	Widely prescribed antibiotic used for pneumonia, chronic bronchitis, syphillis, gonorrhea	Nausea, vomiting if taken systemically
Hydrochlorothiazide	Esidrix, Hydrodiuril	Diuretic often used in treatment of hypertension, premenstrual syndrome	Leg cramps, loss of potassium
Doxycycline hyclate	Doryx, Vibramycin, Vibra Tabs	Tetracycline antibiotic used to treat chlamydia or pelvic inflammatory disease, or prevent travelers diarrhea	Nausea
Ibuprofen	Advil, Motrin, Nuprin	Pain reliever and anti-inflammatory used to treat headaches, cramps, rheumatoid arthritis	Diarrhea, constipation, may counteract benefit of antihypertensives
Erythromycin stearate	E-mycin, Eryc	Broad-spectrum antibiotic useful for those allergic to penicillin or tetracycline	Nausea, diarrhea, rash, itching
Acetaminophen with codeine	Tylenol with codeine, Anacin-3 with codeine	Aspirin substitute used for pain relief	Large doses can be toxic to the livers of people who consume more than 3 or 4 ounces of alcohol daily
Cephalexin	Keflex	Antibiotic used to treat cystitis, bronchitis	Diarrhea
Amitriptyline	Amitril, Elavil, Endep	Tricyclic anti-depressant used in long-term treatment, especially for insomnia	Drowsiness, sweating, dizziness, blurred vision
Furosemide	Lasix	Powerful, fast-acting diuretic used in treatment of hypertension	Dizziness and potassium depletion
Diazepam	Valium	Muscle relaxant that helps relieve nervousness and tension, also used to treat epileptic seizures	Drowsiness and dizziness; drug can be habit-forming if taken for a long time
Phenobarbital	Barbita, Luminal	Anti-convulsant used to prevent epileptic seizures	Drowsiness, clumsiness, dizziness
Hydrocortisone cream	Cortaid, Hytone	In topical form, used for allergies and as anti-inflammatory	In high doses, can induce acne, weight gain

Table 21-1 Continued

Generic Name	Brand Name	Purpose of Drug	Possible Side Effects
Sulfamethoxazole with trimethoprim	Gantanol, Gantanol DS, Bactrim, Septra	Antibacterial used to treat urinary tract infections, gonorrhea, and pneumocystis pneumonia	Nausea, loss of appetite
Dipyridamole	Persantine	Anti-platelet drug usually given with aspirin to "thin" blood of recent heart attack or stroke victims	Nausea
Nitroglycerin	Nitrostat, Nitrodisc	Relief of heart disease symptoms	Headache, flushing, dizziness
Nystatin	Mycostatin, Nilstat	Used to treat thrush and vaginal infections	Nausea and vomiting may occur with high doses taken orally
Triamcinolone	Aristocort, Azmacort, Kenalog	Topical form used to treat eczema, oral form to treat pituitary or adrenal gland disorders	Weight gain, acne, indigestion if taken orally
Propoxyphene napsylate with acetaminophen	Darvon, Dolene	Pain reliever	Dizziness, drowsiness, nausea
Lorazepam	Ativan	Used to treat depression-related anxiety and insomnia	Drowsiness
Imipramine	Tofranil	Tricyclic anti-depressant sometimes used to treat bed-wetting in children	Sweating, dry mouth, blurred vision, dizziness
Thyroid	Armour Thyroid, Thyroid Strong	Used to treat thyroid disorders including goiter	Requires periodic monitoring
Metronidazole	Flagyl, Protostat	Used to treat sexually transmitted diseases and amoebic dysentery	Nausea, loss of appetite, dark urine, abdominal pain
Meclizine	Antivert, Bonine	Antihistamine and anti-emetic used to treat motion sickness and inner ear disorders	Drowsiness, dry mouth
Allopurinol	Lopurin, Zyloprim	Long-term preventive of recurrent attacks of gout	May cause drowsiness; alcohol increases adverse effects of drug
Ferrous sulfate	Feosol capsules	Iron supplement for treatment of anemia	Constipation, diarrhea

Source: *Pharmacy Times; Physicians' Desk Reference; The Essential Guide to Prescription Drugs; The AMA Guide to Prescription and Over-the-Counter Drugs.* From *Washington Post Health*, August 22, 1989, pp. 14–15.

by the U.S. government, at 800-638-6833 (or 800-492-6603 in Maryland).

If your second opinion agrees with the recommendation for surgery, then you can feel more confident in proceeding. If the second opinion conflicts with the first, you may wish to have the physicians confer with each other to clarify the recommendations or you may want to get a third opinion. Disagreements among physicians are usually honest differences of opinion in gray areas of medical knowledge where an expert consensus has not yet been reached. In all cases, you yourself must weigh the opinions carefully, and make the final decision about your treatment.

Although second opinions are most commonly

Welcome!

We are glad you have come to our clinic and hope we can help you get what you need.

Consumer's Rights

As one of our clients, you have choices, rights and responsibilities.

YOU HAVE THE RIGHT TO...

1. Be treated with dignity and respect.
2. Know the names of people serving you.
3. Have privacy and confidentiality of your records.
4. Receive explanations.
5. Receive education and counseling.
6. Review your medical records with a clinician.
7. Consent to or refuse any care or treatment.

Family Planning clients also have the rights to...

8. Decide whether or not to have children and when.
9. Know the effectiveness, possible side effects and problems of all methods of birth control.
10. Participate in choosing a birth control method.

YOU ALSO HAVE THE RESPONSIBILITY TO...

1. Be honest about your medical history.
2. Be sure you understand.
3. Follow health advice and medical instructions.
4. Respect Clinic policies.
5. Report any changes in your health.
6. Keep appointments or cancel at least 24 hours in advance.

When you want to know............ASK
When you have questions...........SPEAK UP
When you have problems...........COMPLAIN
When you like what happens........SMILE

If you have suggestions, compliments, or complaints, please let us know.

Posted prominently in a medical examination room, this statement of consumer's rights and responsibilities serves as a reminder that the patient's relationship with his or her health care providers is one of mutual respect.

sought for elective surgical procedures, you should also consider getting one for any treatment or diagnostic procedure with significant risk or cost.

- *"What are the risks and complications of the surgery?"* All surgical procedures carry some risk. The average risk of death from surgery is about thirteen deaths for every 1,000 operations. Of course, this overall risk will vary depending on the type of operation performed, the surgeon, and your general state of health. You should ask about the **mortality rate** (risk of death) and **morbidity rate** (risk of nonlethal complications). You should also ask how often the surgeon has performed the operation and what his or her personal experience has been with the procedure. Studies show that surgical teams with more experience with an operation tend to have lower rates of complications.

Sometimes an operation can be performed in several different ways using different incisions, techniques, and anesthetics. Discuss these options with your surgeon so that you can better understand your choices.

Some of the risk from a surgical procedure is due to the use of an anesthetic. There are two basic types of anesthesia—general and local. General anesthesia affects our entire body and blocks pain by making you unconscious. Local anesthesia involves injecting a medication that numbs only one area of the body so you remain awake during the operation. There are advantages and disadvantages to each type of anesthesia.

Mortality rate   The number of deaths occurring in the population being studied.

Morbidity rate   The number of illnesses or injuries occurring in the population being studied.

When the Cure Becomes Part of the Problem

A young woman with a sore throat consults her physician. Though her physician diagnoses a mild viral infection, he nonetheless prescribes an antibiotic. A week later the patient develops thrush, a yeast infection of the mouth brought on by the antibiotic. To treat the thrush, the physician prescribes Nystatin solution. Soon thereafter the patient develops stomatitis, a diffuse inflammation of the lining of the mouth, for which her physician prescribes a sulfa drug. One week later the woman's white cell count has dropped to subnormal levels due to suppression of normal bone marrow activity by the sulfa drug. At this point the physician withdraws all treatment. Within two weeks the patient has no more symptoms and white blood cell counts have returned to normal.

What caused a mild infection to spiral out of control? An unnecessary treatment of the original symptom caused a chain reaction of complications that could have had a disastrous outcome. This is a classic example of iatrogenic disease. The word *iatrogenic* comes from the Greek *iatreia,* which means "the art of healing." Hippocrates recognized the hazard of applying this art to excess when he admonished, "as to disease, make a habit of two things—to help or, at least, to do no harm."

Iatrogenesis, or physician-induced disease, is widely prevalent. Consider that 3 to 5 percent of all hospital admissions in the early 1970s were due to a reaction to therapeutic drugs prescribed by physicians. Thirty percent of these patients had a second drug-related reaction while under hospital care. It was reported that in one series of hospital admissions 6 percent of patients admitted for a drug reaction died of further drug-related complications.

Why therapeutic drugs play such a key role in iatrogenesis becomes clear if we look at both doctor and patient behaviors. Physicians, on the average, write prescriptions for 50–75 percent of their outpatients, while inpatients typically receive as many as ten drugs simultaneously. Nearly 90 million new prescriptions for the thirty most commonly used drugs were written in 1988. The typical patient takes three over-the-counter medications in any one month, yet most patients can't identify 60 percent of the drugs they take. To compound matters even more, 40 percent of patients take medications prescribed by two or more physicians, and 12 percent take medications prescribed for someone else.

Drug reactions are but one iatrogenic complication that may lead to hospitalization. Problems resulting from unnecessary outpatient procedures, radiation therapy, and transfusions account for another 1–2 percent of all hospitalizations. Iatrogenic disease often worsens when a patient enters a hospital. A study performed in 1979 at Boston University found a 36 percent incidence of inpatient iatrogenic episodes following admission. About 9 percent of these were considered major, presenting a threat to life or a potential cause of considerable disability. The actual mortality rate was almost 2 percent.

Iatrogenic disease in the elderly warrants special comment. Since the aged often have hearing and vision impairment, as well as compromised function of one or more of their major organs, they are especially vulnerable to iatrogenic complications. One author grouped these complications into four categories, dubbed "the four T's": *tests, treatments, trauma* (such as falling from a bed or wheelchair) and *troubles* (such as confusion, immobilization, malnourishment, or the bed sores, phlebitis, and pneumonia associated with hospitalizing an elderly patient).

What can be done about iatrogenic disease? Many, perhaps most, iatrogenic complications cannot be prevented. They are unpredictable outcomes of indicated treatments or properly performed procedures. But a significant number of iatrogenic complications are preventable. To head off potential iatrogenesis, physicians need to exercise diagnostic and therapeutic restraint, resisting the temptation to order one or another of a vast array of tests and drugs. Patients, on the other hand, should not undermine their physician's restraint by insisting on an antibiotic for every cold or an x-ray for every pain. In preventing iatrogenic illness, less may be better.

Source: Michael Jacobs. 1989. When the Cure Becomes Part of the Problem. *Healthline,* December, pp. 2–3.

Many patients prefer being asleep during the operation so they choose general anesthesia. However, general anesthesia carries a greater risk of heart irregularities and collapse of the cardiovascular system. The risk of death from general anesthesia is estimated somewhere between one in 3,000 to one in 10,000. Local anesthesia is much safer and is now replacing general anesthesia in many types of operations. Be sure to discuss your options in anesthesia with your surgeon.

Blood transfusions may be required during some operations. If you need a transfusion, blood banks have adopted techniques to screen donor blood to ensure its safety. Nevertheless, if an elective operation is planned, ask if you can donate and store some of your own blood in the months preceding the surgery. Then if you need blood during surgery you can receive a transfusion of your own blood. This technique, known as **autologous donation**, reduces the risk even further of developing a transfusion reaction or contracting an infection such as viral hepatitis or AIDS from infected donor blood.

- *"Can the operation be performed on an outpatient basis?"* More than 30 percent of all operations can now be safely performed on an **outpatient** (ambulatory) basis without requiring an overnight stay in the hospital. Ambulatory operative procedures are generally less complex and require less postoperative monitoring. Among the 200 different operations that can now be performed on an ambulatory basis are **vasectomies**, tubal ligations, some hernia repairs, breast biopsies, **dilation and curettage (D&C), tonsillectomies**, cataract surgery, some types of plastic surgery and orthopedic procedures, and scores of other minor surgical procedures.

Outpatient surgery offers many advantages. In most cases, it is less than one-half the cost of comparable in-hospital operations. It prevents some of the family disruption and psychological trauma that often accompany hospitalization. And it decreases the opportunities for the patient to develop a hospital-acquired medical complication such as infection.

- *"What can I expect before, during, and after surgery?"* Knowing what to expect can help you prepare psychologically and physically for the operation. Preparation also appears to decrease postoperative discomfort and need for pain medications and to shorten postoperative hospital stays.

You should also ask about how long it should take you to recover and what you can do to speed recovery. You should also be informed about what to expect after surgery in terms of symptoms and which symptoms might signal a complication and should be reported to your doctor.

You are an important part of the health-care system; not only as a *consumer* of medical care but as a primary health-care *provider*. Managing common medical problems; knowing when and how to self-treat and when to seek professional care; communicating clearly and concisely with your physician; asking questions about medical tests, medications, and surgery; and knowing how to get more information on health topics are some of the essential skills for a health-wise consumer. Developing these skills will not only result in better health care but will also help you develop a real sense of competence and confidence about managing your health.

Autologous donation A process in which a person can receive a transfusion of his or her blood that was previously withdrawn and stored.

Outpatient A person receiving medical attention without being admitted to the hospital.

Vasectomy Surgical cutting of the tube that transports sperm (vas deferens), performed as a method of birth control.

Dilation and curettage (D&C) Scraping of the interior of the uterus, usually performed to diagnose cancer or stop bleeding.

Tonsillectomy Surgical procedure to remove the lymph tissue (tonsils) at the back of the throat.

Summary

- Easy access to health professionals, medical technology, and medications has led people to have less self-confidence in managing their health. On the other hand, the professional health-care system would be overwhelmed if people stopped practicing self-care when appropriate.

Managing Medical Problems

- Self-care involves assessing the body for significant symptoms, which may indicate the need for professional assistance. Symptoms give clues about how well your body is managing an illness on its own.
- Home medical tests, one aspect of self-assessment, al-

low cost savings, convenience, privacy, an increased sense of control, and sometimes more comprehensive information. Especially useful home tests include blood pressure tests, blood glucose monitoring, and pregnancy tests. With all tests, false positives or false negatives are possible.

- Informed self-care requires knowing how to evaluate symptoms so that you don't go to a physician too soon or too late. It's necessary to see a physician if symptoms are severe, unusual, persistent, and recurrent.

- Conditions that require emergency-room treatment include major trauma or injury, such as broken bones or burns; uncontrollable or internal bleeding; intolerable or uncontrollable pain; severe chest pain; severe shortness of breath; and loss of consciousness.

- Because of the triage process, going to an emergency room when it's not an emergency means long waits for treatment as well as high costs.

- When professional advice is required, it's often possible to get it over the phone; visits can be arranged for a convenient time.

- Self-treatment doesn't necessarily require medication. The body can heal itself; or massage, ice or heat, exercises, and relaxation techniques can help.

- Over-the-counter drugs are a necessary and helpful part of self-care but should not be substituted for non-drug coping techniques. Effective use requires (1) reading drug labels and following directions, (2) not exceeding the recommended use, (3) using caution regarding interaction with other medications, (4) selecting products with a single active ingredient, (5) trying to buy generic products, (6) never taking drugs from unlabeled containers, (7) not self-medicating when pregnant or nursing without consulting a physician, (8) disposing of expired medications, (9) storing medicines in a safe place, and (10) using special caution with aspirin for children and adolescents.

- A home medicine kit should contain small quantities of the medicines needed for an individual family as well as essential supplies.

Getting the Most Out of Your Medical Care

- Good communication with the physician and other members of the health-care team is essential. Patients are sometimes afraid to ask questions, and physicians may ignore questions or feel too rushed to answer them adequately. The ideal relationship should be more like a partnership where the physician acts as a consultant and the patient actively participates.

- Preparation for a visit to a physician should include making a written list of questions or concerns and bringing a list of all medications.

- During the visit to the physician, it's important to be open, to ask questions, and request clarification. Repe-

tition of the diagnosis and instructions to check understanding can help ensure good care.

- Diagnoses are normally based on a medical history, physical examination, and tests and procedures.

- The medical history is a description of problems, concerns, and backgrounds. The physician asks questions that will elicit information on the chief complaint, the present illness, the past medical history, all bodily systems, and social history.

- The physical examination, whether complete or limited to one area, consists of inspection, palpation, and auscultation.

- Medical tests account for nearly a third of the national health bill, and patients cannot be passive about their use. Physicians should not use tests as protection against malpractice or as a way to make money; tests should not replace the history and physical exam. Patients should ask questions about the need for the test, the risks, preparation, what the test will be like, and what the results mean.

- Test norms are usually established by testing young, white, healthy volunteers, so they may not be completely valid for everybody and cause false positives.

- Treatments should reflect the wide variety of physical, chemical, and psychosocial factors that cause or aggravate the disease condition. Patients should understand the reasons for treatments, options, risks, and expected benefits. Patients should ask questions about other choices as well as about risks, costs, and expected benefits of the suggested treatment.

- Prescription medicines save lives but also cause problems from drug reactions; physicians can misprescribe or overprescribe drugs, and patients don't always follow instructions, sometimes because they don't understand them. Patients should ask why they need medication, what the medication is supposed to do, how and when to take the medication, what to avoid when taking the medication, what the side effects are, whether a generic is available, and if any written information on the medication is available.

- When surgery is recommended, patients should ask whether it is necessary, what the alternatives are, and what the benefits are. A second opinion is always advisable and is sometimes required by insurance companies.

- All surgical procedures carry risk; some of it is due to general anesthesia. If elective surgery is planned, patients can arrange for autologous donation of blood. More operations can be performed on an outpatient basis, which reduces costs, family disruption, and psychological trauma.

- Knowing what to expect before surgery appears to decrease postoperative discomfort and the need for pain medications as well as to shorten hospital stays.

Take Action

1. Write a self-care medical profile of yourself in your health diary. Include your age and current weight and height; any conditions or diseases you have and the treatments or medications you take for them; any conditions or diseases that run in your family or that are common in your ethnic group; any surgery you have had and the date; the diseases against which you have been immunized and the date of your last tetanus shot; and any drug or food allergies you have. Also include the names and telephone numbers of your health-care practitioners and pharmacy; information about any prescriptions you take, including the prescription number, the number of refills you are allowed, and the telephone number of the pharmacy that filled each one; and information about your health insurance, including your policy number, important details about coverage, and a telephone number for someone who can answer your questions about it. Keep your self-care profile up-to-date and use it for reference when you need it.

2. Examine all the medications in your medicine cabinet. Discard any expired or unlabeled medications. Ask your physician or pharmacist whether you should keep any medications you are uncertain about. Compare the contents of your medicine cabinet with those listed in the box "Your Home Self-care Kit" and expand your supplies if you need to.

3. Before your next visit to your physician, make a *written* list of your concerns. Be prepared to ask questions. After the visit, review how it went—were your concerns satisfactorily addressed? Were you able to communicate your needs? Did you feel involved and in control? What aspects would you like to handle better the next time?

4. Review the box "Medical Tests for Healthy People." Are there any tests you need to have done? If so, make an appointment at your clinic or medical office and have the test done.

Behavior Change Strategy

Complying with Physicians' Instructions

Even though we sometimes have to entrust ourselves to the care of medical professionals, that doesn't mean that we give up responsibility for our own behavior. Following medical instructions and advice often requires the same kind of behavior self-management that's involved in quitting smoking, losing weight, or changing eating patterns. For example, if you have an illness or injury, you may be told to take medication at certain times of the day, do special exercises or movements, attend therapy sessions, or change your diet.

The medical profession recognizes the importance of patient adherence, or compliance, and encourages the use of different strategies to support it, such as the following:

1. Using reminders placed at home, in the car, at work, and so on, that improve follow-through in taking medication and keeping scheduled appointments.
2. Using a diary and other forms of self-monitoring to keep a detailed account of health behaviors, such as pill taking, diet, exercise, and so on.
3. Using self-reward systems so that desired behavior changes are encouraged, with a focus on short-term rewards (such as payment of a sum of money for each week of nonsmoking).

Communication is one of the key requirements of improved adherence. You as the patient must fully understand what needs to be done, and the physician or medical staff member must listen to your personal concerns about the regimen. Sharing information and concerns contributes to a sense of shared responsibility for recovery. Successful medical care involves more than following physicians' orders; it also has to accommodate the individual's habits and preferences. The next time you have to follow a particular regimen or treatment for an illness or an injury, use the suggestions given here and the others found in Chapter 1 to help you comply.

Selected Bibliography

Gartner, Alan, and Frank Riessman. 1977. *Self-help in the Human Services.* San Francisco, Calif.: Jossey-Bass.

Greenfield, Sheldon, Sherrie Kaplan, and John E. Ware. 1985. Expanding patient involvement in care: Effect on patient outcomes. *Annals of Internal Medicine* 102:520–28.

Guide to Clinical Preventive Services: Report of the U.S. Preventive Services Task Force. 1989. Baltimore, Md.: Williams and Wilkins.

Herman, P. G., D. E. Gerson, S. J. Hessel, and others. 1975. Disagreements in chest roentgen interpretation. *Chest* 68:278–82.

Kaplan, Eric B., Lewis B. Sheiner, and others. 1985. The usefulness of preoperative laboratory screening. *Journal of the American Medical Association* 253:3576–81.

Levin, Lowell S., and Ellen L. Idler. 1981. *The Hidden Health Care System.* Cambridge, Mass.: Ballinger.

Louis Harris and Associates. 1983 (March). *Patient Information and Prescription Drugs: Parallel Surveys of Physicians and Pharmacists.* Washington, D.C.: U.S. Food and Drug Administration.

Medical Practices Committee, American College of Physicians. 1981. Periodic health examination: A guide for designing individualized preventive health care in the asymptomatic patient. *Annals of Internal Medicine* 95:729–32.

Runkle, Cecilia, and Catherine Regan. 1985. The role of self-care in medical care. In Wendy Squyres, ed., *Patient Education and Health Promotion in Medical Care.* Palo Alto, Calif.: Mayfield.

Self-medication: The New Era . . . A Symposium (condensation of papers and discussions). 1980 (March 31). Washington, D.C.: The Proprietary Association.

Vickery, Donald M., Howard Kalmer, Debra Lowry, Muriel Constantine, Elizabeth Wright, and Wendy Loren. 1983. Effect of a self-care education program on medical visits. *Journal of the American Medical Association* 250:2952–56.

Williamson, John D., and Kate Kanaher. 1978. *Self-care in Health.* London: Croom Helm.

Recommended Readings

See Appendix III of this chapter for annotated readings.

Taking Your Temperature

Breathing, digesting, moving, even thinking, all generate body heat. Your body temperature reflects your overall body metabolism and muscular activity. Warm-blooded animals have evolved a remarkable mechanism to keep body temperature within a narrow, safe range in spite of considerable variations in environmental temperatures.

Why Performed   It is a good idea to measure your temperature a few times when you are feeling well, to establish your normal baseline. Then if you develop symptoms such as a cough, earache, diarrhea, or skin rash, check your temperature. It can provide a clue about the cause or severity of the symptoms.

Equipment   The most common and least expensive (about $1–2) thermometer is the glass thermometer filled with mercury or a red liquid. There are two types: oral (with a thinner bulb tip) and rectal (with a thicker tip). Plastic fever strips are also available (about $3) containing heat-sensitive liquid crystal that changes color to indicate the temperature. Finally, new electronic thermometers (about $12) show temperature on an easy-to-read-digital display.

Procedure   Oral temperatures should not be measured for at least ten minutes after smoking, eating, or drinking a hot or cold liquid. When using a glass thermometer, first clean it with rubbing alcohol or cool (hot water may break it) soapy water. Then grip the end opposite the bulb and shake vigorously as though trying to shake drops of water off the tip. Shake it down until it reads 95°F or lower. Place the oral thermometer under the tongue and keep your mouth tightly closed around it. Leave the thermometer in place for a *full three minutes*. If you leave it in for only two minutes, nearly one-third of temperature readings will be off by at least a half a degree.

To read the glass thermometer, grip it at the end opposite the bulb and hold it in good light with the numbers facing you. Roll the thermometer slowly back and forth between your fingers until you see the silver or red reflection of the column. Note where the column ends, and compare it with the degrees marked in lines on the thermometer. Each long line is a full degree, and each short line counts for 0.2 (two-tenths) of a degree. Most thermometers have a special mark, usually an arrow, indicating a "normal" temperature of 98.6°F (36.8°C). Most thermometers for home use are calibrated in degrees Fahrenheit (F), but some may have the alternative scale of degrees Celsius (C).

Results   "Normal" temperature varies from person to person, so it is important to know what is normal for you. Your normal temperature will also vary throughout the day, lowest in the early morning and rising by as much as a degree in the early evening. If you exercise or if it is a hot day, your temperature may normally rise. Also, in women body temperature typically varies by a degree or more through the menstrual cycle, peaking around the time of ovulation. Rectal temperatures normally run about 0.5° to 1°F higher than oral temperatures. If your recorded temperature is more than 1.0–1.5°F above your "normal" baseline temperature, you have a fever. Most often fevers are due to an infection, but fevers may also be caused by drug reactions, inflammation, arthritis, hormone abnormalities, cancer, or severe injuries.

Self-exam for Dental Plaque

Dental disease is the most common chronic disease; nearly 95 percent of all Americans suffer from tooth decay (dental caries) and/or gum disease (periodontal disease). The major culprit in both of these preventable diseases is dental plaque, a sticky substance composed of millions of bacteria that accumulates around and between teeth. If not removed by proper daily brushing and flossing, plaque can cause tooth decay, gum infection, and tooth loss.

Why Performed   Plaque is nearly invisible, so how can you know if you are brushing and flossing adequately? Regular dental checkups will help, but you can also test for plaque at home.

Equipment   Disclosing tablets are available in most pharmacies for $2 for 30 tablets. The disclosing tablets contain a harmless red vegetable dye that stains food debris and dental plaque so that you can spot areas not thoroughly cleaned.

Procedure   After brushing and flossing, chew one of the tablets thoroughly, swishing the mixture of saliva and dye over your teeth and gums for about 30 seconds. Then gently rinse your mouth and examine your teeth in the mirror.

Results   Areas of plaque will stain bright red. The stained areas, usually along the gum margins and between teeth, indicate places you missed while brushing and flossing. Don't be discouraged if you "fail" your first few plaque tests with glowing colors. With this feedback, your brushing and flossing techniques will improve until you no longer leave areas of harmful plaque.

Home Blood Pressure Monitoring

Blood pressure is the force exerted against the walls of blood vessels as your heart pumps blood through your body. Your blood pressure changes from day to day, even minute to minute, depending on activity, diet, drugs, and emotions. Even talking has been shown to raise blood pressure. About one in five Americans has high blood pressure (hypertension). If not controlled, it increases a person's risk of stroke, heart failure, kidney failure, and heart attack. Hypertension is discussed more fully in Chapter 15, as is the process of checking your blood pressure.

Why Performed   You should have your blood pressure checked, or check it yourself, at least every two to three years. If it is normal, more frequent testing is not necessary. If it is elevated, you should check with your physician to plan appropriate home blood pressure monitoring and, if necessary, treatment. Self-recording of blood pressure is most useful for people with hypertension or borderline high blood pressure. It can offer a more complete and accurate picture of what your blood pressure is like throughout the day and in different environments, not just the physician's office. It can let you monitor the effects of diet, exercise, weight loss, and

medications on your blood pressure. Many people find that home blood pressure monitoring is sufficient to help them lower their blood pressure to safer levels without medications or with a minimum of medication.

Equipment   There are several types of blood pressure devices: cuffs with a stethoscope, electronic cuffs with built-in microphone, and the newest electronic "mikeless" cuffs. The cost is generally $40–$50, up to $200 for models that inflate automatically and give a printed record. The accuracy of electronic devices for measuring your blood pressure needs to be checked against a standard cuff and stethoscope.

Procedure   The instructions on how to take your blood pressure will vary depending on the type of blood pressure device you use. The basic principles are similar. Wrap the inflatable bag (cuff) firmly around your upper arm. As the cuff is inflated, blood flow to your arm is temporarily blocked. Then, as the cuff is slowly deflated, blood first begins to flow in the arteries when the pressure produced by your heart contracting is high enough to overcome the pressure in the cuff. This higher measurement is called *systolic* and reflects the maximum pressure produced when the heart is contracting. As the cuff continues to deflate, at some point the blood flow through the artery is no longer restricted at all. This pressure is called the *diastolic* pressure and reflects the lowest pressure in the system that occurs when the heart is relaxing. These two pressures are recorded as systolic/diastolic. For example, if your systolic pressure is 122 and your diastolic pressure is 78, your blood pressure would be recorded as 122/78, which is read as "122 over 78." All pressures are expressed in terms of millimeters of mercury (mm Hg) because the original blood pressure devices measured pressure using a column of mercury.

Results   There is no "magic number" for normal blood pressure, but there are some rough guidelines. A systolic pressure below 140 and a diastolic below 90 are considered "normal" even though lower pressures are actually healthier. If you get repeated readings higher than these, you should consult your physician. Also, test the accuracy of your blood pressure device by occasionally bringing it with you to your physician's office. Measure your pressure on your machine and then on the physician's. The readings should match fairly closely. Have a health professional observe and check your technique. Remember, a single measurement of elevated blood pressure does not constitute hypertension. Repeat the procedure if elevated readings are obtained, and check with your physician. Do not adjust your blood pressure medications based on home blood pressure readings without first discussing this more with your physician.

Home Pregnancy Tests

The new home pregnancy test kits are similar to the ones used in physicians' offices and laboratories. They are designed to test for the presence of a hormone in the urine. As explained in Chapter 8, this hormone, called *human chorionic gonadotropin (HCG)*, is produced by the developing placenta and excreted in the urine in increasing amounts during the first weeks of pregnancy. If the hormone is detected in the urine test, it is a sign of pregnancy.

Why Performed When a menstrual period is late, a home pregnancy test can sometimes provide confirmation without having to visit a physician or laboratory. Early confirmation of pregnancy can be very useful. It may allow you to start proper prenatal care right away, during the first month of pregnancy when the risk to the fetus is greatest. Such care includes changes in nutrition and avoidance of cigarettes, drugs, alcohol, and x-ray exposure. On the other hand, if the decision is made to terminate the pregnancy, early detection means a simpler and safer abortion.

Equipment Home pregnancy tests are now available without a physician's prescription in most drugstores and supermarkets. They cost about $10.

Procedure Manufacturers claim that the tests are sensitive enough to detect the pregnancy hormone as early as one day after a missed menstrual period. However, by waiting at least until your period is a week late you improve the accuracy of the test and save money on unnecessary testing. The instructions for the various kits need to be followed exactly: mix the various chemicals together and wait the prescribed amount of time.

Results Results are available in anywhere from a few minutes to an hour or two. Positive and negative results are indicated in different ways depending on the test kit used; a solution may change color, a ring-shaped deposit may form in the bottom of a tube, a dipstick may turn blue, and so on. These tests are not foolproof. They're better at telling you that you are pregnant than in making sure that you are not. A positive test on these tests is 99 to 100 percent accurate, but if the test is negative, there's still a 10 to 20 percent chance that you really are pregnant. So, if your period still hasn't come a week after a negative test, repeat the test. If the problem continues or if you are having lower abdominal pain, see your physician.

Source: Adapted from David S. Sobel and Tom Ferguson. 1985. *The People's Book of Medical Tests* (New York: Summit).

The following self-care guide will help you manage a dozen of the most common symptoms:

- Fever
- Sore throat
- Cough
- Nasal congestion
- Ear problems

- Nausea, vomiting, or diarrhea
- Headache
- Low back pain
- Strains and sprains
- Cuts and scrapes

Each symptom is described here in terms of what's going on in your body. Particular emphasis is given to the fact that most symptoms are part of the body's natural healing response and reflect your body's wisdom in attempting to correct disease. Self-care advice is also given, along with some guidelines as to when to seek professional advice. In most cases, the symptoms are self-limiting; that is, they will resolve on their own with time and simple self-care strategies.

No medical advice is perfect. You will always have to make the decision as to whether to self-treat or get professional help. This guide is intended to provide you with more information so that you can make better, more informed decisions. If the advice here differs from that of your physician, discuss the differences. In most instances, your physician will be best able to customize the advice to your individual medical situation.

The guidelines given here apply to *generally healthy adults*. If you are pregnant, nursing, or have a chronic disease, particularly one that requires medication, check with your physician for special self-care advice appropriate for you. For example, if you have a condition such as inflammatory bowel disease (colitis), your physician should give you specific advice on how to manage diarrhea and when to call for help. Also, if you have an allergy or suspected allergy to any recommended medication, please check with your physician before using it. For guidelines appropriate for children, see *Taking Care of Your Child: A Parent's Guide to Medical Care*, 1990, by Robert H. Pantell, M.D., James F. Fries, M.D., and Donald M. Vickery, M.D. (Reading, Mass.: Addison-Wesley).

If you have several symptoms, read about your main symptom first and then proceed to the lesser symptoms.

Above all, use your common sense. If you are particularly concerned about a symptom or confused about how to manage it, call your physician to get more information.

Fever

A fever is an abnormally high body temperature, usually over 100°F (37.7°C). It is most commonly a sign that your body is fighting an infection. Fever may also be due to inflammation, an injury, or a drug reaction. Chemicals released into your bloodstream during an infection reset the thermostat in the hypothalamus of your brain. The message goes out to your body, "Quick, turn up the heat!" The blood vessels in your skin constrict, you curl up, and throw on extra blankets to reduce heat loss. Meanwhile, your muscles begin to shiver to generate enormous additional body heat. The result is a fever.

Later when your brain senses that the temperature is too high, the signal goes out to increase sweating. As the sweat evaporates, it carries heat away from the body surface.

A fever may not be all bad; it may even help us fight infections by making the body less hospitable to bacteria and viruses. A high body temperature appears to bolster the immune system and may inhibit the growth of infectious microorganisms.

Most generally healthy people can tolerate a fever as high as 103–104°F (39.5–40°C) without problems. Therefore, if you are generally in good health there is little need to reduce a fever unless you are very uncomfortable. The elderly and those with chronic health problems such as heart disease may not tolerate the increased metabolic demand of a high fever, and fever reduction may be advised.

Most problems with fevers are due to the excessive loss of fluids from evaporation and sweating, which may cause dehydration.

Self-assessment

1. If you are sick, take your temperature several times throughout the day.

2. Look for signs of dehydration (excessive thirst; very dry mouth; infrequent urination with dark, concentrated urine; and light-headedness).

Self-care

1. Drink plenty of fluids to prevent dehydration; at least 8 ounces of water, juice, or broth every two hours.
2. Sponge baths using lukewarm water will increase evaporation and help reduce body temperature naturally.
3. Don't bundle up. This decreases the body's ability to lose excess heat.
4. Take aspirin or aspirin substitute (acetaminophen). For adults, two standard-size tablets every 4 to 6 hours can be used to reduce the fever and the associated headache and achiness. Do not use aspirin if you have a history of allergy to aspirin, ulcers, or bleeding problems. In addition, most pediatricians recommend using an aspirin substitute, not aspirin, for fever in children and adolescents. This is because of the finding that some children with chicken pox or influenza when treated with aspirin have developed a life-threatening complication, Reye's syndrome.

When to Call the Physician

1. Fever over 103°F (39.5°C) or 102°F (38.8°C) if over 60 years old
2. Fever lasting more than five days
3. Recurrent unexplained fevers
4. Fever accompanied by rash, stiff neck, severe headache, cough with brown/green sputum, severe pain in flank or abdomen, painful urination, convulsions, or mental confusion
5. Fever with signs of dehydration
6. Fever after starting a new medication

Sore Throat

A sore throat is caused by inflammation of the throat lining due to an infection, allergy, or irritation (especially from cigarette smoke). With an infection, you may also notice some hoarseness from swelling of the vocal cords and "swollen glands," which are enlarged lymph nodes that produce white blood cells to help you fight the infection. The lymph nodes, part of your body's defense system, may remain swollen for weeks after the infection subsides.

Most throat infections are caused by viruses. Your body knows how to fight virus infections, and antibiotics are not necessary or helpful with virus infections. However, about 20–30 percent of throat infections are due to streptoccocal bacteria. This type of bacteria can cause complications such as rheumatic fever and rheumatic heart

disease and therefore should be treated with antibiotics. Strep throat is usually characterized by very sore throat, high fever, swollen lymph nodes, a whitish discharge at the back of the throat, and the absence of other cold symptoms such as a cough and runny nose (which suggest a virus infection). Allergy-related sore throats are usually accompanied by running nose and watery, itchy eyes.

Self-assessment

1. Take your temperature.
2. Look in a mirror at the back of your throat. Is there a whitish, puslike discharge on the tonsils or back of the throat?
3. Feel the front and back of your neck. Do you feel enlarged, tender lymph nodes?

Self-care

1. If you smoke, stop smoking to avoid further irritation of your throat.
2. Drink plenty of liquids to soothe your inflamed throat.
3. Gargle warm salt water (¼ tsp. salt in 4 oz. water) every one to two hours to help reduce swelling and discomfort.
4. Suck on throat lozenges, cough drops, or hard candies to keep your throat moist.
5. Use throat lozenges, sprays, or gargles that contain an anesthetic, to temporarily numb your throat and make swallowing less painful.
6. Try aspirin or aspirin substitute to ease throat pain.
7. For an allergy-related sore throat, try an antihistamine such as chlorpheniramine.

When to Call the Physician

1. Great difficulty swallowing saliva or breathing
2. Sore throat with fever over 101°F (38.3°C), especially if you do not have other cold symptoms such as nasal congestion or cough
3. Sore throat with a skin rash
4. Sore throat with whitish pus on the tonsils
5. Sore throat and recent contact with a person who has had a positive throat culture for strep
6. Enlargement of lymph nodes lasting longer than three weeks
7. Hoarseness persisting longer than three weeks

Cough

A cough is a protective mechanism of the body to help keep the airways clear. There are two types of cough: a dry cough (without mucus) and a productive cough (with mucus). Common causes of cough include infection (viral or bacterial), allergies, and irritation from smoking and pollutants. If you have a cold, the cough may be the last symptom to improve, because the airways may remain irritated for several weeks after the infection has resolved.

Your airways are lined with hairlike projections called *cilia*, which move back and forth to help clear the airways of mucus, germs, and dust. Infections and cigarette smoking paralyze and damage this vital defense mechanism.

Self-assessment

1. Take your temperature.
2. Observe your mucus. A thick green, brown, or bloody mucus suggests a bacterial infection.

Self-care

1. If you are a smoker, stop smoking. Smoking irritates the airways and undermines your body's defense mechanisms, leading to more serious infections and longer-lasting symptoms. Most people do not feel like smoking when they have a cold with a cough. If you want to quit, a cold may provide an excellent opportunity to do so.
2. Drink plenty of liquids (at least six 8-oz. glasses a day) to help thin mucus and loosen chest congestion.
3. Breathe steam through a vaporizer or in a hot shower to help loosen chest congestion.
4. Suck on cough drops, throat lozenges, or hard candy to keep your throat moist and help relieve a dry, tickling cough.
5. If you have a dry, nonproductive cough or the cough keeps you from sleeping, you can use a cough syrup or lozenge that contains the over-the-counter cough suppressant dextromethorphan. Since a cough that produces mucus is protective, it is generally not advised to suppress a productive cough.

When to Call the Physician

1. Cough with thick green, brown, or bloody sputum
2. Cough with high fever—above 102°F (38.8°C)—and shaking chills
3. Severe chest pains, wheezing, or shortness of breath
4. Cough that lasts longer than two weeks

Nasal Congestion

Nasal congestion is most commonly caused by infection or allergies. With infection, the nasal passages become congested due to increased blood flow and mucus production. This congestion is actually part of the body's defense to fight the infection. The increased blood flow raises the temperature of the nasal passages, making them less hospitable to germs. The nasal secretions are rich in white blood cells and antibodies to help fight and neutralize the invading organisms and flush them away. Nasal congestion associated with sore throat, cough, and fever usually indicates a virus infection.

Nasal congestion caused by allergies is often accompanied by a thin, watery discharge, sneezing, itchy eyes, and sometimes a seasonal pattern. In an allergic reaction, the offending allergen (pollen, dusts, molds, dander, and so forth) trigger the release of histamine and other chemicals from the cells lining the nose, throat, and eyes. These chemicals cause swelling, discharge, and itching. Antihistamine drugs block the release of these irritating chemicals.

Self-assessment

1. Take your temperature.
2. Observe the color and consistency of your nasal secretions. A thick green, brown, or bloody discharge suggests a bacterial sinus infection.
3. Tap with your fingers over the sinus cavities above and below the eyes. If this causes increased pain, a bacterial sinus infection may be present.

Self-care

1. If you smoke, stop smoking to prevent continuing irritation of the nasal passages.
2. Use moist heat from a hot shower or vaporizer to help liquify congested mucus.
3. Use a decongestant nasal spray or drops to temporarily relieve congestion. However, if these decongestants are used for more than three days they can cause "rebound congestion" that actually creates more nasal congestion. As an alternative, use saltwater nose drops (¼ tsp. salt in ½ cup of boiled water).
4. Try an oral decongestant such as pseudoephedrine (60 mg every six hours) to help shrink swollen mucous membranes and open nasal passages. In some people, these medications can cause nervousness, sleeplessness, or heart palpitations. If you have uncontrolled high blood pressure, heart disease, or diabetes, check with your doctor before using decongestants.
5. To help relieve nasal discharge and sneezing, try an antihistamine such as chlorpheniramine (4 to 8 mg every eight hours). These medications can cause drowsiness, dry mouth, and excessive drying of the nose and air passages. If you have asthma, glaucoma, or difficulty urinating due to an enlarged prostate gland, check with your doctor before using these medications.

When to Call the Physician

1. Nasal congestion with severe pain and tenderness in the forehead, cheeks, or upper teeth and a high fever (above 102°F or 38.8°C)

2. Thick green, brown, or bloody nasal discharge
3. Nasal congestion and discharge unresponsive to self-care treatment and lasting longer than three weeks

Ear Problems

Ear symptoms include earache, discharge, itching, stuffiness, and hearing loss. They may be caused by problems in the external ear canal, ear drum, middle ear, or Eustachian tube (the passageway that connects the middle ear space to the back of the throat). The ear canal can become blocked by excess wax, producing a sense of the ear being plugged and hearing loss. An infection of the external ear canal due to excessive moisture and trauma is often referred to as "swimmer's ear." It can cause pain, fullness, discharge, and itching. Congestion and blockage of the Eustachian tube by a cold or allergy can result in pain, fullness, and hearing loss. A middle ear infection often produces severe pain, hearing loss, and fever.

Self-assessment

1. Take your temperature. A fever may be a sign of infection.
2. Have someone look into the ear canal with a flashlight or otoscope. Look for wax blockage or a red, swollen canal indicating an external ear infection.
3. Wiggle the outer part of the ear. If this increases the pain, an infection or inflammation of the external canal is the likely cause.

Self-care

1. If blockage of the ear canal with wax is the problem, first try a hot shower to liquify the wax and use a wash cloth to wipe out the ear canal. You can also use a few drops of an over-the-counter wax softener and then flush the canal gently with warm water and a bulb syringe. Do not use sharp objects or cotton swabs; they can scratch the canal or push the wax in deeper.
2. To treat mild infections of the external ear canal, you must thoroughly dry the ear canal. A few drops of a drying agent (Burow's solution) on a piece of cotton gently inserted into the canal can act as a wick to dry the canal.
3. To relieve congestion and blockage of the Eustachian tube, try a decongestant like pseudoephedrine, a nasal spray (but for no longer than three days), or an antihistamine. Hot showers or a vaporizer may help loosen secretions, and yawning or swallowing may help open your Eustachian tube. For a mild plugging sensation without fever or pain, pinch your nostrils and blow gently to force air up the Eustachian tube and "pop" your ears.

When to Call the Physician

1. Severe earache with fever
2. Puslike or bloody discharge from the ear
3. Sudden hearing loss, especially if accompanied by ear pain or recent trauma to the ear
4. Ringing in the ears or dizziness
5. Any ear symptom lasting longer than two weeks

Nausea, Vomiting, or Diarrhea

Nausea, vomiting, and diarrhea usually are defensive reactions of your body to rapidly clear your digestive tract of irritants. These symptoms are most commonly caused by the "stomach flu," a virus infection, but may also be caused by food poisoning, medications, or other types of infection. Vomiting dramatically ejects irritants from your stomach, and nausea discourages eating to allow the stomach to rest. In diarrhea, overstimulated intestines flush out the offending irritants.

The major complications of vomiting and diarrhea are dehydration from fluid losses and decreased intake and the risk of bleeding from irritation of the digestive tract.

Self-assessment

1. Take your temperature. A fever is often a clue that an infection is causing the symptoms.
2. Observe the color and frequency of vomiting and diarrhea. This helps estimate severity of fluid losses and checks for bleeding (red, black, or "coffee grounds" material in stool or vomit).
3. Look for signs of dehydration: very dry mouth, marked thirst, infrequent urination with dark, concentrated urine, and light-headedness.
4. Look for signs of hepatitis, an infection of the liver that produces a yellow color in the skin and white parts of the eyes.

Self-care

1. To replace fluids, take frequent, small sips of clear liquids such as water, non-citrus juice, broths, flat ginger ale, or ice chips.
2. When the vomiting and diarrhea have subsided, you can try nonirritating, constipating foods like the BRAT diet: bananas, rice, applesauce, and toast.
3. For several days avoid alcohol, milk products, fatty foods, aspirin, and other medications that might irritate the stomach. Do not stop taking regularly prescribed medications without discussing this change with your doctor.
4. Medications are not usually advised for vomiting. For diarrhea, over-the-counter medications containing kaolin, pectin, or attapulgite may help thicken the stool.

Medications containing paregoric may help decrease painful intestinal spasms.

When to Call the Physician

1. Inability to retain any fluids for twelve hours, or signs of dehydration
2. Severe abdominal pains not relieved by the vomiting or diarrhea
3. Blood in the vomit (red or "coffee grounds-like" material) or in the stool (red or black, tarlike material)
4. Vomiting or diarrhea with a high fever (above 102°F or 38.8°C)
5. Yellow color in skin or whites of eyes
6. Vomiting with severe headache and history of recent head injury
7. Vomiting or diarrhea that lasts three days without improvement
8. Recurrent vomiting and/or diarrhea
9. If you are pregnant or have diabetes

Headache

Headache is one of the most common symptoms. There are three major types of headache: muscle tension (the most common type), vascular (related to the blood vessels), and sinus (involves blocked sinus cavities). Muscle tension headaches are often due to emotional stress or physical stress such as poor posture. The muscles in the neck, scalp, and jaws tighten, producing a dull, aching sensation or band of tension around the head. Vascular headaches, which include the common migraine, are due to a constriction and then dilation of blood vessels in the head. Vascular headaches are usually severe, one-sided, throbbing headaches often associated with nausea, vomiting, and visual disturbances (flashing lights or stars). Sinus headaches are caused by blockage of the sinus cavities with resulting pressure and pain in the cheeks, forehead, and upper teeth. These headaches are often associated with nasal congestion. Sometimes a combination of these types of headaches will occur. Headache caused by elevated blood pressure is very uncommon and occurs only with very high pressures.

Self-assessment

1. Take your temperature. The presence of fever may indicate a sinus infection. Fever, severe headache, and very stiff neck suggest meningitis, a rare, but serious infection around the brain and spinal cord.
2. Tap with your fingers over the sinus cavities in your cheeks and forehead. If this causes increased pain, it may indicate a sinus infection.
3. For recurrent headaches, keep a headache diary. Re-

cord how often and when your headaches occur, associated symptoms, preceding activities, food and beverage intake.

Self-care

1. Try ice packs or heat on your neck and head.
2. Gently massage the muscles of your neck and scalp.
3. Try deep relaxation or breathing exercises.
4. Take aspirin or aspirin substitute for pain relief.
5. If pain is associated with nasal congestion, try a decongestant medication like pseudoephedrine.
6. Try to avoid emotional stressors and physical stressors (like poor posture and eye strain).
7. Try avoiding certain foods that may trigger headaches. These often include aged cheeses, chocolate, nuts, red wine, alcohol, avocados, figs, raisins, and any fermented or pickled foods.

When to Call the Physician

1. Unusually severe headache
2. Headache accompanied by fever and very stiff neck
3. Headache with sinus pain and tenderness and a fever
4. Severe headache following recent head injury
5. Headache associated with slurred speech, visual disturbance, numbness or weakness in face, arms, or legs
6. Headache persisting longer than three days
7. Recurrent unexplained headaches
8. Increasing severity or frequency of headaches

Low Back Pain

Pain in the lower back is a very common condition that results in large part from our upright posture, which puts tremendous strain on our lower backs. The pain is most often due to a strain of the muscles and ligaments along the spine, which may or may not be triggered by bending, lifting, or other activity. Low back pain can also be due to bone growths (spurs) irritating the nerves as they leave the spine or to pressure from ruptured or protruding discs, the "shock absorbers" between the vertebrae. In addition to back pain, nerve irritation can produce lower leg pain, numbness, tingling, weakness, and loss of bowel or bladder control. Sometimes back pain is actually caused by an infection or stone in the kidney. Fortunately, however, simpler muscular strain is the most common cause of low back pain and can usually be effectively self-treated.

Self-assessment

1. Take your temperature. Back pain with high fever may indicate a kidney or other infection.
2. Check for blood in your urine or frequent, painful urination, which may also indicate a kidney problem.

3. Observe for tingling or pain traveling down one or both legs below the knee with bending, coughing, or sneezing. These symptoms suggest a disc problem.

Self-care

1. Lie on your back or in any comfortable position on the floor or on a firm mattress with knees slightly bent and supported by a pillow. Rest for twenty-four hours or longer if the pain persists.
2. Use ice packs on the painful area for the first twenty-four hours then apply ice or heat.
3. Take aspirin or aspirin substitute for pain relief as needed.
4. After the acute pain has subsided, begin gentle back and stomach exercises. Practice good posture and lifting techniques to protect your back. To learn more about proper back exercises and use of your back, consult a physical therapist or your doctor.

When to Call the Physician

1. Back pain following a severe injury such as an accident or fall
2. Back pain radiating down the leg below the knee on one or both sides
3. Persistent numbness, tingling, or weakness in the legs or feet
4. Loss of bladder or bowel control
5. Back pain associated with high fever (above 101°F or 38.3°C), frequent or painful urination, blood in the urine, or severe abdominal pain
6. Back pain that does not improve after one week of self-care

Strains and Sprains

Missteps, slips, falls, accidents, and athletic misadventures result in a variety of strains, sprains, and fractures. A strain occurs when you overstretch a muscle or a tendon (the connective tissue that attaches muscle to bone). Sprains are caused by overstretching or tearing of ligaments (the tough fibrous bands that connect bone to bone). Depending on the severity and location, a sprain may actually be more serious than a fracture because bones generally heal very strongly while ligaments may remain stretched and lax after healing. After a sprain, it may take six weeks for the ligament to heal.

After most injuries, you can expect pain and swelling. This is the body's way of immobilizing and protecting the injured part so that healing can take place. The goal of self-assessment is to determine whether you have a minor injury that you can safely self-treat or a more serious injury to an artery, nerve, or bone that should be treated by your doctor.

Self-assessment

1. Observe for coldness, blue color, or numbness to the limb beyond the injury. These may be signs of damage to artery or nerve.
2. Look for signs of a possible fracture, which would include misshapen limb, reduced length of the limb on the injured side compared to the uninjured side, inability to move or bear weight, grating sound with movement of injured area, extreme tenderness at one point along the injured bone as you press with your fingers, or a sensation of snapping at time of the injury.
3. Gently move the injured area through its full range of motion. Immobility or instability suggest a more serious injury.

Self-care

1. Immediately immobilize, protect, and rest the injured area until you can bear weight on it or move it without pain. Remember, if it hurts, don't do it.
2. To decrease pain and swelling, immediately apply ice (cold pack or ice wrapped in a cloth) for 15 minutes every hour for the first twenty-four to forty-eight hours. Then apply ice or heat as needed for comfort.
3. Immediately elevate the injured limb above the level of your heart for the first twenty-four hours to decrease swelling.
4. Immobilize and support the injured area with an elastic wrap or splint. Be careful not to wrap so tightly as to cause blueness, coldness, or numbness.
5. Take aspirin or aspirin substitute for pain as needed.

When to Call the Physician

1. An injury that occurred with great force such as a high fall or motor vehicle accident
2. Hearing or feeling a snap at the time of the injury
3. A limb that is blue, cold, or numb
4. A limb that is bent, twisted, or crooked
5. Tenderness at specific points along a bone
6. Inability to move injured area
7. Wobbly, unstable joint
8. Marked swelling of the injured area
9. Inability to bear weight after twenty-four hours
10. Pain that increases or lasts longer than four days

Cuts and Scrapes

Cuts and scrapes are common disruptions of your body's skin. Fortunately, the vast majority of these wounds are minor and don't require stitches, antibiotics, or a physician's care. An abrasion involves a scraping away of the superficial layers of skin. Abrasions, though less serious, are often more painful than cuts because they disrupt more skin nerves. Cuts come in two varieties: lacerations (narrow slices of the skin) and puncture wounds (stabs into deeper tissues).

Normal healing of a cut or abrasion is a wondrous process. After the bleeding stops, small amounts of serum, a clear yellowish fluid, may leak from your wound. This fluid is rich in antibodies to help prevent an infection. Redness and swelling may normally occur as more blood is shunted to the area, bringing white blood cells and nutrients to speed healing. There may also be some swelling of nearby lymph nodes, which are another part of your body's defense against infection. Finally, a scab forms. This is "nature's Band-Aid," which protects the area while it heals.

The main concerns about cuts are the possibilities of damage to deeper tissues and the risk of infection. Damage to underlying blood vessels may lead to severe bleeding as well as blueness and coldness to areas beyond the wound. Injured nerves may produce numbness and loss of ability to move parts of the body beyond the injured area. Damaged muscles, tendons, and ligaments can also result in inability to move areas beyond the cut.

Wound infection usually does not take place until twenty-four to forty-eight hours after an injury. Signs of infection include increasing redness, swelling, pain, pus, and fever. One of the most serious, though fortunately uncommon, complications of cuts is tetanus ("lockjaw"). This bacterial infection thrives in areas not exposed to oxygen, so it is more likely to develop in deep puncture wounds or dirty wounds. Tetanus is very unlikely to develop in minor cuts or wounds caused by clean objects like knives. You need a tetanus shot following a cut under the following conditions:

- If you have never had the basic series of three tetanus immunization injections
- If you have a dirty or contaminated wound and it has been longer than five years since your last injection
- If you have a clean, minor wound and it has been longer than ten years since your last injection

Self-assessment

1. Look for warning signs of complications: persistent bleeding, numbness, inability to move injured area, or the later development of pus, increasing redness, and fever.

2. Measure the size of the cut. If your cut is shallow, less than an inch long, not in a high-stress area (such as a joint, which bends), and you can easily hold the edges of the wound closed, it probably won't need stitches.

Self-care

1. Apply direct pressure over the wound until bleeding is stopped. The only exception is puncture wounds, which should be encouraged to bleed freely (unless spurting a large amount of blood) for a few minutes to flush out bacteria and debris.

2. Try to remove any dirt, glass, or foreign material from the wound with tweezers or by scrubbing.

3. Wash the wound vigorously with soap and water, followed by an application of hydrogen peroxide solution as an antiseptic.

4. If it is an abrasion, cover the area with a Band-Aid until a scab forms. For minor lacerations, close the cut with a butterfly bandage or a sterile adhesive tape (Steristrips), drawing the edges close together but not overlapping. If there is an extra flap of clean skin, leave it in place for extra protection. Do not attempt to close puncture wounds. Instead soak puncture wounds in warm water for 15 minutes several times a day for several days. Soaking helps keep the wound open and thus prevents infection.

When to Call the Physician

1. Bleeding that can't be controlled with direct pressure
2. Numbness, weakness, or inability to move injured area
3. Any large, deep wound
4. A laceration in an area that bends and the edges of the cut cannot be easily held together
5. Cuts on the hands or face unless clean and shallow
6. Contaminated wound in which you cannot remove the foreign material
7. Any human or animal bite
8. If you need a tetanus immunization (see indications noted earlier)
9. Development of increasing redness, swelling, pain, pus, or fever twenty-four hours or more after the injury
10. If the wound is not healing well in three weeks

Books

Bennett, William I., Stephen E. Goldfinger, and G. Timothy Johnson, eds. 1987. *Your Good Health: How to Stay Well, and What to Do When You're Not.* Cambridge: Harvard University Press.

Brody, Jane E. 1982. *Jane Brody's Guide to Personal Health.* New York: Times Books. *A compilation of highly readable newspaper columns on common medical problems and concerns.*

Graedon, Joe, and Teresa Graedon. 1980, 1984, 1986. *The People's Pharmacy.* Vols. 1–3. New York: Avon. *Three lively and highly informative books discussing the pharmacology, profits and politics that affect the drugs we use.*

Griffith, H. Winter. 1985. *Complete Guide to Symptoms, Illness, and Surgery.* Tucson, Ariz.: Body Press. *A mammoth book discussing over 700 symptoms, 500 illnesses, and 160 surgeries.*

Griffith, H. Winter. 1986. *Complete Guide to Prescription and Nonprescription Drugs.* Tucson, Ariz.: Body Press. *A comprehensive guide to side effects, warnings, and precautions for safe use for over 4,000 brand name and generic drugs.*

Inlander, Charles B., and Ed Weiner. 1985. *Take This Book to the Hospital with You.* Emmaus, Pa.: Rodale Press. *The lively and informative guide from The People's Medical Society on how to survive a hospital stay.*

Kemper, Donald W., Kathleen E. McIntosh, and Toni M. Roberts. 1987. *Healthwise Handbook: A Self-care Manual for You.* Boise, Idaho: Healthwise. (P.O. Box 1989, Boise, ID 83701). *Practical, straightforward guidelines on the best home care for*

a variety of common medical problems in adults and children.

Kunz, Jeffrey R.M., ed. 1982. *The American Medical Association Family Medicine Guide.* New York: Random House. *A comprehensive volume discussing more than 650 diseases. Contains ninety-nine question-and-answer charts to help evaluate common medical symptoms and decide when to see the doctor.*

Pantell, Robert H., James F. Fries, and Donald M. Vickery. 1990. *Taking Care of Your Child: A Parent's Guide to Medical Care.* Reading, Mass.: Addison-Wesley. *An indispensable guide for common health problems of children, containing over ninety-five easy-to-use decision charts to help parents decide when to call the doctor and when to treat at home.*

Sehnert, Keith W. and Howard Eisenberg. 1985. *How to Be Your Own Doctor (Sometimes).* New York: Putnam. *The first modern self-care guide offering advice for self-management of the thirty-eight most common illnesses and accidents.*

Sobel, David S., and Tom Ferguson. 1985. *The People's Book of Medical Tests.* New York: Summit Books. *A consumer's guide that answers questions about 200 medical and home diagnostic tests.*

Tapley, Donald F., ed. 1985. *The Columbia University College of Physicians and Surgeons Complete Home Medical Guide.* New York: Crown.

Vickery, Donald M. 1986. *Taking Part: The Survivor's Guide to the Hospital.* Reston, Va.: Center for Corporate Health Promotion. *Using decision-making charts, this book offers a second opinion to help the patient decide whether hospitalization and surgery are necessary for the treatment of twenty common medical problems.*

Vickery, Donald M., and James F. Fries. 1990. *Take Care of Yourself: The Consumer's Guide to Medical Care,* 4th ed. Reading, Mass.: Addison-Wesley. *Over 3 million copies are in print of this excellent self-care guide, which includes over 100 easy-to-follow decision charts outlining when to see the doctor and how to apply safe and effective home treatment*

Wurman, Richard Saul. 1985. *Medical Access.* Los Angeles: Access Press. *A travel guide to medical care containing descriptions of medical tests, surgical procedures, and the most commonly asked consumer health questions.*

Zimmerman, David R. 1983. *The Essential Guide to Nonprescription Drugs.* New York: Harper & Row. *The most comprehensive and authoritative review of the safety and effectiveness of over-the-counter products.*

Newsletters and Magazines

Consumer Reports Health Letter P.O. Box 52148, Boulder, CO 80321

Harvard Medical School Health Letter (P.O. Box 10944, Des Moines, IA 50340)

Healthline (The C. V. Mosby Company, 11830 Westline Industrial Drive, St. Louis, MO 63146-3318)

In Health (formerly *Hippocrates*) (Hippocrates Partners, 475 Gate Five Rd., Suite 225, Sausalito, CA 94965)

Mayo Clinic Health Letter (Mayo Foundation for Medical Education and Research, 200 First Street SW, Rochester, MN 55905)

University of California, Berkeley Wellness Letter (P.O. Box 420148, Palm Coast, FL 32142)

Health Information Centers

Boston Women's Health Collective (445
Mt. Auburn Street, Watertown, MA
02172, 617-924-0271)

Consumer Health Information Research
Institute (3521 Broadway, Kansas
City, MO 64111, 816-753-8850)

Consumer Information Center (Pueblo,
CO 81009 or 18th and E Streets,
N.W., Washington, DC 20405,
202-566-1794)

National Health Information
Clearinghouse (P.O. Box 1133,
Washington, D.C. 20012, 800-336-
4797 or 703-522-2590 in Virginia)

Self-help and Mutual Aid Groups

In the United States alone, over 500,000 self-help groups
and chapters of self-help organizations provide information and peer support for nearly every conceivable
medical condition or problem. There are groups for diabetes, cancer, stroke, heart surgery, Alzheimer's disease,
child abuse, drug abuse, infertility, asthma, cystic fibrosis, nursing mothers, blindness, epilepsy, DES (diethylstilbestrol) exposure, eating disorders, colitis, mental retardation, phobias, sleep disorders, sexual problems,
women's health, and hundreds of others. You can look
in the white pages of the telephone book for your local
chapter or contact one of the following self-help clear-
inghouses for the names of self-help groups in your community.

- National Self-help Clearinghouse (City University of
New York, 33 West 42nd St., New York, NY 10036,
212-840-1258)
- The Self-help Center (Center for Urban Affairs, Northwestern University, 2040 Sheridan Road, Evanston, IL
60201, 312-328-0470)
- Self-help Resource Center (UCLA Psychology Department, 405 Hilgard Avenue, Los Angeles, CA 90024,
213-825-1799, or in California 800-222-5465).

Telephone Hotlines

Acquired Immune Deficiency Syndrome (AIDS): AIDS
Hot Line, 800-342-AIDS (in Hawaii and Alaska, 404-
329-3534 collect), 800-344-SIDA (Spanish), 800-
AIDS-TTY (hearing impaired); Information on clinical
trials of AIDS drugs, sponsored by National Institutes
of Health, 800-874-2572 (9:00 A.M.–7:00 P.M. ET);
Project Inform—information on experimental drugs
for AIDS, ARC, and HIV infection, 800-334-7422
(within California), 800-822-7422 (outside California).

Agoraphobia (fear of open spaces): The Agoraphobia
and Anxiety Program of Temple University, Philadelphia, 215-667-6490.

Alcohol: Al-Anon Family Group Headquarters, 800-
344-2666; National Clearinghouse for Alcohol Information, 301-468-2600; National Council on Alcoholism, 800-NCA-CALL.

Alzheimer's disease: Alzheimer's Disease and Related
Disorders Association, 800-621-0379 (in Illinois, 800-
572-6037), 24 hours.

Anorexia and bulimia: National Association of Anorexia Nervosa and Associated Disorders, 312-831-
3438; Bulimia Anorexia Self-Help (B.A.S.H.), 800-
BASH-STL.

Asthma: National Asthma Center, 800-222-5864.

Battered Victims Services, 800-942-6906, 800-333-
SAFE (Hotlines, referral services).

Blindness: American Council of the Blind, National
Legislative Hotline, 800-424-8666; American Foundation for the Blind, 800-232-5463; The National
Library Service for the Blind (part of the Library
of Congress), 800-424-8567 (in Washington, D.C.
202-287-5100).

Cancer: Cancer Information Service, part of the National Cancer Institute, 800-4-CANCER (in Washington, D.C., 202-636-5700; within Hawaii, 800-542-
1234; within Alaska, 800-638-6070).

Cocaine: Cocaine Abuse Hot Line, 800-COCAINE, 7
days, 24 hours.

Diabetes: Juvenile Diabetes Foundation, 800-223-
1138 (in New York State, 212-889-7575); American
Diabetes Association, 800-232-3472.

Drugs, drug interactions, drug side effects: FDA Center for Drug Evaluation and Research, Legislative,
Professional and Consumer Affairs Branch, 301-295-
8012 (8:00 A.M.–5:00 P.M. ET).

Epilepsy: Epilepsy Foundation of America, 800-EFA-
1000 (outside Maryland).

Food and cosmetics safety: The Consumer Inquiries
Section of the Office of Consumer Affairs of the FDA,
301-443-3170 (8:00 A.M.–5:00 P.M. ET).

Headache: National Headache Foundation, 800-843-
2256 (800-523-8858 within Illinois).

Hearing problems: Dial-a-Hearing Screening Test, part of Occupational Hearing Services, 800-222-EARS (in Pennsylvania, 215-565-6114).

Infertility: Resolve National Phone Counseling Line, 617-643-2424 (M–Th, 9:00 A.M.–12:00 P.M., 1:00–4:00 P.M. EST).

Kidney disease: American Kidney Fund, 800-638-8299 (in Maryland, 800-492-8361; in Washington D.C., 301-986-1444).

Lung disease, respiratory disorders, allergies: Lung Line, sponsored by the National Jewish Center for Immunology and Respiratory Medicine in Denver, Colorado, 800-222-LUNG.

Mental Health: American Mental Health Counselors Association (AMHCA), 800-345-2008.

Premenstrual syndrome: PMS Access, 800-222-4PMS.

Spina bifida: Spina Bifida Association, 800-621-3141 (in Illinois, 312-663-1562).

Sports and sports injuries: Women's Sports Foundation, 800-227-3988.

Sudden Infant Death Syndrome (SIDS): American Sudden Infant Death Syndrome Institute, 800-232-SIDS (in Georgia, 800-847-SIDS).

Surgery: Second Opinion Hot Line, sponsored by the U.S. Government's Department of Health and Human Services, 800-638-6833 (in Maryland, 800-492-6603).

Contents

Making Connections

Even when you take good care of yourself, sooner or later you're bound to have an illness or an injury that requires professional attention. This is why a basic understanding of the health-care system is an essential part of taking charge of your health. To make the decisions that are right for you, you need to know which medical practices are legitimate, how to pay for them, and what to do when you encounter a questionable practice. The scenarios presented on these pages describe situations in which people have to use information, make a decision, or choose a course of action, all related to the health-care system. As you read them, imagine yourself in the situation and consider what you would do. After you finish the chapter, read them again and see if what you've learned has changed how you would think, feel, or act in each situation.

You saw a well-known celebrity on TV last night promoting a new "European formula" hair-replacement product. You're very concerned about your receding hairline and are eager to try any new treatments that promise to slow down hair loss. You're usually skeptical about such products, but since these claims were made on national TV by a well-known person, they must be true, right? Should you call the toll-free number and send in your check?

You decided to try a new physician who was recommended to you, and while you're waiting in the examination room you peruse the diplomas and certificates framed and hanging on the wall. After reading them all you realize that this physician doesn't have an M.D. degree. Instead, he has a D.O.—doctor of osteopathy—degree. Is he a licensed practitioner who will give you reliable, mainstream advice? Can you have confidence in his knowledge and skills? What should you ask him about his training when he comes in?

The Health-Care System

At your new job you're offered a choice between two different health insurance plans. One is described to you as a standard plan that pays 80 percent of most of your medical expenses, including some prescriptions and some office visits. The other one, which would involve a smaller payroll deduction for you, is described as a health maintenance organization based in a downtown clinic. Almost all of your medical expenses would be paid, but you would have to use the staff and facilities available at the clinic. How can you decide which of the two is better for you?

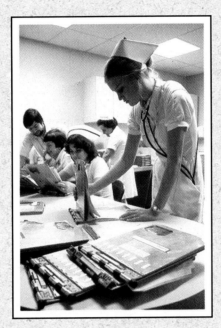

A friend of yours has been diagnosed as having a "systemic yeast infection" by a practitioner she refers to as a clinical ecologist. She says her symptoms were fatigue, fuzzy thinking, intestinal gas, a bloated feeling, and depression. You tell her that you have some of those symptoms on occasion and that you think probably everyone does. She suggests that maybe you have a yeast infection too and urges you to see her practitioner. Should you?

Your grandmother died of cancer in 1978 after several months of taking laetrile, a substance that was touted as a cancer cure at the time. Your grandparents even flew to Mexico to get it when it was illegal in the United States. Although thousands of cancer patients replaced their traditional treatments with laetrile, research finally determined that it was useless against cancer. Now your grandfather has stopped taking his arthritis medication and is wearing a copper bracelet and taking megavitamins instead. He says he's not sure how they work, but he's willing to give them a try. Why isn't he more careful after your grandmother's experience with laetrile? Is there anything you can say to him about his medical choices?

When you seek medical care, how should you go about it? Should you go to a general practitioner? A specialist? A hospital emergency room? An emergicenter? Whom should you see? Of course, the best time to look for a physician is before you are ill.

Most experts believe it is best to have a primary physician who gets to know you and can treat you or coordinate referrals to specialists when needed. Physicians who are board certified in family practice (for adults and children), internal medicine (for adults only), or pediatrics (for children only) are likely to be good choices because they have extensive training in the diagnosis and treatment of general medical problems.

Staff affiliation with a hospital connected with a medical school indicates that a physician is working with up-to-date colleagues and is apt to have up-to-date skills and information. Affiliation with a hospital that trains residents is also favorable. Less certain is affiliation with only privately owned hospitals—especially small ones—unless they are the only ones in the area. Lack of any hospital affiliation may be a sign of substandard care. Information on a physician's credentials may be obtainable from the physician's office, the local medical society, a local hospital, or a directory available at a medical or public library.

When choosing medical care, you should consider such factors as quality of care, cost, convenience, and whether follow-up care is available. Table 22-1 summarizes the advantages and disadvantages of various sources of medical care.

Orthodox Practitioners

Health professionals are regulated by state licensing laws. To become licensed, they must graduate from an accredited professional school, have additional clinical experience, and pass a licensing examination given by a state or national board. This section looks at five types of health professionals who are permitted by law to practice independently in the United States: medical doctors, osteopaths, podiatrists, optometrists, and dentists.

- Medical doctors are **independent practitioners** who hold an M.D. (doctor of medicine) degree from an accredited medical school. Once licensed, they are legally authorized to administer any type of medical or surgical treatment. What they actually do depends on their training, their inclinations, and the available facilities. Because the scope of medicine is so vast, most physicians take additional full-time training after graduation. (A partial list of medical specialties is given in the box "Common Names of Selected Medical Specialties.") Those choosing to become specialists take three or more years of hospital-based specialty training, after when they can become "board certified" by taking a stringent specialty examination. A few specialty boards require periodic recertification to ensure updated skills and knowledge. Some specialists require a referral by a primary physician, while others will also see patients without a referral. To work in a hospital, physicians must apply for staff privileges, which are based on training and experience and are reviewed annually.

- **Osteopathic physicians** are independent practitioners who have received a D.O. (doctor of osteopathy) degree. Osteopathy was founded more than a hundred years ago on an incorrect belief that the main cause of disease was mechanical interference with nerve and blood supply, correctable by spinal manipulation. But as medical science developed, osteopathy gradually incorporated all of its theories and practices. Today, osteopathic practice is virtually identical to medical practice except that osteopaths tend to have greater interest in musculoskeletal problems and manipulative therapy.

- **Podiatrists** are independent practitioners whose care is limited to problems of feet and legs. They are not medical doctors but hold a D.P.M. (doctor of podiatric medicine) degree. The length of their training is similar to that of physicians but emphasizes problems of the feet and legs. Podiatrists can prescribe drugs and do minor surgery in their offices. Those who wish to do major foot surgery must secure hospital privileges.

- **Optometrists** are independent practitioners who are trained to examine the eyes and related structures to detect vision problems, eye diseases, and other problems. They are not physicians but hold an O.D. (doctor of optometry) degree. Most states allow them to use drugs for diagnostic purposes. If they detect eye disease, they are expected to refer the patient to an appropriate physician. However, about half of the states permit them to treat minor ailments.

Independent practitioner A physician or other health professional who is legally permitted to provide health-care services without supervision or direction from another health professional.

Osteopathic physicians Medical practitioners who have graduated from an osteopathic medical school. Osteopathy incorporates the theories and practices of scientific medicine but tends to focus on musculoskeletal problems.

Podiatrists Nonmedical practitioners whose practice is limited to the feet and legs.

Optometrists Nonmedical practitioners who primarily examine the eyes to detect vision problems and prescribe corrective lenses.

Table 22-1 Outpatient health-care facilities

Facility	Advantages	Disadvantages
Medical office	Maximum personal attention. Low cost per visit.	Limited hours.
Multispecialty group practice	Low cost per visit. Consultations may be more readily available.	Same physician may not always be seen (varies with setup of group). May have less choice of consultants.
Student health service	Convenient location. Minimal cost.	Hours and scope of practice may be limited.
Emergicenter	Costs less than hospital emergency room. Open long hours. Convenient appointment times.	Costs more than private office. May not be ideal setup for follow-up care. When care is episodic, doctor does not get to know the patient as an individual.
Hospital emergency room	Open 24 hours a day. Able to handle serious emergencies. Sophisticated equipment available.	Highest cost. Nonemergency cases may not receive much attention. Follow-up care may be minimal. Care is episodic and less personal.
Hospital outpatient clinic	Fees may be reduced for individuals who cannot afford private care.	Patients may have to wait a long time to be seen. Tend to have high staff turnover so different doctors may be seen.
Ambulatory surgical facilities	Surgery costs less than it would in a hospital.	Unsuitable for major surgery.

• **Dentists** form another group of practitioners who can practice without medical supervision. They hold either a D.D.S. (doctor of dental surgery) or D.M.D. (doctor of medical dentistry) degree. Those who wish to become specialists complete two or more years of specialty training after graduation from dental school. Dentists are permitted to perform certain types of surgery and to prescribe a limited number of drugs within the scope of their training.

■ **Exploring Your Emotions**

In general, how do you feel about the orthodox medical practices—confident, reverent, resigned, skeptical, suspicious, apprehensive? How about the unorthodox practices? Why do you think you feel the way you do?

In addition to these independent practitioners, who make up a relatively small percentage of the total number of health-care professionals in the United States, a large body of allied health-care providers deliver care to millions of people. These trained practitioners include registered nurses (R.N.s), licensed vocational nurses (L.V.N.s), registered dietitians (R.D.s), dental hygienists, physical therapists, occupational therapists, laboratory technicians, x-ray technicians, and many others.

Unorthodox Practitioners

The term "orthodox health care" as used in this chapter, refers to the prevention, diagnosis, and treatment of disease based on currently accepted scientific information. Current medical beliefs are based on information gathered by practitioners and researchers throughout the world who share the results of their research and other careful observations. In contrast, the term *unorthodox practitioners* refers to individuals whose philosophy and methods either clash with accepted knowledge about

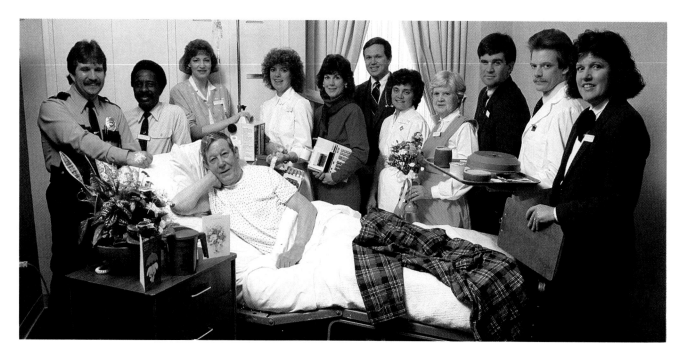

The health care system in the United States includes many different kinds of specialists. This patient is surrounded by the various hospital personnel who provide him with services, both professional and nonprofessional.

health and disease or are both unproven and unlikely. Reliance on unscientific practitioners may delay effective care and often involves financial exploitation.

The Most Common Unorthodox Practices   The ten approaches to health care discussed in this section are based on theories that are unproven or rejected by the scientific community: chiropractic, applied kinesiology, homeopathy, naturopathy, acupuncture, iridology, reflexology, faith healing, chelation therapy, and "clinical ecology." The fact that an approach is unorthodox does not mean that its practitioners never help people or that everything they do should be considered quackery. Many people whose symptoms are bodily responses to tension (such as fatigue or headaches) may lose their symptoms following attention by anyone they believe in. Moreover, many of the practitioners described here might persuade patients to develop healthier living habits. Some also recognize their limitations and refer patients who need it for appropriate medical care.

Many of the practitioners described in this section refer to themselves as "holistic" (or "wholistic"), meaning that they treat the whole patient, giving attention to emotions and lifestyle in addition to physical problems. Good medical doctors have always practiced in this manner. The holistic label is used by a few scientific practitioners who operate wellness clinics. But most "holistic" practitioners use a wide variety of unscientific methods of diagnosis and treatment, including high doses of vitamins.

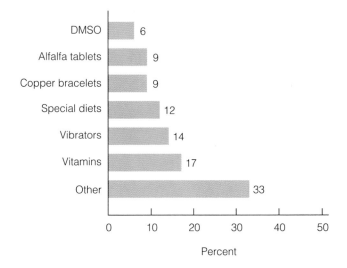

Figure 22-1   Questionable Treatments Used by Arthritis Sufferers. Quacks love arthritis because it can last for years and has no cure. It fluctuates in intensity, so that relief may coincide by chance with a useless treatment. It appears in many forms—and so does arthritis quackery. Americans spend about $500 million each year on worthless treatments such as the ones listed on this chart.

Common Names of Selected Medical Specialties

Allergy and immunology   Subspecialty of internal medicine that deals with allergies and other disorders of the immune system.

Anesthesiology   Administration of drugs to prevent pain or to induce unconsciousness during surgical operations or diagnostic procedures.

Cardiology   Subspecialty of internal medicine that deals with the heart and blood vessels.

Cardiovascular surgery   Surgical treatment of diseases of the heart and blood vessels.

Proctology   Medical and surgical treatment of disorders of the intestines and rectum.

Dermatology   Diagnosis and treatment of skin diseases.

Endocrinology and metabolism   Subspecialty of internal medicine that deals with glandular and metabolic disorders.

Family practice   General medical services for patients and their families.

Gastroenterology   Subspecialty of internal medicine that deals with disorders of the digestive tract (esophagus, stomach, and intestine).

General surgery   Surgery of parts of the body that are not in the domain of specific surgical specialties (some overlapping areas).

Geriatrics   Subspecialty of family practice and internal medicine that deals with the medical problems of the elderly.

Hematology/oncology   Subspecialty of internal medicine concerned with blood disorders and cancers.

Internal medicine   Diagnosis and nonsurgical treatment of internal organs of the body of adults.

Nephrology   Diagnosis and treatment of kidney diseases.

Neurology   Diagnosis and nonsurgical treatment of diseases of the brain, spinal cord, and nerves.

Neurosurgery   Diagnosis and surgical treatment of diseases of the brain, spinal cord, and nerves.

Nuclear medicine   Use of radioactive substances for diagnosis and treatment.

Obstetrics and gynecology   Care of pregnant women and disorders of the female reproductive system.

Ophthalmology   Medical and surgical care of the eye, including the prescription of glasses.

Orthopedics   Care of diseases of the muscles, and diseases, fractures, and deformities of the bones and joints.

Otolaryngology   Care of diseases of the head and neck except for those of the eyes or brain.

Pathology   Examination and diagnosis of organs, tissues, body fluids, and excrement.

Pediatrics   Care of children from birth through adolescence. Subspecialties include allergy, cardiology, hematology/oncology, nephrology, and surgery.

Physiatry   Treatment of convalescent and physically handicapped patients.

Plastic surgery   Surgery to correct or repair deformed or mutilated parts of the body, or to improve facial or body features.

Psychiatry   Treatment of mental and emotional problems.

Pulmonary disease   Subspecialty of internal medicine that deals with diseases of the lungs.

Radiology   Use of radiation for the diagnosis and treatment of disease.

Rheumatology   Subspecialty of internal medicine that deals with arthritis and related disorders.

Urology   Treatment of male sex organs and urinary tract and female urinary tract.

Unorthodox methods are sometimes called "alternative" approaches to health care. However, this term can be misleading because it wrongly implies that the methods are *equivalent* or equally logical choices—which they are not (see Figure 22-1 for examples of unorthodox treatment for arthritis).

• **Chiropractic** is based on the teachings of Daniel David Palmer, a "magnetic healer" who concluded in 1895 that the main cause of disease is misplaced spinal bones. He theorized that these partial dislocations interfere with the flow of "nerve energy" from the brain to the rest of the body and that spinal manipulation

---

Chiropractic   A system of health care based on the premise that misalignments of the vertebrae contribute to most diseases and ailments.

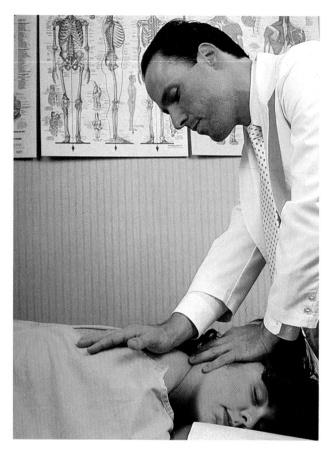

Chiropractic is based on the theory that disease results from misplaced spinal bones; it can be used to alleviate backaches and other musculoskeletal problems. This chiropractor is manipulating his patient's spine to realign the vertebrae and increase their mobility.

can restore the vertebrae to their proper places, enabling the body to heal itself.

Chiropractors today are licensed in all 50 states, and most of their schools are accredited. They can be classified into two main groups, "mixers" and "straights." Mixers, the larger group, acknowledge that germs, hormones, and other factors play a role in disease, but regard mechanical disturbances of the spine as the major underlying cause. In addition to manipulation, mixers use physical therapy methods and may prescribe food supplements. Straights still cling to Palmer's original doctrines and tend to confine themselves to manual

manipulation of the spine. Chiropractors are not licensed to prescribe drugs or perform surgery. A small number of chiropractors completely reject Palmer's theories and limit their practice to musculoskeletal disorders that have been medically diagnosed.

Most people who consult chiropractors suffer from backaches or other musculoskeletal disorders. Properly applied, manipulation can benefit people with back pain caused by lack of mobility of bony segments of the spine. Chiropractors often help people, but many of them encourage their patients to come weekly or monthly for "preventive maintenance" of their spine, a practice that has no medical justification. Chiropractors have also been criticized for inappropriately prescribing high doses of vitamins and for overuse of x-rays.

- **Applied kinesiology** is based on the notion that every organ dysfunction is accompanied by a specific weak muscle. Its proponents, most of whom are chiropractors, also claim that nutritional deficiencies, allergies, and other adverse reactions to food substances can be detected by placing substances in the mouth so that the patient salivates. "Good" substances will lead to increased strength in specific muscles, whereas "bad" substances will cause specific weaknesses. Treatment of muscles diagnosed as "weak" may include special diets, food supplements, acupressure, and/or spinal manipulation. These concepts do not conform to accepted scientific beliefs about the nature of health and disease, and critics believe that any apparent beneficial results are the result of patient suggestibility.
- **Homeopathy** is based on the theories of Samuel Hahnemann (1755–1843), a German physician. Hahnemann was justifiably alarmed about bloodletting, leeching, purging, and other medical procedures of his day that did far more harm than good. He was also critical of medications such as calomel (mercurous chloride), which was given in doses that caused mercury poisoning. Instead, he proposed his "law of similars"—that the symptoms of disease can be cured by substances that produce similar symptoms in healthy people. The word *homeopathy* is derived from the Greek words *homeo* ("similar") and *pathos* ("suffering" or "disease").

Hahnemann believed that diseases represent a disturbance in the body's ability to heal itself and that only a small stimulus is needed to foster the healing process. After experimenting on himself and others, he

---

Applied kinesiology A treatment method based on the theory that organ dysfunction is accompanied by muscle weakness that may be correctable by nutritional methods.

Homeopathy A treatment method based on the theory that tiny doses of certain substances can exert powerful effects within the body.

Naturopathy A treatment approach based on the belief that the basic cause of disease is violation of nature's laws.

Acupuncture A technique based on the theory that insertion of needles into points on the skin can restore health.

Acupressure (Shiatsu) A technique based on the theory that pressing on various body parts can restore health.

Iridology A diagnostic method based on the theory that each area of the body is represented by a corresponding area in the eye.

Signs of Quality Care

- Does the office appear to be run efficiently?
- Were you given adequate time to describe your problem?

- Did the physician seem thorough?
- Did the physician seem receptive to your concerns?

- Were your questions answered?
- Did you receive sufficient explanation of your problem and any recommended treatment?

---

concluded that the smaller the dose, the more powerful the effect—just the opposite of what pharmacologists believe today.

Homeopathic remedies are plant products, minerals, or other substances diluted to an extreme degree. The dilution of some preparations is so great that no molecule of original substance remains. But Hahnemann believed that vigorous shaking with each step of dilution leaves behind a spirit-like essence that cures by restoring the body's "vital force" to normal.

As scientific drug use developed, homeopathy declined sharply, particularly in America, where its schools either closed or converted to modern methods. But a few hundred physicians trained in modern methods have kept the practice alive in this country by taking courses here or abroad or by training with a practicing homeopath.

Homeopathic remedies were recognized as drugs by the 1938 amendment to the Federal Food, Drug, and Cosmetic Act. Unlike most other drugs, homeopathic remedies have been allowed to remain on the market without proof of their effectiveness being presented to the FDA. They can be obtained from practitioners and are also available without a prescription from health food stores, pharmacies, and manufacturers. These products appeal primarily to people who are afraid of doctors or of taking more potent drugs.

- **Naturopathy** is based on the idea that disease is caused by a violation of nature's laws. Naturopaths say that diseases are the body's effort to purify itself and that cures result from "increasing the patient's vital force by ridding the body of toxins." Naturopathic treatment can include "natural food" diets, vitamins, herbs, tissue minerals, cell salts, manipulation, massage, remedial exercise, diathermy, colonic enemas, acupuncture, reflexology, hypnotherapy, and homeopathy. Radiation may be used for diagnosis but not for treatment. Drugs are forbidden except for compounds that are components of body tissues. Naturopaths, like many chiropractors, believe that most diseases are within the scope of their practice. Naturopaths are licensed in a few states, and one of their two schools is accredited.
- **Acupuncture**, a technique dating from ancient China, involves the insertion of needles into the skin, or mus-

cles or tendons beneath, at one or more "acupuncture points." These points, said to represent various internal organs, are generally located along "meridians" on the surface of the body. Proponents claim that good health is produced by a harmonious mixture of yin and yang and that stimulation of acupuncture points can balance them so that internal organs can return to normal function. Similar claims are made for **acupressure (Shiatsu)**, but no needles are used.

Acupuncture defines the body according to systems that have no relation to established facts about body physiology. "Meridians" and acupuncture points on the surface of the body cannot actually be seen or measured. They are part of the mystical ancient Chinese way of looking at the body, health, disease, and nature. Although there is no evidence that acupuncture can affect the course of any physical illness, it may produce temporary pain relief. It probably works either by suggestion or by triggering release of the body's own morphine-like drugs, known as endorphins. The American Medical Association Council on Scientific Affairs has recommended that acupuncture for pain relief be regarded as experimental and performed only in medical research settings. However, some states license nonmedical acupuncturists.

- **Iridology** was devised more than a hundred years ago by Ignatz von Peczely, a Hungarian physician. It is based on the belief that each area of the body is represented by a corresponding area in the iris of the eye (the colored area surrounding the pupil). Iridologists claim that states of health and disease can be diagnosed from the color, texture, and location of various pigment flecks in the eye and that "imbalances" can be treated with vitamins, minerals, herbs, and similar products. According to a leading proponent, "Nature has provided us with a miniature television screen showing the most remote portions of the body by way of nerve reflex responses."

Iridologists use elaborate charts that supposedly show where various organs are represented in the eye. The American Medical Association Council on Scientific Affairs has noted that these charts are similar in concept to those used years ago in "phrenology," the pseudoscience that related protuberances of the skull

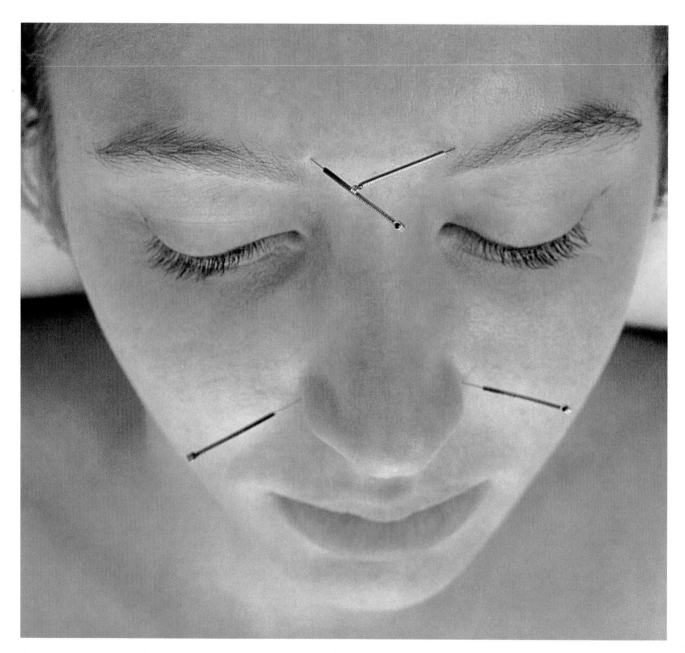

Acupuncture is based on the theory that illness results from an imbalance of vital energy flowing through the body along twelve meridians, each of which corresponds to a vital organ. The acupuncturist inserts needles at certain points along the meridians and rotates the ends to stimulate the energy flow. This woman is undergoing treatment for hay fever.

to the mental faculties and character of the individual. Of course, medical doctors can diagnose a few conditions by examining the interior of the eye with an ophthalmoscope, but that is not what iridologists do.

- **Reflexology,** also known as "zone therapy," is based on the theory that pressing on certain areas of the hands or feet can help relieve pain and remove the underlying cause of disease in other parts of the body. Proponents claim that: (1) the body is divided into ten

zones that begin or end in the hands and feet, (2) each organ or part of the body is represented by an area on the hands and feet, (3) the practitioner can diagnose abnormalities by feeling the feet, and (4) massaging or pressing each area can stimulate the flow of energy, blood, nutrients, and nerve impulses to the corresponding body zone. Reflexologists also claim that their techniques have been effective against anemia, arthritis, asthma, cataracts, deafness, diabetes, heart disease, high blood pressure, kidney disease, and many other health problems.

Acupressure, iridology, and reflexology are utilized by some licensed practitioners (mainly chiropractors and naturopaths) as well as by bogus "nutritionists" and other unlicensed practitioners. In most states, unlicensed individuals who use these methods could be convicted of practicing medicine without a license, but few are ever prosecuted.

- **Faith Healing**, a practice based on the belief that prayer and other rituals can heal, has existed since ancient times. The idea that demons cause disease was accepted by ancient practitioners but still is prevalent today among segments of the American public. In the United States, several religions include faith healing as part of their dogma, and many evangelistic healers have attracted large followings.

Few scientific attempts have been made to evaluate faith healing. Although testimonials abound, it is difficult and time-consuming to investigate such claims. Many cures attributed to faith healing are cases in which the ailment simply runs its natural course and the person recovers as he or she would have anyway. In one extensive study, Dr. William A. Nolen examined many people who had supposedly been "miraculously healed" and found that not one had been helped. A more recent investigation led by magician James Randi found that several prominent healers were outright frauds.

- **Chelation therapy** involves intravenous administration of a synthetic amino acid called EDTA into the bloodstream, where it supposedly cleans out unwanted minerals from various parts of the body before exiting through the kidneys. It is used most often in cases of heart disease, but its promoters also claim it is effective against kidney disease, arthritis, Parkinson's disease, multiple sclerosis, emphysema, and many other serious diseases. However, no controlled trial has shown that chelation can help any of these conditions. A course of treatment consisting of 20 to 50 injections can cost thousands of dollars, and serious complications have been reported.

- **Clinical ecology** is practiced by a few hundred medical and osteopathic physicians. It is not a recognized specialty but is based on the notion that hypersensitivity to common foods and chemicals can cause depression, difficulty in thinking, headaches, muscle and joint pains, and many other common symptoms. Clinical ecologists speculate that the immune system is like a barrel that continually fills with chemicals until it overflows, leading to multiple symptoms. Much of their diagnosis is based on the provocation-neutralization test in which suspected substances are administered under the tongue or injected into the skin. If symptoms occur, the test is considered positive and the patient is diagnosed as suffering from "environmental illness." Steps are recommended to prevent or reduce contact with the substances involved—through dietary restriction and various environmental changes. Many clinical ecologists claim their patients are suffering from hypersensitivity to the common yeast *Candida albicans*. The American Academy of Allergy and Immunology, which is the nation's largest professional organization of allergists, considers clinical ecology a form of "poor medical practice" and regards the concepts of "environmental illness" and **candidiasis hypersensitivity** as "speculative and unproven."

Evaluating Unorthodox Practices   Given the relatively advanced state of medical science and the fairly high level of consumer awareness among Americans, why do unorthodox practices persist—and even thrive? Promoters of quackery appeal to people in many ways. They offer hope to people who feel desperate. They exploit any strains in the relationship between patient and physician, promising to cure those who are dissatisfied with the course of their treatment. They take advantage of current health threats—in another era it was typhoid fever; today it's AIDS. They attack the medical establishment, suggesting that it is trying to suppress effective treatments or that physicians and scientists have other ulterior motives. They foster anxiety and doubt by suggesting that many people have problems that are actually uncommon, such as vitamin deficiencies and low blood sugar. And they promise new, quick, or easy ways to attain vitality, vigor, strength, energy, youthful looks, and much more.

How can you protect yourself against quackery? Most important maintaining an appropriate level of suspicion. For example, don't assume that health claims made in advertisements or on radio or television talk shows must be true or would not have been allowed. This is not necessarily the case. If you wish to take advantage of the

---

Reflexology   A treatment method based on the theory that pressing on certain areas of the hands or feet can help relieve pain and remove the underlying cause of disease in other parts of the body.

Chelation therapy   An intravenous treatment claimed to provide various health benefits by removing unwanted substances from the body.

Clinical ecology   A treatment approach based on the concept that multiple symptoms can be triggered by hypersensitivity to common foods and chemicals when the immune system becomes "overloaded."

Candidiasis hypersensitivity   A "fad diagnosis" based on the unscientific concept that hidden allergies to yeast can cause a wide spectrum of symptoms.

best that medical science can offer and to avoid being led astray, it is necessary to make reasoned, informed decisions about what to believe. Many resources exist to help people assess the claims made for a product or treatment. You can consult a physician, registered dietitian or other reputable professional; do some reading at a public library (preferably with some professional guidance); contact a consumer group or local health organization; or ask your insurance company whether they will pay for the treatment. The specific strategies listed in the box entitled "Ten Ways to Avoid Being Quacked" will help you know what to do the next time you encounter a treatment that seems too good to be true.

Protection against quackery isn't just the individual's responsibility, of course. At the community, state, and national level, protection may be provided by various agencies; we turn to this topic next.

Consumer Protection Agencies

Legal protection against health frauds and quackery is based on a framework of federal and state laws. Professional and voluntary agencies can sometimes apply pressure to wrongdoers. Educational information is available from many sources.

Federal Agencies   In addition to its mission to protect our food supply, the U.S. Food and Drug Administration (FDA) has jurisdiction over advertising of prescription drug products and labeling of nonprescription products and health devices. It is illegal to market a product without FDA approval (which usually means that the agency considers it safe and effective). When the FDA learns that a product is being marketed with unapproved claims, it can issue a warning letter, seize the product, or obtain an injunction. Criminal prosecution is also possible but rarely occurs.

The FDA has a very active public educational program. Its magazine, *FDA Consumer,* provides excellent coverage of health, nutrition, and safety issues. Its Office of Consumer Affairs distributes pamphlets, sponsors talks and conferences, and answers individual inquiries. Its field offices, located in major cities throughout the country, distribute educational materials, answer inquiries, and provide speakers.

The Federal Trade Commission (FTC) has jurisdiction over interstate advertising of all health products and services except for prescription drugs. However, it rarely takes action against licensed health practitioners because they are subject to supervision by state licensing boards. When the FTC becomes aware of wrongdoing, it can obtain a cease-and-desist order, which, if violated, can trigger penalties up to $10,000 a day for each violation.

The U.S. Postal Service has jurisdiction over the sale of products or services by mail. When misleading mail-order promotions are detected, the agency can seek voluntary discontinuation or obtain administrative permission to intercept orders and return them to the senders. After a scheme has been stopped, a promoter who resumes similar activity can be fined up to $10,000 per day.

■ **Exploring Your Emotions**

How do you feel about some of the claims made on TV and radio and in the print media for health-related items? Do you think it's OK for manufacturers to deliberately mislead consumers about their products? Whose responsibility is it to evaluate such claims?

Although actions by federal agencies can be extremely powerful and put illegal operators out of business, federal enforcement has serious limitations. Some illegal schemes are never detected, while others are detected long after their promoter has done considerable harm. In some cases, offenders can remain in business for years by appealing to federal courts. For example, it took the FTC sixteen years to force the makers of Carter's Little Liver Pills—which cannot benefit the liver—to remove the word "liver" from their product. Most important, the number of illegal schemes is so great that federal agencies do not have sufficient resources to act against all they detect.

State and Local Agencies   Licensed practitioners are regulated by state boards that can conduct investigations into alleged wrongdoing. When an offense takes place, the practitioner can be ordered to take corrective action and can be placed on probation or have his or her license suspended or revoked.

State attorneys general have jurisdiction over illegal health activities such as illegal representations by unlicensed practitioners, marketing of unapproved drugs, and false advertising. In cases involving individual victims, local district attorneys may have primary jurisdiction.

The extent to which individual states protect their residents from quackery and health fraud depends on the strength of their laws and resources allotted to the problem. While some states conduct extensive investigations and prosecute many promoters of quackery, others do virtually nothing.

Professional and Voluntary Organizations   Professional groups such as state and local medical societies can often help individuals check the reputation of practitioners or products. These groups can also investigate accusations of unethical and unprofessional conduct and

Ten Ways to Avoid Being Quacked

Promoters of quackery know how to appeal to every aspect of human vulnerability. What sells is not the quality of their products but their ability to influence their audience. Here are ten strategies to avoid being quacked:

- *Remember that quackery seldom looks outlandish.* Its promoters often use scientific terms and quote (or misquote) from scientific references. Some actually have reputable scientific training but have diverged from it.
- *Ignore any practitioner who says that most diseases are caused by faulty nutrition or can be remedied by taking supplements.* Although some diseases are related to diet, most are not. Moreover, in most cases where diet actually is a factor in a person's health problem, the solution is not to take vitamins but to alter the diet.
- *Be wary of anecdotes and testimonials.* If someone claims to have been helped by an unorthodox remedy, ask yourself and possibly your physician whether there might be another explanation. Most single episodes of disease recover with the passage of time, and most chronic ailments have symptom-free periods. Most people who give testimonials about recovery from cancer have undergone effective treatment as well as unorthodox treatment, but give credit to the latter. Some testimonials are complete fabrications.
- *Be wary of pseudomedical jargon.* Instead of offering to treat

your disease, some quacks will promise to "detoxify" your body, "balance" its chemistry, release its "nerve energy," "bring it in harmony with nature," or correct supposed "weaknesses" of various organs. The use of concepts that are impossible to measure enables success to be claimed even though nothing has actually been accomplished.

- *Don't fall for paranoid accusations.* Unorthodox practitioners often claim that the medical profession, drug companies, and the government are conspiring to suppress whatever method they espouse. No evidence to support such a theory has ever been demonstrated. It also flies in the face of logic to believe that large numbers of people would oppose the development of treatment methods that might someday help themselves or their loved ones.
- *Forget about "secret cures."* True scientists share their knowledge as part of the process of scientific development. Quacks may keep their methods secret to prevent others from demonstrating that they don't work. No one who actually discovered a cure would have reason to keep it secret. If a method works—especially for a serious disease—the discoverer would gain enormous fame, fortune, and personal satisfaction by sharing the discovery with others.
- *Be wary of herbal remedies.* Herbs are promoted primarily through literature based on

hearsay, folklore, and tradition. As medical science developed, it became apparent that most herbs did not deserve good reputations, and most that did were replaced by synthetic compounds that are more effective. Many herbs contain hundreds or even thousands of chemicals that have not been completely cataloged. While some may turn out to be useful, others could well prove toxic. With safe and effective treatment available, treatment with herbs rarely makes sense.

- *Be skeptical of any product claimed to be effective against a wide range of unrelated diseases—particularly diseases that are serious.* There is no such thing as a panacea or "cure-all."
- *Ignore appeals to your vanity.* One of quackery's most powerful appeals is the suggestion to "think for yourself" instead of following the collective wisdom of the scientific community. A similar appeal is the idea that although a remedy has not been proven to work for other people, it still might work for you.
- *Don't let desperation cloud your judgment.* If you feel that your physician isn't doing enough to help you, or if you have been told that your condition is incurable and don't wish to accept this fate without a struggle, don't stray from scientific health care in a desperate attempt to find a solution. Instead, discuss your feelings with your physician and consider a consultation with a recognized expert.

A Quack for All Seasons

Different groups of people are vulnerable to exploitation and health fraud for different reasons. Some examples:

Teenagers may be in the prime of life, but they are still vulnerable to quackery. They love what is new and different. They're insecure about physical appearances. They want quick results. In our era of dual-career or single-parent families, they have plenty of opportunities to shop. Credit cards make

buying easier. Teens thus become special targets for bogus muscle-builders and tanning methods.

Adults past age 65 make up 12 percent of the U.S. population—and 60 percent of health fraud victims. Older people have more extensive health needs. They grew up in a less skeptical era and, if they are confined to home care, have less opportunity to do comparison shopping.

Ethnic minorities may be less familiar with legitimate medicine. Language barriers can lead to isolation. Some quacks have posed as "government inspectors," ordering new immigrants to pay for worthless treatments.

Source: Quackery: It's Alive and Well, but Threatening Your Health—and Pocketbook. *Mayo Clinic Health Letter,* June 1988.

---

can sometimes persuade wrongdoers to take corrective action. Professional societies can reprimand or expel members. Hospital officials can reduce, suspend, or revoke a practitioner's privileges at their particular hospital. But practitioners who neither belong to a professional group nor work in a hospital are unlikely to be affected by the disciplinary efforts of these organizations.

Local Better Business Bureaus investigate unethical business practices but rarely get involved in disputes involving licensed practitioners. The National Council of Better Business Bureaus investigates and publishes occasional reports about quack products and their promotion. BBB's National Advertising Division investigates questionable product advertising and can sometimes persuade offending advertisers to stop.

The National Council Against Health Fraud is a membership organization of more than 1,500 persons concerned about quackery and health frauds. It sponsors meetings, publishes a newsletter and position papers, distributes other publications, helps victims obtain redress, and operates an information clearinghouse for individuals, government agencies, and media representatives. Information and advice are also available from many local, state, and national professional and voluntary organizations.

Table 22-2 lists places where you can obtain information or complain about questionable health matters. Remember that people who make appropriate complaints may not only help themselves, but may also help to protect others.

Health Insurance

Health insurance enables people to budget in advance for health-care costs that may otherwise be unpredictable and ruinously high. Hospital care costs hundreds of dollars a day, and surgical fees can cost thousands. So health insurance is important for almost everyone.

Types of Policies   There are three basic types of health insurance coverage: basic, major medical, and comprehensive.

■ **Exploring Your Emotions**

Do you believe that physicians and hospitals have a responsibility to treat and care for patients who can't pay? Do you think medical care is a right or a privilege? What is the basis for your beliefs and opinions?

Basic protection includes expenses for hospital, surgical, and medical care. Hospital benefits may provide payment of a specific amount for a specified number of days, or full charges may be paid for daily room, board, routine nursing services, and intensive care up to a maximum number of days. Coverage may also be provided for various inpatient and outpatient services such as laboratory tests, x-ray films, medications, and physical therapy. Visits to physicians' offices are not usually covered.

Basic protection   Insurance that includes hospital, surgical, and medical care.

Table 22-2 Where to complain or seek help	
Problem	**Agencies to Contact***
False advertising	FTC Bureau of Consumer Protection Regional FTC office National Advertising Division, Council of Better Business Bureaus Editor or station manager of media outlet where ad appeared
Product marketed with false or misleading claims	Regional FDA office State attorney general State health department Local Better Business Bureau Congressional representatives
Bogus mail-order promotion	Chief Postal Inspector, U.S. Postal Service Editor or station manager of media outlet where ad appeared
Improper treatment by licensed practitioner	Local or state professional society (if practitioner is a member) Local hospital (if practitioner is a staff member) State licensing board National Council Against Health Fraud Task Force on Victim Redress
Improper treatment by unlicensed individual	Local district attorney State attorney general National Council Against Health Fraud Task Force on Victim Redress
Advice needed about questionable product or service	National Council Against Health Fraud Local, state, or national professional or voluntary health groups

*Addresses
FTC Bureau of Consumer Protection, Washington, DC 20580. Tel. 202-326-2222.
National Advertising Division, Council of Better Business Bureaus, 845 Third Avenue, New York, NY 10022. Tel. 212-753-1358.
FDA, 5600 Fishers Lane, Rockville, MD 20857. Tel. 301-295-8024.
Chief Postal Inspector, U.S. Postal Service, Washington, DC 20260. Tel. 202-268-4267.
National Council Against Health Fraud, P.O. Box 1276, Loma Linda, CA 92354. Tel. 714-824-4690.
NCAHF Task Force on Victim Redress, P.O. Box 33008, Kansas City, MO 64114. Tel. 816-444-8615. For regional offices of
   federal agencies consult the telephone directory under U.S. Government.

Major medical insurance (also called "extended benefit" or "catastrophic coverage") is designed to help protect against medical expenses resulting from prolonged illness or serious injury. These contracts generally include a deductible clause, a co-insurance provision, high maximum limits, and coverage of a broad spectrum of services not included under basic coverage. Typically they pay 80 percent of covered services after a $100 deductible. Psychiatric benefits are usually more limited than others. **Comprehensive major medical insurance** policies integrate basic and major medical insurance into one program.

Health insurance policies may be sold to groups or individuals. Group policies generally offer more coverage and cost less than individual policies. Most people are insured through a group policy obtained through their place of employment. Because the extent and type of covered services varies widely from contract to contract, policies should be read carefully to understand what protection they provide.

Government Programs   In many states, certain categories of people who are unable to afford health care are eligible for **Medicaid**, a state-run, federally subsidized program that covers a broad spectrum of services.

Individuals who are chronically disabled or have reached age 65 are eligible for **Medicare**, a federal program composed of two parts. Part A provides hospital

---

Major medical insurance   Insurance designed to help protect against medical expenses resulting from prolonged illness or serious injury.

Comprehensive major medical insurance   Policies that combine basic and major medical insurance into one program.

Medicaid   Federally subsidized state-run plan of health care for indigent people.

Medicare   Federal health insurance program for people 65 or older and for certain disabled younger people.

Patient's Bill of Rights

The American Hospital Association presents a Patient's Bill of Rights with the expectation that observance of these rights will contribute to more effective patient care and greater satisfaction for the patient, the physician, and the hospital organization. Further, the Association presents these rights in the expectation that they will be supported by the hospital on behalf of its patients, as an integral part of the healing process. It is recognized that a personal relationship between the physician and the patient is essential for the provision of proper medical care. The traditional physician-patient relationship takes on a new dimension when care is rendered within an organizational structure. Legal precedent has established that the institution itself also has a responsibility to the patient. It is in recognition of these factors that these rights are affirmed.

1. Patients have the right to considerate and respectful care.

2. Patients have the right to obtain from their physicians complete current information concerning their diagnosis, treatment, and prognosis in terms patients can be reasonably expected to understand. When it is not medically advisable to give such information to patients, the information should be made available to an appropriate person on their behalf. They have the right to know by name the physician responsible for coordinating their care.

3. Patients have the right to receive from their physician information necessary to give informed consent prior to the start of any procedure and/or treatment. Except in emergencies, such information for informed consent should include but not necessarily be limited to the specific procedure and/or treatment, the medically significant risks involved, and the probable duration of incapacitation. Where medically significant alternatives for care or treatment exist, or when patients request information concerning the medical alternatives, patients have the right to such information. Patients also have the right to know the name of the person responsible for the procedures and/or treatment.

4. Patients have the right to refuse treatment to the extent permitted by law, and to be informed of the medical consequences of that action.

5. Patients have the right to every consideration of their privacy concerning their own medical-care program. Case discussion, consultation, examination, and treatment are confidential and should be conducted discreetly. Those not directly involved in their care must have the permission of patients to be present.

6. Patients have the right to expect all communications and records pertaining to their care be treated confidentially.

7. Patients have the right to expect that within its capacity a hospital must make reasonable response to the request of patients for services. The hospital must provide evaluation, service, and/or referral as indicated by the urgency of the case. When medically permissible, patients may be transferred to another facility only after they have received complete information and explanation concerning the needs for and alternatives to such a transfer. The institution to which a patient is to be transferred must first have accepted the patient for transfer.

8. Patients have the right to obtain information as to any relationship of their hospital to other health-care and educational institutions insofar as their care is concerned. Patients have the right to obtain information as to the existence of any professional relationships among individuals by name, who are treating them.

9. Patients have the right to be advised if the hospital proposes to engage in or perform human experimentation affecting their care or treatment. Patients have the right to refuse to participate in such research projects.

10. Patients have the right to expect reasonable continuity of care. They have the right to know in advance what appointment times and physicians are available and where. Patients have the right to expect that the hospital will provide a mechanism whereby they are informed by their physician or a delegate of the physician of the patients' continuing health-care requirements following discharge.

11. Patients have the right to examine and receive an explanation of their bill regardless of the source of payment.

12. Patients have the right to know what hospital rules and regulations apply to their conduct as patients.

No catalog of rights can guarantee for patients the kind of treatment they have a right to expect. A hospital has many functions to perform, including the prevention and treatment of disease, the education of both health professionals and patients, and the conduct of clinical research. All these activities must be conducted with an overriding concern for patients, and, above all, the recognition of their dignity as human beings. Success in achieving this recognition assures success in the defense of the rights of the patients.

American Hospital Association

insurance financed through Social Security taxes. Part B helps pay for medical services and is financed through monthly premiums paid by those who wish to subscribe. Private insurance companies also sell "medigap" policies to supplement Medicare coverage.

Under Medicare, physicians who "accept assignment" are paid directly by the government and may not bill the patient for the difference between their usual fee and the amount the government pays (except for amounts that involve deductibles and co-insurance).

Prepaid Group Plans   Most insurance contracts permit the policyholder complete freedom to decide where to obtain treatment. Because health-care costs have been rising, insurance companies, hospitals, and private groups have been marketing plans aimed at controlling these costs. The physicians in these plans must agree to certain cost controls, and the patients are restricted in their choice of physicians.

Health maintenance organizations (HMOs) are comprehensive programs in which physicians agree to accept a monthly fee **(capitation)** per patient or to charge for actual services rendered according to a fee schedule that is usually lower than the physicians' standard fees. Many HMOs hold back a percentage of the fees until the end of the plan year. Then, if the plan meets its financial goals, the withheld funds will be distributed according to the agreement between the plan and the physicians. This type of arrangement is designed to encourage physicians to avoid unnecessary services. The physicians belonging to the HMO may be located in their own offices or at a central facility where the physicians are salaried. Under HMO programs, patients can choose their primary physician from a list of participating physicians and need a referral by the primary physician for services by specialists to be covered.

Preferred provider organizations (PPOs) are programs in which participating physicians and hospitals agree to accept fixed fees that are usually 15 to 20 percent less than their usual fees. Patients can go to any provider, but use of nonparticipating providers results in considerably higher cost to the patient.

Choosing a Policy   Choosing health insurance can be complicated because there are many types of plans and contracts can vary greatly from company to company and even within the same company.

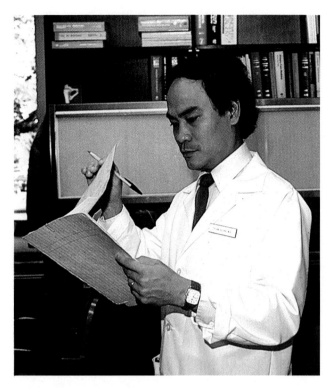

Physicians who work for a health maintenance organization are often located in a central facility and receive a salary rather than fees from patients. One advantage of HMOs for physicians is that they are relieved of having to maintain a private practice. The advantage of HMOs for patients is that their medical care is all prepaid.

Colleges typically provide outpatient health services through a student health service. Some also require students to purchase additional insurance to cover hospitalization or other outside services. Students who are still covered under their family's policy may not be required to purchase additional insurance. It is usually most economical to remain covered under a family policy as long as possible rather than obtaining a separate policy of one's own.

After college it is usually best to see whether group coverage is available through work or membership in an organization. If you work for a large company, several plans may be available. If no group coverage is available, contact Blue Cross/Blue Shield and agents for several other insurance companies. After discussing your needs with them, obtain a copy of each policy that sounds suitable, read them carefully, and be sure you understand

---

Health maintenance organization (HMO)   A prepaid health plan in which patients receive health care from designated providers.

Capitation   Payment to health providers according to number of patients they agree to serve rather than amount of service rendered.

Preferred provider organization (PPO)   A prepaid insurance plan in which providers agree to deliver services for discounted fees. Patients can go to any provider, but using nonparticipating providers results in higher costs to the patient.

Glossary of Health Insurance Terms

Because health insurance policies are legal contracts, they use precise legal language. Some of these terms appear in all policies, while others appear just in some. Understanding them will help you figure out how a policy works and what it actually covers. Following are terms not defined elsewhere in this chapter.

Assignment of benefits By signing a form (usually the insurance claim form), you authorize the insurance company to pay the physician directly. Otherwise payment must be made directly to you. Most physicians will ask you to sign the form if you don't want to pay your bill before the insurance company pays its share.

Co-insurance An arrangement whereby you and the insurance company share costs. Typically, the insurer pays 75 to 85 percent of covered costs and you pay the rest. Some policies set an upper limit to co-insurance expense, after which the company pays all additional charges.

Conversion privilege A provision that enables those insured by group contracts to obtain an individual policy under various circumstances, such as leaving the job that provided the group coverage.

Coordination of benefits A provision that prohibits you from collecting identical benefits from two or more policies, thereby profiting when you are ill. After the primary company pays, other companies will calculate their coverage of the remainder. All group policies contain a coordination clause, but most individual policies do not.

Deductible The amount you must pay before the insurance company starts paying.

Endorsement or rider An attachment to the basic insurance policy that changes its coverage.

Exclusions Specified conditions or circumstances for which the policy does not provide benefits.

Grace period The number of days that you may delay payment of your premium without losing your insurance.

Guaranteed renewability A policy where the company agrees to continue insuring you up to a certain age (or for life) as long as you pay the premium. Under this provision, the premium structure cannot be raised unless it is raised for all members of a group or class of insured, such as all people living in your state with the same kind of policy.

Inpatient services Services received while hospitalized.

Notice of claim Written notice the company must receive when a claim exists. Typically it must be received within twenty days or as soon thereafter as reasonably possible.

Outpatient services Services obtained at a hospital by people who are not confined to the hospital.

Participating physician A physician who agrees to abide by the rules of a plan in return for direct payment by the insurance company. The agreement includes acceptance of a fixed fee schedule, a monthly fee per eligible patient, or other fee limitation.

Preexisting condition A health problem you had before becoming insured. Some policies exclude these conditions, while others do not.

Provider Any source of health-care services, such as a hospital, physician, pharmacist, or laboratory.

Reasonable charge The amount a company will pay for a given service based on what most providers charge for it.

Waiting period A specified time between issuance of a policy and coverage of certain conditions. Typically there are waiting periods for preexisting conditions and maternity benefits.

---

what they say. If you want both basic and major medical coverage, it is often best to get both from the same company to avoid gaps in coverage. However, your aim should be to insure mainly against the most serious types of losses. In the long run, it is more economical to absorb the cost of minor medical expenses as part of your overall budget. "Dread disease" policies that cover only one disease, such as cancer, are inadvisable, and other types of overlapping policies should also be avoided. Mail-order policies that pay a daily amount generally have low limits and a waiting period, which make them unsuitable for basic coverage. The following questions are designed to help you choose the most appropriate insurance for you.

- What services are covered? Different policies may cover any of the following:

    Inpatient hospital costs

    Surgical costs, including anesthesia

    Inpatient medical services

    Physicians' office visits

    X-ray examinations

Quality Care Eludes Many Americans

The American health-care system is in critical condition, according to the National Committee for Quality Care, a coalition of health and hospital systems and companies. The deterioration they warn about is not simply part of a "disturbing future." It is going on now. Some of the evidence for these conclusions includes the following:

- Some hospitals have been closing, squeezed by tighter payments from the government and private insurers. In 1988 there were 50,000 fewer hospital beds than there were in 1983. A study in eight rural Florida counties with no hospitals found that both infant mortality and the death rate from accidents were higher than in rural counties with hospitals.
- Physicians are disappearing in some areas, sometimes because a hospital has disappeared, sometimes because they are either quitting medicine or abandoning some practices—especially obstetrics and to some extent neurosurgery—because of high malpractice premiums.
- Partly because of much-advertised pressures on physicians, partly because of the crushing cost of medical school and the

fact that other fields promise quicker returns, the number—and, some say, the quality—of medical school applicants is declining. Where there were five applicants for every place in the mid-1970s, in 1988 there were two.
- There is a serious shortage of nurses to care for hospital patients. One reason is the failure to pay better salaries, which the hospitals say they can't afford. Some hospitals fail to fill 20 percent of their nursing slots.
- At the same time, hospitals need more nurses to deliver new life-saving medical technologies. In the past, hospitals tried to hire one nurse for every two patients; in 1988 they tried to hire almost two per patient, but finding them was difficult. Hospitals often cope by hiring many part-time nurses and shifting nurses from ward to ward, day by day. Nursing homes tend to have an especially hard time hiring qualified nurses.
- The cost of health care is continuing to rise, and patients are being forced to shoulder a growing percentage of their medical and hospital bills. More employers are requiring increased employee contributions. Health insurance premiums went up

sharply in 1987, with increases of 33 percent common.
- The number of uninsured Americans is 35 to 37 million, and millions of others are inadequately insured. Medicare, intended to protect the elderly, finances less than 50 percent of this group's health bills. Medicaid, the program for the poor, is covering less than 40 percent of the poverty population.
- Nearly 39 million Americans have trouble getting necessary health services; nearly half of them said the reason was financial. The number of children going unvaccinated is on the increase. So is the number of babies born to women getting late or no prenatal care. So is infant mortality in some states or cities.

It may be that only aggressive action on the part of the federal government can resolve these difficulties. As Congress struggles with controversial and expensive bills to provide Americans with adequate health care, individuals continue to make do as best they can—and turn increasingly to self-care.

Adapted from Quality of Care Eludes Many Americans. *Washington Post Health*, February 9, 1988, p. 8.

Outpatient diagnostic tests

Medications

Physical therapy

Maternity fees

Private-duty nursing

Psychiatric services

Skilled nursing home care

- Which of these services am I most likely to need?

- Are there exclusions for any preexisting conditions?
- How do the various policies compare in cost?
- Are the deductible and co-insurance provisions suitable?
- Are the maximum limits high enough?
- Will I be able to see the physicians I prefer?
- Does my present physician participate?

Most of the time, you can take care of yourself without personally consulting an expert. You can learn to manage stress, eat well, get adequate exercise, minimize contact with contagious disease, and so on. When you do need professional care—and Chapter 21 provides guidelines to help you identify those situations—you can continue to take responsibility for yourself by making reasoned decisions about the care and insurance you obtain.

Because so many people are involved in the health-care field, of course, and because human knowledge has its limits, you are bound to have a frustrating or unpleasant experience now and then, as can happen in any other area of your life. Take setbacks in stride and be persistent about getting what you need—within the bounds of practices based on scientific fact.

Summary

- When seeking medical care, people usually should find a primary physician, who can refer them to specialists when necessary; in most cases, physicians should be affiliated with hospitals that are connected to medical schools or that train residents.

Orthodox Practitioners

- Medical doctors have degrees from accredited medical schools and are licensed to administer medical and surgical treatment; specialists have additional training and can become board-certified.
- Osteopathic practice has incorporated all of the theories and practices of medicine, though osteopaths usually have more interest in musculoskeletal problems and manipulative therapy.
- Podiatrists specialize in the care of feet and legs; they can prescribe drugs and do surgery.
- Optometrists examine the eyes to detect vision problems and eye diseases. They may use drugs for diagnostic purposes but need to refer patients with eye disease to a physician.
- Dentists are permitted to perform certain types of surgery on the mouth and to prescribe certain drugs within the scope of their training.
- Other trained practitioners include registered nurses, licensed vocational nurses, dietitians, dental hygienists, physical therapists, occupational therapists, laboratory technicians, and x-ray technicians.

Unorthodox Practitioners

- Unorthodox practice consists of philosophies or methods that clash with accepted knowledge or are unproven and unlikely. Unorthodox practitioners sometimes help people by helping them relieve stress, by giving them attention, and by persuading them to develop healthier living habits—not because the unorthodox theories are valid.
- Holistic practitioners pay attention to emotions and lifestyle as well as to physical problems; good medical practice has always been holistic.
- Chiropractic is based on the idea that the main cause of disease is misplaced spinal bones and that spinal manipulation can enable the body to heal itself.
- Applied kinesiology rests on the idea that every organ dysfunction is accompanied by a specific weak muscle; its practitioners also believe they can diagnose nutritional deficiencies by placing substances in the mouth so that the patient salivates.
- Homeopathy is based on the belief that the symptoms of disease can be cured by substances that produce similar symptoms in healthy people and that the smaller the dose, the more powerful the effect; homeopathic remedies are diluted to an extreme degree.
- Naturopathy is based on the idea that violations of nature's laws cause diseases, which are the body's effort to purify itself. Naturopathic treatment purports to rid the body of toxins.
- Acupuncture involves the insertion of needles into the skin, muscles, or tendons at various points said to represent internal organs. Acupressure is a similar technique that doesn't use needles. Acupuncture may temporarily relieve pain, perhaps by triggering the release of endorphins.
- Iridology is based on the belief that areas of the body are represented by corresponding areas in the iris of the eye and that diseases can be diagnosed from the color, texture, and location of various flecks in the eye.
- Reflexology is based on the theory that pressing on certain areas of the hands or feet can remove underlying causes of disease in other parts of the body.
- Faith healing is based on the belief that prayer and other rituals can heal; it is a part of some organized religions. The scientific investigations that have been carried out fail to substantiate faith healing claims.
- Clinical ecology is based on the notion that hypersensitivity to common foods and chemicals can cause depression, headaches, and other symptoms.
- Promoters of unorthodox methods exploit others by offering hope to the desperate, taking advantage of current health threats, attacking the medical establishment, fostering anxiety, and promising "quick fixes."
- Protection against quackery is ensured by maintaining a level of suspicion and by reading or seeking out information from qualified groups.

Consumer Protection Agencies

- The federal government offers protection against false advertising, mislabeling, and fraudulent mail-order schemes through the FDA, FTC, and U.S. Postal Service.

- State boards investigate alleged wrongdoing by licensed practitioners, and state attorneys general have jurisdiction over illegal health activities.
- Professional groups can help consumers check reputations and can investigate charges against members. Hospitals can restrict a practitioner's privileges. Better Business Bureaus and the National Council Against Health Fraud can provide information to consumers.

Health Insurance

- Basic health insurance includes expenses for hospital, surgical, and medical care. Coverage may include not only hospitalization but also laboratory tests, x-rays, medicines, and physical therapy.
- Major medical insurance protects against medical expenses resulting from prolonged illness or serious in-

jury. These policies usually pay 80 percent of a broad range of services after a deductible has been paid.

- Comprehensive policies combine basic and major medical policies. Group policies usually offer more coverage and cost less than individual policies.
- Government programs include Medicaid, for the poor, and Medicare, for those who are 65 or chronically disabled. Part A of Medicare pays for hospital services, and Part B (paid for by subscribers) pays for other medical services.
- In health maintenance organizations (HMOs), physicians agree to accept a monthly fee per patient or to use a lower fee schedule than usual. With preferred provider organizations, participating physicians agree to accept lower fees; patients can go to any provider.
- Group insurance usually offers the best coverage. Choice of a policy should depend on services covered, services needed, exclusions, deductibles, maximum limits, and choice of physicians.

Take Action

1. Visit the student health center or another health-care facility, and write a brief evaluation of the quality and kinds of services available. Consider such things as hours, waiting time, health literature available, scope of services, availability of specialists, and so on. Try to determine where there is room for improvement and make recommendations. Give your evaluation to the manager of the facility and ask for a response.

2. Talk to a hospital official to get some idea of hospital-care costs in your community. Then find out what health insurance programs are available for college students. Which one or ones would you recommend? Which would you not recommend?

3. Talk to a practitioner of one or more of the unorthodox practices described in this chapter. Ask what training they have, what conditions they treat most often, how they make diagnoses, what treatments they give, and whether they have any pamphlets you can read. Make a list of the questions you have about these practices and where you would go to find the answers.

Selected Bibliography

American Heart Association. 1987. *Questions and Answers About Chelation Therapy.* Dallas: American Heart Association.

Barrett, S., ed. 1980. *The Health Robbers—How to Protect Your Money and Your Life,* 2nd ed. Philadelphia: Stickley.

Randi, J. 1989. *The Faith Healers.* Buffalo, N.Y.: Prometheus.

Stalker, D., and Glymour, C., eds. 1985. *Examining Holistic Medicine.* Buffalo, N.Y.: Prometheus Books.

Recommended Readings

Barrett, S., and the editors of *Schemes, Scams, and Frauds.* Consumer Reports

Books. 1990. *Health.* New York: Consumer Reports Books. *A comprehensive discussion of current forms of quackery and how to avoid them.*

Barrett, S., and Cassileth, B. R. 1990. *Dubious Cancer Treatment.* Tampa, Florida: The American Cancer Society, Florida Division, Inc. *A report on "alternative" methods and the practitioners and patients who use them.*

Brody, J. 1982. *Jane Brody's Guide to Personal Health.* New York: Times Books. *A guide to health strategy based on the author's newspaper columns.*

Butler, K., and Rayner, L. 1990. *The New Handbook of Health and Preventive Medicine.* Buffalo, N.Y.: Prometheus Books. *A comprehensive discussion*

of disease prevention and treatment plus tips on avoiding quackery.

Cornacchia, H., and S. Barrett. 1989. *Consumer Health—A Guide to Intelligent Decisions,* 4th ed. St. Louis: Times-Mirror/Mosby. *A comprehensive guide to the health marketplace.*

Herbert, V., and S. Barrett. 1981. *Vitamins and "Health" Foods: The Great American Hustle.* Philadelphia: Stickley/Lippincott.

Inglis, B., and R. West. 1983. *The Alternative Health Guide.* New York: Knopf. *Seventy "alternative" therapies from the viewpoint of two proponents.*

Jarvis, W. T. *Quackery and You.* 1985. Washington, D.C.: Review and Herald Publishing Association. *A 32-page booklet of basic facts about quackery.*

Contents

Making Connections

Even the healthiest lifestyle can't protect you from the possibility of disability or premature death if you're involved in an accident. Luckily, most accidents are far from "accidental," and there are many things you can do to avoid becoming an accident statistic. The scenarios presented on these pages describe situations in which people have to use information, make a decision, or choose a course of action, all related to accidents and safety. As you read them, imagine yourself in each situation and consider what you would do. After you've finished the chapter, read the scenarios again and see if what you've learned has changed how you would think, feel, or act in each situation.

Your mother-in-law never wears a safety belt in her car or in anyone else's, even though most other people she knows do. She says she doesn't ever want be trapped in a burning car or one that plunges into water. Is she right about the risks? Is it safer to wear a safety belt or not to wear one?

You're driving home from school for Thanksgiving vacation in a freezing rain. As you're negotiating a curve in the road, the rear end of your car starts to fishtail, and then the rear wheels start skidding out to the left. One of your passengers says, "We're skidding—step on the brakes." The other one says, "No, steer into it—turn the wheel to the left." What should you do?

23
Accident Prevention

As you were riding your bike the other day, you came to an intersection with good visibility in all directions. You could see that nothing was coming and intended to ride straight through, but your friend started braking for the stop sign. "It's clear," you call to her. "You don't need to stop." She stopped briefly anyway before continuing through the intersection. Should you have stopped too, or was she being overly careful?

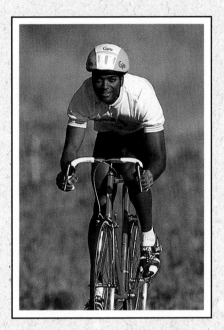

You've been enjoying a visit from your sister and her 2-year-old, who live in another state. While you're sitting out back drinking lemonade and talking, the toddler plays nearby and explores the shrubs and bushes. Suddenly he appears in front of you clutching a fistful of bright orange berries. There are orange stains around his mouth, too, and you realize he's been eating a plant he found in your yard. Your sister jumps up in alarm and asks you what kind of berries they are. You have no idea, but you tell her you're sure there wouldn't be anything dangerous growing in your yard. She's not reassured. Is there some action you should take?

You recently started jogging and have been following a popular jogging path around campus. Most of the route is along walking and bike paths, but in a few places it runs along main roads. You notice that some people jog with the traffic and some jog against it. Why? Which way should you jog?

Accidents are the leading cause of death among all people in the United States aged 1 to 37 and the third leading cause overall, following cardiovascular disease and cancer. Last year alone, the cost of accidents in the United States was over $140 billion. **Motor vehicle accidents** were responsible for nearly 50 percent of this total cost, followed by **work-related accidents** at 33 percent, **home accidents** at 10 percent, and **public accidents** (accidents in public places not involving motor vehicles) at 7 percent.

These figures strongly indicate that accidents are a serious risk for many people and that no one is "immune." The National Traffic Safety Institute, for example, estimates that half of all Americans will be involved in a serious car crash during their lives or have an immediate family member involved in one. Ironically, most people feel safe when they are at work, in their homes, or on the road. Believing that accidents happen to "the other guy," they increase their risks by ignoring safety precautions, taking chances, working at dangerous jobs, or driving under the influence of alcohol or drugs. Males are particularly vulnerable, accounting for about 69 percent of all accidental deaths, but accidental death rates are increasing for women too, as they enter new occupations and begin taking similar risks. Through all the statistics and accident scenarios run the inconsistency and unpredictability of human nature.

Many people these days are more aware of health issues and are taking better care of themselves. But this awareness has to extend to safety too; otherwise improvements in health make little sense. Safety and health go hand in hand, and many of the same sensible attitudes, responsible behaviors, and informed decisions that protect your health can improve your chances of avoiding accidents. This chapter explains how you can protect yourself and those around you from becoming the victims of serious or fatal accidents.

What Causes Accidents?

Have you ever had a series of mishaps and wondered if you were "accident prone"? Have you ever thought there might be some hidden self-destructive streak in yourself or in someone you knew who seemed to have more accidents than other people? This is probably not the case. Accidents occur under certain circumstances rather than to certain people. The term *accident proneness* was coined in 1926 by some researchers who thought that certain personality traits might predispose some people to have more accidents. Sigmund Freud and other early psychiatric investigators believed that accidents resulted from unconscious motivations and hidden desires for self-punishment. Researchers tested these theories for years without finding any strong evidence for them.

■ **Exploring Your Emotions**

Do you know anyone who seems to have more than the average number of accidents? If so, what do you think accounts for this pattern?

Although people with particular personality traits do not necessarily have more accidents, higher accident rates are associated with certain attitudes and behaviors. The **social pathology theory** of accident causation is based on the notion that accidents reflect how much responsibility a person takes for his or her life. Studies indicate that significant relationships exist between accidents and the tendencies to reject social constraints, exert inadequate self-control, disregard the rights and opinions of others, and express hostility and aggression. When people trust to luck or take chances to prove themselves, they tend to have more accidents. When they take more responsibility for their actions, they have fewer accidents.

But what about the vast majority of accidents, in which irresponsible attitudes don't seem to play a part? **Multiple causation theory** proposes that accidents are caused not by a single event or factor but by a combination of human and environmental factors working together in a dynamic interaction. Human factors are inner conditions or attitudes that lead to an unsafe state, whether physical, emotional, or psychological (see Table 23-1). Environmental factors are external conditions and circumstances—poor visibility due to snow or fog, a defective

---

Motor vehicle accidents Injuries and deaths involving motor vehicles in motion, both on and off the highway or street. Examples include collisions between vehicles, collisions with objects, noncollision accidents, and pedestrian accidents.

Work accidents Injuries and deaths that arise out of and in the course of gainful work. Examples include falls, electric shocks, exposure to radiation and toxic chemicals, burns, cuts, back sprains, and loss of fingers or other body parts in machines.

Home accidents Injuries and deaths that occur in the home and on home premises to occupants, guests, domestic servants, and trespassers. Examples include falls, burns, poisonings, suffocations, shootings, drownings, and electric shocks.

Public accidents Injuries and deaths that occur in public places or places used in a public way, not involving motor vehicles. Most sports and recreation deaths and injuries are included. Examples include falls, drownings, shootings, burns, and temperature exposures.

Social pathology theory The notion that accidents reflect a person's attitude toward life.

Multiple causation theory The idea that accidents are caused by several factors that dynamically interact.

V I T A L   S T A T I S T I C S

Accident Facts

Did you know that . . .

- On the average there are 11 accidental deaths and about 1,040 disabling injuries every hour during the year.
- A motor vehicle death occurs every 11 minutes.
- An injury occurs in the home every 9 seconds.

- Nearly 67 percent of all motor vehicle accidents cite improper driving as the error, with speeding being the type most often recorded.
- Use of safety belts can reduce the number of serious injuries by at least 50 percent and the number of fatalities by 60 to 70 percent.

- Drinking alcohol is identified as a factor in 50 to 55 percent of all fatal motor vehicle accidents.

Source: National Safety Council. 1989. *Accident Facts*, (Chicago: National Safety Council).

tool or machine, a child running into a street, a poorly marked curve in a road. According to multiple causation theory, human and environmental factors together create the conditions for an accident.

Human Factors in Accidents   Many different human factors can contribute to accidents. Physically, people have different levels of skill at different activities, and knowing one's own limits is an important step toward safe behavior. Sometimes people have accidents because they try to do something beyond their capabilities, such as riding a bicycle on a busy street or swimming across a lake. People also have natural physical limits in strength, endurance, sensory abilities, and so on. And as people age, physical abilities decline and vision and hearing often become impaired, sometimes without the in-

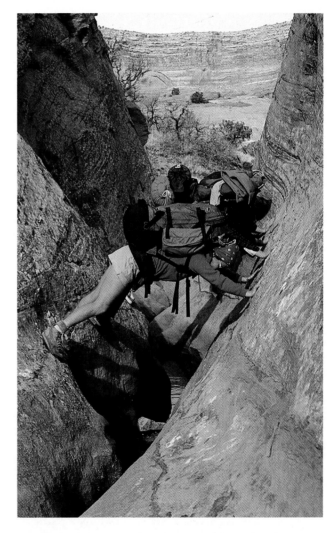

An accurate assessment of one's own physical skills and limitations is an important factor in accident prevention. Many people wouldn't want to try the tricky maneuver these hikers have mastered.

Table 23-1 Examples of human and environmental factors in accidents

Human Factors	Environmental Factors
Physical incapability	Imperfect weather conditions
Poor visual acuity	Overcrowded conditions
Stress and fatigue	Defective equipment
False sense of security	Inadequate law enforcement
Distractibility	Nonsupportive social environment
Lack of knowledge	Inadequate legislation
Poor attitudes	Lack of safety education programs
Bad habits	

dividual's realizing the full extent of impairment. Older people may also have heart irregularities, balance problems, slower reflexes, and other conditions that can contribute to a fall or other type of accident.

■ **Exploring Your Emotions**

When you have an accident, do you ever feel you somehow "willed" it or wanted to get hurt? If so, what is the basis for your feelings?

Physical impairments are also produced by various drugs. Alcohol, a factor in at least half of all auto crashes, affects reason, judgment, and coordination. Marijuana affects perception, reaction time, and coordination. Cocaine initially enhances alertness and then, about twenty minutes later, lets the user down with a resulting loss of attention and judgment. A recent study revealed that almost one out of every four drivers between the ages of 16 and 45 who were killed in automobile accidents in New York City had taken cocaine. About half of those using cocaine had also used alcohol. Even legal drugs, both over-the-counter and prescription medications, can produce dizziness, drowsiness, distorted perceptions, and other potentially dangerous side effects. And, of course, people can be distracted by naturally occurring physical conditions like hunger, physical exhaustion, or illness.

A variety of psychological factors can also play a role in accidents, including knowledge, awareness, attitudes, beliefs, and emotions. Knowledge is critical. People need to know what is safe and what is unsafe, and, surprisingly, this is not always obvious. Sometimes people act on the basis of inadequate or inaccurate information. For example, a person who believes that safety belts trap people in cars when an accident occurs and who consequently decides not to wear a safety belt is acting on an inaccurate belief. No study has shown a higher incidence of injury for accident victims wearing safety belts than for those who don't wear safety belts, yet this misconception persists. Safety belts actually help a person retain control of the vehicle and reduce the likelihood of being thrown out of the car or against an object inside the car and knocked unconscious.

Awareness is another crucial ingredient in accidents and their prevention. Sometimes the potential for a serious accident exists, but a person is unaware of the danger. A person who rides a motorcycle without a helmet, for example, may think safety equipment is unnecessary simply because he or she has never been involved in an accident. The longer the person goes without having an accident, the more the unsafe behavior and beliefs are reinforced. The person may develop a false sense of se-

curity and begin to take even more risks, until eventually the wrong combination of circumstances conspires to produce an accident.

Unsafe attitudes, often based on mistaken beliefs, are another factor in accidents. An unsafe attitude common among many teenagers and young adults comes from the belief that they are special and that bad things happen only to others. They have a "personal fable" about themselves and believe they are exempt, immune, even immortal. They know that drinking impairs their ability to drive, for example, but they think that only other people have accidents. They know that engaging in horseplay around water can be dangerous, but they think that only others get hurt diving into pools. (Other common beliefs are that they can smoke without damaging their lungs and have unprotected sexual intercourse without getting pregnant.) Attitudes like these, by no means limited to adolescents, can lead to risk taking and ultimately to accidents.

■ **Exploring Your Emotions**

Do you have a tendency to blame other people for things that happen to you? Do you ever take risks driving because you consider yourself an excellent driver who can handle virtually any situation?

Emotions and general psychological state also have a part in accidents. When you're angry or tired after work, impatient to finish mowing the lawn so you can watch your favorite television program, or stressed out by worry and lack of sleep, you may be easily distracted and unable to perceive events objectively and clearly. You may act on impulse or make a choice you would never make in a calmer frame of mind. Any or all of these "human, all-too-human" factors may be at work when an accident occurs.

Environmental Factors in Accidents   Environmental factors play important roles in accidents too. They may be natural (weather conditions, an earthquake), societal (stop-and-go traffic, a drunk driver), work-related (defective equipment, unsafe facilities), home-related (throw rugs, faulty wiring), or any of a variety of other dangerous conditions. Although changes in attitude and behavior are crucial to accident prevention, making the environment safer is also an important aspect of safety.

Sometimes, environmental hazards arise when new technological advances create unforeseen and unknown dangers. As knowledge and awareness increase, safety devices are developed and safety measures are introduced that control the dangers inherent in the technology. In

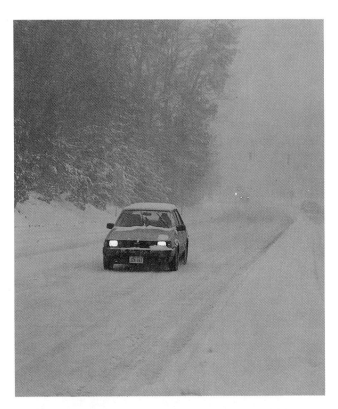

Weather is a crucial environmental factor in motor vehicle accidents. The slippery road surfaces and poor visibility of snow storms require slower, more defensive driving.

some cases, however, people try to outsmart or bypass safety features, particularly in the workplace. They may fail to wear protective clothing because it impedes their movement or is uncomfortable, or they may figure out faster but more dangerous ways to operate machinery. The issue then arises of whether people have the right to act unsafely or whether they can be forced to be safe. In the workplace, employers have the responsibility to enforce safety regulations. In the public arena, laws requiring people to wear safety belts or helmets are based on the belief that the government has the right to enforce a certain level of safety among the members of a society.

When an Accident Occurs   When unsafe states (the human factors) and unsafe conditions (the environmental factors) interact, an accident is very often the result. At a critical moment, the individual must frequently make a decision that influences the outcome of the situation.

If the decision is a good one, the accident may be avoided and the person may learn something from the experience. If the decision is not as good, or if the accident is unavoidable at this point, someone may be injured or killed.

Again, it is important to realize that accidents do not "just happen." In fact, some people question the very definition and concept of "accident," which implies random forces beyond our control. With hindsight, we can almost always pinpoint the internal and external factors that combined to cause an accident. It may be a left-handed worker using a tool designed for the right-handed and beginning a new job without adequate supervision. It may be an inexperienced driver maneuvering a tricky mountain road in a rainstorm. Or it may just be a distracted pedestrian thinking about what to buy for dinner and twisting an ankle on the curb. Knowing that hazards exist in everyday life is in itself an important step toward accident prevention.

Types of Accidents and Ways to Prevent Them

Accidents are generally categorized into four general types—motor vehicle accidents, home accidents, work accidents, and public accidents. The greatest number of accidental deaths occur in motor vehicle accidents, but the greatest number of disabling injuries occur in home accidents (see Table 23-2). In each of these arenas, the action you take can mean the difference between injury or death and no accident at all.

Motor Vehicle Accidents   Nearly three-fourths of all motor vehicle accidents are caused by bad driving; speeding is the most often recorded error. Most people do not truly understand the safety implications of speeding. As speed increases, the motor vehicle's momentum and force of impact increase; simultaneously, the time allowed for the driver to react *decreases*. A car traveling at a speed of 30 miles per hour is traveling at a speed of 44 feet per second! If you are the driver, your **reaction time** must be within three-fourths of a second and you must react correctly in order to stop that vehicle within 80 feet. Moreover, these figures assume that conditions are ideal; wet pavement, decreased visibility, driving under the influence of drugs or when half asleep, and additional

Reaction time   The time it takes for a person to react to what he or she has seen or heard. In a driving situation, the time required for the driver to release the accelerator and apply the brake.

V I T A L S T A T I S T I C S				
Table 23-2 Accidental deaths and injuries in the United States in 1988				
	Deaths	% Change from 1987	Deaths per 100,000 People	Disabling Injuries
Motor vehicle	49,000	+1.0	19.9	1.8 million
Work	10,600	−5.0	4.3	1.8 million
Home	22,500	+5.0	9.2	3.4 million
Public	18,000	+3.0	7.3	2.3 million
All classes*	96,000	+2.0	39.1	9.1 million

Source: National Safety Council. 1989. *Accident Facts.* (Chicago: National Safety Council), p. 3.

*Deaths and injuries for the four separate classes total more than the national figures because of rounding and because some deaths and injuries are included in more than one class.

passengers in your car increase the stopping distance significantly.

Speed limits are posted to establish (1) the safest *maximum* speed limit (2) for a given area (3) under *ideal* conditions. Such laws are meant to enhance safety, not infringe on your driving rights. If you consistently find that you need to speed to get where you're going on time, allow more time for traveling. By leaving ten or fifteen minutes earlier, you can relieve a lot of the pressure and compulsion to speed. Reduced speed also gives you control of your vehicle and increased time to react to any emergency situation.

■ Exploring Your Emotions

Some otherwise mild-mannered people become hostile and aggressive behind the wheel of a car. Does this ever happen to you? If so, what do you think accounts for it?

A second factor that contributes to injury and death in motor vehicle accidents is the decision not to wear safety belts. Most people understand that restraint systems such as safety belts offer protection in an accident. What most people do not realize is that failure to wear them doubles your chances of being hurt in a crash. Using safety belts could reduce the number of serious injuries by at least 50 percent and the number of fatalities by 60 to 70 percent in motor vehicle mishaps. If you use a system that combines a lap and shoulder belt, your chances of survival are three to four times better than a person who rides beltless.

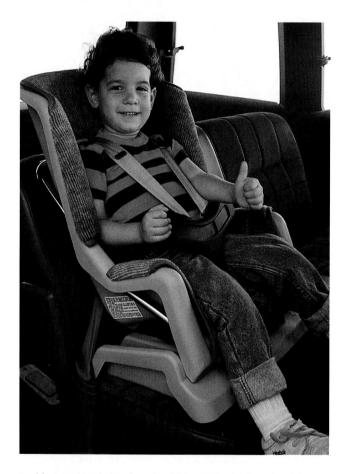

Buckling up is a habit that should begin in childhood and last a lifetime. Many states require special car seats like this one, secured to the seat with the auto safety belt, for children 4 years old or younger.

Second collision The collision that occurs when the occupants of a motor vehicle collide with the car interior and/or are ejected from the vehicle.

Myths about Safety Belts

Myth   If I wore a seat belt, I might get trapped in my car if it caught on fire or were submerged in water.

Fact   In reality, only one-half of 1 percent of motor vehicle accidents involve fire or submersion. If that does happen, safety belts will help prevent you from being knocked unconscious, so you will be able to escape from your car.

Myth   I would be better off if I were thrown clear of the car in a crash.

Fact   The chances of being killed are twenty-five times greater if you're thrown out of the vehicle. Hitting a tree or the pavement causes severe injuries, which wouldn't occur if you stay buckled inside the car. Also, people who are thrown out of their cars are sometimes crushed or hit by their own vehicles or those of others.

Myth   I can brace myself in an accident, so I don't need to bother with a safety belt.

Fact   The force of an impact at just 10 mph can be equivalent to catching a 200-pound bag of cement thrown from a 10-foot ladder. At 35 mph the force of impact is even more brutal. There's no way your arms and legs can brace against that kind of force—even if you could react in time.

Myth   A safety belt couldn't possibly hold me in place during a sudden stop or accident. When I yank it by hand, it doesn't work.

Fact   Most safety belts are designed to automatically lock when the car stops suddenly or changes directions quickly. Belts normally expand and contract to allow freedom of movement.

Myth   I'm not going far or driving fast, so I don't need to wear a safety belt.

Fact   It is wise to wear a safety belt no matter where you are going since 75 percent of all crashes occur within 25 miles of home. Most deaths and injuries (80 percent) occur in automobiles traveling less than 40 mph. People have been killed in accidents at crash speeds of less than 12 mph.

Myth   Pregnant women are not supposed to wear safety belts.

Fact   According to the American Medical Association, both a pregnant woman and her unborn child are much safer with belts than without, provided the lap belt is worn as low as possible on the pelvic area.

Myth   I am a good driver, so I will never be in an accident. I don't need to wear a safety belt.

Fact   Safety belts are the most effective defense against a drunken driver. No matter how well you drive, you can't control what other drivers are going to do. A typical American is almost certain to be involved in a traffic crash during his or her lifetime, according to the University of Michigan's Transportation Research Institute. Regardless of driving skills, everyone faces a one-in-fifty chance of dying and a 50 percent probability of suffering a disabling injury from an auto accident.

Source: *Buckle Up*, 1987, a publication of Traffic Safety Now, Inc., Detroit, Michigan.

Most people who don't use safety belts don't understand their value (see the box "Myths about Safety Belts"). Safety belts work at the time of the "second collision." If a car is traveling at 55 mph and hits another vehicle, first the car must stop and then the occupants must stop because they are also traveling at the same speed. The **second collision** occurs when an occupant hits something inside the car, like the steering column, dashboard, or windshield. Using a safety belt helps prevent that second collision from occurring; the safety belt also spreads the stopping force over the body to reduce the likelihood of injury. (It also keeps occupants from being thrown out of the car.)

People give lots of reasons for not wearing their safety belts. Typical responses include discomfort, lack of mobility, wrinkling of clothes, fear of getting trapped in the car, the belief that safety belts do not work, the admission that safety belt use has not become a habit, and having air bags as an automatic protection device installed in their motor vehicle. All those answers can be easily countered by the facts. It would be wonderful if you could know in advance when you were going to be involved in an accident situation, whether a collision with another car or just stopping suddenly to avoid hitting a child who has run into the street to retrieve a ball. But you can't know in advance. Furthermore, relying on air

Drive Like a Pro

Along with safe cars, safety belts, air bags, and sobriety, driving skills are an important element in motor vehicle safety. Learn to drive defensively, avoiding dangerous situations and reacting intelligently in a crisis. To find out how well you drive already, try this defensive-driving quiz. (Some questions have more than one correct answer.)

1. The safest way to brake is
   a. as fast as possible.
   b. as far in advance as possible.

2. In moderate town traffic, with another car at a safe distance in front of you, you're being tailgated. What do you do?
   a. Tap the brakes and start to slow down—gradually, keeping an eye on the rearview mirror.
   b. Increase your speed to the allowable limit.
   c. Try to pass the car in front of you.
   d. Pull over to the right.

3. You're heading toward a green light at an intersection. A woman (not in the crosswalk and walking against the light) steps off the curb and starts across without looking. Your first move is to
   a. sound the horn but don't give in. A little scare will do her good.
   b. change lanes to avoid her.
   c. begin braking, anticipating a full stop if necessary, and sound the horn.

4. Preparing to change lanes on a multilane highway, which of the following should you do?
   a. Check your rearview mirror.
   b. Check your side mirror.
   c. Take your eyes off the road momentarily and glance at the lane you're planning to move into.

d. Turn on your directional signal.
e. Be aware of what traffic in front of you is doing.

5. You've swerved to the right to avoid a collision on a two-way highway, and your right wheels drop off the pavement and are riding on the shoulder. To get back on the road you
   a. accelerate, cutting the wheel to the left.
   b. don't brake, but take your foot off the accelerator. Hold the wheel steady. When the car slows, check the traffic and steer back onto the pavement.
   c. brake sharply and try to pull off the road altogether. When you've got the car under control, pull onto the road again.

6. On a two-way highway, in what's clearly marked as a no-pass zone with limited visibility, a car pulls out to pass you, and you wonder if he's going to make it. Your best move is to
   a. speed up, hoping he'll duck behind you.
   b. ignore him—it's his problem.
   c. reduce your speed so he can get around you faster.

7. The most important factor in defensive driving is
   a. quick reflexes.
   b. anticipating trouble.
   c. skill at vehicle handling.
   d. strict observation of the law.

8. You're most likely to go into a skid
   a. in a steady downpour.
   b. in the first few minutes of a light rain.

9. Which of the following road conditions up ahead should tell you to reduce your speed?

a. A deep pothole.
b. Leaves on the pavement.
c. Any bridge, when the temperature is just above freezing.

10. Your car is skidding (see diagram). What's the safest reaction?

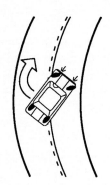

a. Turn the wheel to the right.
b. Turn the wheel to the left.
c. Brake as hard as possible and avoid turning the wheel until you've stopped the car.

11. In two-way highway traffic, an oncoming car suddenly pulls into your lane. What action do you take?
   a. Brake hard and sound your horn.
   b. Move quickly into the left lane.
   c. Blow your horn, and head to the shoulder.

12. The best position for your hands on the steering wheel is
   a. at 10 and 2 o'clock position.
   b. at 8 and 4 o'clock.
   c. wherever you're most comfortable.
   d. at 9 and 3 o'clock.

13. True or false: Underinflated tires are safer, particularly in hot weather.

Drive Like a Pro (continued)

14. You realize you're heading into a curve too fast. Therefore you should
   a. brake sharply.
   b. brake gradually.
   c. avoid braking but take your foot off the accelerator.

Answers

1. (b) A basic principle of defensive driving is never to get into a situation that calls for slamming on the brakes. This can throw you into a skid and injure you and your passengers. Good braking technique: pump the brakes, reapplying as you come to a full stop. However, according to Professor Donald Smith, Highway Traffic Safety Program, Michigan State University, if you are forced to brake fast and have disc brakes, "threshold" braking is the best technique: push the brake just short of locking and hold it there.

2. (a) and **(d)**, depending on circumstances. If the tailgater is daydreaming, tapping your brakes (and activating the brake lights) should wake him up. If he's being aggressive, you've politely signaled him to let up. If he doesn't stop tailgating, pull over as soon as you can and let him pass.

3. (c) Always yield the right of way to pedestrians, even when they're in the wrong. Let them know you're there. A diversionary swerve could put you in the path of an oncoming car. Also, pedestrians might dart into your path.

4. (all) All steps are essential, but some people forget (c). You always have a blind spot (about a car length behind you on either side) and may not be able to see an overtaking vehicle in either mirror. Always glance over your shoulder before making your move. The signal light (turned on several seconds in advance) will help protect you as well.

5. (b) Braking hard or jerking the wheel can cause you to skid into oncoming traffic. Don't brake but do reduce your speed and stay on a steady course. Then, after checking traffic, make a sharp quarter turn to the left to put yourself back on the road, then straighten out.

6. (c) Passing is always a cooperative venture. If this reckless driver has a head-on collision, you might be hurt, too.

7. (b) Obeying the law and vehicle-handling skills are all important. But anticipating trouble up ahead, and acting to prevent it, can make the speed of your reflexes far less important and thus may prevent many collisions.

8. (b) A little water plus the oil and dirt on the road form a slick film. A heavy rain will wash it clean. Be extra careful during the first half hour of a rainfall.

9. (all) The pothole may only jar you, but it could damage your car or even cause you to lose control. Leaves can send you into a skid. And even though there's no ice on the road, a bridge is about 6° F colder than a highway and may be hazardous when the road is not.

10. (b) Turn the wheel straight down your lane. That is, if your rear wheels are skidding left, as in the diagram, turn with the skid—that is, to the left. Don't brake, as this increases skidding.

11. (c) Don't move left, which could put you in someone else's pathway. Always move right when heading off the road.

12. (d) And some expert drivers recommend that you hook your thumbs lightly over the horizontal spokes. This gives you a feel for the front tires and is a good way to get a quick grip if you strike a pothole.

13. False. An underinflated tire is more likely to skid, whether in hot weather or on wet or icy pavement. Because underinflation allows a tire to "flap" slightly and thus to create more heat, it's also likelier to blow out. Even for desert driving, keep tires at the recommended maximum air pressure, and check them weekly. The number should be printed on the side of the tires; or check the instruction manual if the car still has its original tires.

14. (b) Take your foot off the accelerator, and brake before you get into the curve, but gradually release brakes as you get into it. Once you're rounding the curve, accelerate. This will help you steer safely around it and onto the straightaway.

Adapted from Driving like the pros, *University of California, Berkeley, Wellness Letter*, October 1989.

bags is not the solution because they encourage a "false sense of security." Currently, most cars equipped with air bags are designed to provide protection only in frontal collisions (not side, rear, or rollover crashes). Since air bags deflate immediately after detonation, they are also less effective in multiple collisions. Air bags are most effective when used in combination with safety belts. Developing the habit of buckling up puts you one step ahead. Taking three seconds for that one click can mean the difference, but you must take *responsibility* for that decision. Safety belts save lives—it's as simple as that.

Another major cause of motor vehicle accidents is the unsafe behavior of drinking and driving. As mentioned earlier, alcohol is identified as a factor in at least half of all fatal motor vehicle accidents. Alcohol-impaired driving is illegal in all states because it threatens the health and safety of many people, both directly and indirectly. People who have a few drinks at a party may feel relaxed and less inhibited initially, but alcohol works to depress the central nervous system and slow down body functions. It affects the brain first in terms of reason and caution, then in terms of judgment, and finally in terms of motor skills. Unfortunately, most people do not realize what is happening to them until they reach the third phase of motor skill impairment. The impaired person who continues to drive is not in control and is taking a major risk. The same is true of the other psychoactive drugs. (Refer to Chapters 10 and 11 for full discussions of the effect of all these substances on users.)

The environment is another factor that affects motor vehicle accidents. Weather is an obvious problem, because of its unpredictability. When weather deteriorates, you must drive more defensively. You need to increase the distance at which you follow another car in traffic and reduce speed to compensate for hazards. Of course, you also need to have your car in good working order. People typically take care of the obvious needs like tires, gas, and oil, but it's easy to forget the simple things like replacing windshield wipers, at least until it starts to rain and you find out they don't work. Regular inspection and maintenance checks make sense if you expect your vehicle to perform well.

Road type and location also influence the likelihood of injury or fatality in an accident. Many people travel on rural highways because they think they can drive at faster speeds without getting caught. Consequently, the fatality rates on rural highways are much higher. Contrary to common belief, interstate highways are much safer for a number of reasons; for example, visibility is increased, all travel is in one direction, and fewer incidents require driving adjustments. If you have a choice, it makes more sense to travel on the interstate. Moreover, about 75 percent of all motor vehicle accidents occur within 25 miles of home, where the driver is probably more familiar with the driving terrain and on roadways with speed limits of less than 40 miles per hour. Often the driver mistakenly believes that safety measures are not warranted for a quick trip to the store or for a short ride of a few blocks to a friend's house. The facts prove otherwise.

Home Accidents   Contrary to common belief, one of the most dangerous places to be is at home. One obvious reason is that many people spend a major portion of their day at home, often alone. The majority of deaths in the home involve accidents classified as falls, fires and burn-related accidents, poisoning by solids and liquids, and suffocation by ingested objects.

■ **Exploring Your Emotions**

Have you ever had a serious accident? What were the contributing factors? How did it change your feelings and behavior about safety?

Falls are second only to motor vehicle accidents in terms of causing deaths. About 85 percent of the fatal falls involve people 45 years of age and older, but falls are the fifth leading cause of accidental death for all people under 25 years of age. Most falls occur as a result of common activities in the home, with nearly two-thirds of the deaths occurring from falls at floor level rather than at a height. In most cases it is the person's difficulty in adjusting to different degrees of traction, rather than the slipperiness of the surface, that causes the fall. A rug, a bathtub, or some characteristic of the floor itself is often a factor in falls in the home. Large rugs tend to be safer, but small rugs can be used if they have cork or rubber backing to help reduce slippage. Waxed floors should be avoided, since they can be dangerously slippery, and toys and other objects on the floor, which create tripping hazards, should be picked up. Falls in the bathroom can be prevented by using nonslip applications on the bottom of the tub or shower and installing handrails on the walls. Outside the house, dangerous surfaces created by ice, snow, or rough ground should be alleviated for your own safety and that of your guests.

Ladders and stairs are also common sources of accidents in the home. People tend to get hurt using the stairs when the lighting is poor, a firm handrail for support is missing, or inappropriate footwear is worn. All of these potential problems are correctable. Height also becomes a concern when people stand on chairs or unstable objects rather than using stepladders or stepstools. When you use a stepladder, make sure the spreader brace is in the locked position and never stand higher than the third step from the top. If you use a straight ladder the "4 to 1" rule (setting the ladder base out one foot for every

Special Precautions for the Young and Old

Anyone can have an accident, but the very young and the very old are at special risk. Babies and children—especially inquisitive, irrepressible toddlers—easily get in trouble when the environment hasn't been adapted to their needs and limitations. About 4,000 children under 4 years of age die in accidents each year in the United States, the victims of falls, burns, chokings, poisonings, and a variety of other dangers. Follow these guidelines to protect children in your home:

- Never leave a baby unattended on a bed or table or in a crib with the side down. Even newborns can move reflexively and plunge over the edge.
- Place gates at the tops and bottoms of stairs and in doorways to areas that are off limits to children. Place barriers around stoves, floor grates, and radiators.
- Keep all medicines, poisons, and household chemicals in locked cabinets or places inaccessible to children. Buy medicines in the smallest available quantity, and keep purses out of children's reach.
- When driving, strap infants and toddlers into government-tested car seats. Never hold a child in your lap while a car is moving.
- Keep small objects out of reach of children under age 3, and don't give them raw carrots, hot dogs, nuts, popcorn, or hard candy. Balloons pose a serious choking hazard for young children.
- Inspect toys carefully for small parts that could come loose and be put in the mouth.
- Inspect hand-me-down furniture to make sure it's free of lead-based paint and other hazards, such as spaces where a child's head could become stuck.
- Set your hot water heater no higher than 120°F and keep children out of the kitchen where they might be burned by spills.
- Use plastic covers over electrical outlets.
- Keep the number of the poison control center near your telephone, and keep a bottle of ipecac syrup on hand to induce vomiting if so instructed by the poison center or a physician.

At the opposite end of the spectrum, the elderly are also vulnerable to accidents, especially accidental falls. Every year, about a quarter of all people over age 70 take a fall, many of them serious enough to require hospitalization. Of those hospitalized, only half regain their former level of independence. The most severe common injury from a fall is a hip fracture; about 170,000 people over age 65 suffer hip fractures ever year in the United States.

Elderly people are at risk for falls for a variety of reasons. May have become unsteady on their feet or have impaired vision, hearing, memory, mental status, or mobility. Some suffer from arthritis, osteoporosis, or inner ear problems that affect balance. In some cases, medications cause problems, such as incoordination, weakness, light-headedness, or dizziness. Often, accidents occur from a combination of infirmity and environmental hazards—poor vision and dim lighting, weak legs and ill-fitting shoes, uncertain balance and a loose rug.

Up to half of all falls can be prevented with some practical changes in the home environment. The following guidelines can help you make your home a safer place:

- Be sure stairs are well lighted and have secure bannisters or handrails. Bright tape applied to the first and last steps can help a person with a vision problem.
- Cover raised thresholds in doorways with carpet. Fasten area rugs to the floor with tape or tacks and avoid throw rugs. Keep electrical cords out of the way. Keep objects off the floor.
- Put a light switch by the door of every room so no one has to cross a dark room to turn on a light. Avoid placing furniture where it obstructs a path across a room or creates a hazard.
- Put a nonskid mat near the bathtub and another near the toilet. Install handrails by the tub so no one will be tempted to grab onto a towel bar.
- Use nonskid floor wax, and wipe up floor spills immediately.
- Keep furniture, floors, stairs, and walkways in good repair.

The best protection against a fall is to be in good overall health. Studies show that elderly people who recover most rapidly from a fall are in good physical condition before the accident. It makes sense then not only to improve environmental conditions but also to encourage people to take care of themselves at all stages of life.

Adapted from Judy Schickedanz, Karen Hansen, and Peggy Forsyth, 1989, *Understanding Children* (Mountain View, Calif.: Mayfield); Preventing falls at home, *Mayo Clinic Health Letter,* March 1988; and All fall down, *Harvard Medical School Health Letter,* December 1989.

Home maintenance offers endless opportunities for accidents, especially for older people. This man may be used to doing repairs around the house and not be aware of changes in his physical capabilities.

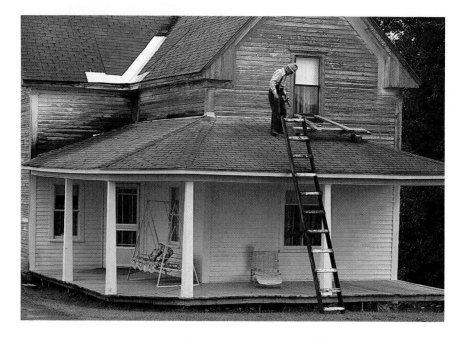

four feet of height) is also a safe procedure to follow. When using a ladder you should use both hands when climbing and not reach too far to either side.

Fires pose another safety problem in the home. Most people do not really appreciate or understand the dangers associated with fires. To burn a fire requires (1) a source of ignition, (2) fuel, and (3) oxygen. If any one component can be eliminated, fire can be prevented. Each year approximately 80 percent of fire deaths and 65 percent of fire injuries occur in the home. Fire ignition of furniture, combustible liquid or gas, and bedding account for 60 percent of the cases. Two-thirds of all home fires begin in the living room and bedroom. Many are caused by careless actions such as smoking in bed or leaving a cigarette burning in an ashtray.

Most people are inadequately prepared to handle fire-related situations, especially those in the home. Such preparation includes planning escape routes, installing fire and smoke detection devices at every floor level of the home, and practice using fire-extinguishing devices. You should not wait until the time of a fire emergency to consider such actions. When a fire does occur, the important point to remember is to get out of the house as quickly and safely as possible.

Since smoke is the largest single cause of death and injury in fires, you should also know how to avoid smoke inhalation. The simplest method is to crawl along the floor away from the heat and smoke and cover your mouth, ideally with a wet cloth. If trapped in a burning building, signal for help with a white cloth. If you must try to extinguish a fire, you should be aware that fires are classified into four categories—Class A (wood, cloth, and paper), Class B (flammable liquids such as greases,

gasoline, and lubricating oils), Class C (electrical equipment), and Class D (combustible metals). Fire extinguishers labeled "ABC" are effective against the three kinds of fire you're likely to encounter in your home and are available in many stores.

Accidental poisonings pose another health and safety threat in the home. Statistics reveal that the home is the site for about 80 percent of the deaths by poisonous solids and liquids and over 60 percent from poisonous gases and vapors. A majority of the cases involve children under age 5, although the 15–24 and 25–44 age groups have shown increased death rates in recent years. Over 2 million poisonings occur every year, with about 90 percent due to accidental exposures. Poisons come in many forms and are not harmful in every case. For example, medications are safe when used as prescribed, but overdoses and incorrectly combining medications with another substance may result in accidental poisoning.

Your home may contain a multitude of potentially poisonous substances (see Table 23-3). Solid and liquid forms include medications (aspirin, prescriptions, vitamins and minerals, and over-the-counter drugs), cleaning agents (furniture polish, oven cleaner, bleach, toilet bowl cleaners, and detergents), petroleum-based products (kerosene, gasoline, and antifreeze), insecticides and herbicides, other household items (cosmetics, nail polish and remover, room deodorizers, and floor polishes), and poisonous plants (see Table 23-4). The most common type of poisoning by gases is due to carbon monoxide poisoning, such as that emitted by motor vehicle exhaust. Other types commonly result from improper ventilation and incomplete combustion involving furnaces, kerosene heaters, and cooking appliances.

What Should You Do in Case of Poisoning?

Millions of poisonings occur in the United States every year, most of them involving small children. Do you know what to do if someone in your home is poisoned? The single most important step you can take to prevent a poisoning injury or death is to go to the telephone book right now, look up the Poison Control Center located in your area, and write the number down where you will be able to find it in an emergency. Poison Control Centers exist in many areas of the United States to provide immediate and authoritative advice on how to handle poisonings. They are staffed by poisoning specialists who answer the telephone twenty-four hours a day, seven days a week. If you cannot locate a Poison Control Center, write down the number of the nearest hospital emergency room, physician, or paramedic service.

If you are faced with a case of poisoning, take the following emergency steps and then call the poison center or, preferably, have somone else call the poison center while you stay with the victim.

• Swallowed poison

1. Do *not* follow emergency instructions on labels of containers; they may be old or incorrect.

2. Give water immediately, except in these important cases: the person is unconscious, having convulsions, or cannot swallow; you don't know what the person swallowed; the person swallowed a strong acid or alkali (toilet bowl cleaner, rust remover, chlorine bleach, dishwasher detergent, etc.) or a petroleum product (kerosene, gasoline, furniture polish, lighter fluid, paint thinner, etc.)

• Inhaled poison

1. Get the person to fresh air immediately.

2. Open doors and windows.

• Poison on the skin

1. Remove contaminated clothing and flood skin with water for 10 minutes.

2. Wash skin gently with soap and water and rinse.

• Poison in the eye

1. Flood the eye with lukewarm water poured from a glass held 2 or 3 inches from the eye. Continue for fifteen minutes.

2. Have the person blink as much as possible while flooding the eye. Do not force the eyelid open.

When you contact the poison control center, be prepared to provide the following information: (1) the age and weight of the victim; (2) the name of the product involved; (3) how much was taken; and (4) when it was taken. The poison specialist may recommend that you induce vomiting. Keep a bottle of syrup of ipecac on hand in your home for this purpose. Syrup of ipecac is a harmless substance (except, of course, that it makes you vomit) available at your pharmacy. The poison center will tell you what dose to give. Do not induce vomiting unless instructed to do so; some products do more damage to the throat, esophagus, or lungs if they are vomited. If the person vomits, keep his or her head lower than the rest of the body so that choking on the vomit doesn't create another emergency.

If the victim is unconscious, maintain an open airway by tipping the head back or turning the person on his or her side. If the victim is having convulsions, loosen tight clothing but do not attempt to restrain him or her. In either of these cases, seek medical attention immediately by calling the paramedics, ambulance, fire department, or other rescue personnel for transportation to the hospital. Take the poison container with you to the hospital for inspection.

When someone has been poisoned, an immediate response can make the difference between life and death. Be sure that you know what to do, whom to call, and where to go before you find yourself in an emergency situation. More important, poison-proof your home and educate the members of your household, including small children, so that poisonings don't occur in the first place.

Adapted from *Emergency Action for Poisoning*, Central-Coast Counties Regional Poison Control Center, 751 S. Bascom Ave., San Jose, Calif. 95128.

Table 23-3 Chemical hazards in the home

Product	Possible Hazards	Disposal Suggestions	Precautions and Substitutes
Aerosols	When sprayed, contents are broken into particles small enough to be inhaled. Cans may explode or burn.	Put *only* empty cans in trash. Do not burn. Do not place in trash compactor.	Store in cool place. Propellant may be flammable. Instead: use nonaerosol products.
Batteries: mercury button type	Swallowing one may be fatal if it leaks. *Toxicity 5**	Throw in trash.	No substitutes.
Bleach: chlorine	Fumes irritate eyes. Corrosive to eyes and skin. Poisonous if swallowed. *Toxicity 3**	Use up according to label instructions.	*Never mix with ammonia!* Instead: use nonchlorine bleach or other laundry additive, sunlight, lemon juice.
Detergent cleaners	All are corrosive to some degree. Eye irritant. Toxicity varies. *Toxicity 2–4**	Use up according to label instructions or give away. May be diluted and washed down sink.	Instead: use the mildest product suitable for your needs. Liquid dishwashing detergent is mildest, laundry detergent is moderate, automatic dishwasher detergent is harshest.
Disinfectants	Eye and skin irritant. Fumes irritating. Poisonous if swallowed. *Toxicity 3–4**	Use up according to label instructions or dilute and pour down drain.	Some may contain bleach, others ammonia—*Do not mix!* Instead: use detergent cleaners whenever possible.
Drain cleaners	Very corrosive. May be fatal if swallowed. Contact with eyes can cause blindness.	Use up according to label instructions.	Prevention best; keep sink strainers in good condition. Instead: use plunger, plumber's snake, vinegar and baking soda followed by boiling water.
Flea powders, sprays, and shampoos	Moderately to very poisonous. *Toxicity 2–4**	Use up or save for hazardous waste collection day.	*Do not use dog products on cats.* Vacuum house regularly and thoroughly. Launder pet bedding frequently.
Insect and pest sprays	All are poisonous, some extremely so. May cause damage to kidneys, liver, or central nervous system. Toxicity varies from product to product.	Use very carefully and according to label instructions. Save for hazardous waste collection day.	Instead: do not attract insects; keep all food securely covered, practice good sanitation in kitchen and bathrooms, remove trash every night.
Medicines: unneeded or expired	Frequently cause child poisonings	Flush down sink or toilet.	Check contents of medicine chest regularly. Old medications may lose their effectiveness but not necessarily their toxicity.
Metal polishes	May be flammable. Mildly to very poisonous. *Toxicity 2–4**	Use up according to label instructions or give away.	Use only in well-ventilated area. Instead: substitute vinegar and salt or use baking soda on damp sponge.
Mothballs	Some are flammable. Eye and skin irritant, poisonous, may cause anemia in some individuals.	Use up according to label instructions or give away.	Do not use in living areas. Air out clothing and other items before use. Clean items before storage. Instead: use cedar shavings or aromatic herbs.

Product	Possible Hazards	Disposal Suggestions	Precautions and Substitutes
Oven cleaner	Corrosive. Very harmful if swallowed. Irritating vapors. Can cause eye damage. *Toxicity 2–4**	Use up according to label instructions or give away. Save for hazardous waste collection day.	Do not use aerosols, which can explode and are difficult to control. Instead: use paste. Or heat over to 200 degrees, turn off, leave small dish of ammonia in oven overnight, then wipe oven with damp cloth and baking soda. Do not put baking soda on heating elements.
Toilet bowl cleaner	Corrosive. May be fatal if swallowed. *Toxicity 3–4**	Use up according to label instructions or wash down the sink or toilet with lots of water.	Ventilate room. Instead: use ordinary cleanser or detergent and baking soda.
Window cleaner	Vapor may be irritating. Slightly poisonous. *Toxicity 2**	Use up according to label instructions or give away.	Ventilate room. Instead: spray on vinegar, then wipe dry with newsprint.
Wood cleaners, polishes, and waxes	Fumes irritating to eyes. Product harmful if swallowed. Eye and skin irritant. Petroleum types are flammable.	Use up according to label instructions or save for hazardous waste collection day.	Do not use aerosols. Use only in well-ventilated areas. Instead: use lemon oil or beeswax.

*General Toxicity Ratings

Number rating	1	2	3	4	5	6
Toxicity rating	Almost nontoxic	Slightly toxic	Moderately toxic	Very toxic	Extremely toxic	Super toxic
Lethal dose for 150 lb. adult	More than 1 quart	1 pint to 1 quart	1 ounce to 1 pint	1 teaspoon to 1 ounce	7 drops to 1 teaspoon	Less than 7 drops

Source: *National Safety Council*

Work Accidents   Since 1912, when industrial records were first kept in the United States, the work site has become a much safer place, as evidenced by a reduction in the accidental death rate of nearly 76 percent. That figure becomes even more impressive when one realizes that the size of the work force has more than doubled and production has increased more than tenfold. One very significant factor to account for such a marked decline in accidents has been the Occupational Safety and Health Act of 1970. As a result of that act, the Occupational Safety and Health Administration (OSHA) was created within the U.S. Department of Labor to ensure a safer and healthier environment for workers. Inspections, more detailed recordkeeping, and penalties for noncompliance have probably been most responsible for the changes.

■ **Exploring Your Emotions**

How do you feel about safety devices on appliances and tools? Do you ever try to circumvent them?

Laborers have the occupation with the highest risk of injury or illness. Although laborers make up less than half of the work force, they account for over 75 percent of all work-related injuries and illnesses. Such jobs usually involve extensive manual labor and lifting, neither of which is addressed in OSHA safety standards. Consequently, back problems are the most frequently cited injury and account for over 20 percent of work injuries. For guidelines on safe lifting techniques, see the box "Protect Your Back When Lifting." Skin disorders account

Table 23-4 Common poisonous plants

This list of easily accessible poisonous plants in one or more regions of the United States is not exhaustive. There are many more plants that cause serious or fatal poisoning when ingested, especially by children.

FLOWER GARDEN PLANTS

Plant	Toxic Part	Symptoms
Azalea	All parts	Produces nausea and vomiting, depression, difficult breathing. May be fatal.
Daffodil, Narcissus	Bulb	Nausea, vomiting, diarrhea. May be fatal.
Delphinium	Seeds, young plants	Stomach upset, nervous excitement or depression if eaten in large quantities. Toxicity decreases with age of plant.
Foxglove	Leaves, seeds	One of the sources of the drug digitalis, used to stimulate the heart. In large amounts, causes dangerously irregular heartbeat and pulse, usually digestive upset and mental confusion. May be fatal.
Hyacinth	Bulb	Nausea, vomiting, diarrhea. May be fatal.
Iris (Blue Flag)	Underground stems	Severe, but not usually serious, digestive upset.
Jonquil	Bulb	Nausea, vomiting, diarrhea. Convulsions and death if eaten in large quantities.
Larkspur	Seeds, young plants	Digestive upset, nervous excitement, depression. May be fatal.
Lily-of-the-valley	Leaves, flowers	Irregular heartbeat and pulse, usually accompanied by digestive upset and mental confusion.
Morning glory	Seeds	Produce LSD-like effects but can cause death from severe mental disturbances.
Oleander	Leaves, branches	Dizziness, nausea, irregular heartbeat. May be fatal.
Peony	Roots	Juice can cause paralysis.

VEGETABLE GARDEN PLANTS

Plant	Toxic Part	Symptoms
Potato	All green parts	Cardiac depression. May be fatal.
Rhubarb	Leaf blade	Kidney damage. Large amounts of raw or cooked leaves can cause convulsions, coma, followed rapidly by death.
Tomato	Green parts	Cardiac depression. May be fatal.

HOUSE PLANTS

Plant	Toxic Part	Symptoms
Caladium	Leaves, roots	Irritation of mouth, tongue, and throat. Difficult breathing, nausea, vomiting, and diarrhea.
Castor bean	Seeds	Burning of mouth and throat, excessive thirst, convulsions. One or two seeds are near the lethal dose for adults.
Dumbcane (Dieffenbachia)	All parts	Intense burning and irritation of the mouth and tongue. Death can occur if base of tongue swells enough to block the air passage of the throat.
Elephant ear philodendron	All parts	Intense burning and irritation of mouth and tongue. Death can occur if base of tongue swells enough to block the air passage of the throat.
Mistletoe	Berries	Acute stomach and intestinal irritation with diarrhea and slow pulse. May be fatal.
Poinsettia	Leaves/stems	Severe irritation to mouth, throat, and stomach.

ORNAMENTAL PLANTS

Plant	Toxic Part	Symptoms
Golden chain	Beanlike capsules in which seeds are suspended	Severe poisoning. Excitement, staggering, convulsions, nausea, and coma. May be fatal.
Lantana (Red sage, wild sage)	Green berries	Affects lungs, kidneys, heart, and nervous system. Grows in southern U.S. and in moderate climates. May be fatal.
Magnolia	Flower	Headache and depression.
Rhododendron (Western azalea)	All parts	Nausea, vomiting, depression, difficult breathing, prostration, and coma. May be fatal.
Wisteria	Seeds, pods	Mild to severe digestive upset.
Yellow jessamine	Berries	Digestive disturbance and nervous symptoms. May be fatal.
Yew	All parts, except fleshy red pulp of fruit	Foliage more toxic than berries. Convulsions with rapid death.

TREES AND SHRUBS

Plant	Toxic Part	Symptoms
Apple	Seeds	In quantity (50 or more), cyanide poisoning. May be fatal.
Black locust	Bark, sprouts, foliage, seeds	Children have suffered nausea, weakness, and depression after chewing the bark and seeds.
Cherry	Leaves, twigs, seeds	Contains a compound that releases cyanide when eaten. Difficult breathing, excitement, paralysis of voice, and prostration. May be fatal.
Elderberry	All parts, especially roots	Nausea and digestive upset.
Oak	Foliage, acorns	Affects kidneys gradually. Symptoms appear only after several days or weeks. Takes a large amount for poisoning.
Peach	Leaves, twigs, seeds	Contains a compound that releases cyanide when eaten. Difficult breathing, excitement, paralysis of voice, and prostration. May be fatal.

WILD PLANTS

Plant	Toxic Part	Symptoms
Buttercup	All parts	Irritant juices may severely injure the digestive system.
Jack-in-the-pulpit	All parts	Intense irritation and burning of mouth and tongue.
Jimson weed (Thorn apple)	All parts	Abnormal thirst, distorted sight, delirium, incoherence, and coma. May be fatal.
Mushrooms (Fly agaric and amanita)	All parts	Stomach cramps, thirst, difficult breathing. Fatal. *Avoid all wild mushrooms unless positive of their identity.*
Nightshade	All parts	Intense digestive disturbances and nervous symptoms. May be fatal.
Poison hemlock	All parts	Digestive disturbances. May be fatal.
Poison ivy, oak, sumac	All parts	Itching, burning, redness.
Skunk cabbage	Leaves, rhizomes	Burning and swelling of mouth, tongue, and throat. Large quantities may cause stomach and intestinal irritation.

Source: Adapted from *Poisonous Parts of Common House and Garden Plants*, Central-Coast Counties Regional Poison Control Center, 751 S. Bascom Ave., San Jose, Calif. 95128.

TACTICS AND TIPS

Protect Your Back When Lifting

Almost everyone has to lift a heavy object at one time or another. Doing it the right way can protect your back from serious injury. Follow these simple rules:

- Know your own strength and don't try to lift beyond it. Get help if necessary.
- Avoid bending at the waist. Try to remain in an upright—but not stiffly straight—position. If you need to lower yourself to grasp the object, crouch down. Bending at the knees and hips rather than at the waist is the key to safe lifting.
- Get a firm footing, with feet about shoulder width apart. Get a firm grip on the object with the palms of your hands. If the object or your hands are slippery, wipe them off.

- Lift gradually, keeping your arms straight. Avoid quick, jerky motions, which put a strain on your muscles. Lift by standing up or by pushing up with your leg muscles.
- Don't twist. Twisting is a common and dangerous cause of injury when you're moving something. If you have to turn with the object, change the position of your feet.

- Keep the object close to your body. Your ability to lift safely will be greatly increased.
- Put the object down gently, reversing the rules for lifting.
- Plan ahead. Make sure doors are open and your pathway is clear before you pick up the object.

Back injuries are among the most common, painful, and long-lasting of all the injuries you can sustain. If you hurt your back when you're young, you may have a "bad back" your whole life. It pays to take precautions to make sure your back will be there when you need it.

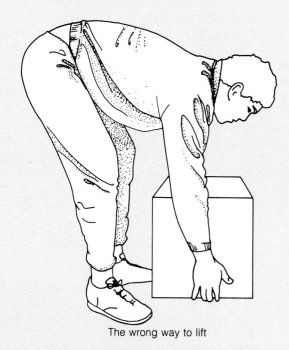

The wrong way to lift

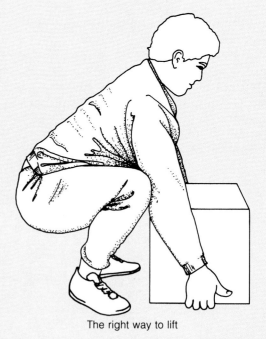

The right way to lift

for nearly 40 percent of occupational illnesses reported. These disorders are becoming an increasing concern due to the introduction of more chemicals and hazardous materials at the work site. A third area of concern is the worker's experience. Data show that more than 40 percent of work-related injuries and illnesses involve workers on the first year of a job. More advanced technology is making many jobs more demanding and increasing the need for training and education programs for workers.

Public Accidents   Public accidents are defined as injuries and deaths that occur in public places not involving a motor vehicle. Most sports and recreational accidents are included in this category. The death rate from public accidents has declined by 73 percent in the United States since 1912. Falls are the primary cause of death in public accidents, followed by drownings. The highest number of drownings occur in the 15–44 age group, with rates higher than average for all age groups under 25 years of age. Over 80 percent of all public drowning victims are males and involve swimming or playing in the water. Most drownings can be attributed to a person's lack of swimming skill, being chilled by water whose temperature is less than 70°F, and/or excessive consumption of alcohol. Swimming alone is irresponsible and can obviously lead to problems if help is needed. All these factors can be countered by education, increased awareness of the associated dangers, and increased individual responsibility for taking precautions.

Jogging is another popular recreational activity that can be made safer by following a few simple precautions. Risks associated with jogging include cramps, exhaustion, and heatstroke (see the box "Avoiding Heat Stress"). The greatest danger facing a jogger is motor vehicles. Surprisingly, most jogging accidents involve more "experienced" runners, many of whom believe they deserve to be part of the traffic flow and have equal rights to share the roadway.

To be safe, joggers should avoid busy roadways whenever possible, but if that isn't possible, they should at least run against the flow of traffic rather than with it. They should also avoid running when visibility is poor, wear bright, light-colored, or reflective clothing, and not use stereo headphones, which can block out sounds and distract the user from hazards.

Pedestrian safety is another area of personal concern. Each year about 18 percent of all motor vehicle deaths involve pedestrians and another 100,000 people are injured each year as a result of such accidents. As would be expected, most pedestrian accidents occur in urban settings. The young and the elderly are involved most often, but it is important to note that alcohol contributes to nearly 25 percent of the adult pedestrian deaths. The most unsafe pedestrian behavior is crossing between streets or intersections, whether walking or darting into traffic. Poor decision making accounts for the biggest problem, not the traffic situation itself.

Pedestrian safety can be improved by following the guidelines given for joggers, as well as by crossing at the corner in designated walk areas and not darting into traffic. Hitchhiking places a person in a potentially dangerous situation. Drivers have difficulty seeing pedestrians and joggers, especially after dark, unless they are wearing very light-colored clothing and/or are carrying an object that reflects light. Pedestrians, joggers, and drivers all need to accept responsibility for safety.

Bicycling is now popular with over 125 million people, ranging from preschoolers to the elderly, who ride them for transportation, recreation, and fitness. As more riders have entered the traffic flow, more accidental deaths and injuries have occurred. Research indicates that these accidents are primarily the result of not knowing or misunderstanding of the rules of the road, failure to follow laws and ordinances, and/or inexperience and lack of skill in traffic conditions. A bicyclist can improve the safety situation by first of all realizing that bicycles are legally considered vehicles that must obey local and state ordinances. Cyclists should always ride with the traffic flow (not against it), know and use proper hand signals, ride defensively (never assume drivers see them), properly maintain their bike, wear safety equipment (including helmets, gloves, and proper footwear), and use the bicycle paths whenever available.

Sports also contribute to the public accident statistics, especially since more people are participating in community, recreational, and intramural activities to improve their health and physical fitness. Regardless of the sport, following certain guidelines can reduce the incidence of accidental injuries and deaths. They include developing the skills to enhance safer participation, recognizing and guarding against hazards associated with each activity, making sure facilities are safe, following the rules, and promoting good sportsmanship. It is also important to include appropriate exercises for conditioning, "warm up," and "cool down". Another critical factor is the use of proper safety equipment (such as helmets for football, hockey, and baseball; eye protection for racquetball, handball, squash, and basketball; knee and elbow pads for volleyball, skateboarding, and soccer; mats for gymnastics and wrestling; appropriate footwear for each particular sport or activity). None of these suggestions will eliminate all dangers from sports and recreational activities (nor were they meant to), but these practices will enhance safety by encouraging self-responsibility for each participant.

Firearms pose a significant threat to the 15–24 age group, with most fatalities involving males who are cleaning or handling guns they thought were unloaded. People

Proper safety equipment reduces the incidence of public accidents. Head and face protection is the main concern for these baseball players.

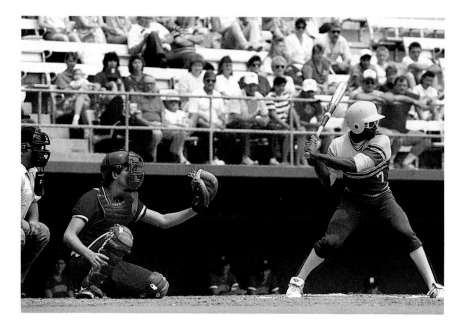

who use firearms should (1) never point a loaded gun at something they do not intend to shoot; (2) store unloaded firearms under lock and key (in a place separate from the ammunition); (3) always inspect firearms carefully before handling; and (4) behave in the safe and responsible manner advocated in firearms safety courses.

Keeping Yourself Safe and Assisting Others

By following the safety and prevention guidelines described in this chapter, you can avoid many accidents on the road, at home, at work, and in public places. But there are a few more steps you can take to protect yourself from injury as well as to provide assistance to others in case of accident.

One area of personal concern is assault. The incidence of physical assault and of sexual assault and rape increases in our society every year. Both men and women are threatened by these incidents. As a first step, never assume that you could not be the victim of an assault. Then, protect yourself by taking action that is appropriate for your campus or community. Avoid walking alone, especially after dark; become more aware of your surroundings, including possible escape routes and sources

of help in an emergency; and consider changing your routes to and from class or work so a would-be assailant won't be able to count on your routines. If there have been assaults in your area, check with the police or other authorities about specific precautions you should take. For a full discussion of how to avoid rape and what to do if you can't, see Chapter 5.

Another situation that can lend itself to possible assault is a mechanical breakdown of your car. If you drive your own car, and especially if you travel long distances, make sure you know what to do in case of a road emergency. Keep your car in good working order, check your spare tire and jack before long trips, have an emergency kit in your car, and know how to change a flat tire. Sometimes it makes more sense to sit in your car and wait for assistance than to set out in search of help. Plan ahead what you will do in an emergency before it happens.

Not all dangerous situations involve a personal threat to you; sometimes another person requires emergency assistance. If you are prepared to provide help, you can improve someone else's chances of surviving or of avoiding the serious consequences of an accident. A course in **first aid**, such as those offered by the American Red Cross, can help you respond appropriately when someone is injured. One important benefit of first aid training is that you learn what *not* to do in certain situations. For

First aid   Emergency care given to an ill or injured person until medical care can be obtained.

Avoiding Heat Stress

In summer's sometimes sizzling temperatures and stifling humidity, you may not always be able to "sweat it out." Excessive heat can subject your body to hazardous stress. Its potential toll is a spectrum of ills ranging from mild discomfort to life-threatening heatstroke.

You can protect yourself with commonsense approaches. But if heat stress strikes, be alert to its signs and act quickly to cool down.

How Your Body Cools Itself

Your body maintains its normal temperature of 98.6° F by radiating heat from its core outward to your skin's surface, where breezes of air help transfer it into the atmosphere. However, this process works well only when the temperature of the air is equal to or lower than that of your body.

As air temperature rises, or when your body produces more heat during exertion, your brain triggers an increase in blood flow to your skin. This increases your sweat production, which helps drive away heat through evaporation of the moisture. When the humidity is less than 75 percent, this is the principal way your body cools itself. At a higher humidity, evaporation of sweat diminishes rapidly, stopping completely when the humidity exceeds 90 percent.

When it's both hot and humid, it becomes more difficult for your body to release the heat that builds up. As a result, your body temperature can climb. Initially, you may be only mildly uncomfortable. You may feel dizzy, headachy, and tired.

Heat cramps represent the mildest form of heat stress. They are most often seen in poorly conditioned athletes who drink inadequate amounts of liquids before and during strenuous exercise. If relief from the heat is not obtained, heat exhaustion and heatstroke may follow.

Heat exhaustion results when your heart, circulatory system, and central nervous system fail to respond to heat stress. In the early stages, heat exhaustion causes nausea, vomiting, and muscle aches.

Heat exhaustion quickly can progress to *heatstroke*, a condition in which the temperature-regulating center in your brain shuts down. At this point, your body temperature soars. This can lead to severe, even fatal, brain, liver, or kidney damage.

Commonsense Approaches You Can Use to Beat the Heat

When the temperature pushes into the 90s or above and the humidity becomes oppressive, be alert for heat-related illness. Here are several suggestions:

- *Limit your activity*—Reserve vigorous exercise for the early morning or evening. If you participate in outdoor sports events,

---

Heat stress: The degrees of danger Recognizing the early signs of heat-related illness and acting quickly can prevent a mild reaction from becoming a fatal response. Here are the three degrees of heat stress, how to recognize them, and the steps you should take:

Condition	How to Recognize It	What to Do
Heat cramps	Painful muscle spasms, sweaty skin, normal body temperature.	1. Sit or lie down in the shade. 2. Drink cool water. 3. Stretching muscles may help. Do not massage.
Heat exhaustion	Profuse sweating, clammy or pale skin, dizziness, nausea, vomiting, headache, muscle aches, rapid pulse, thirst, normal or slightly elevated body temperature.	1. When mild, treat the same as for heat cramps. 2. If persistent headache and vomiting, or confusion, gently apply wet towels and call for emergency help.
Heatstroke	Unconsciousness (or, if conscious: confused, staggered walk, agitated); hot, dry skin *or* (rarely) sweating; rapid pulse; body temperature of 105° F or higher.	1. Move person to a reclining position in the shade. 2. Call for emergency help. 3. If the person is conscious, offer sips of cool water. 4. Fan the person and sponge with cold water. An ice bath may be necessary.

Source: *Mayo Clinic Health Letter*, July 1989.

Avoiding Heat Stress (continued)

"acclimatize" yourself by gradually building up your tolerance to heat with exercise in similar conditions over five to six weeks.
- *Drink plenty of liquids*—Choose from water, fruit or vegetable juices. Shun beverages containing alcohol or caffeine. They can dehydrate your body. A general rule: Drink at least 1½ times the amount that quenches your thirst.
- *Avoid the sun*—When outdoors, wear a wide-brimmed hat or carry an umbrella.

- *Keep rooms cool*—Open your windows on opposite sides of rooms to encourage cross ventilation. Use fans to pull cooler air into rooms. Pull shades over sunny windows. If you have air conditioning, set the thermostat between 75° and 80° to both cool and help dehumidify the air. If you cannot cool your home, go to an air-conditioned public place such as a library or shopping mall.

- *Select the right clothing*—Wear lightweight, loose-fitting clothes that breathe. Light-colored clothes reflect heat. Take frequent cool showers or baths.

    Another practical point to remember: On a hot day, *never* leave children or pets in a car with the windows rolled up. The temperature within the vehicle can quickly become life-threatening.

---

example, a person with a suspected neck or back injury should not be moved unless other life-threatening conditions exist. A knowledgeable person can assess emergency situations accurately before acting. An emergency first aid guide is provided inside the back cover of this book.

Choking is a common emergency situation that caused 5,000 accidental deaths per year before the **Heimlich maneuver** was introduced in 1974. Today, many choking victims can be saved with this simple procedure (see Figure 23-1). Until 1986, the Red Cross recommended blows to the upper back for choking, but since then it has adopted the Heimlich maneuver (which it also calls "abdominal thrusts") as the easiest and safest thing to do when an adult is choking.

Finally, emergency rescue techniques can save the lives of heart attack and accident victims who have stopped breathing or whose hearts have stopped beating. Pulmonary resuscitation (also known as rescue breathing, artificial respiration, or mouth-to-mouth resuscitation) is used when a person is not breathing (see Figure 23-1). **Cardiopulmonary resuscitation (CPR)** is used when a pulse can't be found. Training is required before a person can perform CPR. Courses, again, are offered by the Red Cross.

■ **Exploring Your Emotions**

How do you feel about being trained to handle emergency situations by taking courses in CPR or first aid? Does it make you feel more confident and in control to know you could help? Or does it feel like a possibly frightening responsibility? What is the basis for your feelings?

Like other kinds of behavior, avoiding and preventing accidents and acting safely involve choices you make every day. If you perceive something to be a serious personal threat—whether physically or psychologically, socially or economically—you tend to take action to protect yourself. Ultimately, your goal is healthy, safe behavior. You can motivate yourself to act in the safest way possible by increasing your knowledge and level of awareness, by examining your attitudes to see if they're realistic, by knowing your capacities and limitations, by adjusting your responses when environmental hazards exist, and, in general, by taking responsibility for your actions. You can't eliminate all risks and dangers from your life—no one can do that—but you can improve your chances of avoiding accidents and living to a healthy, ripe old age.

Heimlich maneuver   A maneuver developed by Henry J. Heimlich, M.D., to help force an obstruction from the airway.

Cardiopulmonary resuscitation (CPR)   Emergency first aid procedure that combines artificial respiration and artificial circulation. It is used in first aid emergencies where breathing and blood circulation have stopped.

American Red Cross

TO SAVE A LIFE

RESCUE BREATHING

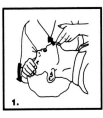

IF VICTIM APPEARS TO BE UNCONSCIOUS, TAP VICTIM ON THE SHOULDER AND SHOUT "ARE YOU OKAY?"

1. Apply the major force with the hand on the forehead.
- Place fingertips under the bony part of the jaw.
- Support and lift the jaw with your fingertips. Avoid closing the mouth.
- Do not push the soft tissues of the throat; it may block the airway.

If necessary, pull the lower lip down slighty, with your open thumb to keep the mouth open.

2. Look, listen and feel for breathing for 3-5 seconds.

3.
- If the person is not breathing, pinch nose closed.
- Place your mouth tightly around victim's mouth and blow into his mouth.
- Give two full breaths

Stop blowing when victim's chest has expanded.
- Turn head and listen for exhalation.
- Give 1 breath every 5 seconds.

4. INFANTS AND SMALL CHILDREN
- Tilt head slightly.
- Cover & seal nose with your mouth.
- Blow shallow breaths.
- Give 1 breath every 3 seconds.

FIRST AID FOR CHOKING

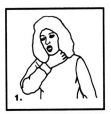

1. ASK:
"ARE YOU CHOKING?"
If victim cannot breathe, cough, or speak...
GIVE THE HEIMLICH MANEUVER.
Stand behind the victim. Wrap your arms around the victim's waist.

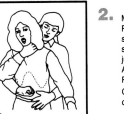

2. Make a fist with one hand; PLACE your FIST (thumbside) against the victim's stomach in the midline just ABOVE THE NAVEL AND WELL BELOW THE RIB MARGIN.
Grasp your fist with your other hand.

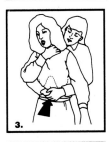

3. PRESS INTO STOMACH WITH A QUICK UPWARD THRUST.
REPEAT IF NECESSARY.

4. IF A VICTIM HAS BECOME UNCONSCIOUS:
Sweep the mouth.

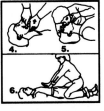

5. Attempt rescue breathing.

6. Give 6 - 10 abdominal thrusts.
Repeat Steps 4, 5, and 6 as necessary.

TO CONTROL BLEEDING

2. If bleeding continues, apply PRESSURE on the supplying artery.

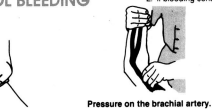

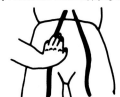

1. Apply DIRECT PRESSURE and elevate.

Pressure on the brachial artery.

Hand pressure on the femoral artery.

Figure 23-1   Rescue breathing and first aid for choking—procedures recommended by the Red Cross.

Summary

- Accidents are the third leading cause of death in the United States and the leading cause for those between ages 1 and 37. The same attitudes, behaviors, and decisions that protect health can improve a person's chances of avoiding accidents.

What Causes Accidents?

- Accidents occur under certain circumstances, not because of accident proneness or personality traits.
- Higher accident rates are associated with certain attitudes and behaviors. According to the social pathology theory, the more responsibility people take for their lives, the fewer accidents they have.
- According to multiple causation theory, accidents are caused by a dynamic interaction of human and environmental factors.
- One human factor is level of skill; people have accidents when they try to do something beyond their capabilities and natural physical limits.
- Psychoactive drugs (including alcohol, cocaine, and marijuana) and prescription and over-the-counter medications can impair ability and judgment and lead to motor vehicle accidents.
- Having correct knowledge about safety is essential; acting on misinformation can lead to injury.
- Awareness of risks is crucial to preventing accidents, and lack of awareness often reinforces unsafe behavior and beliefs. Unsafe attitudes lead to risk taking; people may believe they are exempt from the rules that protect others against injury.
- Emotions and psychological states like anger, fatigue, impatience, and stress make people unable to perceive events objectively or clearly.
- Environmental factors may be natural, societal, work-related, or home-related; making the environment safe is important to safety.
- Environmental hazards can be a result of technological advances. It's dangerous to bypass safety features, fail to wear safety equipment, or figure out faster ways to operate equipment. Employers have the responsibility to enforce safety regulations; the government has the right to enforce a certain level of safety among the members of a society.
- An accident is often the result of interaction between human factors and environmental factors. Sometimes an individual can make a decision that will help avoid an accident; the wrong decision can lead to injury or death.

Types of Accidents and Ways to Prevent Them

- Bad driving, especially speeding, causes three-fourths of all motor vehicle accidents. As speed increases, momentum and force of impact increase, and reaction time needed to stop a car within a given distance decreases.
- Speed limits establish the safest *maximum* speed limit for a given area under ideal conditions. At times, driving more slowly is advisable.
- Failure to wear safety belts doubles the chances of being hurt in a crash. Safety belts prevent a *second collision*, an occupant's hitting something inside the car, like a dashboard; safety belts also spread the stopping force over the body.
- Air bags provide protection in frontal collisions but not in other kinds of collisions; they are also less effective in multiple collisions.
- Alcohol is a factor in at least half of all fatal motor vehicle accidents. Alcohol slows down body functions; it affects reason and caution, judgment, and motor skills.
- Because of its unpredictability, weather is an environmental factor that affects motor vehicle accidents. In bad weather, driving defensively and making sure the vehicle is well-maintained are especially important.
- Interstate highways are safe places to drive, partly because of increased visibility and one-way travel. Most accidents occur within 25 miles of home and on roadways with speed limits of less than 40 mph.
- Many accidents happen at home, partly because people spend so much time there. Falls usually occur as a result of common activities in the home.
- Nearly two-thirds of fall-related deaths are a result of falls at floor level rather than from a height. These falls are caused by difficulty in adjusting to degrees of traction. Small rugs, waxed floors, slippery bathtubs, as well as ice, snow, and rough ground can lead to falls.
- Stairs are a problem when lighting is poor, handrails are missing, or footwear is inappropriate. Using chairs or other objects rather than stepladders or stepstools leads to dangerous situations. The "4 to 1" rule should be followed when using straight ladders.
- Approximately 80 percent of fire deaths and 65 percent of fire injuries occur in the home. Fires require a source of ignition, fuel, and oxygen.
- Being prepared for fire emergencies means planning escape routes, installing fire and smoke detection devices, and knowing how to use fire-extinguishing devices. The most important thing to remember is to get out of the house as quickly and safely as possible.

- In a fire, smoke inhalation can be avoided by crawling along the floor and covering the mouth. Fire extinguishers that are labeled ABC are effective against home fires.
- Most home poisonings involve children under age 5. The home can contain many poisonous substances. Carbon monoxide causes most poisonings by gas; other cases of poisoning by gas result from improper ventilation and incomplete combustion.
- Partly because of the Occupational Safety and Health Act of 1970, the work site has become much safer. OSHA requires inspections, detailed recordkeeping, and penalties for noncompliance.
- Most work-related injuries involve extensive manual labor and lifting. Back problems are most common, and skin disorders are increasing because of chemical and hazardous substances. Workers are especially at risk for accidents during their first year on the job. Training and education programs are helpful in reducing risk.
- Since 1912 the death rate from public accidents—those that occur in public places not involving a motor vehicle—have declined by 73 percent. Sports and recreational accidents fall into this category; falls and drownings are the major causes of death.
- Jogging can be made safer by avoiding busy roadways, running against the flow of traffic, wearing clothes that add to visibility, and not using stereo headphones.
- Pedestrian accidents often involve the young and the elderly; alcohol contributes to 25 percent of pedestrian deaths. The most unsafe pedestrian behavior is crossing between streets or intersections. Hitchhiking creates a potentially dangerous situation.

- Most bicycling accidents are the result of not knowing or misunderstanding the rules of the road, failure to follow the law, and lack of experience in traffic conditions.
- The risk of injuries and deaths in sports can be reduced by developing skills, recognizing hazards, making sure facilities are safe, promoting good sportsmanship, and using proper equipment. Participants must take responsibility for personal safety.
- Firearms accidents are especially prevalent in the 15–24 age group, often as a result of cleaning a gun that is thought to be unloaded.

Keeping Yourself Safe and Assisting Others

- Assault is a matter of personal safety; people should never assume they can't be victims and should take action appropriate for their community. People become vulnerable to assault when they travel in vehicles that break down.
- By taking first aid courses people can learn how to help others who are injured in an accident.
- Using the Heimlich maneuver can prevent accidental deaths due to choking.
- Pulmonary resuscitation and cardiopulmonary resuscitation can help save the lives of those who have stopped breathing or whose hearts have stopped beating.
- People make choices every day that help them avoid and prevent accidents.

Take Action

1. In your health diary, list the positive behaviors that help you avoid or prevent accidents and keep yourself safe. What can you do to reinforce and support these behaviors? Then list the behaviors that block your safe behaviors or that put you at risk of having an accident. How can you change one or more of them?

2. Look up the nearest Poison Control Center in your telephone book and post the number near

your telephone. Contact the center and ask them to send you information and literature on poisonings. Read it carefully so you know what to do in such cases as an accidental overdose with a prescription or an OTC drug or an accidental ingestion of a drain cleaner by a child.

3. Contact your local fire department and obtain a checklist for fire safety procedures. What would you do if a fire started in your home? What types of evacuation

procedures would be necessary? Do a practice fire drill at home to see what problems might arise in a real emergency.

4. Contact the Red Cross in your area and ask about first aid and CPR classes. These courses are usually given frequently and at a variety of convenient times and locations. They can be invaluable in saving lives. Consider taking one or both of the courses.

Behavior Change Strategy

Adopting Safer Habits

Why do you have accidents? What are the human and environmental factors that contribute to them? Identifying those factors is one step toward making your lifestyle safer. Changing unsafe behaviors *before* they lead to accidents is an even better way of improving your chances.

For the next seven to ten days, keep track of any mishaps or accidents you are involved in, recording them on a daily accident behavior record like the one shown in Chapter 1 for eating behavior. Count each time you cut, burn, or injure yourself, fall down, run into someone, or have any other accident, no matter how trivial. Also record any risk-taking behaviors, such as failing to wear your seat belt or bicycle helmet, drinking and driving, exceeding the speed limit, putting off home or bicycle repairs, and so on. For each entry (accident or incidence of unsafe behavior), record the date, time, what you were doing, who else was there and how you were influenced by him or her, what your motivations were, and what you were thinking and feeling at the time.

At the end of the monitoring period, examine your data. For each incident, determine both the human factors and the environmental factors that contributed to the accident or unsafe behavior. For example, were you tired? Distracted? Did you not realize this situation was dangerous? Did you take a chance? Did you think this accident couldn't happen to you? Was visibility poor? Were you using defective equipment? Then consider each contributing factor carefully, determining why it existed and how it could have been avoided or changed. Finally, consider what preventive actions

you could take to avoid such incidents or change your behaviors in the future. Refer to the behavior change aids and techniques described in Chapter 1, such as recruiting a buddy, asking family and friends for support, using a role model, and so on.

As an example, let's say that you usually ride your bicycle without wearing your helmet (an unsafe behavior) and that several factors contribute to this behavior—you don't really think helmets are necessary, you only go on short trips, you never know where your helmet is when you're leaving the house, most people you know don't wear them, they're not legally required, and so on. One of the contributing factors to your unsafe behavior is inadequate or inaccurate knowledge (you don't think helmets are necessary). You can change this factor by obtaining accurate information about bicycle accidents and helmets. If you do some library research, you might run across the following facts:

- Every year, nearly 50,000 bicyclists suffer serious head injuries.
- Every year, there are approximately 1,300 bicycle-related fatalities, almost all of them involving head injuries.
- 95 percent of all bicycle accidents involve a collision between a bike and a car.
- A helmet can reduce your risk of serious head and brain injury by almost 90 percent should you be involved in a bicycle accident.
- Nearly half of all accidents resulting in head and brain injuries cause no damage to the bicycle.
- On a concrete surface, a fall from a distance of less than 1 foot can cause a concussion.

This is the kind of information that you often read in the paper *after* a serious accident has occurred, when everyone feels vulnerable and is sensitized to the need for safe habits. But you can become knowledgeable about safety without waiting for someone you know to be injured. Just acquiring information about bicycle accidents may lead you to examine your beliefs and attitudes about helmets and motivate you to change your behavior. You may decide that it's worth it to you to wear your helmet.

Once you're committed, you can use behavior change techniques to build a new habit. Put a picture of a bicycle racer wearing a helmet on your mirror. Get in the habit of keeping your helmet with your bike. Recruit a buddy from among your friends—someone who is aware of the risks involved in not wearing a helmet and willing to start wearing one. Others may even follow your example. If this happens, you will have influenced one of the environmental factors that contributed to your behavior—the fact that other people you knew didn't wear helmets. In the process, you may have become a role model for someone else. By changing this behavior, you have reduced the chances that you will ever suffer a head injury in a bicycle accident.

Every accident and unsafe behavior will have its own contributing factors, both human and environmental. Once you've analyzed them, you can find ways to change the cues and interrupt the behavior chains that lead to them and that reinforce them once they've occurred. If you often forget to wear your safety belt, put a sign in your car to remind yourself to buckle up, and ask your friends to remind you when you're in their car. If you have accidents in the kitchen, make a list of behaviors that can prevent accidents and put it on your refrigerator. It might include putting away knives and sharp tools, wiping up wet spots on the floor, sweeping up glass right away if something breaks, remembering to turn off the oven, and unplugging extension cords from the wall when they're not being used.

A personal contract can provide an added incentive to an accident prevention program. If there is a behavior you particularly want to change, draw up a contract specifying in detail the target behavior of concern, such as keeping within the speed limit when you drive or avoiding a convenient shortcut through a wooded area at night. Have a friend witness your contract, and devise a reward system to reinforce your successes. As with

any behavior, it may take some time to break old habits and develop new, safer patterns that fit in with your daily living patterns. But if it seems as if it's not worth the effort, remind yourself that all it takes is one serious accident to cost you your future or your life.

Selected Bibliography

Are you accident-prone? 1989. *University of California, Berkeley, Wellness Newsletter*, November.

Bever, D. L. 1987. *Safety: A Personal Focus*. St. Louis: Times Mirror/Mosby.

Florio, A. E., W. F. Alles, and G. T. Stafford. 1979. *Safety Education*. 4th ed. New York: McGraw-Hill.

National Highway Traffic Safety Administration. 1982. *The Automobile Safety Belt Fact Book*. Washington, D.C.: U.S. Department of Transportation.

National Research Council. 1985. *Injury in America: A Continuing Health Problem*. Washington, D.C.: U.S. Department of Transportation.

National Safety Council. 1989. *Accident Facts*. Chicago: National Safety Council.

Oldenburg, D. 1989. Henry Heimlich: Still maneuvering. *Washington Post Health*, October 10.

Sleet, D., et al. 1984. Automobile occupant protection: An issue for health educators? *Health Education* 15(5): 54–56.

Recommended Readings

Baker, S. P., and S. P. Teret. 1981 (March). Freedom and protection: A balancing of interests. *American Journal of Public Health* 71(3):295–97. *Addresses the issue of "freedom of choice" in safety matters relative to the costs to society as a whole.*

Baughman, W. Henry. 1988. *First Aid for Injuries and Illness*. (Published and sold by author.)

Keates, R. 1988. Preventing eye injuries: Some questions and answers. *Physician and Sports Medicine* 16(8): 122–24, 126. *Addresses the problem of eye injuries and ways to prevent them.*

Morehouse, C. et al. 1983. Critical areas in sports safety. *Journal of Physical Education, Recreation, and Dance* 54(6): 45–55. *An overview of sports-related safety concerns and suggestions for minimizing risks.*

Perin, M. J., W. L. Stohler, and W. G. Faraclas. 1984. *None for the Road*. Dubuque, Ia: Kendall/Hunt. *Discusses the problems associated with "driving under the influence" and recommends strategies for changing this pattern of behavior.*

Strasser, Maryland K., and James E. Aaron. (latest edition) *Fundamentals of Safety Education*, New York: Macmillan.

Sweeting, R. L. 1990. *A Values Approach to Health Behavior*. Champaign, Ill.: Human Kinetics Books. *This textbook focuses on self-concept as the core of all health behavior, with specific reference in one chapter to examples pertinent to safety and security issues.*

Thygerson, Alton L. 1977. *Accidents and Disasters: Causes and Countermeasures*. Englewood Cliffs, N.J.: Prentice-Hall.

Thygerson, Alton L. (latest edition) *Safety: Principles, Instruction, and Readings*. Englewood Cliffs, N.J.: Prentice-Hall.

Thygerson, A. 1989. *First Aid Essentials*. Boston: Jones and Bartlett. *This textbook stresses the importance of first aid and provides information essential for skill development and training.*

Wasserman, R. et al. 1988. Bicyclists, helmets and head injuries: A rider-based study of helmet use and effectiveness. *American Journal of Public Health* 78(9): 1220–1. *Provides research findings documenting head trauma resulting from bicycle accidents; emphasizes the importance of wearing helmets.*

Contents

Making Connections

Because of the intimate relationship between human beings and their environment, even the healthiest lifestyle can't protect a person from the effects of polluted air, contaminated water, or a nuclear power plant accident. Many of the health challenges of the next century will involve cleaning up and protecting the environment in order to maintain and improve the quality of life on earth. The scenarios presented on these pages describe situations in which people have to use information, make a decision, or choose a course of action, all relating to environmental health. As you read them, imagine yourself in each situation and consider what you would do. After you've finished the chapter, read the scenarios again and see if what you've learned has changed how you would think, feel, or act in each situation.

You were driving a friend home one hot day recently and turned on the air conditioner in your car. "Why don't we just open the windows?" your friend asked. "You don't want to make the hole in the ozone layer worse, do you?" You like the comfort and convenience of automobile air conditioning—is there something wrong with it? What does it have to do with ozone?

You're moving out of your apartment and would like to get rid of a lot of the things you've accumulated under the sink for the past year—oven cleaner, bathroom tile cleaner, flea powder, bicycle chain lube, and several other items. A lot of the labels say you should dispose of empty containers by wrapping them in several layers of newspaper and throwing them in the trash, but they don't say what to do with half-full containers or leftover contents. Can you wrap them up and throw them in the trash anyway? Should you dump the liquids down the drain and then wrap and throw away the containers? How can you find out the best way to dispose of these products?

Environmental Health

You're planning a backpacking trip with some friends and go to a camping store to get some equipment. Once you're there you find a huge selection of camping foods—individually foil-wrapped freeze-dried dinners, sauces for noodles, packets of instant oatmeal, hot chocolate, and dehydrated soup. As you're counting out the number of items you'll need for the trip, one of your friends comes over and says, "Let's not get this stuff. You're paying for all the wrapping. Let's get bigger quantities at the super-market and pack it ourselves in plastic containers." It seems a shame not to take advantage of these convenient packages, pre-pared especially for backpacking. Are they a good idea, or does your friend have a point?

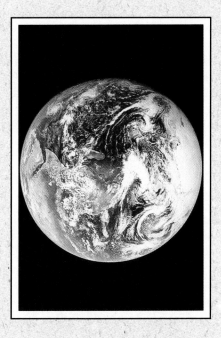

Your grandparents told you they would help you buy a car next year, and they'd like you to get a big eight-cylinder model, which they think is safer. When you tell them you'd really like to get something a little more fuel-efficient, your grandfather says, "Haven't you heard? The energy shortage is over. There's plenty of gasoline now. Just look at the prices. A gallon of gas costs less than a gallon of milk." You know gas prices are down, but does that mean people don't have to conserve any more? And what about air pollution? Isn't that im-portant any more either?

Your roommate says his parents are doing some home improve-ments to lower the levels of radon inside their house. They're install-ing a ventilation system in their basement and resealing the base-ment walls and floor. Your room-mate says they're worried about getting cancer by being exposed to radon in the soil, though he's not sure exactly what the connection is. Your parents live in the same state as his parents. Should they be making the same kinds of home improvements? How can they find out if radon is affecting their health?

Earth Day 1990 reminded us once again of our intimate relationship with all that surrounds us—our environment. Once we struggled against the environment on a daily basis in order to survive; now we realize that our survival as a species may entail protecting the environment from the by-products of our own modern way of life. We are acutely aware that what we do on an everyday basis may very well have a long-term impact on the environment and ultimately on planetary life.

How does the environment affect our health? In the past, our main environmental health concern was the transmission of infectious diseases. Now our attention is focused on the possible snowballing effects of environmental degradation on human health and life—the effects of ozone depletion, global warming, acid rain, and other modern phenomena. In health terms, we are concerned about cancer, birth defects, and the many ways that environmental poisons can cause injury and illness. But we are also aware of our responsibility to future generations and to other forms of life. The quality of life on the planet depends on our actions now.

There is no doubt that the visible environment is cleaner today than it was twenty years ago, at least in the United States. Federal laws have established standards and set goals that have reduced pollution and resulted in cleaner air and water. Our task now is to make similar inroads into solving the less visible and more difficult problems that remain. Individuals can contribute to this effort in many ways. This chapter explains what's involved in environmental health issues and suggests ways that you can make a difference in the future of the planet.

Why Are Environmental Problems More Serious Now?

Environmental health problems aren't new, but the problems we face today are more serious and broader in scope than any that human beings have had to face before. One reason for this is the sheer number of people living on the planet and their concentration in urban areas. In the past, people typically lived in small, relatively isolated, self-sufficient groups. Each group drew its food and water from its environment and disposed of its wastes without infringing on the environment of another group. With industrialization, urbanization, and population growth, these simple approaches became unworkable. One can hardly imagine every family in Los Angeles, for example,

having its own well, septic tank, garbage incinerator, and plot of land on which to grow food.

World population continues to grow, despite efforts to slow or stop it. The growth rate in 1989, 1.8 percent, was slightly higher than the rate in 1988. According to Worldwatch Institute, the population of the world will increase from 5 billion now to 9 billion by the year 2030 if present trends continue (see Figure 24-1). A result both of health improvements over the past fifty years and of women's lack of access to contraception in many countries, the increase places tremendous burdens on farmlands and other natural resources. Several European countries have stabilized their populations, but the United States and most of the rest of the world's nations have not.

A second reason for the severity of our environmental problems is that modern technology, while increasing our standard of living and even our life span, produces many harmful by-products. When these by-products are concentrated in the environment, they are much more dangerous than any naturally occurring hazard. Our power sources, for example, with the exception of solar and water-generated electricity, are not clean. They produce air-polluting emissions ranging from sulfur dioxide to radiation, and more people than ever are using them (see Figure 24-2). Motor vehicles produce vast quantities of carbon monoxide, hydrocarbons, and other pollutants. Through technology, human beings make a far greater impact on the environment, in a shorter period of time, than they ever could before. Once, it took a worker a day to cut down a dozen trees for lumber; new equipment allows that same worker to clear more than an acre in a day.

The combination of densely populated urban societies and modern technology means that people and environments all over the world are interconnected in highly complex ways. Acid rain, caused by emissions from electric power plants and motor vehicles, threatens forests, lakes, and wildlife hundreds of miles from the source of emissions. Jungles and rain forests are being destroyed to provide lumber and grow food for people living in other countries and on other continents. Rain forest clearing and other environmentally unsound practices may be contributing to global climate and atmospheric changes that threaten to change human life and health on a scale never before imagined.

The grim news today shouldn't blind us to the significant progress that has been made in environmental health over the years, as mentioned earlier. No one is suggesting

---

DDT   A common insecticide now stringently controlled in the United States.

Malaria   An often-fatal mosquito-borne disease marked by chills and fever.

Typhus   A louse-born fever disease associated with crowding and poor sanitation.

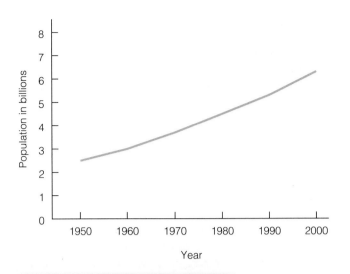

Figure 24-1   World population growth. Population is still exploding. 1.6 billion people have been added since Earth Day 1970; we'll reach 10 billion within a century.

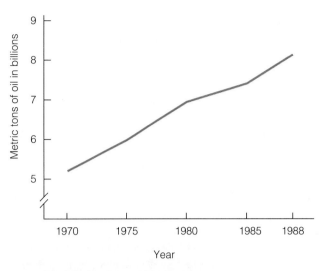

Figure 24-2   World Energy Use. Energy consumption is still rising, despite conservation. Steep increases are expected in the Third World as it develops.

that we return to the "good old days," because many environmental conditions were worse in the past, including air and water quality, sanitation, and food and drug safety. But we do have to take steps to conserve our planet. Unfortunately, there are no simple solutions; there are always trade-offs. In looking at environmental issues today, we have to weigh the costs and benefits of various practices and decide which ones are worth the price.

The case of **DDT** provides a good example of this decision-making process. Recognized as a powerful pes-

ticide in 1939, DDT was extremely important in efforts to control such widespread insect-borne diseases as **malaria**, yellow fever, **typhus**, and bubonic plague. DDT spraying virtually eradicated malaria in many tropical countries by 1950 and increased crop yields in other countries, including the United States. But in 1962, biologist Rachel Carson questioned the safety of DDT in her book *Silent Spring,* leading to recognition of the fact that the pesticide disrupts the life cycles of birds, fish, and reptiles. It was also found to build up in the food chain, increasing in concentration as larger animals ate smaller

Environmental Index: The World

- Net increase in world population each hour: 11,000.
- Years it took to build a population of 2 billion people: 4 million.
- Years it took to add the second 2 billion people: 45.
- Years it will take to add the third 2 billion: 22.
- Proportion of deaths caused by air pollution in Hungary: 1 in 17.
- Number of Americans who breathe unhealthy air: 150 million.

- Number of acres protected under the U.S. Wilderness Act: 91 million.
- Number of acres of pristine wilderness without protection: almost 100 million.
- Percentage decline in world rhinoceros population since 1970: 84.
- Number of dolphins killed each year by tuna-fishing boats: 129,000.

- Number of plastic containers dumped in the ocean by ships each day: 639,000.
- Number of U.S. species listed as endangered: 531.
- Number for which a recovery plan has been developed: 284.
- Number of listed species that are actually recovering: 16.
- Number that have been removed from the list because they recovered: 2.

ones (a process known as *biomagnification*). Its exact effects on humans have never been determined. DDT was banned in the United States in 1972 despite its effectiveness as an insecticide and its obvious contribution to human health—the cost was too great.

■ Exploring Your Emotions

Does your community have curbside recycling or a recycling center? If so, do you recycle? What inconveniences do you (or would you) put up with in order to recycle? Do you think it's worth it?

Many hard decisions like this face us in the years ahead. We will have to seek a balance among various competing interests. We may decide that preventing starvation is worth the price of using chemical fertilizers on food, or that ensuring fresh food and safe drugs is worth the price of paper and plastic packaging. At the same time, we may decide that some environmental hazards are too dangerous or contribute only to convenience. As a society and as individuals, we can make changes in our attitudes and behaviors that will improve the quality of life on the planet for everyone.

Classic Environmental Health Concerns

The field of environmental health was not always focused on pollution and other typical concerns of today. It originally grew out of efforts to control communicable diseases in the nineteenth century. The discovery by Louis Pasteur and others that many diseases are caused by microorganisms led to the acceptance of the germ theory of disease and then to a variety of efforts to prevent disease transmission Certain insects and rodents were found to carry microorganisms that cause disease in humans, and campaigns were undertaken to eradicate or control these animals hosts, or *vectors*. It was also recognized that pathogens could live and be transmitted in sewage, drinking water, and food. These discoveries led to the development of such practices as systematic garbage collection, sewage treatment, water protection, food inspection, and the establishment of public health enforcement agencies.

These successful efforts to control and prevent communicable diseases changed the health profile of the developed world (see Chapter 1). We no longer worry about contracting cholera, typhoid fever, plague, diphtheria, or any of a variety of other diseases that once killed whole populations. But that doesn't mean that no efforts are required to keep these diseases under control. In fact, a huge, complex health system is constantly at work behind the scenes attending to the details of these traditional concerns. Every time this system is disrupted, danger recurs. Every time a flood, a hurricane, an earthquake, a tornado, or some other natural disaster damages a community, these areas again become of prime importance. And every time we venture beyond the boundaries of our everyday world, whether traveling to a less developed country or camping in a wilderness area, we are reminded of the importance of these basics—clean water, sanitary waste disposal, safe food, and insect and rodent control.

Clean Water   Few parts of the world have adequate quantities of safe, clean drinking water, and yet few things are as important to human health. What we take for granted each time we turn on a faucet is really a product of the great revolution in human understanding of disease transmission that occurred in the nineteenth century. In 1854, John Snow showed a relationship between contaminated well water and **cholera** in London. Other researchers followed, proving that several infectious diseases could be transmitted by water. Until this time, people could only guess that their health depended partly on the quality of their drinking water.

In the latter half of the nineteenth century, the United States and Great Britain both began building complex water systems that brought clean water to cities, right into buildings. Governments took on the role of inspecting water, and in most instances governments provided it too. As a result, the incidence of cholera, typhoid fever, and other water-borne diseases fell sharply by 1900 and remains virtually nil today in areas that have municipal water supplies.

Many cities still rely at least in part on wells that tap local groundwater, but often they have to find lakes and rivers to supplement wells. Because such surface water is more likely to be "dirty"—contaminated with both organic matter and disease-causing microorganisms—it is

---

Cholera   An acute infectious disease characterized by severe diarrhea, vomiting, muscle cramps, and dehydration, caused by an organism often transmitted in contaminated drinking water.

Fluoridation   The addition of fluoride to the water supply, which reduces tooth decay.

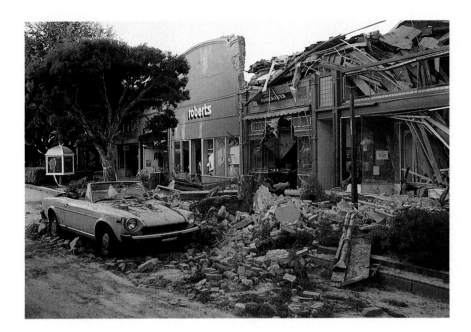

We often take for granted the well-organized system responsible for environmental health in our society, but natural disasters remind us of its fragility. The 1989 Loma Prieta earthquake destroyed buildings in California, touched off fires, and temporarily disrupted essential services. In less well developed countries, earthquakes can mean contaminated water, spoiled food, and sewage disposal problems.

purified in water treatment plants before being piped into the community. At treatment facilities, the water is subjected to a variety of physical and chemical processes, including screening, filtration, and disinfection (often with chlorine), before it is introduced into the water supply system. In many communities, the water is also treated with fluoride (**fluoridation**), which reduces tooth decay by 60 to 65 percent. In most areas of the United States, water systems have adequate, dependable supplies, are able to control water-borne disease, and provide water without unacceptable color, odor, or taste.

As we move toward the year 2000, water has once again become a worldwide environmental concern, although the reasons are different from those of a century ago. Water pollution from sewage and from many industrial sources has been controlled in the United States and some other countries, but many supplies of water, both on the surface and in the ground, are becoming polluted with hazardous chemicals. Manufacturing and agriculture are responsible for part of this toxic waste, but the accumulated hazardous waste from individual households also contributes to the problem. Increased incidence of cancer is just one of the health problems associated with chemical pollution of the water supply.

Water shortages are also a growing concern. Some parts of the United States are experiencing rapid population growth that outstrips the ability of local systems to provide adequate water to all. Many proposals are being discussed to relieve these shortages, including long-distance transfers (similar to those that already exist in some parts of the country) from the Great Lakes to the Southwest.

Worldwide, only about 35 percent of the population has an adequate water supply, according to the World Health Organization. Groundwater pumping and the diversion of water from lakes and rivers for irrigation are reducing the amount of water available to local communities even more. In the Soviet Union, for example, the Aral Sea, once the fourth largest body of fresh water in the world, has lost two-thirds of its volume to irrigation since the 1960s. The affected people of central Asia have to deal not only with a severe shortage of water for everyday use but also with the unforeseen health consequences of environmental degradation, including sharp increases in respiratory diseases and throat cancers linked to dust storms from the dry seabed.

Problems of this scope obviously demand long-range solutions on both the national and the international level. Whatever the outcome of plans to address these problems, two actions are now being implemented. One involves minimizing pollution of all waters with hazardous wastes. All freshwater supplies must be treated as if they will be needed as a source of drinking water in the future. In the United States, the Environmental Protection Agency (EPA) sets limits for the presence of toxic substances in drinking water, and many countries regulate the discharge of industrial wastes into waterways.

The second action involves a rethinking of our water distribution system. Most cities usually have just one system that provides "treated" water to homes, industry, and agriculture alike. However, much of that water doesn't have to be made as pure and safe as drinking water. The water you use to wash a car or water a lawn doesn't have to meet the same standards as the water you drink. As

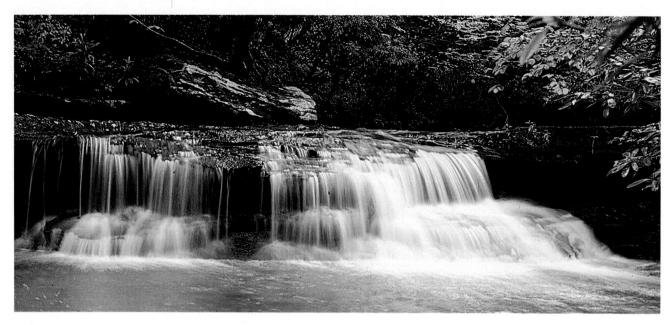

Water is a precious resource that has to be protected from both wasteful use and pollution. Many American rivers are cleaner than they were twenty years ago, but groundwater contamination from toxic wastes is a growing threat.

treatment becomes more expensive and as the cleanest water becomes scarcer, cities may have to develop several levels of distribution based on intended use, which may be less costly than treating all water.

Waste Disposal   Humans generate large amounts of waste, which must be handled in an appropriate manner if the environment is to be safe and sanitary. Some of this waste is sewage composed of human excrement, some is garbage from food materials, and some is solid waste, a by-product of our "throw-away" society. This last category, consisting of packaging, newspapers, "junk mail," insulated fast food wrappers, aluminum cans, and other trash, accounts for an ever-growing proportion of the solid waste generated in the United States.

Sewage   One of the great advances in public health in the last 150 years was the development of safe and relatively inexpensive ways to dispose of human wastes. Prior to the mid-nineteenth century, many people contracted the great killing diseases, such as typhoid and cholera, as well as disabling diseases like hepatitis A, by direct contact with fecal matter, which was simply disposed of at random. Very little effort was made to separate sewage from sources of drinking water or from human habitation.

In the United States, the development of the outhouse, or privy, did much to control diseases like hookworm. This parasite, prevalent in the South, can be contracted by walking barefooted on grass or soil contaminated by fecal matter. People were taught how to build sanitary outhouses and how to locate them so they wouldn't contaminate potential water sources. As plumbing moved indoors, sewage disposal became more complicated. In rural areas the **septic system**, a self-contained sewage disposal system for one family, worked quite well; today, many rural homes still rely on this system.

Different approaches became necessary as urban areas developed. Many early cities developed on rivers. The inhabitants got their drinking water upstream and dumped their sewage downstream. For small populations, this tended to work fairly well as long as the cities were sufficiently separated. If they are not overloaded by organic wastes, rivers and lakes can "clean themselves" fairly well through the processes of dilution and bacterial action. But as cities grew, governments began to regulate waste disposal just as they regulated water supplies. City and state health departments are responsible for these services in most areas in the United States today.

Most cities have sewage treatment systems that separate fecal matter from water in huge tanks and ponds and stabilize it so that it cannot transmit infectious diseases. Once treated and biologically safe, the water is released back into the environment. The sludge that remains behind may be spread on fields as fertilizer if it is free from **heavy metal** contamination, or it may be burned or buried. Heavy metals, such as lead, zinc, cadmium, copper, and tin, can be incorporated into the food chain and cause illness and death. Recent studies indicate that even more care than was once thought necessary must be taken to prevent these chemicals from being released into the environment when sludge is burned or buried.

■ Exploring Your Emotions

There is no doubt that disposable diapers have a tremendous convenience advantage over cloth diapers, but they are quickly filling landfills and have even been banned at some disposal sites. If you had to choose between disposable and cloth diapers, which would you choose? Why?

Many cities have now begun to treat sewage further to remove heavy metals and other hazardous chemicals. This action has resulted from many studies linking exposure to such chemicals as mercury, lead, and **polychlorinated biphenyls (PCBs)** with long-term health consequences, including cancer and central nervous system damage. Sewage treatment systems that collect and concentrate these chemicals from an entire city should not dump them back into the environment where they might contaminate a present or future water source. The technology to effectively remove heavy metals and chemicals from sewage is still developing, and the costs involved are immense.

Solid Waste   Solid waste disposal in the United States has changed drastically in the last thirty years. Until then, a primary component of household solid waste was garbage—food and cooking wastes—which had to be disposed of in a way that would not spread disease. Governments developed health regulations about feeding garbage to pigs to prevent **trichinosis** (a worm disease transmitted to humans through poorly cooked pork) as well as regulations about garbage cans designed to minimize the number of insects or animals attracted to them. Usually, garbage was carted to the town dump out at the edge of town, burned, and never thought about again.

Technology has altered that practice. The bulk of the organic food garbage produced in American kitchens is now dumped in the sewage system by way of the mechanical garbage disposal. The garbage that remains is not very hazardous from the standpoint of infectious disease, since there is very little food waste in it, but it

does represent an enormous disposal and contamination problem.

Since the 1960s much of this solid waste has been buried in **sanitary landfill** disposal sites. Careful site selection and daily management are an essential part of this approach to disposal. First, a thorough study is done of the site to make certain that it is not near groundwater, streams, or any other source of water that could be contaminated by leakage from the landfill. Soil composition under and around the site is studied to make certain that materials cannot leach, or seep, from the area. Sometimes protective liners are used around the site, and nearby monitoring wells are now required in most states. Layers of solid waste are covered with thin layers of dirt on a regular basis until the site is filled. Some communities then plant grass and trees and convert the site into a park. Landfill is very stable; almost no decomposition occurs in the solidly packed waste.

Burying solid waste in sanitary landfills has several disadvantages. Much of this waste contains chemicals, ranging from leftover pesticides to nail-polish remover to paints and oils, which should not be released indiscriminately into the environment. Despite precautions, buried contaminants do leak into the surrounding soil and groundwater. Possible contamination, along with unpleasant sights and smells, makes burial politically unpopular and inspires the NIMBY (Not in My Backyard) syndrome—no one wants a disposal site near his or her home.

Burial is also expensive and requires huge amounts of space. Over two-thirds of the country's landfills have closed since the late 1970s, and one-third of those remaining will be full by 1994. At the same time that disposal is becoming more restricted, the amount of garbage is growing all the time. The average American produces more than one ton of solid waste per year, up 80 percent since 1960 and expected to rise another 20 percent by 2000. Our throw-away society uses ever more disposable products, ranging from plastic ketchup bottles to disposable diapers to overpackaged products of every kind.

The biggest single component of this trash (41 percent by weight) is paper products, a share fed by junk mail, glossy mail-order catalogs, and computer printouts. Yard waste is the next biggest source by weight (18 percent before recycling), followed by metals (8.7 percent), glass (8.2 percent), food (7.9 percent), plastics (6.5 percent),

---

Septic system   A self-contained sewage disposal system for one family, used in rural areas.

Heavy metal   A metal with a high specific gravity, such as lead, copper, or tin.

Polychlorinated biphenyl (PCB)   An industrial chemical used as an insulator in electrical transformers and linked to cancers in humans.

Trichinosis   A parasite-caused disease once commonly transmitted through poorly cooked pork.

Sanitary landfill   A special disposal site for solid wastes where there is some assurance that groundwater will not become contaminated.

Many existing landfills are reaching their limits at the same time that people are becoming more resistant to the opening of new ones in their communities. The solution to the waste problem lies in less consumption of disposal items and more recycling.

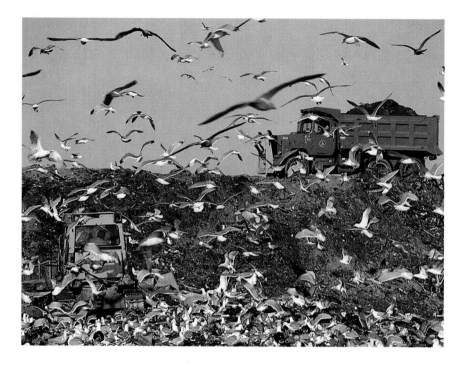

and wood (3.7 percent). A small but highly visible (and indestructible) component of trash is polystyrene foam, appearing as fast-food containers, meat trays, styrofoam cups, and packaging materials. About 1 percent of the solid waste is toxic. Burning, as opposed to burial, reduces the bulk of this solid waste, but it may release hazardous material into the air. The ultimate solution to this problem is to reduce packaging and consume less.

Solid waste is not limited to household products. Manufacturing, mining, and other industries all produce large amounts of potentially dangerous materials that cannot simply be dumped. The experiences of communities like Love Canal near Buffalo, New York, and Times Beach, Missouri, demonstrated clearly the dangers of careless disposal of toxic wastes. At Love Canal, toxic industrial wastes had been dumped into a waterway for years until, in the 1970s, nearby residents began to suffer from associated birth defects and cancers. At Times Beach, oil contaminated with **dioxin**, a highly toxic chemical, was spread on roads instead of being dumped in a landfill. In both cases, human health was affected, government had to step in, people had to move from homes, and huge costs were incurred.

■ Exploring Your Emotions

Are you ever tempted to throw toxic substances down the drain or in the trash? If so, what do or can you tell yourself in order to resist?

Because of the expense and potential chemical hazards posed by any form of solid waste disposal, many communities today encourage individuals and businesses to recycle their trash. Some cities offer curbside pickup of recyclables; others have recycling centers to which people can bring their waste. These materials are not limited to paper, glass, and cans but also include such things as discarded tires and used oils. By following recommended disposal procedures and by participating in recycling, people can reduce the spread of chemical contamination, slow the rate at which natural resources are consumed, reduce the cost of solid waste disposal, and help the nation gain time to develop more environmentally efficient methods of disposal and packaging.

Food Inspection Today we take for granted that the food we buy in grocery stores and in restaurants is safe to consume. This has not always been the case. At the turn of the century, tremendous pressure was put on the government to set minimum standards in all areas of food preparation and handling, resulting in the Pure Food and Drug Act of 1906. Illness and death associated with foodborne disease and toxic food additives has decreased substantially ever since. However, we are now becoming more concerned with the long-term health consequences of the foods we eat, either because of chemical contamination or because of characteristics of the foods themselves (as discussed in Chapters 12, 15, and 16, on nutrition, cardiovascular disease, and cancer).

Most people would be surprised at the number of agencies that inspect food at the various points of production. On the federal level, the Department of Agriculture inspects grains and meats, the Department of Commerce inspects some fish, and the Food and Drug Administration is responsible for ensuring the wholesomeness of foods and regulating the chemicals that can be used in food, drugs, and cosmetics. On the state level, public health departments inspect dairy herds, milking barns, storage tanks, tankers that transport milk, and processing plants. Local health departments inspect and license restaurants.

Considering the number of meals eaten outside the home and the number of meals prepared at home with purchased food, it is remarkable how few instances there are of food-borne illness or death. The food distribution system in the United States is very safe and efficient. Recalls of ice cream, cheese, and tuna in recent years have usually been based on a potential for illness because of processing error, not on actual illness or death. In fact, most food-associated illnesses are caused by contamination in the home, such as from salmonella bacteria or from **staphylococcus** poisoning (see Chapter 12). It is estimated that each person in the United States suffers an average of two to three episodes of food poisoning every year, although these episodes are usually assumed to be caused by a twenty-four-hour virus.

Insect and Rodent Control We have known for only a hundred years that insects and rodents could transmit disease. For centuries, people believed that bad odors, or **miasmas,** caused many diseases, such as yellow fever and malaria, two diseases that may have accounted for more deaths in human history than any other cause. In fact the very word *malaria* derives from the Greek for "bad air." This ignorance not only shortened human lives but also limited technological development. For example, several thousand people died of these two diseases during the construction of the Panama Canal. Not until the role of mosquitoes was determined and methods were developed to control them could the canal be completed.

We now realize the great number of illnesses that can be transmitted to humans by animal and insect vectors. In recent years we have seen outbreaks of **encephalitis** transmitted by mosquitoes, **Lyme disease** from ticks in the Northeast, Midwest, and Pacific states (see Chapter

18), **Rocky Mountain spotted fever** from another type of tick in the Southeast, and **bubonic plague** from fleas on rodents in the West. Rodents carry forms of typhus, tapeworms, and even **salmonella.** Constant vigilance is necessary to minimize illness associated with insects and rodents. Disability and death from these diseases is prevented by spraying insecticides, wearing protective clothing, and exercising reasonable caution in infested areas.

Pollution

As mentioned earlier, the classic environmental health concerns aren't just historical. They still have the potential to cause serious problems today under certain circumstances. They also take on added significance as population growth and new technology put new twists on old problems. For example, antibiotics added to cattle and poultry feed have minimized the risk of contracting bacterial infection from consuming contaminated meat, but the overuse of antibiotics may be fostering the development of more resistant strains of bacteria, a potentially more serious problem (see Chapter 18).

At the same time, new problems are arising, and some long-standing problems are gaining increased public attention. Many of these modern problems are problems of pollution. The term *pollution* has come to refer to any unsightly, noisy, smelly nuisance in our surroundings. When we are also talking about health risks, the level of concentration of a particular pollutant becomes very important. In typical concentrations, many environmental pollutants don't seem to harm our general health in the short term. The long-term effects are harder to evaluate.

Air Pollution Air pollution is not a human invention or even a new problem. The air is "polluted" naturally with every forest fire, pollen bloom, and dust storm, as well as with countless other natural pollutants. To these natural sources, human beings have always contributed the by-products of their activities. During the Industrial Revolution, English cities had far more daily air pollution than we can observe or even imagine today. However, two recent developments have changed our attitudes to-

---

Dioxin A powerful chemical found in herbicides and linked to human cancers.

Staphylococcus A bacterium found on the skin that can cause food-borne infections if allowed to multiply in bland foods.

Miasma Bad-smelling air, which was thought to cause disease before germ theory became accepted.

Encephalitis An inflammation of the brain sometimes caused by insect-borne diseases.

Lyme disease A disease spread by a deer tick that can lead to fever and arthritis-like conditions if untreated.

Rocky Mountain spotted fever A wood-tick-borne disease causing high fevers and found primarily in the Southeast.

Bubonic plague A virulent infectious disease carried by rodents and insects, marked by characteristic discolored swellings. One of the great plagues of the European Middle Ages.

Salmonella infection An often food-borne bacterial infection caused by eating food contaminated with fecal matter, such as improperly cleaned and cooked chicken.

ward air pollution. First, we are living long enough to experience both the short-term and the long-term health consequences. Second, increased population growth, combined with more industrialization using old technologies, concentrates the problems and makes them more visible and possibly more dangerous.

■ Exploring Your Emotions

If a friend told you he could get you a smog certificate without your having to get your car fixed, what would you do? Would the convenience be worth the pollution?

Air pollution can be more than just unsightly; it can cause illness and death if pollutants become concentrated for a period of several days or weeks. The first such incidents came in the Meuse Valley in Belgium in 1930 and in Donora, Pennsylvania, in 1948. In the latter incident, over 10 percent of the population of the town ended up in hospitals due to a stagnant air mass. Public awareness increased when London (1952) and New York City (1963) experienced air pollution disasters that made thousands ill and caused hundreds of premature deaths, primarily among those who already had respiratory problems. Increased amounts of carbon monoxide and airborne acids and decreased amounts of oxygen all put excess strain on people suffering from **congestive heart failure** and **chronic obstructive pulmonary diseases,** such as chronic bronchitis or emphysema, as well as on the very young and the elderly.

Before an air pollution emergency can occur, three conditions must be present. First, there must be a source of pollution. Today, this is most frequently the burning of fossil fuels, such as coal in industry or gasoline in cars. Second, there must be a topographical feature, such as a mountain range or a valley, that prevents the prevailing winds from pushing stagnant air out of the region. Third, there must be a weather event called a **temperature inversion.**

A temperature inversion occurs when there is little or no wind and a layer of warm air traps a layer of cold air next to the ground. Normally, the sun heats the earth, making the air closest to the ground warmer than that just above it. Warm air rises and is replaced by cooler air, which in turn is warmed and rises, thereby producing a natural vertical circulation. This circulation, combined with horizontal wind circulation, prevents pollutants from reaching dangerous levels of concentration.

When there is a temperature inversion, this replacement and cleansing action cannot occur. The effect is like covering an area with a dome that traps all the pollutants and prevents vertical dispersion. If this condition persists for several days, the buildup of pollutants may reach dangerous levels and threaten people's health. Many cities have plans for shutting down certain industries and even curtailing transportation if unsafe levels are approached. Most states also have "clean air" legislation, which has improved air quality in the last twenty years in American cities.

The disasters of the 1950s and 1960s involved a human-made form of air pollution called smog. There are two types of smog, London-type smog and Los Angeles-type smog, distinguished primarily by the source of the pollution. **London-type smog** results from the burning of fossil fuels such as coal. At one time coal was the major source of heat for homes as well as the major energy source for factories. A very serious problem arose when a lengthy temperature inversion occurred in the winter months in an area where coal was being burned. Now that many homes and factories use oil, steam, gas, and electricity, this source of pollution has been minimized in developed countries. However, coal burning is increasing in the developing countries.

Los Angeles-type smog (also known as **photochemical smog**) is a more complex phenomenon. Here the source of pollution is primarily motor vehicle exhaust that contains oxides of nitrogen. When sunlight acts on these products (a photochemical reaction), the result is a characteristic brown smog. Large cities with a high ratio of cars to people and with poorly developed public transportation are more likely to experience Los Angeles-type smog. The health effects are very similar to London-type smog—eye irritation, impairment of respiratory and cardiovascular functioning in vulnerable individuals, and cancers.

Congestive heart failure   A condition in which the heart cannot pump enough blood leading to a buildup of fluid in the tissues.

Chronic obstructive pulmonary disease   A general term for respiratory diseases such as emphysema and chronic bronchitis, in which airways are narrowed and oxygen intake is reduced.

Temperature inversion   A weather condition in which a cold layer of air becomes trapped by a warm layer so that pollutants cannot be dispersed.

London-type smog   An air pollution problem caused by coal burning.

Los Angeles-type smog   An air pollution problem caused by the burning of transportation fuels in combination with sunlight.

Photochemical smog   Another term for Los Angeles-type smog; caused by sunlight (hence "photo") reacting with transportation fuels (hence "chemical").

Greenhouse effect   Warming of the earth due to a buildup of carbon dioxide.

Carbon monoxide (CO)   A gas produced by combustion that combines with hemoglobin in human blood more readily than oxygen, causing shortness of breath or even suffocation.

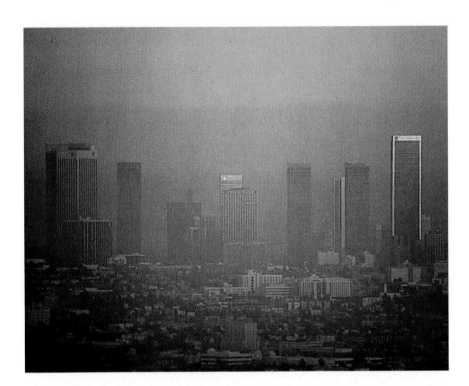

Smog tends to form over Los Angeles because of the natural geographical features of the area and because of the tremendous amount of motor vehicle exhaust in the air. The health effects of smog are most noticeable in people who already have some respiratory impairment.

Concern about air pollution in the 1960s led to the establishment of the U.S. Environmental Protection Agency, which has the task of setting standards and monitoring pollution levels. The ten-year trend (trend considered for ten-year time periods) has been fairly encouraging. The EPA reports improved air quality as measured by decreased levels of smog and several airborne chemicals in many areas. How this improvement translates specifically into improved health status has yet to be determined.

In recent years, however, new atmospheric problems have surfaced that may have long-range effects on the planet, its climates, and its inhabitants. These are the "greenhouse effect," increased amounts of carbon monoxide in the air, depletion of the ozone layer, and acid rain. Because these problems are global and involve the ecology of the whole planet, there are many unknowns. Experts really don't know exactly what kind of climate changes may occur, for example, or what further effects such changes may have, or even whether some unknown or overlooked factors will get into the act and produce some completely different result (see the box "Climate Variables Keep the Experts Guessing").

The Greenhouse Effect and Global Warming   Normally, carbon dioxide and other natural gases in the atmosphere act as a blanket around the earth (or as the glass in a botanical greenhouse, thereby giving the name **greenhouse effect**), intensifying the heat of the sun and trapping it close to the surface of the planet. Levels of green-house gases, especially carbon dioxide, appear to be rising, most likely from the combustion of oil, gasoline, coal, and natural gas, as well as from forest fires. And, deforestation (often by burning) is reducing the number of trees available to convert carbon dioxide into oxygen.

Many experts predict that this increase in greenhouse gases will cause temperatures on earth to rise and climates all over the planet to become warmer. Such a temperature rise, they say, would melt polar ice caps and raise the level of the sea, affecting seacoasts and food-producing areas of the world. Some experts predict a rise of 4–7°F worldwide in the next seventy years; others predict a milder warming trend of 1–2°F. Whatever the outcome, the full implications of this type of climate change are unknown.

Carbon Monoxide   A second problem associated with air pollution is an increase of **carbon monoxide** (CO), a product of combustion and one of the most toxic components of both smog and automobile exhaust. When breathed, carbon monoxide combines more readily with hemoglobin in blood than does oxygen. Less oxygen gets to the tissues, causing shortness of breath and other signs of oxygen deprivation. People suffering from respiratory and circulatory diseases are at risk in high-carbon-monoxide environments. A recent study demonstrated that people with heart disease are at significant risk when smokers are present in a closed room. Because of this evidence, airlines have banned smoking on domestic flights.

Climate Variables Keep the Experts Guessing

Even sophisticated formulas used to predict the greenhouse effect and other possible climate changes can't take all of nature's forces into account. Some variables may offset global warming; others may quicken it.

The following factors are cited by experts as "silver linings," variables that may delay the greenhouse effect:

Clouds: Higher temperatures increase evaporation and hence clouds, which are made of water vapor and help cool the planet.

Volcanoes: Eruptions spew tiny particles into the atmosphere that deflect sunlight, causing cooling.

Plankton: Warmth and extra carbon dioxide might promote the growth of these tiny marine organisms, which absorb CO_2 and take it out of circulation.

Oceans: Their heat-absorbing capacity might delay warming for more than a century.

The following factors are cited by other experts as cause to "start building an ark," because they could hasten global warming once it began:

Sea ice: Once it starts to melt, less sunlight will be reflected away, increasing the warming.

Acid rain: Sulfur dioxide, which causes acid rain, also cools the earth. Controlling acid rain might thus accelerate the greenhouse effect.

Permafrost: Warming might melt the frozen soil, releasing buried methane—a greenhouse gas.

Soil: Warming ordinary soil would increase the rate at which bacteria convert dead organic matter into CO_2, intensifying the human-caused greenhouse effect.

Whatever the exact dimensions of the greenhouse effect, it seems clear that global warming is a definite possibility in the years ahead. Some countries are already taking steps to mitigate climate changes, such as researching ways to recycle carbon dioxide and developing energy sources to replace fossil fuels. In the meantime, science, industry, and government are all watching the weather carefully to see what happens next.

Adapted from Keeping a weather eye on the mercury, *Newsweek*, November 20, 1989.

To control the release of carbon monoxide and other chemicals into the air, the federal government has established emission control standards for cars. The catalytic converter on cars significantly reduces CO emissions. Driving less is another way of reducing air pollution generated by motor vehicles.

The Ozone Layer   A third air pollution problem is the apparent thinning of the **ozone layer** of the atmosphere, a fragile, invisible layer that shields the surface of the earth from the sun's ultraviolet rays. Since 1983 scientist have observed the seasonal appearance and growth of a "hole" in the ozone layer over Antarctica and, more recently, over the Arctic and other areas of the earth. This is of concern because without the ozone layer to absorb radiation from the sun, life on earth would be impossible.

According to the Environmental Protection Agency, a 1 percent drop in ozone could result in 20,000 additional cases of skin cancer in the United States per year. Cataracts and blindness are other possible health risks.

Speculations about the cause of these holes range from weather patterns and volcanic eruptions to the release of **chlorofluorocarbons (CFCs)**. CFCs are versatile chemicals appearing in both liquid and gaseous form. They are used as coolants in refrigerators and in home and automobile air conditioners; as foaming agents in foam packaging and foam insulation; as propellants in some kinds of aerosol sprays (most such sprays were banned in 1978); and as solvents in the electronic industry. When CFCs are released on earth, they slowly drift up into the atmosphere where sunlight breaks them down, releasing chlorine. Chlorine destroys ozone molecules.

Ozone layer   A layer of oxygen molecules in the upper atmosphere that screens out ultraviolet rays from the sun.

Chlorofluorocarbons (CFCs)   Chemicals used as spray-can propellants, refrigerants, and industrial solvents, implicated in the destruction of the ozone layer.

Acid rain   Precipitation with a low pH (acid) caused by rain forming with products of industrial combustion to form acids such as sulfur dioxide. Acid rain is harmful to forests and lakes, which cannot tolerate changes in acidity/alkalinity.

What You Can Do to Save the Ozone Layer

When a health issue involves the health of the planet, people often feel that there's little they can do to change the course of events. The depletion of the earth's protective ozone layer is one of these mega-issues. While most of the measures needed to safeguard the ozone layer involve nations and industries, there are significant steps you can take—as an individual consumer and as a member of a society.

The stratospheric ozone layer is being destroyed in large part by chlorofluorocarbons, or CFCs. The United States remains the leading producer and consumer of CFCs. By following these steps, you can help reduce the American contribution to the destruction of the ozone layer:

• Have your car's air conditioner carefully serviced. *Auto air conditioners are the single largest source of CFC emissions in the U.S.* Don't simply refill your leaky air conditioner; if you don't have the leak fixed, the CFCs you add will end up in the air. Go to a service station equipped to recycle the refrigerant (this costs an additional $35 to $55); otherwise the CFCs will be vented into the atmosphere. In Los Angeles, an ordinance requiring service stations to recycle CFCs is expected to go into effect by January 1, 1990; it will

also ban the sale of small cans of refrigerant, which allow people to "top off" their car air conditioners instead of repairing leaks. Car air conditioners using less-harmful refrigerants are expected to be available in the mid-1990s. (Home air conditioners contain coolants that are far less ozone-depleting.)

• Avoid products made of plastic foam (polystyrene), such as fast food containers, egg cartons, Styrofoam cups, and foam trays for meats. Although many of these products are now made from less-damaging compounds, you can't tell which are which, so limit your use of them. They also add to the waste disposal problem, since they are virtually indestructible.

• Don't use foam plastic insulation in your home, unless it is made with ozone-safe agents. Or use fiberglass, gypsum, fiberboard, or cellulose insulation.

• Don't buy a halon fire extinguisher for home use.

• Check labels on aerosol cans. VCR-head cleaners, boat horns, spray confetti, photo-negative cleaners, and drain plungers are still allowed to contain the most dangerous CFCs. Many cans say if they contain CFCs, but such labeling isn't required.

• When buying a refrigerator, choose an energy-efficient model:

it may contain as little as half the CFCs. Thus when the fridge wears out and you dump it, fewer CFCs will be released. All refrigerators sold in the United States contain CFCs. To keep your fridge in the best working order, clean the coils regularly; that way it may last until CFC-free models are developed, or at least until recycling programs for CFCs are available.

• If you feel strongly, write to your senator and representative and to the president urging them to protect the ozone layer by tightening regulations on CFCs and halons, speeding up their elimination, mandating warning labels on products containing them, and pressing other nations to take such steps.

Substitutes for CFCs may add to the cost of many products, be less efficient, and have other drawbacks, at least at first. This may be hard to accept, especially since CFC emissions are invisible, and most of the damage they cause may not become evident for decades. But the steps we take now to protect the ozone layer will benefit our grandchildren.

Adapted from what you can do to save the ozone layer, *University of California, Berkeley, Wellness Letter*, October 1989.

Western nations have committed themselves to a 50 percent reduction in CFC manufacturing by the year 2000, and DuPont, the principal CFC manufacturer, has said it will stop production by then. But in developing nations, where food spoilage is a critical problem, the trade-off between affordable refrigeration and ozone protection is a more difficult and complex issue. To help

reduce the American contribution to the destruction of the ozone layer, see the suggestions given in the box "What You Can Do to Save the Ozone Layer."

Acid Rain   A by-product of many industrial processes, **acid rain** occurs when atmospheric pollutants combine with moisture in the air and fall to earth as highly acidic rain or snow. It occurs especially when coal containing large amounts of sulfur is burned and sulfur dioxide, sulfur trioxide, nitrogen dioxide, nitric acid, and other chemicals are released into the atmosphere. These concentrations can be carried great distances by the prevailing winds and form a highly acidic mixture containing sulfuric acid and nitric acid. Most of the pollutants in acid rain are produced by coal-burning electric power plants. Other sources include motor vehicles and certain industrial activities, such as smelting.

Many trees and some aquatic life can tolerate only a very narrow range of acidity and are either damaged or killed by acid rain. Currently, acid rain seems to be affecting forests and lakes in Canada, the northeastern United States, and some areas of Europe (see Figure 24-3). The known risk at the moment is an esthetic one: we want to protect the environment from destruction. The potential risk to human life is that the food chain may be endangered in the long term.

New federal legislation revising the Clean Air Act of 1970 is designed to reduce acid rain and toxic air emissions from cars, trucks, and factories. It cuts new car pollution to 2 percent of what was allowed in 1970, extends auto emission controls to trucks, and reduces industrial emissions by three-quarters. The hoped-for result is a 50 percent reduction in acid rain and a restoration of damaged lakes and forests in the eastern United States.

Chemical Pollution   Chemical pollution is by no means a new problem. The ancient Romans were plagued by lead poisoning, which damages the central nervous system, because they stored sugar solutions in lead containers. Two hundred years ago in Europe, the phrase "mad as a hatter" came from the hatters' practice of cleaning felt hats with mercury—which also destroyed the central nervous system.

The difference today is that new chemical substances are constantly being created and introduced into the environment, whether as pesticides, herbicides, solvents, cleaning fluids, flame retardants, or any of hundreds of other products. We have many more chemicals, in more concentrated forms and in wider use, and larger numbers of people are exposed and potentially exposed to them than ever before.

Chemical pollutants have been responsible for several environmental disasters. The cases of Love Canal, New York, and Times Beach, Missouri, involving dioxin and other toxic chemicals, were mentioned earlier in this chapter. The Hudson River in New York and the Housatonic River in Massachusetts have both been contaminated with polychlorinated biphenyls (PCBs), carcinogenic compounds used in the manufacture of electrical appliances. In 1984, thousands of people in Bhopal, India, were killed and injured when a powerful chemical used in manufacturing the insecticide Sevin was released from a plant. Catastrophes illustrate the short-term potential for disaster, but the long-term health consequences may be just as deadly. The following are brief descriptions of just a few current problems.

Asbestos   A mineral-based compound, asbestos was widely used for fire protection and insulation in buildings until the late 1960s. It was often applied to pipes, metal supports, and ceilings. When first introduced, asbestos was hailed as a great advance in fire safety of buildings. As long as it stayed where it was applied and its protective coating was not disturbed, there was no problem. However, the microscopic asbestos fibers that are released into the air when this material is applied or when it later deteriorates or is damaged can lodge in the lungs, inflaming them. This condition, known as **asbestosis,** can result in lung cancer over a period of years. Similar conditions are risks in the coal mining industry, from coal dust (black lung disease), and in the textile industry, from cotton fibers (brown lung disease).

Media and public awareness led to a 1987 federal law requiring that asbestos be removed from public buildings, including schools. Unfortunately, removal creates the very conditions in which asbestos is most dangerous, so it has to be done carefully by trained workers. In homes, asbestos insulation that is inside walls or covered with intact sheathing around pipes is best left alone. If small areas of crumbling asbestos insulation are found, they can sometimes be sealed with plaster rather than removed. Professional help is required to remove it.

Lead Poisoning   Modern concerns about lead poisoning focus primarily on children in urban settings. When lead is ingested, it can damage the central nervous system, cause mental retardation, hinder oxygen transport in the blood, and create digestive problems. Many people mistakenly think that this problem is past. Studies by state health departments and the Centers for Disease Control indicate that lead poisoning continues to be a serious problem among children living in older, deteriorating buildings in inner cities.

Children are exposed to lead in two ways. The first is

Asbestosis   A lung condition caused by inhalation of microscopic asbestos fibers, which inflames the lung and can lead to lung cancer.

Formaldehyde   A powerful disinfectant gas often used in solution for germ control but also given off by some synthetic building materials.

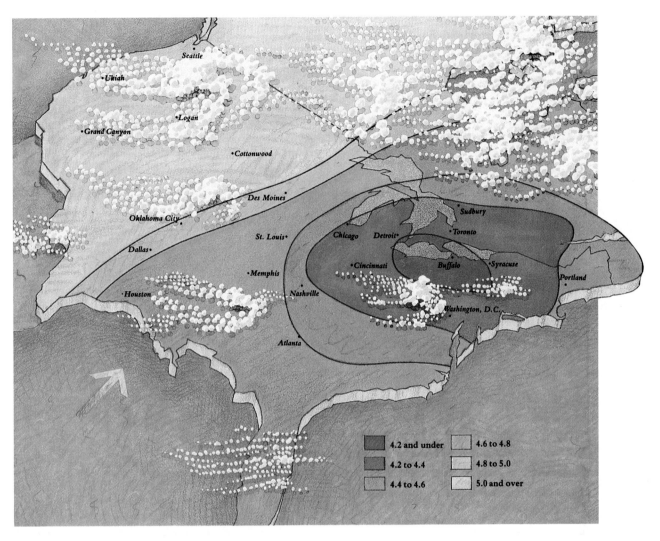

Figure 24-3   Acid rain in the United States. On the 14-point pH scale of acidity and alkalinity, a perfectly neutral sample of water would have a 7.0 rating. Unpolluted rainwater, which registers a pH of 5.6, may be described as slightly acidic because of the combination of carbon dioxide with water vapor. A one-point increase in acidity on this logarithmic scale means a tenfold boost in that critical measurement, so a pH of 4.10, for example, indicates that rainfall is 31.6 times more acidic than normal.

by chewing on surfaces, such as window sills, painted before 1960, when most house paints were lead-based. The second is by playing in dirt near heavily traveled roadways. Since leaded gasoline was used for so many years, the soil near highways is contaminated with lead. Legislation phasing out the use of leaded fuels will minimize this problem in the future.

Pesticides   Pesticides are used primarily for two purposes—to prevent the spread of insect-borne disease and to maximize food production by killing insects that eat crops. Both uses have risks as well as benefits. As mentioned earlier, DDT was extremely effective in controlling the mosquitoes that carry malaria and in increasing crop yields, but its damaging effects were greater than its benefits. Currently, it is clear that food would not be as plentiful or as cheap if pesticides weren't used to control insects. The cost may come in the long-range health consequences of pesticide residues in food chains. Almost all the pesticide hazards to date have been a result of overuse or abuse.

The list of real and potential chemical pollution problems may well be as long as the list of known chemicals. To the preceding list we can add recent concern about mercury in fish, **formaldehyde** in synthetic building materials, and other by-products of our industrial age. As

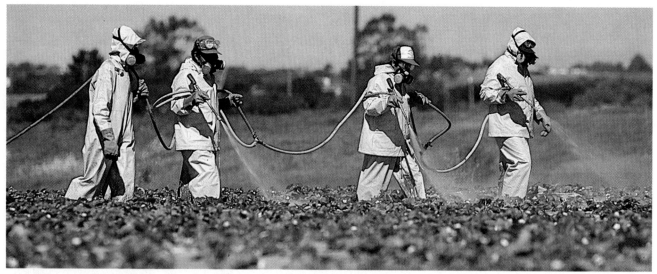

Although some pesticide residues may remain in or on produce when it reaches the consumer, the most serious health effects of pesticides are seen in agricultural workers. Special clothing and equipment help protect these workers from toxic chemicals as they spray strawberries.

mentioned earlier, hazardous wastes are also found in the home and should be handled and disposed of properly. They include automotive supplies (motor oil, antifreeze, transmission fluid), paint supplies (turpentine, paint thinner, mineral spirits), art and hobby supplies (oil-based paint, solvents, acids and alkalis, aerosol sprays), insecticides, batteries, and household cleaners containing sodium hydroxide (lye) or ammonia. These chemicals are dangerous when inhaled or ingested, when they contact the skin or the eyes, or when they are burned or dumped. Many communities provide guidelines about approved disposal methods for household chemicals and have special hazardous waste collection days. (Refer to Table 23-3 in Chapter 23 for a summary of disposal guidelines for some hazardous wastes.)

■ **Exploring Your Emotions**

Some developing nations want to "catch up" with the West by using the same kind of industrial practices that developed nations have used to get where they are. They are cutting down forests to raise cattle for beef, using pesticides that have been banned in the West on their export crops, and polluting their water and air with industrial and agricultural wastes. Do you think it's fair to expect them to be environmentally conscious when the developed nations weren't? Can you make a convincing case for or against their continuing use of these practices?

In our society we seem to introduce a chemical, sing high praise about its contribution to our lifestyle, and then discover a negative health consequence. After a pe-

riod of time we either find a substitute or develop a safer way of using that chemical. We usually don't retreat from technological advances because we don't want to give up their contributions to our way of life. Thus far in history, it appears that the benefits of new chemicals generally outweigh their costs or risks.

Radiation   Many people are afraid of **radiation**, in part because they don't understand what it is. Basically, radiation is energy. It can come in different forms, such as ultraviolet rays, microwaves, or x-rays, and from different sources, such as the sun, uranium, and nuclear weapons. Although radiation can't be seen, heard, smelled, tasted, or felt, its health effects can include **radiation sickness** and death at high doses and chromosome damage, sterility, tissue damage, cataracts, and cancers at lower doses. Currently, health concerns about radiation center on nuclear weapons and nuclear energy, medical uses of radiation, and sources of radiation in the home and workplace.

Nuclear Weapons and Nuclear Energy   Although the superpowers have entered negotiations aimed at slowing down the arms race, huge stockpiles of nuclear weapons pose a health risk of the most serious kind to all species. Public health associations have stated that in the event of an intentional or accidental discharge of these weapons, both "health" and "public" would become meaningless words. In even the most conservative estimates of a "limited" nuclear war, the casualties would run into the hundreds of thousands or millions. Reducing these stockpiles is a challenge and a goal for the 1990s.

Nuclear power-generating plants also pose health

problems. When **nuclear power** was first developed as an alternative to oil and coal, it was promoted as clean, efficient, inexpensive, and safe. In general, this has proven to be the case. Power systems in several parts of the world rely on nuclear generating plants. However, despite all the built-in safeguards and regulating agencies, accidents in nuclear power plants do happen, and the consequences of such accidents are far more serious than similar accidents in other types of power-generating plants. The accidents at Three Mile Island in 1979 and at Chernobyl in the U.S.S.R. in 1986 demonstrated the potential for disaster that exists at nuclear plants.

An additional, enormous problem is disposing of the radioactive wastes these plants generate. They cannot be dumped in a sanitary landfill because the amount and type of soil used to cap a sanitary landfill is not sufficient to prevent radiation exposure. Because many of these landfills are converted into park land once they are filled, and because we might lose track of which ones have radioactive wastes, these sites can't be used even for low concentrations of radioactive wastes. Deposit sites have to be developed that will be secure not just for a few years but for tens of thousands of years—longer than the total recorded history of human beings on this planet. To date, no storage method has been devised that can provide infallible, infinitely durable shielding for nuclear waste.

Medical Uses of Radiation   Another area of concern is the use of radiation in medicine, primarily the x-ray. The development of machines that could produce images of the internal bone structure was a major advance in medicine, and applications abounded. Chest x-rays were routinely given to screen for tuberculosis, and children's feet were even x-rayed in shoe stores to make sure their new shoes fit properly. But as is so often the case, this advance was not without a cost. As time passed, studies revealed that x-ray exposure is cumulative and that no exposure is absolutely safe.

Early x-ray machines are no longer used because of the high amounts of radiation they give off. Each "generation" of x-ray machines has used less radiation more effectively. From a personal health point of view, individuals should never have a "routine" x-ray examination. Each x-ray exam should have a definite purpose, and its benefits and risks should be carefully weighed. Many

health professionals are beginning to recommend that records of all x-ray exposures be kept for every individual, the same way a record of vaccinations is kept.

Radiation in the Home and Workplace   Recently, there has been concern about the electromagnetic radiation associated with such common modern devices as microwave ovens, computer video display terminals (VDTs), microwave telephones, and even high voltage power lines. We know that these forms of radiation do have effects on health. For example, new bone growth at the point of a fracture can be stimulated by a slight electric current. But current research is contradictory and inconclusive about the health effects of this type of radiation.

Another recent area of concern is **radon**, a form of radiation that is found in certain soils, rocks, and building material (see Figure 24-4). An unknown number of homes have been built on or with these substances. Well-insulated homes retain radon and allow higher concentrations to develop. Radon gas increases the incidence of lung cancer. Most state health departments can now test for radon gas concentrations, but the short- and long-term health consequences of radon are still unknown. For a closer look at radon and other hazards in the home, see the box "Indoor Air Pollution."

Noise Pollution   We are increasingly aware of the health effects of loud or persistent noise in the environment. Concerns focus on two areas, hearing loss and stress. Prolonged exposure to sounds above 80–85 **decibels** (a measure of the volume of sound) can cause permanent hearing loss. The scream of an infant, the noise in a machine shop, and freeway traffic sounds can all exceed the safe range. The two most common sources of excessive noise, however, are the workplace and rock concerts. The Occupational Safety and Health Administration sets legal standards for noise in the workplace, but no laws exist regulating noise levels at rock concerts, which often exceed OSHA standards for the workplace.

Most hearing loss occurs in the first two hours of exposure, and hearing usually bounces back within two hours after the noise stops. But if exposure continues or is repeated frequently, hearing loss can be permanent. The employees of a club where rock music is played loudly are at much greater risk than the patrons of the club, who might be exposed for only two hours at a time.

Radiation   Electromagnetic rays such as light or particles given off from a source.

Radiation sickness   An illness marked by low white blood counts, nausea, and death from an overexposure to nuclear radiation.

Nuclear power   Use of controlled nuclear reactions to produce steam, which in turn drives turbines to produce electricity.

Radon   A naturally occurring radioactive gas that is emitted from rocks and natural building materials and that can become concentrated in insulated homes, causing lung cancer.

Decibel   A unit for expressing the relative intensity of sounds; 0 is least perceptible, and 130 is the average pain level.

Figure 24-4 Possible radon hot spots. Shaded areas on the map show the government's best guess about the places where radon may be a problem, based on the location of uranium-bearing rock formations. Even if you live in one of these areas, your home's radon level may still be low; local geological variations and the characteristics of the house are also important factors.

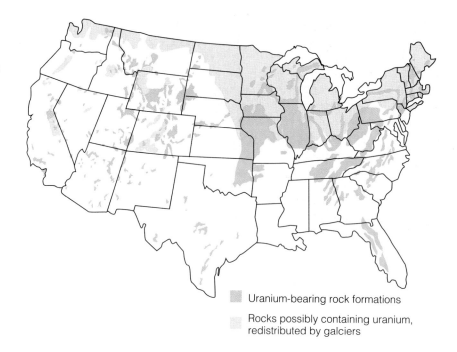

Uranium-bearing rock formations

Rocks possibly containing uranium, redistributed by galciers

Another possible effect of exposure to excessive noise is **tinnitus,** a condition of more or less continuous ringing or buzzing in the ears.

■ **Exploring Your Emotions**

Do you like to listen to loud music? If so, does it change your feelings about it to know you could be damaging your hearing? Do you think you'll make any changes?

Excessive noise is also an environmental stressor, producing the typical stress response described in Chapter 2—faster heart rate, increased respiration, higher blood pressure, and so on. A chronic and prolonged stress response can have serious effects on health. To prevent hearing loss and protect their general well-being, people should limit the length of time they're exposed to loud noise and avoid repeated exposures.

What Can You Do?

Every aspect of your health is influenced in some way by the environment around you. In the past, when infectious diseases were the most common cause of death, health advances came from efforts in the classic areas of environmental health. Today, with most deaths caused by chronic degenerative diseases like heart disease and cancer, most health advances have to come from lifestyle changes—and from improvements in the quality of the global environment.

Faced with a vast array of confusing and complex ecological issues, you as an individual may feel overwhelmed. You may conclude that there isn't anything you can do about global problems. But this isn't true. An estimated 200 million people around the world participated in Earth Day 1990 activities, planting trees, learning how to recycle, protesting industrial pollution, and letting politicians know they wanted leadership on environmental issues and environmentally sound laws. If every one of those people made individual changes in his or her life, the impact would be tremendous.

At the same time, it's important to recognize that large corporations and manufacturers are the ones primarily responsible for the environmental degradation constantly going on all over the world. Many of them have jumped on the "environmental bandwagon" with public relations and advertising campaigns designed to make them look good, but they haven't changed their practices. To influence them, people have to become educated, demand changes in production methods, and elect people to office who will put environmental concerns first and business profits second.

Large-scale changes and individual actions complement each other. What you do every day *does* count;

Tinnitus Ringing in the ears, a condition that can be caused by excessive noise exposure.

Trichloroethane A propellant in some aerosol spray cans that can cause dizziness, irregular respiration, and heartbeat.

Paradichlorobenzene A chemical found in some air fresheners and mothballs, linked to cancer in animals.

Indoor Air Pollution

If you think housework is killing you, you may be right. Your home could be harboring such potentially dangerous pollutants as asbestos, radon gas, benzene, and many more.

Some of these trigger allergic responses. Others have been linked to cancer in laboratory animals. Still others have been documented as causing human cancer. In fact, the U.S. Environmental Protection Agency has reported that toxic chemicals found in the home are three times more likely to cause cancer than outdoor airborne pollutants, even in areas near chemical plants.

In well-ventilated homes these indoor pollutants are found at very low levels. But as people try to save energy by adding insulation and weatherstripping to their homes, they are also trapping these unwanted hazards inside.

And chemical exposure can be cumulative: inhaling a single pollutant may not make you sick, but the more chemicals you are exposed to, the greater the chance of your health suffering.

You may bring some of these chemicals home with you. For instance, you are exposed to benzene vapors every time you fill up at a service station. The vapors get in your clothes and are later released into the air at home. Tetrachloroethylene follows you home from the dry cleaners, clinging to newly cleaned clothes.

Other indoor health hazards may be built into your home. One of the most widely publicized is asbestos. Commonly found in home insulation or wrapped

around pipes in a basement or crawl space, asbestos is made up of tiny mineral fibers that, when released into the air and inhaled, can trigger cancer.

Radon gas is another indoor pollutant that may be causing health problems. A colorless, odorless gas, radon is produced by the radioactive decay of uranium found in different amounts in soil and rocks all over the world. When radon gas is released into the atmosphere, it dissipates harmlessly. It becomes a hazard only when it seeps into a closed structure, such as a home, and then can be a very real hazard indeed. Radioactive particles become attached to dust particles in the air and are readily inhaled. When they enter the lungs, these particles release small bursts of energy that can damage lung tissue and lead to disease after many years of exposure. The Centers for Disease Control estimate that as many as 5,000 to 20,000 excess lung cancer deaths each year are attributable to radon gas. Smoking significantly increases the risk of suffering the harmful effects of radon. The risk of lung cancer from smoking and radon exposure combined is much greater than from either alone.

Radon seeps into homes through cracks in foundations and basement walls. It can also be released into the air in small amounts through running water, such as in showers or washing machines. Until 1989, the EPA set 4 picocuries per liter of air as a safe level for radon in the home, but then reduced it to "background levels,"

about 0.5 to 0.7 picocuries per liter, or "as low as practicable." Radon levels are known or suspected to be high in areas where uranium-bearing rock formations are prevalent. In the United States, these areas tend to be in the Northeast and Midwest, but there is great variation in radon levels from one house to another even in these areas.

Homeowners can test their homes for radon levels with test kits purchased at the hardware store. If levels are found to be high, they can contact their state health department for help in bringing the levels down. These steps usually involve sealing cracks and openings, venting basements, and circulating the air in the house. (The EPA publishes a booklet entitled *Radon Reduction Methods*, which you can obtain from state health offices or the EPA's Office of Radiation Programs, Radon Division, 401 M Street, SW, Washington, D.C. 20460.)

While asbestos and radon are two of the better-known indoor environmental dangers, dozens of others may be lurking undetected in your home. Here are some you should be aware of.

Carbon monoxide is produced when carbon-bearing fuels—petroleum products and wood—are burned. Improperly vented gas appliances, woodburning stoves and kerosene heaters, as well as simple tobacco smoke, all raise indoor carbon monoxide levels. It can also enter your house when a vehicle is idling in an attached garage or near the house. At moderate levels, carbon monoxide

Indoor Air Pollution (continued)

can cause headaches and irregular heartbeat. At higher levels, it can cause loss of consciousness and death.

Formaldehyde gas seeping from resins used in manufacturing particle board, plywood paneling, and some carpeting and upholstery can cause headaches, dizziness, nausea, rashes, and eye and throat irritation. Some studies have linked formaldehyde exposure to cancer.

Found in some air fresheners and in moth ball crystals, **paradichlorobenzene** has been linked to cancer in laboratory animals.

Trichloroethane is an ingredient in some aerosol sprays. Prolonged exposure can cause dizziness and irregular breathing.

Removing the sources of these indoor air pollutants can sometimes be a costly and complicated business. Fortunately you can protect yourself to a large extent by using a little common sense.

- Be sure your house is adequately ventilated, including the basement. This will keep down levels of indoor airborne pollutants.
- Follow manufacturer's directions when using a product that emits pollutants. Use the proper protective equipment. Be sure your work space is very well ventilated—opening a window may not be adequate to safely work with some products. Install an exhaust fan, or, if possible, move the project outside. Note whether the product should be kept away from heat sources.
- Keep paints and cleaning solvents in the original, tightly sealed containers and store them in cool, well-vented areas. Discard partially empty containers unless you're sure you'll use the rest of the product soon.
- Clean air conditioners, air ducts, air filters, heat exchangers, and humidifiers regularly. They are

all potential sources of allergens or disease-producing organisms.
- If you have gas appliances, check them regularly to make sure the pilot lights are burning with a clear blue flame. Burning gas produces small amounts of carbon monoxide and other harmful by-products, and when the pilots aren't burning cleanly, they give off even more pollutants. If you're buying new gas appliances, you might want to consider ones with spark ignition systems, which eliminate the need for pilot lights.

Sources: Adapted from Mitch Coleman, Air pollution: The inside story, *Family Safety & Health*, Winter 1986–87, pp. 5–6; Radon in the home, *Mayo Clinic Health Letter*, December 1988; and Should you test for radon? *Hippocrates*, September/October 1989, p. 65.

there are many actions you can take to "save the world." The following is just a sampling of some of the ways that you can make a difference.

Conserving Energy, Improving the Air

- Cut back on driving. Ride your bike, walk, use public transportation, or carpool in a fuel-efficient vehicle. Keep your car tuned up and well maintained. Using less oil and gasoline conserves nonrenewable energy resources and reduces air pollution.
- Use less electricity and less heat. Make sure your home is well insulated; use insulating shades and curtains to keep heat in in winter and out in summer.
- Replace incandescent light bulbs with compact fluorescent bulbs (not fluorescent tubes). They cost more initially but save you money over the life of the bulb. They produce a comparable light, last longer, and use about one-third to one-quarter of the energy of a regular bulb. By using less electricity, they contribute to lower carbon dioxide emissions from electric power plants.
- Plant trees. Because they recycle carbon dioxide, trees

work against global warming. They also provide shade and cool the air, so less air conditioning is needed.

Saving Water

- Take showers, not baths, to cut water consumption. Don't let water run when you're not actively using it while brushing your teeth, shaving, or hand-washing clothes. Don't run a dishwasher or washing machine until you have a full load.
- Install sink faucet aerators and water-efficient showerheads, which use two to five times less water with no noticeable decrease in performance.
- Put a displacement device in your toilet tank to reduce the amount of water used with each flush. A plastic bottle or bag filled with water works well.

Reducing Garbage and Toxic Wastes

- Buy products with the least amount of packaging you can, or buy products in bulk. Buy recycled and recyclable products; avoid disposables. For example, buy large jars of juice, not individually packaged juice drinks.

T A C T I C S   A N D   T I P S

Making Your Letters Count

It only takes a few minutes to write to an elected official, but it can make a difference on an environmental issue you care about. When elected officials receive enough letters on a particular issue, it will influence their votes—they want to be reelected and your vote counts!

To help give your letter the greatest possible impact:

- Use your own words and your own stationery.
- Be concise, but try to write more than just one or two sentences. A one-page letter is a good length.
- Identify your subject clearly—refer to legislation by its name or number.

- Discuss only one issue in each letter—different issues are handled by different staff members, so stick to one subject to ensure your letter goes to the right person.
- Ask the legislator to do something specific—to vote a particular way on a particular bill, request hearings, cosponsor a bill, etc.
- Ask for a reply.
- Try not to use form letters.
- Don't be unnecessarily critical. Never threaten or insult.

To find out the current status of legislation pending in the House or Senate, call the legislative status line: (202) 225-1772.

Your phone book has addresses of all state and local representatives. United States senators and representatives can be reached at the following addresses:

The Honorable _____
United States Senate
Washington, DC 20510

Dear Senator _____

The Honorable _____
U.S. House of Representatives
Washington, DC 20515

Dear Representative _____

_____
Adapted from Russell Wild (ed.). 1990. *The Earth Care Annual 1990*. Emmaus, Pa.: National Wildlife Federation and Rodale Press.

- To store food, use glass jars and waxed paper rather than plastic wrap. Reuse plastic bags.
- Recycle your newspapers, glass, cans, paper, and other recyclables. Start a compost pile for your organic garbage if you can.
- When buying products, read labels and try to buy the least toxic ones available.
- Dispose of your household hazardous wastes properly. If you're not sure whether something is hazardous or don't know how to dispose of it, contact your local environmental health office or health department.

Preserving Wildlife and the Natural Environment

- Snip or rip plastic six-pack rings. When seabirds and animals get them stuck on their necks or bills, they can strangle or starve to death.
- Don't buy products made from endangered species, such as furs or ivory. Avoid tropical hardwoods.
- When you're hiking or camping, don't leave anything behind, not even soapsuds in lakes or streams.

Beyond Individual Actions . . .

- Make sure your friends and family are informed and knowledgeable about environmental issues. Share what you learn.
- Join, support, or volunteer your time to organizations working on environmental causes that are important to you.
- Contact your elected representatives and communicate your concerns. For guidelines on how to be heard, see the box "Making Your Letters Count."

These are just a few of the steps you can take to improve the quality of the environment. Assuming responsibility for your actions in relation to the environment isn't very different from assuming responsibility for your own health behaviors. It involves knowledge, awareness, insight, motivation, and commitment. You can also use the same strategies to change your behaviors in relation to the environment that you use to change your health behaviors. And as with personal health behaviors, the crucial step is to get started, today. Let the size and scope of the problems be a call to action, not an excuse for apathy.

The environment is no longer as threatening to humans as it was once. Our attitude toward it is changing; we realize we have to modify our own attitudes and behaviors to protect it. We are also realizing that we are not the only species with a right to inhabit the planet. We hold the world in trust for future generations and for other forms of life. Our responsibility is to pass on to the next generation an environment no worse, and preferably better, than the one we enjoy today.

Summary

- The survival of the human species may entail protecting the environment from the by-products of the modern way of life.

Why Are Environmental Problems More Serious Now?

- With industrialization, urbanization, and population growth, environmental problems have become more serious and broader in scope. World population growth has placed increased burdens on farmlands and other natural resources.
- The by-products of a modern technological society—like sulfur dioxide emissions and radiation—are more dangerous than naturally occurring hazards.
- The combination of increased population and modern technology has created interconnections among people and environments all over the world. Environmentally unsound practices can contribute to global climate and atmospheric changes.
- Many environmental conditions, like water and air quality, sanitation, and food and drug safety, were worse in the past. The costs and benefits of practices that might harm the environment need to be weighed in order to make decisions.

Classic Environmental Health Concerns

- In the nineteenth century, controlling communicable diseases was more important than controlling pollution. This concern led to government involvement in garbage collection, sewage treatment, water protection, and food inspection and also changed the health concerns of the developed world.
- The relationship between contaminated water and cholera and other infectious diseases was first understood in the nineteenth century.
- Surface water used in municipal systems must be purified because it's likely to be contaminated with organic matter and disease-causing microorganisms. Physical and chemical treatment processes may be supplemented with fluoridation to help prevent tooth decay.
- Concerns with water today center on hazardous chemicals from industry and households as well as on shortages because of increased population and excessive irrigation. To solve these problems, all freshwater supplies must be treated as if they will be used as a source of drinking water and water distribution systems must be restructured.
- Since septic systems and sewage treatment systems have been developed, diseases like typhoid and cholera have virtually disappeared in the developed world. Although rivers and lakes can purify themselves when not overloaded, population growth has made sewage treatment necessary.
- Sewage treatment today needs to deal with heavy metals and hazardous chemicals; they cannot be dumped back into the environment.
- Solid waste disposal used to be a matter of disposing of food and cooking wastes in a way that prevented disease and minimized the insects or animals attracted to them.
- The sanitary landfills that are used today for solid waste disposal are subject to careful site selection and daily management. Burial of waste is expensive and requires much space.
- The amount of garbage is growing all the time, and paper is the biggest component. About 1 percent is toxic. Burning can reduce bulk but may release hazardous material into the air.
- Recycling of trash can help solid waste disposal problems by reducing the spread of chemical contamination, slowing the consumption rate of natural resources, and reducing the cost of solid waste disposal.
- Illness and death associated with food-borne disease and toxic food additives have decreased substantially since implementation of the Pure Food and Drug Act in 1906. Concern today centers on long-term health consequences because of chemical contamination or the characteristics of the foods themselves.
- A number of federal, state, and local agencies inspect food at the various points of production; most food-associated illnesses are caused by contamination in the home.
- It became known only a hundred years ago that insects and rodents could transmit many diseases. Disability and death can be prevented by spraying insecticides, wearing protective clothing, and being careful in infested areas.

Pollution

- In terms of health risks, the level of concentration of a particular pollutant becomes very important. Long-term effects of many seemingly harmless pollutants are difficult to evaluate.
- The air has always been polluted as a result of natural processes, but human beings contribute the by-products of their activities. People today live long enough to experience the long-term health consequences of air pollution, and increased population and industrialization make the problems more visible and dangerous.

- Increased amounts of carbon monoxide and airborne acids and decreased amounts of oxygen are especially stressful to those with heart and lung problems. Air pollution emergencies occur when (1) fossil fuels are burned, (2) a topographic feature prevents prevailing winds from pushing stagnant air away, and (3) a temperature inversion exists.
- Temperature inversions prevent the vertical circulation of air that, along with horizontal wind circulation, prevents pollutants from building up.
- Smog is human-made air pollution caused by burning fossil fuels (London-type) or by motor vehicle exhausts containing oxides of nitrogen (Los Angeles-type). The EPA sets standards and monitors pollution levels.
- Atmospheric problems like the greenhouse effect, increased carbon monoxide, depletion of the ozone layer, and acid rain are global problems, involving the ecology of the entire planet.
- Carbon dioxide and other natural gases act as a "greenhouse" around the earth, intensifying the heat of the sun and trapping it close to the surface. Levels of these gases are rising as is deforestation; as a result, temperatures could rise and the climate could become warmer.
- Levels of carbon monoxide are increasing as a result of combustion and automobile exhaust. Emission controls on cars significantly reduce CO levels.
- The ozone layer shields the earth's surface from the sun's ultraviolet rays, but a "hole" has been found seasonally since 1983. One cause is the release of chlorofluorocarbons, which break down into chlorine in the atmosphere; chlorine destroys ozone molecules.
- Acid rain occurs when atmospheric pollutants (especially those resulting from burning high-sulfur coal) combine with moisture in the air and become highly acidic rain or snow. Because many trees and some aquatic life can tolerate only a very narrow range of acidity, they are damaged or killed by acid rain. The food chain is potentially at risk.
- Chemical pollution, not a new problem, is more serious today because new chemical substances are constantly being created and introduced into the environment; in addition, more people are exposed to these chemicals.
- Asbestos can protect against fire, but if its fibers are released into the air, they can cause serious lung damage. Lead poisoning is mainly a problem for children in urban areas who chew on old painted surfaces or play in dirt near heavily traveled roadways. Ingestion of lead can damage the central nervous system and hinder oxygen transport in the blood.
- Pesticides prevent the spread of insect-borne diseases and kill insects that eat crops; hazards are usually a result of overuse or abuse.
- Other chemical pollutants include mercury, formaldehyde, and hazardous wastes found in the home.
- Radiation—from the sun, uranium, or nuclear weapons, for instance—can cause radiation sickness, chromosome damage, and cancers, among other health risks.
- Casualties from even a limited nuclear exchange would be as high as millions of people. Accidents at nuclear power plants are potentially disastrous, and disposal of their radioactive waste is another major problem, so far not resolved. Exposure to medical x-rays is cumulative, and no exposure is absolutely safe.
- Research into the health hazards of electromagnetic radiation associated with common household appliances is inconclusive. Radon, found in certain soils, rocks, and building materials, can concentrate in homes; it increases the incidence of lung cancer.
- Loud or persistent noise can lead to hearing loss and/or stress; the two most common sources of excessive noise are the workplace and rock concerts.

What Can You Do?

- Most health advances today must come from lifestyle changes and improvements in the global environment. The impact of personal changes made by every concerned individual could be tremendous.

Take Action

1. Do an inventory to find out what hazardous chemicals you have in your household. Read the labels for disposal instructions. If there aren't any instructions, call your local health department and ask how to dispose of specific chemicals. Also ask if there are hazardous waste disposal sites in your community or special pickup days. If possible, get rid of some or all of the hazardous wastes in your home.

2. Investigate the recycling facilities in your community. Find out how materials are recycled and what they are used for in their recycled state. If recycling isn't available in your community, contact your local city hall to find out how a recycling program can be started.

3. Contact your local health department to find out if radon is a problem in your part of the country. If it is, ask health officials how they advise people to deal with it. Investigate the radon test kits available in local hardware stores. Which ones do the store personnel recommend?

4. Find out where your community gets its drinking water and how it disposes of its garbage and sewage. Is adequate water available even in dry years? Do disposal companies expect any problems with closing landfills in the near future? Is sewage adequately treated?

5. Junk mail is an environmental hazard coming and going—millions of trees are cut down to produce the paper it's printed on, and millions of pieces of junk mail clog the nation's landfills. Keep your name from being sold to any more mailing list companies by writing to Mail Preference Service, Direct Marketing Association, 6 East 43rd Street, New York, N.Y. 10017. Recycle the junk mail you still get; newsprint can be recycled with newspapers,

paper and envelopes (without windows) with paper.

6. Keep track of exactly how many bags (or gallons) of trash your household produces per week. Is it more or less than the national weekly average of 6.73 bags (87.5 gallons) per three-person household? In either case, try to reduce it by recycling, composting, and buying and using fewer disposable products.

Selected Bibliography

Buried alive. 1989. *Newsweek*, November 27.

Easterbrook, Gregg. 1990. Everything you know about the environment is wrong. *The New Republic*, April 20.

Freed, Virgil H. 1986. Hazards in the physical environment. In V. W. Holland, R. Detels, and G. Knox, eds., *The Oxford Textbook of Public Health*, Vol. 1. Oxford: Oxford University Press.

How we're killing our world. 1990. *San Jose Mercury News*, April 8.

Is it all just hot air? 1989. *Newsweek*, November 20.

Okun, Daniel A. 1986. Water and waste disposal. In Maxcy-Rosenau, ed., *Public Health and Preventive Medicine*, 12th ed. Norwalk, Conn.: Appleton-Century-Crofts.

Revell, P., and C. Revelle, 1984. *The Environment: Issues and Choices for Society*. Boston: Willard Grant Press.

Waldron, H. A. 1986. The control of the physical environment. W. W. Holland, R. Detels, and G. Knox, eds., *The Oxford Textbook of Public Health*, Vol. 2. Oxford: Oxford University Press.

Recommended Readings

Carson, Rachel. 1962. *Silent Spring*. Boston: Houghton Mifflin. *The classic that awakened people to the dangers of wide-scale insecticide spraying.*

Chiras, Daniel D. 1985. *Environmental Science: A Framework for Decision-Making*. Menlo Park, Calif.: Addison-Wesley, 1985. *Basic textbook on environmental health. Includes a good section on ethics.*

Dubos, Rene. 1986. *Man, Medicine, and Environment*. New York: Praeger. *A landmark book, written by a highly respected scientist, that focused scientific concern on environmental issues.*

The Earth Works Group. 1989. *50 Simple Things You Can Do to Save the Earth*. Berkeley, Calif.: Earthworks Press. *Full of useful information, practical advice, sources, and resources, this slim volume is an indispensable guide to improving the environment. Includes names and addresses of organizations that can provide further information on specific issues. Several other similar books are also available.*

Ehrlich, Paul R. 1990. *The Population Explosion*. New York: Ballantine Books. *An update of Ehrlich's landmark 1971 book calling attention to the problems associated with population growth.*

Murphy, E. M. 1983. *The Environment to Come: A Global Survey*. Washington, D.C.: The Population Reference Bureau. *A prediction of future trends in the environment.*

Index

Streptococci, 502
Stress, 22-47
    and aging, 526
    anxiolytic drugs for, 291-292
    body response to, 24-28
    and caffeine, 41
    coping with, 37-43, 44
    definition, 24, 25
    emotional responses to, 29-30
    exercise and, 39, 41
    and exhaustion, 25, 27
    and hormones, 24, 26-27
    and immune system, 30-31, 515
    levels, 25
    mobilization for, 27-29
    and nutrition, 41-42
    and overweight, 41, 351
    and personality type, *see* Type A/B behavior
    post-traumatic, 64
    premenstrual, 96-97
    relaxation techniques, 38-41
    role in disease, 30-32
    signals, 29t
    and social support systems, 33, 36
    sources, 24
    stages, 25
    and time management, 37-38
    test anxiety, 44-46
    and weight control, 350
Stressors, 24, 25
Stress response, 24-25, 670
Stress test, 385, 419
"Stress vitamins," 42
Stroke, 235, 409, 421-422
Student health services, 72, 607t
Students Against Driving Drunk (SADD), 264
Stupor, 254, 255
Sucrose polyester; *see* Olestra
Suction curettage, 182
Sudden infant death syndrome (SIDS), 238
Sugar, 319, 320, 344-345
Suicide, 57, 58, 543-544
    barbiturate overdose, 280
    danger signals, 58
    myths about, 61
    reasons for, 543-544
Sulfites, 328
Sun protection factor (SPF), 446, 447
Sunscreens, 445, 446, 447, 457
Surety bond, 545
Surgeon General reports
    on AIDS, 464, 465, 472
    on nutrition, 302, 319, 320
    on smoking, 228, 233
Surgery, 582, 585, 587
    for abortions, 182, 183
    anesthesia for, 587
    breast cancer, 441
    elective, 582
    for sterilization, 150-152
    heart, 420, 421
    outpatient, 587, 607t
    risks, 584-585, 587
    second opinions on, 582, 584
Surrogate motherhood, 197, 198
Swimmer's ear, 597
Sympathetic nervous system, 26
Synesthesia, 289
Synovial fluid, 390, 391
Syphilis, 206, 472, 474-475
Systematic desensitization, 45-46, 66, 67
Systole, 408, 413
Systolic blood pressure, 415

T-cells, 31, 466, 467, 495, 496, 487, 498-499, 515
Tanning salons, 445, 446
"Tar," in cigarette smoke, 230
Target behavior, 8-9
Target heart rates, 385
Telephone hotlines, 470, 485, 584, 602-603
Temperature inversion, 662
Teratogen, 206

Test anxiety, 44-46
Testes, 82-83, 85
Testicle self-examination, 448
Testimonials, 615
Testosterone, 91, 94
Tetanus, 501, 501t
Thalidomide, 206
THC (tetrahydrocannabinol), 287
Thrombus, 410-411
Thrush, 512, 513
Time management, 37-38
Tinnitus, 670
Tobacco
    carcinogens in 230, 233
    characteristics of users 225, 228-229
    politics, 239, 241-242
    prevalence of use, 229, 229t, 230t
    reasons for use, 224-229
    smokeless; *see* Smokeless tobacco
    warnings required, 240t
    See also Cigarettes; Smoking
Tobacco-free society, aiming toward, 222-248
Tobacco Institute, 239
Tolerance (to drugs), 260, 275, 289
Tonsillectomy, 587
Tooth decay, 591
TOPS (Take Off Pounds Sensibly), 364-365t
Toxemia of pregnancy, 202
Toxic psychosis, 290, 291
Toxic shock syndrome, 145
Training
    for athletic skills, 389, 391, 394
    periodization of, 386
Training effect, of exercise, 381, 384-386
Tranquilizers, 279, 291
Transient ischemic attack (TIA), 422, 423
Transsexualism, 114, 115
Transvestism, 114, 115
Treadmill test, 385, 419
Treponema pallidum, 474
Triage, 567
Trichinosis, 514, 659
Trichloroethane, 670, 672
Trichloroethylene, 671
Trichomoniasis, 95, 482-483, 513
Tubal sterilization, 151-152, 587
Tuberculosis, 501t, 506
Tumor(s)
    benign, 434, 435
    malignant, 435; *see* Cancers
    primary, 434, 435
Type A/B behavior, 31-32, 34-36, 423-424, 426
Typhus, 501t, 506, 654, 655

Ulcers, peptic, 232, 236
Ultrasound, 194, 455
Umbilical cord, 202, 204, 212
Unconscious mind, 68
Uniform Anatomical Gift Act, 547
Uniform Donor Card, 547, 548
Unorthodox practices, 607-613
Urethra, 81, 83, 85
U.S. Dietary Guidelines, 313, 319
U.S. government agencies; *see* individual
    agencies
U.S. Recommended Daily Allowances (U.S.
    RDAs), 316, 325
Uterus, 196, 204

Vaccines, 500-501, 501t
Vacuum aspiration, 182
Vagina, 81-82
Vaginal ring, 153
Vaginismus, 98, 100
Vaginitis, 95
Valium (diazepam), 262, 279, 280
Varicella zoster, 480
Vasa deferentia, 85, 150, 151
Vasectomy, 150-151, 587
Vasocongestion, 88, 98
Vasoconstriction, 282, 283
Vegetarian diets, 303, 322-324, 451

Vena cava, 407
Venereal diseases (VD); *see* Sexually transmissible diseases
Ventricles, 407-408
Venules, 408
Very low density lipoproteins (VLDL), 412
Viruses, 508-513
    and cancer, 444, 482, 513
    common cold, 510
    herpes; *see* Herpes infections
    structure and life cycle, 509
Vitality, 4
Vitamin(s), 302, 310, 311t, 312
    A, and cancer, 449, 452t
        toxicity during pregnancy, 310
    B6, toxicity, 310
    B12, 310, 323
    C, and cancer, 449, 452t
        and the common cold, 511
    deficiency diseases, 310, 323
    E, and cancer, 449, 451, 452t
    estimated safe and adequate intakes,
        (ESADDI), 312
    food sources of, 311t
    functions of, 311t
    losses during food preparation, 312
    niacin, 310
    and pregnancy, 206, 330
    recommended amounts, 311t
    supplementation, need for, 329-330
    toxicity of large doses, 310, 330, 570
Vomiting, self-treatment, 597-598
Voyeurism, 114, 115
Vulva, 80

Walking for fitness, 381
Water purification, 656-658
Water, 302
Weight assessment. 352-357, 354t
Weight control, 340-373
    amphetamines and, 284
    behavior modification for, 347
    crash diets, 363
    desirable weight, 319
    and eating habits, 347, 363
    and emotions, 350, 352
    and exercise, 347-348, 348t, 350, 351, 358,
        362, 378, 381
    evaluation of programs, 367
    fad diets, 362
    fasting, 363
    and lifestyle, 342-344, 351, 360
    myths and facts, 358, 363
    resources for help, 360-368
    tips for achieving, 360, 361
    very-low-kcalorie diets, 362-363, 366
    weight-loss clinics, 364-365t
    See also Obesity
Weight Watchers, 363, 364-365t
Wellness profile, 6-7
Wellness, achieving, 7-18
    as health goal, 4-6
White blood cells, 495, 496
"Will, living," 552, 553
Will, need for, 545-546
Withdrawal symptoms, 260, 275
    from alcohol, 260
    from amphetamines, 286
    from caffeine, 287
    from nicotine, 224-225
    from opiates, 274-275
    from Valium, 280
Women Organized Against Rape, 118, 119
World Health Organization, 4, 316, 466, 657
Worms, parasitic, 514

X and Y chromosomes, 90-91
X rays, medical use, 454

Yeast infection, 95, 137

Zone therapy; *see* Iridology